FOOD ALLERGY
AND
INTOLERANCE

To DB and CBC

FOOD ALLERGY
AND
INTOLERANCE

JONATHAN BROSTOFF

MA DM FRCP FRCPath
Reader in Clinical Immunology
and Honorary Consultant Physician
Department of Immunology
Middlesex Hospital and Medical School
London

STEPHEN J. CHALLACOMBE

PhD BDS MRCPath
Reader in Oral Immunology
and Honorary Consultant
Department of Oral Immunology and Microbiology
United Medical and Dental Schools of
Guy's and St Thomas' Hospitals, London

79334

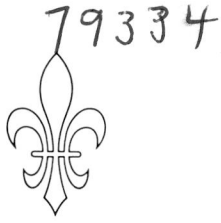

Baillière Tindall
LONDON PHILADELPHIA TORONTO
MEXICO CITY SYDNEY TOKYO HONG KONG

| Baillière Tindall | 33 The Avenue |
| W. B. Saunders | Eastbourne, East Sussex BN21 3UN, England |

West Washington Square
Philadelphia, PA 19105, USA

1 Goldthorne Avenue
Toronto, Ontario M8Z 5T9, Canada

Apartado 26370—Cedro 512
Mexico 4, DF Mexico

ABP Australia Ltd, 44–50 Waterloo Road
North Ryde, NSW 2113, Australia

Ichibancho Central Building, 22–1 Ichibancho
Chiyoda-ku, Tokyo 102, Japan

10/fl, Inter-Continental Plaza, 94 Granville Road
Tsim Sha Tsui East, Kowloon, Hong Kong

First published 1987

Typeset, printed and bound in Great Britain by
Butler and Tanner Ltd, Frome and London

British Library Cataloguing in Publication Data

Food allergy and intolerance.
  1. Food allergy
  I. Brostoff, Jonathan   II. Challacombe,
  Stephen J.
  616.97′5   RC596
ISBN 0-7020-1156-8

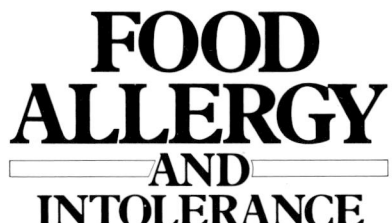

FOOD
ALLERGY
⊏AND⊐
INTOLERANCE

Contents

PART I. BASIC MECHANISMS

SECTION A. NORMAL STRUCTURE AND FUNCTION

SECTION B. SPECIALIZED CELLS OF THE GUT

SECTION C. SPECIALIZED SECRETIONS OF THE GUT

SECTION D. ANTIGEN HANDLING

PART V. TREATMENT OF FOOD ALLERGY

Contributors

Kjell Aas MD
Professor, Medical School, University of Oslo; Voksentoppen (Rikshospitalet), University Hospital, Ullveien 14, Voksenkollen, Oslo 3, Norway.

Virginia Alun Jones MB BChir
Clinical Research Fellow, Addenbrooke's Hospital, Department of Gastroenterology, Hills Road, Cambridge CB2 2QQ, UK.

P. Asquith MD, FRCP
Consultant Physician and Gastroenterologist, Honorary Senior Lecturer in Medicine and Immunology, Departments of Medicine and Immunology, University of Birmingham; Director of the Alistair Frazer and John Squire Metabolic and Clinical Investigation Unit.

David J. Atherton MA, MB, FRCP
Consultant Paediatric Dermatologist, Hospital for Sick Children, Great Ormond Street, London WC1, UK.

Nathan Becker MD
Assistant Clinical Professor of Medicine, University of California, San Francisco, Parnassus Avenue, San Francisco, California 94117, USA; Mount Zion Hospital, Ralph K. Davies Medical Center and St. Luke's Medical Center, San Francisco, California.

A. Dean Befus PhD
Professor, Department of Microbiology and Infectious Diseases, University of Calgary, Health Sciences Centre, 330 Hospital Drive N. W., Alberta, Canada T2N 4NI.

Iris R. Bell MD, PhD
Adjunct Assistant Professor, Department of Psychiatry, University of California, San Francisco, California; Langley Porter Psychiatric Institute, University of California, 401 Parnassus Avenue, San Francisco, California 94143, USA.

John Bienenstock FRCP, FRCP(C)
Professor and Chairman, Department of Pathology, 1200 Main Street West, Hamilton, Ontario, 8N 3Z5, Canada; McMaster University Medical Center, Chedoke McMaster Hospital, Hamilton, Ontario, Canada.

Angus Graham Bird BM BCh, MD, MRCP, MRCPath
Senior Lecturer in Immunology, University of Newcastle Upon Tyne; Consultant Immunologist, Newcastle General Hospital, Westgate Road, Newcastle Upon Tyne, NE4 6BE, UK.

Dale E. Bockman PhD
Professor and Chairman of Anatomy, Department of Anatomy, Medical College of Georgia, Augusta, Georgia 30912, USA.

F. J. Bourne BVetMed, PhD, MRCVS
Professor of Veterinary Medicine, Department of Veterinary Medicine, University of Bristol, Bristol BS18 7DU, UK.

Per Brandtzaeg PhD
Professor of Pathology, The Medical Faculty, University of Oslo, Norway; Chief, Laboratory of Immunohistochemistry and Immunopathology (LIIPAT), The National Hospital, Rikshospitalet, 0027 Oslo 1, Norway.

Jonathan Brostoff MA, DM, FRCP, FRCPath
Reader in Clinical Immunology, Department of Immunology, Arthur Stanley House, Middlesex Hospital Medical School, 40–50 Tottenham Street, London W1P 9PG, UK; Honorary Consultant Physician, Middlesex Hospital.

Ollie Dawkins Brown MEd, MS
WJR & Associates Inc., dba/EHC-Dallas, 8345 Walnut Hill Lane, Suite 205, Dallas, Texas 75231, USA.

S. J. Challacombe PhD, BDS, MRCPath
Reader in Oral Immunology, Consultant in Diagnostic Microbiology and Immunology, Honorary Consultant in Oral Medicine and Microbiology, United Medical and Dental Schools, Guy's Hospital, London SE1 9RT, UK.

John Richard Clamp MD, PhD, FRCP, FRCS
Professor, Department of Medicine, University of Bristol; Consultant, Bristol Royal Infirmary, Bristol BS2 8HW, UK.

Sylvia S. Crago PhD
Research Assistant Professor, Department of Cell Biology, University of New Mexico School of Medicine, Albuquerque, New Mexico 87131, USA.

Charlotte Cunningham-Rundles MD, PhD
Assistant Professor, Department of Medicine, Memorial Sloan-Kettering Cancer Center, New York, New York 10021, USA.

Morrell H. Draper OBE, MB BS, PhD, FRSE
Formerly with the International Programme on Chemical Safety (IPCS), World Health Organization, Geneva; sometime Senior Lecturer in Physiology, University of Edinburgh; Senior Medical Officer, Department of Health and Social Security, Division of Medical Aspects of Chemical Contamination of the Environment, Food and Smoking.

Joseph Egger MD
Kinderklinik, Dr. von Haunersches Kinderspital der Universität München, Lindwurmstrasse 4, 8000 Munich 2, FRG.

Ronald Finn MD, FRCP
Consultant Physician, Royal Liverpool Hospital, Prescot Street, Liverpool L7 8XP, UK; Lecturer in Clinical Medicine, University of Liverpool, Liverpool.

R. P. K. Ford MD, FRACP
Senior Lecturer, Christchurch Clinical School, Otago University, New Zealand; Community Paediatrician, Reserve Bank Building, 158 Hereford Street, Christchurch, New Zealand.

A. W. Frankland MA, DM, BCh
Consulting Allergist, Guy's Hospital, London SE1, UK.

David L. J. Freed MD
Allergy Specialist, Beaumont Hospital, Bolton, BL6 4LA, UK.

Oscar L. Frick MD, PhD
Professor of Pediatrics, University of California, San Francisco, San Francisco, California, 94143 USA; Attending Physician, University of California, San Francisco, Medical Center, San Francisco.

Lionel Fry BSc, MD, FRCP
Consultant Dermatologist, Department of Dermatology, St. Mary's Hospital, Praed Street, London W2 1NY, UK.

John W. Gerrard DM, FRCP(C)
Professor Emeritus, Department of Paediatrics, Room 1201, New Mall, University of Saskatchewan, Saskatoon, Saskatchewan, S7N 0X0, Canada; Active Staff, University Hospital, Saskatoon.

Randall M. Goldblum MD
Professor, Division of Immunology/Allergy, Department of Pediatrics, University of Texas Medical Branch, Galveston, Texas 77550, USA.

Armond S. Goldman MD
Professor, Division of Immunology/Allergy, Department of Pediatrics, University of Texas Medical Branch, Galveston, Texas 77550, USA.

Antony J. Ham Pong MB BS
Clinical Lecturer in Pediatrics, University of Ottawa, Ottawa, Ontario, K1N 6N5 Canada; Associate Active FPAFF, Children's Hospital of Eastern Ontario, Ottawa.

D. J. Hendrick MD, FRCP, MFOM
Honorary Lecturer in Medicine and Occupational Health, University of Newcastle Upon Tyne; Consultant Physician, Newcastle General Hospital, Westgate Road, Newcastle Upon Tyne, NE4 6BE, UK.

John Oakley Hunter MA, MD, FRCP
Associate Lecturer, University of Cambridge, Cambridge; Consultant Physician, Addenbrooke's Hospital, Hills Road, Cambridge CB2 2QQ, UK.

Anand G. Kantak MD
Assistant Professor, Department of Pediatrics, University of Missouri, Columbia, Missouri 65211, USA.

George F. Kroker MD, FACA
Allergy Associates of La Crosse Ltd., 615 South 10th Street, P.O. Box 2408, La Crosse, Wisconsin 54602–2408, USA; St. Francis Medical Center, La Crosse, Wisconsin.

Michael E. Lamm MD
Professor and Chairman of Pathology, Case Western Reserve University School of Medicine, 2085 Adelbert Road, Cleveland, Ohio 44106, USA; Director, Department of Pathology, University Hospitals of Cleveland.

Tor Langeland MD
Department of Dermatology, Rikshospitalet, University Hospital, Oslo 1, Norway.

John L. Laseter PhD
President and Chief Executive Offier, Enviro-Health Systems, Inc., 990 North Bowser Road, Suite 800, Richardson, Texas 75081, USA.

Jonathan Leonard BSc, MD MRCP(UK)
Senior Registrar in Dermatology, St. Mary's Hospital, Praed Street, London W2 1NY, UK.

Alan Scott Levin MD
Adjunct Associate Professor, Department of Dermatology, University of California, San Francisco, San Francisco, California 94143, USA.

Colin H. Little MB BS, MRCP(UK), FRACP
26 Erin Street, Richmond 3121, Australia.

Christopher Mallinson FRCP
Consultant Physician, Lewisham and North Southwark Health Authority, Lewisham Hospital, High Street, London SE13 6LH, UK.

L. McEwen MA, BM BCh(Oxf.)
London Medical Centre, 144 Harley Street, London W1N 1AH, UK.

N. Mike MB, MRCP
Medical Registrar, Metabolic Unit, East Birmingham Hospital, Bordesley Green East, Birmingham B9 5ST, UK.

Melody J. Milam PhD
Fort Worth Psychological Center, 5508 Dunham, Fort Worth, Texas 76114, USA.

B. G. Miller BSc, PhD
Research Fellow, Department of Veterinary Medicine, University of Bristol, Bristol BS18 7DU, UK.

Joseph B. Miller MD
The Miller Center for Allergy, 273 Azalea Road, Three Office Park, Suite 110, Mobile, Alabama 36609, USA; Consultant to the Department of Pediatrics, University of South Alabama College of Medicine, Mobile, Alabama.

D. A. Moneret-Vautrin MD
Professor of Internal Medicine, Clinical Immunology and Allergology, Service de Médecine D, CHU Brabois, Route de Neufchâteau, Vandoeuvre-lès-Nancy, 54511 France.

Jean Monro MB BS, LRCP, MRCS
Medical Director, Allergy and Environmental Medicine Clinic, The Nightingale Hospital, 19 Lisson Grove, London NW1; Medical Director, Allergy and Environmental Medicine Clinic, 10 St. John's Road, Boxmor, Hemel Hempstead HP1 1JR, UK.

Allan McI. Mowat BSc, MB ChB, PhD, MRC
Senior Clinical Fellow, Department of Bacteriology and Immunology, Honorary Senior Registrar in Immunology, Western Infirmary, Glasgow G11 6NT, UK.

D. M. V. Parrott PhD, DSc, FRCPath, FRSE
Gardiner Professor, University of Glasgow; Head of Department, Bacteriology and Immunology, Western Infirmary and Gartnavel General Hospitals, Glasgow G11 6NT, UK.

Elide Pastorello MD
Research Assistant, Internal Medicine, 2nd Clinic, University of Milan, Via F. Sforza 35, Milan, Italy.

Fred L. Pearce PhD
Reader, Department of Chemistry, University College, London WC1 0AJ, UK.

D. J. Pearson MB, PhD, MRCP
Senior Lecturer in Medicine, University of Manchester, Manchester; Honorary Consultant Physician, University Hospital of South Manchester, Manchester, UK.

Z. Pelikan MD
Director, Department of Allergology and Immunology, Institute of Medical Sciences 'De Klokkenberg', Galderseweg 81, 4836 AE Breda, The Netherlands.

Alan Phillips BA(Hons)
Electron Microscopist, Queen Elizabeth Hospital for Children, Hackney Road, London E2 8PS, UK.

Julia M. Phillips-Quagliata PhD
Associate Professor of Pathology, Department of Pathology, New York University School of Medicine, 550 First Avenue, New York, New York 10016, USA.

Michael Pike MB, MRCP
Research Fellow, Institute of Child Health, 30 Guilford Street, London WC1N 1EH, UK; Senior Registrar in Paediatrics, Queen Mary's Hospital for Children, Carshalton, and St. George's Hospital, Tooting.

Michael John Radcliffe MB, MRCGP
General Practitioner, The Medical Centre, Hythe, Southampton, SO4 52B, UK.

Doris J. Rapp BA, MA, MD
Clinical Associate Professor of Pediatrics, State University of New York at Buffalo, 3435 Main Street, Buffalo, New York 14214, USA; Courtesy Staff at Buffalo Children's Hospital, DeGraff Memorial Hospital and Kenmore Mercy Hospital.

William J. Rea MD, PA, FACS, FACA
WJR & Associates Inc., dba/EHC-Dallas, 8345 Walnut Hill Lane, Suite 205, Dallas, Texas 75231, USA.

K. J. B. Rix MPhil, MD, CBiol, MRCPsych
Senior Lecturer in Psychiatry, University of Leeds, Leeds; Consultant Psychiatrist, Department of Psychiatry, St. James's University Hospital, Leeds LS9 7TF, UK.

Duncan Alexander Findlay Robertson BSc, MD, MRCP
Lecturer in Medicine, Southampton University, Southampton; Senior Registrar, Southampton General Hospital, Tremona Road, Southampton, SO9 4XY, UK.

Bogdan Romanski
Professor Dr. hab. med., Professor at Medical Academy in Bydgoszcz, Poland; Chairman and Head of Department of Allergology and Internal Medicine, Medical Academy Hospital, Bydgoszcz, Poland; National Consultant of Allergology in Poland.

Mark G. P. Saifer PhD
Vice President and Research Director, DDI Pharmaceuticals, Inc., Mountain View, California, USA.

Phyllis L. Saifer MD, MPH
Allergy and Environmental Medicine Private Practice, 3031 Telegraph Avenue, Berkeley, California 94705, USA; President Elect and Newsletter Editor, American Academy of Environmental Medicine.

Douglas H. Sandberg MD
Professor of Pediatrics, University of Miami School of Medicine; University of Miami Jackson Memorial Medical Center, Miami, Florida 33101, USA.

Douglas B. Seba PhD
P.O. Box 23737, Washington, DC 20024, USA.

F. Shakib PhD
Head of Immunology Division, Midlands Asthma and Allergy Research Association, 12 Vernon Street, Derby DE1 1FT, UK.

John G. Shields PhD
Research Fellow, Department of Immunology, Institute of Child Health, University of London, 30 Guilford Street, London WC1N 1EH, UK.

Roy G. Shorter MD, FRCP, FACP, FRCPath
Professor of Medicine and Pathology, Mayo Medical School, Rochester, Minnesota 55905, USA.

John F. Soothill MA, MB, FRCP, FRCPath
Emeritus Professor of Immunology, Institute of Child Health, London University, Guilford Street, London WC1N 1EH, UK; Honorary Consultant Immunologist, Hospital for Sick Children, Great Ormond Street, London.

Donald E. Sprague MD, PA
WJR & Associates Inc., dba/EHC-Dallas, 8345 Walnut Hill Lane, Suite 205, Dallas, Texas 75231, USA.

C. R. Stokes BSc, PhD
Research Fellow, Department of Veterinary Medicine, University of Bristol, Bristol BS18 7DU, UK.

Stephan Strobel MD, PhD
Lecturer in Paediatric Immunology, Department of Immunology, Institute of Child Health, University of London, 30 Guilford Street, London WC1N 1EH, UK; Honorary Consultant in Infectious Diseases and Immunology, Hospital for Sick Children, Great Ormond Street, London.

Thomas B. Tomasi MD, PhD
Distinguished University Professor and Chairman, Department of Cell Biology, University of New Mexico School of Medicine, Albuquerque, New Mexico 87131, USA.

W. Allan Walker MD
Professor of Pediatrics, Harvard Medical School; Chief, Combined Program in Pediatric Gastoenterology and Nutrition, Children's Hospital, 300 Longwood Avenue, Boston, Massachusetts 02115, USA.

John Walker-Smith MD(Sydney), FRCP(Lon.) FRCP(Ed), FRACP
Professor of Paediatric Gastroenterology, Queen Elizabeth Hospital for Children, Hackney Road, London E2 8PS, UK.

Richard K. Winkelmann MD, PhD
Professor of Dermatology, Mayo Medical School, Rochester, Minnesota; Consultant in Dermatology, Mayo Clinic, Rochester, Minnesota 55905, USA.

Jan Wojtulewski MRCP
Consultant Physician, Department of Rheumatology, Eastbourne District General Hospital, King's Drive, Eastbourne, Sussex, BN21 2UD, UK.

Derek G. Wraith MD, FRCP
Honorary Consultant Physician, Allergy Clinic, St Thomas' Hospital, London SE1 7E11, UK, Churchill Hospital Oxford, and London Allergy Clinic.

Ralph Wright MA, MD, DPhil, FRCP
Professor of Medicine, Southampton University, Southampton; Professor of Medicine, Southampton General Hospital, Tremona Road, Southampton, SO9 4XY, UK.

L. J. F. Youlten MB BS, PhD
Honorary Lecturer in Medicine and Clinical Pharmacology, United Medical and Dental Schools of Guy's and St. Thomas' Hospitals, London; Honorary Consultant in Applied Pharmacology, Guy's Hospital, London SE1 9RT, UK.

Carlo Zanussi MD
Chief of Department, Internal Medicine, 2nd Clinic, University of Milan, Via F. Sforza 35, Milan, Italy.

Preface

As all who deal in the field will know, food allergy is an exciting, challenging, exasperating and sometimes controversial subject. Its study should be a clinical science with diagnosis based on a combination of clinical observations and scientific investigations.

The study of food allergy is incomplete without a fundamental knowledge of how food is processed by the body, in both normal and abnormal conditions, and of how the majority of us are tolerant from an immunological point of view of large quantities of foreign protein to which the body is exposed each day. This is a triumph of the body's adaptation to man's eating habits. It is when this tolerance is broken that maladaptation and disease occur.

The field of food allergy has generally been considered to be a clinical art rather than a laboratory science. There is more than an element of truth in this since clinical observations have often not been supported by reliable diagnostic tests or even laboratory data. This has led to scepticism of some of the clinical associations, especially when the mechanisms of any proposed food allergies are not understood.

Clinical pragmatism is accepted as fundamental in most of the major specialties, but food allergy seems to be an exception. Here there has been a strong tendency for the conventional physician to say that if the mechanism is not understood then food allergy does not exist, especially if the symptoms of the patient do not fit into a conventional diagnostic pigeonhole. This is of course unacceptable.

Clinical medicine is the practice of an art which combines clinical ability with sound judgement based on experience and an understanding of the scientific basis of the specialty. To make a diagnosis certainly requires clinical skill but does not necessarily need a complete understanding of the mechanisms underlying the disease process or an exact understanding of the aetiology. Clinical observation comes before scientific understanding and this is highlighted by many of the names that we give diseases such as Intrinsic Asthma, Essential Hypertension, Minimal Change Nephropathy, Nummular Eczema, and Irritable Bowel Syndrome. These are labels of ignorance and are hardly enlightening as to mechanism or cause.

In this book we have attempted to provide a scientific basis for the clinical observations of food allergy and intolerance. The importance attached to understanding the basic mechanisms underlying food allergy is, we hope, emphasized by a comprehensive review of the structure and function of the gut, its immune cells and secretions, the mechanisms of normal antigen handling, and the contribution that animal models can make to our understanding. This section also emphasizes the fact that, under normal conditions, processing of antigens in the gut may lead to protective effects at distant sites, especially with regard to secretory immunity and oral tolerance.

Certain food allergens have now been chemically characterized, and in the second section of the book the relevance of these in food allergic disease and as models for yet uncharacterized antigens or allergies is discussed.

A major part of the book is devoted to end-organ effects of food allergy or intolerance. Our objective has been to review the evidence for the involvement of reactions to foods in the manifestation of disease at different sites and in different organs. We have brought together a group of scientists and clinicians whose main aim is to help us understand the immunopathological and other processes in our patients. Their points of view are diverse and some are considered unorthodox. There is no suggestion that, because we have invited particular authors to contribute to our book, we necessarily agree with their view. Occasionally the reverse is true! Differing views in clinical medicine are more the rule than the exception, but we hope that these chapters provide the link between clinical art and laboratory science.

A thread running through all these chapters and those in Parts IV and V is that the cornerstone of diagnosis of food intolerance is the removal of that food from the patient's diet with concomitant improvement (or not) of the patient's symptoms and their reappearance on adding that food back—preferably in a double-blind manner. At the clinical level, the effect of the manoeuvre is all that matters to the patient— the mechanism is irrelevant. However, the more that is understood about mechanisms the closer we come to diagnostic tests, and the value of in vivo or in vitro tests in diagnosis has been critically reviewed.

The objective of increased understanding of food allergic disease must be the application of this knowledge to the treatment and prevention of disease in the patient. Antigen avoidance, hyposensitization, the usefulness of drugs and immunological intervention are all discussed in the final section. The prevalence of food allergy in the population is unknown, but it is possible that it may be as high as that of classical atopy (about 15%). It should be one of the easiest diseases to treat (by avoidance), which should therefore obviate the need for treatment with drugs.

We hope that the emphasis placed in this book on the correct methods for the diagnosis of food allergy may result in fewer patients being classified as food allergic without good evidence; but in contrast we hope too that increased understanding of food allergy will make physicians more aware that at least some of their polysymptomatic patients may have an organic basis for their complaints.

For many of the reasons outlined above, we feel that this is an exciting book which we hope will be found useful, stimulating and challenging. Increased understanding of the mechanisms of antigen handling, more accurate clinical diagnosis and the rapid development of laboratory tests all suggest that the extent of the role of food allergy or intolerance in disease will become even clearer in the near future.

As a postscript we would like to refer our readers to the words of Sir Peter Medawar (see p. 1017) which encapsulate what we must all be striving for.

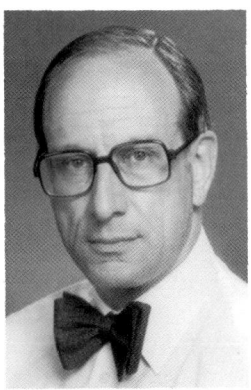 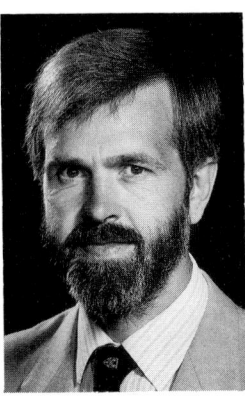

Jonathan Brostoff
Stephen Challacombe

Acknowledgements

We thank the staff of Baillière Tindall for their very great help and support and in particular Rosemary Deane, David Dickens, Cliff Morgan and Prue Theaker, and also David Inglis for his occasional Solomon-like intervention.

There is something fascinating about science. One gets such wholesale return of conjecture out of such a trifling investment of fact.

Mark Twain

SYMPATHY FOR EDITORS

I note what you say about your aspiration to edit a magazine. I am sending to you by this mail a six-chambered revolver. Load it and fire every one into your head. You will thank me after you get to Hell and learn from other editors how dreadful their job was on earth.

H. L. Mencken   *Letter to William Saroyan, January 25, 1936*

Why do we Eat?

Although physiologists have described a number of possible mechanisms that can operate to drive an individual to seek food, it is doubtful if any of these are of much importance in the life of those living in affluent Western societies. Here, with a wide variety of attractive foods freely available, eating would seem to be governed by social custom rather than necessity. The characteristic pattern of three meals a day, interspersed with midmorning and afternoon coffee or tea (or 'coke') breaks, and possibly even a last nibble before bed, scarcely leaves any time for classical hunger to develop. Indeed, the fact that most individuals maintain a reasonably constant, albeit often excessive, weight despite the frequency of presentation of ample portions of attractive foods, directs attention to the reasons for a person desisting from eating further at a particular meal, i.e. the attainment of satiety.

Although the three meal pattern, as mentioned, would obviously preclude many of the classical hunger drive mechanisms, the matter may not be so simple. Many people working in the business and professional sectors adopt a rather different meal habit. Breakfast for them may consist merely of a cup of coffee, and so they go from their evening meal to the midday meal, a matter of some 17–18 hours, without significant food or concern about its absence. Such a prolonged abstinence should call into play classical hunger mechanisms, particularly as normal carbohydrate reserves should be exhausted. Clearly the particular eating habit and a metabolic adjustment can override the effect of the physiological stimuli to the hypothalamic hunger centres that would be expected in a person not accustomed to such an eating pattern.

In considering such mechanisms and their overriding, it is salutary to consider what drastic changes have taken place in the eating habits of the affluent in a relatively short time compared to the tens of thousands of years of existence wherein the dominant pattern of eating was firstly governed by the limits of hunter-gatherer societies and then by the greatly improved food situation provided by the larger agrarian societies. However, for the vast majority of mankind, even at best, food was usually in short supply, ranging from subsistence to the occasional modest surplus. This remains true today probably for the majority of the peoples of the earth. But for some hundreds of millions of people who now make up the burgeoning affluent society the situation is quite different. For them ample supplies of a wide variety of attractive foods are freely available. It needs to be appreciated that this situation is in reality a dramatically new development in human affairs. In fact its full flowering has only occurred during the past few decades, although the seeds were planted in the latter part of the eighteenth century, when the Industrial Revolution began. The first century of this was primarily concerned with the development of large-scale industries and thus the development of great wealth for relatively few. The welfare of the many was not considered a matter of importance by governments. In matters of nutrition, the factory workers, formerly farm workers, were in many areas markedly worse off. The twentieth century saw the shift in Western societies from a dominance of heavy industries to light industries and, of particular importance, an enormous expansion of the so-called service industries. This has produced an unprecedented growth of the middle classes. Their relative wealth, wider spread within society and their wider aspirations have led to their designation as the affluent society, an important new subclassification of populations. Little noticed during these developments was another revolution, at first apparently wholly beneficial, but now in question, namely intensive animal husbandry or factory farming.

The Second World War necessitated moving millions of soldiers great distances, particularly the deployment of United States forces to Europe and the Pacific fighting areas. The supply of food to these soldiers was a major and critical problem. This was largely solved by scientists who, by applying genetic and physiological knowledge with the financial resources available due to the exigencies of war, managed to transform and amplify the production of eggs and poultry meat. Thus modern intensive farming came into being, the greatest transformation in farming practice since the introduction of the sowing and harvesting of crops. In the postwar years intensive farming techniques were rapidly developed and soon eggs from 'battery hens' dominated the marketplace and the luxury roast chicken was transformed into the ubiquitous and cheap 'broiler' chicken. Labour-intensive factory farming methods now dominate the production of animal protein. Turkeys, ducks, pigs, calves, beef and even fish can now be raised on a vast scale. Not only has production been intensified but also marketing, and not only of meat and poultry. The supermarket chains with their huge turnovers of all kinds of foods depend themselves upon the mass production of food products, many in the form of so-called 'convenience' foods. The mass production of foodstuffs depends upon a complex technology which necessitates the use of a wide range of chemicals such as preservatives, emulsifiers, stabilizers, antioxidants, flavourings and colourings. In all it has been estimated that over 2000 such non-nutritive food additives are used in the manufacture and marketing of foodstuffs. The supermarket is not the only source of 'convenience' foods. The complex social changes that have accompanied the growth of the service industries has produced a situation where, in order to afford the consumer products manufactured by the consumer society, it is now common for both husband and wife to be wage earners. Hence the role of the wife as a preparer of meals from carefully selected raw materials has diminished as the availability of tasty takeaway meals from a wide variety of small restaurants has increased. Thus the latter part of the twentieth century has seen fundamental changes in nutrition and life styles. These have come about mainly because of economic factors, i.e. the wider disposition of wealth in societies and the consequential forces of the marketplace, with little consideration for actual human needs.

It comes as no surprise, therefore, that affluent societies can be characterized by an apparent increase in susceptibility to certain diseases, particularly chronic diseases such as atherosclerosis, cardiovascular diseases, diabetes and some forms of cancer, and there is growing awareness of the possibility that underlying some of these manifestations of disease is an increase in autoimmune dysfunction. Thus, just as there are the diseases of destitution, so there are the diseases of affluence. Nutritional and environmental factors, particularly overnutrition and stress, are increasingly implicated; but which stress factors are important, and which particular nutrients are in excess remain matters of considerable controversy. Apart from the above considerations the affluent society is also exposed, possibly even more so in some cases, to the increasing pervasiveness of toxic chemicals in the domestic and general environments. Thus although the reasons for the ill-health characteristic of an affluent society are undoubtedly multifactorial there remains the concern that the basis of good health and the resistance to disease factors resides in proper nutrition and that, in the midst of apparent plenty, this is just what many people do not achieve. Thus the question—Why do we eat?—asked in the context of an affluent society needs serious consideration because it seems that, in a situation of free choice, many people are not selecting the correct mix of foods needed to supply all the molecules in the right balance necessary to maintain adequately a healthy body.

The human metabolic machinery is highly evolved and dependent upon a constant supply of molecules, some of them extremely complex. These in turn are synthesized from simple organic and mineral substances by less evolved organisms. Recent advances in molecular biology have provided new insights into not only the incredible complexity of these metabolic processes but, perhaps of greater practical significance, the extraordinary rapidity of turnover of the constituents of many important systems. Some idea of this can be gained from the magnitude of overall protein turnover, which is some 200 g per day in an adult weighing 65 kg. This is over five times the daily protein requirement. This is, however, only a crude estimate of activity. A more meaningful idea of the intensity of synthetic activity is given by the turnover of tissues. For example, the entire mucosa of the gastrointestinal tract is renewed in one to two days, and it has been estimated that some one million B lymphocytes are produced each second. This represents, among other molecules such as DNA and RNA, the daily synthesis of about 25 g of highly specialized proteins, particularly enzymes, to which can be added about 10 g of serum albumin and 2 g of fibrinogen with probably at least this amount of immunoglobulins. These few examples show that, quite apart from the activity of the liver and secretory glands, there is an enormous turnover of complex molecules each second needed for the maintenance of basic metabolic and protective functions.

Thus one essential aspect of eating can be easily identified. This is the supply of the raw materials needed to maintain the highly specialized metabolic activity of the vital tissues. The quantities needed are not large; for example, some 30 g of protein should suffice to supply the amino acid requirement—that is about one medium steak. However, at the level of the vital 'core' tissues it is the quality of the input that matters not the quantity. In particular it is the crucial supply of micronutrients that must be maintained, because many of them, for example vitamin C, cannot be stored in the body. Although knowledge of the importance of many micronutrients, such as the vitamins and trace elements, has been known for decades, their mode of action at the molecular level remains in many cases obscure, as does their requirement particularly when the dynamics of supply are considered in a situation of metabolic stress. Another aspect of eating that has been well publicized in a calorie-conscious age is the need for energy to drive the biological machine. This is the function of the fats and carbohydrates of the diet. However, this simple statement is proving extemely difficult to translate into quantitative practical terms such as what kind, how much and in what ratios. One of the problems of the affluent society is the question of so-called empty calories that come from excess consumption of energy-rich foods, especially alcoholic beverages. It is held by some that prolonged excess consumption results in endocrine and metabolic changes that underlie the diseases of affluence.

It is now appreciated that food contains, in addition to its useful constituents, useless and even potentially dangerous substances and, even though these latter may be in minute quantities, their low-level prolonged intake can result in serious diseases such as cancer. Such toxic molecules are widespread in natural products, for example the aflatoxins, and some may be produced by the process of cooking itself, particularly grilling and toasting. Human metabolic processes have evolved to detoxify many of these substances. Such detoxifications do, however, depend upon a supply of specialized intracellular molecules, such as glutathione, and these in turn depend upon a suitable supply of substrate molecules from the diet. In addition it is now known that certain micronutrients such as vitamin C, vitamin E and β-carotene play a crucial role as anti-carcinogens. A further problem in this context arises from the ubiquity of the products of the chemical industry in the domestic and general environments, a phenomenon of the mid-twentieth century. Toxicologists have discovered that a few widely used chemicals were, rather surprisingly, carcinogens. The identification of vinyl chloride monomer, the basis of the plastic polythene, as a carcinogen was the first intimation of the possible dangers of new classes of man-made molecules. Since that discovery many potentially dangerous chemicals have been identified and eliminated. However there are thousands of chemicals in common use about which little is known toxicologically. There is concern that some of these may produce health effects as yet unidentified because the possibility is not considered, despite the growing evidence from animal studies.

The intracellular detoxification of molecules is one aspect of the defence system of the body against foreign material. Molecules too large to enter cells, macromolecules or microorganisms that gain entrance to the body are dealt with, not always effectively, by the incredibly complex and dynamic immune system. The turnover of its constituents is enormous and is obviously dependent for full efficiency on an adequate and continuing supply of substrate molecules. Thus it can be seen that the diet must provide in addition to the molecules needed for vital functions, maintenance and energy, a further and variable supply of key molecules for the 'non-nutritive' functioning of the defence systems of the body.

The importance of nutritional factors in the disease of affluence seems obvious. Thus the question—Why do we eat?—is not trivial. It is necessary to understand why people choose to eat what they eat, and in so doing fail to obtain what they need. It is also obvious that nutritional science has at present no satisfactory understanding of what should constitute an adequate diet. It is to be hoped that the wider perspectives that have come about because of the great advances in molecular biology will stimulate scientists and clinicians to pay greater attention to human nutrition, particularly as what seems apparent in the adult must also have implications for infants, children, the pregnant and the aged.

Morrell Draper

PART I

BASIC MECHANISMS

1

SECTION F. MODEL SYSTEMS OF ANTIGEN HANDLING

SECTION A
NORMAL STRUCTURE AND FUNCTION

Chapter 1
The Structure and Organization of Lymphoid Tissue in the Gut

D. M. V. Parrott

Introduction

Large numbers of lymphocytes, macrophages, eosinophils, mast cells, plasma cells and various types of antigen-presenting cells are distributed throughout the mucosal surfaces of the gut. There are, therefore, all the cellular components required for the induction and implementation of the whole spectrum of immune responses. Some of these cellular components are organized into discrete lymphoid organs, whilst other cell types, e.g. IgA-secreting plasma cells and some phenotypes of intraepithelial lymphocyte, are found only in the mucosa. The purpose of this introductory chapter is to describe functional anatomy of the lymphoid tissue of the gut tract and to point out the strategic placement of various organs or cell types especially during development.

STRUCTURE OF THE LYMPHOEPITHELIAL ORGANS

The lymphoepithelial structures of the gut differ from other lymphoid organs in that they lack a defined capsule or afferent lymphatics but are distinguished by their covering epithelium which facilitates antigen sampling.

This contrasts with the remainder of the epithelium of the gut which forms a barrier to large particles, organisms and undigested macromolecules. The lymphoepithelial structures of gut-associated lymphoid tissues (GALT) include tonsils, Peyer's patches, appendix, caecal patches and colonic patches, which are common to several species including man, rabbit, rat, mouse, hamster, dogs and monkeys [8, 72]. Other species have additional but comparable tissue such as the sacculus rotundus in the rabbit and the caecal tonsil in the bird.

There are similar lymphoepithelial structures in the respiratory tract. These include the adenoids and the bronchus-associated lymphoid tissues [6].

Structure of Peyer's patches

Correlation between the structure and function of the lymphoepithelial organs is most easily understood by examining Peyer's patches since these are present in all mammals and have been the focus of most experimental work.

They were first described by Peyer in 1667 and are present from the duodenum to the ileum but are more numerous and larger in the distal than in the proximal intestine. The number of Peyer's patches varies according to species, from around 12 in the mouse, 20 in the rat to 200 in man [14, 93]. In sheep [82] and pigs [7] there are two separate categories of Peyer's patch: those (approximately 25–35

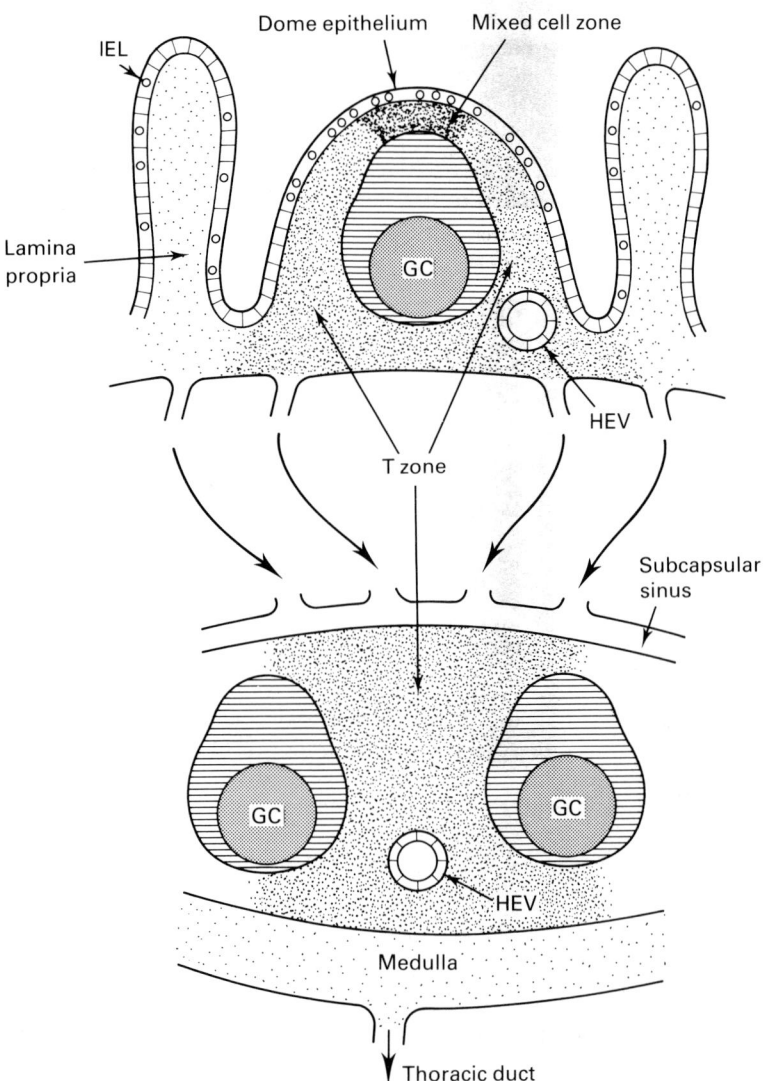

Fig. 1.1 Diagram of the structure of a Peyer's patch and a mesenteric lymph node. HEV = high endothelial walled venule, GC = germinal centre.

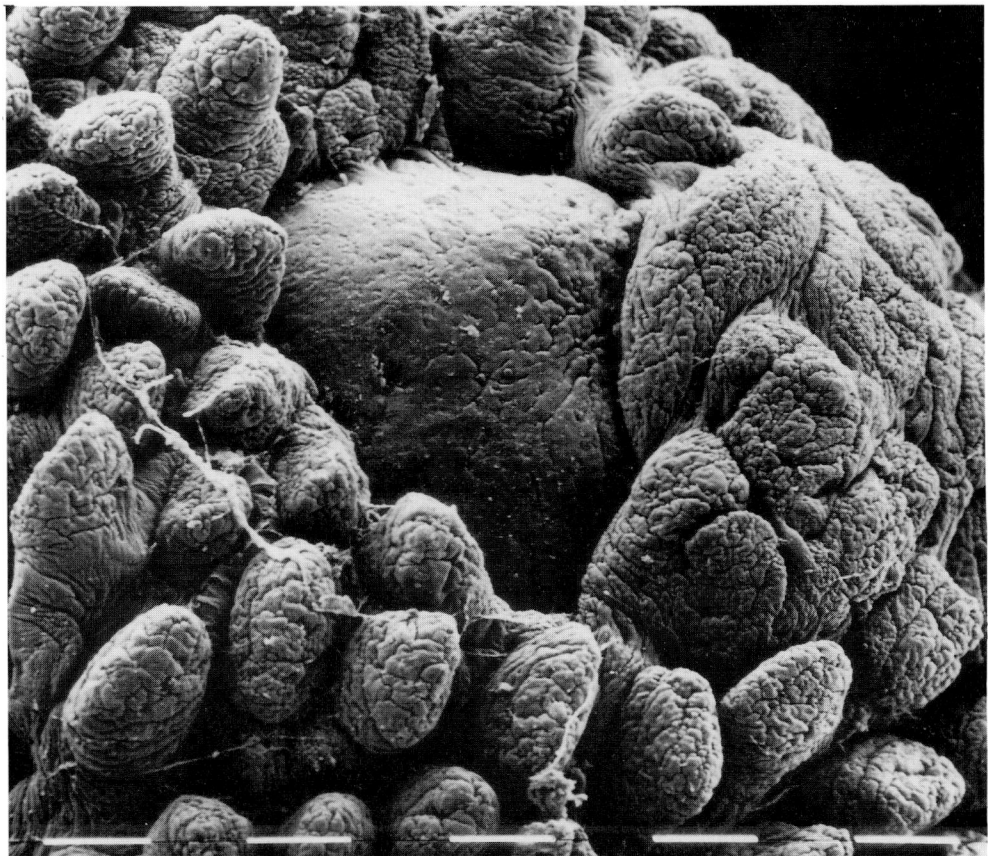

Fig. 1.2 (a) Scanning electron micrograph of a Peyer's patch. This preparation was made four days after a primary infection with *T. spiralis* and there is patchy villous atrophy to the right of the dome area.

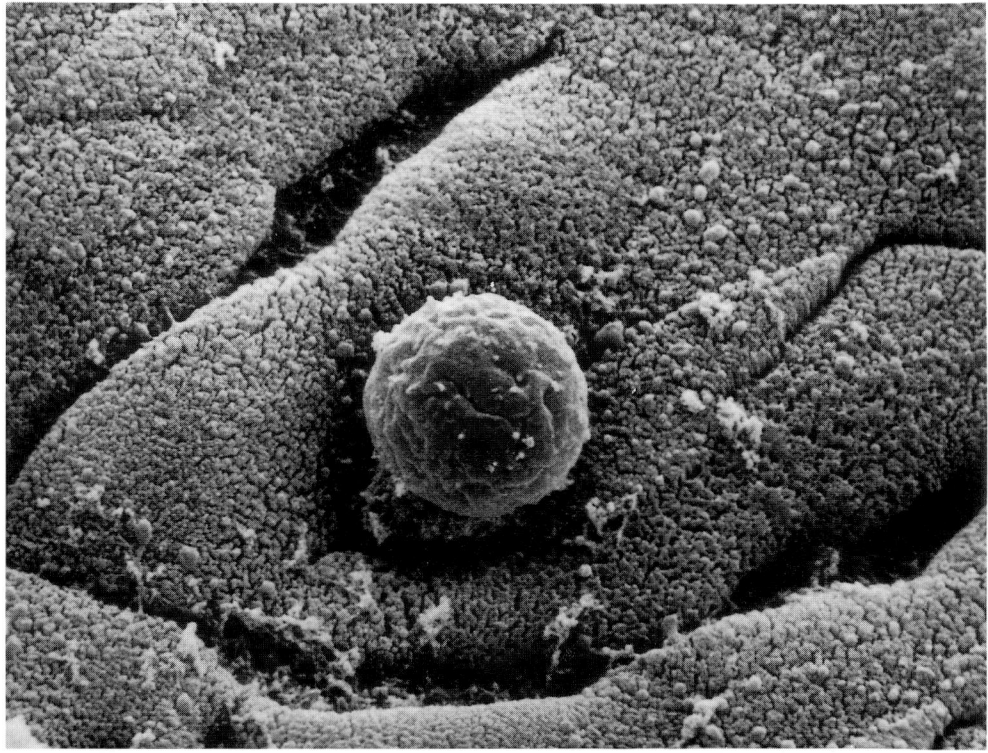

Fig. 1.2 (b) Higher power electron micrograph of the dome epithelium. A lymphocyte has been extruded.

in number and comparatively small) that are distributed along the jejunum and proximal ileum and persist throughout life; and one very large ileocaecal patch which extends for up to 2.5 metres along the terminal ileum but which involutes at about one year of age.

Peyer's patches extend through the lamina propria and submucosa of the small intestine and are usually composed of several nodules of lymphocytes though individual single nodules do occur, and they are almost always only one nodule thick (Figs. 1.1 and 1.2). Crypts and villi are sparse in the overlying epithelium of Peyer's patches and that part of the epithelium which is immediately above the nodules is heavily infiltrated with lymphocytes and is known as the dome area (Fig. 1.1). The epithelium of the dome is cuboidal rather than columnar and there are few, if any, goblet cells [25].

Follicle-associated epithelial cells

Within the epithelium are modified cells, called follicle-associated epithelial (FAE) cells in mouse Peyer's patches [10] and M or microfold cells in human Peyer's patches [71] (see Chapter 4). These cells have short, irregular microvilli and numerous tubules, vesicles and vacuoles in the apical cytoplasm. The FAE cells have been demonstrated to transport inert particles such as carbon particles and ferritin as well as microorganisms. An example of the efficiency of FAE cells is demonstrated by the experiments of Wolf et al [106] who inoculated reovirus type 1 into mouse ileum and observed a preferential adherence of viral particles to the surface of FAE cells. Within one hour, virus particles had been transported through FAE cells to the strategically placed subepithelial layer. This layer has some of the characteristics of a traffic area with an open-work pattern of reticulum [76] containing small T and B lymphocytes, plasma cells, macrophages and dendritic cells (Fig. 1.1) (see below and Chapter 4) and has all the cellular components to be an important site of interaction with antigen. The nodules and germinal centres are composed primarily of B cells and the interfollicular corridors between are occupied by T cells [21]. Prominent postcapillary high endothelial-walled venules (HEV) are located in the interfollicular zones which provide an entry pathway for circulating T and B lymphocytes [21, 74, 76].

In this chapter, most emphasis will be placed on Peyer's patches and on the organization of the lymphoid elements of the intestine. It is, however, worth reflecting that the route of sensitization to food antigens is not certain, and, although it may be reasonable to assume that sensitization takes place where digested food is absorbed, i.e. in the intestine, a role for other tissues higher in the gastrointestinal tract or even the upper respiratory tract cannot be excluded. A potentially important tissue is, therefore, the tonsillar tissue.

Tonsils

In humans, the palatine tonsils which lie between the palatine arches at the junction of the mouth and pharynx are the first lymphoepithelial organs of the gut tract to come into contact with food and other ingested materials. The external surface of the tonsils, unlike Peyer's patches and appendix, is covered by several layers of squamous epithelium [18] infiltrated with lymphocytes. There are crypts which penetrate deeply into tonsil tissue and these crypts facilitate the interaction of luminal contents with lymphocytes and macrophages [45]. Studies in pigs have shown that antigens, including horseradish peroxidase and bacteria, can be transported from the pharynx into the tonsil [105]. These antigens stimulate germinal centre formation in both tonsil tissue and draining lymph nodes.

Two other potentially important lymphoepithelial tissues are the appendix and colonic lymphoid patches.

The appendix

The appendix lies at the junction of the small intestine and the colon. It is a blind diverticulum from the caecum, lined with colonic epithelium and studded with lymphoid follicles. It is seen only in rabbits, anthropoid apes, gibbons and man. The appendix has many structural characteristics in common with Peyer's patches [10, 72, 75, 96] with a clearly defined dome, nodular aggregates of B lymphocytes and a T dependent area sandwiched between adjacent nodules [75, 96] (see Fig. 1.3a–c). The dome epithelium is non-columnar, lacking goblet cells and containing large numbers of intraepithelial lymphocytes (Fig. 1.3a–c). Soluble and particulate antigens, Indian ink and even intact bacteria pass freely through the dome epithelium [10, 90]. The appendix epithelium of both humans and rabbits contains cells with short irregular microvilli and pinocytotic properties similar to the FAE cells in Peyer's patches [10, 72].

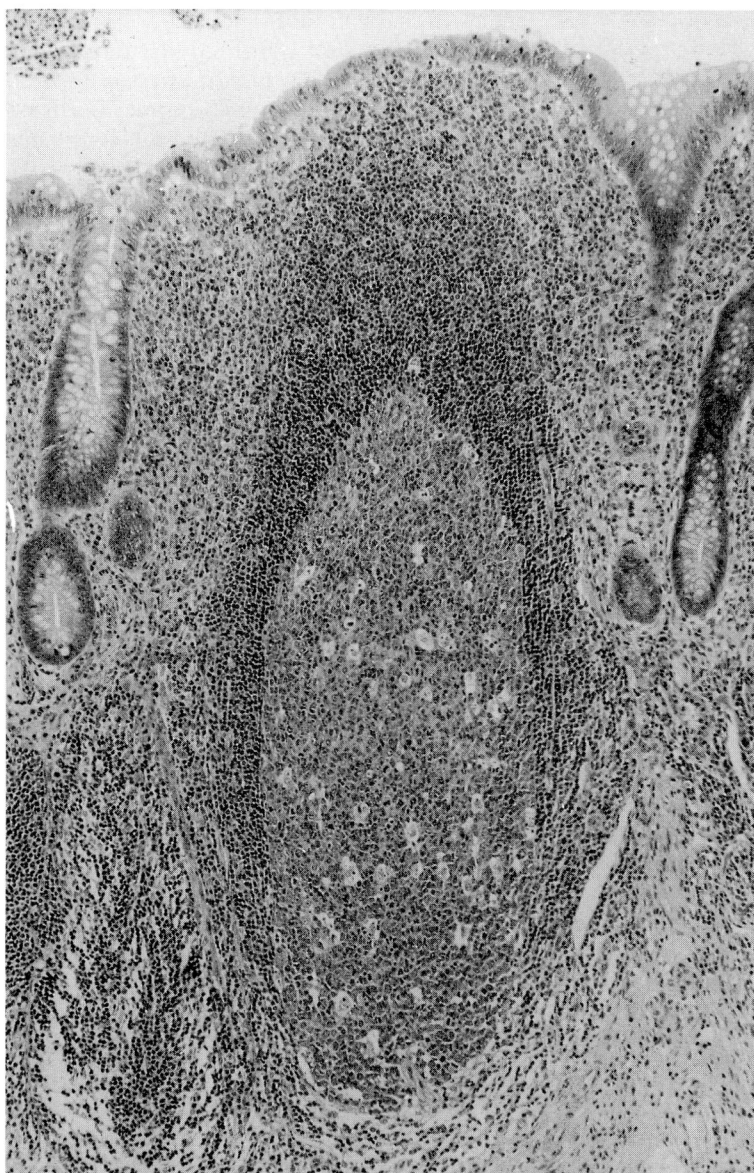

Fig. 1.3 (a) Lymphoid nodule in human appendix. A prominent reactive nodule with many tingible body macrophages is surrounded by a mantle of lymphocytes which merges with the mixed cell zone beneath the dome epithelium. There are many IEL in the dome epithelium but no goblet cells. Goblet cells are prominent in the adjacent crypts. Haematoxylin and eosin × 100.

Colonic lymphoid patches

Bland and Britton [8] have recently carried out a detailed study of the antigen-sampling structures known as colonic lymphoid patches in the rat. These patches are very similar to Peyer's patches and appendix in that the nodules are separated from the gut lumen by follicle-associated epithelium which lacks goblet cells. The FAE cells preferentially take up ferritin and Indian ink and are capable of lysing bacteria, but have normal microvilli unlike the microfold cell which is present in the FAE of Peyer's patches.

The phenotypes of lymphocytes in GALT

The proportion of T:B lymphocytes varies according to organ and the age of the animal. For example, there are approximately 61% of T cells in the human tonsil [45] compared with 20–30% of T cells in rodent Peyer's patch [49, 78] (Table 1.1). In the unusual ileocaecal Peyer's patches of sheep [82] and pigs [7], T lymphocytes account for only 1–2% of the total lymphocyte population though jejunal Peyer's patches of the same species contain 25% of T cells. In the newborn mouse or rat, T lymphocytes account for almost all the lym-

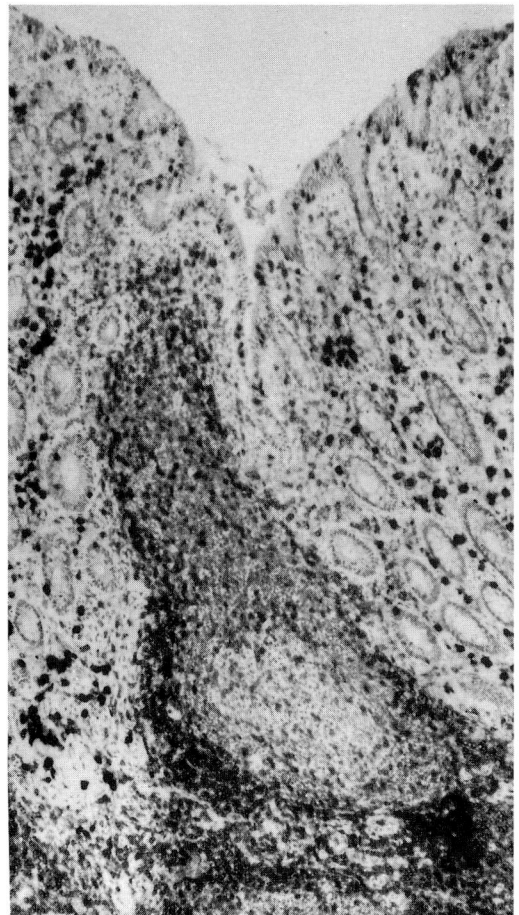

Fig. 1.3 (b) Cryostat section of a human appendix stained with a pan T cell monoclonal antibody (UCH T₁). A rim of T cells can be seen around the lymphoid nodule plus a few T cells within the nodule. These merge with a sheet of cells below the T dependent area. Many intraepithelial lymphocytes (IEL) are also stained. Immunoperoxidase × 100.

phocytes that can be found in Peyer's patches [74,104] (Fig. 1.4), but in adult animals with large follicles and germinal centres with their surrounding corona of lymphocytes B cells almost always predominate [76]. T cells stained with the monoclonal antibody W3/13 (a pan T cell marker) are found in the interfollicular (T dependent area) of rat Peyer's patches [53,104]. There are a few T cells in the dome area, in the lumenal pole of the germinal centre and scattered in the corona. The antibody (W3/13) does not stain many of the cells in the intraepithelial position of the dome. These cells do, however, stain with W3/25 which stains both macrophages and helper T cells. A mixture of cell types in the epithelium covering the human appendix has also been described recently by Spencer et al [96] who found T cells predominantly of the suppressor type together with 4–5% of B cells. Spencer et al [96] and Janossy et al [45] both emphasize the predominance of helper T cells over suppressor T cells in human appendix and tonsil. In the human appendix follicle, the only T cells present are of the helper phenotype and in the T cell areas, the ratio of helper to suppressor cells is 8:1. In the human tonsil, the helper to suppressor ratio is 3.5:1 and in mouse and rat Peyer's patch tissue (Table 1.1) there is a similar numerical predominance of helper T cells.

Immunoglobulin-producing cells in GALT

Although the GALT contains very large numbers of surface Ig-bearing cells, the statement is often made, most frequently in respect

Fig. 1.3 (c) Cryostat section of the mixed cell zones and dome epithelium stained with monoclonal antibody to B cells. Numerous B cells are present in the mixed cell zone. A cluster of stained cells (presumably B cells) is evident in the dome epithelium but not amongst intraepithelial lymphocytes in the crypt epithelium. Immunoperoxidase × 350. (Fig. 1.3a–c reproduced from [96] by kind permission of Dr Jo Spencer and the editors of *Gut*.)

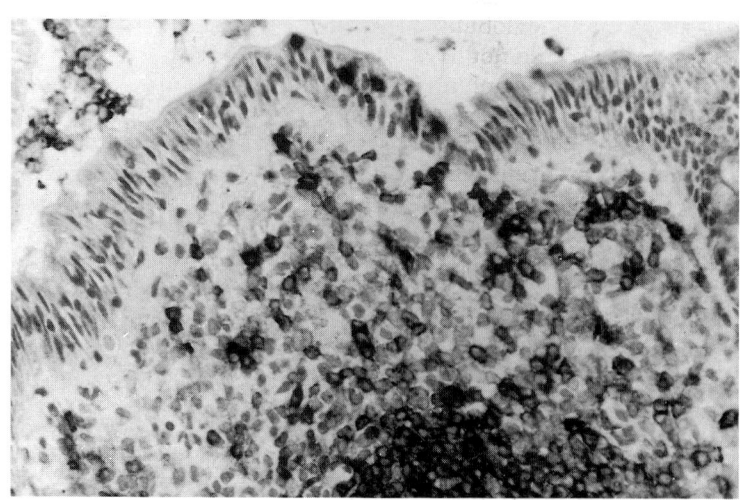

Table 1.1   Cell surface characteristics of lymphoid and antigen-presenting cells in the intestinal mucosal system.

(a) **Lymphoid**

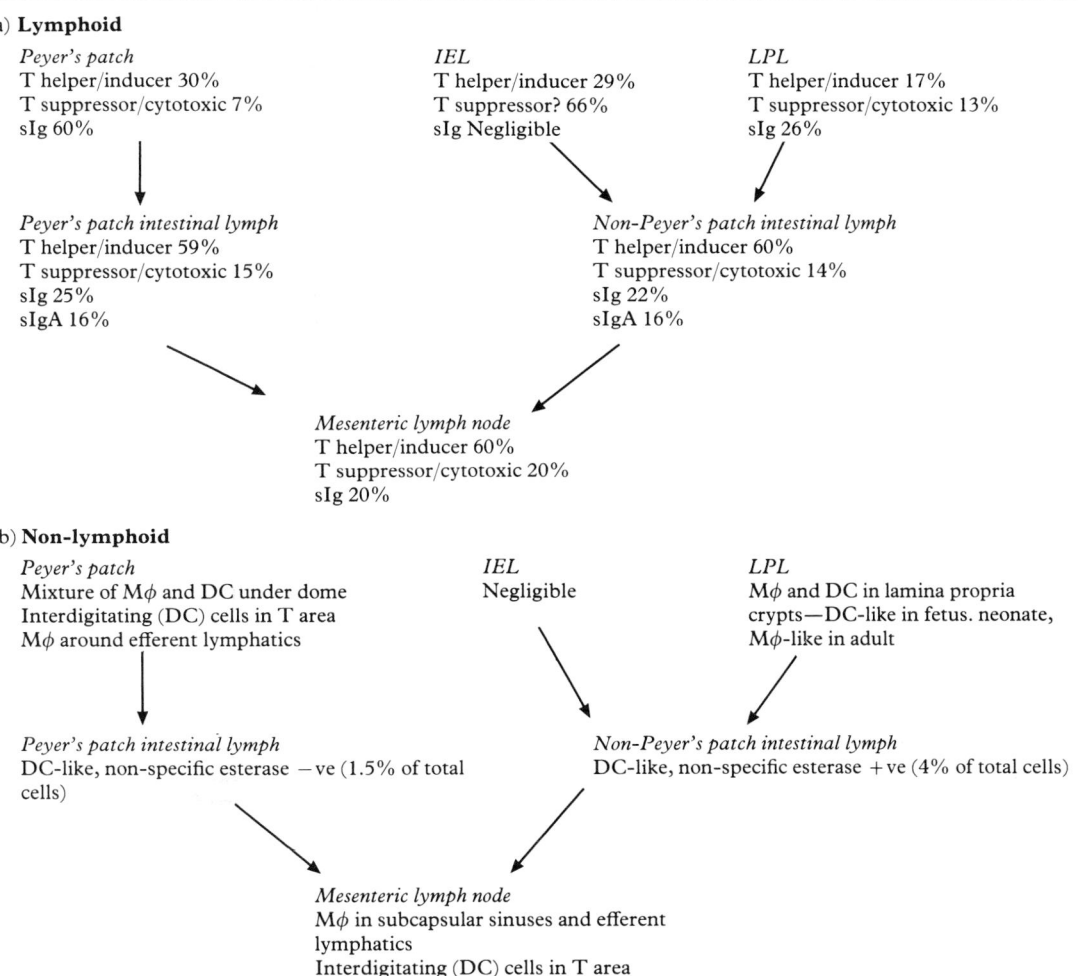

Peyer's patch
T helper/inducer 30%
T suppressor/cytotoxic 7%
sIg 60%

IEL
T helper/inducer 29%
T suppressor? 66%
sIg Negligible

LPL
T helper/inducer 17%
T suppressor/cytotoxic 13%
sIg 26%

Peyer's patch intestinal lymph
T helper/inducer 59%
T suppressor/cytotoxic 15%
sIg 25%
sIgA 16%

Non-Peyer's patch intestinal lymph
T helper/inducer 60%
T suppressor/cytotoxic 14%
sIg 22%
sIgA 16%

Mesenteric lymph node
T helper/inducer 60%
T suppressor/cytotoxic 20%
sIg 20%

(b) **Non-lymphoid**

Peyer's patch
Mixture of Mφ and DC under dome
Interdigitating (DC) cells in T area
Mφ around efferent lymphatics

IEL
Negligible

LPL
Mφ and DC in lamina propria
crypts—DC-like in fetus. neonate,
Mφ-like in adult

Peyer's patch intestinal lymph
DC-like, non-specific esterase −ve (1.5% of total cells)

Non-Peyer's patch intestinal lymph
DC-like, non-specific esterase +ve (4% of total cells)

Mesenteric lymph node
Mφ in subcapsular sinuses and efferent lymphatics
Interdigitating (DC) cells in T area

Data from [35, 49, 53, 78, 98, 104].
Mφ = macrophage(s); DC = dendritic cell(s).

of Peyer's patches, that the GALT does not contain immunoglobulin-producing cells. These structures do not have areas comparable to the medulla of lymph nodes or the red pulp of the spleen where plasma cells accumulate. The human tonsil, however, contains fairly large numbers of cells which have cytoplasmic immunoglobulin, the most predominant class being IgG followed by IgA, IgM and IgD [47]. The appendix and Peyer's patches do have some plasma cells which are to be found in T areas [53,76] and occasionally in the dome [75,76], and the absence of specific antibody-forming cells after oral stimulation is striking [5]. It has been reported that immunoglobulin-producing cells do appear transiently in Peyer's patches between four and five weeks of age but then disappear [36].

The resolution of this particular problem is still to be found but it is almost certainly not due to inadequate numbers of helper T cells or of antigen-presenting cells (see below), nor to abnormally large numbers of suppressor cells, at least as far as can be deduced from phenotype expression.

The phenotype of mucosal leukocytes

Large numbers of leukocytes inhabit all the mucosal tissues of the gut tract but as with the gut-associated lymphoid tissues, most experimental studies have been directed towards one part of the tract, namely the small intestine, on the tacit assumption that the small intestine is representative of the whole. There are two distinct and separate populations: those clo-

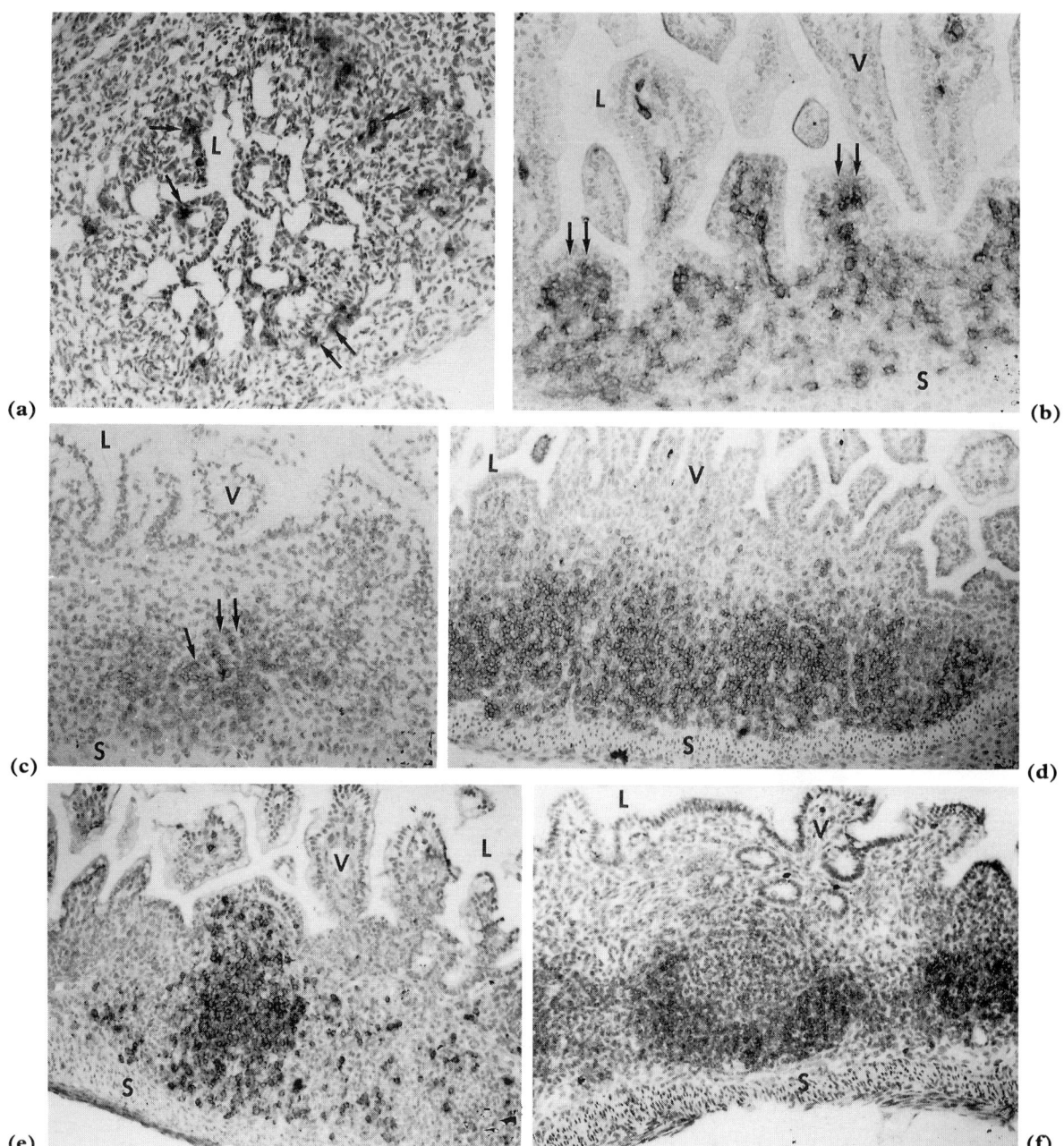

Fig. 1.4 The ontogeny of rat Peyer's patches. (a) Gut of 16-day-old fetus. Numerous Ia-positive cells (arrows). (b) Peyer's patch at 20 days gestation. Note the dome-shaped epithelium (arrows) and accumulations of Ia-positive dendritic cells. (c) Peyer's patch at day of birth. Scattered W3/13 positive cells (T cells). (d) Peyer's patch at four days after birth. T lymphocytes form a broad band near the serosal side. (e) Peyer's patch eight days after birth with nodule containing numerous sIgM cells. (f) At eight days after birth, T lymphocytes are present in a horseshoe-shaped area beneath the nodules of sIgM cells. Cryostat sections stained with MRC-Ox 3 mouse anti-rat Ia serum (a, b) or with mouse anti-rat T cell (W3/13) (c, d). × 200. L = gut lumen, S = serosal side, V = villus.

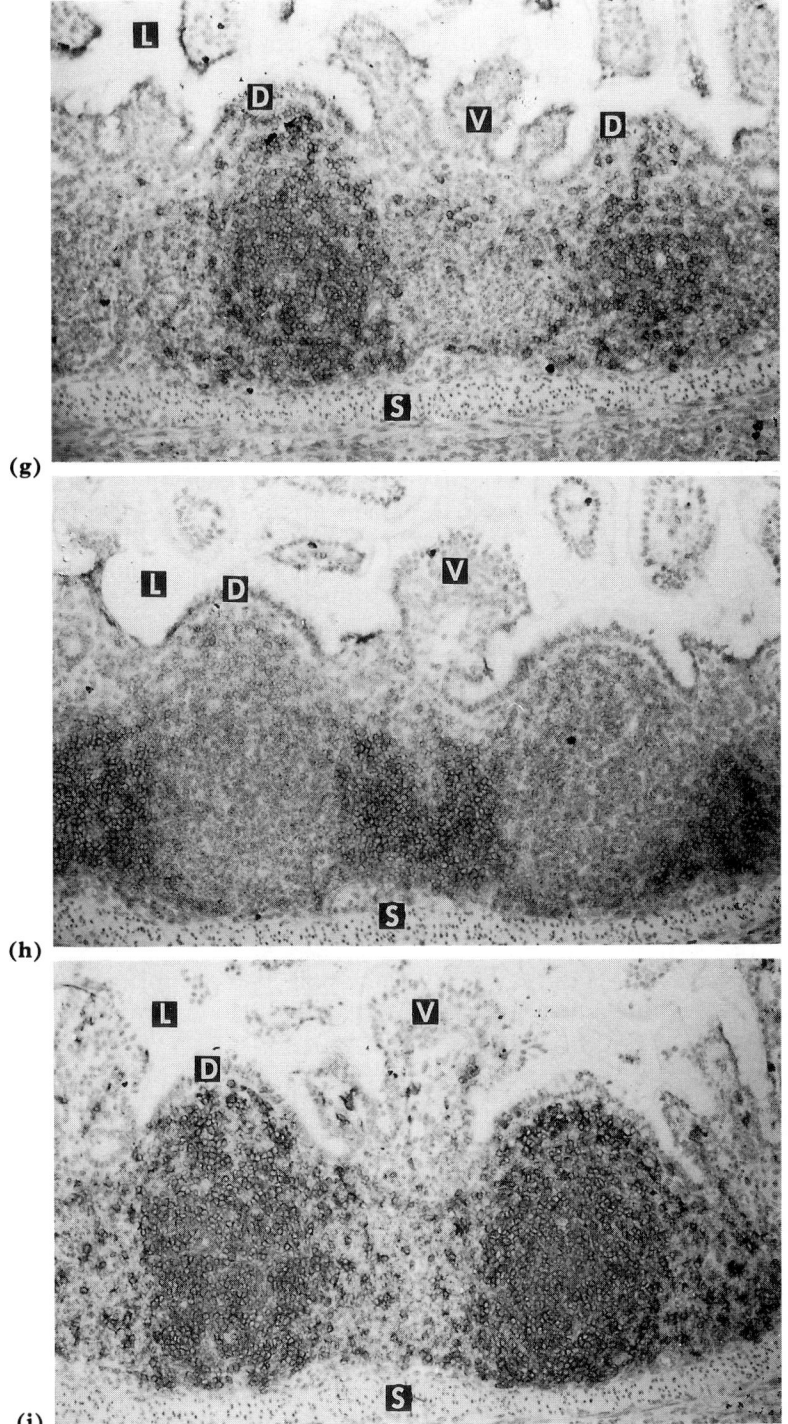

(g)

(h)

(i)

Fig. 1.4 (g–i) Peyer's patches of 12-day-old rats. Cryostat sections stained with (g) goat anti-mouse sIgM, (h) mouse anti-rat T cell (W3/13) (i) MRC-Ox 3 mouse anti-rat Ia serum. × 200. L = gut lumen, D = dome, S = serosal side, V = villus.

Note: Peyer's patches are beginning to assume adult morphology although there are no germinal centres yet. T cells are pushed into an interfollicular site by developing nodules. sIg cells are still mostly IgM. Villi still contain only Ia-positive cells—there are no T cells or Ig containing cells.

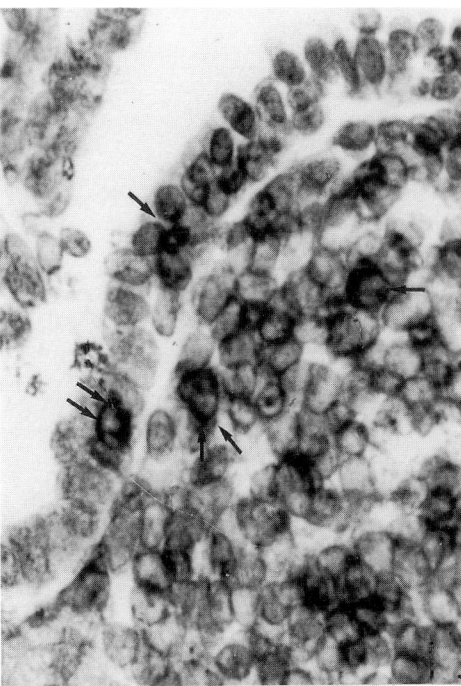

Fig. 1.4 (j) Ia-positive dendritic cells (arrows) between the epithelial cells of the dome and in the subepithelial mixed cell of the Peyer's patch of a 12-day-old rat (× 500). (Fig. 1.4a–j reproduced from [104] by kind permission of the authors and the editor of *Immunology*.)

sest to antigenic challenge and sited between the epithelial cells, and the so-called intra-epithelial lymphocytes (IEL) once considered to be all T lymphocytes [27] but which recent data indicate may be much more heterogeneous than previously supposed [24, 78]. There may be a few mast cells, very few macrophages and virtually no Ig+-bearing cells amongst IEL [19], though there may be isolated antigen-presenting cells [53] (Fig. 1.4j). The cells on the lamina propria are separated from the surface epithelium and include large numbers of plasma cells, T and B lymphocytes, some macrophages, granulocytes and mast cells. Plasma cells are usually considered to be the major cell type in the lamina propria, but even in situ this is probably not true, there being roughly equal numbers of lymphocytes and plasma cells in the lamina propria. In preparing suspensions of lamina propria lymphocytes almost all plasma cells are lost [19, 49] and the representation of different subsets of T cells may also be changed [87]. Methods of isolating IEL and lamina propria lymphocytes (LPL) have facilitated studies of phenotype and function but they do change the proportions of different cell types found.

The morphology and histochemistry of intraepithelial lymphocytes

IEL are located amongst the epithelial cells, above the basal lamina, and they are intimately related to lumenal antigen [27]. It has been known for many years that their numbers are a sensitive reflection of external stimuli [29]. A variable proportion are thymus-independent, very few have surface immunoglobulin and although the majority carry surface antigens associated with T lymphocytes they are morphologically and functionally very heterogeneous. Up to 60% of IEL in mice, depending upon strain, contain distinct cytoplasmic granules that stain with Giemsa or Astra blue [78]. Similar granules in IEL have also been found in rats and rabbits, and somewhat smaller ones in humans [2, 34]. The presence of these granules has given rise to theories that granular IEL may be natural killer (NK) cells or mast-cell precursors (see later chapters). But although mouse IEL do express some NK activity they are functionally very different from spleen NK cells and lack AsGM and NK1 surface antigens [100]. Furthermore, HNK 1+ cells have rarely [11, 86] been identified in tissue sections of human bowel though since not all human NK cells express HNK antigen it is unwise to assume that no NK activity is present in human intestinal mucosa [101].

Expression of T cell surface antigens

The expression of T cell surface antigens on IEL has recently aroused considerable interest. In 1981, Selby and his co-workers [88] made the unexpected observation in sections of human biopsy material that the majority of IEL expressed the phenotype of a cytotoxic/suppressor T 8+. Since then, there have been much more extensive observations by flow cytometry on isolated preparations of mouse IEL [24, 78] and fluorescence analysis of isolated preparations of mouse, rat and human IEL and histological sections of human material [11, 86] with appropriate monoclonal antibodies. Several unusual findings have emerged when comparing IEL with either lymph nodes or Peyer's patch lymphocytes and indeed with lamina propria lymphocytes (LPL).

Mouse and rat IEL. In mouse lymph nodes [78] or Peyer's patches virtually all T cells stain with both Thy 1 and Lyt 1, whereas a

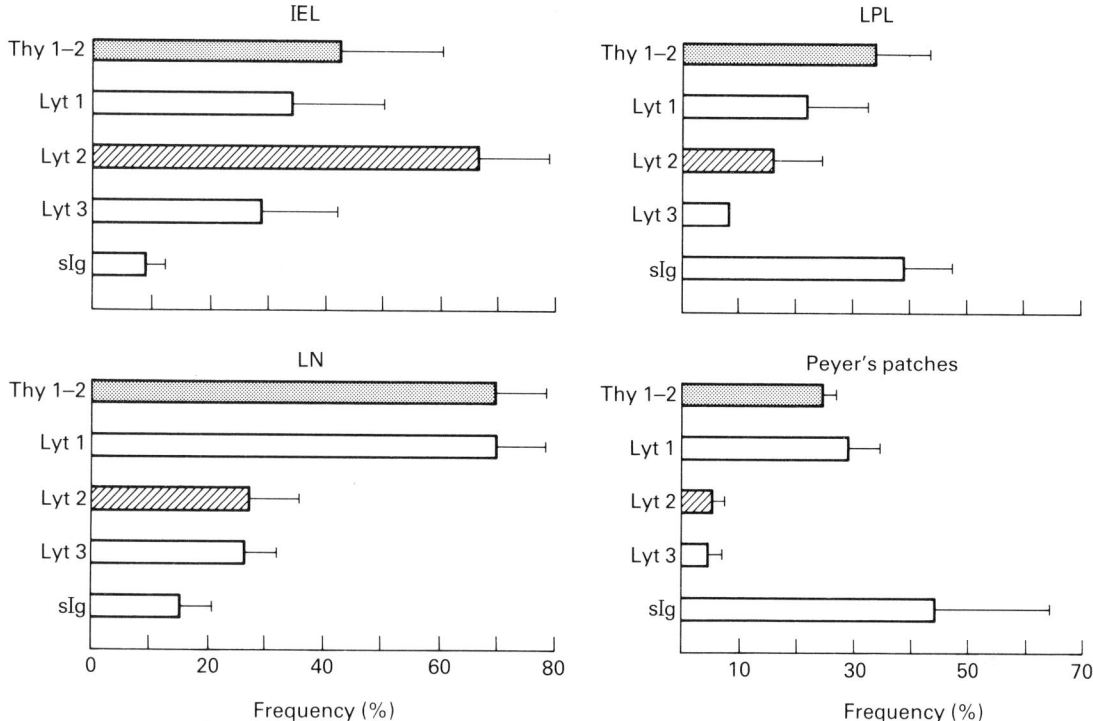

Fig. 1.5 The frequency (%) of cells carrying various membrane antigens, determined by immunofluorescence staining with monoclonal antibodies in CBA/C mice. The results are mean $\pm$ SD from between 5–12 separate pools of cells. Attention is drawn to the results of Thy 1-2 (stippled) and Lyt 2 (cross-hatched). (From [78], reproduced by kind permission of the editors of *Ann NY Acad Sci*.)

minority of cells stain for Lyt 2 and Lyt 3 in addition to Thy 1 and Lyt 2 (Fig. 1.5). Lymph nodes from nude mice contain minimal numbers of cells with any T cell markers. The distribution of staining amongst IEL is very different for lymph nodes and Peyer's patches. There are Thy 1+ cells that do not stain for Lyt 1 and there are Lyt 2+ cells which do not stain for Lyt 3, Thy 1 or Lyt 1. The Thy 1− Lyt 1−2+3− cells are especially obvious amongst IEL from nude mice because of the very low numbers of cells carrying any other T cell marker [78].

A comparable cell type possessing markers associated with suppressor cells but lacking a pan T cell marker has also been found in rat IEL [49]. It has been suggested [24, 78] that this type of IEL is a novel cell type and is probably not a T lymphocyte. In mice, the heterogeneity of IEL extends further for there are both Thy 1− and Thy 1+ cells with granules, and although the majority of Lyt 2+ have granules there are, nevertheless, significant numbers of Lyt 2+ cells without granules.

Human IEL. Selby and his colleagues [86] have carefully examined sections of human small and large intestine stained with monoclonal antibodies and they considered that since all IEL carry one pan T cell marker (HuTLA), the majority of IEL in man are T lymphocytes. The majority of IEL (over 80%) from both small and large intestine also carry OKT 8 marker though only one-third of these react with anti-Leu 1 antibody which is directed towards an antigen found on peripheral T cells. It would appear, therefore, that in humans as well as rodents, there is a variable expression of pan T cell markers on IEL. There is also a predominance of cells carrying markers which are associated with suppressor activity though whether these cells function as suppressor cells is far from clear [34]. It is clear, however, that not only are IEL morphologically and phenotypically very heterogeneous but they are also functionally very heterogeneous and do not fit neatly into patterns of phenotype and function which have been deduced by studies of blood or lymph node lymphocytes.

The phenotype of lamina propria lymphocytes (LPL)

Suspensions of lamina propria lymphocytes (LPL) contain many more cells which stain for surface Ig than for IEL (Fig. 1.5) [24, 78]. In the mouse LPL, these include cells bearing surface IgM, IgG and IgD and large numbers of cells bearing only IgA [15, 102]. In LPL, very few B lymphocytes have C3 receptors [19, 102]. There are also lymphoid cells containing immunoglobulin, again mostly IgA. The staining of T cells in LPL does show some variation. Using anti-Thy 1-2 and complement cytotoxicity, it was deduced that 75–80% of LPL carry T cell markers [19]. Similarly, high numbers of cells carrying T cell markers have been found in human intestinal LPL [87] but estimations using flow cytometry are somewhat lower, i.e. 30–40% (Fig. 1.5) [24, 78].

LPL T lymphocytes do, however, have the usual pattern of dominance of helper over suppressor phenotype. In mice, most cells stained for Thy 1^+ and Lyt 1^+ with a minority staining for Lyt 2 and Lyt 3 as well. Nevertheless, there are cells that stain for Thy 1-2 but not Lyt 1 and cells that stain for Lyt 2 but not Lyt 3. The unusual phenotype Thy 1^- Lyt 1^- Lyt 2^+ Lyt 3^- characteristic of IEL is only very rarely seen in LPL suspensions. In sections and suspensions of human intestine and colon T cells of the helper type predominate (OKT 4^+) [11, 86, 88]. It is interesting to speculate briefly on the possible function of this substantial population of helper T cells though as yet there are comparatively few experimental studies. Most immunoglobulin secretory cells are already committed to isotype and specificity before arriving in the mucosa. LPL T cells (mouse and human) have nevertheless been shown capable of stimulating immunoglobulin synthesis in peripheral blood B lymphocytes [23] but help was not restricted to particular isotypes and was seen for IgA, IgM and IgG. It could be that they are required for antigen-specific B cell expression after secondary challenge. Alternatively, their function could be related to cell-mediated immunity (see below).

MACROPHAGES, ANTIGEN-PRESENTING CELLS AND DENDRITIC CELLS

The siting of antigen-presenting cells in the gut

There are two broad classes of cells involved in the processing and presentation of antigen-inflammatory macrophages and dendritic-type cells. Macrophages have endocytic and microbicidal capabilities, are usually positioned to scavenge and clear antigen and are a major first line of defence. By contrast, the dendritic type of cells which function as accessory cells and are a requirement for the stimulation of many lymphocyte responses are likely to be poised near recirculating lymphocytes and are accessible to antigen that escapes macrophage clearance. For example, the macrophages are concentrated on the red pulp of the spleen and the sinuses of lymph nodes whilst dendritic cells are concentrated on the white pulp of the spleen and the cortex of the lymph nodes. The expression of Class II antigens on macrophages is variable in rats and mice but increases considerably under stimuli; it is usually present in inflammatory macrophages in humans. Class II antigens are almost always present on antigen presenting/accessory/dendritic cells.

The identification of the siting of macrophages versus dendritic cells is, therefore, a very important consideration in terms of mucosal immunity. In achieving a nice balance between clearance of antigen load and initiating immune defensive reaction without initiating destructive immune reaction, the correct strategic placement of different cell types is especially important in processing food antigens.

The presence of follicle-associated epithelium in the dome areas of GALT has already been mentioned in the previous section but there are also both macrophages and dendritic cells in mucosa and various GALT. However, it has proved more difficult to differentiate clearly between macrophages and dendritic/accessory cells in the gut tract than in other lymphoid tissue.

Peyer's patch and other GALT

It has been known for some time that there are macrophages with phagocytic properties in Peyer's patches [9, 46]. There are also obvious tingible body macrophages in germinal centres. The macrophage-like cells under the dome (and occasionally in the epithelium itself) are however heterogeneous [53, 91] being strongly acid phosphatase and non-specific esterase (NSE) positive with only slight Ia membrane staining. There are also cells which are stongly Ia positive in the T cell areas with weak acid phosphate and NSE staining. They are non-adherent and have the characteristics of dendritic (or interdigitating) cells which behave functionally as dendritic cells released from other lymphoid tissues [95]. Immunohistochemical studies on the human appendix have also shown large numbers of HLA-DR stained cells in both T and dome areas [96]. Follicular dendritic cells are present in germinal centres of rat Peyer's patches. These are yet another type of accessory cell which appear to be involved in the presentation of antigen to germinal centre B cells and are different from other dendritic cells in possessing Fc receptors, in being very adherent and in having a variable expression of Ia antigens [39]. The existence of these cells in the human tonsil has been known for some time [94] but only recently have they been isolated from human tonsils and adenoids and are now therefore available for in vitro functional testing.

Intestinal mucosa

Rat macrophage-like cells. It is only recently that the macrophage-like cells which are present in the intestine have been differentiated into macrophages and dendritic-like cells [53, 104]. Mayrhofer et al [53] have described abundant Ia$^+$ cells in the lamina propria of the rat intestine. They are large, with dendritic morphology. Between the crypts and lower one-third of the villi the cells have little cytoplasm but those in the upper two-thirds of the villi have long cytoplasmic processes which appear to extend to the basement membrane and between overlying epithelial cells. In the adult rat these Ia$^+$ cells carried the antigen W3/23$^+$ and therefore resembled macrophages. In the fetus and neonatal rat these cells (see below) are however W3/23$^-$ and are more like dendritic cells.

Human macrophage-like cells. Selby et al [89] have examined sections of human intestine and colon for the presence of macrophages and dendritic-type cells which are both HLA-DR$^+$ in humans. They found that 80–90% of HLA-DR staining cells in the lamina propria of the intestine are small stellate-shaped cells with the staining characteristics of interdigitating/dendritic cells (strong membrane adenosine triphosphatase activity), whilst in the colon the majority of cells (60–70%) are large round cells with the staining characteristics of macrophages (strong acid phosphatase and non-specific esterase).

Ontogeny of intestinal lymphoid and non-lymphoid cells in the intestine

The first cells of immunological importance to appear in the gut tract are Ia-positive dendritic cells which appear in the fetal rat at 16 days of gestation and that is well before other lymphoid cells and Peyer's patches can be identified [104] (Table 1.2, Fig. 1.4). By 18 days of gestation, there are numerous Ia-staining cells, particularly in the proximal intestine, and this is followed two days later by their appearance in the distal intestine [53]. Areas destined to be Peyer's patches can be identified by cuboidal epithelium and primitive dome structures by 20 days gestation in the rat [104] and at birth in the mouse and the rabbit [74]. Wilders et al [104] comment on the apparent correlation between the development of cuboidal epithelium and the concentration of dendritic cells.

Table 1.2   The ontogeny of intestinal lymphoid and antigen-presenting cells in rodents.

Days of gestation	
16	Ia$^+$ dendritic cells appear
18	Numerous Ia$^+$ DC in proximal intestinal mucosa
20+	Numerous Ia$^+$ DC in distal intestinal mucosa. Primitive cuboidal epithelium and concentration of DC in Peyer's patches
Birth + days	
2–4	T lymphocyte in Peyer's patches. HEV identifiable
8–10	B lymphocyte in Peyer's patches—mostly sIgM, few sIgA or sIgE
14	IgA-producing cells in mucosa. IEL appear. DC in mucosa begin to acquire macrophage characteristics. Expression of Ia$^+$ in villous epithelial cells
28	Germinal centres in Peyer's patches appear

Data from [15, 29, 53, 104]

T lymphocytes can be identified within a few days of birth in both the mouse and rat [53, 104]. B lymphocytes appear by eight days, and by two weeks of age Peyer's patches begin to assume adult form [29]. It is only at this time that immunoglobulin-producing cells [15] and intraepithelial lymphocytes [29] appear elsewhere in the mucosa but it is not until four to five weeks after birth that the numbers approach those found in the adult. Organized nodules of lymphocytes, however, can be seen well before birth in some species. The sheep fetus has both jejunal Peyer's patches and a large ileal caecal patch which is already well developed by 120 days of gestation [82]. A few lymphocytes can also be identified in the lamina propria and in the intraepithelial position [81] but plasma cells do not appear until directly after birth. There are nodular aggregates of lymphocytes in the human appendix at about 140 days of gestation [72] and Ia-staining cells in clusters at about the same time [60].

Dendritic cell–lymphocyte sequence. Wilders et al [104] and Mayrhofer et al [53] both emphasize the fact that Ia^+ dendritic cells (DC) colonize both Peyer's patches and lamina propria of the intestine before the appearance of lymphocytes and before exposure to antigen in the gut lumen, a point which is further emphasized by the appearance of dendritic cells in antigen-free gut grafts implanted under the kidney capsule [53]. From two weeks after birth Ia^+ dendritic cells in the lamina propria of rats begin to assume some of the characteristics of macrophages [53, 104] (e.g. increasing acid phosphatase activity), and in the adult many cells would appear to be classical macrophages.

The situation in Peyer's patches is different from that in the lamina propria in that clearly identifiable dendritic cells remain into adult life, being present in the dome area and within the epithelium and as interdigitating cells in the T dependent areas [53, 104]. In the adult rat there are also obvious macrophages especially in the dome area [9, 91].

The lifespan of effector cells within the intestinal mucosa

The preceding descriptions of the structure and arrangement of the various lymphoid populations tend to give a misleading static picture as most of the effector cells are short-lived or mobile or both. IgA plasma cells have a half-life of 4–7 days [52] and must be constantly replaced by B lymphoblasts. IEL are also short-lived cells which have an equally short stay within the epithelium itself [51]. Most IEL will rejoin the general circulation via the lacteals but some may be shed into the gut lumen [73]. Cell traffic studies have shown that the length of stay of most lymphocytes in the gut tract is measured in hours rather than days [38, 66]. Isotope studies of dendritic cells in afferent lymph draining the intestine have shown that these cells spend only 3–5 days in the mucosa [80]. All of the observations imply that there must be a very efficient system for the replacement and control of effector cells in order that mucosal immunity should be sustained.

THE DELIVERY OF CELLS TO AND FROM THE GALT AND MUCOSAL TISSUES

There is substantial evidence that Peyer's patches have a major role in supplying T cells [35, 84] and IgA precursors [16, 79, 85] which populate the intestinal mucosa (see Chapter 3). It would seem likely that the other components of GALT also preferentially supply their local mucosal tissue but the available experimental data are less conclusive than those for Peyer's patches. Craig and Cebra [17] have shown that the appendix contributes to the supply of IgA-forming cells. There is circumstantial evidence from studies on the reduced response to Salk vaccine in subjects after tonsillectomy [61] that the tonsils may serve to populate the upper gastrointestinal tract with immunoglobulin-producing cells. The mid and distal parts of the mouse colon and rat colon are presumably supplied by colonic patches [8] which are drained by the pancreatic and caudal nodes and not by the mesenteric node [8]. This correlates with evidence [79] that drainage of the thoracic duct, whilst causing a profound effect on depression of lymphoid cell populations in the intestinal mucosa, has little effect on the numbers of cells in the colonic mucosa.

Entry and exit routes of the intestine

The various GALT not only have effective means of sampling lumenal antigen and appropriate microenvironments for the interaction of antigen-presenting cells with lymphocytes, they also have very efficient mechanisms for the extraction of lymphocytes from the circulating blood. Recently it has been calculated that Peyer's patches extract lymphocytes from the blood just as efficiently as lymph nodes and between 1 in 4 and 1 in 10 of all lymphocytes in the blood which perfuses the Peyer's patches will gain access to the tissue [63, 66]. The means by which this efficiency is achieved is almost certainly due to the presence in all the GALT of postcapillary venules with high endothelial walls and there are numerous cell traffic studies including the early important studies of Gowans and Knight [33] which show that the route of entry of lymphocytes into Peyer's patches [21, 33, 74, 76] is by way of the high endothelial venule (HEV).

Microvascular pattern of Peyer's patches. Bhalla and co-workers [4] have described the microvascular pattern of rat Peyer's patches and this appears to be a modification of the fountain pattern seen elsewhere in the intestine [54]. Ascending arterioles pierce each germinal centre and feed a sub-dome-epithelium network of capillaries; these descend over the surface of the follicle and interconnect with baskets of capillaries beneath adjacent crypts before flowing into the HEV in the T areas.

Role of HEV in GALT. The molecular basis for the interaction of lymphocytes with HEV is not yet fully understood but is the subject of experiments using techniques developed by Woodruff and by Butcher and their colleagues. These workers have studied the binding of lymphocytes to HEV in vitro. In rats, a factor is present in thoracic duct lymph which can block the binding of lymphocytes to lymph node HEV in vitro [12]. Treatment of thoracic duct lymphocytes with the non-opsonizing fragment of an antibody against this factor selectively decreases the in vivo accumulation of lymphocytes in lymph nodes but not Peyer's patches [13]. Gallatin and his co-workers [31] have developed an antibody which recognizes a surface component on lymphocytes. Treatment of lymphocytes with this antibody inhibits both the binding of the cells to peripheral lymph node HEV in vitro and the accumulation of the cells in peripheral lymph nodes in vivo. In contrast, antibody pretreatment of lymphocytes has no effect on the interaction of the cells with Peyer's patch HEV in vitro, or their accumulation in Peyer's patches in vivo [31]. These studies indicate that there may be differences in cell surface structures between HEV in GALT and other

lymph nodes and these investigations will undoubtedly be pursued further.

Other very pertinent observations are those of Ottaway [62], who has shown that T lymphocytes have vasoactive peptide (VIP) receptors, and incubation of T lymphocytes in VIP selectively inhibits the uptake of lymphocytes into both Peyer's patches and mesenteric lymph nodes but not other tissues [62]. He has speculated that VIP may be available locally from nerve endings [63] within the microvasculature of lymphoid tissue including the HEV, and that T cells recognize and respond to the specific neurophysiological signals which facilitate their uptake into Peyer's patches and mesenteric lymph nodes.

Entry and exit in non-GALT mucosa

It is important to realize that HEV are not present in mucosal tissues outside of the GALT [43, 74, 76]. In the intestine, each villus is supplied by a central ascending arteriole which runs unbranched to the villus tip; there it divides into two arcade vessels that descend on the lateral margins of the villus [54]. These arcade vessels give rise to a subepithelial capillary system. It is presumably at this point that lymphocytes and other effector cells enter into each villus. Autoradiographic studies [56] have indicated that more cells emerge in the basal lamina propria near the crypts than higher up the villi. The capillaries eventually drain into venules but, unlike those in Peyer's patches, these venules do not have the pseudocolumnar appearance of HEV and are not adapted to the efficient extraction of lymphocytes from the perfusing blood.

Efficiency of lymphocyte uptake. The efficiency of uptake of either lymphocytes or lymphoblasts into the intestine is an order of magnitude less than into either Peyer's patches or mesenteric lymph nodes [63, 66] so that only one or two in 100 lymphocytes gain access to the intestine from the perfusing blood. There is, nevertheless, a substantial daily flux of lymphocytes through the non-lymphoid areas of the intestine as well as lymphoid areas of the intestine, as can be seen by examining peripheral lymph draining directly from the intestine wall [37, 98]. Observations in which the mesenteric lymph node chain has been removed from sheep or rats have provided information on the total output of lymph from the intestine and direct evidence that intravenously injected labelled lymphocytes and

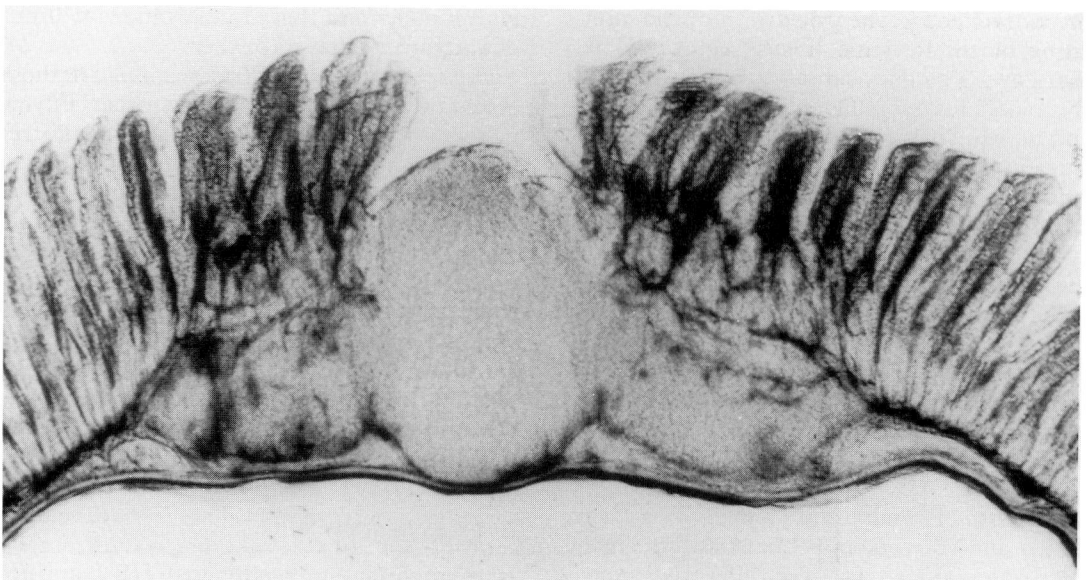

Fig. 1.6 Lymphocyte drainage from rat Peyer's patch tissue and individual lacteals from villi. (Reproduced by kind permission of Dr AO Anderson.)

lymphoblasts can be recovered from draining intestinal lymph [37, 38].

Comparison with GALT areas. The only way in which the output of lymph from non-lymphoid parts of the intestine can be compared with lymph draining Peyer's patches is by cannulation of individual lymphatics (Fig. 1.6) [98]. The findings by Steer [98] in rats show that there are approximately 10 times as many cells in the lymph leaving the gut in an area containing a Peyer's patch compared with an equivalent area lacking a Peyer's patch. The total area of intestine occupied by Peyer's patch tissue is, however, only one-twentieth or less of the total intestine so that the total daily flux of lymphocytes through the intestine is at least as great through non-lymphoid as lymphoid areas [63, 98]. Identification of entry and exit points is important for investigating the transit of lymphocytes and non-lymphoid cells but there are, nevertheless, other physiological and structural factors which control the populating of the gastrointestinal tract with effector cells; these include blood flow, availability of appropriate cells and retention of selected populations.

Blood flow to the intestine

It is known that blood flow controls the accumulation of small lymphocytes in lymph nodes, including the mesenteric lymph node

[40, 64]. Blood flow also controls the accumulation of lymphoblasts in the small intestine [65, 67]. There are regional differences in the distribution of mesenteric lymphoblasts, more

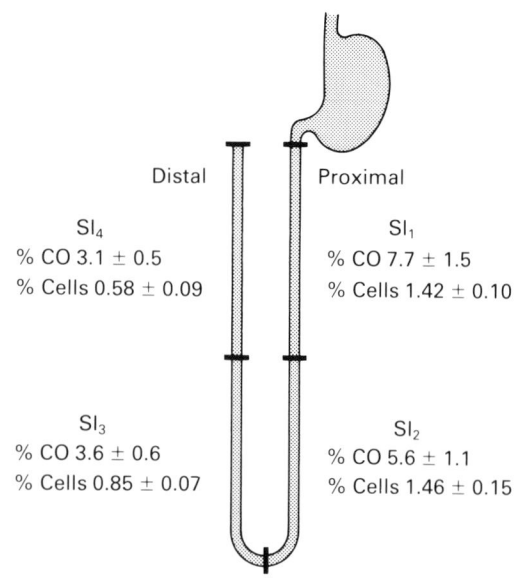

Distal   Proximal

SI_4
% CO 3.1 ± 0.5
% Cells 0.58 ± 0.09

SI_1
% CO 7.7 ± 1.5
% Cells 1.42 ± 0.10

SI_3
% CO 3.6 ± 0.6
% Cells 0.85 ± 0.07

SI_2
% CO 5.6 ± 1.1
% Cells 1.46 ± 0.15

Total Small Intestine % CO 20.9 ± 2.4
% Cells 4.22 ± 0.23

Fig. 1.7 The relationship between blood flow and the delivery of lymphoblasts to the mouse small intestine (SI). The percentage of the cardiac output (CO) received by the proximal intestine is higher than that received by the distal intestine and the 24-hour localization of iododeoxyuridine ([125]IUdR)-labelled mesenteric lymphoblasts is proportional to the blood flow. (Data from [65], reproduced by kind permission of Dr CA Ottaway.)

being localized in the proximal than the distal region of the intestine. These regional differences are directly related to blood flow [65] (Figs. 1.7 and 1.8). The correlation of the accumulation with blood flow applies to both T and B lymphoblasts [65] and to the colon as well as the intestine. Expansion of blood flow is an important way in which lymph nodes

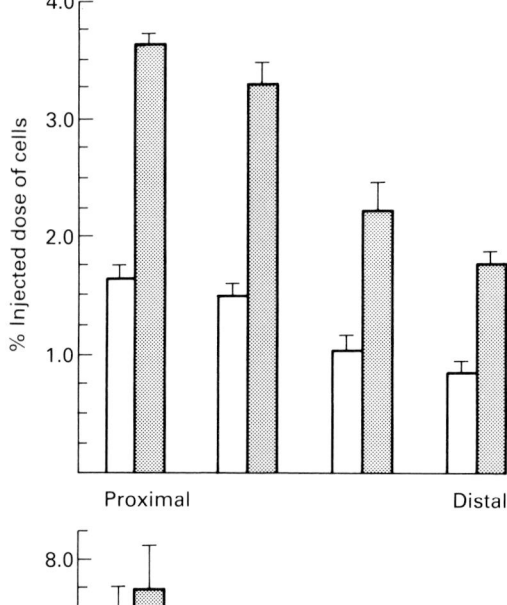

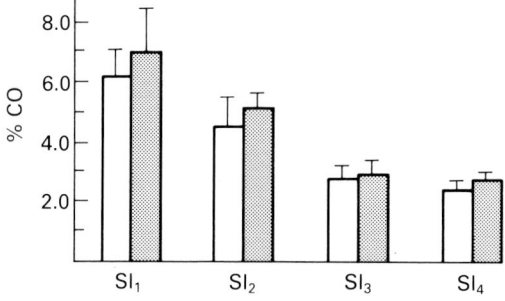

Fig. 1.8 A comparison of the 24-hour localization of unseparated ^{125}IUdR-labelled mesenteric lymphoblasts (open areas) and nylon wool separated (T cell enriched) ^{125}IUdR-labelled mesenteric lymphoblasts (stippled areas). More lymphoblasts localize in the proximal than the distal intestine and more T lymphoblasts localize than unseparated lymphoblasts. Both are related to cardiac output. SI = Small intestine. (Data from [67], reproduced by kind permission of the editors of *Gut*.)

respond to an antigenic stimulus [40, 64]. There are arteriovenous connections in lymph nodes [40], in Peyer's patches [4] and in intestinal villi [54]. In lymph nodes, these connection shunts can direct part of the incoming blood directly into the HEV and bypass capillaries [40], and the acute changes in blood and increased delivery of small lymphocytes are believed to be due to increased flow through these shunts.

Effect of infection. In mice undergoing acute enteritis in response to *Trichinella spiralis* infection, mesenteric lymph node blood flow increases within three days of infection [68] and this is accompanied by an increase in uptake of small lymphocytes [83]. There is not, however, a comparable acute increase in blood flow to the intestine [69] or Peyer's patches [68] early in infection though hyperaemia does develop from five days onwards [70]. An increase in blood flow cannot, therefore, account for the increase in lymphoblast localization seen in the intestine at early stages in *T. spiralis* infection [69, 70, 83, 84], though increased blood flow to the intestine could occur in response to other antigenic or inflammatory stimuli.

Recently, a method [41] has been developed for examining blood flow to individual rat villi. It has been shown that the peptide hormone glucagon increases villus blood flow whilst vasopressin dramatically decreases blood flow [41]. Whether the transient changes caused by these hormones would affect delivery has not been tested but they could be precipitating factors preceding local pathological change.

Availability of cells

The concentration of cells in the delivering blood is also an important consideration. The localization of mesenteric lymphoblasts is directly related to the numbers of cells transferred [56]. The numbers of cells arriving does ultimately depend on the number produced and on the integrity of the pathway from Peyer's patches through mesenteric lymph node to thoracic duct and the circulatory blood [79, 85]. Some cells may enter the mucosa directly from Peyer's patches but this short cut only leads to villi in the immediate vicinity of Peyer's patches [76]; the main traffic route is through the mesenteric lymph node. There is good evidence that the mesenteric node is an important site in the differentiation of IgA-producing cells as well as T lymphoblasts destined for the gut [35, 84, 85].

Cells in mesenteric lymph. The mesenteric node receives an equivalent number of lymphocytes including sIgA-bearing cells from the non-lymphoid areas of the intestine and from Peyer's patches (Table 1.1). Some are also received from the proximal colon in addition to a very large number of lymphocytes coming directly from the blood through the HEV. These converging streams of lymphocytes do affect the total flux of lymphocytes through the mesenteric node [92] but there is so far little information as to whether the differentiation of lymphocytes is influenced by meeting up in the mesenteric node (Fig. 1.1).

Phenotypically different antigen-presenting cells also arrive at the mesenteric nodes from lymphoid and non-lymphoid areas of intestine [80] together with some free antigen meeting lymphocytes from the blood stream. There will also be IgA-producing cells, activated T cells and free IgA in the lymph which could inhibit further secretion of IgA. It would be surprising if efferent lymph from the intestine did not contain pharmacologically active components such as prostaglandin E_2 which can influence the exit of cells from a lymph node [42]. Yet animals from which the mesenteric lymph node chain is removed recover rapidly and have no reported deficiences of mucosal immunity provided lymphatic continuity is re-established [38, 80]. Possibly the lack of a mesenteric node as a site of differentiation and antigen presentation is compensated for by the lack of suppressor effects.

The microenvironments of selection and retention

Peyer's patches, like the mesenteric node and other lymphoid tissues, have clearly defined areas in which T and B cells are segregated from one another (Fig. 1.1) which recent findings have shown are characterized by different types of antigen-presenting cells (see above and Table 1.1). Interactions of lymphocytes with antigen-presenting cells are known to be vital events in the initiation of immune responses [103] but such interactions may also be important mechanisms whereby lymphocytes are retained in organized lymphoid tissue [20, 77]. An extension to this hypothesis is to suggest that during the process of differentiation and activation of lymphocytes to lymphoblasts, the lymphocytes lose their receptors which recognize the microenvironment of

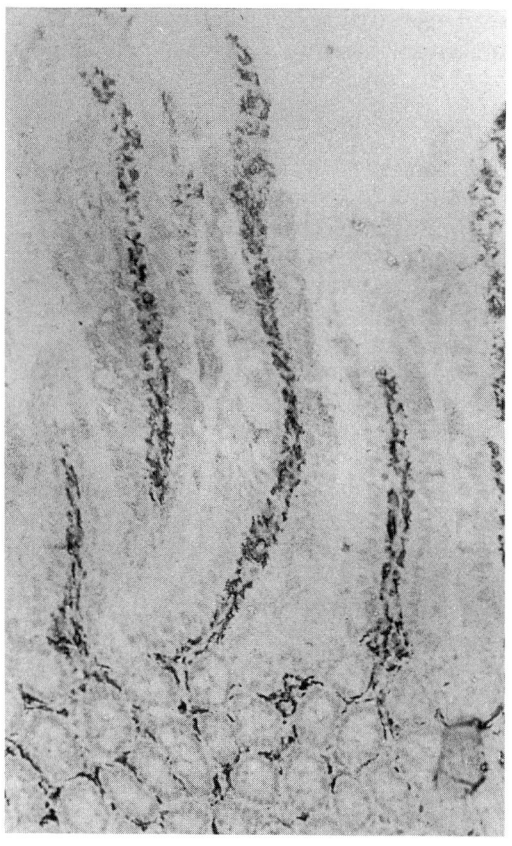
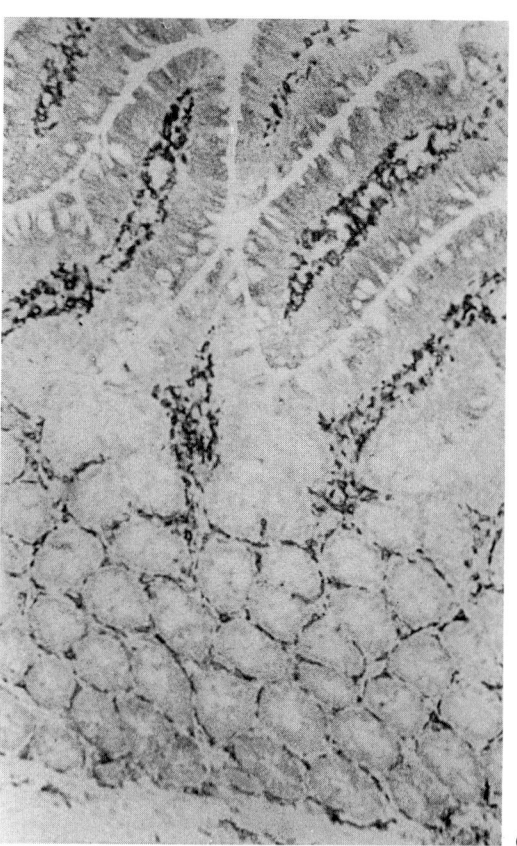

(a)   (b)

Fig. 1.9 Induction of Ia antigen in epithelia of rat small intestine during infection with *T. spiralis*. Ia antigen localized on cryostat sections by immunoperoxidase staining. (a) Normal rat. MRC-Ox 4 antibody stains cells in the lamina propria and between the crypts heavily. There is very weak patchy staining in the upper two-thirds of the villi. (b) Rat 12 days after infection with 500 *T. spiralis* larvae. MRC-Ox antibody give heavier staining of the epithelium than in normal rats. (Reproduced by kind permission of Dr Neil Barclay.)

organized lymphoid tissue (whether Peyer's patches, mesenteric lymph node or other GALT) and are released into the lymph to start on their journey to the mucosae.

Properties of microenvironment. The microenvironment which arriving lymphoblasts and other cells recognize within the gut mucosa must be different from that in organized lymphoid tissue since the cell types which reside, albeit temporarily, in the mucosa are very different from those in organized tissue. The mucosal microenvironment must not only facilitate the retention of IgA-producing cells and gut-primed T cells whilst relinquishing small lymphocytes and lymphoblasts from peripheral sources [33, 35, 38, 66, 84, 85] but it must also provide the means by which the motley assortment of cells which comprise the intraepithelial lymphocytes can cross the basal lamina and slot in between the crypt epithelial cells [27, 51].

It is an intriguing coincidence that during development, the dendritic cell and Ia$^+$-staining cells in the lamina propria undergo subtle changes and become more macrophage-like at about the same time that T cells and IgA-producing cells appear in the lamina propria of the intestine [53, 104] (Table 1.2). Furthermore, intraepithelial lymphocytes also increase in number coincidentally as the villus epithelial cells begin to express Ia antigen [53] (Fig. 1.9a, b); whether either of these coincidental events indicates that Ia$^+$ cells are the major microenvironmental components involved in selection and retention of lymphoid cells in the mucosa as well as in the organized lymphoid tissues awaits further investigation.

THE EFFECT OF THE ANTIGENIC CONSTITUENTS OF DIET ON THE STRUCTURE OF THE GUT TRACT

The number of effector cells and the size of the GALT in adult animals are a reflection of the continuous bombardment with antigenic stimuli including food, microorganisms, nematodes and so on, which the gut tract normally receives. In fact, the structure of the gut is abnormal when deprived of normal stimulation. The upper part of the intestine is relatively free of bacteria and it is generally considered that the presence of large numbers of IgA-producing cells (which are greatest in the proximal part of the intestine) and the diminution in number in the ileum and large intes-

tine are a reflection of the antigenic components of food [44, 48].

Germ-free animals. Mice which are raised under germ-free conditions are deprived of normal gut flora but eat food which retains antigenic moieties even if it is sterilized; in spite of this there are few IEL [26] or plasma cells in the intestine of germ-free mice, and Peyer's patches remain undeveloped with few germinal centres [15]. The total amount of Peyer's patch tissue is significantly less in germ-free than conventional animals but the patch tissue nevertheless contains surface immunoglobulin-bearing cells. Their isotype expression, is, however, different in germ-free compared with conventional animals and there are fewer surface IgM (sIgM) cells, more sIgA and large numbers of sIgE cells present, an isotype which is very rarely seen in conventional Peyer's patches [22]. Durkin and her colleagues [22] have speculated that the normal intestinal flora inhibits the expression of IgE isotype. In germ-free mice, intestinal villi are abnormally long and crypt cell production is very low [1]. The musculature of the colon is poorly developed and fails to function efficiently.

Separated areas of the gut. Sections of gut which are separated from the rest of the gut, such as in an isolated loop of intestine [81], or when the normal continuity of the rabbit appendix is interrupted [97] or when a graft of fetal gut is implanted under the kidney capsule, also have very reduced numbers of IEL, plasma cells and very small lymphoid nodules without germinal centres [29, 76]. Placing germ-free animals in a normal environment [15] or feeding them unsterilized food and reestablishing the continuity of the gut to isolated loops brings about a prompt return towards normal appearance [81]. The separation of gut loops and preparation of gut grafts have been seen to be useful tools in demonstrating that the uptake of lymphoblasts [29, 76, 81] and dendritic cells [53] is not dependent upon the presence of luminal antigen. However, such preparations are structurally abnormal, they may lack lymphatic drainage which inhibits egress [76], there is accumulation of cell debris, a reduction in villus height and progressive atrophy [81].

Elemental diet. A more physiological approach to studying the effects of food antigens on the structure of the gut tract can be achieved by

Table 1.3 Effects of an elemental diet on the gastrointestinal tract of mice.

Tissue	Diet	Weight (mg)	Cardiac output (%)	Localization of mesenteric lymphoblasts†
Intestine	P	1406 ± 62	14.9 ± 1.5	5.0 ± 0.3
	E	1343 ± 95	14.9 ± 2.3	4.8 ± 0.5
Caecum	P	208 ± 30	1.8 ± 0.6	0.49 ± 0.7
	E	133 ± 21	0.9 ± 0.3	$0.24 \pm 0.05 \star$
Large intestine	P	419 ± 35	4.0 ± 0.4	0.73 ± 0.35
	E	$349 \pm 41 \star$	$2.8 \pm 0.8 \star$	0.53 ± 0.19
Mesenteric lymph node	P	184 ± 37	0.74 ± 0.26	0.73 ± 0.35
	E	$132 \pm 26 \star$	$0.40 \pm 0.10 \star$	$0.53 \pm 0.12 \star$

Mice were weaned on to either pellet (P) or elemental diet (E) and maintained for a few weeks before experimentation.
Statistically significant differences between mice fed a normal pellet diet and an elemental diet: $\star P < 0.05$, †% injected dose recovered at 24 h.
Data from [67].

weaning suckling mice on to an elemental diet [67]. Such a procedure eliminates exposure to food antigens whilst at the same time maintaining exposure to normal intestinal flora [67]. Mice fed for some weeks on an elemental diet retain a normal growth rate but the size of the caecum and large intestine as well as the mesenteric lymph and spleen is substantially reduced. These reductions in size are accompanied by decreases in blood flow and corresponding decreases in the localization of lymphoblasts to the affected tissues [67] (Table 1.3). There is not, however, any significant reduction in the total weight of the small intestine, in the numbers of IEL [26] or any overall reduction in blood flow or delivery of lymphoblasts, though there are minor changes in the distal region of the intestine [67]. These results demonstrate that food antigens do not affect the delivery or uptake of cells to the intestine and that the distribution of IgA plasmablasts [15, 44, 48] in the intestine is the reflection of the delivery of IgA-secreting lymphoblasts by the perfusing blood [64, 67].

Effect of immune responses

The induction of a variety of cell-mediated immune responses at the local level in the intestine brings about a spectrum of changes which are in many respects the opposite of those observed in the gut deprived of lumenal stimulation. There are increases in crypt cell production rate, in crypt length and in numbers of IEL. These changes were first attributed to cell-mediated immune mechanisms in experiments on allograft rejection [30] and have since been observed in the intestine in rats and mice undergoing graft-versus-host reaction [28], protozoan and nematode infections

[28] and in hypersensitivity reactions to food protein antigens [57]. There may also be additional changes, including an increase in goblet cells [55], villous atrophy [28, 30, 50] (Fig. 1.2a) and increased expression of Ia antigen by villous epithelial cells (Fig. 1.9b) [3]. The close similarity of all of these changes with those present in food-sensitive enteropathies will be described extensively in Chapters 30 and 33.

All of the experimental studies have implicated T lymphocytes as the major cells involved in the intestinal changes, but more recent work has examined the events and subsets of lymphocytes involved in greater detail [58, 59, 99]. Mice fed ovalbumin normally develop tolerance to that antigen, but interference with the suppressor system by treatment with cyclophosphamide abrogates tolerance and precipitates increases in crypt cell production and numbers of IEL on challenge with ovalbumin [99]. Stimulation of the reticuloendothelial system, including presumably antigen-presenting cells, by injection of oestrodiol also abrogates tolerance and stimulates crypt cell production and numbers of IEL on challenges with ovalbumin [58].

Possible role of T cells in crypt cell regulation. Recently, Mowat and his colleagues [59], using the induction of graft-versus-host reaction in F_1 hybrid mice as a model of intestinal change, have examined the phenotype of T cells responsible for intestinal alterations and the region of the MHC which stimulates them. They have shown that T cells of the helper subset recognizing incompatibility at the Ia region of the H_2 are responsible for the observed increases in crypt cell production rate and numbers of IEL. There are also preliminary indications that suppressor T cells may be activated by Class I antigens and the I-J region and that these cells will down-regulate crypt cell production.

The crypt cell production rate is a very sensitive barometer of intestinal change induced by immune mechanisms; there is too little production in the germ-free animal and too much during local cell-mediated immune reactions. It is tempting to speculate that the function of the large numbers of helper T cells in the lamina propria is not only to help antibody production but also to maintain crypt cell production, to influence the differentiation of crypt cells into Paneth cells, goblet cells or villus columnar cells, as well as to control the expression of Ia antigen by the release of appropriate lymphokines. If one extends the speculation, then the function of the cells bearing the suppressor phenotype amongst the IEL is, therefore, to suppress crypt cell production and to inhibit differentiation.

CONCLUDING REMARKS

In this chapter, attention has been drawn to the fact that, although there are a substantial number of investigations directed towards Peyer's patch tissue, there is still remarkably little information about the functional structure of other gut-associated lymphoid tissues or indeed the contribution which 'intermediate' structures such as the mesenteric lymph nodes make towards mucosal immunity, other than as convenient sources of lymphoblasts. There is now some understanding of the contribution which regional blood flow makes to the distribution of effector cells. There are ways of calculating the relative efficiency of uptake of cells into the mucosa or into the GALT and we now have monoclonal antibodies which can identify receptors on HEV. The structures which comprise the essential microenvironments for selection, retention and interactions of effector cells have still to be identified in the mucosa, though there are promising developments in respect of antigen-presenting cells, especially in the neonate. The notion that the multiplication and differentiation of epithelial cells covering the surface of the intestinal mucosa are normally regulated by immune mechanisms is especially relevant to problems of structural change in food allergy.

REFERENCES

1 Abrams GD, Bauer N, Sprinz H: Influence of the normal flora on mucosal morphology and cellular renewal in the ileum. A comparison of germ-free and conventional mice. Lab Invest 1963; 12:355–64.

2 Austin LL, Dobbins WO III: Intraepithelial leucocytes of the intestinal mucosa in normal man and in Whipple's disease: a light and electron microscopic study. Dig Dis Sci 1982; 27:311–20.

3 Barclay AN, Mason DW: Induction of Ia antigen in rat epidermal cells and gut epithelium by immunological stimuli. J Exp Med 1982; 156:1665–76.

4 Bhalla DK, Murakami T, Owen RL: Microcirculation of intestinal lymphoid follicles in rat Peyer's patches. Gastroenterology 1981; 81:481–91.

5 Bienenstock J, Dolezel J: Peyer's patches: lack of specific antibody-containing cells after oral and parenteral immunization. J Immunol 1971; 4:938–45.

6 Bienenstock J, Johnston N: A morphologic study of rabbit bronchial lymphoid aggregates and lymphoepithelium. Lab Invest 1976; 35:343–8.

7 Binns RM, Licence ST: Patterns of migration of labelled blood lymphocyte subpopulations. Evidence for two types of Peyer's patch in the young pig. Adv Exp Med Biol 1985; 186:661–8.

8 Bland PW, Britton DC: Morphological study of antigen-sampling structures in the rat large intestine. Infect Immun 1984; 43:693–9.

9 Bockman DE, Boydston WR, Beezhold DH: The role of epithelial cells in gut-associated immune reactivity. Ann NY Acad Sci 1983; 409:129–44.

10 Bockman DE, Cooper MD: Pinocytosis by epithelium associated with lymphoid follicles in the bursa of Fabricius, appendix and Peyer's patches: an electron microscope study. Am J Anat 1973; 136:455–77.

11 Cerf-Bensussan N, Schneeberger EE, Bhan AK: Immunohistologic and immunoelectron microscopic characterization of the mucosal lymphocytes of human small intestine by the use of monoclonal antibodies. J Immunol 1983; 130:2615–22.

12 Chin Y-H, Carey GD, Woodruff JJ: Lymphocyte recognition of lymph node high endothelium. I. Inhibition of in vitro binding by a component of thoracic duct lymph. J Immunol 1980; 125:1764–9.

13 Chin Y-H, Carey GD, Woodruff JJ: Lymphocyte recognition of lymph node high endothelium. IV. Cell surface structures mediating entry into lymph nodes. J Immunol 1982; 129:1911–5.

14 Cornes JS: Number, size and distribution of Peyer's patches in the human small intestine. Gut 1965; 225–33.

15 Crabbe PA, Nash DR, Bazin H et al: Immunohistochemical observations on lymphoid tissues from conventional and germ-free mice. Lab Invest 1970; 22:448–57.

16 Craig SW, Cebra JJ: Peyer's patches: an enriched source of precursors for IgA-producing immunocytes in the rabbit. J Exp Med 1971; 142:1550–63.

17 Craig SW, Cebra JJ: Rabbit Peyer's patches, appendix and popliteal lymph node B lymphocytes. A comparative analysis of their membrane immunoglobulin components and plasma cell precursor potential. J Immunol 1975; 114:492–502.

18 Curran RC, Jones EL: Immunoglobulin-containing cells in human tonsils demonstrated by immuno-

histochemistry. Clin Exp Immunol 1977; 28: 103-15.

19 Davies MDJ, Parrott DMV: Preparation and purification of lymphocytes from the epithelium and lamina propria of murine small intestine. Gut 1981; 22:481-8.

20 de Sousa MAB: Lymphocyte circulation—experimental and clinical aspects. Chichester: Wiley and Sons, 1981; 1-259.

21 de Sousa MAB, Parrott DMV, Pantelouris EM: The lymphoid tissues in mice with congenital aplasia of the thymus. Clin Exp Immunol 1969; 4:637-44.

22 Durkin HG, Bazin H, Waksman BH: Origin and fate of IgE-bearing lymphocytes. I. Peyer's patches as differentiation site of cells simultaneously bearing IgA and IgE. J Exp Med 1981; 154:640-8.

23 Elson CO, Weiserbs DB, Ealding W et al: T helper cell activity in intestinal lamina propria. Ann NY Acad Sci 1983; 409:230-7.

24 Ernst PB, Befus AD, Bienenstock J: Leukocytes in the intestinal epithelium: an unusual immunological compartment. Immunol Today 1985; 22:50-6.

25 Faulk WP, McCormick JN, Goodman JR et al: Peyer's patches: morphologic studies. Cell Immunol 1970; 1:500-20.

26 Ferguson A: Models of intestinal hypersensitivity. Clin Gastroenterol 1976; 5:271-88.

27 Ferguson A: Intraepithelial lymphocytes of the small intestine. Gut 1977; 18:921-37.

28 Ferguson A, MacDonald TT: Effect of delayed hypersensitivity on the small intestine. Ciba Foundation Symposium 46, Immunology of the Gut. Amsterdam: Elsevier/North-Holland, 1977, 305-27.

29 Ferguson A, Parrott DMV: The effect of antigen deprivation on thymus dependent and thymus independent lymphocytes in the small intestine of the mouse. Clin Exp Immunol 1972; 12:477-88.

30 Ferguson A, Parrott DMV: Histopathology and time course of rejection of allografts of mouse small intestine. Transplantation 1973; 15:546-54.

31 Gallatin WM, Weissman IL, Butcher EC: A cell-surface molecule involved in organ-specific homing of lymphocytes. Nature 1983; 304:30-4.

32 Ginsel LA, Liepman HP, Waterman IT: Light and electronmicroscopical studies on the distribution of various cell types in the sigmoid colon of normal subjects and in patients with Crohn's disease. In: Pena HS, Waterman IT, Booth CC, Strober W, eds. Recent advances in Crohn's disease. Recent developments in gastroenterology, Vol 1. The Hague: Martinus Nijhoff, 1981;124-30.

33 Gowans JL, Knight EJ: The route of recirculation of lymphocytes in the rat. Proc R Soc (B) 1964; 59:257-82.

34 Greenwood JH, Austin LL, Dobbins WO III: In vitro characterization of human intestinal intraepithelial lymphocytes. Gastroenterology 1983; 85: 1023-35.

35 Guy-Grand D, Griscelli C, Vassali P: The mouse gut T lymphocyte, a novel type of T cell: nature, origin and traffic in mice, in normal and gvh conditions. J Exp Med 1978; 148:1661-77.

36 Haaijman JJ, Schiut HRE, Hijmans W: Immunoglobulin-containing in different lymphoid organs of the CBA mouse during its life-span. Immunology 1977; 32:427-34.

37 Hall JG: An essay on lymphocyte circulation and the gut. Monogr Allergy 1980; 16:100-11.

38 Hall JG, Hopkins J, Orlans E: Studies on the lymphocytes of sheep. III. Destination of lymph borne immunoblasts in relation to their tissue of origin. Eur J Immunol 1977; 7:30-7.

39 Heinen E, Lilet-Lederg C, Marsh DY et al: Isolation of follicular dendritic cells from human tonsils and adenoids. II. Immunocytochemical characterization. Eur J Immunol 1984; 14:267-73.

40 Herman PG, Ursunomiya R, Hessel SJ: Arteriovenous shunting in the lymph node before and after antigenic stimulus. Immunology 1979; 36:793-7.

41 Hollinger CH, Radzymer M, Knoblauch M: Effects of glucagon, vasoactive intestinal peptide and vasopressin on villous microcirculation and superior mesenteric artery blood flow of the rat. Gastroenterology 1981; 85:1036-43.

42 Hopkins J, McConnell I, Pearson JD: Lymphocyte traffic through antigen-stimulated lymph nodes. II. Role of prostaglandin E_2 as a mediator of cell shutdown. Immunology 1981; 42:225-31.

43 Husband AJ: Kinetics of extravasation and redistribution of IgA-specific antibody containing cells in the intestine. J Immunol 1982; 128:1355-9.

44 Husband AJ, Gowans JL: The origin and antigen-dependent distribution of IgA containing cells in the intestine. J Exp Med 1978; 148:1146-60.

45 Janossy G, Tidman N, Selby WS et al: Human T lymphocytes of inducer and suppressor type occupy different microenvironments. Nature 1980; 288:81-4.

46 Joel DD, Laissue JA, Lefevre ME: Distribution and fate of ingested carbon particles in mice. J Reticuloendothel Soc 1978; 24:477-87.

47 Korsfad FR, Brandtzaeg P: Immune systems of human nasopharyngeal and palatine tonsils: histomorphometry of lymphoid components and quantification of immunoglobulin-producing cells in health and disease. Clin Exp Immunol 1980; 39:361-70.

48 Lange S, Mygren H, Svennerholm A et al: Antitoxic cholera immunity in mice: influence of antigen deposition on antitoxin containing cells and selective immunity in different parts of the intestine. Infect Immun 1980; 28:17-23.

49 Lyscom N, Brueton MJ: Intraepithelial, lamina propria, and Peyer's patch lymphocytes of the rat small intestine: isolation and characterization in immunoglobulin markers and receptors of monoclonal antibodies. Immunology 1982; 45:775-83.

50 Manson-Smith DF, Bruce RG, Parrott DMV: Villous atrophy and expulsion of intestinal *Trichinella spiralis* are mediated by T cells. Cell Immunol 1979; 47:285-92.

51 Marsh MD: Studies of intestinal lymphoid tissue. II. Aspects of proliferation and migration of epithelial lymphocytes in the small intestine of mice. Gut 1975; 16:674-82.

52 Mattioli CA, Tomasi TB: The lifespan of IgA plasma cells from the mouse intestine. J Exp Med 1973; 138:452-60.

53 Mayrhofer G, Pugh CW, Barclay AN: The distribution, ontogeny and origin in the rat of Ia-positive cells with dendritic morphology and of Ia antigen epithelia, with special reference to the intestine. Eur J Immunol 1983; 13:112-22.

54 Miller DS, Rahman MA, Ranner R et al: The vascular architecture of the different forms of small intestinal villi in the rat (*Rattus norvegicus*). Scand J Gastroenterol 1969; 4:477-82.

55 Miller HRP, Nawa Y: Immune regulation of intestinal goblet cell differentiation. Specific induction of non-specific protection against helminths? Nouv Rev Fr Hematol 1979; 21:31-45.

56 Mirski SE, McDermott MR, Befus AD et al: Selec-

tive localisation of mesenteric lymphoblasts in mucosal tissues: Effects of altering the number of donor lymphoblasts. Immunology 1981; 43:669-75.

57 Mowat AMcI, Ferguson A: Hypersensitivity in the small intestinal mucosa. V. Induction of cell-mediated immunity to a dietary antigen. Clin Exp Immunol 1981; 43:574-82.

58 Mowat AMcI, Parrott DMV: Immunological responses to fed protein antigen in mice. IV. Effects of stimulating the reticuloendothelial system on oral tolerance and intestinal immunity to ovalbumin. Immunology 1983; 50:547-54.

59 Mowat AMcI, Borland A, Parrott DMV: Pathogenesis of the intestinal phase of the graft-versus-host reaction in F₁ hybrid mice. Adv Exp Biol Med 1985; 186:531-8.

60 Natali PG, Russo C, Ng AK et al: Otogeny of human Ia antigens. Cell Immunol 1982; 73:385-96.

61 Ogra PL: Effect of tonsillectomy and adenoidectomy on nasopharyngeal antibody response to polio virus. New Eng J Med 1971; 284:59-64.

62 Ottaway CA: In vitro alteration of receptors for vaso-reactive intestinal peptide changes in the in vivo localization of mouse T cells. J Exp Med 1984; 160:1054-69.

63 Ottaway CA: Lymphoid cell migration in the intestine in health and disease. In: Losowsky M, Heatley RV, eds. Gut defences in clinical practice. Edinburgh: Churchill Livingstone (in press).

64 Ottaway CA, Parrott DMV: Regional blood flow and its relationship to lymphocyte and lymphoblast traffic during a primary immune reaction. J Exp Med 1979; 150:218-30.

65 Ottaway CA, Parrott DMV: Regional blood flow and the localization of lymphoblasts in the small intestine of the mouse. I. Examination of the normal small intestine. Immunology 1980; 41:955-61.

66 Ottaway CA, Parrott DMV: A method for the quantitative analysis of lymphoid cell migration. Immunol Lett 1981; 2:283-90.

67 Ottaway CA, Parrott DMV: Regional blood flow and the localization of lymphoblasts in the small intestine of the mouse: effect of an elemental diet. Gut 1981; 22:376-82.

68 Ottaway CA, Parrott DMV: The role of blood flow in the distribution of lymphocytes and lymphoblasts in vivo. Microcirc Rev 1982; 1:134-44.

69 Ottaway CA, Bruce RG, Parrott DMV: The in vivo kinetics of lymphoblast localization on the small intestine. Immunology 1983; 49:641-8.

70 Ottaway CA, Manson-Smith DF, Bruce RG et al: Regional blood flow and the localization of lymphoblasts in the small intestine of the mouse. II. The effect of a primary infection with *Trichinella spiralis*. Immunology 1980; 41:963-71.

71 Owen RL, Jones AL: Epithelial cell specialization within Peyer's patches: an ultrastructural study of intestinal lymphoid follicles. Gastroenterology 1974; 66: 189-203.

72 Owen RL, Nemanic P: Antigen processing structures of the mammalian intestinal tract: an SEM study of lymphoepithelial organs. Scan Electron Microsc 1978; 11:367-78.

73 Owen RC, Nemanic PC, Stevens DP: Ultrastructural observations on giardiasis on a murine model. I. Intestinal distribution attachment and relationship to the immune system of *Giardia muris*. Gastroenterology 1979; 76:757-69.

74 Parrott DMV: The gut as a lymphoid organ. Clin Gastroenterol 1976; 5:211-28.

75 Parrott DMV: The gut-associated lymphoid tissues and gastrointestinal immunity. In: Ferguson A, MacSween RNM, eds. Immunological aspects of the liver and gastrointestinal tract. Lancaster: MTP, 1976:1-32.18.

76 Parrott DMV, Ferguson A: Selective migration of lymphocytes within the mouse small intestine. Immunology 1974; 26:571-88.

77 Parrott DMV, Wilkinson PC: Lymphocyte locomotion and migration. Prog Allergy 1981; 28:193-284.

78 Parrott DMV, Tait C, MacKenzie S et al: Analysis of the effector functions of different populations of mucosal lymphocytes. Ann NY Acad Sci USA 1983; 490:307-20.

79 Pierce NF, Gowans JL: Cellular kinetics of the intestinal immune response to cholera toxoid in rats. J Exp Med 1975; 142:1550-63.

80 Pugh CW, MacPherson GG, Steer HW: Characterisation of non-lymphoid cells derived from rat peripheral lymph. J Exp Med 1983; 157:1758-79.

81 Reynolds JD, Morris B: The influence of gut function on lymphoid cell populations in the intestinal mucosa of lambs. Immunology 1983; 49:501-9.

82 Reynolds JD, Pabst R, Bordman G: Evidence for the existence of two distinct types of Peyer's patches. Adv Exp Biol Med 1985; 186:101-10.

83 Rose ML, Parrott DMV, Bruce RG: Migration of lymphoblasts to the small intestine. I. Effect of *Trichinella spiralis* infection on the migration of mesenteric lymphoblasts in syngenic mice. Immunology 1976; 31:723-30.

84 Rose ML, Parrott DMV, Bruce RG: Migration of lymphoblasts to the small intestine. II. Divergent migration of mesenteric and peripheral immunoblasts to sites of inflammation in the mouse. Cell Immunol 1976; 27:36-46.

85 Roux ME, McWilliams M, Phillips-Quagliata J, Lamm ME: Differentiation pathway of Peyer's patch precursors of IgA plasma cells in the secretory immune system. Cell Immunol 1981; 61:141-53.

86 Selby WS, Janossy G, Bofill M et al: Lymphocyte subpopulations in the human small intestine. The findings in normal mucosa and in the mucosa of patients with adult coeliac disease. Clin Exp Immunol 1983; 52:219-28.

87 Selby WS, Janossy G, Bofill M et al: Intestinal lymphocyte subpopulations in inflammatory bowel disease: an analysis by immunohistological and cell isolation techniques. Gut 1984; 25:32-40.

88 Selby WS, Janossy G, Goldstein G et al: T lymphocyte subsets in human intestinal mucosa: the distribution and relationship to MHC-derived antigens. Clin Exp Immunol 1981; 44:453-8.

89 Selby WS, Poulter LW, Hobbs S et al: Heterogeneity of HLA-DR-positive histiocytes in human intestinal lamina propria: a combined histochemical and immunohistological analysis. J Clin Pathol 1983; 36:379-84.

90 Shimiza Y, Andrew W: Studies on the rabbit appendix. I. Lymphocyte-epithelial relations and the transport of bacteria from human to lymphoid nodule. J Morphol 1967; 123:231-50.

91 Sminia T, Wilders MM, Janse EM et al: Characterization of non-lymphoid cells in Peyer's patches of the rat. Immunobiology 1983; 164:136-43.

92 Smith ME, Ford WL: The recirculating lymphocyte pool of the rat. A systemic description of the migrating behaviour of recirculating lymphocytes. Immunology 1983; 43:83-94.

93 Sobhon P: The light and electron microscopic studies

of Peyer's patches in non-germ free adult mice. J Morphol 1971; 457–82.

94 Sordat B, Moser R, Gerber H et al: Differentiation pathway within germinal centers of human tonsils. Adv Exp Med Biol 1969; 5:73–83.

95 Spalding DM, Koopman WJ, Eldridge JH et al: Accessory cells in murine Peyer's patch. I. Identification and enrichment of a functional dendritic cell. J Exp Med 1983; 157:1649–59.

96 Spencer J, Finn T, Isaacson PG: Gut-associated lymphoid tissue: a morphological and immunocytochemical study of the human appendix. Gut 1985; 26: 672–9.

97 Stramignoni H, Mollo F, Rua S et al: Development of the lymphoid tissue in the rabbit appendix isolated from the intestinal tract. J Pathol 1969; 99:265–70.

98 Steer H: Analysis of the lymphocyte content of rat lacteals. J Immunol 1980; 125:1845–8.

99 Strobel S, Mowat AMcI, Drummond H et al: Immunological responses to fed protein antigen in mice. II. Oral tolerance for CMI is due to activation of cyclophosphamide-sensitive cells by gut-processed antigen. Immunology 1983; 49:451–6.

100 Tagliabue A, Befus AD, Clark DA et al: Characteristics of natural killer cells in the murine intestinal epithelium and lamina propria. J Exp Med 1982; 155:1785–96.

101 Targan S, Britvan L, Kendall R et al: Isolation of spontaneous and interferon inducible natural killer like cells from human colonic mucosa: lysis of lymphoid and autologous epithelial target cells. Clin Exp Immunol 1983; 54:14–22.

102 Tseng J: Expression of immunoglobulin isotypes by lymphoid cells isolated from the lamina propria of mouse small intestine. Ann NY Acad Sci 1983; 409:885–6.

103 Unanue ER: The regulatory role of macrophages in antigenic stimulation—part two: symbiotic relationship between lymphocytes and macrophages. Adv Immunol 1981; 31:1–136.

104 Wilders MM, Sminia T, Janse EM: Ontogeny of non-lymphoid and lymphoid cells in the rat gut with special reference to large mononuclear Ia-positive dendritic cells. Immunology 1983; 50:303–14.

105 Williams DM, Rowland AC: The palatine tonsils of the pig—an afferent route to the lymphoid tissue. J Anat 1972; 113:131–7.

106 Wolf JL, Rubin DH, Finberg R et al: Intestinal M cells: a pathway for entry of reovirus into the host. Science 1981; 212:471–2.

Chapter 2
Basic Functions of the Gut

C. N. Mallinson

Introduction

This chapter is intended to provide a summary of current understanding of human gastrointestinal physiology. The research of the past 20 years has enlarged this knowledge immensely, making the job of compression into a short chapter correspondingly difficult. For this reason a large number of broad statements of orthodoxy have been made largely without references. The interested or sceptical reader will find fuller reviews, meticulously referenced, in the general reading suggested in refs. 3, 10, 13, 48, particularly ref. 10 which comprises a series of extremely good review articles covering all the main areas of gastrointestinal physiology.

The function of the gut is to absorb nutrients. This is achieved by the coordinated activity of motility, secretion and absorption.

The introduction of food into the stomach and the expulsion of waste from the colon are purely motor activities, and the oesophagus and anorectal apparatus have no secretory or absorptive functions. The stomach, pancreas and biliary apparatus and the very proximal small intestine are the main secretory organs of the gut, rendering a randomly mixed diet absorbable. Coordination of motor function is integrated with secretion and consequent digestion to this end. The first 100 cm of the small intestine are highly adapted to absorption of nutrients, and the terminal part of the small intestine and the entire colon are involved in reclaiming the large amount of fluid and electrolytes secreted during the digestive period into the proximal gut in response to a meal.

While it is rather artificial to consider these three processes separately in the light of inextricably integrated function, it remains still the only clear way of presenting the known facts.

MOTILITY

It is the motor activity of the gut which, self-evidently, is responsible for the passage of contents throughout the gut. This is rapid in the oesophagus, whereafter contents are held up in the reservoir of the body of the stomach and are progressively liquidized by the gastric antrum. The antrum also sieves liquid through the remaining solid matter and is responsible for a continuous slow rate of gastric emptying. This continues for 1.5–2 hours after a standard meal. The small intestinal contents pass down to the ileocaecal valve more or less steadily over the succeeding 2–6 hours (Table 2.1). There is evidence that the ileocaecal valve acts as a brake, holding up ileal contents temporarily as well as acting as an antireflux valve. Colonic contents move irregularly towards the rectum over the next 12 hours undergoing prolonged periods of mixing between brief periods of movement.

Table 2.1 Transit of contents through different parts of the gastrointestinal tract.

Segment	Range of transit time
Oesophagus	4–8 seconds
Stomach	1–2 hours
Small intestine	2–6 hours
Colon	12–24 hours

GASTROINTESTINAL MUSCLE

The inherent contractile property of gastrointestinal smooth muscle upon which all this activity depends is modified by neural and humoral influences resulting in different patterns of motor activity which differ again in the fasting and the fed state.

The fasting gut

In the fasting state the oesophagus shows tonic contraction in the upper and lower sphincter and flaccidity of the body. The proximal part of the stomach, the body, exhibits low-grade tonic contraction while the gastric antrum, duodenum and small intestine show slow-wave myoelectric depolarization which is only occasionally accompanied by contraction.

Slow-wave activity

In vitro and in vivo the gastric antrum shows slow-wave activity at a rate of 3 cycles/minute, the duodenum at 12 cycles/minute and the ileum 6–8 cycles/minute (Fig. 2.1). Only when excitation reaches a critical level either spontaneously or under the influence of extrinsic neural or humoral conditions does the slow

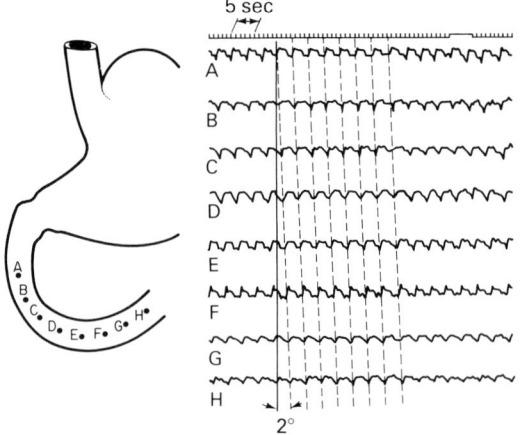

Fig. 2.1 Slow waves recorded simultaneously from closely spaced electrodes in the unanaesthetized cat. Eight monopolar AC-amplified records are shown as recorded from eight chronically implanted needle electrodes spaced uniformly 1 cm apart along the duodenum. Slow-wave configuration is between that of the actual signal and its second derivative. The last few slow waves, at the right, carry spike bursts. Dashed lines are drawn through corresponding slow-wave cycles from each record. The angle, 2°, between these lines and the solid line, the common time-base, is a function of the apparent velocity of spread of slow waves and of the paper speed of the recording polygraph. From Christensen [5], with permission.

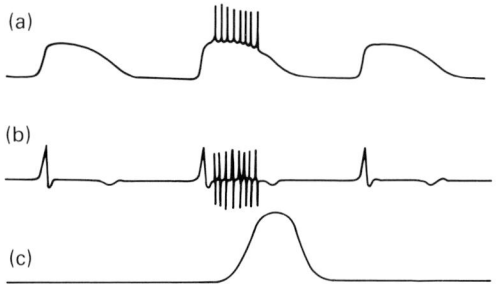

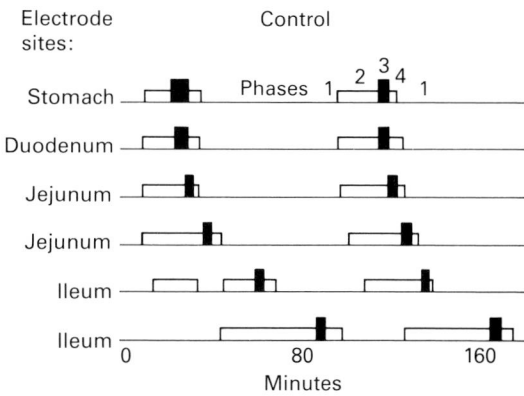

Fig. 2.2 Diagram of time relations between slow waves, spike bursts, and contractions. Curve A represents the electromyogram of a single smooth muscle cell, recorded with an intracellular microelectrode. Curve B represents the electromyogram recorded from several cells by a large extracellular volume-recording electrode. Curve C shows tension in the muscle mass. All three traces are drawn to a common time-base. In A, three slow waves appear as a monophasic depolarization from a stable maximal value, the resting membrane potential. Observe that the rate of depolarization is faster than the rate of repolarization. In B, the slow waves appear with two components, an initial biphasic spike, which represents depolarization, and secondary slower biphasic signal, representing repolarization. The trace shown in B approximates the second derivative of the trace shown in A. The second of the three slow waves bears a burst of spikes, appearing on the plateau of the slow wave. The tension record, in C, shows a contraction beginning during the spike burst, and apparently initiated by it. From Christensen [5], with permission.

Fig. 2.3 Phases of the interdigestive myoelectric complex at multiple recording sites in the dog. Phase 1 has slow waves with no action potentials. In Phase 2 there are an increasing number of slow waves with action potentials. In Phase 3 each slow wave has action potentials. Phase 4 shows a steady diminution in the number of slow waves with action potentials. From [13], with permission.

wave coincide with muscular contraction. At this point spike potential is also recorded. In the fasting state approximately 10–30% of slow wave is accompanied by contraction and spike potentials while the proportion rises sharply after eating (Fig. 2.2). Contraction does not occur without a slow wave and thus the intrinsic frequency of slow-wave activity of a particular part of the gut imposes an upper limit on the maximum frequency of contraction. This is of great importance in the small intestine where true peristalsis does not occur but where the greater frequency of contraction in the proximal part of the intestine than the distal results in a caudal movement of gut contents even in the absence of peristalsis.

Migrating motor complexes [6, 50]

In the fasting state the slow-wave pattern is modified at approximately 100-minute intervals by a 40-minute period of inertia followed by a 30–40-minute period of irregular increased activity and then a 5- or 6-minute period of organized contraction accompanied by spike potentials. This entire sequence of events is termed the migrating motor complex

(MMC) and appears to start in the gastric antrum and sweep over the duodenum, jejunum and ileum to the ileocaecal valve (Fig. 2.3). The MMC is accompanied by a short burst of gastric, pancreatic and biliary secretion. It appears, among other properties, to have a housekeeping function in cleansing the gut of debris and basal secretions, and the absence of MMC certainly allows bacterial overgrowth in the proximal small intestine. The MMC is initiated by a sequence of neural events accompanied by the secretion of the peptide motilin. The propagation of MMC does not depend on motilin and is neurally organized.

The fed state

Feeding abolishes MMC completely and is associated with increased excitation, presumably mediated by extrinsic autonomic nervous activity which is largely cholinergic and possibly by autonomic nerves secreting a transmitter substance which is neither acetylcholine or noradrenaline. In the gastric antrum, spike potentials rapidly increase in frequency and soon coincide with every slow wave, to a maximum of 3 cycles/minute. Meanwhile activity is also increased in the duodenum and small intestine. The result is a more rapid transfer of contents down the small intestine.

Stomach and small intestine. Motor activity in the stomach and the small intestine in the fasting and fed state is greatly reduced by ablation of extrinsic autonomic nerves and ganglion-blocking drugs. It is also influenced in widely different ways by major alterations of the ionic milieu and by the presence of certain hormonal polypeptides, at least in pharmacological doses.

The colon. The myoelectrical activity of the colon is more complicated than that of the stomach and small intestine. There are two frequencies of slow activity, 2–3 cycles/minute and 6–10 cycles/minute, the latter being associated with propulsion of contents and the former probably originating in the longitudinal muscle. Only recently has it been possible to correlate in man the observations of movement of contents, alteration of intraluminal pressure and myoelectrical activity. So far the only generalization to be made is that feeding increases all forms of myoelectrical and motor activity, both mixing and propulsive.

OESOPHAGEAL FUNCTION [36]

The upper oesophageal sphincter is tonically contracted until the subject either swallows, belches or vomits. The relaxation of the upper oesophageal sphincter is followed by an orderly peristaltic contraction of the circular muscle of the body of the oesophagus; this can be recorded manometrically as a single high monophasic wave passing without a break over the junction between the striated muscle of the upper few centimetres of the oesophagus into the smooth muscle of the main part of the body of the oesophagus as far as the lower oesophageal sphincter (Fig. 2.4). The velocity of the wave is increased by warm contents and

decreased by cold and the amplitude increases caudally and is directly related to the size of the bolus swallowed. Acid in the body of the oesophagus has no effect on motor activity but does so when instilled below the upper oesophageal sphincter to increase its tone. In experiments in which a large bolus was tethered in the oesophagus the circular muscle contracted strongly to expel the bolus towards the stomach and this caudal direction of peristalsis is preserved even in isolated segments of the oesophagus [5].

Stimulus-response pattern

The stimulus-response pattern in the body of the oesophagus is described as on-off, which indicates that the peristalsis does not begin for an appreciable pause until the end of the stimulus however prolonged that may be (Fig. 2.5). This pattern is preserved in the face of oesophageal transection and is only disrupted by nerve toxins such as tetrodotoxin. Otherwise ephedrine reduces peristaltic amplitude and force while cholinergic drugs increase amplitude alone. Acute hypercalcaemia reduces peristalsis in the striated muscles of the oesophagus and increases it in the smooth muscle. Calcium-blocking drugs appear to reduce peristaltic contraction in the condition of a diffuse oesophageal spasm. Thus the control and initiation of peristalsis are clearly neural. There is evidence that peristalsis is modified by local factors within the lumen and a high degree of autonomy exists in the isolated or transected oesophagus.

Lower oesophageal sphincter [14]

In 1956 manometric methods confirmed what radiologists had long realized, that there is a sphincter-like zone of increased pressure at the lower end of the oesophagus which prevents reflux of gastric contents upwards. This sphincter relaxes when swallowing occurs before the arrival of the bolus at the lower end of the oesophagus. This antireflux sphincter is of great clinical importance in the prevention of oesophagitis and has attracted a large amount of research work. This has to be read with great care to avoid undue extrapolation from the results of experiments using different techniques and different animal species.

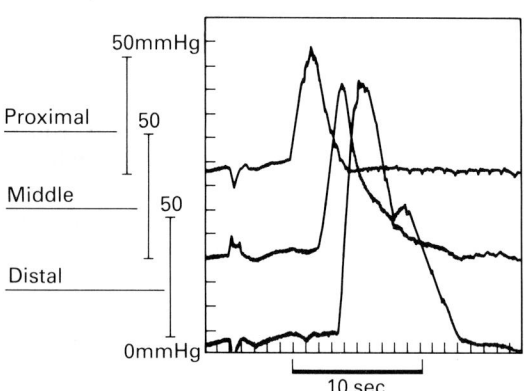

Fig. 2.4 Normal peristalsis in the body of the oesophagus. A Honeywell probe with recording tips 5 cm apart is in the body of the oesophagus. A small jog in the baseline of all three tracings is a movement artifact signalling the onset of deglutition. A high monophasic wave is recorded sequentially by the three tips. From [48], with permission.

Sphincter pressure. The sphincter is dynamic, asymmetrical and exerts a variable pressure between swallows. The values of this pressure vary greatly, depending on the methods used to elicit it. On swallowing the pressure falls to a level which is still higher than that in the oesophagus or stomach, and oesophageal contents require active peristalsis to pass into the stomach (Fig. 2.5). While gravity is an important aid to the transit of oesophageal contents in species which eat in an upright position, it is by no means indispensable as the oesophageal function of the grazing giraffe illustrates so vividly.

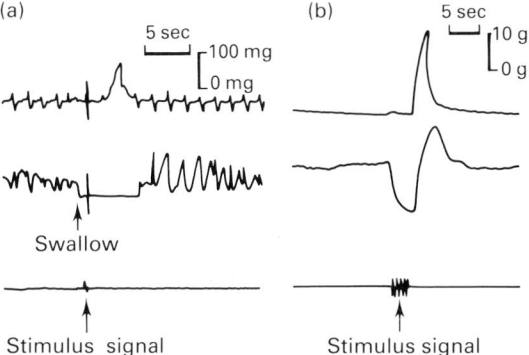

Fig. 2.5 Normal peristalsis in the body of the oesophagus (upper tracing) and lower oesophageal sphincter relaxation (lower tracing) in the opossum are shown in the left (a). The response of strips of opossum oesophageal circular smooth muscle from the body of the oesophagus (upper tracing) and the lower oesophageal sphincter (lower tracing) to electrical field stimulation are shown on the right (b). It can be seen that the patterns in vivo and in vitro are similar. The fluctuations in resting pressure measured manometrically in the lower oesophageal sphincter are due to movement of the sensing orifice with the sphincter. They are invariably seen if a high-fidelity recording system is used. From [13], with permission.

Changes in sphincter tone. The basal tension in the lower oesophageal sphincter is reduced by hypoxia, calcium antagonists and pharmacological levels of glucagon, secretin, gastric inhibitory peptide (GIP) and vasoactive intestinal peptide (VIP) (Table 2.2). The tension is increased by raising intra-abdominal pressure, the infusion of acid immediately below it, and by gastrin in pharmacological doses. No effect is seen after the common clinical form of vagotomy which may be too low to eliminate all

Table 2.2 Tension in lower oesophageal sphincter.

Decreased by:	Increased by:
Calcium antagonists	Raised intraabdominal pressure
Glucagon	Acid infusion
Secretin	Gastrin
GIP	
VIP	
	No effect:
	Atropine (in man)

vagal fibres supplying the sphincter. There is no correlation between lower oesophageal sphincter tone and blood levels of any known gastrointestinal hormone. This does not, however, exclude the possibility that one or more such peptides do play an important paracrine effect, achieving high local concentrations near the sphincter which are not reflected in blood levels.

Atropine has a marked effect on the tone of the sphincter in the cat, very little in man and none in the opossum—one of the most studied mammals with regard to the oesophagus.

Relaxation of the oesophageal sphincter. The relaxation of the lower oesophageal sphincter is triggered by swallowing, belching or vomiting, and by distension of the oesophageal body; it is probably innervated sympathetically. Relaxation is blocked by general nerve toxins such as tetradotoxin, and by hexamethonium ganglion blockers, but it is not blocked by adrenergic or cholinergic blockade. The neurotransmitter for relaxation has been ascribed to different peptides but VIP is the current candidate.

THE STOMACH

The stomach stores a meal, liquefies it, empties it in a controlled fashion and acidifies it. At the same time gastric secretion adds pepsins and gastric intrinsic factor to the luminal contents, and the surface secretion of mucus and bicarbonate protects the gastric mucosa from the effects of acid and peptic digestion, as well as corrosive or abrasive ingested matter.

Motor function

The fasting stomach. The proximal two-thirds of the stomach by volume, the body, exhibits no peristaltic activity and remains tonically contracted in the fasting state. The distal stomach exhibits the cyclical slow-wave electrical depolarizations described above, 10–30% of which are taken up as contractions organized as peristaltic waves gathering speed as they move distally towards the pylorus. A pacemaker for slow-wave activity appears to be located in the mid part of the greater curve of the stomach.

The effects of eating and storage. Cannon observed that the proximal stomach acts as a

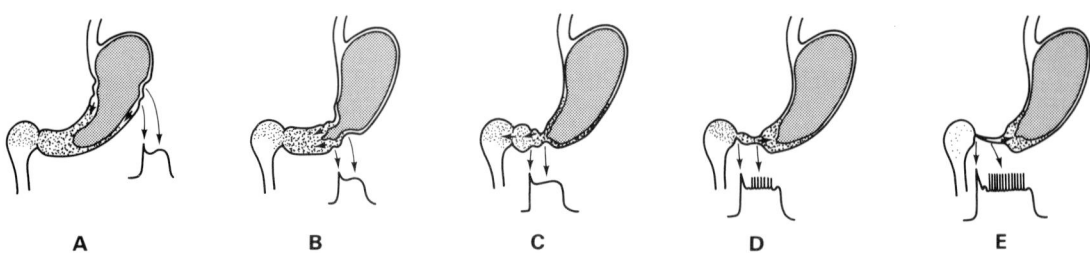

Fig. 2.6 Schema of gastric processing and emptying of solid food. Intracellular electrical potentials, gastric contractions and the effects of contraction on gastric contents are diagrammed. In panel A, solid food fills the proximal stomach and corpus. Gastric peristalsis begins with gentle contractions of the corpus. Paced by the electrical slow wave, the wave of contraction travels distally, compressing and kneading the solid food and breaking off small pieces (panel B). These pieces are propelled into the antrum by progressively stronger waves, and small particles of food are accelerated through the still open pylorus by the force of contraction (panel C). Antral contraction proceeds, and food is squirted through the narrowing pylorus and through the central orifice of the contraction wave (panel D). The pylorus closes during the terminal antral contraction (panel E), and all material is forced back to the corpus. Another wave then starts in the corpus, and the cycle is repeated. This pattern of activity results in the mixing and grinding of solid food and in the selective passage of small food particles into the duodenum. From [48], with permission.

reservoir and storage area by relaxing in direct relation to the volume of the meal consumed without any increase in intragastric pressure. Isotopic studies confirm that the major part of the meal is stored in the proximal part of the stomach while very small amounts remain in the antrum. The volume of the body of the stomach diminishes exponentially as emptying proceeds while the antral portion remains constant in volume until the stomach is nearly empty (Fig. 2.6).

The liquidizer. The distal stomach is cone shaped and during the postprandial period exhibits vigorous peristalsis at 3 cycles/minute. Peristalsis only results in material passing the pylorus if it coincides with duodenal peristalsis. Thus the majority of peristaltic waves occur against a 'closed' pylorus. The cone shape and the peristaltic activity of the antrum serve to produce a shearing and streaming effect on the contents with the observed result that solid particles are reduced to a diameter of 1 mm or less, and not until then do solid particles usually pass the pylorus under normal circumstances (Fig. 2.6).

The control of receptive relaxation of the body of the stomach is under vagal control with vagovagal reflexes also involved. Truncal vagotomy largely abolishes this function and partly explains the sense of fullness commonly experienced after this operation. The regulation of mixing and grinding and the critical particle size of solids is poorly understood, but truncal vagotomy reduces this activity greatly and also permits larger particles to pass into the small intestine. In addition it also reduces the basal MMC activity and the stomach in consequence often retains moderate volumes

of food residue of high bacterial content long after eating.

Gastric emptying [39]

The study of gastric emptying has been comprehensive; it was originally undertaken with liquid meals and, more recently, using isotopic methods, with mixed meals of liquid and solid.

In any phase the gastric emptying of its contents occurs exponentially in relation to the volume introduced into the stomach. The rate of emptying is inversely related to the nutritional density of the gastric contents, their osmolarity, acidity and the particle size of any solids present (Fig. 2.7). Thus fats are, molecule for molecule, more effective in slowing gastric emptying than protein or carbohydrate. The emptying of mixed meals of solids and liquids is complex; liquids appear to empty before solids and solids depend upon the rate at which they can be reduced to 1 mm diameter particles. Solids, moreover, are emptied at

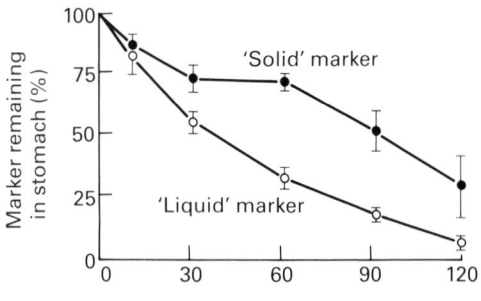

Time (min) after ingestion of meal

Fig. 2.7 Gastric emptying of solid and liquid phase meal markers. Liquids empty more rapidly than simultaneously ingested solids. From Heading et al [22], with permission. © Williams & Wilkins, 1976.

a comparatively steady rate which is presumably directly related to antral activity.

The regulation of gastric emptying. This appears to be under neural control and is rapidly adjusted to the nature of the contents entering the upper few centimetres of the small intestine. The observations on gastric emptying can best be explained by postulating the presence of postpyloric receptors in the mucosa of the duodenum and jejunum deep to the brush border enzyme. Such receptors have never been isolated anatomically. One example of their activity is in the slowing of emptying by glucose and starch. Sequential meals of isocaloric content empty at the same rate in the normal individual although starch has negligible osmolarity and glucose a high osmolarity. The suggestion is that the starch stimulates the slowing of emptying after it has been digested, and absorbed as glucose. In support of this suggestion is the observation that, in patients with severe pancreatic insufficiency where starch is not digested, the slowing of emptying by starch is lost while that by glucose is preserved [33].

Central nervous system effects. Apart from the nature of the gastric and small intestinal contents there are central areas in the cortex and brain stem, and possibly the spinal cord, which can effect gastric motility. Gastric emptying is slowed in patients in extreme pain or distress, and subclinical nausea induced pharmacologically slows gastric emptying even if the patient does not appreciate the nausea; this is restored to normal by centrally acting antiemetic drugs.

The role in this context of gastrointestinal peptide hormones is not clear. When given exogenously in pharmacological doses they may modify gastric emptying but their physiological role is uncertain.

Gastric secretion

The fasting stomach. The stomach secretes at an extremely low rate in the resting state even in stage III of the interdigestive cycle. Basal acid output is almost undetectable in the majority of normal subjects. Failure of this suppression is held to account for the increased basal acid secretion seen in certain patients with duodenal ulcer disease.

The effects of feeding. The anticipation of a meal and the postprandial phase is marked by an intense period of secretory activity of acid, electrolytes and macromolecules.

Acid secretion. The quantitation of acid secretion has been exhaustively studied partly because of accessibility and partly because of the undoubted importance of acid in the genesis of peptic ulceration. While several steps are poorly understood it is clear that gastric acid secretion is carried out exclusively by the parietal cell of the gastric glands and recently an enzyme unique to this cell has been isolated near the secretory surface. The enzyme is an acid/potassium ATPase which is probably the immediate mediator of acid secretion into the lumen of the gastric gland accelerating a one-to-one exchange of hydrogen for potassium ions, a process accompanied by striking morphological alterations of the secretory surface membrane.

Peak and basal secretion [2]

Basal secretion may represent the intrinsic activity of the parietal cell mass with minimal stimulation or it may be the result of parietal cell activity subjected to specific inhibitory mechanisms.

Stimulated acid secretion, however, is closely related to the parietal cell mass of the individual, and the peak that can be achieved by maximal pharmacological stimulation is definitely so related; in particular, it is directly related to body weight. Peak secretion is relatively constant from day to day and is nearly equal to the acid secretion seen in the first postprandial hour after an agreeable meal in pleasant surroundings. Parietal cell mass and peak acid output is greatly increased in patients with prolonged hypergastrinaemia, hypercalcaemia and in experimental animals with hyperhistaminaemia. Loss of vagal tone by vagotomy or cholinergic blockade, or reduced gastrin secretion, reduce peak acid output by approximately 70–75%. A natural example of reduced acid secretion is seen in patients with reduced parietal cell mass as a result of an autoimmune process, namely pernicious anaemia.

The response to food [10]

The response to food occurs in anticipation, a vagally mediated response known as the cephalic phase of secretion [43]. This is abolished by vagotomy. The gastric phase of secretion depends upon food entering the stomach and the intestinal phase of secretion

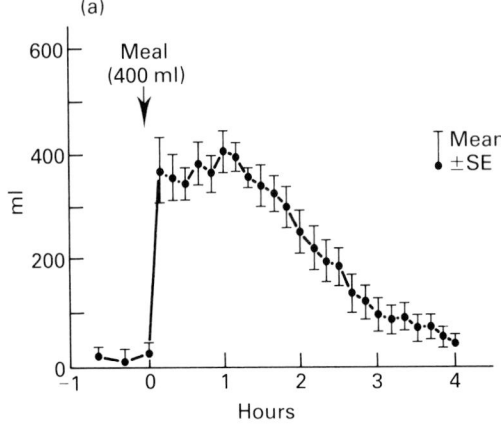

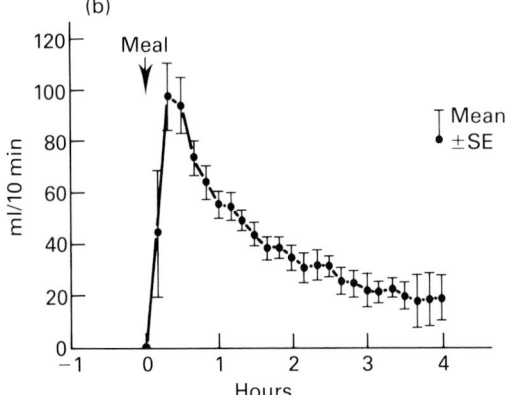

Fig. 2.8 (a) Postprandial volume of gastric contents. (b) Volume of gastric contents emptied into the duodenum after a meal. The intragastric volume is constant during the first hour after a meal during which period gastric secretion and emptying rates are at a peak but offset each other. As secretion declines intragastric volume also falls and pH, not shown, stays steady. From Malagelada et al [34], with permission.

upon food entering the intestine. Thought, sight, smell or chewing of appetizing food produces a sharp increase in acid secretion from the basal level and an elevation of serum gastrin. This appears to be mediated by hypothalamic vagal centres relayed by preganglionic fibres to the various parasympathetic plexuses grouped around the routes of the major blood vessels to the gut. Thus as food enters the stomach it already contains acid. Gastric secretion continues at a higher level for an hour or two following a substantial meal, presumably partly by continued vagal activation but also under the influence of vagovagal reflexes in response to distension of the proximal part of the stomach (Fig. 2.8).

Vagal impulses. In addition to the neural stimulation of secretion, vagal impulses sensitize

the antral gastrin-secreting cells to the arrival of protein-containing or alkaline material in the antrum resulting in the release of antral gastrin. This circulates back to the parietal cells and enchances vagally mediated acid secretion. The extent to which histamine itself is involved in physiological gastric secretion has been highlighted in the past 15 years by the effective reduction of acid secretion by H_2-receptor blockers.

Effect of food on acid secretion. Fig. 2.9 demonstrates the diminishing effect of an emptying meal on the acidification of the gastric contents [34]. As the meal diminishes in volume acid

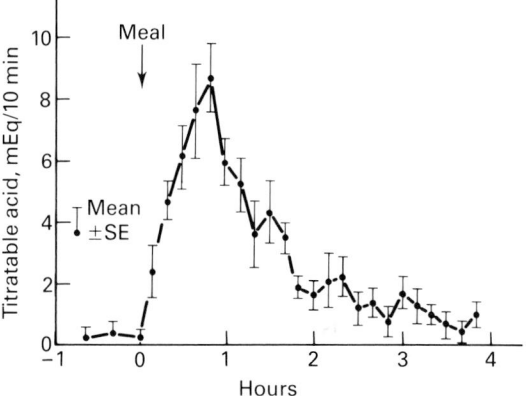

Fig. 2.9 Postprandial gastric acid output in man showing the cephalic phase, the peak secretion and the lesser phase of secretion after 2 hours. From Malagelada et al [34], with permission.

secretion diminishes in absolute amount but is enough to keep the pH of the reducing volume of the contents low. In the normal subject secretion and acidity of gastric contents fall to basal levels within approximately 2 hours of eating.

Macromolecules

The stomach secretes macromolecules in the form of mucus and gastric intrinsic factor.

The surface cells and the neck cells of the gastric mucosa secrete mucopolysaccharide and, for the most part, mucus glycoproteins. The latter contain antigens in common with the red blood cell surface antigens belonging to the ABH Lewis blood group system. The role of mucus glycoproteins in protecting the gastric mucosa from acid peptic digestion and from the effects of local trauma to the mucosa is suspected though unproven (Fig. 2.10) (see Chapter 10). Mucus secretion also provides

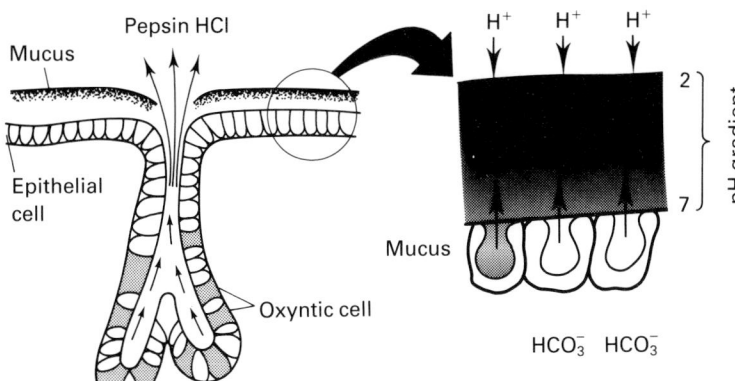

Fig. 2.10 Diagrammatic representation of the gastric epithelium showing the relationship between mucus and bicarbonate secretion by the surface cells which are probably protected against pepsin and hydrochloric acid secreted by glands. From Rees and Turnberg [42], with permission.

the mechanism for trapping an unstirred layer over the surface of the stomach which may in turn hold sodium bicarbonate secreted by the surface cells. This amounts to 10% of gastric ion secretion and would thus provide a high concentration of sodium bicarbonate to neutralize acid impinging on the gastric surface itself [42].

Pepsinogens

Pepsinogens are secreted by the chief cells of the gastric glands. Six or eight pepsinogens are recognized which are converted, at various pHs, to active pepsin. Pepsinogens are polypeptides with high molecular weight of 42 000 or so and are activated usually at a pH of less than 5. The N-terminal part may be recapped at higher pH thus rendering the pepsin inactive again but at a pH of greater than 6 pepsin is held to be irreversibly inactivated.

Active pepsins have several functions, the principal one being to initiate the hydrolysis of proteins in the gastric contents both at the terminal bonds and at the bonds within the molecule, thus creating large numbers of medium-sized polypeptide fragments. Loss of pepsin secretion such as occurs in pernicious anaemia or after gastrectomy does not create clinically ineffective protein digestion given the large reserves of the pancreas and small intestinal mucosa for proteolysis. The regulation of pepsin secretion is closely connected to that of acid and is under the influence of vagal stimulation and gastrin. Somatostatin, prostaglandins and H_2-receptor blockers all inhibit pepsin secretion.

THE SMALL INTESTINAL LUMEN

The absorption of nutrients by the small intestine is the raison d'être of the gastrointestinal tract. The ingestion of a meal provokes intense activity in pancreatic secretion, bile flow, and intraluminal digestion of complex nutrients during the first hour (Fig. 2.11). Over the next 2–6 hours the contents pass down the small

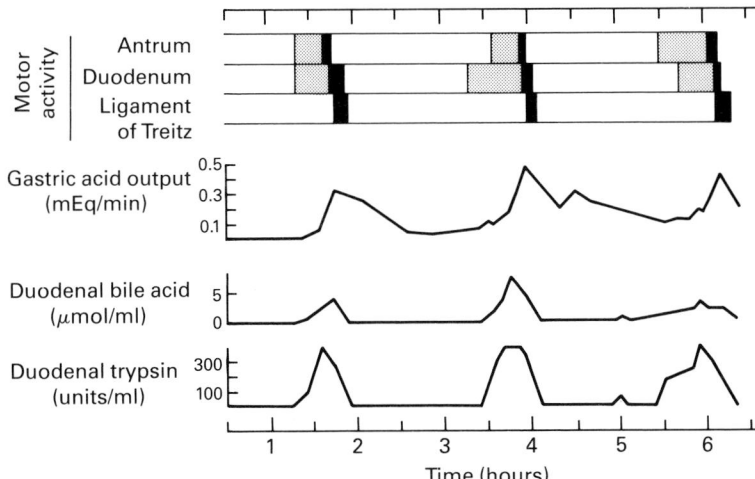

Fig. 2.11 Phases of interdigestive motor activity in association with gastric acid output and duodenal secretion of trypsin and bile acids. Regular recurring interdigestive motor activity: phase I, white portion; phase II, stippled portion; phase III, solid black portion. From Keane et al [28], with permission.

intestine, and by the first hundred centimetres the major nutritional part of the meal is absorbed. The remainder of the small intestine serves to reclaim the large volume of secreted fluid and electrolyte. The terminal ileum is highly specialized in having an ileocaecal sphincter, and also as being the specific site for absorption of vitamin B_{12} and bile salts.

Pancreatic secretion following a meal [18]

The details of the biochemical steps involved in the pancreatic secretion of enzyme, water and sodium bicarbonate, which are its principal products, have been the object of intensive study for 50 years, and are summarized in several reviews. The burden of this work is that the acinar cells of the pancreas synthesize and secrete pancreatic enzyme into the ductules of the gland, largely under the stimulation of vagal cholinergic fibres and of cholecystokinin, which is secreted by the mucosa of the duodenum and jejunum. The large volume (approximately 1 litre/day) of water containing isosmotic sodium bicarbonate is secreted mainly by the ductular cells of the pancreas under the influence of secretin in conjunction with cholecystokinin, and is largely independent of vagal fibres but probably much influenced by enteropancreatic neural reflexes.

The pancreas in the fasting state secretes very little. A small amount of water, bicarbonate and enzyme is secreted in phase II and phase III of the interdigestive cycle.

In response to a meal there is a cephalic phase of pancreatic secretion, vagally mediated and abolished by vagotomy, which may amount to 25% of the total output [45]. This is further augmented upon the arrival of food in the stomach, probably mediated through vagovagal reflexes.

Enzyme secretion

The greater part of enzyme secretion, however, is stimulated by the arrival of nutrients in the duodenum and upper jejunum which is rapidly followed by the release of the peptide hormone cholecystokinin. While this is secreted more abundantly in response to hypercalcaemia and the ingestion of solubilized fat, mixed meals even in the absence of fat provide a near-maximal stimulation of pancreatic enzyme secretion. Moreover, this secretion is greatly in excess of any possible requirements provoked by the ingestion of a single meal [18].

Nature of enzymes. The 8 g or so of enzyme protein secreted each day is composed of a mixture of hydrolases which are responsible for proteolysis, lipolysis and starch hydrolysis. Bond-splitting of numerous fat-soluble vitamin esters and other lipid esters also possibly occurs without specific hydrolases. The proteolytic enzyme trypsin and the phospholipases are secreted in an inactive form and are only activated within the gastrointestinal lumen under normal circumstances. The remainder are secreted in their active forms.

The secretion of water and bicarbonate has long been attributed to the release of secretin by acid in the duodenum. However, it is now

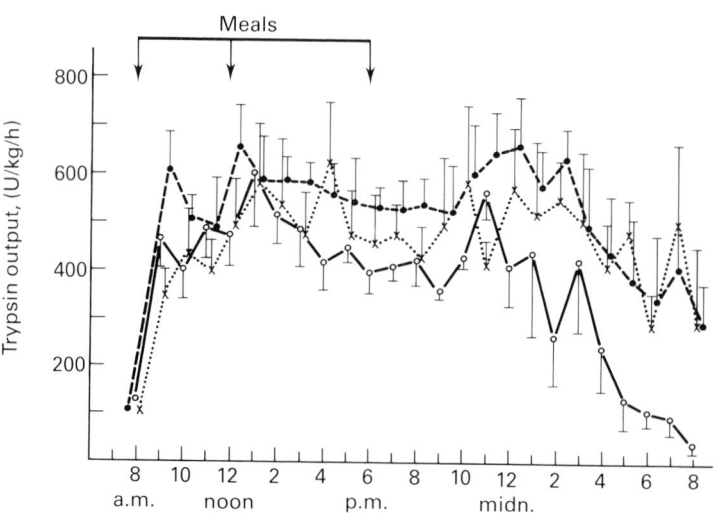

Fig. 2.12 Trypsin secretion into the duodenum (mean ± s.e.) in 18 healthy people ingesting three equicaloric liquid meals. (○), 20 cal/kg; (●), 30 cal/kg; (x), 40 cal/kg. From Brunner et al [4], with permission.

doubtful whether this alone accounts for the secretion of these substances, and the additive effect of cholecystokinin and enteropancreatic reflexes is almost certain to be involved [51].

Rates of secretion. Following a meal there is a peak of secretion within the first 45 minutes followed by a plateau of high secretion until the duodenum is empty of nutritional contents. Thereafter secretion dwindles, more by reduction of stimulation than by any specific inhibitory action, although pancreatic polypeptide does inhibit enzyme secretion and may do so physiologically (Fig. 2.12).

Biliary secretion

Bile is a complex solution of water and electrolytes, bilirubin, cholesterol and phospholipid in micellar solution with a critical concentration of bile salts. Again the control of the synthesis and secretion of bile has been the subject of intensive study which has been reviewed elsewhere. In the context of digestion, the fasting subject shows a steady secretion of bile which is largely diverted to the gall bladder, which has a capacity in man of approximately 30 ml. During the interdigestive phases II and III up to 10 ml of bile are secreted into the gut by the gall bladder accompanied by a brief burst of motor activity in the gall bladder and bile duct.

There is little or no cephalic phase of gall bladder emptying which nevertheless begins rapidly after the ingestion of a meal under the influence of cholinergic nerve fibres and cholecystokinin, a potent stimulator of gall bladder emptying. At the same time the sphincter of Oddi at the lower end of the common bile duct opens and remains so until the end of the postprandial period approximately 2 hours later. Hepatic bile subsequently by-passes the gall bladder during the postprandial period and passes directly into the duodenum.

Bile acids

The synthesis, secretion and enterohepatic circulation of the bile acid pool has also received detailed attention [29]. Three bile acids are synthesized by the liver, secreted into the bile and are responsible for the solubilization, in the bile, of cholesterol and phospholipids and are essential to their excretion. Bile acids play an intrinsic part in the secretion of bile by the hepatocytes. In the gut, bile acids are responsible for the solubilization of lipids and hence the absorption of dietary lipid and fat-soluble vitamins. They also have an effect in stimulating pancreatic secretion.

In brief, conjugated bile acids remain in the small intestinal lumen until they reach the terminal ileum where there appears to be a specific receptor site for their absorption. Recirculation occurs through the portal blood to the liver and re-secretion by the hepatocytes (Fig. 2.13). In experimental studies in man the total bile acid pool circulates at least twice per meal. Bile acid synthesis is limited, in contrast to the exuberant overproduction of pancreatic enzymes for example. The by-passing of the gall bladder in the postprandial phase, the easy passage of bile from liver to duodenum and the storage of bile in the gall bladder between meals can all be interpreted as creating an economical system for obtaining the best benefit from a limited resource. Nevertheless, with modern food and cooking, removal of the gall

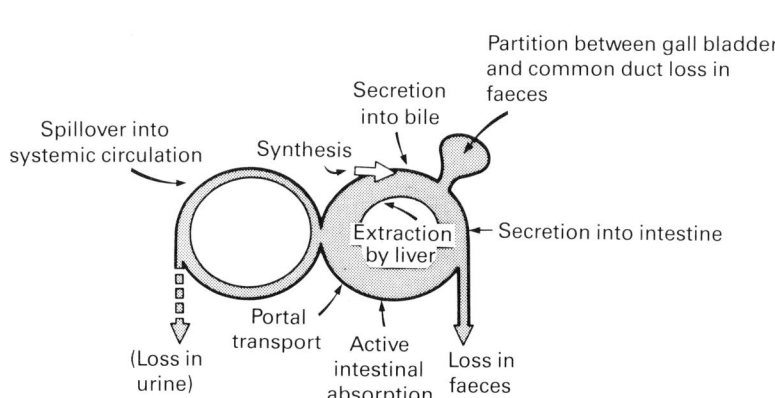

Fig. 2.13 Schematic depiction of the enterohepatic circulation of bile acids in man. Gall bladder filling is determined by contraction of the sphincter of Oddi (not shown). The movement of the enterohepatic circulation is largely mediated by intestinal motility. The serum level of bile acids is determined by the fraction of bile acids returning from the intestine that are removed by the liver. In healthy man, individual bile acids are eliminated from the body only in faeces. The composition of the circulatory bile acids reflects hepatic synthesis from cholesterol and bacterial formation of secondary bile acids that are absorbed from the distal intestine (not shown). From [48], with permission.

bladder does not have any obvious adverse effects on the digestion or absorption of fats.

Intraluminal digestion

Very little of the nutrient content of a normal diet is in the form of material that can be absorbed unchanged by the small intestine. High-energy foods such as protein, starches, fat and even vitamins require to be broken down into simpler molecules before absorption can occur. It is the process of intraluminal digestion in the upper small intestine which results in the enterocyte being presented with absorbable fragments (Fig. 2.14).

Proteins in the diet are already partially fragmented by the activity of gastric pepsin; lipids may be partly digested within the gastric lumen under the influence of lingual lipase, while starch may have been partly digested by salivary amylase in the mouth during chewing. Nevertheless, the burden of hydrolysis falls upon pancreatic enzymes.

Nature of protein digestion

Protein digestion, under the influence of trypsin and carboxypepsidases, proceeds both at the terminal linkages of the protein molecules and at the internal bonds. This provides an efficient means of breaking the proteins into oligopeptides. Trypsinogen is converted to active trypsin by the intervention of intestinal enterokinase. The rare congenital absence of this enzyme greatly reduces protein digestion in the sufferer. Starches are digested by pancreatic amylase at the α-linkages. This leaves the branch chains of the amyloses unbroken and produces fragments of finite size known as limit dextrins.

Fat digestion

Fat digestion is more complex [25]. Pancreatic lipase requires the presence of a colipase to function at the neutral pH of the duodenal contents. Moreover, the presence of a critical concentration of bile salt is important to ensure the solubilization of the digestion products into micelles. Pancreatic lipase hydrolyses the bond between fatty acid and glycerol in the 1-position on the glycerol molecule, but internal rearrangement of the residual diglyceride permits hydrolysis to continue, resulting in monoglyceride and fatty acid both of which are incorporated into the micelle. While

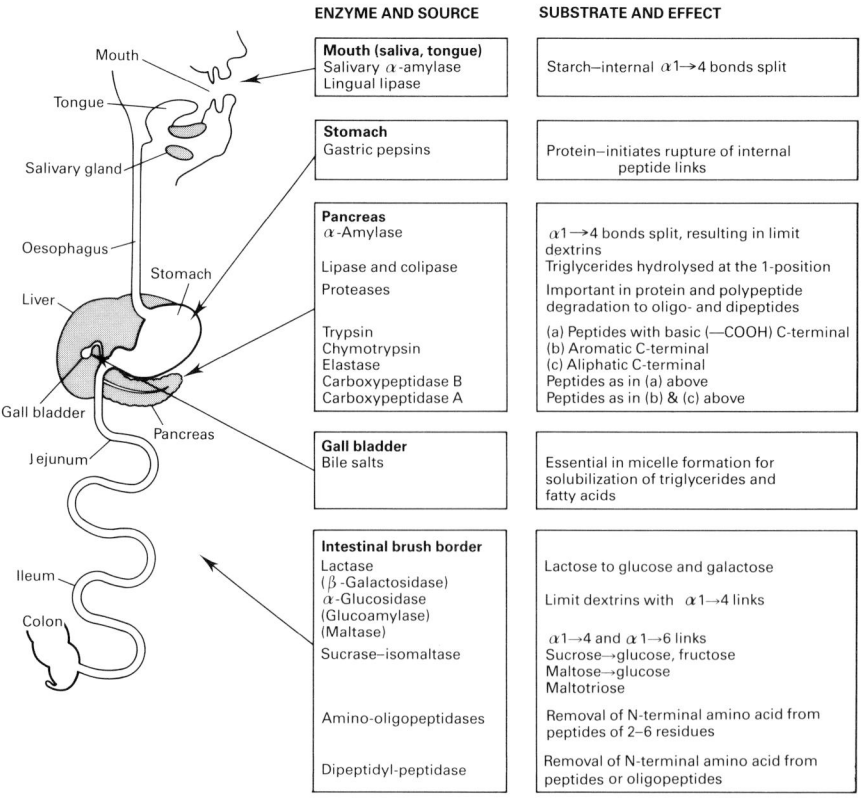

Fig. 2.14   Main sites of enzyme activity.

a certain amount of lipid can be absorbed in the total absence of pancreatic enzyme or bile acid this is greatly reduced in either case with the result of fat malabsorption. The fat-soluble vitamins are similarly incorporated (after de-esterification by pancreatic enzyme) in the centre of micelles whence they are presented to the surface of the enterocyte.

Rates of intraluminal digestion

The process of intraluminal digestion is complex but it is nevertheless extremely rapid and the rate of absorption and the appearance of the products of absorption in the circulation are just as rapid if the native dietary elements are presented to the intestine as when the primitive amino acids, peptides or monosaccharides are administered. Thus intraluminal digestion presents no limiting factor in absorption provided the enzymes and the milieu and bile salt concentration are all adjusted to a minimum critical requirement (Fig. 2.14).

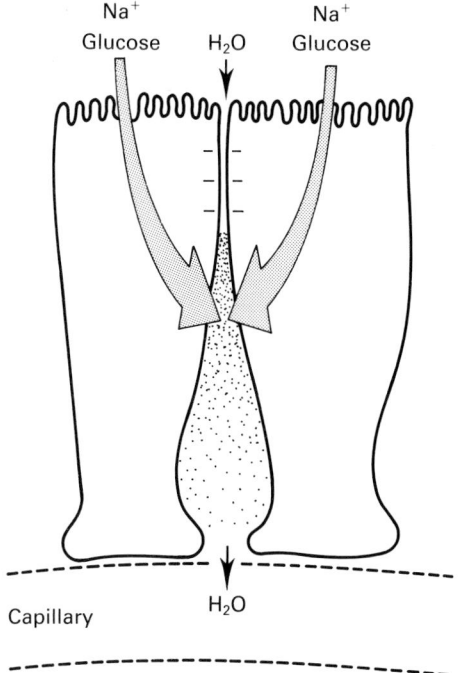

Fig. 2.15 A diagram of the hypothesis of fluid absorption involving the transport of sodium and glucose into the cell and the subsequent pumping of sodium into the intercellular space. Water is shown to pass through the tight junction between the cells into the lateral space. The increase in hydrostatic pressure in the lateral space so created encourages fluid to move in the direction of least resistance into the capillary. From [3], with permission.

The function of the small-intestinal cell—the enterocyte

The surface of the enterocyte is formed into microvilli covered by a bimolecular lipid membrane in which are borne a variety of mucosal enzymes, principally peptidases and carbohydrases. So-called tight junctions exist between the apical borders of the enterocyte, but as shown in Fig. 2.15, the basal parts of the enterocytes are separated to surround the lateral intercellular spaces. The base of the cell is contiguous with capillary endothelium while the intercellular spaces communicate more generally with lymphatic channels.

Digestion at the brush border membrane

Disaccharides and small oligosaccharides resulting from intraluminal digestion of starch are presented to the brush border surface by the movements of the bulk phase in the lumen [46]. The enterocytes can only absorb monosaccharide, and the brush border carbohydrases (as shown in Fig. 2.16) are responsible

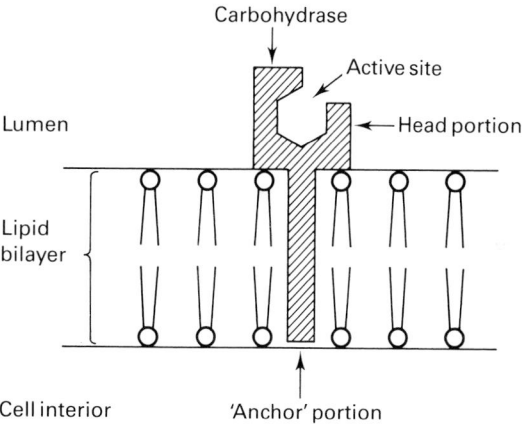

Fig. 2.16 Diagram of the integration of brush border carbohydrases into lipid cell membrane. The tail within the membrane anchors the head portion which 'projects' into the lumen. From [3], with permission.

for completing the digestion of the oligosaccharides. Thus the important dimer sucrase-isomaltase is responsible for approximately 90% of the maltase activity of the intestine, and also for splitting sucrose into glucose and fructose. In comparison, lactase is responsible for splitting lactose into glucose and galactose and is important principally in neonatal life during milk-feeding. In large ethnic groups lactase is regressive thereafter and its absence is only a disadvantage in those habituated to the consumption of large quantities of milk in adult life.

Peptidases also abound in the brush border calyx, but they function in a more obscure fashion and are discussed below [9]. The enzyme enterokinase is also found in the brush border membrane but the principal site of trypsinogen activation is nevertheless probably in the bulk phase in the lumen where enterokinase is also present in soluble form.

The unstirred layer. Even when the bulk phase luminal contents are energetically stirred at the interface with the cell membrane, a still, unstirred layer of fluid exists. This is the case in the small intestine as well as in the remainder of the gut, and has proved of importance in the study of molecular absorption. The thickness of the unstirred layer has a considerable effect on the dynamics of absorption, and the possibility that a considerably lower pH obtains in the unstirred layer than in the bulk phase has influenced interpretation of the absorption of folic acid at least.

INTESTINAL CELLULAR ABSORPTION

In this context the transfer of material across the intestinal cell membrane from the lumen is referred to as absorption and the transfer from the cell into the lumen as secretion [47].

Such transfer may be effected by a variety of mechanisms such as cytosis, diffusion, active transfer and carrier-mediated transfer.

Cytosis

Cytosis is the transfer of discernible particulate matter or solutions within vesicles produced by cell membranes. Secretion in this manner is typified by the secretion of pancreatic enzymes. The transfer of long-chain lipid from the enterocyte into the lateral intercellular space in the form of chylomicrons is another example, and vitamin B_{12}–intrinsic factor complexes are absorbed by micropinocytosis.

Passive diffusion

Diffusion is the random movement of a substance due to thermal agitation. In solution substances disperse by diffusion until an even distribution is achieved. The nature of diffusion implies that back-diffusion is bound to

occur, although, in many natural systems in which a diffusion is responsible for the transfer of material across a membrane, back-diffusion is often reduced by some form of trapping mechanism on one side of the membrane. If this results in a reduced concentration of the original substance then diffusion will proceed apparently directionally and may mimic an actively assisted process.

This is particularly apposite in the instance of non-ionic diffusions. A number of lipid-soluble substances are weak acids or bases, as are most pharmacological preparations. Thus a weak acid in solution and largely dissociated on one side of a membrane will diffuse steadily and continuously across that membrane if the physicochemical environment on the far side removes undissociated acid by trapping it or rendering the milieu on the far side more alkaline.

Active transfer

A substance may be moved by active transfer against an electrical or chemical gradient (electrochemical). The implication is that the cell participates in active transfer by devoting metabolic energy to regulate and influence the rate and direction of transfer. The resulting transfer is greater than could be expected from the existence of the known chemical potential, osmotic, hydrostatic and electrical forces. In practice it is often difficult to distinguish between passive transfer assisted by a trapping mechanism and an active transfer system.

Carrier-mediated transfer

Hexoses, amino acids and certain ions appear to be transferred by specific carriers which act as a ferry shuttling across the lipid cell membrane. Carrier-mediated transfer exhibits several characteristics: the rate of transfer exhibits saturation with increasing concentration of substrate, it exhibits competition when substances of similar structure are present, it is highly specific and also inhibitable. Moreover, the transfer rate of substances is higher than can be predicted by simple physicochemical characteristics.

Water absorption [30]

Approximately 1.5 litres of water are ingested daily, a further 8–10 litres of fluid enter the gut via secretion daily and a mere 0.1 litre leaves in the stool, the remainder being absorbed largely by the small intestine. The reserve for the absorption of water is large in that under steady-state conditions the limit appears to be 20 litres and the colon alone can absorb 6 litres of isotonic normal saline.

The orthodox view of water absorption is that it is secondary to the absorption of sodium and glucose. These solutes are absorbed across the cell membrane and are then concentrated in the lateral intercellular space. As shown in Fig. 2.15, this establishes a hypertonic zone in the space, and water moves into this directly through pores in the so-called tight junctions between the cells. Thus water does not traverse the lipid cell membrane but by-passes it. The flow of water into the hypertonic zone increases the hydrostatic pressure in the space, and the capillary flow or the lymphatic flow at the base of the space provides the route of least resistance through which water and sodium and glucose pass. One objection to this hypothesis is that in the jejunum at least the tight junctions are calculated to be large and permeable and would permit more back-flow than is actually observed.

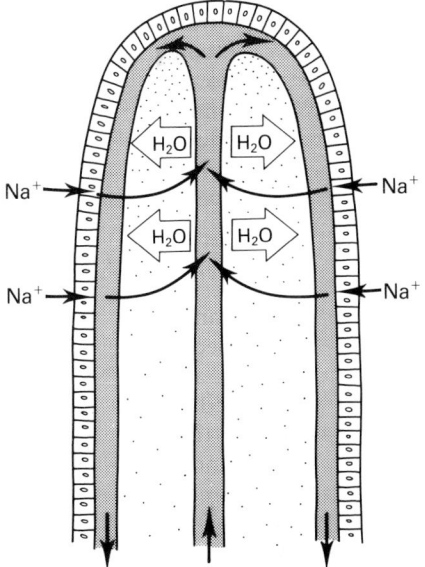

Fig. 2.17 A diagram of the counter-current hypothesis for fluid absorption from the small intestine. Active transepithelial absorption of sodium establishes a sodium gradient between the peripheral capillary and the central artery. This results in a cross-diffusion of sodium from capillary to artery, while water travels in the opposite direction from artery to capillary. This effect is multiplied towards the villus tip until very large osmotic gradients are built up. From Hallback et al [21], with permission. © 1978 by The American Gastroenterological Association.

Countercurrent hypothesis. An alternative hypothesis proposes a countercurrent mechanism in the cells at the tip of the villus (Fig. 2.17). This theory has the advantage of explaining why 50% of net water absorption occurs via the lymph while blood flow in the villus is 500 times greater than lymph flow. It is possible that a combination of these mechanisms occurs in the jejunum.

The presence of pores in the tight junctions is postulated as a result of observed data concerning absorption in the jejunum, ileum and colon. In the proximal small intestine the pores are apparently larger than in the ileum and in the colon they are smaller than either [11]. Water absorption is extremely rapid in the jejunum and slower in the ileum, but active cellular intervention appears to account for the observation that fluid can be absorbed from a more dilute intraluminal solution, thus against a higher concentration gradient. In the colon the channels are apparently tightest and transit is slow, one result being that water is extracted from progressively drier material against an ever steeper concentration gradient.

Electrolyte absorption

In the jejunum sodium absorption is linked to the absorption of non-ionic substances such as sugars, peptides and amino acids, all of which have an active carrier transport mechanism. Sodium appears to travel on the same carrier and increases the sodium concentration of the cell. However, the low concentration is maintained by an intracellular sodium pump acting at the lateral intercellular membrane creating the high concentration in the lateral intercellular space. The subsequent passage of water into the lateral space as described above is accompanied by sodium chloride. Thus the energy for the process is generated at the lateral membrane sodium pump. Sodium absorption may also occur in the absence of non-electrolyte by an active sodium–hydrogen exchange pump.

In the ileum there is little non-electrolyte remaining in the lumen and the major sodium absorption path is by a neutral sodium–hydrogen exchange pump coupled to a pump exchanging intracellular bicarbonate for chloride which is largely cleared from the luminal contents. As shown in Fig. 2.18, the colon absorbs sodium and water in a different fashion, is entirely dependent on an intracellular pump mechanism and could be regarded as adapted to the extraction of sodium from very low con-

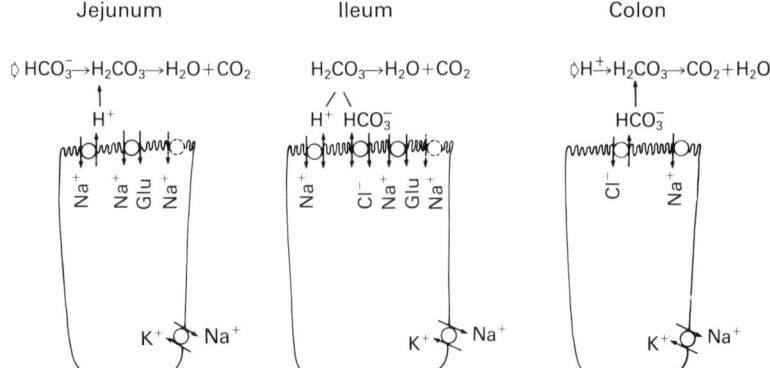

Fig. 2.18 Diagrams of the carrier-mediated mechanisms thought to exist for the absorption of sodium, potassium and chloride across the mucosal and basolateral membranes in the human jejunum, ileum and colon. From [3], with permission.

centrations (15 mmol/l) into a cell cytosol of greatly higher concentration.

Transport of potassium across the small intestinal epithelium behaves throughout as though it were a passive process accompanying the diffusion of water into the intercellular space by solvent drag.

Failure of water and electrolyte absorption

While the osmolality of the small intestinal contents undergoes periodic change during the process of intraluminal digestion [40], the combination of pancreatic and biliary secretion and the rapid removal of osmotically active small molecules by intestinal absorption appears to result in a remarkably steady level of 300–325 mosmol/kg. Indeed, osmotically induced secretion of water by the intestine is difficult to sustain, possibly because the lateral intercellular spaces collapse and do not permit further secretion. In vivo hydrostatic pressure applied to the serosal surface of the intestine inhibits absorption and increases secretion, but this does not have a counterpart in vitro.

In pathological states there are several mechanisms of failure of water and electrolyte absorption resulting in more or less liquid stools of increased volume. For example, in coeliac disease in which the mucosal architecture is grossly disturbed, experimental evidence suggests that the pores in the tight junctions of the jejunum are smaller than normal and sodium and chloride absorption is decreased, throwing an increased burden on the ileum and colon. Conversely, in proximal colonic resection, excessive bile salt leakage into the colon reduces the absorptive capacity of the right colon and increases the absorptive work of the distal colon, often beyond its capacity which is in any case less than that of the right colon.

Active secretion of water and electrolytes

Cholera toxin, a well-researched substance, alters the permeability of the mucosal membrane to chloride which passes into the lumen. This is compensated by the entry of further chloride from the circulation into the cell accompanied by sodium. While the chloride enters the lumen through the mucosal membrane, sodium is pumped into the lateral space and is thence extruded together with water into the lumen. The result is the well-recognized diarrhoea containing a high concentration of sodium chloride. This abnormality is probably localized to the crypts of the villi leaving the mature absorptive cells of the villus relatively unaffected. This would explain why the oral ingestion of water, sodium chloride and glucose provides a mechanism whereby these substances can be absorbed effectively and offset the massive secretory losses, thus providing effective treatment.

Secretagogues

There are several agents which act as intestinal secretagogues, all of them by apparently increasing intracellular levels of calcium. Cholera toxin and VIP activate via a surface receptor, adenylate cyclase, thus leading to the formation of cyclic AMP. This is believed to be followed by the release of calcium from intracellular stores and also increases the uptake into the cell from extracellular fluid, as illustrated in Fig. 2.19.

Other secretagogues including serotonin act differently, by inducing hydrolysis of phospholipid in the cell membrane and enabling calcium to enter via the channels so formed. The effect of calcium, by whatever means it is increased in the cytosol, is apparently to induce specific chloride loss into the lumen

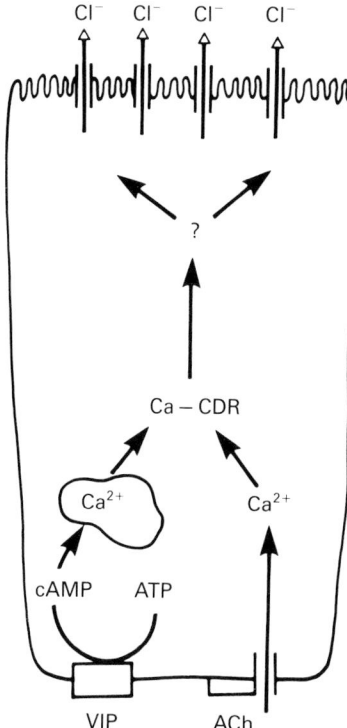

Fig 2.19 A diagram of the proposed intracellular mechanism via which secretagogues exert their effect on the enterocyte by promoting chloride secretion across the cell membrane and increasing intracellular calcium. From [3], with permission. CDR = calmodulin.

through the surface membrane with the consequences described above.

Transmitter substances. Table 2.3 shows the numerous transmitter substances that inhibit epithelial absorption or increase fluid and electrolyte secretion. VIP and serotonin are both well-recognized transmitter substances found

Table 2.3 Possible transmitter substances that may act on the intestinal epithelium to reduce or increase absorption or secretion of fluid and electrolytes.

Reduce absorption, increase secretion	Increase absorption, reduce secretion
Muscarinic agonists	Catecholamines
VIP	Dopamine
Angiotensin (high dose)	Angiotensin (low dose)
Secretin	Enkephalins
Serotonin	Somatostatin
Bombesin	Prostacyclin
Substance P	
Neurotensin	
ATP	
Gastrin	
Cholecystokinin	
Bradykinin	
Histamine	
Prostaglandins	

in abundance in enteric neurons. Both are released by vagal stimulation, and induce intestinal secretion, and in both excessive secretion by endocrine tumours induces watery diarrhoea although much more severely in the case of VIP-secreting tumours.

Histamine is present in the large mass of mast cells in the gut. Its principal action in inducing diarrhoea is probably by altering capillary permeability, although it also has a direct effect on inhibiting the chloride–bicarbonate exchange in the ileum resulting in more acidic small-intestinal contents. In the context of this chapter the actions of histamine are particularly relevant in patients with established food allergy and of course the rare disease of systemic mastocytosis.

Prostaglandins

These substances stimulate intestinal secretion by direct action on the cell membrane to induce cyclic AMP. Vagal stimulation may release them as well as mucosal injury or excessive distension of the gut. Their precise physiological and pathological role is yet to be delineated.

Bile acids and hydroxy fatty acids

Non-physiological concentrations of bile acids released into the colon as a result of small bowel disease or resection impair colonic absorption, or may even stimulate secretion by stimulating production of cyclic AMP. Hydroxy fatty acids are formed by bacterial degradation of fat and have a similar effect. The factors influencing secretion into the intestine are summarized in Table 2.3.

The absorption of sugars [15, 46]

Glucose and galactose are absorbed via an active carrier system in the brush border membrane of the enterocyte. As outlined above, absorption is accompanied by absorption of sodium across the cell membrane which occurs down its concentration gradient into the cells. The concentration gradient for sodium is maintained by the active pumping of sodium into the lateral intercellular space in exchange for potassium; the energy for this is provided by the hydrolysis of ATP.

Fructose appears to enter the mucosal cell by facilitated diffusion independent of sodium transport.

Disorders of carbohydrate absorption are very rarely caused by glucose or galactose malabsorption. However, such a condition does occur and is a striking vindication of the carrier-mediated transport hypothesis in the congenital disease of glucose–galactose malabsorption.

The cellular absorption of lipid [16]

Lipid in micellar solution impinges on the lipid membrane of the cell but it is unknown how it emerges from the centre of the micelle. Emerge it does, however, and the empty micelle returns through the unstirred layer to the lumen to take up more lipid and thus further economize on bile salt reserves. The absorption of dietary lipid in the form of monoglyceride and fatty acid is by passive diffusion across the lipid membrane of the cell. However, the concentration gradient is enhanced by the presence, immediately beneath the membrane, of the fatty-acid-binding protein in the cytosol of the enterocyte. Apart from binding absorbed fatty acid and enhancing the rate of absorption thereby, it also transports the fatty acid to the smooth endoplasmic reticulum whereupon the absorbed fat is re-esterified to triglyceride which appears first in the smooth endoplasmic reticulum near the apex of the enterocyte, thus providing a further mechanism for maintaining the concentration gradient of fatty acid across the luminal membrane.

The triglyceride passes slowly through the endoplasmic reticulum to become associated with the Golgi apparatus. Here the triglyceride is enveloped in lipoprotein, the envelope of the lipoprotein being synthesized in the rough endoplasmic reticulum (Fig. 2.20). The chylomicrons thus formed pass through a microtubular system to the lateral basal part of the cell membrane where the chylomicron membrane fuses with the cell membrane and the whole microvesicle thus formed passes by the process of exocytosis into the lateral space and thence to the lymphatics.

Medium-chain triglyceride provides a small percentage of dietary fat in humans and is of interest because it can be absorbed without first being solubilized into micelles. It appears to diffuse through the cytosol without metabolic conversion and passes without chylomicron formation through the basal membrane into the portal circulation. Thus patients with incurable forms of malabsorption of long-chain triglyceride, such as occasionally occurs in congenital abnormality of β-lipoprotein, can be nourished with medium-chain triglyceride.

Absorption of peptides and amino acids [20]

In contrast to carbohydrate which is absorbed entirely as monosaccharide, the majority of the products of protein digestion are probably absorbed as peptides. The original work suggesting this showed that an oral load of glycine

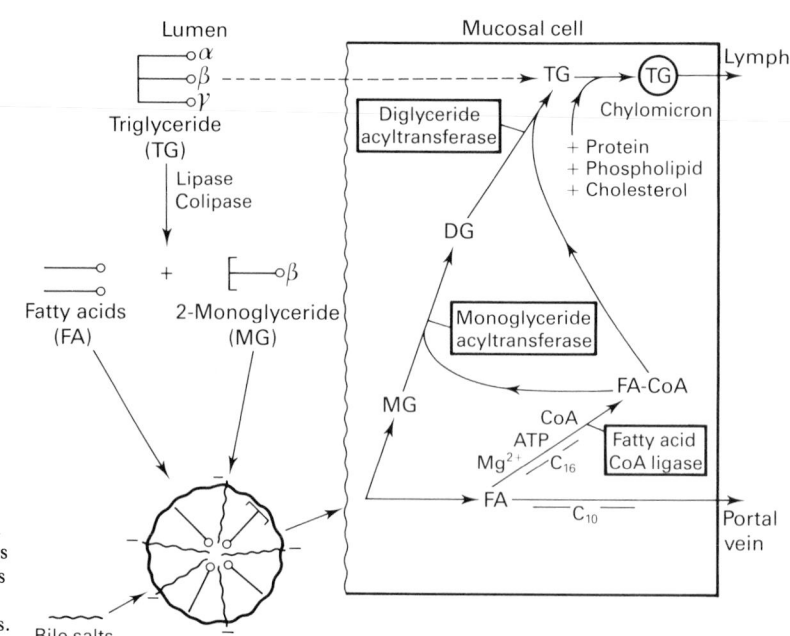

Fig. 2.20 Diagrammatic representation of fat digestion and absorption. Abbreviated structures and names are given. DG indicates diglyceride. C_{10} and C_{15} denote carbon chain length of amino acids. From [48], with permission.

delivered as dipeptide or tripeptide was absorbed more rapidly than glycine itself. More striking evidence came from studies of patients with Hartnup disease in which there is an intestinal transport defect for neutral amino acids [35], and in cystinuria in which there is a transport defect for dibasic amino acids [37]. In these patients the absorption of the affected amino acids was rendered normal if they were presented to the gut as dipeptides.

Following these observations a consistent line of work using intestinal perfusion in man has supported the belief that protein is preponderantly absorbed in peptide form by mechanisms independent of those resulting in single amino acid transport (Fig. 2.21) [23].

acids, the dibasic amino acids and the dicarboxylic amino acids.

The absorption of whole protein

In nutritional terms the absorption of whole protein is a negligible contribution. But, as is discussed comprehensively elsewhere in this book, there is convincing evidence that whole protein is indeed absorbed in sufficient quantity to be antigenically significant. Certainly there is nothing to suggest that whole protein cannot be shielded from intraluminal and membrane digestion by travelling in the centre of small food particles, associated with fibre strands, or simply escape digestion by an

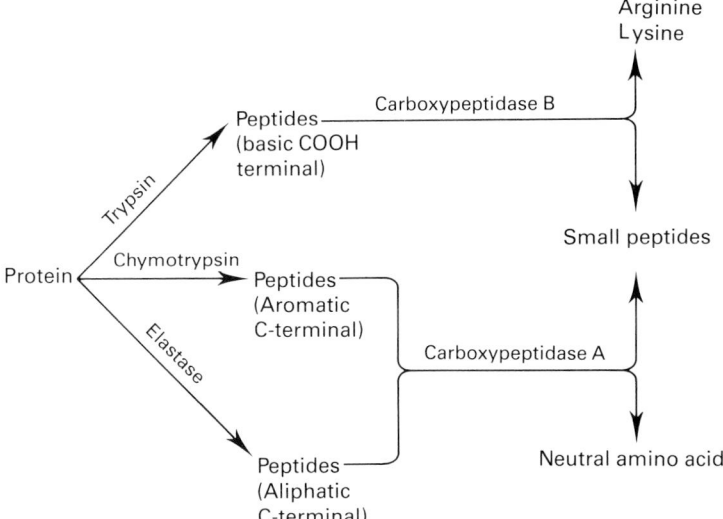

Fig. 2.21 Sequence of events leading to hydrolysis of dietary protein by intraluminal proteases. The fate of the final oligopeptide and amino acid products depends on the intestinal epithelial cell. From [48], with permission.

The intestinal brush border is rich in peptidases; however, these have a greater affinity for certain dipeptides than others, and it appears that dipeptides with high affinity for peptidases are likely to undergo mucosal hydrolysis followed by absorption as individual amino acids. Dipeptides with a low affinity for such peptidases are absorbed intact. Existing evidence, while not comprehensive, suggests that unhydrolysed dipeptides and tripeptides are absorbed by an energy- and sodium-dependent carrier mechanism which is saturable. There is conflicting evidence as to whether there is a single peptide carrier or multiple specific carriers.

As with glucose, amino acid absorption is mediated by a sodium-dependent carrier-mediated mechanism. Three major groups of amino acids appear to have group-specific active transport systems: the neutral amino

accident in mixing. Likewise the constant turnover of cell material with the implication of momentary gaps in the enterocyte lining makes it entirely possible for whole protein of large size to be absorbed haphazardly between enterocytes.

Vitamin absorption

Fat-soluble vitamins. Fat-soluble vitamins, A, D, K, E, are all absorbed from micellar solution in the proximal small intestine. Like a long-chain triglyceride they are extruded into the lymphatic channels in chylomicrons. They are present in small amounts in the diet, and, although they are only required in very small amounts to maintain adequate supplies, any prolongation of absolute bile salt deficiency such as occurs in biliary obstruction results in almost complete absorptive failure. The appearance of deficiency then depends upon body stores, which are small for vitamin K, highly variable for vitamin D and almost inexhaustible for vitamin A.

Water-soluble vitamins. The water-soluble vitamins are absorbed by a variety of mechanisms. Ascorbic acid and pyridoxine are both absorbed by passive diffusion. Niacin and thiamine are absorbed by a sodium-dependent active-transport system, while the absorption mechanisms for biotin, riboflavin and pantothenic acid are unknown. Nevertheless, even severe small-intestinal disease does not lead to significant deficiency, which is almost invariably due to dietary deficiency.

Vitamin B₁₂

Vitamin B_{12} has been the subject of intensive study and has a unique mode of absorption.

Cooking and gastric digestion release vitamin B_{12} from the animal foodstuffs in which it is largely found. It is promptly bound to the glycoprotein intrinsic factor (IF) secreted by the gastric parietal cell. The B_{12}-IF complex is resistant to tryptic digestion in the intestinal lumen where it stays until it is absorbed at highly specific receptor sites in the epithelium of the last few centimetres of the ileum (Fig. 2.22). The complex is extremely large and is thought to be absorbed by endocytosis.

Following one exposure to vitamin B_{12} the ileum is blocked to further absorption for 4 hours or more. During this time intrinsic factor is digested from vitamin B_{12} by lysosomal enzymes in the cytosol and vitamin B_{12} reappears in portal blood after several hours bound to a different carrier protein, transcobalamin II, which is probably synthesized within the ileal enterocyte. The peak blood level after absorption of 8–12 hours represents a uniquely prolonged latency for any absorbed substance. Vitamin B_{12} deficiency does not

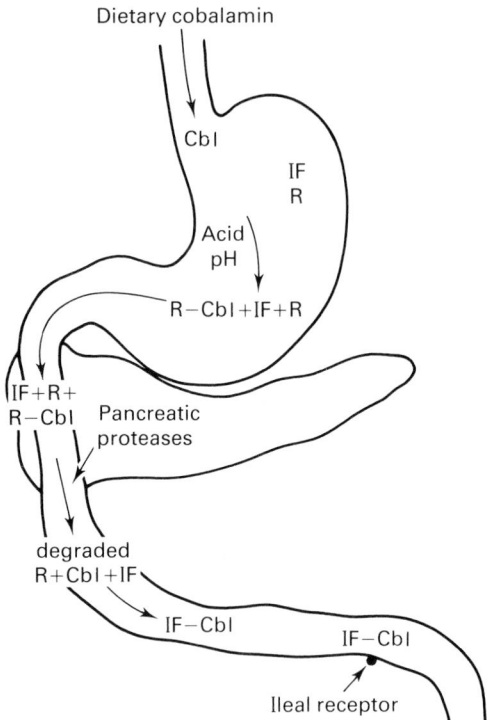

Fig. 2.22 Absorption of cobalamin (Cbl) requires proteolysis and intrinsic factor (IF). The mass of intrinsic factor secreted is far in excess of that needed for binding the available cobalamin. R protein derived from saliva is also present in great abundance. More R protein and cobalamin are added from biliary secretions into the duodenum. Note that cobalamin (Cbl) binds initially to R protein in the stomach at acid pH. Only after R protein is degraded by proteases does Cbl bind IF. After Cbl is absorbed in the ileum, it is bound to transcobalamin II and perhaps TC I and III. From [48], with permission.

enhance vitamin B_{12} absorption in the ileum and ileal resection is followed by permanent failure of B_{12} absorption, which is not corrected by the adaptation of more proximal gut. Other types of deficiency are outlined in Table 2.4. Enterohepatic circulation occurs resulting in 1–40 μg of vitamin B_{12} per day being avail-

Table 2.4 Abnormalities in cobalamin absorption producing deficiency.

Physiological step	Disorder
Impaired food digestion	Gastrectomy, achlorhydria
Decreased intrinsic factor secretion	Pernicious anaemia, gastrectomy
Impaired transfer to intrinsic factor	Pancreatic insufficiency, Zollinger–Ellison syndrome
Abnormal intrinsic factor	Decreased ileal binding
Competition for uptake	Bacterial overgrowth
Impaired attachment to ileal receptor	Ileal disease or resection
Impaired passage through the ileal cell	Familial cobalamin malabsorption
Impaired uptake into blood	Transcobalamin II deficiency

From [48], with permission.

able for reabsorption since it is bound to free intrinsic factor in the gut.

Folic acid (folate)

Folate occurs naturally in a wide variety of food, particularly offal, nuts and greens. While the average Western diet contains six times the requirement, folate is easily denatured by cooking, storing or leaching out by large volumes of water during food preparation. Absorption appears to take place in the proximal small bowel after conversion of the numerous polyglutamates in the diet to the single, fully reduced monoglutamate derivative. Absorption may be by passive diffusion—at least it is unsaturable.

The absorption of minerals

Iron absorption [26]

This important mineral is present in excess in the Western diet, but as a rule only 10% of the dietary supply is absorbed. Worldwide the combination of dietary deficiency, multiple child-bearing and chronic intestinal parasitic infestations make iron deficiency one of the commonest diseases of the world. A major interest in iron absorption is that it appears to be controlled by body stores. An increased supply of oral iron in excess of body requirements leads to a proportional fall in absorption which, however, does not fall to zero. Ferric iron present in food is reduced to ferrous iron by gastric digestion; this is then bound to mucoproteins in the gastric juice. Reducing substances and low pH favour conversion to ferrous iron which is absorbable,

while the higher pH prevailing in the stomach immediately after food or in pancreatic juice favours the ferric state which forms insoluble hydroxide. Absorption is more complete from animal food than from vegetable food which contains more binding material. Inorganic iron is better absorbed than haem iron and is then best absorbed in the fasting state or 1 hour after food when gastric contents are usually acidified.

Absorption is by an active transport system in the brush border membrane whence it is transferred slowly across the enterocyte attached to a carrier protein (Fig. 2.23). The extreme slowness of absorption may result in a substantial proportion of absorbed iron being lost into the gut by desquamation of the mature enterocyte from the villus tips. Certainly the suggestion is that increased rate of desquamation as seen in coeliac disease is partly responsible for the iron deficiency seen in this condition. This represents one mechanism whereby excessive iron absorption may be blocked. Nevertheless, it does not explain the comparatively exact control whereby the amount of iron entering the portal blood is approximately relevant to the body's requirements, and is increased in deficiency states.

The absorption of calcium, magnesium, zinc and copper

Although calcium, magnesium, zinc and copper are all divalent ions, their absorption, transport and excretion differ in many ways. The subject is comprehensively reviewed elsewhere [1, 19, 49] but is too detailed for further consideration here.

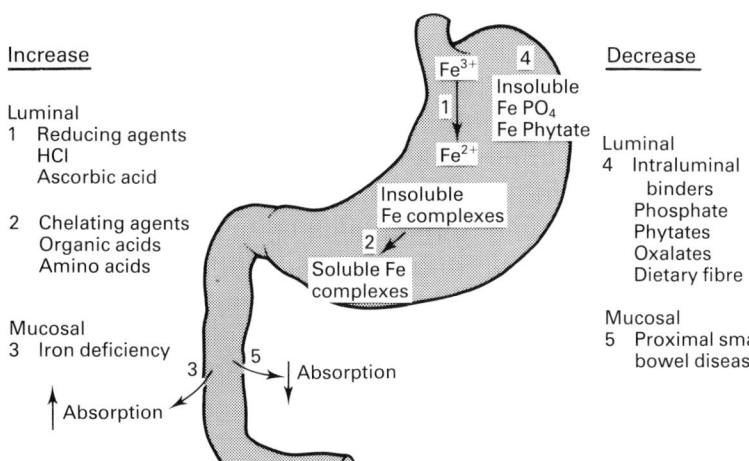

Increase

Luminal
1 Reducing agents
  HCl
  Ascorbic acid

2 Chelating agents
  Organic acids
  Amino acids

Mucosal
3 Iron deficiency

Decrease

Luminal
4 Intraluminal
  binders
  Phosphate
  Phytates
  Oxalates
  Dietary fibre

Mucosal
5 Proximal small
  bowel disease

Fig. 2.23 Factors that affect iron absorption. Non-haem iron absorption is affected both by intraluminal factors (1, 2, and 4) and by the total iron body content (3) as well as by small bowel disease (5). Haem iron absorption is altered only by those factors that affect the mucosa itself (3 and 5). From [48], with permission.

COLONIC FUNCTION

The colon is unique in absorbing water and sodium against high concentration gradients and doing so from increasingly drier luminal contents. Moreover, the motor function of the colon is specifically adapted to slowing the progress of its contents, mixing them thoroughly and pushing the semisolid contents of the left colon in an orderly fashion towards the rectum and eventual defecation [41].

Absorption and secretion

The ileum discharges approximately 1500 ml of liquid into the colon per 24 hours, containing approximately 200 mmol of chloride and 50 mmol of bicarbonate [27]. The faeces contain a mere 100 ml of water and as little as 4 mmol of sodium and perhaps 24 mmol of chloride and 20 mmol or so of potassium.

The active absorption against unprecedentedly high concentration gradients occurs mainly in the right colon [24], although it is a common observation that stool neglected in the left colon becomes progressively drier, presumably as a result of sodium and water absorption, as well as evaporation.

Sodium

As illustrated in Fig. 2.18, the mechanism of sodium and secondarily of water absorption in the colon is different from that in the small intestine. Sodium is absorbed actively by a sodium-activated membrane-bound ATPase. This is independent of hydrogen ion exchange, and it is also independent of non-ionic absorption, e.g. by glucose or amino acid, neither of which enhance sodium and water absorption by the colon. Chloride is more readily absorbed than bicarbonate by passive diffusion at high luminal concentration and by active exchange of bicarbonate below 24 mmol/l.

Potassium

Potassium may be actively secreted into the colon to a concentration of 100 mmol/l, although usually a much lower concentration is found.

Effect of mineralocorticoids. The colon is unusual in the gut in responding to the influence of mineralocorticoids and antidiuretic hor-

mone in increasing sodium and hence water absorption in conditions of hypovolaemia or mineralocorticoid administration as, for example, in corticosteroid treatment. Conversely, the diarrhoea seen in Addison's disease may represent a failure of mineralocorticoid influence on the colon.

Bidirectional fluxes. The colon mucosa like the rest of the gut exhibits bidirectional fluxes of all these substances and under normal conditions is strongly in favour of absorption overall. However, there are strict limitations on the capacity of the colon for absorption of water and an ileal input of greater than 3 litres/day usually results in liquid stool; likewise no more than approximately 450 mmol of sodium or chloride can be absorbed per day. Thus overloading and consequent salt and water loss occurs readily in the face of failure of small bowel absorption. The small intestine has a far greater capacity for adaptation to a high fluid input than the colon, and the capacity of the ileum for taking over almost the entire colonic function in the case of ileostomy is well established [27]. This is not so in the case of resection of both ileum and colon when adequate absorption of nutrients is seen, but no adaptation of excessive water and electrolyte is possible, and long-term intravenous water and electrolyte repletion is required. It is not certain whether the diarrhoea caused by VIP, serotonin and cholera toxin are the result of the action of these substances on colonic mucosa as well as the small intestine or are due simply to an excessive amount of water and electrolyte entering the colon from above.

Colonic absorptive function is summarized in Fig. 2.24.

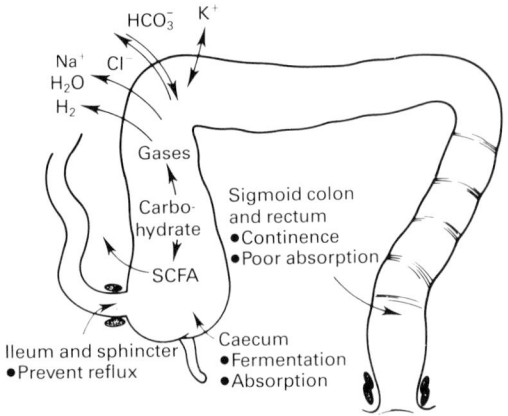

Fig. 2.24 Function of the large bowel (SCFA = short-chain fatty acids). From [28a], with permission.

Motor function

Transit through the colon has been studied using barium, the passage of radiopaque markers [24] and isotopically labelled meals, as well as by using radiotelemetering capsules. The latter are capable of recording pressures generated in the colonic lumen in a more realistic fashion than the traditional intraluminal tubes inserted via the rectum. The overall transit rate for colonic contents averages 12 hours for caecum to rectum but is very variable and much modified by activity, discomfort, and regular feeding. Progress is intermittent and achieved by two or three mass movements each day, imperceptible to the subject but striking on radiological visualization when a transfer of a large bulk of colonic contents through 30 cm can happen in a few seconds. It is this progression that is much influenced by the combination of eating and exercise.

Segmental movement

The principal movement of the colon is, however, segmentation which appears to have the function of holding up the passage of contents and mixing them thoroughly [38, 44]. This is largely achieved by a series of circular muscular contractions creating the familiar haustra of radiological imaging. The haustrations are not permanent but change as successive circular contractions occur. This is apparently an effective method for mixing the thickening contents of the colon and it is particularly prominent in the right and transverse colon. Segmentation is associated with the generation of high intraluminal pressure and the slowing of transit encourages greater contact of the bulk phase with the mucosa. Transit is slow in the right colon, tends to be faster in the transverse and left colon which is the site of mass movement, and is then slow again in the sigmoid.

ANORECTAL FUNCTION [13]

This has been the subject of numerous papers and reviews. In brief, the rectum is a short terminal portion of the colon which exhibits greater sensitivity to distension than the colon proper. It ends at the proximal part of the anal canal to which it is held at an angle of 80° (Fig. 2.25), largely as a result of the sling action of the puborectalis part of the levator ani. The anal canal is held gently shut by the

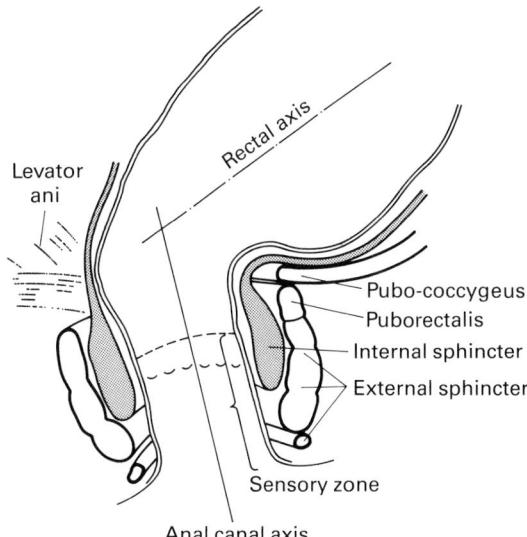

Fig. 2.25 Diagram of a longitudinal section of the anorectum showing the angulation at the pelvic floor between rectum and anal canal and the disposition of the muscles. The zone of somatic sensation in the anal canal is also indicated. From [13], with permission.

internal and external sphincters (Fig. 2.25). There is a low resting pressure within the canal (10-20 mmHg) which is unaffected by ablation of local nerves or cord section, and a ring of high pressure (50-100 mmHg) within the anal canal at the point where the internal and external sphincters overlap (see Fig. 2.25). This high pressure is abolished by ablation of local parasympathetic autonomic nerves and is largely the result of internal sphincter activity.

Sensation

The rectum is usually empty and out of mind; it imparts a transient sense of distension at volumes of 80-120 cm³, very much smaller volumes than are sensed by the remainder of the colon. The sensation of distension is continuous but resistible between 200 and 300 cm³, and irresistible above 400 cm³ at which volume explosive defecation occurs.

Anal sensation, on the other hand, is that of normal skin with the capacity to discriminate effectively between contact with gas, fluid or solid.

Anorectal reflexes

Three reflexes combine to maintain anal continence interrupted by flatus and by controlled defecation.

The accommodation reflex of the rectum permits increasing volumes of contents to be

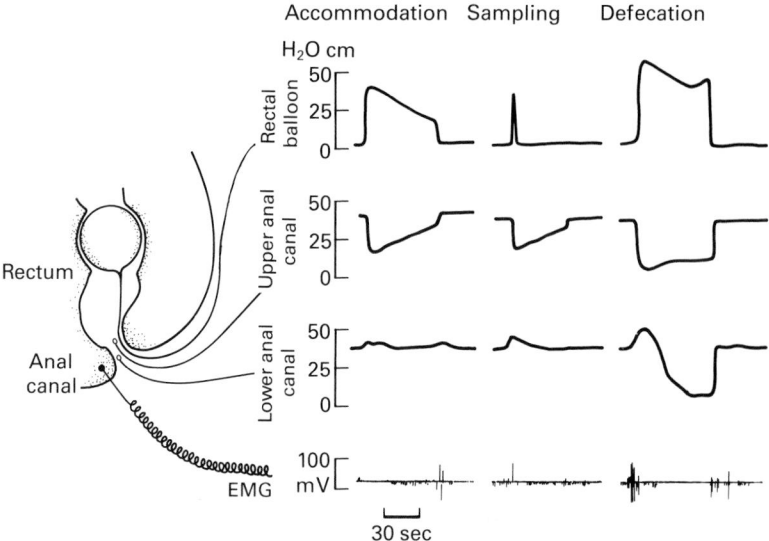

Fig. 2.26 Diagram of manometric measurements during three reflexes involving the anorectum. From [13], with permission.

tolerated unconsciously until a critical volume is reached of approximately 200–300 ml, which varies between individuals and tends to decline with age and most mucosal, muscular or neurological diseases affecting the rectum.

The sampling reflex of the anus which is illustrated in the tracing in Fig. 2.26 occurs when any transient increase in rectal contents occurs de novo. The upper anal sphincter relaxes, the rectal contents descend into the canal and are sampled by the sensitive mucosa. Gas alone is usually permitted to escape by further relaxation of the anus, liquid imparts a burning desire to defecate, which may have to be consciously countered by an extra voluntary squeeze of the anal sphincter, and solid may be expelled or pushed back into the rectum by a sudden squeeze of the sphincter. This sampling reflex, all important to continence, is preserved even with sleeve resection of the anorectal mucosa, and is probably conveyed from sensory nerve endings in the levator ani and the myenteric nerve plexus in the rectal wall. It is not abolished by cord section or pudendal nerve block.

Defecation

The defecation reflex is induced by increasing the volume of rectal contents whereby accommodation is overcome and a rapid sequence of anal relaxation, increased abdominal pressure and relaxation of the puborectalis results in the expulsion of rectal contents. Controlled defecation in the appropriately conditioned person is the result of released cortical inhibition and a voluntary increase in the intra-abdominal pressure. The assumption of the sitting, and even more so, the squatting position, helps to straighten out the anorectal angle which also facilitates the passage of the rectal bolus through the anus.

It follows that anorectal function is impaired by abnormalities in the consistency of the colonic contents, the musculature of the rectum and the pelvic floor, the sensory or motor innervation or by anatomical abnormalities of the anus or rectum.

DIARRHOEA

This is the frequent passage of loose stools, and, by definition, more than three per day. The clinician would separate patients with diarrhoea and normal stool weight of 200 g/day from the rest. The former group represent poorly coordinated motor function and seldom prove to have organic disease of severity unless there is clear evidence of rectal mucosal inflammation. The passage of frequent loose stools of increased weight may represent failure of fluid and electrolyte absorption, steatorrhoea or spontaneous purgation with unabsorbed bile salts, hydroxy fatty acids or, as in the widely prevalent microbiological infestation, infective diarrhoea. Alternatively, diarrhoea may be the result of resection, in which case it is particularly common in ileal and right-sided colonic resection. The diarrhoea associated with inflammatory bowel disease probably represents a contribution from several of these factors plus disorderly motor function.

There is no simple guide to the diagnosis of diarrhoea and in many cases the answer is not clear even after the most intensive investigation. In patients who are convinced of an allergic basis to their diarrhoea careful exclusion studies may show, initially, a response to certain dietary elements, but subsequent re-challenge with the patient unaware of the introduction of the offending item has often cast doubt on the value of the diet. Finally, the possibility of laxative abuse must ever be borne in mind even in the most plausible patient.

GASTROINTESTINAL BACTERIA [12]

Shortly after birth the gastrointestinal tract of mammals becomes rapidly colonized by a complex mixture of bacteria and possibly of viruses. While the germ-free state is no bar to good health, and indeed confers an increase in the size of the villi of the small intestine, it is a difficult state to maintain and confers no benefit except under highly unusual circumstances such as severe immune deficiency. The flora of the gastrointestinal contents is derived from ingested food [32]. Food is seldom completely sterile, and is incompletely sterilized by the gastric secretion. Thus, after eating, the upper small intestinal contents are transiently colonized by over 100 bacterial species. However, with increasing gastric secretion the gastric and jejunal contents rapidly become sterile in the postprandial hours. It is in the lower small intestine that the ingested bacteria proliferate and even more so when this flora moves on into the colon with its slow-moving contents. A high proportion of faecal dry weight is bacterial in origin and, moreover, a large proportion of the increased stool weight consequent upon increased fibre intake is due to increased bacterial proliferation in the colon.

Role of bacteria

It is not clear whether the presence of this mass of bacteria represents a well-adjusted symbiosis in the face of inevitable contamination or whether biological advantage is conferred. There is some evidence to suggest that a stable mixed flora in the lumen and subsequently attached to the mucus of the gastrointestinal tract confers additional protection against infection by *Salmonella, Cholera* and *Candida albicans.*

The suggestion has been made that the presence of bacteria in the gut primes immunological surveillance and could thus be considered advantageous. However, the presence of a normal flora may backfire in hypovolaemic shock, intestinal perforation, and inflammatory bowel disease. Moreover, in experimental animals the germ-free state appears to confer added protection against certain viral infections including hepatitis B.

GASTROINTESTINAL GAS [31]

The gastrointestinal tract contains, fasting or fed, approximately 200 ml of gas even in subjects complaining of excessive wind. There is, however, a wide difference between normal subjects in the rate of transfer of gas through the gut from 200 to 2000 ml day, with a mean of 600 ml/day. The mean number of passages of flatus is 15 per day with an extrapolated mean volume of 40 ml per emission. Many foods have been blamed for increasing the volume of intestinal gas but alone amongst them the bean has been carefully studied with the conclusion, unsurprising to cinema enthusiasts, that a diet containing 50% of its calories as pork and beans results in an increase of hourly basal flatus volume from 15 to 150 ml.

The composition of intestinal gas is a highly variable mixture of nitrogen, carbon dioxide, hydrogen, oxygen and methane.

Origins of gas

Swallowed air is the major contributor to gas in the upper gut, but the composition is modified partly by the eructation of the major part of the swallowed air and then by diffusion of gas into and out of the gut through the intestinal mucosa and, finally, by the products of bacterial decomposition of food residues in the colon.

Nitrogen varies from 90% to 10% of the intestinal gas but is usually the predominant component. Oxygen may vary from 5% to 50% but is usually in very low concentration. Carbon dioxide, resulting from the reaction of gastric acid and pancreatic bicarbonate, is high in the duodenum but is rapidly absorbed unless rates of transit are high. The major component of hydrogen and methane is from bacterial activity in the colon.

The importance of intestinal gas in symptomatology is great but very few scientific studies have been made in this enigmatic field.

The prime apologist for scientific flatology is Levitt whose writings on the subject combine scientific exactitude with the best English in the gastrointestinal literature [31].

REFERENCES

1 Alcock N, MacIntyre I: Interrelation of calcium and magnesium absorption. Clin Sci 1962; 22:185-93.

2 Baron JH: Studies of basal and peak acid output with an augmented histamine test. Gut 1963; 4:136-44.

3 Bouchier IAD, Allan RN, Hodgson HJF, Keighley MRB, eds: Textbook of gastroenterology. London: Baillière Tindall, 1984.

4 Brunner H, Northfield TC, Hofmann AF et al: Gastric emptying and secretion of bile acids, cholesterol, and pancreatic enzymes during digestion. Duodenal perfusion studies in healthy subjects. Mayo Clin Proc 1974; 49:851-60.

5 Christensen J: The controls of oesophageal movement. Clin Gastroenterol 1976; 5(1):15-28.

6 Code CF, Schlegel JR: The gastrointestinal interdigestive housekeeper: motor correlates of the interdigestive myoelectric complex of the dog. In: Daniel EE et al, eds. Proceedings of the Fourth International Symposium on Gastrointestinal Motility. Vancouver: Mitchell Press, 1973:631-4.

7 Christensen J: The controls of gastrointestinal movements: some old and new views. N Engl J Med 1971; 285:85.

8 Craft IL, Geddes D, Hyde CW et al: Absorption and malabsorption of glycine and glycine peptides in man. Gut 1968; 9:425-37.

9 Crane CW: Some aspects of protein absorption and malabsorption. In: Girdwood RH, Smith AN, eds. Malabsorption. Edinburgh: Edinburgh University Press, 1969:33.

10 Curr Opinion Gastroenterol 1985; I (1-6).

11 Davis GR, Santa Ana CA, Morawski SG, Fordtran JS: Permeability characteristics of human jejunum, ileum, proximal colon and distal colon. Results of potential difference measurements and unidirectional fluxes. Gastroenterology 1982; 83:844-50.

12 Drasan BS, Shiner M, McLeod GM: Studies on the intestinal flora. I. The bacterial flora of the gastrointestinal tract in healthy and achlorhydric persons. Gastroenterology 1969; 56:71-9.

13 Duthie ML, Wormsley KG, eds: Scientific basis of gastroenterology. Edinburgh: Churchill Livingstone.

14 Edwards DAW: The anti-reflux mechanism, its disorders and their consequences. Clin Gastroenterol 1982; 11(3): 479-96.

15 Fordtran JS: Stimulation of active and passive absorption by sugars in the human jejunum. J Clin Invest 1975; 55:728-37.

16 Gangl A, Ockner RK: Intestinal metabolism of lipids and lipoproteins. Gastroenterology 1975; 68:167-86.

17 Go VLW, DiMagno EP: Assessment of exocrine pancreatic function by duodenal intubation. Clin Gastroenterol 1984; 13:701-15.

18 Go VLW, Hofmann AF, Summerskill WHJ: Simultaneous measurements of total pancreatic, biliary, and gastric outputs in man using a perfusion technique. Gastroenterology 1970; 58:321-8.

19 Golden MH, Golden BE: Trace elements. Potential importance in human nutrition with particular reference to zinc and vanadium. Br Med Bull 1981; 37: 31-6.

20 Gray GM, Cooper HL: Protein digestion and absorption. Gastroenterology 1971; 61:535-44.

21 Hallback DA, Hulten L, Jodal M et al: Evidence for the existence of a countercurrent exchanger in the small intestine of man. Gastroenterology 1978; 74:683-90.

22 Heading RC, Tothill P, McLoughlin GP, Shearman DJC: Gastroenterology 1976; 71:45.

23 Hellier MD, Holdsworth CD, Perrett D: Dibasic amino acid absorption in man. Gastroenterology 1973; 65:613-8.

24 Hinton JM, Lennard-Jones JE, Young AC: A new method for studying gut transit times using radio opaque markers. Gut 1969; 10:842-7.

25 Hofmann AF, Borgstrom B: The intraluminal phase of fat digestion in man: the lipid content of the micellar and oil phase of intestinal content obtained during fat digestion and absorption. J Clin Invest 1964; 43: 247-57.

26 Jacobs A, Worwood M: Iron metabolism, iron deficiency and overload. In: Hardisty RM, Weatherall DJ, eds. Blood and its disorders, 2nd ed. Oxford: Blackwell Scientific Publications, 1982:149-97.

27 Kanaghinus T, Lubran M, Coghill NF: The composition of ileostomy fluid. Gut 1963; 4:322-38.

28 Keane FD, Dozois RR, Go VLW, DiMagno EP: Interdigestive canine pancreatic juice composition and pancreatic reflux and pancreatic sphincter anatomy. Dig Dis Sci 1981; 26:577-84.

28a Kerlin P, Phillips SF: Absorption of fluids and electrolytes from the colon with reference to inflammatory bowel disease. In: Allan R, Keighley M, Hawkins C, Alexander-Williams J, eds. Inflammatory bowel diseases. Churchill Livingstone.

29 Krag E, Phillips SF: Active and passive bile acid absorption in man. Perfusion studies of the ileum and jejunum. J Clin Invest 1974; 53:1686-94.

30 Krejs GJ, Fordtran JS: Physiology and pathophysiology of ion and water movement in the human intestine. In: Sleisenger MH, Fordtran JS, eds. Gastrointestinal disease. Philadelphia: WB Saunders, 1978:297-335.

31 Levitt MD: Volume and compositions of human intestinal gas determined by means of an intestinal washout technique. N Engl J Med 1971; 284:1394.

32 Mackowiak PA: The normal bacterial flora. N Engl J Med 1982; 307: 83-93.

33 Mallinson CN: The gastric emptying of starch and glucose in patients with pancreatic insufficiency. Gut 1968; 9:737.

34 Malagelada JR, Longstreth GF, Summerskill WHJ, Go VLW: Measurement of gastric functions during digestion of ordinary solid meals in man. Gastroenterology 1976; 70: 203-10.

35 Matthews DM, Adibi SA: Peptide absorption. Gastroenterology 1976; 71: 151-61.

36 Meyer GW, Castell DO: Physiology of the oesophagus. Clin Gastroenterol 1982; 11(3): 439-51.

37 Milne MD, Asatoor AM, Edwards KDG, Loughridge LW: The intestinal absorption defect in cystinuria. Gut 1961; 2:323-37.

38 Misiewicz JJ: Colonic motility. Gut 1975; 16:311-4.

39 Moromtz M, Cook DJ, Collins PJ et al: The application of techniques using radionuclides to the study of gastric emptying. Surg Gynecol Obstet 1982; 155:737-44.

40 Parsons DS, Wingate DL: The effect of osmotic gradients on fluid transfer across rat intestine in vitro. Biochim Biophys Acta 1961; 46:170-83.

41 Read NW: The relationship between intestinal motility and intestinal transport. Clin Res Rev 1981; 1 (suppl 1): 73-81.

42 Rees WDW, Turnberg LA: Mechanisms of gastric mucosal protection: a role for the mucus–bicarbonate barrier. Clin Sci 1982; 62:343-8.

43 Richardson CT, Walsh JH, Cooper KA et al: Studies on the role of cephalic-vagal stimulation in the acid secretory response to eating in normal human subjects. J Clin Invest 1977; 60:345-441.

44 Ritchie JA: Colonic motor activity and bowel function. 1. Normal movement of contents. Gut 1968; 9:442-56.

45 Sarles H, Dani R, Preselin G, Souville C, Figarella C: Cephalic phase of pancreatic secretion in man. Gut 1968; 9:214-21.

46 Silk DBA, Dawson AM: Intestinal absorption of carbohydrate and protein in man. Int Rev Physiol 1979; 19:151-204.

47 Sladen GE: Methods of studying intestinal absorption. In: McColl I, Sladen GE, eds. Methods of studying intestinal absorption in man. London: Academic Press, 1975:1-50.

48 Sleisinger MH, Fordtran JS, eds. Gastrointestinal disease. Philadelphia: WB Saunders, 1983.

49 Sternlieb I: Gastrointestinal copper absorption in man. Gastroenterology 1967; 52:1038-41.

50 Vantrappen GR, Peeters TK, Janssens J: The secretory component of the interdigestive migrating motor complex in man. Scand J Gastroenter 1979; 14:663-7.

51 Wormsley KG: Pancreatic function tests. Clin Gastroenterol 1972; 1:27-42.

Chapter 3
Circulation and Differentiation of Lymphocytes in Gut-associated Lymphoid Tissue and Mammary Glands

Julia M. Phillips-Quagliata and Michael E. Lamm

Introduction

All mucosae are potentially at risk of infection by viruses or invasion by the microorganisms which thrive on their moist surfaces, but the intestinal and respiratory tracts are especially vulnerable because they have large surface areas and actively sample the environment. The problem of protecting these and distant mucosae has been solved during the evolution of contemporary mammals by the development of a complex mucosal immune system. This interdigitates with the systemic immune system but has features peculiar to its function in relation to mucosal sites. The mucosa-associated lymphoid tissue (MALT), especially the gut-associated lymphoid tissue (GALT), is so constructed that it can, as it were, spot-check the secretions bathing the mucosa, mount an immune response against antigens presented in sufficient concentration, and then, via the bloodstream, deliver to both local and distant mucosae effector cells and antibodies capable of warding off a potentially invasive organism. In the special case of the GALT, the ability to develop local responses has evidently been coupled with the ability to suppress induction of systemic responses to the same antigen. This presumably reflects the adaptive advantage of preventing, as far as possible, systemic immunization against any food antigens which reach the blood circulation.

Four key features of the mucosal immune system distinguish it from the systemic immune system:

1 It has the ability to survey antigens in the fluids *outside* the body, i.e. in the intestinal or bronchial secretions. Only those antigens which tend to adhere to epithelia, thus displaying a property essential to an invasive microorganism, are likely to be efficiently

taken up into the mucosal immune system. In the systemic immune system, by contrast, all foreign macromolecules reaching the body fluids stand a good chance of being filtered out by either the spleen or regional lymph nodes, and of initiating an immune response.

2 Its effector cells are distributed throughout the lamina propria of the mucosae at sites distant from the organized lymphoid structures in which the proliferation and maturation of their precursors took place. Dissemination of effector cells during the response to infection at one mucosal site has the potential to offer antigen-specific protection to hitherto uninfected and even distant mucosae. This could serve to reduce the impact of transmission of an infectious agent from one mucosa in the body to another.

3 Its major immunoglobulin class is the secretory form of IgA (SIgA), in contrast to the systemic immune system in which IgG predominates. SIgA is particularly well adapted to functioning in the intestinal fluids because of its relative resistance to proteolytic digestion.

4 Its effector cells and epithelium interact in producing effector molecules which can be delivered to the external surface rather than to the circulatory system. The prime example of this interaction is seen in the production of SIgA by the combined efforts of plasma cells and epithelial cells (see Chapter 9). A second example of cooperation between mucosal effector cells and mucosal epithelial cells is seen in the case of augmented mucus secretion by goblet cells in response to an immune reaction elicited by worm infestation (see Chapter 10).

ANATOMY OF THE MUCOSAL IMMUNE SYSTEM

The major elements of the mucosal immune system are: (a) the lymphoid nodules of the GALT and bronchus-associated lymphoid tissue (BALT) in which commitment to IgA production and/or eventually to seeking mucosa apparently takes place [6, 7, 11, 12, 29, 30, 62, 64, 65]; (b) the regional lymph nodes in which IgA-committed and/or mucosa-committed lymphocytes proliferate and mature to a blast stage at which they are capable of migrating into lamina propria [21, 43]; (c) the efferent lymphatics, thoracic duct and blood circulation by which the blasts are delivered to the lamina propria [20, 21, 24, 56]; and (d) the lamina propria itself.

The central organs of the mucosal immune system are lymphoid follicles scattered singly or in clusters in the lamina propria of the in-

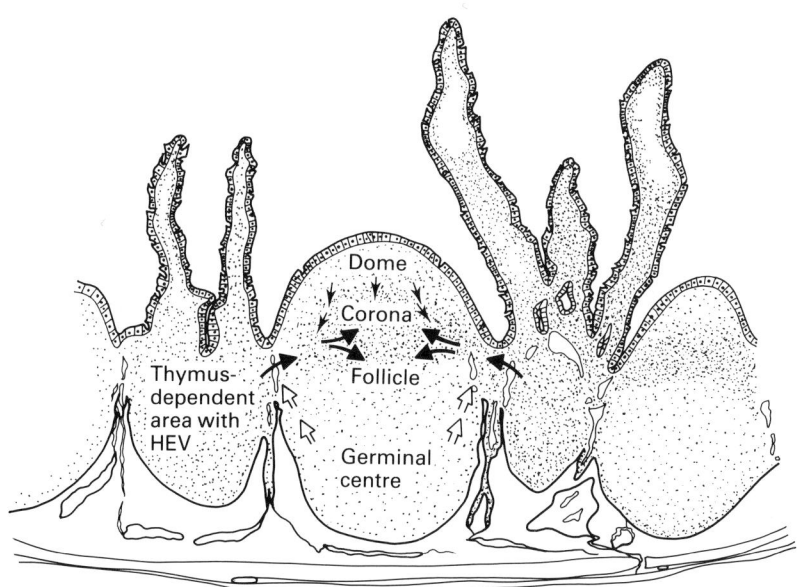

Fig. 3.1 Drawing of a section of a Peyer's patch (simplified from a photomicrograph). Small black arrows indicate presumed direction of flow of fluid and antigen via the epithelium overlying the dome towards the lymphatic plexus surrounding the lymphoid nodule; large black arrows indicate apparent migration pathways of lymphocytes from the HEV, located in the thymus-dependent areas, through the dome and corona of the nodule; open arrows indicate probable direction of movement of mitotic cells away from the germinal centre, where DNA synthesis occurs, towards the lymphatic plexus.

testine and bronchial tree. Discrete lymphoid nodules and organs of the mucosal immune system, including the tonsils, adenoids, Peyer's patches and appendix, are made up of large clusters of such follicles (Fig. 3.1). The follicle-associated epithelium is generally modified compared to the regional glandular epithelium, lacking a glycocalyx, having fewer goblet cells and having large numbers of specialized epithelial cells with short, irregular microvilli (see Chapters 1 and 4). These last cells have a marked capacity to transport macromolecules from the lumen of the mucosal organ and to release them into the interstitial fluids bathing the macrophages and lymphocytes in the loose connective tissue of the 'dome' immediately beneath the epithelium.

Antigen access and the lymphatic system

Mucosal lymphoid follicles differ from the lymphoid follicles of lymph nodes in that they have no organized afferent lymphatic system. The fluid that percolates down through the domes towards the follicles presumably subserves the function of afferent lymph. During its passage the macromolecular material originally derived from the lumen of the mucosal organ is taken up by macrophages in the domes and lymphoid follicles. Some of it is presumably processed and presented to lymphocytes by antigen-presenting cells known to be present, at least in the best-studied of the mucosal lymphoid organs—the Peyer's patches [34, 66]. Precisely where antigen presentation takes place is unknown. The follicular fluid eventually collects in a plexus of lymphatics surrounding each follicle and from there it passes into a network of lymphatics lying in the wall of the mucosal organ. Here it is mixed with the lymph from the mucosa surrounding the follicle or group of follicles. The mixed lymph passes into the afferent lymphatics of a regional lymph node: in the case of the small intestine, the mesenteric lymph nodes and in the case of the lungs and bronchi, the mediastinal (bronchial) lymph nodes.

The absence of an afferent lymphatic system capable of conducting fluids, antigens and lymphoid cells laterally from the surrounding mucosa to mucosal lymphoid follicles is, in a sense, surprising. A priori, one might expect that antigen pinocytosed by columnar absorptive cells or microorganisms entering the lamina propria through the epithelium would be passed to the nearest Peyer's patch where a local immune response could be initiated. A consideration of the microanatomy of the intestinal lymphatic system suggests, however, that except in the case of villi immediately overlying the thymus-dependent areas of the patch this generally does not occur. Any antigen which enters the body through intestinal villi is likely to pass by way of lymphatics directly to mesenteric lymph nodes where it may induce a systemic immune response or, if it enters the capillaries, by way of the portal system to the liver, where it may become tolerogenic (see Chapters 11 and 14).

Immunization and the mucosal immune system

Neither of these routes of antigen access is appropriate for immunization of the mucosal immune system. Efficient immunization, resulting in eventual delivery of antibody-forming cells to the lamina propria, *requires* that at some stage antigen be presented through the agency of the mucosal lymphoid follicles. For example, experiments involving instillation of antigen into isolated lengths of small intestine (Thiry–Vella loops) with or without Peyer's patches have shown that these lymphoid aggregates are essential for the appearance of specific antibody-forming cells at both local and distant mucosal sites [7, 27, 59]. Whether this is because the antigens used in the experiments efficiently penetrate the body from the lumen of the small intestine only via the specialized follicle-associated epithelial cells of the Peyer's patch, or because the Peyer's patch is the only site at which T and B precursor cells capable of eventual mucosal migration can be immunized, is not clear. Probably both the antigen-sampling ability of Peyer's patch epithelial cells and the unique populations of lymphoid cells contained in Peyer's patches are crucial.

Optimal priming. The best method thus far described for immunizing the mucosal immune system to provide an IgA antibody response in the small intestine is first to prime with antigen via the intraperitoneal route and then to boost with antigen via the intraduodenal route [56], although this may not apply to all antigens. The advantages of the intraperitoneal priming may be: (a) to permit B and T cell activation and memory cell generation to occur without interference from suppressors, which form a major obstacle to direct priming via the enteric route (see Chapter 14); the majority of the antigen-reactive cells that populate the Peyer's patches will then be memory cells that can respond to the intra-duodenal antigenic challenge before interfering suppressor cells are induced; (b) to permit expansion within the lymph nodes draining the peritoneal cavity, primarily the mediastinal lymph nodes, of a population of antigen-specific cells with the capacity both to traffic through MALT, including the Peyer's patches, and subsequently, at the later plas-mablast stage, to extravasate from blood into the lamina propria.

LYMPHOCYTE MATURATION IN THE MUCOSAL IMMUNE SYSTEM

Both GALT and BALT are greatly enriched relative to spleen and peripheral lymph nodes in cells with the potential to populate the lamina propria at mucosal sites with IgA plasma cells [11, 12, 64, 65]. There are, however, relatively few IgA-bearing or -containing cells in nodules such as Peyer's patches [2, 16, 42], except in the germinal centres [5]. It generally takes about a week from the time of cell transfer for IgA-secreting cells to become evident in the intestine of irradiated recipients of Peyer's patch or BALT cells [11, 12, 64, 65]. Presumably these plasma cells are the progeny of B cells initially stimulated by environmental antigens in the BALT or GALT of the donor animals. Whether they are actually derived from the germinal centre cells is not known.

Cell transfer studies

In repopulation studies in irradiated rabbits, it has been shown that the majority of Peyer's patch precursors of donor IgA plasma cells found in the spleen seven days after transfer are contained in a population that is μ-chain negative [30] and that includes α-chain-bearing cells [29]. In repopulation studies in irradiated mice [70], by contrast, resting IgM-IgD double-bearing cells were shown to be the major precursors of the IgA plasma cells appearing in the lamina propria 12 days after intravenous transfer of normal or lymphoblast-depleted populations from Peyer's patches. These populations apparently have a greater capacity to expand and fill the lamina propria than Peyer's patch IgA-bearing cells, which are the more immediate precursors of mouse lamina propria IgA plasma cells [62, 70].

Migration of Peyer's patch cells

When radiolabelled mouse Peyer's patch cells are transferred intravenously into syngeneic recipients, very few of them are found in the lamina propria of the small intestine 24 hours later [62]. Many of the cells are too immature or too large and are lost in the liver and lungs after intravenous transfer; the surviving cells presumably require time to differentiate and mature before they can settle in the lamina propria. Some of them undoubtedly do so in the spleen [69]; others accumulate and mature in the mesenteric lymph nodes to which they are carried in intestinal lymph after traversing the walls of the blood vessels in the small intestine [62]. Whether they leave the blood in the Peyer's patches or in the lamina propria is not clear. Over 90% of the IgA-containing radiolabelled blasts that can be found in sections of the small intestine, cut through Peyer's patches 30 minutes after intravenous injection of Peyer's patch cells, appear in the Peyer's patch portion of the section [54]. This suggests that Peyer's patch blasts that are capable of migrating into MALT tend to do so via the high endothelial venules (HEV) of the patch rather than through the walls of blood vessels in the lamina propria (Fig. 3.1).

Lamina propria cells

There is, however, sufficient lamina propria down the length of the intestine relative to the mass of Peyer's patch tissue to allow for the possibility that many of the Peyer's patch-derived blasts that arrive in the mesenteric lymph nodes do so by traversing vessels in the lamina propria at large. The fact that lamina propria-seeking cells can be shown to be present in the initial labelled Peyer's patch population suggests that some of the patch cells are not only precommitted to eventually seeking lamina propria but are actually able to do so before leaving the patch. One problem with this interpretation, however, is that Peyer's patch cell populations could be contaminated with lamina propria-derived cells. Radiolabelled lamina propria cells can themselves return to lamina propria after intravenous injection [71]. Whether this merely illustrates their retention of the ability to recognize lamina propria after they have settled there or whether there is a population of cells that recirculates through lamina propria is not clear.

Role of mesenteric lymph nodes

The mesenteric lymph node is the site at which expansion and maturation of GALT-derived, lamina propria-seeking lymphocyte populations normally take place. The ability to migrate directly from the blood circulation to the lamina propria of the gut seems to be a property expressed largely or only by DNA-synthesizing cells which are concentrated in mesenteric lymph nodes [21, 40, 43] and which, maturing under physiological conditions, would normally leave the mesenteric lymph nodes in their efferent lymph and pass via the thoracic duct into the bloodstream [20, 24, 56]. The majority of the lamina propria-seeking cells bear surface IgA [21, 43, 44], lack complement receptors [43] and, as they come to maturity, contain increasing concentrations of intracytoplasmic IgA [43, 76]. There are also, however, populations of lamina propria-seeking GALT-derived T lymphoblasts [21, 22, 53, 60, 67] and IgG-committed B lymphoblasts [40] which follow the same route.

The extent to which localization of circulating GALT-derived lymphoblasts occurs in sites such as the intestine is influenced by regional blood flow [49], but it is not influenced initially by the presence of specific antigen locally [21, 23, 26, 53]. When antigen is absent, however, specific antibody-containing cells that initially become localized tend to disappear from intestinal lamina propria [26]. When antigen is present, antibody-containing cells not only remain but apparently proliferate within the lamina propria [26, 39].

THE IgA CELL CYCLE AND THE COMMON MUCOSAL IMMUNE SYSTEM

The circular route followed by GALT-derived IgA-committed B lymphocytes in the course of their normal maturation and migration back to the lamina propria of the small intestine has been called the IgA cell cycle [37]. However, there are considerable similarities between GALT and BALT and these two more central lymphoid organs contain cells capable of populating the lamina propria of irradiated animals at either site with IgA plasma cells [64, 65]. This observation has led to the suggestion that there might be a common mucosal immune system [40], an idea that finds support in the demonstration that lymphocytes from mesenteric lymph nodes are capable of selective lodging in lactating mammary glands [40, 63], uterine cervix [40], salivary and lacrimal glands [46] as well as intestinal [21, 40, 43] and bronchial lamina propria and lungs [40]. There is, however, some specificity in localization, for cells from bronchial lymph nodes localize poorly in the small intestine, tending, instead, to migrate to the lungs [40], while cells from mesenteric lymph nodes localize in the small intestine to a greater extent than in the lungs. Furthermore, specific antibody-containing cells that appear in thoracic duct lymph after localized immunization of rat duodenum or colon, when transferred to normal recipients lodge preferentially in the jejunum if they were induced by intraduodenal immunization and in the colon if induced by intracolonic immunization [55]. This suggests a remarkable regional specificity in localization even within the gastrointestinal tract.

REGULATION OF MIGRATION AND DIFFERENTIATION IN THE MUCOSAL IMMUNE SYSTEM

Three special properties of mucosal B lymphocyte populations distinguish them from B cells functioning in the systemic immune system. The first is their ability, during their resting stages, to traffic through mucosal lymphoid follicles where appropriate antigenic stimulation can take place. The second is their ability on reaching the plasmablast stage to migrate to lamina propria and become secretory cells at that site. The third is their tendency to become committed to IgA production. Mucosal T cells apparently share with mucosal B cells the ability to traffic through mucosal lymphoid follicles and, on reaching effector cell stages, to populate the lamina propria. They do not, of course, become committed to IgA production. Presumably all three properties are independently controlled. Their tendency to be expressed together in mucosal B lymphocyte populations may be the result of either selective or inductive influences.

High endothelial venules (HEV)

For traffic through mucosal lymphoid follicles to occur, lymphocytes must leave the blood circulation by migrating through HEV in the local thymus-dependent areas. Small recirculating lymphocytes discriminate between HEV in Peyer's patches and peripheral lymph nodes by means of distinct surface glycoproteins which promote binding of the lymphocytes to HEV at one or the other site [4, 8, 9, 17]. Some lymphomas and, in all probability, their normal lymphocyte counterparts, bind to only one kind of HEV; others can evidently bind to either, so must bear both moieties [4]. Cells contained within Peyer's patches predominantly bear Peyer's patch HEV-binding moieties [4], but cells bearing these moieties can be found in all lymphoid organs, especially among B lymphocyte populations [68]. On the whole, T cells bind preferentially to and migrate through HEV of peripheral lymph nodes rather than Peyer's patches, but some Lyt $2,3^-$ T cells in all lymphoid organs can migrate into Peyer's patches and do so much more efficiently than Lyt $2,3^+$ T cells [36]. Taken together, these observations are consistent with the idea that Peyer's patches contain mixed populations of lymphocytes, many of which may be uniquely committed to life in MALT, but others of which can recirculate

through all lymphoid tissues. This could be predicted, since it has been known for years that a single shielded Peyer's patch can repopulate all the lymphoid tissues of an irradiated animal [28].

Migration to lamina propria

The mechanism of effector cell migration into lamina propria, which lacks HEV, is not understood. It could involve endothelial cell-surface interaction molecules, such as are involved in migration through HEV, or might involve responses to local chemotactic factors. Evidently the expression of appropriate receptors or factors by lamina propria is constitutive in the small intestine but under hormonal control in the mammary gland [74] and in the female genital system [41]. The expression of appropriate molecules by B lymphocytes appears to be cell-cycle dependent, being principally observed in blasts.

Two hypotheses accounting for the commit-

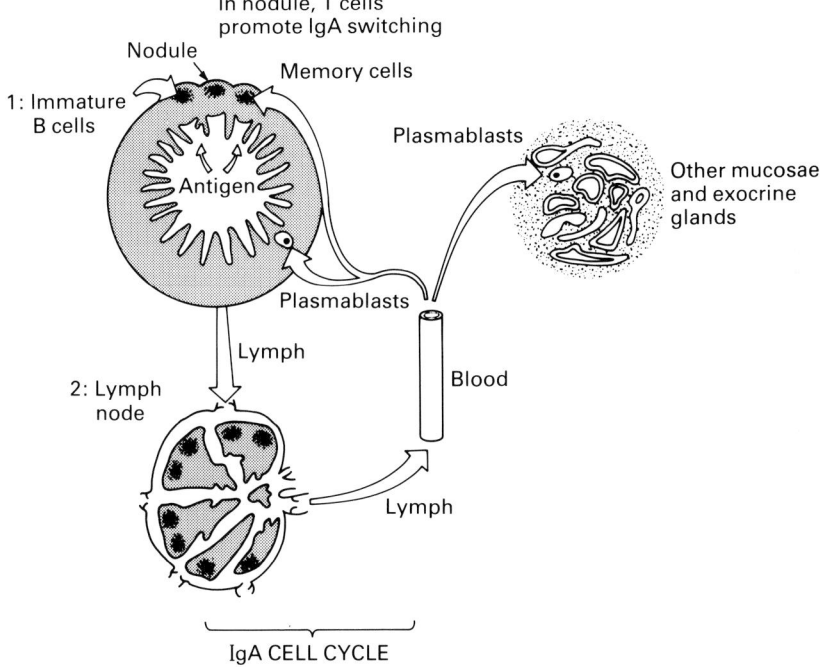

Fig. 3.2 Hypothetical *instructive* scheme for the expansion and maturation of lamina propria-seeking plasmablasts under the influence of inductive signals supplied primarily by MALT nodules. According to both this and the selective scheme shown in Fig. 3.3, memory cells would recirculate through all lymphoid tissues for which they have appropriate HEV-binding moieties. They would, however, be most likely to re-encounter their specific antigen in the MALT nodules and draining lymph nodes nearest to the site of their original stimulation. 1: Immature B cells with MALT nodule HEV-binding moieties extravasate in nodule. Antigen priming and initial clonal expansion take place here. IgA 'switch' T cells promote commitment to IgA. Other signals induce eventual development of lamina propria-seeking capacity by plasmablasts. 2: Further differentiation takes place in draining mesenteric or mediastinal lymph node. Mature cells leave in lymph; plasmablasts migrate to lamina propria; memory cells recirculate.

ment of B lymphocytes in mucosal lymphoid nodules to seeking lamina propria and to producing IgA have been considered [54]. Neither of these hypotheses has yet been excluded and elements of both may be true.

The first hypothesis (Fig. 3.2) suggests that inductive signals are delivered to the lymphocytes in mucosal lymphoid nodules. The lymphocytes preferentially switch to IgA, perhaps under the influence of a unique population of T cells such as has recently been described [31, 32]. Under the influence of another, unknown, inductive signal they become capable, on reaching the effector cell stage, of migrating through or being retained in lamina propria. If this hypothesis is true, then to account for jejunal versus colonic homing specificity [55] the lamina propria specificity of the lymphocytes must relate in some unknown way to their MALT HEV-binding specificity.

The second hypothesis (Fig. 3.3) suggests that selective influences are at work. Lymphoblasts which already express, as a result of random genetic events, elements necessary for seeking lamina propria pass from blood through lamina propria and thence, via afferent lymphatics, into draining lymph nodes. Here they are expanded by exposure to antigen. The expanded populations leave in the efferent lymph and reach the blood circulation. Cells which, on a stochastic basis, express appropriate mucosal HEV-binding elements are then selected out of the expanded populations as they pass in the blood through mucosal lymphoid nodules. Re-exposure in the nodules to the same antigens results in further expansion of the antigen-reactive pool and so the population in MALT becomes skewed in favour of having the ability to seek the lamina propria at the lymphoblast stage and to recirculate through mucosal lymphoid nodules at the resting memory cell stage. Expansion of jejunum-seeking versus colon-seeking populations by local immunization is well explained by this hypothesis.

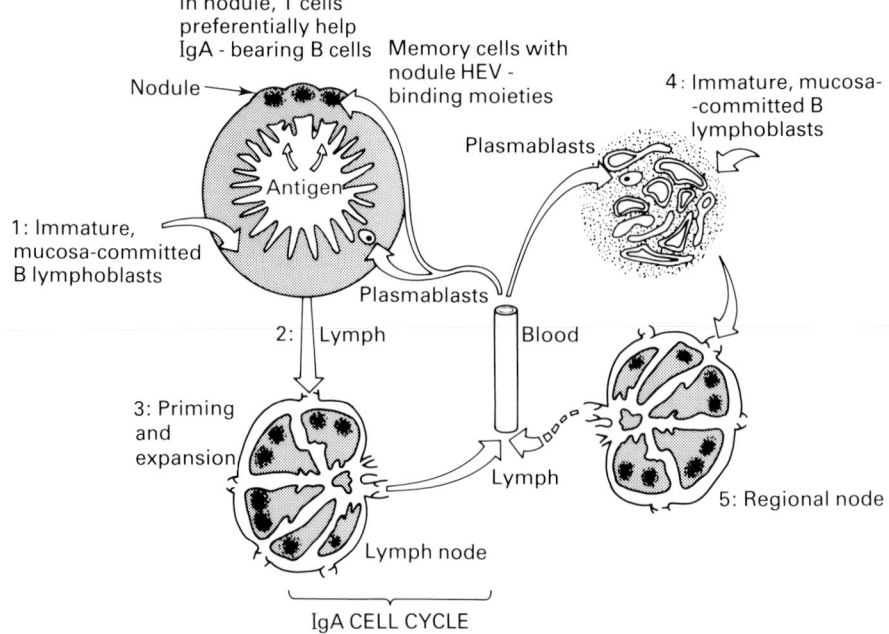

Fig. 3.3 Hypothetical scheme for the expansion and maturation of lamina propria-seeking plasmablasts under the influence of *selective* forces operating first in the lymph nodes draining mucosal sites and subsequently in the MALT nodules. (See also Fig. 3.2.) 1: Immature, mucosa-committed B lymphoblasts extravasate from blood and pass into lymph within lamina propria of GALT or BALT. 2: They rapidly enter draining mesenteric or mediastinal lymph nodes along with antigen and MALT nodule-derived blasts and small recirculating lymphocytes. 3: Priming and initial expansion of mucosa-committed clones takes place in lymph node. Secondary expansion of memory cells occurs both here and in MALT nodule where T cells preferentially help IgA-bearing cells. 4: Immature, mucosa-commited B lymphoblasts can also extravasate in other mucosae and exocrine glands. 5: Without strong antigenic stimulation, expansion of the population is minimal in regional nodes; no special help for IgA is available.

Commitment to IgA

Commitment to IgA of the majority of the B cells in MALT could also be a selective process. It could result from expansion and differentiation of B cells that spontaneously become committed to IgA in the presence of both T helper cells capable of recognizing surface IgA [15, 33, 35] and specialized antigen-presenting cells [66]. There is increasing evidence that T cells uniquely capable of helping IgA responses do exist [15, 31–33, 35] and that their distribution is skewed in favour of GALT [1, 14]. What controls this segregation pattern is unknown. It is clear that shortly after antigen priming, antigen-specific T helper cells capable of helping IgA production are as plentiful in peripheral lymph nodes as in Peyer's patches [1]. It is possible that selection in GALT by soluble IgA itself, interacting with T cells randomly expressing Fcα receptors, results in gradual accumulation of T cells capable of delivering increased help to IgA-bearing B cells.

THE MAMMARY GLAND IN THE CONTEXT OF MUCOSAL IMMUNITY

The immune components of the mammary gland and its secretory products—colostrum and milk—provide passive protection to the suckling offspring and also defend against infections within the mammary gland itself. A number of constituents may play a role but the best understood are the milk immunoglobulins. This section will emphasize what is known about the kinds of immunoglobulins in human colostrum and milk, their specificity as antibodies and their cellular and humoral origins. Studies in animals that are pertinent to the situation in humans will be mentioned.

Mammals vary in how passive immunity is transferred from mother to offspring. In humans, and some other species, there is an important transport of maternal IgG to the fetus via the placenta. This IgG, reflecting the recent systemic antigenic stimulation of the mother, offers protection for several months after birth while the infant's own IgG system is still immature. In humans there is no analogous mechanism to that obtaining in the placenta for active transport of IgG from the serum or extracellular fluid to external secretions such as milk, and IgG therefore affords little in the way of protection to the intestinal tract of the infant. For those mammals in which significant amounts of IgG are present in milk early in lactation, the immature intestinal tract of the offspring permits ingested IgG to be absorbed into the systemic circulation. Again, this IgG is derived from the mother's serum pool and is not geared to mucosal immunity.

Human milk

Human milk, however, contains little IgG at any time. Throughout lactation the antibodies in human milk are principally IgA and reflect the mother's mucosal, mainly intestinal, immune system; i.e. they have specificity for the antigens of microorganisms resident in the mother's intestinal tract. After ingestion, the antibodies are not absorbed from the infant's gastrointestinal tract but instead afford local protection there against endemic microorganisms, including potential pathogens. This linkage between the intestinal immune system of the mother and that of the offspring via IgA provides a built-in protective mechanism for the immunologically naive infant whose intestinal tract is suddenly exposed to an onslaught of microorganisms and foreign macromolecules. In those areas of the world where modern methods of sanitation and public health are deficient, this passively acquired protection is likely to be especially important [18].

Acquisition of IgA antibody in milk

The question of the mechanism by which milk acquires IgA with specificity for intestinal microorganisms now arises. One potential source is the serum pool of the mother from which milk IgA might be derived by selective pumping. This IgA could be synthesized and secreted by intestinal plasma cells and reach the mammary gland via the general circulation, a route that would certainly account for its specificity, as antibody, for intestinal antigens. Since, however, only the dimeric form of IgA can actively pass through epithelial cells into exocrine secretions such as milk, and since human serum IgA is predominantly monomeric, this route is not likely to be very significant in humans. The major source of IgA in human milk is the abundant plasma cells within the mammary gland [3, 57]. In rodents, which contrast with humans in having appreciable proportions of dimeric IgA in their serum, the situation is somewhat different. In mice, transport of IgA from serum appears to be significant early in lactation, but by a week after onset local production predominates [25]. In rats, on the other hand, dimeric IgA is not effectively transported from serum into milk [13].

Cell migration

To account for the specificity of IgA produced in the mammary gland for intestinal microorganisms, it could be postulated that the antigens somehow reached the mammary gland. There is scant evidence for this. On the other hand, lymphocytes are known to circulate and recirculate. Lymphocytes originally sensitized in the gut to local antigens could migrate to the mammary gland, differentiate into plasma cells and secrete IgA antibodies that enter the milk, a scheme which eliminates the problem of having to explain how lymphoid cells already in the mammary gland could be stimulated there by the antigens of intestinal microbes. Support for this scheme will now be reviewed.

Lactating animals and humans exposed to intestinal antigens can be shown to have specific IgA antibodies in milk in the absence of serum antibodies of any class [19, 45]. The preferred explanation was migration of sensi-

tized lymphocytes from gut to mammary gland with subsequent local synthesis of IgA (Fig. 3.4). Studies of humans and of many animal species have disclosed marked increases in the number of plasma cells in the mammary gland during pregnancy and lactation compared with the usual low levels prevailing in the non-pregnant state [3, 57, 73]. In the instances in which the nature of the plasma cells in the mammary gland was studied, they were shown to be IgA producers.

Animal models

The mouse seems to be an appropriate model for providing insights into the immunology of human milk. In mice there is a marked increase in the number of IgA plasma cells per unit area of tissue during pregnancy and lactation. Moreover, this increase is under hormonal control [74]: oestrogen, progesterone and prolactin enhance the number of IgA plasma cells in the mammary glands of virgin female mice, and testosterone given to naturally lactating females depresses it. In vitro, the above hormones (plus insulin) can promote the differentiation of murine mammary epithelial cells to the point where they selectively bind and internalize dimeric IgA [72].

More direct evidence of B lymphocyte traffic between gut and mammary gland, the so-called enteromammary axis, has been provided by experimental studies in mice. When mesenteric lymph node cells, as representative of GALT, were injected intravenously into lactating mice, they evidenced a much greater tendency than did lymphocytes from peripheral lymphoid tissue to reach the mammary gland [40, 63]. Furthermore, those mesenteric node cells that did reach the lactating mammary gland were overwhelmingly IgA producers a day after cell transfer. In another series of experiments, antigen was given to mice in the drinking water before and during pregnancy and during lactation in order to stimulate an intestinal immune response; the lactating mammary glands then contained numerous antigen-specific IgA plasma cells [75].

The idea that antigen-specific lymphocytes can migrate from the GALT to the mammary gland (via the mesenteric lymphatic system, thoracic duct and blood) is supported by studies of cells transferred from the mesenteric nodes of such orally sensitized donors to lactating recipients that have not been exposed to the particular antigen: antigen-specific IgA

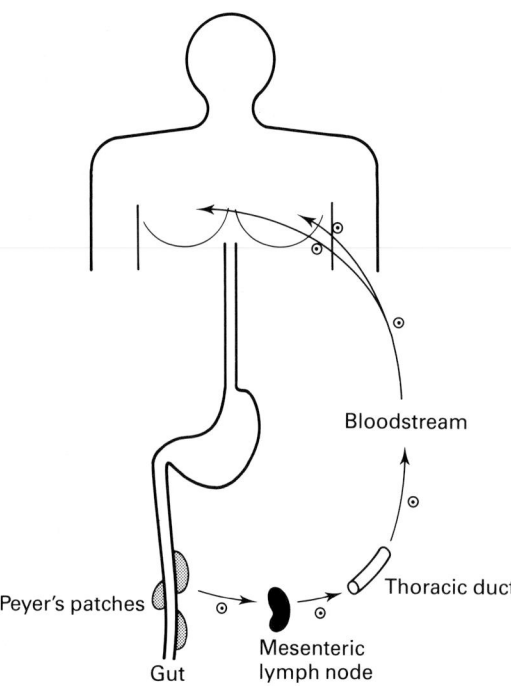

Bloodstream

Peyer's patches

Thoracic duct

Mesenteric lymph node

Gut

Fig. 3.4 Enteromammary circulation of lymphocytes. On contact with antigen, IgA precursor cells are stimulated to leave the Peyer's patches and migrate to the mammary glands where dimeric IgA is secreted.

plasma cells of mesenteric node origin are rapidly and preferentially observed in the recipients' mammary glands, showing that the cell migration is both selective for cells making IgA and not directed by antigen previously absorbed and trapped in the mammary gland. Evidence has also been obtained that the migrating cells in question occur in a highly restricted subpopulation of lymphocytes, one that bears cell surface IgA, but not IgM or IgG, and lacks the C3 complement receptor found on most mature B cells [63].

Summary

There is much species-to-species variation in both the absolute and relative amounts of the different immunoglobulin classes in mammary secretions and the routes and mechanisms by which they are transported. For IgA, the important variables appear to be the level of dimeric IgA in serum, the number of plasma cells within the mammary gland and the amount of available secretory component, the cell surface receptor required for the selective transport across mammary epithelial cells of dimeric IgA, whether it is locally produced or serum-derived. In the case of human milk it is abundantly clear that the important immunoglobulin is secretory IgA. Although there is little direct experimental evidence to indicate how much of this IgA is locally produced versus transported from serum, in the authors' opinion available evidence favours local synthesis by plasma cells derived from gut precursors as the dominant source. It should be kept in mind that since much of the dimeric IgA in serum in all mammals is the product of plasma cells resident in the gut, species to species or time to time variations in relative transport of serum or locally produced IgA do not affect the important principle that the IgA in milk reflects the mother's intestinal immune experience.

T cells in mammary glands

The situation with regard to the origin of the T cells in the mammary gland is less clear. There is some evidence suggesting that T cells in the mammary gland do not merely mirror T cells in the blood circulation, and may therefore be a selected subset. For example, in women, T cell responses to mitogens and antigens differ among populations from blood and milk [47, 51], as do the ratios of helper to suppressor cells [58]. In mice, the species in

which much of the evidence for the homing of IgA B cells from the GALT to the mammary gland has been obtained, there is good evidence for a gut-associated T cell with a similar life cycle to that of the B cells participating in mucosal immune responses [22]. Nevertheless, when T cell homing to the lactating mammary gland was specifically addressed in rats, the tendency of T cells from peripheral lymph nodes to migrate to the lactating mammary gland after intravenous injection fully equalled that of cells from the gut-associated mesenteric nodes [38]. The authors concluded that the rat discloses no preferential migration of T cells from the GALT to the mammary gland. It may be that the origins of plasma cells and of T cells in the mammary gland do indeed differ or that species differences, rats versus mice, exist. Another possibility is that although T cell migration to the mammary gland occurs from both gut-associated and peripheral lymphoid tissues, the mechanisms are different, with T cells going from the former as part of a generalized mucosal associated lymphoid system and from the latter as a manifestation of the tendency of some T cells to go to skin, the tissue of origin of the mammary gland [52, 61].

Cells in milk and colostrum

Milk and colostrum, as well as lactating mammary glands, contain appreciable numbers of leukocytes, but in colostrum only 5-10% are lymphocytes and none are plasma cells [10]. The lymphocytes, mostly T cells, are about equally divided between helper and suppressor cells [58]. It should be kept in mind that the representation and function of immunocytes in the mammary gland and in milk are not necessarily similar. Most of the cells selectively homing to the mammary gland in cell transfer studies in mice appear to be B cells, in particular, precursors of IgA plasma cells [63], whereas in milk, at least in humans, most of the lymphocytes are T cells [58]. The function of the B cells/plasma cells is clearly to produce IgA antibodies, which in humans at any rate would be expected to be more important in offering passive protection against infections to the offspring than in actively protecting the mammary gland itself. The T cells in the mammary gland, which in the rat are mostly the helper phenotype [50], could be expected to promote IgA antibody secretion and possibly aid in host defence within the mammary gland. It has also been suggested by several groups that T cells in milk could have a functional role in cellular immunity within the offspring (e.g. [48]).

Acknowledgements

The authors' research has been supported by NIH grants AI-20786 and CA-32582.

REFERENCES

1 Arny M, Kelly-Hatfield P, Lamm ME, Phillips-Quagliata JM: T cell help for the IgA response: the function of T cells from different lymphoid organs in regulating the proportions of plaque-forming cells expressing various isotypes. Cell Immunol 1984; 89: 95–112.

2 Bienenstock J, Dolezel J: Peyer's patches: lack of specific antibody-containing cells after oral and parenteral immunization. J Immunol 1971; 106: 938–45.

3 Brandtzaeg P: The secretory immune system of lactating human mammary glands compared with other exocrine organs. Ann NY Acad Sci 1983; 409: 353–81.

4 Butcher EC, Scollay RG, Weissman IL: Organ specificity of lymphocyte migration: mediation by highly selective lymphocyte interaction with organ-specific determinants on high endothelial venules. Eur J Immunol 1980; 10: 556–61.

5 Butcher EC, Reichert RA, Coffman RL et al: Surface phenotype and migratory capability of Peyer's patch germinal center cells. Adv Exp Med Biol 1981; 149: 765–72.

6 Cebra JJ, Cebra ER, Clough ER et al: IgA commitment: models for B-cell differentiation and possible roles for T cells in regulating B-cell development. Ann NY Acad Sci 1983; 409: 25–37.

7 Cebra JJ, Kamat R, Gearhart P et al: The secretory IgA system of the gut. Ciba Foundation Symposium 46 (new series) Immunology of the Gut. Amsterdam: Elsevier/North-Holland, 1977; 5–22.

8 Churi YH, Carey GD, Woodruff JJ: Lymphocyte recognition of lymph node high endothelium. IV. Cell surface structures mediating entry into lymph nodes. J Immunol 1982; 131: 1368–74.

9 Churi YH, Rasmussen R, Cakiroglu AG, Woodruff JJ: Lymphocyte recognition of lymph node high endothelium. VI. Evidence of distinct structures mediating binding to high endothelial cells of lymph nodes and Peyer's patches. J Immunol 1984; 133: 2961–5.

10 Crago SS, Prince SJ, Pretlow TG et al: Human colostral cells. I. Separation and characterization. Clin Exp Immunol 1979; 38: 585–97.

11 Craig SW, Cebra JJ: Peyer's patches: an enriched source of precursors for IgA-producing immunocytes in the rabbit. J Exp Med 1971; 134: 188–200.

12 Craig SW, Cebra JJ: Rabbit Peyer's patches, appendix and popliteal lymph node B lymphocytes: a comparative analysis of their membrane immunoglobulin components and plasma cell precursor potential. J Immunol 1975; 114: 492–502.

13 Dahlgren U, Ahlstedt S, Hedman L et al: Dimeric IgA in the rat is transferred from serum into bile but not into milk. Scand J Immunol 1981; 14: 95–8.

14 Elson CO, Heck JA, Strober W: T cell regulation of murine IgA synthesis. J Exp Med 1979; 149: 632–43.

15 Endoh M, Sakai H, Nomoto Y et al: IgA-specific helper activity of T_α cells in human peripheral blood. J Immunol 1981; 127: 2612–9.

16 Faulk WP, McCormick JN, Goodman JR et al: Peyer's patches: morphologic studies. Cell Immunol 1971; 1: 500–20.

17 Gallatin WM, Weissman IL, Butcher EC: A cell sur-

face molecule involved in organ-specific homing of lymphocytes. Nature 1983; 304: 30–4.

18 Glass RI, Svennerholm A-M, Stoll BJ et al: Protection against cholera in breast-fed children by antibodies in breast milk. N Engl J Med 1983; 308: 1389–92.

19 Goldblum RM, Ahlstedt S, Carlsson B et al: Antibody-forming cells in human colostrum after oral immunization. Nature 1975; 257: 797–8.

20 Gowans JL, Knight EJ: The route of recirculation of lymphocytes in the rat. Proc R Soc Lond (Biol) 1964; 159: 257–82.

21 Guy-Grand D, Griscelli C, Vassalli P: The gut-associated lymphoid system: nature and properties of the large dividing cells. Eur J Immunol 1974; 4: 435–43.

22 Guy-Grand D, Griscelli C, Vassalli P: The mouse gut T lymphocyte, a novel type of T cell. Nature, origin and traffic in mice in normal and graft-versus-host conditions. J Exp Med 1978; 148: 1661–77.

23 Hall JG, Hopkins J, Orlans E: Studies on the lymphocytes of sheep. III. Destination of lymph-borne immunoblasts in relation to their tissue of origin. Eur J Immunol 1977; 7: 30–7.

24 Hall JG, Parry DM, Smith ME: The distribution and differentiation of lymph-borne immunoblasts after intravenous injection into syngeneic recipients. Cell Tissue Kinet 1972; 5: 269–81.

25 Halsey JF, Mitchell C, Meyer R, Cebra JJ: Metabolism of immunoglobulin A in lactating mice: origins of immunoglobulin A in milk. Eur J Immunol 1982; 12: 107–12.

26 Husband AJ: Kinetics of extravasation and redistribution of IgA-specific antibody-containing cells in the intestine. J Immunol 1982; 128: 1355–9.

27 Husband AJ, Gowans JL: The origin and antigen-dependent distribution of IgA-containing cells in the intestine. J Exp Med 1978; 148: 1146–60.

28 Jacobson LO, Marks EK, Simmons EL, Gaston EO: Immune response in irradiated mice with Peyer's patch shielding. Proc Soc Exp Biol Med 1961; 108: 487–93.

29 Jones PP, Cebra JJ: Restriction of gene expression in B lymphocytes and their progeny. III. Endogenous IgA and IgM on the membranes of different plasma cell precursors. J Exp Med 1974; 140: 966–76.

30 Jones PP, Craig SW, Cebra JJ, Herzenberg LA: Restriction of gene expression in B lymphocytes and their progeny. II. Commitment to immunoglobulin heavy chain isotype. J Exp Med 1974; 140: 452–69.

31 Kawanishi H, Saltzman L, Strober W: Characteristics and regulatory function of murine Con A-induced, cloned T cells obtained from Peyer's patches and spleen: mechanisms regulating isotype-specific immunoglobulin production by Peyer's patch B cells. J Immunol 1982; 129: 475–83.

32 Kawanishi H, Saltzman L, Strober W: Mechanisms regulating IgA-class specific immunoglobulin production in murine gut-associated lymphoid tissues. I. T cells derived from Peyer's patches which switch sIgM B cells to sIgA B cells in vitro. J Exp Med 1983; 157: 433–50.

33 Kiyono H, Cooper MD, Kearney JF et al: Isotype

specificity of helper T cell clones: Peyer's patch Th cells preferentially collaborate with mature IgA B cells for IgA responses. J Exp Med 1984; 159: 798–811.

34 Kiyono H, McGhee JR, Wannemuehler MJ et al: In vitro immune responses to a T cell-dependent antigen by cultures of disassociated murine Peyer's patch. Proc Natl Acad Sci USA 1982; 79: 596–600.

35 Kiyono H, Phillips JO, Colwell DE et al: Isotype-specificity of helper T cell clones: Fcα receptors regulate T and B cell collaboration for IgA responses. J Immunol 1984; 133: 1087–9.

36 Kraal G, Weissman IL, Butcher EC: Differences in in vivo distribution and homing of T cell subsets to mucosal vs. nonmucosal lymphoid organs. J Immunol 1983; 130: 1097–102.

37 Lamm ME: Cellular aspects of immunoglobulin A. Adv Immunol 1976; 22: 223–90.

38 Manning LS, Parmely MJ: Cellular determinants of mammary cell mediated immunity in the rat. I. The migration of radioisotopically labelled T lymphocytes. J Immunol 1980; 125: 2508–14.

39 Mayrhofer G, Fisher R: IgA-containing plasma cells in the lamina propria of the gut: failure of a thoracic duct fistula to deplete the numbers in rat small intestine. Eur J Immunol 1979; 9: 85–91.

40 McDermott MR, Bienenstock J: Evidence for a common mucosal immunologic system. I. Migration of B immunoblasts into intestinal, respiratory and genital tissues. J Immunol 1979; 122: 1892–7.

41 McDermott MR, Clark DA, Bienenstock J: Evidence for a common mucosal immunologic system. II. Influence of the estrous cycle on B immunoblast migration into genital and intestinal tissues. J Immunol 1980; 124: 2536–9.

42 McWilliams M, Lamm ME, Phillips-Quagliata JM: Surface and intracellular markers of mouse mesenteric and peripheral lymph node and Peyer's patch cells. J Immunol 1974; 113: 1326–33.

43 McWilliams M, Phillips-Quagliata JM, Lamm ME: Characteristics of mesenteric lymph node cells homing to gut-associated lymphoid tissue in syngeneic mice. J Immunol 1975; 115: 54–8.

44 McWilliams M, Phillips-Quagliata JM, Lamm ME: Mesenteric lymph node B lymphoblasts which home to the small intestine are precommitted to IgA synthesis. J Exp Med 1977; 145: 866–75.

45 Montgomery PC, Rosner BR, Cohn, J: The secretory antibody response. Anti-DNP antibodies induced by dinitrophenylated type III pneumococcus. Immunol Commun 1974; 3: 143–56.

46 Montgomery PC, Ayyildiz A, Lemaitre-Coelho IM et al: Induction and expression of antibodies in secretions: the ocular immune system. Ann NY Acad Sci 1983; 409: 428–39.

47 Ogra SS, Ogra PL: Immunologic aspects of human colostrum and milk. II. Characteristics of lymphocyte reactivity and distribution of E-rosette forming cells at different times after the onset of lactation. J Pediatr 1978; 92: 550–5.

48 Ogra SS, Weintraub D, Ogra PL: Immunologic aspects of human colostrum and milk. III. Fate and absorption of cellular and soluble components in the gastrointestinal tract of the newborn. J Immunol 1977; 119: 245–8.

49 Ottaway CA, Bruce RG, Parrott DMV: The in vivo kinetics of lymphoblast localization in the small intestine. Immunology 1983; 49: 641–8.

50 Parmely ML, Manning LS: Cellular determinants of mammary cell-mediated immunity in the rat: kinetics of lymphocyte subset accumulation in the rat mammary gland during pregnancy and lactation. Ann NY Acad Sci 1983; 409: 517–32.

51 Parmely MJ, Beer AE, Billingham RE: In vitro studies on the T-lymphocyte population of human milk. J Exp Med 1976; 144: 358–70.

52 Parrott DMV: Source, identity, and locomotor characteristics of lymphocyte populations migrating to mammary glands: problems and predictions. In: Ogra PL, Dayton DH, eds. Immunology of breast milk. New York: Raven Press, 1979; 131–41.

53 Parrott DMV, Ferguson A: Selective migration of lymphocytes within the mouse small intestine. Immunology 1974; 26: 571–88.

54 Phillips-Quagliata JM, Roux ME, Arny M et al: Migration and regulation of B-cells in the mucosal immune system. Ann NY Acad Sci 1983; 409: 194–202.

55 Pierce NF, Cray WC Jr: Determinants of the localization, magnitude and duration of a specific mucosal IgA plasma cell response in enterically immunized rats. J Immunol 1982; 128: 1311–5.

56 Pierce NF, Gowans JL: Cellular kinetics of the intestinal immune response to cholera toxoid in rats. J Exp Med 1975; 142: 1550–63.

57 Pumphrey RSH: A comparative study of plasma cells in the mammary gland in pregnancy and lactation. Symp Zool Soc Lond 1977; 41: 261–76.

58 Richie ER, Bass R, Meistrich ML, Dennison DK: Distribution of T lymphocyte subsets in human colostrum. J Immunol 1982; 129: 1116–9.

59 Robertson SM, Cebra JJ: A model for local immunity. Ric Clin Lab 1976; 6 (suppl) 3: 105–19.

60 Rose ML, Parrott DMV, Bruce RG: Migration of lymphoblasts to the small intestine. II. Divergent migration of mesenteric and peripheral immunoblasts to sites of inflammation in the mouse. Cell Immunol 1976; 27: 36–46.

61 Rose ML, Parrott DMV, Bruce RG: The accumulation of immunoblasts in extravascular tissues including mammary gland, peritoneal cavity, gut and skin. Immunology 1978; 35: 415–23.

62 Roux ME, McWilliams M, Phillips-Quagliata JM, Lamm ME: Differentiation pathway of Peyer's patch precursors of IgA plasma cells in the secretory immune system. Cell Immunol 1981; 61: 141–53.

63 Roux ME, McWilliams M, Phillips-Quagliata JM et al: Origin of IgA-secreting plasma cells in the mammary gland. J Exp Med 1977; 146: 1311–22.

64 Rudzik O, Perey DYE, Bienenstock J: Differential IgA repopulation after transfer of autologous and allogeneic rabbit Peyer's patch cells. J Immunol 1975: 114: 40–4.

65 Rudzik O, Clancy RL, Perey DYE et al: Repopulation with IgA-containing cells of bronchial and intestinal lamina propria after transfer of homologous Peyer's patch and bronchial lymphocytes. J Immunol 1975; 114: 1599–604.

66 Spalding DM, Williamson SI, Koopman WJ, McGhee JR: Preferential induction of polyclonal IgA secretion by murine Peyer's patch dendritic cell–T cell mixtures. J Exp Med 1984; 160: 941–6.

67 Sprent J: Fate of H-2-activated T lymphocytes in syngeneic hosts. 1. Fate in lymphoid tissues and intestines traced with ^{3}H-thymidine, ^{125}I-deoxyuridine and ^{51}chromium. Cell Immunol 1976; 21: 278–302.

68 Stevens SK, Weissman IL, Butcher EL: Differences in the migration of B and T lymphocytes: organ-selective localization *in vivo* and the role of lymphocyte-endothelial cell recognition. J Immunol 1982; 128: 844–51.

69 Tseng J: Transfer of lymphocytes of Peyer's patches

between immunoglobulin allotype congenic mice: re-population of the IgA cells in the gut lamina propria. J Immunol 1981; 127: 2039–43.

70 Tseng J: A population of resting IgM-IgD double-bearing lymphocytes in Peyer's patches: the major pre-cursor cells for IgA plasma cells in the gut lamina propria. J Immunol 1984; 132: 2730–5.

71 Tseng J: Repopulation of the gut lamina propria with IgA-containing cells by lymphoid cells isolated from the gut lamina propria. Eur J Immunol 1984; 14: 420–5.

72 Weisz-Carrington P, Emancipator S, Lamm ME: Binding and uptake of immunoglobulins by mouse mammary gland epithelial cells in hormone-treated cultures. J Reprod Immunol 1984; 6: 63–75.

73 Weisz-Carrington P, Roux ME, Lamm ME: Plasma cells and epithelial immunoglobulins in the mouse mammary gland during pregnancy and lactation. J Immunol 1977; 119: 1306–9.

74 Weisz-Carrington P, Roux ME, McWilliams M et al: Hormonal induction of the secretory immune system in the mammary gland. Proc Natl Acad Sci USA 1978; 75:2928–32.

75 Weisz-Carrington P, Roux ME, McWilliams M et al: Organ and isotype distribution of plasma cells pro-ducing specific antibody after oral immunization: evi-dence for a generalized secretory immune system. J Immunol 1979; 123: 1705–8.

76 Williams AF, Gowans JL: The presence of IgA on the surface of the rat thoracic duct lymphocytes which contain internal IgA. J Exp Med 1975; 141: 335–45.

SECTION B
SPECIALIZED CELLS OF THE GUT

Chapter 4
Gut-associated Macrophages

Dale E. Bockman

Introduction

Macrophages occur in large quantities in the gut. They are the predominant cell type in the lamina propria immediately beneath the epithelium lining the gastrointestinal tract. They are located in solitary lymphoid follicles, in Peyer's patches and in the appendix. They may be found, in smaller numbers, within the epithelium.

The functions of macrophages in the gut may be generalized or specific. As examples of general activity, particulate material which has penetrated the epithelial barrier, or effete lymphocytes in the lamina propria and epithelium, may be phagocytosed. On the other hand, gut-associated macrophages may be mediators and regulators of quite specific immune reactivity. They do not exist and function alone.

They release substances which affect other cells involved in the immune response, and react to other cells and their products. These interactions may modulate the environment by affecting circulation and coagulation. Generalized and specific activity usually occur simultaneously in vivo.

A complete understanding of normal and pathological responses to antigens in the gut, including food antigens, must encompass the functions which are performed by gut-associated macrophages. However, most of the studies which have revealed the functional capabilities of macrophages in the last several years have been performed not on those from the gut, but on those from adherent cells of lymph nodes, spleen, peritoneal cavity and lungs. Therefore, this chapter will begin with a consideration of some characteristics of macrophages in general, and then proceed to macrophages in the gastrointestinal tract proper. It has become evident that Peyer's patches are important sites for the handling of gut antigens, so the role of macrophages in these areas will be emphasized.

It would seem that a well-rounded approach to the function of gut-associated macrophages must include the study of some cells and organs which do not fit under the headings macrophage or gut. Therefore the parallel and associated functions of neutrophils and eosinophils will be touched upon where appropriate. Similarly, macrophages associated with the mammary glands will be discussed because of the obvious association with gastrointestinal function.

Finally, some discussion of macrophage involvement in selected diseases and disorders of the gastrointestinal tract will be undertaken for the purpose of trying to establish some generalizations which might be helpful when applied to the problems of food intolerance and allergy.

CHARACTERISTICS OF MACROPHAGES

General features

A number of characteristics which commonly are used to identify macrophages may be described, but it should be noted that even these basic characteristics may vary with time and conditions. Macrophages are large mononuclear cells. They adhere to glass or plastic surfaces, and are capable of considerable phagocytic activity. In routine histological sections, a large, slightly irregular nucleus is surrounded by abundant, pinkish, granular cytoplasm which may have numerous vacuoles or inclusions. Many dense granules are evident in the cytoplasm upon examination by phase contrast microscopy. Transmission electron microscopy clearly shows a heterogeneous population of granules dispersed among cytoplasmic membranes and mitochondia, and frequently among phagocytic vacuoles and phagolysosomes. These granules are lysosomes, and a lysosomal enzyme marker, acid phosphatase, usually may be detected in macrophages by biochemical or cytochemical techniques. Other common characteristics of macrophages are positive reactions for non-specific esterase and adenosine triphosphatase (ATPase) [53, 84]. Active macrophages have a characteristic appearance when viewed by

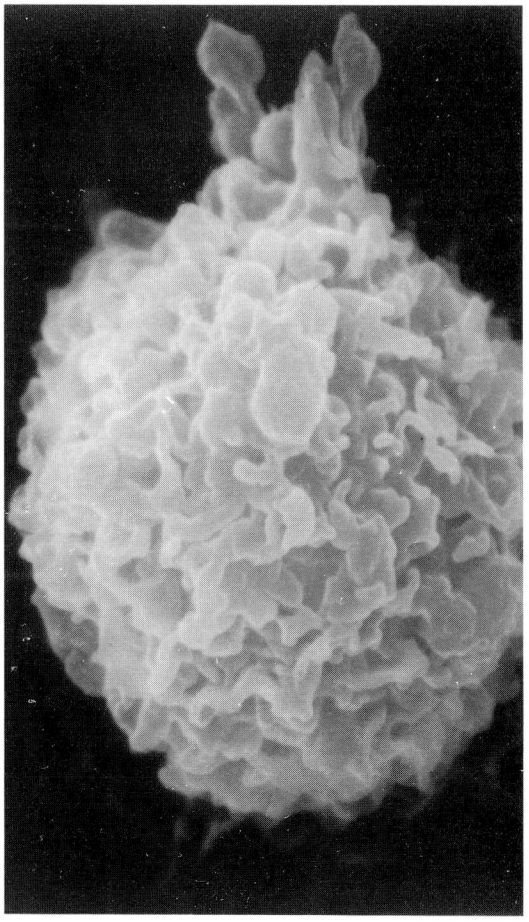

Fig. 4.1 Scanning electron micrograph of a macrophage from the peritoneal cavity of a rat. The surface membrane is highly convoluted or ruffled. × 15 000. Reproduced from [11] with kind permission of the editor of the *Journal of the Reticuloendothelial Society*.

scanning electron microscopy (Fig. 4.1), due to elaborate folding or ruffling of the cell membrane, and sometimes to the extension of filamentous protrusions.

Heterogeneity of macrophages

Heterogeneity among macrophages is produced because they have a large number of characteristics which are acquired or lost with time, in response to multiple stimuli present in the local microenvironment, during differentiation of their cell line. Macrophages normally are not replenished by cell division in situ, but by the differentiation of cells which arise elsewhere and are transported to the site of activity. Monocytes are produced from more primitive cells in the bone marrow, enter the bloodstream for transport and differentiate into macrophages in the connective tissues [17, 19, 89]. Macrophages may differentiate further into epithelioid cells and giant cells. Monocytes and macrophages have in common a number of morphological characteristics (ruffling of surface membrane, lysosomes, pinocytotic vesicles, shape and structure of nucleus) and functional capabilities. There also are differences. For example, compared with human resident peritoneal macrophages, human monocytes are smaller, more adherent to glass, more capable of intracellular killing of *Salmonella typhimurium* and have less acid hydrolase content [39].

Activated macrophages

Macrophages acquire heightened activity and distinct morphological and functional characteristics when stimulated ('activated') by a variety of agents. Macrophages harvested from animals combatting infection or stimulated by the proper agents display an increased capacity for phagocytosis, ruffling of the surface membrane, increased adherence and spreading on a glass or plastic surface, increased numbers of phagolysosomes and endocytic vesicles, altered metabolism and increased secretions [18, 44, 52, 63, 64]. Living or dead microbes, endotoxins, foreign serum proteins, immune complexes and lymphokines are among the agents capable of initiating these kinds of changes. The resulting activated macrophages express more microbicidal activity than non-stimulated ones. Although a large number of functional properties usually are changed simultaneously during this process, it cannot be assumed that the presence of one necessarily indicates the presence of the others. Again, there is heterogeneity.

Phagocytosis

The process of phagocytosis consists of two separable steps. The first is attachment to the cell membrane. The second is internalization. These processes are illustrated in Figs. 4.2 and 4.3. Attachment may occur without internalization. Reynolds et al [70] reported, for example, that although human alveolar macrophages bound complement-coated erythrocytes to their surface, they did not internalize them. During phagocytosis, potent oxidizing agents such as superoxide, hydrogen peroxide and hydroxyl radical, which may be effective in killing internalized organisms and breaking down ingested and surrounding material, may be released rapidly [63].

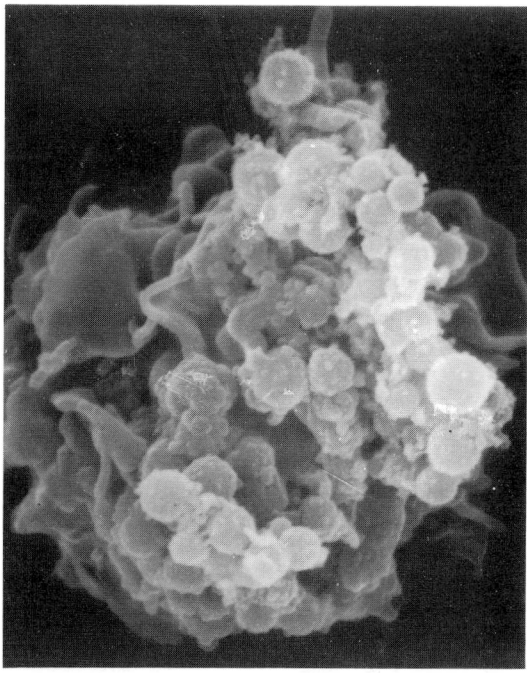

Fig. 4.2 Scanning electron micrograph of rat peritoneal macrophage after ferritin-coated zymogen granules have been added to the culture medium and become attached to the cell membrane. × 7000. Reproduced from [11] with kind permission of the editor of the *Journal of the Reticuloendothelial Society*.

Degradation of antigen

The end stage of breakdown finds the bulk of the material degraded to non-antigenic fragments, but some antigen remains undegraded. Some of this may be released into the environment and some may be found on the surface membrane of the macrophages. For continued reactivity to the antigen, there is an essential interaction between macrophages and T lymphocytes. This process may be referred to as antigen presentation, and the macrophages are said to be carrying out accessory cell function. For a complete discussion of this interaction, see the review by Unanue [88].

Interaction between macrophages and lymphocytes

The interaction of macrophages and lymphocytes is controlled by the I region of the major histocompatibility complex (the HLA-D region in man). The products of this region, which are detectable on the cell surface, are called Ia antigens (DR antigens in man). Macrophage–lymphocyte cooperativity is dependent upon the presence of these antigens. Not

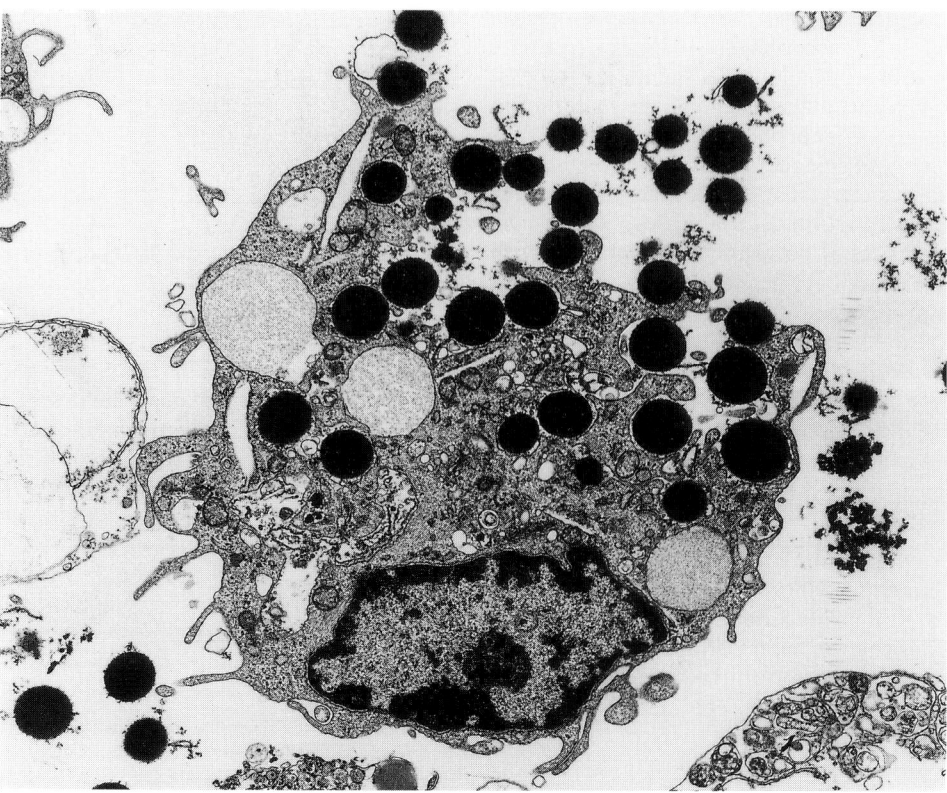

Fig. 4.3 Transmission electron micrograph of a macrophage which has been incubated with ferritin-coated zymogen granules. Both surface adherence and internalization are obvious. × 9000. Reproduced from [11], with kind permission of the editor of the *Journal of the Reticuloendothelial Society*.

all macrophages have Ia antigens at a particular time, and the antigens may be lost with time, so the maintenance of a population of Ia-positive macrophages in any area requires the continued replenishment through immigration of new monocytes.

Secretory products of macrophages

Additional interactions between macrophages and lymphocytes, and between macrophages and many other elements in their environment, are mediated through secretory products. Nathan et al [63] have listed over 50 secretory products of mononuclear phagocytes. Some of these are shown in Table 4.1. Regulation is extensive and complex. Macrophages secrete both lymphocyte-activating factors and factors inhibiting replication of lymphocytes. Cell products of lymphocytes (lymphokines) may stimulate macrophages to secrete such diverse products as lysosomal enzymes, interferon, collagenase and plasminogen activator [88]. Macrophage secretory products may promote replication of myeloid and erythroid precursors, fibroblasts and endothelial cells.

Table 4.1 Factors secreted by macrophages.

Induced by lymphokines
Lysosomal enzymes
Interferon
Collagenase
Plasminogen activator
Acting on other cells
Myeloid precursors
Erythroid precursors
Fibroblasts
Endothelial cells
Biologically active factors
Prostaglandins
Collagenase
Elastase
Plasminogen activator
Lysozyme
Complement factors
Interferon
Biological inhibitors
α_2-macroglobulin
α_1-antitrypsin inhibitor

Secreted prostaglandins may affect circulation. Secreted collagenase and elastase may lyse their connective tissue substrates, and plasminogen activator may lead to the formation of plasmin to lyse fibrin. On the other hand, macrophages may secrete α_2-macroglobulin, which inhibits collagenase, elastase and plasmin. Macrophages secrete lysozyme which causes bacterial breakdown, interferon which inhibits viral replication, many complement factors and α_1-antitrypsin inhibitor. The endogenous pyrogen (IL-1) which they secrete produces fever and causes granulocytes to release lactoferrin.

Surface membrane of macrophages

The surface membranes of macrophages present a heterogeneous array of substances which contribute to their functional characteristics and provide markers for their presence and activity. Plasma membrane ectoenzymes, such as 5'-nucleotidase, are quantifiable and usually decrease markedly with activation [18, 52]. Laminin and fibronectin are detectable on the surface of macrophages and may be important in cell–cell and cell–matrix adhesive properties [40, 93].

Surface receptors

Receptors for the Fc portion of immunoglobulin, for the C3b fragment of complement and for lactoferrin are on the macrophage membrane [63, 70, 90]. The binding of lactoferrin to the membrane may modulate macrophage secretion and thus play a role in immune regulation [63]. Binding of IgG through its Fc receptor is important in phagocytosis of particles coated with IgG (opsonization). Complement binding may augment opsonization in some cases. Receptors for IgE [13, 37] on macrophages may assist adhesion and killing of parasites.

Receptors for IgA

It is likely that macrophages have receptors for IgA on their surface as well. Fanger et al [27, 28] have demonstrated IgA receptors on monocytes, and it would be unlikely that they would be lost, especially on those macrophages which exist in an IgA-rich milieu like the gastrointestinal tract. IgA has been shown to opsonize for bactericidal activity of monocytes [34, 54, 55]. Opsonization by IgA does not, however, seem to be nearly as vigorous or as important as that by IgG [51]. Mestecky et al [57] have pointed out that the function of IgA does not rely on opsonization. Reynolds et al [70] found that *Pseudomonas* coated with IgA was not ingested by alveolar macrophages, whereas those organisms coated with IgG were ingested. They therefore suggest lack of IgA receptors on alveolar macrophages. Regional variation in the quantity of IgA receptor remains a possibility which must be kept in mind [27]. There appears to be an absence of receptors for IgM on macrophage membranes [70, 89].

Surface antigens. A large number of membrane components of macrophages may be grouped under the general designation of surface antigens. These range from well-characterized components like the Ia antigens already discussed, through those characterized by molecular weight and general biochemical constitution but with unknown function, to those about which little is known. Surface antigens are identified by the use of specific antibodies, frequently monoclonal antibodies. Subpopulations of mononuclear phagocytes may be identified through the profiles of surface antigens present, sometimes in combination with other characteristics. Some antigens reflect the differentiative steps achieved by mononuclear phagocyte cell lines, and marked heterogeneity among these cells is evident [3, 30].

MACROPHAGES IN THE LAMINA PROPRIA

The lamina propria is a solid cellular mass in which the most conspicuous cell type is the macrophage [25, 82]. The macrophages collect mainly in the upper 100–150 μm of the mucosa so that they, along with fibroblasts, are prominent in the subepithelial region, and thus are quite evident between crypts and in villous apices in the small intestine, and immediately beneath the lining epithelium in the colon [20, 25, 72]. Collan [20] has shown that many macrophages immediately beneath the epithelium may insert long pseudopodia through the basal lamina into the epithelial layer proper and there make contact with intraepithelial lymphocytes. Macrophages occasionally are found within the epithelial layer [81, 82]. Other cell types which make up the lamina propria with macrophages include plasma cells, lymphocytes, mast cells and eosinophils. Close associations and contacts between macrophages and some of these cells have been demonstrated by electron microscopical study, showing the possibility of interactions which may depend on cell–cell contacts [20, 23].

Morphology of lamina propria macrophages

Macrophages in the lamina propria have a heterogeneous morphology, dependent upon their developmental and functional history. Some may be similar to monocytes, others may display the features of mature phagocytes. Cytoplasmic granules (Fig. 4.4) and vacuoles are prominent with study by phase microscopy

[32, 96] and by electron microscopy [23, 87]. Dead cells and degenerating cell fragments commonly are seen in phagolysosomes, indicating that in situ phagocytosis and breakdown of lymphocytes and other cells is a normal function of gut-associated macrophages [20, 72].

Ingestion of antigens. Phagocytosis and pinocytosis of foreign material may be demonstrated as well. Ferritin, a large protein molecule with micelles of iron, administered by either subcutaneous of intraepithelial injec-

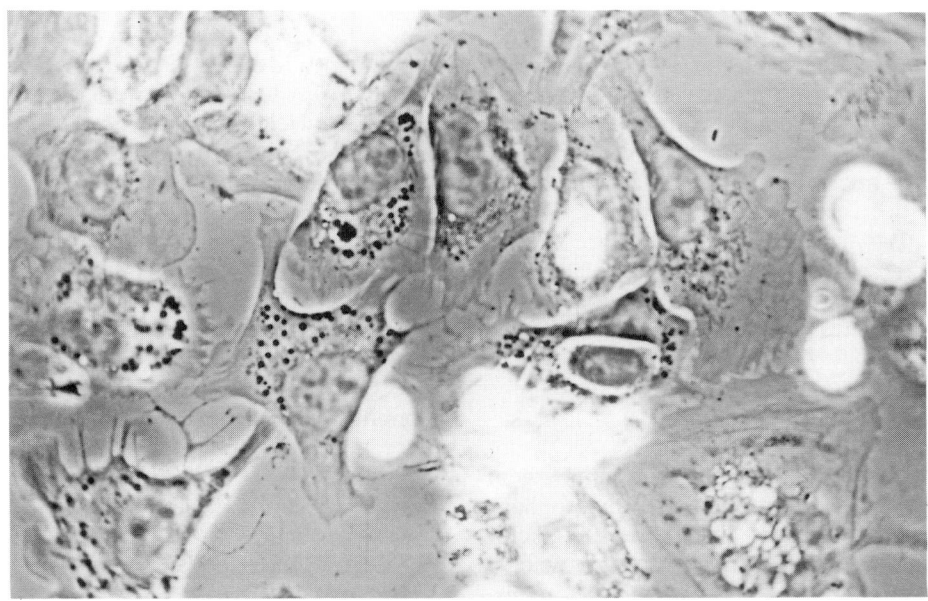

Fig. 4.4 Human intestinal macrophage after 24 hours in culture. The cytoplasm contains many phase-dense granules, and cellular extensions are prominent. Reproduced from [96], with kind permission of Elsevier Science Publishing Co., Inc. Copyright 1983 by the American Gastroenterological Association.

(a)   **(b)**

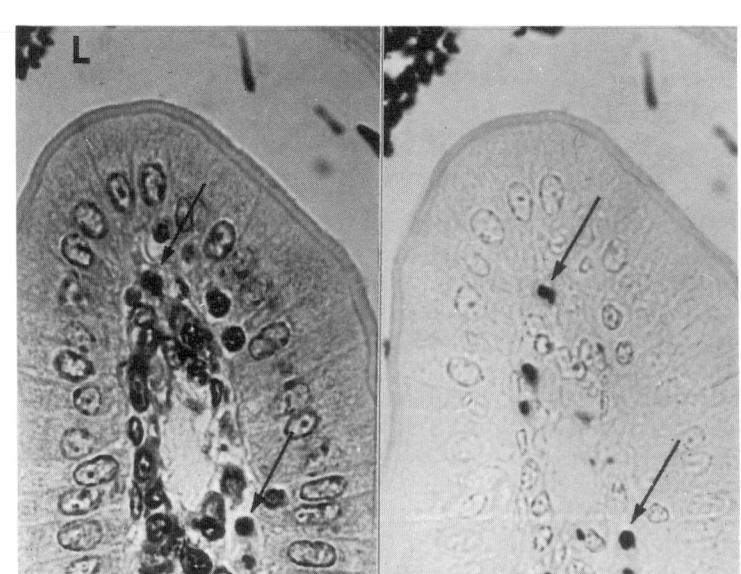

Fig. 4.5 Intestinal villus from hamster after previous intraperitoneal injections of ferritin. Paraffin section is treated with Prussian blue reagents to reveal the iron moiety of ferritin. The arrows point to macrophages containing ferritin. (a) Photographed with regular light; (b), photographed with red to emphasize the location of blue reaction product. × 760. Reproduced from [9], with kind permission of the editor of the *Anatomical Record*, a publication of the Wistar press.

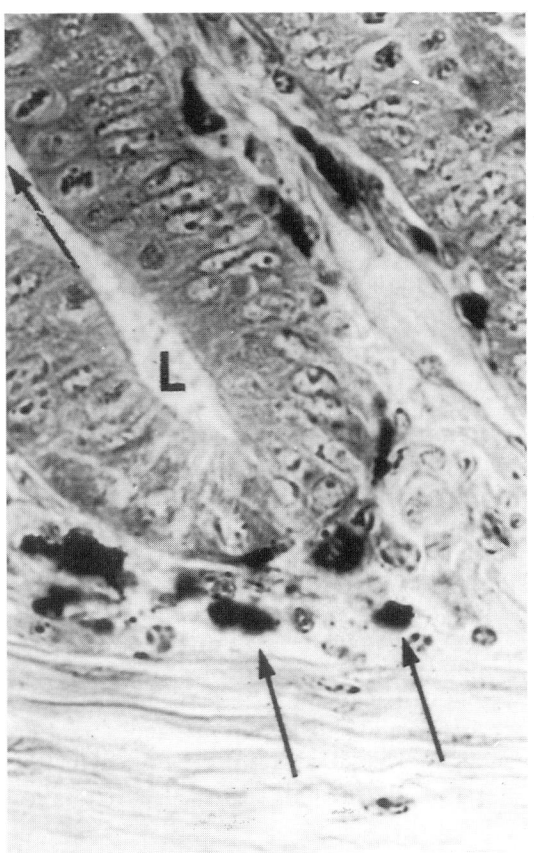

Fig. 4.6 Intestinal crypt region after intraperitoneal injections of ferritin and localization of ferritin with the Prussian blue reaction. Arrows indicate ferritin-laden macrophages. × 1050. Reproduced from [9], with kind permission of the editor of the *Anatomical Record*, a publication of the Wistar Press.

tion, is taken up and concentrated within macrophages in intestinal villi and surrounding intestinal crypts (Figs. 4.5 and 4.6). Bovine serum albumin may be demonstrated in lamina propria macrophages after two days of feeding with this substance [2].

Isolation of lamina propria macrophages. Lamina propria macrophages have been isolated and characterized only recently. Golder and Doe [32] characterized macrophages from human colon after ethylenediaminetetraacetic acid (EDTA) and enzyme dispersal, collection by Percoll density gradients, then adherence to plastic. Winter et al [96] prepared their cells by adherence to coverslips coated with fibronectin. The cells thus isolated were capable of phagocytosis mediated by Fc receptors, had receptors for complement, were positive for Ia antigens and non-specific esterase, were negative for peroxidase, synthesized complement

and secreted lysozyme. Thus they had many of the basic characteristics described previously for macrophages derived from other sites.

Responsiveness of lamina propria macrophages

Macrophages in the lamina propria are demonstrably responsive to luminal contents. Takeuchi et al [82] studied the response of the intestinal mucosa in guinea pigs made susceptible to infection with *Shigella flexneri* by starvation. Macrophages increased in size and number, became quite active phagocytically, and along with other inflammatory cells, breached the epithelium. Donnellan [25] studied colonic mucosa from patients during chronic colonic obstruction. Although there was absence of apparent bacterial invasion, macrophages were markedly increased. Lamina propria macrophages then must be considered as constantly interacting with material from the lumen of the gastrointestinal tract and the cells which are involved both in specific immune responses and in generalized inflammatory responses.

CELLS AND ORGANS WHICH MAY INTERACT WITH MACROPHAGES

When considering the normal function and protective reaction involving macrophages of the gastrointestinal tract, it seems judicious to include a consideration of certain additional cells and organs.

Polymorphonuclear leukocytes

Eosinophils and neutrophils (polymorphonuclear leukocytes) normally are found in gut mucosa. They are most prominent in the lamina propria, but occasionally may be found within the epithelium under normal conditions [20, 81, 82]. The number and apparent activity of these granulocytes may increase dramatically with inflammation.

Both types of granulocytes may phagocytose material under proper conditions. Eosinophils may phagocytose antigen–antibody complexes. They have receptors for IgE on their surface and have been shown to phagocytose microfilariae of *Dipetalonema*, mediated through IgE antibodies, and to degranulate on the ingested material [37]. This did not, however, kill the microfilariae, whereas macrophages killed and degraded them after phagocytosis mediated by the same antibody.

Surface receptors. The surface receptors for immunoglobulins on neutrophils are somewhat similar to those on macrophages, in that receptors for IgA and IgG, but not IgM, are present [27, 33]. IgG may opsonize for phagocytosis by neutrophils from peripheral blood.

IgA opsonization

Coating erythrocytes with IgA causes binding to peripheral blood neutrophils, but not internalization. IgA has been shown to augment the phagocytosis mediated by IgG in some studies, but inhibit IgG opsonization in others [95]. Furthermore, neutrophils from the oral cavity carry out phagocytosis mediated by IgA alone, indicating the possibility that environmental effects (such as high concentrations of IgA) may increase the number of IgA receptors on the cell surface, thus modulating reactive capability [27]. This raises the possibility that neutrophils in the IgA-rich environment of the gut lamina propria might be able to carry out IgA-mediated phagocytosis.

Fixed macrophages

Drainage from the gastrointestinal tract via blood and lymph leads to the liver and to mesenteric lymph nodes. Particulate and soluble material, free in the fluid or associated with cells, may be intercepted in these locations. Kupffer cells dispersed along the sinusoids of the liver are highly phagocytic and form an important part of the system of mononuclear phagocytes. Mesenteric lymph nodes also contain a plethora of phagocytes, and in addition may serve as a location for a stage in maturation of lymphocytes which have been stimulated in the gastrointestinal tract.

MACROPHAGES IN GALT

The unit of organization of gut-associated lymphoepithelial tissue (GALT) is the lymphoid follicle. Lymphoid follicles occur singly along the gastrointestinal tract (solitary follicles or nodules), and in addition may be grouped together in large numbers up to the highly organized arrays present in Peyer's patches and appendix. Solitary follicles take up and respond to luminal contents, and are similar morphologically to the follicular units in more complex GALT [41, 45].

Distribution of macrophages

Macrophages are prominent in GALT [21, 29, 36, 50, 51, 74, 77]. They are found

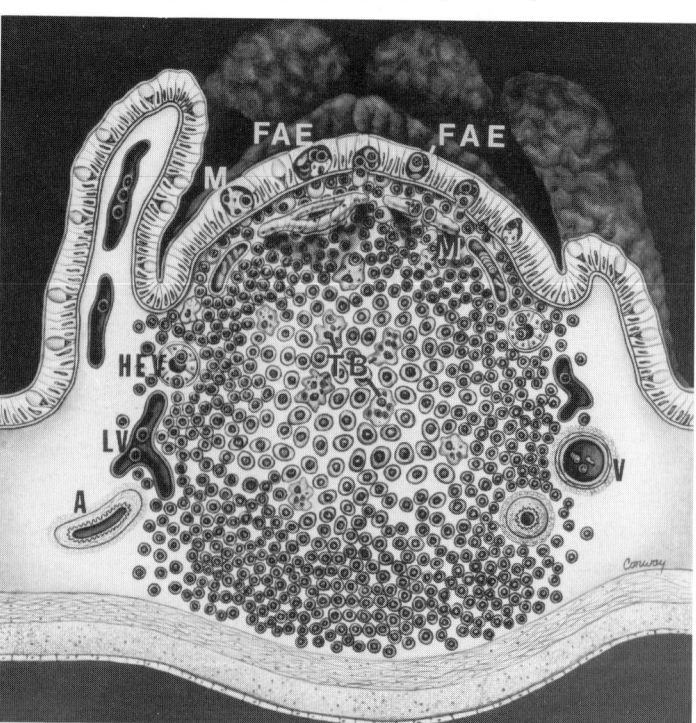

Fig. 4.7 Pictorial representation of some pertinent features of Peyer's patch. Tingible body macrophages (TB) are prominent in the germinal centre. Macrophages (M) are located within and beneath the epithelium; some are associated closely with follicle-associated epithelial (FAE) cells. A, artery; V, vein; LV, lymphatic vessel; HEV, high endothelial venule. Reproduced from [5], with kind permission of Pergamon Press.

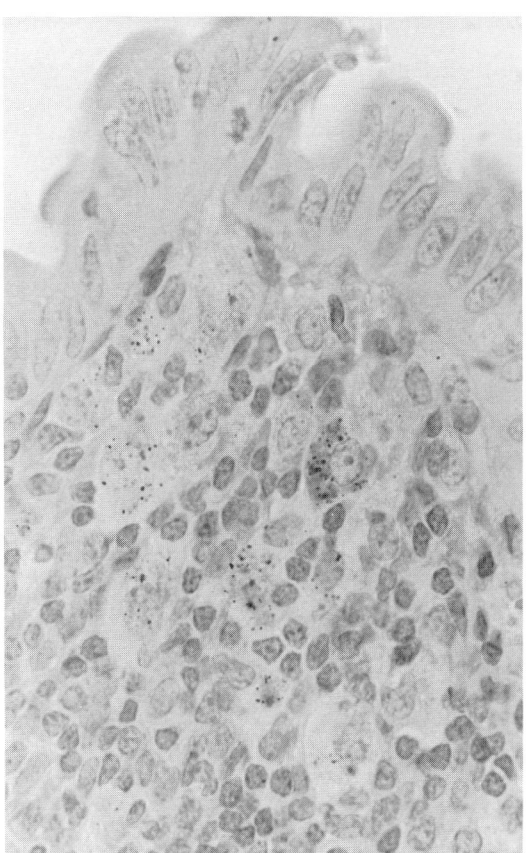

Fig. 4.8 Light micrograph of portion of mouse Peyer's patch after ingestion of Fe₂O₃. The small dense particles are localized within macrophages in the dome area. Provided through the courtesy of Drs ME LeFevre and DD Joel.

throughout each follicle. Within the germinal centre, numerous so-called tingible body macrophages are usually concentrated (Fig. 4.7). These are macrophages with many engulfed cells, mostly lymphocytes in various stages of breakdown, in their cytoplasm. The disintegrating cellular products stain densely. Other macrophages are found closer to the periphery of the follicle. There is a concentration of macrophages in the subepithelial region of each follicle (Fig. 4.8), and some may be found within the epithelial layer proper [1, 5, 7, 21, 66, 91].

Responsiveness of GALT macrophages

The macrophages in GALT obviously are responsive to the contents of the intestinal lumen. There are fewer macrophages in GALT of germ-free animals compared with conventional animals [85]. When luminal contents are transmitted through the specialized follicle-associated epithelium (FAE) [8, 10] or breach the epithelial barrier they are likely to be taken up by macrophages. Naturally occurring bacteria in the lumen of the rabbit appendix penetrate the epithelium to be taken up by intraepithelial macrophages (Fig. 4.9) or by subepithelial macrophages [6, 10, 74].

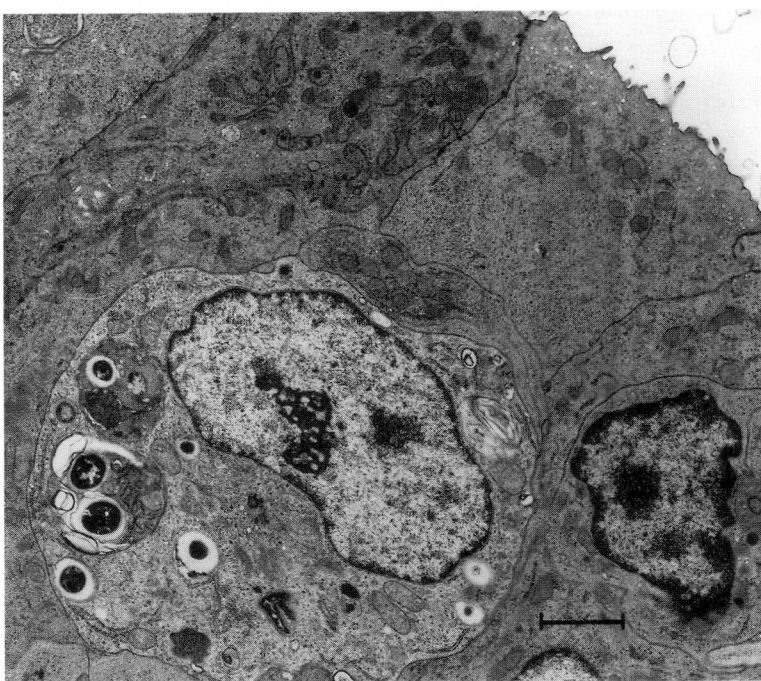

Fig. 4.9 Electron micrograph of an intraepithelial macrophage in rabbit appendix. Phagocytosed bacteria are evident in the cytoplasm. × 3700. Reproduced from [7], with kind permission of the editor of *Scanning Electron Microscopy*.

Ingestion of carbon particles

Macrophage activity in GALT has been demonstrated clearly by Joel et al [41] and Hammer et al [36] by histological examination at various times after gavage or long-term feeding (in drinking water) of carbon particles. The carbon was taken up to a much greater extent in lymphoid follicles (solitary follicles and follicles in Peyer's patches) than in the remaining intestine (Figs. 4.10 and 4.11). Sub-epithelial macrophages with engulfed carbon particles were identified on the second day of gavage. After chronic ingestion for two months, concentrations of carbon were heaviest in the subepithelial region and toward the periphery of the serosal pole of each follicle, but carbon-containing macrophages were present throughout the follicle. Many tingible body macrophages had carbon particles in the

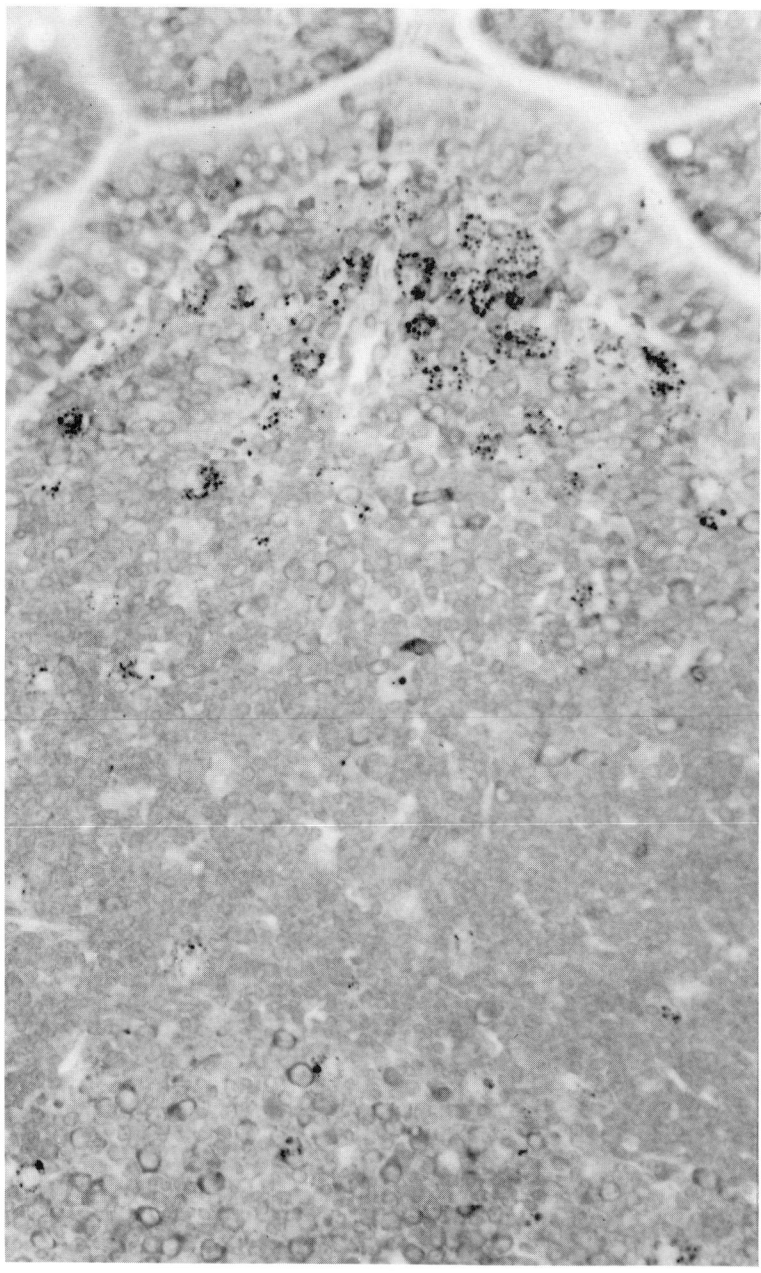

Fig. 4.10 Peyer's patch follicle from mouse after ingestion of carbon particles. The dense particles are concentrated in macrophages in the dome. Compare with particles in Fig. 4.12. Provided through the courtesy of Drs ME LeFevre and DD Joel.

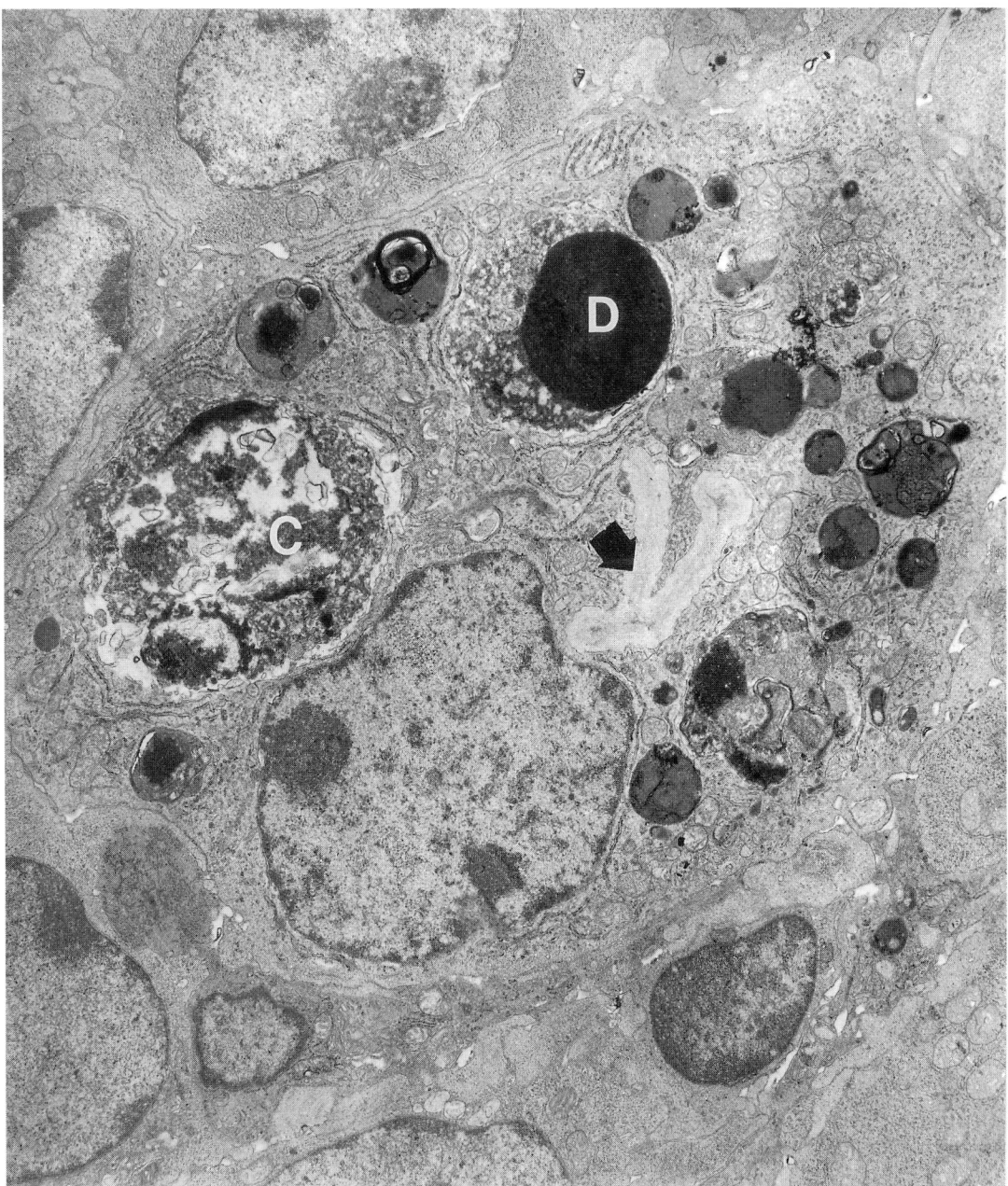

Fig. 4.11 Electron micrograph of macrophage in dome of mouse Peyer's patch follicle. Fluffy masses of carbon (C), and cellular debris (D) are seen in the cytoplasm. The configuration at the arrow indicates vigorous uptake activity. Provided through the courtesy of Drs R Hammer, ME LeFevre and DD Joel.

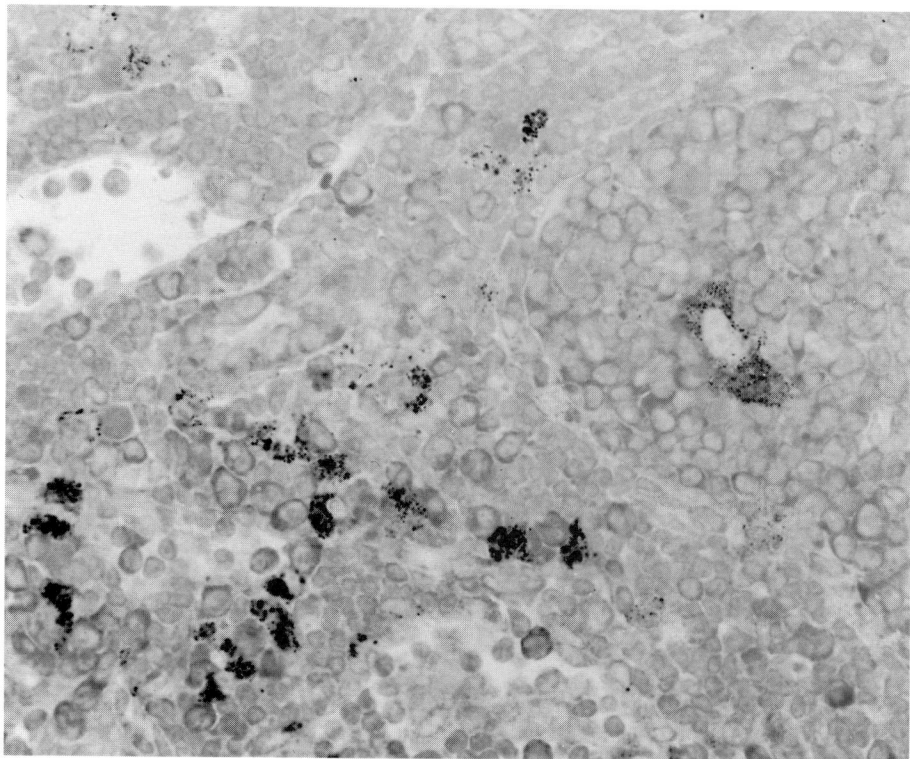

Fig. 4.12 Dense accumulations of carbon particles are seen in a mesenteric lymph node from a mouse after long-term ingestion of carbon. Provided through the courtesy of Drs ME LeFevre and DD Joel.

cytoplasm in addition to the degenerating cells. Carbon-particle-laden macrophages were identified in mesenteric lymph nodes (Fig. 4.12). After cessation of carbon feeding, clearance of carbon from the subepithelial zone took over two months. Carbon particles could be identified in the dome epithelium 40 days after termination of carbon exposure. It is possible that this carbon was in intraepithelial macrophages, but the histological technique did not allow this to be verified or denied.

Uptake of organic material by Peyer's patch macrophages has been demonstrated in several studies. Kimura [46] studied rabbit Peyer's patches after intravenous immunization with a bacterial antigen and subsequent oral administration of killed bacteria. The number of intraepithelial macrophages increased, and phagocytosed bacteria could be found in the intraepithelial and subepithelial macrophages of immunized animals, but not of controls.

Intraepithelial macrophages may phagocytose and degrade cells which they encounter in the epithelial layer, including plasma cells (Fig. 4.13). Ferritin, administered as a tracer in the intestinal lumen, may be transmitted through follicle-associated epithelium (FAE) cells to the intracellular space, where intraepithelial macrophages may internalize it (Fig. 4.14).

Experimental infection with Giardia. Owen et al [67] studied the reaction by Peyer's patches in mice experimentally infected with *Giardia muris.* These organisms inserted themselves between epithelial cells near dying and desquamating columnar cells. Macrophages beneath the basal lamina extended pseudopods into the epithelial layer to engulf the *Giardia.* Some macrophages entered the epithelium for phagocytosis. Macrophages containing remnants of digested organisms could be identified deep in the follicle dome.

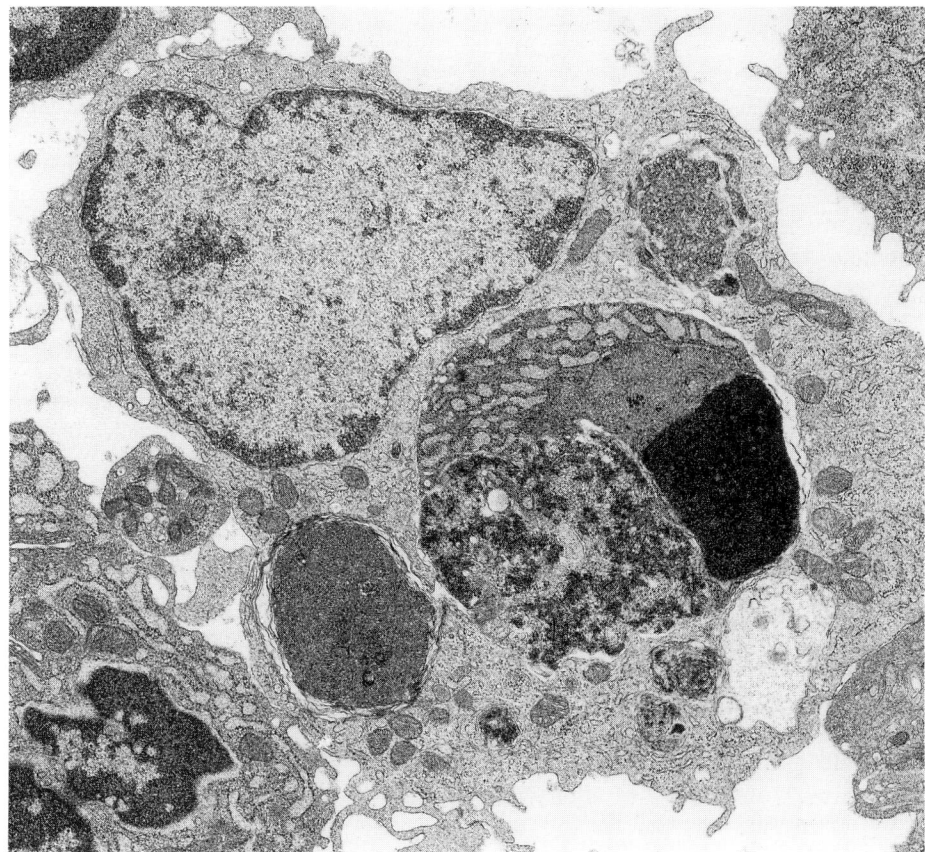

Fig. 4.13 Electron micrograph of macrophage within the epithelium covering a dome in a rat Peyer's patch. Cellular debris, including the remnants of a plasma cell, are seen in the cytoplasm. × 9000. Reproduced from [49], with kind permission of the editor of *Cell and Tissue Research*.

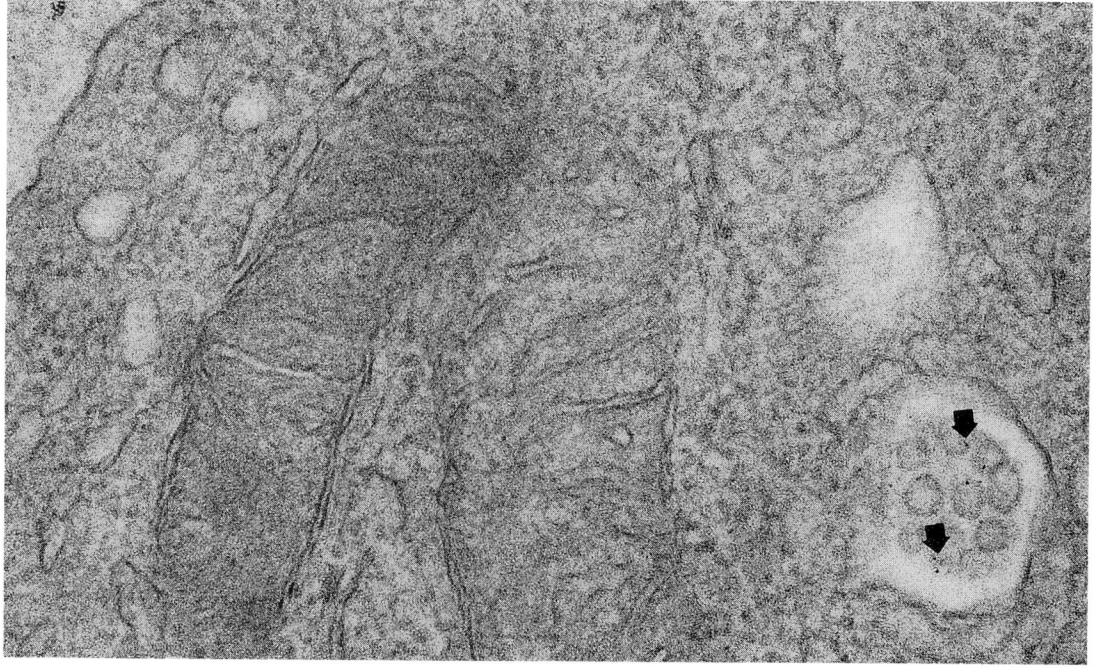

Fig. 4.14 Part of an intraepithelial macrophage from a rat given ferritin in the gut lumen 1 hour prior to sacrifice. Tiny dense dots representing ferritin molecules are seen in the intercellular space (upper left) and in a multivesicular body (arrows). × 57 000. Reproduced from [49], with kind permission of the editor of *Cell and Tissue Research*.

Accessory cell function in Peyer's patches

Peyer's patch macrophages are capable of accessory cell function. There is ample evidence, however, that differences exist between Peyer's patches and other lymphoid organs with respect to the methods necessary to prepare functional macrophages, the in vitro techniques necessary to reveal those functions and perhaps in the nature of the accessory cells.

Antigen presentation: differences from other macrophages

Kagnoff and Campbell [42] prepared cells from spleen and Peyer's patches similarly, by mechanical disruption, to compare the capabilities of each to produce antibodies to erythrocytes in vitro. While spleen cells could perform this function, Peyer's patch cells could not, until adherent peritoneal cells or 2-mercaptoethanol were added. Cytotoxic allograft reactions in vitro also were deficient. Similarly, spleen cells, but not Peyer's patch cells, could display antibody-dependent cell-mediated cytotoxicity [43]. It was suggested that Peyer's patches were deficient in an accessory cell type or types necessary for the generation of these activities.

Tomasi and co-workers [86] found adherent cells from Peyers patches could not present antigens such as ovalbumin, human γ-globulin or purified protein derivative to sensitized lymph node cells, whereas adherent cells from spleen, lymph node and peritoneal exudate induced marked stimulation, indicating antigen presentation. Low density Peyer's patch cells were capable of presenting poly(L-glutamine:L-alanine:L-tyrosine) to T cells, although less efficiently than spleen cells. Low density spleen cells were said to have large numbers of cells (40% or more) with the morphological characteristics of dendritic cells, while Peyer's patch low density cells had less than 5%. Steinman and Cohn [80] reported that dendritic cells occupied 1.0–1.6% of total nucleated cells in spleen and 0.1–0.2% in Peyer's patches.

Complete accessory cell function?

Evidence for more complete accessory cell function has been presented by other workers. Richman et al [71] compared Peyer's patch macrophages with spleen macrophages in their ability to present ovalbumin to primed lymph node cells. Macrophages prepared from Peyer's patches by collagenase digestion were able to present antigen at least as well as those from spleen. Cells prepared from Peyer's patches not incubated with collagenase frequently were unable to present antigen. Furthermore, these workers demonstrated that Peyer's patch macrophages from animals fed ovalbumin could stimulate primed lymph node cells without the need for antigen to be added in vitro.

Other clear evidence that the macrophages of Peyer's patches show accessory cell function has come from study of the cell populations after dispersal of tissue by a neutral protease [47, 59]. In vitro cultures prepared in this manner demonstrated plaque-forming cell responses similar to those in spleen cell cultures. Priming mice orally with sheep erythrocytes prior to in vitro exposure to sheep erythrocytes produced high IgA plaque-forming cell responses. The enzymatic extraction of Peyer's patches produced greater than 10-fold higher numbers of esterase-positive macrophages than conventional methods.

Heterogeneity of Peyer's patch macrophages

Peyer's patch macrophages are heterogeneous in a number of ways, as judged by characteristics such as adherence, expression of Ia antigens, non-specific esterase and phagocytosis [26, 48, 49, 68]. Accessory cell function may be carried out by Peyer's patch cells which are low density, non-adherent and lack Fc receptors [78, 86]. It seems quite possible that the macrophages (in the broad sense of the term) in GALT may differ from their counterparts in other lymphoid organs because of a heterogeneity generated by the extent of differentiation of characteristic features, interacting with the local microenvironment. It also should be kept in mind, as elucidated by Challacombe [15], that the nature of the antigen may well have an effect on the reactivity by GALT.

MACROPHAGES ASSOCIATED WITH MAMMARY GLANDS

Milk and colostrum have remarkably large quantities of IgA and many cells. IgA antibodies and cellular immunity may be transferred from the mother through colostrum and milk to the offspring soon after birth [65]. The cells in colostrum and milk include macrophages, neutrophils, lymphocytes and epithelial cells [22, 38, 73, 75]. Total leukocyte counts in early postpartum colostrum range from 500 to 8000 per mm³. Macrophages and neutrophils are the predominant cell types. Eosinophils are seen occasionally.

Colostral and milk macrophages

Colostral and milk macrophages range from 8 to 40 μm in diameter; most are mononuclear, but the larger ones may be multinucleate and have ingested cellular material in their cytoplasm [38]. Leukocytes penetrate the epithelium of mammary gland to gain access to the lumina of the alveoli and ducts even before lactation begins (Fig. 4.15) [73]. The cytoplasm of many of the macrophages becomes filled with numerous, rather uniform, fat droplets (Fig. 4.16). Neutrophils also display lipid-containing vacuoles. Colostral macrophages are positive for non-specific esterase and acid phosphatase. Many do not adhere to glass readily [22]. They are phagocytic, capable of including newly presented material in the cytoplasm along with the numerous lipid droplets [38]. Breast milk macrophages have demonstrable Ia (DR) antigens on their surfaces [4]. Macrophages and lymphocytes may be shown to interact by cell–cell contact [22, 76]. Milk macrophages have been shown to act as accessory cells in T cell proliferative responses [60]. While they are deficient in sti-

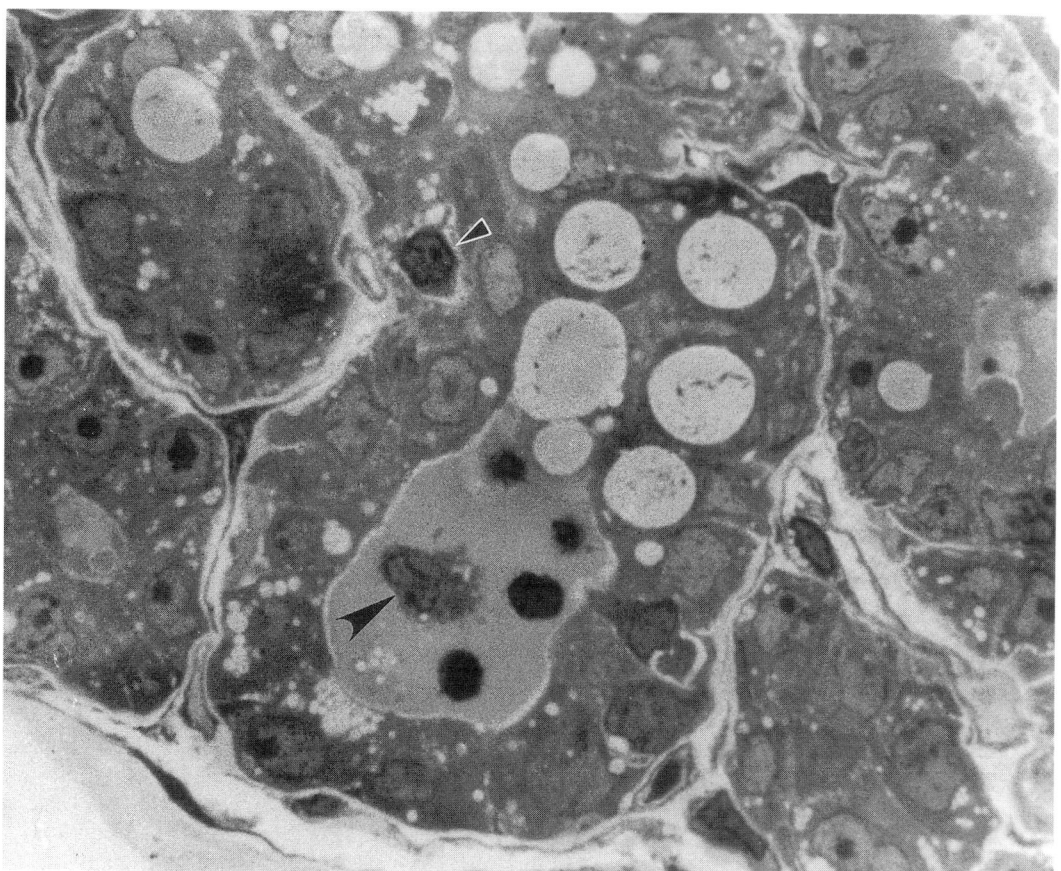

Fig. 4.15 Light micrograph showing a portion of human mammary gland late in pregnancy. A macrophage is present in the alveolar lumen (large arrow). Leukocytes are migrating through the epithelium (small arrow). × 1000. Reproduced from [73], with kind permission of the editor of *Biology of Reproduction*.

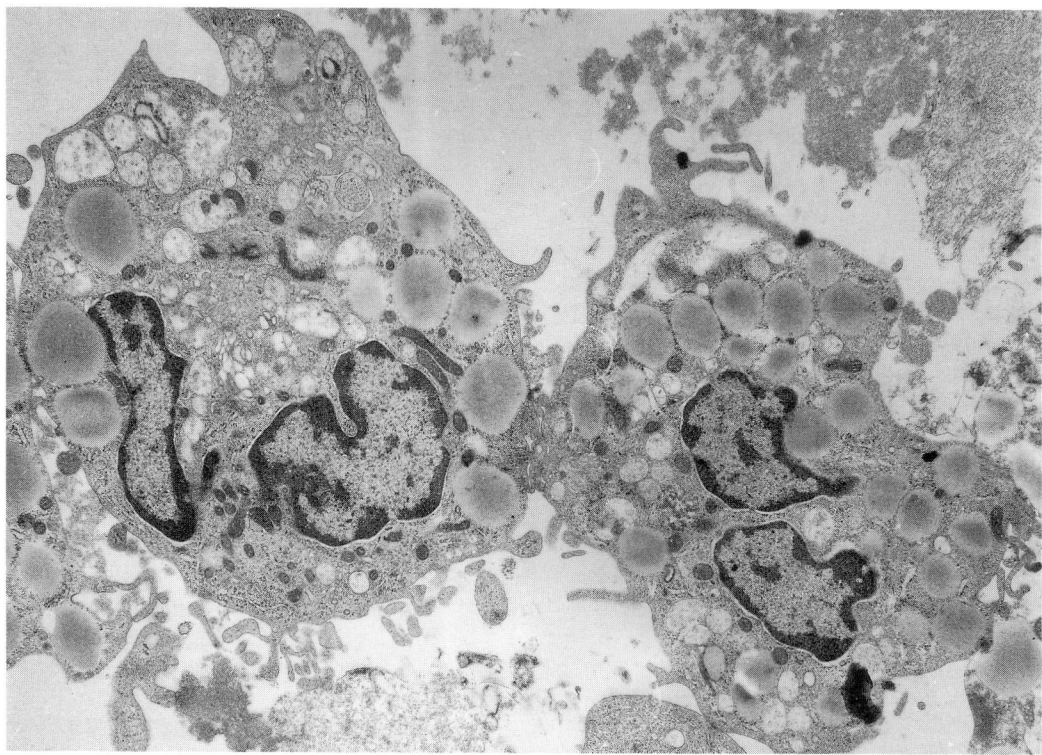

Fig. 4.16 Electron micrograph of macrophages from milk of rat. Fat vacuoles are prominent in the cytoplasm. × 10 500. Provided through the courtesy of Dr L Seelig.

mulating tumoricidal activity [4], they may mediate antibody-dependent cytotoxicity [56].

Mammary gland macrophages

Macrophages from the mammary glands contain large quantities of IgA which is released during phagocytosis [69, 92]. It has been suggested, in fact, that macrophages may be important in the mammary glands as transporters of immunoglobulin [69]. This possibility has not been ruled out, but the coincidental appearance of immunoglobulins with secretory component in macrophages has been advanced as an argument for the case that uptake occurred after transport of IgA through epithelial cells [22]. Brandtzaeg [12] reported that he found no evidence for a significant role of macrophages in the translocation of IgA into colostrum in the mammary gland tissue taken from a woman early in her eighth month of pregnancy. Some intraepithelial and intraluminal IgA-positive macrophages were found in ducts adjacent to occasional interlobular accumulations of macrophages in the mammary gland tissue taken from a woman who had been breast feeding regularly for eight months.

Summary. Although macrophages from the mammary gland obviously have characteristics which allow them to participate in immune reactivity, the full extent of their role in protection of the infant is not yet appreciated. Part of this activity may take place in the gut lumen. Colostrum and milk have non-immunological protective factors as well. The non-specific defence factors, lysozyme and lactoferrin, must be derived, at least in part, from the macrophages and neutrophils.

MACROPHAGE INVOLVEMENT IN DIGESTIVE SYSTEM DISEASES

Macrophages clearly are involved in a number of disease processes associated with the digestive system. LeFevre et al [51] have reviewed some of these relationships in the small intestine. Macrophages certainly may be affected by materials introduced orally. For example, long-term use of anthraquinone laxatives may cause marked accumulation of brownish lipofuscin-bearing macrophages in the gut mucosa, a condition known as melanosis coli

[94]. Bacterial toxins, as well as pathogenic microorganisms, may be reacted to by macrophages immediately upon passing the epithelial barrier.

Focal role of GALT

It is interesting that GALT seems to be an initial focus for some intestinal diseases. Tubercle bacilli seem to establish the initial lesions in lymphoid follicles [83]. It is likely that the earliest lesions of Crohn's disease (regional enteritis) are in solitary lymphoid follicles and Peyer's patches [35,61]. Carter and Collins [14] observed that Peyer's patches seemed to be intimately involved in the establishment of the primary focus of infection by *Salmonella enteritidis* in mice.

Uptake by macrophages is not sufficient for protection, however, for it does not necessarily signify the killing of the organisms [37]. Live tubercle bacilli may be carried by macrophages until cell-mediated immunity is induced [51]. The characteristic bacilli of Whipple's disease [24] may crowd the cytoplasm of gut-associated macrophages and not be killed. Although macrophages may be shown to degrade viruses very rapidly [31], they also may be the vector for virus replication and spread.

Epithelioid and giant cells

The reaction carried out by macrophages in gastrointestinal diseases frequently involves the formation of epithelioid cells and giant cells. Sarcoidosis has been described as a high turnover granuloma of macrophages and their derivatives, although the stimulus for this turnover remains a mystery [79]. The characteristic lesions of intestinal tuberculosis are granulomas. Examination of surgical specimens from patients with ulcerative colitis and Crohn's disease usually will reveal granulomas composed of epithelioid and giant cells [62]. Production of these lesions through recruitment of monocytes is followed by differentiation in situ into macrophages which fuse with each other to form multinucleated giant cells [58]. Figure 4.17 shows a granuloma in the small intestine.

Although the stimulus for granuloma formation is the bacillus in the case of tuberculosis, the stimulus is not known for ulcerative colitis and Crohn's disease. It would seem reasonable that some inciting agent which affects macrophages would be involved.

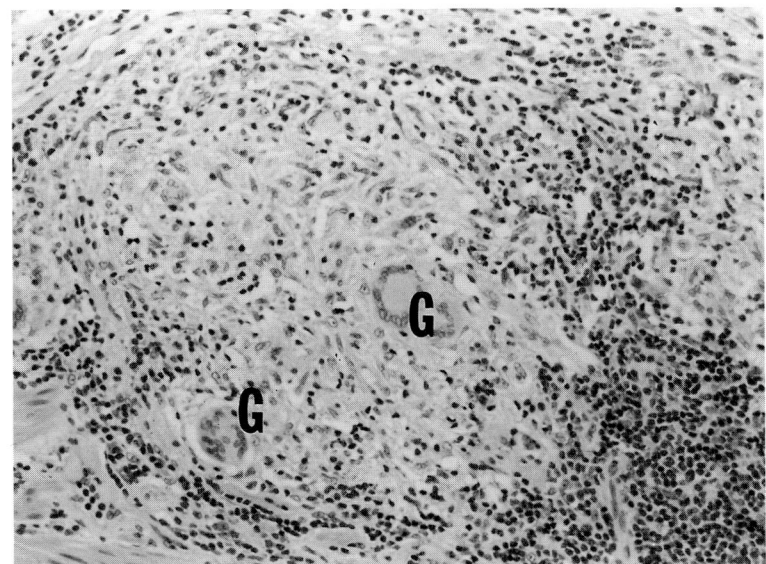

Fig. 4.17 Granuloma from human small intestine. Multinucleated giant cells (G) are surrounded by epithelioid cells. Lymphocyte infiltration is greatest at lower right. Provided through the courtesy of Dr Luther Mills.

Conclusions

There can be little doubt that gut-associated macrophages are active participants in gastrointestinal function. Reaction to the contents of the gut lumen begins with macrophages once the material has traversed the epithelial barrier. Depending upon the nature of the material and the previous experience and capabilities of the responding macrophages, the reaction may take many directions. It may be immunologically specific or generalized. It may provide immediate protection or delayed reactivity, or be the focus of continuing difficulty.

Despite the obvious involvement of macrophages in the well-being of the gastrointestinal tract and the whole organism, we are only now learning enough about their characteristics and behaviour to think about manipulating conditions to enhance protection. Macrophages from the lamina propria of the gut only recently have been prepared successfully for in vitro study. Although macrophages in Peyer's patches certainly are important in day-to-day gut immunity, their characteristics and capabilities, and therefore their true functions, remain uncertain. Indeed, the macrophages which are studied as though coming from Peyer's patches in reality are only enriched for true follicular macrophages, because the current technique of dissecting grossly visible Peyer's patches includes villi and crypts along with the follicles. Lamina propria macrophages are thereby mixed with follicular macrophages.

It is particularly striking to note the paucity of our detailed knowledge about the role which macrophages play in food intolerance and immunity to foods. Most of the information available now centres on changes in general microscopic morphology of the mucosa, such as decrease in the height of villi.

Through application of recently developed techniques, and by approaching the problems with a clear understanding of the capacities displayed by macrophages studied in other connections, it should be possible to develop precise understandings rapidly, and this should provide a good platform for suggesting those factors which must be included in the manipulation necessary for the best approach to food intolerance and immunity.

Acknowledgement

Supported by Fogarty Senior International Fellowship TW00789, NIH, for work in INSERM Unité de Recherche de Pathologie Digestive, Marseille, France (Professor Henri Sarles, Director).

REFERENCES

1 Abe K, Ito T: Fine structure of the dome in Peyer's patches of mice. Arch Histol Jpn 1978; 41:195-204.

2 Bienenstock J, Dolezel J: Peyer's patches: lack of specific antibody-containing cells after oral and parenteral immunization. J Immunol 1971: 106:938-45.

3 Biondi A, Rossing TH, Bennett J, Todd RF III: Surface membrane heterogeneity among human mononuclear phagocytes. J Immunol 1984; 132:1237-43.

4 Biondi A, Peri G, Colombo J et al: Antibody-dependent and independent cytotoxicity of human mononuclear phagocytes: defective stimulation of tumoricidal activity in milk macrophages. Clin Exp Immunol 1982; 50:701.

5 Bockman DE: Range of function of gut-associated lymphoepithelial tissue. In: Solomon JB, ed. Aspects of developmental and comparative immunology I. Oxford: Pergamon Press, 1980; 273-7.

6 Bockman DE: Functional histology of appendix. Arch Histol Jpn 1983; 46:271-92.

7 Bockman DE, Boydston WR: Participation of follicle associated epithelium (FAE), macrophages, and plasma cells in the function of appendix. Scan Electron Microsc 1982; 3:1341-50.

8 Bockman DE, Cooper MD: Pinocytosis by epithelium associated with lymphoid follicles in the bursa of Fabricius, appendix, and Peyer's patches. An electron microscopic study. Am J Anat 1973; 136:455-78.

9 Bockman DE, Winborn WB: Light and electron microscopy of intestinal ferritin absorption. Observations in sensitized and non-sensitized hamsters (*Mesocricetus auratus*). Anat Rec 1966; 155:603-22.

10 Bockman DE, Boydston WR, Beezhold DH: The role of epithelial cells in gut-associated immune reactivity. Ann NY Acad Sci 1983; 409:129-43.

11 Bockman DE, Lause DB, Doran JE, Waldrep JC: Preparation of protein-coated zymogen granules for use in studies of phagocytosis, vascular distribution and adherence techniques. J Reticuloendothel Soc 1979; 26:539-48.

12 Brandtzaeg P: The secretory immune system of lactating human mammary glands compared with other exocrine organs. Ann NY Acad Sci 1983; 409:353-82.

13 Capron A, Dessaint J-P, Capron M: Specific IgE antibodies in immune adherence of normal macrophages to *Schistosoma mansoni* schistosomules. Nature 1975; 253:474-5.

14 Carter PB, Collins FM: The route of enteric infection in normal mice. J Exp Med 1974; 139:1189-203.

15 Challacombe SJ: Salivary antibodies and systemic tolerance in mice after oral immunization with bacterial antigens. Ann NY Acad Sci 1983; 409:177-92.

16 Chin KN, Hudson G: Ultrastructure of Peyer's patches in the normal mouse. Acta Anat (Basel) 1971; 78:306-18.

17 Cohn ZA: The structure and function of monocytes and macrophages. Adv Immunol 1968; 9:163-214.

18 Cohn ZA: The activation of mononuclear phagocytes: fact, fancy and future. J Immunol 1978; 121:813-6.

19 Cohn ZA, Hirsch JG, Fedorko ME: The in vitro differentiation of mononuclear phagocytes. IV. J Exp Med 1966; 123:747-57.

20 Collan Y: Characteristics of nonepithelial cells in the epithelium of normal rat ileum. Scand J Gastroenterol [Suppl 18] 1972; 7:1-66.

21 Crabb ED, Kelsall MA: Organization of the mucosa and lymphatic structures in the rabbit appendix. J Morphol 1940; 67:351-67.

22 Crago SS, Prince SJ, Pretlow TG et al: Human colostral cells. I. Separation and characterization. Clin Exp Immunol 1979; 38:585-97.

23 Deane HW: Some electron microscopic observations of the lamina propria of the gut, with comments on the close association of macrophages, plasma cells and eosinophils. Anat Rec 1964; 149:453-74.

24 Dobbins WO, Kawanishi H: Bacillary characteristics in Whipple's disease: an electron microscopic study. Gastroenterology 1981; 80:1468-75.

25 Donnellan WL: The structure of the colonic mucosa. The epithelium and subepithelial reticulohistiocytic complex. Gastroenterology 1965; 49:496-514.

26 Eldridge JH, Lee, Y, Kiyono H et al: Peyer's patch accessory cells bear Ia. Ann NY Acad Sci 1983; 409:819-21.

27 Fanger MW, Goldstine SN, Shen L: The properties and role of receptors for IgA on human leukocytes. Ann NY Acad Sci 1983; 409:552-62.

28 Fanger MW, Shen L, Pugh J, Bernier GM: Subpopulations of human peripheral granulocytes and monocytes express receptors for IgA. Proc Natl Acad Sci USA 1980; 77:3640-44.

29 Faulk WP, McCormick JN, Goodman Jr et al: Peyer's patches: morphologic studies. Cell Immunol 1970; 1:500-20.

30 Flotte TJ, Springer TA, Thorbecke GJ: Dendritic cell and macrophage staining by monoclonal antibodies in tissue sections and epidermal sheets. Am J Pathol 1983; 111:112-24.

31 Friend DS, Rosenau W, Winfield JS, Moon HD: Uptake and degradation of T2 bacteriophage by rat peritoneal macrophages. I. Electron microscopic and immunologic studies. Lab Invest 1969; 20:275-82.

32 Golder JP, Doe WF: Isolation and preliminary characterization of human intestinal macrophages. Gastroenterology 1983; 84: 795-802.

33 Goldstine SN, Tsai A, Kemp CJ, Fanger MW: Role of IgA antibody in phagocytosis by human polymorphonuclear leukocytes. Ann NY Acad Sci 1983; 409:824.

34 Griffiss JM: Biologic function of the serum IgA system: modulation of complement-mediated effector mechanisms and conservation of antigenic mass. Ann NY Acad Sci 1983; 409:697-707.

35 Hadfield G: The primary histological lesion of regional ileitis. Lancet 1939; ii:773-5.

36 Hammer R, Joel DD, LeFevre ME: Ultrastructure of macrophages of the murine Peyer's patch dome. Exp Cell Biol 1983; 51:61-9.

37 Haque A, Ouaissi A, Joseph M et al: IgE antibody in eosinophil- and macrophage-mediated in vitro killing of *Dipetalonema viteae* microfilariae. J Immunol 1981; 127:716-25.

38 Ho FCS, Wong RLC, Lawton JWM: Human colostral and breast milk cells. A light and electron microscopic study. Acta Paediatr Scand 1979; 68:389-96.

39 Hoover DL, Ganguly R, Foss JF: Microbicidal capacity and acid hydrolase content of human blood monocytes and peritoneal macrophages. J Reticuloendothel Soc 1982; 31:99-105.

40 Hopper KE, Geczy CL, Davies WA: A mechanism of migration inhibition in delayed-type hypersensitivity reactions. I. Fibrin deposition on the surface of elicited peritoneal macrophages in vivo. J Immunol 1981; 126:1052-8.

41 Joel DD, Laissue JA, LeFevre ME: Distribution and fate of ingested carbon particles in mice. J Reticuloendothel Soc 1978; 24:477–87.

42 Kagnoff MF, Campbell S: Functional characteristics of Peyer's patch lymphoid cells. I. Induction of humoral antibody and cell-mediated allograft reactions. J Exp Med 1974; 139:398–406.

43 Kagnoff MF, Campbell S: Antibody-dependent cell-mediated cytotoxicity. Comparative ability of murine Peyer's patch and spleen cells to lyse lipopolysaccharide-coated and uncoated erythrocytes. Gastroenterology 1976; 70:341–6.

44 Karnovsky ML, Lazdins JK: Biochemical criteria for activated macrophages. J Immunol 1978; 121:809–13.

45 Keren DF, Holt PS, Collins HH et al: The role of Peyer's patches in the local immune response of rabbit ileum to live bacteria. J Immunol 1978; 120:1892–6.

46 Kimura A: The epithelial-macrophagic relationship in Peyer's patches: an immunopathological study. Bull Osaka Med Sch 1977; 23:67–91.

47 Kiyono H, McGhee JR, Wannemeuhler MJ et al: In vitro immune responses to a T cell-dependent antigen by cultures of dissassociated murine Peyer's patch. Proc Natl Acad Sci USA 1982; 79:596–600.

48 Krco CJ, Challacombe SJ, Lafuse WP et al: Expression of Ia antigens by mouse Peyer's patch cells. Cell Immunol 1981; 57:420–6.

49 Lause DB, Bockman DE: Heterogeneity, position, and functional capability of the macrophages in Peyer's patches. Cell Tissue Res 1981; 218:557–66.

50 LeFevre ME, Joel DD: The Peyer's patch epithelium: an imperfect barrier. In: Schiller M, ed. Toxicology of Intestinal Function. New York: Raven Press, 1984; 45–46.

51 LeFevre ME, Hammer R, Joel DD: Macrophages of the mammalian small intestine: a review. J Reticuloendothel Soc 1979; 26:553–73.

52 Lemaire G, Drapier J-C, Tenu J-P et al: Stimulation of several functional properties of macrophages after injection of a suspension of killed streptococci. J Reticuloendothel Soc 1982; 32:87–99.

53 Li CY, Lam KW, Yam LT: Esterases in human leukocytes. J Histochem Cytochem 1973; 21:1–12.

54 Lowell GH, Smith LS, Griffiss JM, Brandt BL: IgA-dependent monocyte-mediated antibacterial activity. J Exp Med 1980; 152:452–7.

55 Lowell GH, Smith LS, Griffiss JM, Brandt BL: Antibody-dependent mononuclear cell-mediated anti meningococcal activity. Comparison of the lytic effects of convalescent and post-immunization immunoglobulins G, M and A. J Clin Invest 1980; 66:260–7.

56 Mandyla H, Xanthou M, Maravelias C et al: Antibody-dependent cytotoxicity of human colostrum phagocytes. Pediatr Res 1982; 16:995.

57 Mestecky J, Kutteh WH, Brown TA et al: Function and biosynthesis of polymeric IgA. Ann NY Acad Sci 1983; 409:292–305.

58 Meunet G, Bitzi A, Hammer G: Macrophage turnover in Crohn's disease and ulcerative colitis. Gastroenterology 1978; 74:501–3.

59 Michalek SM, McGhee JR, Kiyono H et al: The IgA response: inductive aspects, regulatory cells, and effector functions. Ann NY Acad Sci 1983; 409:48–71.

60 Mori M, Hayward AR: Phenotype and function of human milk monocytes as antigen presenting cells. Clin Immunol Immunopathol 1982; 23:94.

61 Morson BC: Regional enteritis (Crohn's disease). Skandia International Symposia 1970; 15–33.

62 Morson BC: Regional enteritis (Crohn's disease). Part I. Pathology. In: Bockus HL, ed. Gasteroenterology, Vol. 2, Philadelphia: WB Saunders, 1976; 550–61.

63 Nathan CF, Murray HW, Cohn ZA: The macrophage as an effector cell. NEngl J Med 1980; 303:622–6.

64 North RJ: The concept of the activated macrophage. J Immunol 1978; 121:806–9.

65 Ogra SS, Weintraub D, Ogra PL: Immunologic aspects of human colostrum and milk. III. Fate and absorption of cellular and soluble components in the gastrointestinal tract of the newborn. J Immunol 1977; 119:245–8.

66 Owen RL: Macrophage function in Peyer's patch epithelium. Adv Exp Med Biol 1982; 149:507–13.

67 Owen RL, Allen CL, Stevens DP: Phagocytosis of *Giardia muris* by macrophages in Peyer's patch epithelium in mice. Infect Immun 1981; 33:591–601.

68 Pappo J, Ebersole J, Taubman M, Smith D: Isolation and characterization of M cells and macrophages in rat Peyer's patches. Fed Proc 1982; 41:434.

69 Pittard WB, Polmar SH, Fanaroff AA: The breast milk macrophage: a potential vehicle for immunoglobulin transport. J Reticuloendothel Soc 1977; 22:597–603.

70 Reynolds HY, Atkinson JP, Newball HH, Frank MM: Receptors for immunoglobulin and complement on human alveolar macrophages. J Immunol 1975; 114:1813–20.

71 Richman LK, Graeff AS, Strober W: Antigen presentation by macrophage-enriched cells from the mouse Peyer's patch. Cell Immunol 1981; 62:110–8.

72 Sawicki W, Kucharczyk K, Szamska K, Kujawa M: Lamina propria macrophages of intestine of guinea pig. Gastroenterology 1977; 73:1340–4.

73 Seelig LL Jr, Beer AE: Intraepithelial leukocytes in the human mammary gland. Biol Reprod 1981; 24:1157–63.

74 Shimizu Y, Andrew W: Studies on the rabbit appendix. I. Lymphocyte-epithelial relationships and the transport of bacteria from lumen to lymphoid nodule. J Morphol 1967; 123:231–50.

75 Smith CW, Goldman AS: The cells of human colostrum. I. In vitro studies of morphology and functions. Pediatr Res 1968; 2:103–9.

76 Smith CW, Goldman AS: Interactions of lymphocytes and macrophages from human colostrum: characteristics of the interacting lymphocyte. J Reticuloendothel Soc 1970; 8:91.

77 Sobhon P: The light and the electron microscopic studies of Peyer's patches in non-germ-free adult mice. J Morphol 1971; 135:457–82.

78 Spalding DM, Koopman WJ, McGhee JR: Identification of a nonadherent accessory cell in murine Peyer's patches. Ann NY Acad Sci 1983; 409:880–1.

79 Spector WG: Epithelioid cells, giant cells, and sarcoidosis. Ann NY Acad Sci 1976; 278:3–6.

80 Steinman RM, Cohn ZA: Identification of a novel cell type in peripheral lymphoid organs of mice. I. Morphology, quantification, tissue distribution. J Exp Med 1973; 137:1142–62.

81 Takeuchi A, Jervis HR, Sprinz H: The globule leukocyte in the intestinal mucosa of the cat: a histochemical, light and electron microscopic study. Anat Rec 1969; 164:79–100.

82 Takeuchi A, Sprinz H, LaBrec EH, Formal SB: Experimental bacillary dysentery. An electron microscopic study of the response of the intestinal mucosa to bacterial invasion. Am J Pathol 1965; 47:1011–44.

83 Tandon HD, Prakash A: Pathology of intestinal tuberculosis and its distinction from Crohn's disease. Gut 1972; 13:260–9.

84 Tew JG, Torbecke GJ, Steinman RM: Dendritic cells in the immune response: characteristics of recommended nomenclature (A report from the Reticuloendothelial Society Committee on Nomenclature). J Reticuloendothel Soc 1982; 31:371–80.

85 Tlaskalova-Hogenova H, Sterzl J, Stepankova R et al: Development of immunological capacity under germfree and conventional conditions. Ann NY Acad Sci 1983; 409:96–113.

86 Tomasi TB, Barr WG, Challacombe SJ, Curran G: Oral tolerance and accessory-cell function of Peyer's patches. Ann NY Acad Sci 1983; 409:145–63.

87 Trier JS, Phelps PC, Rubin CE: Electron microscopy of mucosa of small intestine. J Am Med Assoc 1963; 183:768–74.

88 Unanue ER: The regulatory role of macrophages in antigenic stimulation II. Symbiotic relationship between lymphocytes and macrophages. Adv Immunol 1981; 31:1–136.

89 van Furth R: Origin and kinetics of mononuclear phagocytes. Ann NY Acad Sci 1976; 278:161–75.

90 Vray B, Hrabak A, Coquette A: Expression of Fc and C3b receptors and intracellular distribution of bacteria in rat macrophages. Adv Exp Med Biol 1982; 141:567–73.

91 Watanabe Y, Tashiro Y: An electron microscopic observation of the lymphoid tissue from the rabbit appendix. Recent Adv Respir Res 1971; 10:51–80.

92 Weaver EA, Goldblum RM, Davis CP, Goldman AS: Enhanced immunoglobulin A release from human colostral cells during phagocytosis. Infect Immun 1981; 34:498–502.

93 Wicha MS, Huard TK: Macrophages express cell surface laminin. Exp Cell Res 1983; 143:475–90.

94 Wijesinha SS, Steer HW: Observations on the immunocytes and macrophages in megacolon. Dis Colon Rectum 1982; 25:312–20.

95 Wilton JMA: Suppression by IgA of IgG-mediated phagocytosis by human polymorphonuclear leucocytes. Clin Exp Immunol 1978; 34:423–8.

96 Winter HS, Cole FS, Huffer LM et al: Isolation and characterization of resident macrophages from guinea pig and human intestine. Gastroenterology 1983; 85:358–63.

Chapter 5
Intestinal Mast Cells in Pathology and Host Resistance

Dean Befus, Fred Pearce and John Bienenstock

Introduction

Until recently the roles of mast cells have received little consideration in discussion of intestinal immunity and pathology. However, understanding of mast-cell biology is evolving rapidly and mast cells, because of their virtually ubiquitous distribution throughout the body, responsiveness to diverse stimuli and content of potent mediators, are involved in most, if not all, inflammatory responses and pathological conditions. One central theme of current research is that mast-cell populations are composed of functionally distinct subtypes. This is perhaps not surprising if one considers the lymphocyte as an analogy. The best examples of mast-cell heterogeneity involve comparisons between intestinal mucosal and peritoneal mast cells in the rat [6, 15, 28, 50, 75]. These differences in mast-cell characteristics have important implications in the pathogenesis and treatment of intestinal and other diseases.

Despite considerable information to the contrary, mast cells are still widely viewed with the conceptual restrictions that solely consider their role in IgE-mediated immediate hypersensitivity reactions. However, it is clear that in addition to immediate reactions, mast cells are involved in late phase components of allergic reactions [53, 106], delayed onset hypersensitivity [3] and regulation of many immune responses [8]. Moreover, mast cells can be cytotoxic [31, 43] or can potentiate eosinophil [18] or macrophage cytotoxic actions [27]. Many different cells can respond to mast-cell mediators. For histamine, one of the many mast-cell mediators, at least two receptor types have been recognized (H_1, H_2) and these are expressed on a variety of cells including lymphocytes, macrophages, neutrophils, basophils, eosinophils, smooth muscle and parietal cells [7, 9]. If one considers other mediators including prostaglandins and leukotrienes, there must be few cell types which are not directly or indirectly influenced by local mast-cell secretions.

The major clinical interests in mast cells have been restricted to allergic reactions [145], parasitic infections [2, 9, 76], mastocytosis, inflammatory conditions such as inflammatory bowel disease [145] and pulmonary fibrosis [39, 42, 57]. In this brief synopsis of mast-cell biology, their characteristics will be reviewed including: mediators, secretory stimuli and ontogeny, differentiation and proliferation. These aspects will be discussed in view of present knowledge of mast-cell heterogeneity and intestinal diseases. We will identify the rapidly changing frontiers of mast-cell research but also will seek to highlight fundamental gaps in our understanding.

APPROACHES TO STUDYING MAST CELLS

Mast-cell heterogeneity

Much of the information which forms the basis of our understanding of mast cells has been derived from studies of rat peritoneal mast cells (Fig. 5.1) and the human peripheral blood basophil. As will be clear from the information to be presented, the characteristics and functions of mast cells vary markedly depending upon the tissue of origin, and species. Moreover, the relationship between mast cells and basophils, both ontogenetically and functionally, is not well understood. Therefore one must be cautious in any extrapolation from studies on rat peritoneal mast cells and human basophils to mast-cell function in intestinal or other diseases of man.

Techniques for mast-cell isolation

To understand more completely the nature and extent of mast-cell heterogeneity and to determine the characteristics of mast cells from different sites (Fig. 5.1), procedures have been developed to isolate cells from different tissues by enzymatic and mechanical means. In some studies at least, successful attempts have been made to enrich mast cells to near homogeneity so that more precise biochemical definition of their properties could be conducted. Intestinal mucosal mast cells have been isolated from rats and man and have been

extensively characterized in the former [13, 64, 88, 89, 113, 114]. Recently, isolated rat intestinal mucosal mast cells have been purified by a combination of procedures based on density and size and it has been confirmed that their unique functional properties are endogenous to the cell and not merely the result of modulation by some other cell types present in the cell suspension [63]. Characterization of isolated human intestinal mast cells has begun [10, 33], although methods for enrichment to near homogeneity are not yet available. Perhaps the combined procedures utilizing cell density and size which have been successfully used for the purification of rat intestinal mucosal mast cells [63], or elutriation, which has been so successful in the enrichment of human lung mast cells [109], will be approriate to purify human intestinal mast cells.

In vitro mast-cell culture

Another approach to studying mast-cell subtypes has been the use of in vitro culture procedures in the rat, mouse and man. In the rat, two mast-cell subtypes have been cultured; one from the thymus, which has characteristics of peritoneal mast cells [49], and another from mesenteric lymph nodes or bone marrow with characteristics of intestinal mucosal mast cells [24, 41]. The growth of the latter is dependent upon a T cell-derived factor(s) which can be generated from the mesenteric lymph node cells of parasitized rats by mitogen or parasite antigens [24, 41]. In the mouse, thymic mast cells similar to peritoneal mast cells can be cultured [36], and mast cells which may be analogous to rat intestinal mucosal mast cells can be cultured from bone marrow, lymph nodes, fetal liver, spleen and the gut mucosa [30, 40, 98, 107, 122]. These cultured mast cells preferentially synthesize the proteoglycan chondroitin sulphate E [99] rather than heparin, and when challenged with antigen to which they have been sensitized by IgE antibody they generate relatively large amounts of leukotriene, LTC_4 [98]. Whether they have an in vivo correlate such as the intestinal mucosal mast-cell subtype, or represent an in vitro anomaly, remains to be established [12, 50].

In man, culture procedures for mast cells are beginning to be developed [22, 24] but as yet they are not widely available and the nature of the cultured cells has not been defined in the context of in vivo equivalence. However, in vitro culture approaches promise to be very useful in the ultimate dissection of mast-

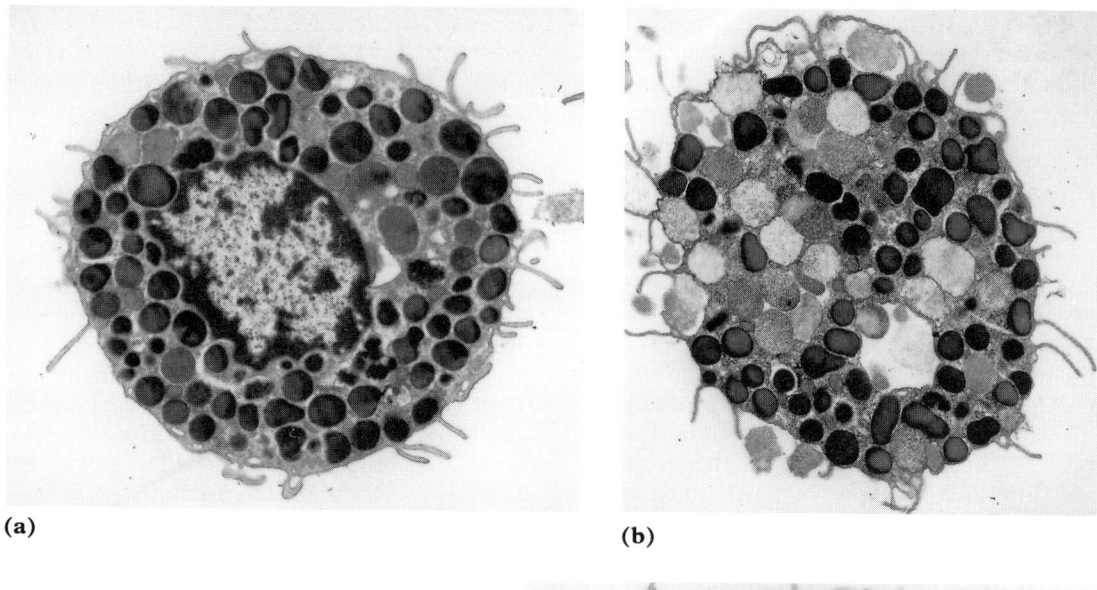

(a)

(b)

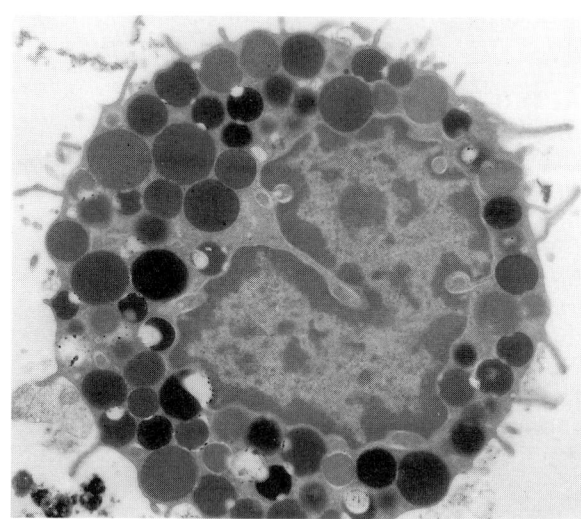

Fig. 5.1 Rat mast cells in various phases of degranulation following activation with specific allergen: (a) peritoneal mast cell in early phase of activation, note variability in granule density; (b) peritoneal mast cell in later phase of exocytosis; (c) isolated intestinal mucosal mast cell, note partial degranulation and lobed nuclear structure. Peritoneal mast cells have an average diameter of 18 μm, whereas intestinal mucosal mast cells are smaller (approximately 12 μm in diameter).

(c)

cell heterogeneity in humans as well as in other species.

MAST-CELL STRUCTURE AND CONTENTS

Proteoglycans

Mature mast cells contain many electron-dense granules (Fig. 5.1) and are easily recognized using dyes such as toluidine blue which can exhibit binding to the proteoglycan constituents of the granules, revealed as metachromasia. The abundance of different proteoglycans varies in different mast-cell populations (Table 5.1). For example, in human lung and in mouse and rat peritoneal mast cells heparin is the major constituent [74], whereas it is absent in rat intestinal mucosal mast cells or those cultured from rat bone marrow. In the mouse, mast cells cultured from bone marrow, fetal liver and immunized lymph node [100] do not contain heparin but contain chondroitin sulphate E [99, 100] and may be analogous to the intestinal mucosal mast-cell subtype best characterized in the rat which contains the proteoglycan, chondroitin sulphate di B (Stevens, Lee, Befus, et al, unpublished observations). Regardless of their precise nature in mast-cell subtypes, these proteoglycans are major constituents of granules and their polyanionic character is important in interactions with other preformed, stored granule moieties.

Table 5.1 Mast-cell heterogeneity: comparisons of different species and anatomical sites.

Characteristic	Mast-cell type			
	Rat		Human	Mouse
	Peritoneum	Gut mucosa	Gut/lung	Bone marrow culture
Histochemistry				
Formalin* sensitivity	−	+	+ and −	+
Staining pH	Up to 7	< 1	Up to 7; < 1	< 1
Proliferation				
Thymus dependency	−	+	?	+
Mediators				
Histamine (pg/cell)	8–24	1–2	1–2	0.1–1.0
Serotonin	+	+	−	+
Arachidonic acid metabolites	PGD$_2$	?	LTC$_4$, PGD$_2$	LTB$_4$, LTC$_4$, PGD$_2$
Proteoglycans	Heparin	Chondroitin sulphate di B	Heparin	Chondroitin sulphate E
Neutral proteases	Chymase I, carboxypeptidase	Chymase II	Tryptase	?

* Mast cells fail to stain by routine techniques when tissues are fixed in formalin.

Biological effects of heparin and chondroitin sulphate

Both heparin and chondroitin sulphate can regulate the alternative pathway of complement activation [140]. Similarly, heparin and chondroitin 6-sulphate inhibit blastogenic responses of lymphocytes to certain mitogens [34]. Heparin will inhibit phagocytosis of unopsonized bacteria by rabbit polymorphonuclear leukocytes [132] and will also inhibit various neutrophil-derived enzymes including acid-glycerophosphatase, acid *p*-nitrophenylphosphatase, *β*-glucuronidase and *N*-acetyl-*β*-D-glucosaminidase (e.g. [138]). Such inhibitory effects of mast-cell-derived proteoglycans may be relevant in modulating tissue damage mediated by eosinophil major basic protein (MBP, [37]) and also the killing of parasites such as the worm *Schistosoma mansoni* [17] and the protozoan *Trypanosoma cruzi* [59]. Recent suggestions that heparin stimulates angiogenesis [5] and thus may facilitate neovascularization of tissues and even tumours [95] defines new exciting lines of mast-cell research.

Mediators

Other preformed moieties stored in mast cells [6, 110] are listed in Table 5.2. Another group of mediators is synthesized de novo by mast cells following activation and these include the cyclooxygenase and lipoxygenase metabolites of arachidonic acid, namely prostaglandins and leukotrienes respectively [110, 124], as well as the phospholipid, platelet-activating factor [83, 110] (Table 5.2).

Table 5.2 Mast-cell mediators.

Preformed	Newly synthesized
Heparin	Platelet-activating factor
Chondroitin sulphate	Arachidonic acid metabolites:
Histamine	(a) Cyclooxygenase pathway—PGD$_2$
Serotonin	(b) Lipoxygenase pathway—LTB$_4$, LTC$_4$
Neutrophil chemotactic factor	
Eosinophil chemotactic factor	
Neutral proteases	
Acid hydrolase	
Peroxidase	
Superoxide dismutase	

Proteases

In addition to the distinct proteoglycan content of at least some mast-cell subtypes, the protease content also distinguishes intestinal mucosal from peritoneal mast cells in the rat [60, 110, 142] (Table 5.1). The serine protease of the intestinal mucosal mast cell (RMCP-II) differs from the serine protease (RMCP-I) found in mast cells in the peritoneal cavity and elsewhere in pH optimum, molecular weight and structure (about 75% amino acid homology). Moreover, RMCP-II is released upon intestinal mast cell activation and can be detected in the circulation [110]. Interestingly there is a marked elevation in serum levels of RMCP-II immediately preceding and during the dramatic loss of worms from the intestine of rats infected with the nematode *Nippostrongylus brasiliensis* [143] suggesting that this enzyme and probably many other mast-cell components are active in generating the microenvironment which leads to worm expulsion. The precise roles of these distinct serine proteases are unknown, although it is interesting that RMCP-II apparently degrades the basal lamina underlying the intestinal epithelium. The pathological implications are obvious.

Histamine and serotonin

Histamine

The many actions of histamine have perhaps received more study than those of any other mast-cell-derived mediator. Because of the abundance of literature in this field [7, 8, 70, 118], the roles of histamine will not be extensively reviewed here. In brief, histamine plays diverse roles, including in gastric acid secretion, chemotaxis, modulation of the microcirculation, influence on fibroblast growth, function as a neurotransmitter, activation of both suppressor and contrasuppressor lymphocytes, induction of auto-anti-idiotypic regulatory antibodies, regulation of alkali secretion in the ileum and even inhibition of lysosomal enzyme release from neutrophils [16, 35, 58, 70, 118, 127].

Serotonin

Another mast-cell amine, serotonin, has received less attention than histamine, although its functions may be as diverse. For example, serotonin stimulates water and sodium secretaion in the jejunum and ileum [25, 61], stimulates smooth muscle contraction in sites such as the rat intestine [11], appears to be important in the killing of fibrosarcoma targets by mast cells [31], inhibits lectin-stimulated lymphocyte proliferation [119] and decreases the expression of IL-2 (interleukin-2) receptors on at least some lymphocytes [119].

Late phase reaction factors

In the last 10 to 12 years, prolonged inflammatory reactions (4–24 hours), in addition to immediate reactions (0.5–1 hour) have been shown to be associated with mast-cell secretion [54]. These late phase reactions can be elicited in rat skin by injection of isolated inflammatory factors derived from purified mast-cell granules. Late phase reactions are complement independent, characterized by an influx of neutrophils initially and monocytes subsequently, and can be markedly diminished in magnitude using a combination of H_1 and H_2 histamine antagonists or corticosteroids [54]. Attempts to define the mediators of late phase reactions derived from mast-cell granules have established that both low and high molecular weight moieties have activity [54, 82]. The low molecular weight moiety consists of 12 amino acids and has a molecular weight of 1407. The larger moiety remains to be characterized. How these factors relate to neutrophil and eosinophil chemotactic factors present in mast cells is unclear at present.

Arachidonic acid metabolites

Heterogeneity of mast-cell mediators

It is not known whether all the other mediators described above are present in all mast-cell subtypes. Rat intestinal mucosal mast cells are known to contain histamine, serotonin, a form of chondroitin sulphate and RMCP-II, but convincing evidence does not exist regarding other preformed mediators, including the mediators of late phase reaction and chemotaxis. No studies of arachidonic acid metabolism or platelet-activating factor have been conducted on purified mast cells derived from the intestinal mucosa, so their repertoire of prostaglandins, leukotrienes and platelet-activating factor is unknown. However, evidence from cultured murine bone marrow-derived mast cells which may be analogous to intestinal mucosal mast cells shows that leukotriene, LTC_4, is a major arachidonic acid metabolite and prostaglandin, PGD_2, is also produced [98], but in lesser amounts. The spectrum of leukotriene and prostaglandin metabolities of arachidonic acid that are or may be produced by mast cells as well as many other cell types is large and their potential activities have been widely reviewed (e.g. [38, 66, 81, 104]). For example, LTC, LTD and LTE are highly potent mediators of smooth muscle contraction in sites such as vessels or bronchi, whereas LTB is chemotactic for and activates neutrophils and eosinophils, and suppresses T lymphocytes.

Effect of leukotrienes on intestinal function

To date there have been fewer studies of the effects of leukotrienes on intestinal functions than on respiratory or vascular physiology, but undoubtedly this will be corrected in the near future. At a recent meeting on intestinal immunity and inflammation it was reported that the mucosal extracts from patients with ulcerative colitis have elevated levels of LTB_4 and corresponding neutrophil chemotactic activity. This is reminiscent of reports of enhanced prostanoid synthesis in active Crohn's disease [144]. Such alterations in arachidonic acid metabolism could be highly relevant in control of mucus secretion by mast cells or other cells [69, 116], especially given the diversity of mediators that influence goblet cells, and evidence that histamine and LTC_4 interact in some manner to enhance mucus release [52].

Effect of mucus on parasitic nematode larvae. The biological activities of such mediators in host resistance may be significant as shown by recent studies of the inhibitory effect of mucus on parasitic nematode larvae [26]. The inhibitory activity was associated with components that have leukotriene-like properties. However, the origins of various arachidonic acid metabolites will be difficult to determine in vivo, so before the role of mast cells in normal intestinal physiology or disease can be clarified, it is essential that isolated and purified mast cells be studied and the mediator content or potential synthetic pathways be defined.

STIMULI FOR MAST-CELL ACTIVATION

Stimulation by antibody and T cell factor

The list of stimuli which induce mast-cell activation and secretion is long and keeps growing [62] (Table 5.3). It is well known that antigen induces mediator secretion from mast cells sensitized with specific IgE antibodies and that IgG antibody is also active in this system under certain conditions [48, 123]. More recently it has been established that an antigen-specific T cell factor also induces mast-cell secretion [4], but that the mechanism of exocytosis differs from IgE-mediated secretion [130] and involves preferential release of serotonin, at least in the mouse [130]. This T cell-mediated mast-cell activation has been investigated most extensively in delayed onset hypersensitivity reactions [131] and obviously its relevance to other immune and inflammatory responses must be defined. Furthermore, as identified above with regard to mediator content, whether various mast-cell subtypes are equally responsive to this T cell-derived secretagogue remains to be studied. By possible analogy, T cell-dependent differentiation and proliferation to date appears to be subtype restricted and has served as a marker to distinguish intestinal mucosal (T cell-dependent) from other (T cell-independent) mast cells [12, 50].

Other selected secretagogues

For experimental purposes secretagogues such as 48/80, concanavalin A, dextran, polylysine and ionophores have been widely studied [62] (Table 5.3), although their direct relevance in vivo is questionable. Nevertheless, they have

Table 5.3 Mast-cell heterogeneity in the rat: factors which induce mediator secretion.

Factor	Mast-cell source	
	Peritoneum	Intestinal mucosa
Antigen, anti-IgE	+ +	+ +
Neutrophil cationic protein, C3a, C5a dextran	+ +	?
48/80, bee venom 401	+ +	0
T cell factor	+ +	?
Ionophores	+ +	+/+ +
Substance P	+ +	+
VIP, somatostatin, bradykinin, neurotensin	+ +	0
Dynorphin, β-endorphin, α-neoendorphin	+ +	0

facilitated study of calcium flux and other biochemical pathways implicated in secretion, and raised questions about chemical basicity as a common factor responsible for the activity of many secretagogues. Furthermore, 48/80 is the most widely studied secretagogue that defines functionally distinct (responsive, e.g. peritoneal; unresponsive, e.g. intestinal mucosal) mast-cell subtypes at least in the rat [87]. Complement fragments C3a and C5a induce mediator release from some mast-cell populations (e.g. chopped rat lung) but not others [86, 105], despite the presence of C3 receptors on at least one unresponsive mast-cell subtype (rat peritoneum, [117]). Neutrophil-derived cationic protein activates some mast cells [96], but comparative studies with various subtypes have not been conducted.

Neuropeptides

Over the last decade various workers studying rat peritoneal mast cells have established that various neuropeptides/hormones induce mediator release and thus must be involved in nervous–immune/inflammatory–endocrine systems communication. Peptides with secretagogue activity include vasoactive intestinal peptide (VIP), neurotensin, substance P, somatostatin, bradykinin, adrenocorticotrophic hormone and parathormone [32, 51, 85, 113]. Recent studies comparing mast-cell subtypes in the rat [113, 115] indicate that only substance P induces mediator release from intestinal mucosal mast cells, despite the large array of peptide hormones which stimulate peritoneal mast cells (Table 5.3).

Neurotensin

There are however reports from a single laboratory [111, 112] that neurotensin stimulates mast-cell degranulation in the human jejunal mucosa. These studies were conducted using histological analysis of tissues treated in vitro with neurotensin and other agents, and employed fixation procedures which would allow detection of only one mast-cell subtype, namely the so-called connective tissue type mast cell. Whether human intestinal mucosal mast cells respond to neurotensin, unlike rat intestinal mucosal mast cells, has not been determined. Moreover, this could not be adequately assessed using histological analysis on formalin-fixed tissues; mediator release in vitro using isolated cells would be more convincing. Alternatively, pharmacological approaches using in vitro preparations of intestinal tissue may be helpful. For example, neurotensin excitation of canine gastric smooth muscle has been shown to be mediated by mast cells using such approaches [68].

Opiate peptides

The opiate peptides, dynorphin, α-neoendorphin and β-endorphin also induce histamine secretion from rat peritoneal mast cells [114, 126], but none has secretagogue activity on isolated rat intestinal mucosal mast cells [114]. The underlying mechanisms of this differing responsiveness among mast cells, as well as its clinical and biological significance require study.

Innervation of mast cells

Recent reports suggest that the direct innervation of mast-cell subtypes occurs [80, 139]. It is not known whether such nerves are cholinergic, adrenergic or peptidergic. The relevance of nerve–mast cell interactions remains to be defined. Evidence that both histamine and serotonin can act as neurotransmitters [134], as well as recent results which imply that histamine release can be a 'learned' response [102], predict that studies of nerve–mast cell interactions will have significant impact upon concepts central to mast-cell biology in health and disease.

EFFECTS OF ANTIALLERGIC COMPOUNDS ON MAST-CELL SUBTYPES

From a therapeutic standpoint it is essential to know if a particular antiallergic drug is efficacious against all mast cells or is restricted in its antisecretory action to only a certain subtype. The corollary is that if a local mast-cell subtype is relevant in a particular disease state, then drugs which modulate its activity must be identified and carefully analysed as a therapeutic measure. Most extensive studies to date have been conducted in the rat [88, 89] where it has been determined that many drugs which inhibit peritoneal mast-cell secretion (e.g. disodium cromoglycate, AH9679, theophyline) are without effect on intestinal mucosal mast cells (Fig. 5.2). Doxantrazole [89] and the flavonoid, quercetin [88], inhibit antigen-induced histamine release by both

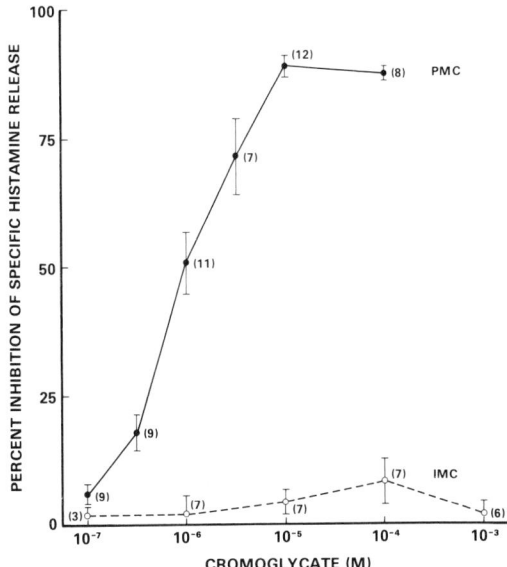

Fig. 5.2 Effect of disodium cromoglycate on antigen-induced (20 WE/ml) histamine release from rat peritoneal mast cells (PMC) (●) and intestinal mucosal mast cells (IMC) (○). Values are mean ± SEM for the number of experiments noted: unblocked releases were 38.5% ± 1.7 (●) and 26.0% ± 2.3 (○). From Pearce et al [89]

[71] has opened new avenues of research because this binding moiety is quintessential for mast-cell exocytosis [72, 73]. Additionally, it has been proposed that cromoglycate acts to inhibit mediator release by inducing the early phosphorylation of an endogenous, secretion-regulating 78 kDa protein [129, 137]. It will be enlightening to determine whether mast-cell subtypes such as the rat intestinal mucosal mast cell or the mouse peritoneal mast cell [65] which are not inactivated by cromoglycate, possess the binding protein or undergo cromoglycate-induced phosphorylation events. Thus, antiallergic drugs such as cromoglycate provide potentially powerful tools to determine the biochemical pathways of mediator secretion and mast-cell heterogeneity.

ONTOGENY, DIFFERENTIATION AND PROLIFERATION

As early as day 16 in utero the rat embryo contains detectable mast cells in the region of the developing spinal cord [20]. Subsequently, mast cells are seen widely distributed throughout the embryo and newborn [20, 133]. The distribution and abundance of mast cells changes in various organs within the first week after birth [133] but the significance of this is unknown. An interesting example which highlights our present ignorance of mast-cell function is the change with age in mast-cell number in specific localities in the rat brain [94] that can be modified by merely handling the newborn [93]. For the intestine, a detailed analysis of the ontogeny of mast cells and RMCP-II in young rats showed that levels are low at birth and progressively increase to reach maximum normal levels by 6 weeks of age [141].

Helminth infection

Infection with many helminth parasites induces a dramatic T cell-dependent proliferation of intestinal mucosal mast cells [2, 28, 75, 76]. It appears that the mast-cell precursors involved in this intestinal mastocytosis probably originated in the bone marrow as a pluripotent stem cell but can be found in the intestinal mucosa, draining mesenteric lymph nodes, thoracic duct lymph and even the spleen probably as a committed, but relatively undifferentiated mast-cell progenitor [40, 107]. Their frequency in Peyer's patches is low.

mast-cell subtypes. To date no drug has been identified which inhibits only the rat intestinal mucosal cell and is impotent against the rat peritoneal mast cell.

Drug effects on human intestinal mast cells

Isolated, but not purified, human intestinal mast cells which contain two histochemically different subtypes, can be inhibited by high doses of theophylline (preincubation 10^{-2} M, 20 min) but are largely unresponsive to the antiallergic actions of disodium cromoglycate (approximately 20% inhibition). Whether this low-level inhibition by disodium cromoglycate represents potent inhibition of a minor mast-cell subtype in the mixture, or merely experimental variability, will only be determined when distinct subtypes can be purified and studied separately. The development of antiallergic drugs specific for different human mast-cell subtypes may have great therapeutic importance and will also aid in understanding the role of mast-cell subtypes in disease processes.

Cromoglycate-binding protein

Recent evidence that rat mast cells and basophils possess a cromoglycate-binding protein

IL-3 production

Parasitic infection stimulates the production of interleukin-3 (IL-3) which is a multipotent haemopoietic growth factor [47,84], and acts both as a mast-cell differentiative and proliferative factor; numbers of mast-cell progenitors in thoracic duct lymph rise and these appear to localize in the intestinal lamina propria where IL-3 and other factor(s) facilitate their local differentiation [40, 107]. The T cell dependency of this mastocytosis lies in IL-3 and perhaps other factor production, but not in the origin of the precursor. Mast-cell precursors in culture studies have been identified as Thy 1^-, Lyt 1^-, Lyt 2^-, Lyt 5^+, H2-K$^+$, H2-D$^+$ and Ia$^+$ [29, 79, 107]. The mast-cell precursor in the intestine is not a so-called 'granulated lymphocyte' which is so common in the intestinal epithelial leukocyte population [29].

Pluripotent stem cell differentiation

Schrader [108] recently reviewed in detail the information that demonstrates that both the typical, apparently thymus-independent connective tissue mast cell and the so-called atypical, thymus-dependent mucosal mast cell are derived from the pluripotent haemopoietic stem cell (Fig. 5.3). It appears that this stem cell can be influenced by the multipotent growth factor, IL-3, but that subsequently progenitors committed to one mast-cell lineage or the other arise, and only one of these, namely the atypical, mucosal-type is still strongly influenced by a thymus-dependent factor(s) (IL-3) for proliferation.

Thymus dependency of connective tissue mast cell

The question of whether the connective tissue type mast cell is under thymus-dependent influence had not been studied until recently under conditions where it was proliferating in vivo. However, using congenitally athymic nude rats we have established that hyperplasia of connective tissue type mast cells in the lungs of rats with bleomycin-induced pulmonary fibrosis is thymus-independent ([39], Goto, Bienenstock, Befus, unpublished observations). In the further dissection of the possibility that distinct mast-cell progenitors are committed to separate lineages, both in vitro and in vivo studies will be essential. The elegant in vivo studies of Sonoda and co-workers [120, 121] on mast-cell reconstitution experiments in mast-cell-deficient mice, together with culture studies comparing progenitors, growth-regulating factors and functional qualities of cultured cells will go a long way in the delineation of differentiation pathways and functional heterogeneity of mast cells. Undoubtedly, microenvironmental factors selectively induce the expression of distinct portions of the genome in a committed progenitor, leading to phenotypic heterogeneity (Fig. 5.1). The use of monoclonal antibodies [21, 55, 56] and other newer biochemical and molecular approaches will also provide essential components in unravelling the complexities we now recognize.

Mucosal mast cells and globule leukocytes: ontogeny

One question that has received considerable attention has been the relationship between

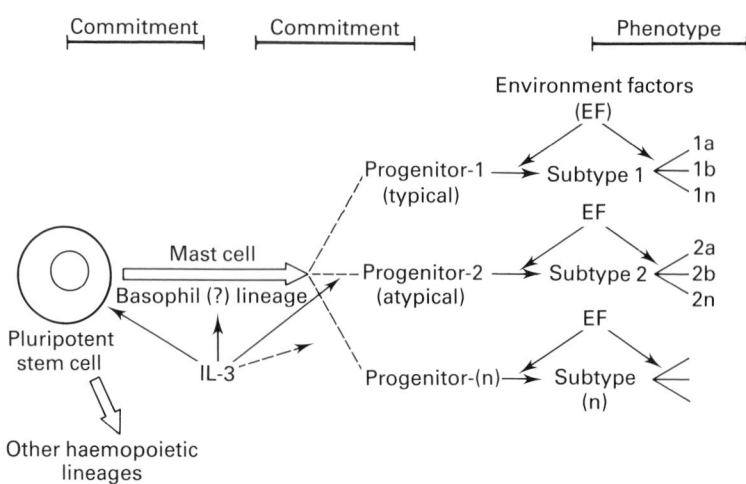

Fig. 5.3 Model of mast-cell differentiation, proliferation and heterogeneity. It is proposed that mast-cell subtypes arise from pluripotent stem cells in bone marrow. A range of factors including IL-3 and as yet unknown local environmental components regulate proliferation and the expression of portions of the genome, ultimately producing mast-cell subtypes.

mucosal mast cells and globule leukocytes. The latter are abundant in the intestinal epithelium under certain circumstances such as during some parasitic infections in some species. Murray et al [78] proposed that globule leukocytes are derived from mucosal mast cells which had degranulated. However, Ruitenberg and co-workers [101] on the basis of inconsistencies in the temporal relationships between the numbers of mast cells and globule leukocytes, proposed that they are independently derived cell types. This conflict appears to be resolved at least for the parasitized sheep intestine by the recent studies of Huntley et al [46] which clearly demonstrate that cells in transition between mast cells and globule leukocytes can be identified and all three cell types share a number of common characteristics including glycosaminoglycan, surface and cytoplasmic immunoglobulin, serine esterase and dopamine (Table 5.4). Whether cells in other tissues or species which have been labelled globule leukocytes (e.g. [90]) have a similar origin and life history remains to be established.

Table 5.4 Relationships between intestinal mucosal mast cells and globule leukocytes in sheep.

Property	Cell type*		
	MMC	TC	GL
Glycosaminoglycan	+ +	+	±
Immunoglobulin			
Surface	+ +	+ +	+ +
Cytoplasmic	+	+	+
Serine esterase	+	+	+
Dopamine	+	+	+

* MMC = mucosal mast cell; GL = globule leukocyte; TC = transitional cell, intermediate between MMC and GL in size, granule morphology and staining properties. Data taken from Huntley et al [46].

MAST-CELL FUNCTION

It is obvious that the role of the mast cell in any inflammatory disease or infection will be difficult to define, in large part because the potential activities are so diverse. Many mediators may influence smooth muscle in the vasculature or elsewhere, and both histamine and serotonin may also be neurotransmitters, thereby modifying local nervous activity. Lymphocytes, macrophages, neutrophils, eosinophils, platelets, fibroblasts and certain bone marrow stem cells are also targets of certain mediators. The range of activities could include alterations in blood flow, vascular and epithelial permeability, pain, mucus production and secretion, motility, inflammatory cell recruitment and function, differentiation, fibroblast proliferation, connective tissue turnover, etc. In the gastrointestinal tract it is probable that any pathological condition, directly or indirectly, activates mast-cell-dependent networks. The relative importance of mast-cell activation in the underlying pathophysiology of each condition will need to be carefully researched.

Diseases with mast-cell involvement

Some diseases in which intestinal mast cells have been implicated in pathogenesis include coeliac disease [125], food allergy [103], graft-versus-host reactions [77], inflammatory bowel disease [67], ulceration [1] and cancer [128]. In recent studies of intestinal immediate hypersensitivity reactions ('food allergy') marked changes in epithelial cell function have been defined [92], and the fact that these changes can be inhibited by doxantrazole [91], the antiallergic compound which blocks intestinal mucosal mast cells [89], suggests that direct or indirect communication occurs between mast cells and absorptive–secretory epithelial cells. It is interesting, albeit difficult, to explain that disodium cromoglycate, although poorly absorbed by the intestinal tract [14], is potent in treating some patients with immune-mediated food allergy [23]. Whether this involves inhibition of secretion from one mast-cell subtype in the human gut (see above), or the other activities of cromoglycate [14] remains to be established. The role of mast cells in the pathophysiology of some diarrhoeal diseases has yet to be explored.

Mast cells and fibrosis

Another communication network involving mast cells which is just beginning to be explored is that of the fibroblast and complexities of fibrosis. Undoubtedly, many cell types are involved including macrophages and lymphocytes [45]. Granuloma and fibrosis are prominent features of Crohn's disease and in involved areas mast cells and histamine levels are elevated. Granuloma formation in *Schistosoma mansoni* infection involves delayed onset hypersensitivity reactions and after some time the magnitude of the granulomatous reaction is modulated by suppressor T cells [19].

It is interesting that: (a) intestinal granulomata are smaller than those in the liver [135]; (b) mast cells are important in delayed onset hypersensitivity [3]; (c) mast cells are abundant in granulomata [136]; and (d) histamine H_2 antagonists inhibit the T suppressor cell modulation of the granulomatous response, suggesting that mast-cell-derived histamine activates the modulating suppressor T cells [136].

Other studies show that mast cells interact directly with fibroblasts [97] or alternately act through macrophages to modulate fibroblast characteristics [58]. Such studies are important for the understanding of intestinal, pulmonary and other fibrotic diseases.

Cytolytic function of mast cells

In addition to the role mast cells play in modulating the activities of a variety of cell types by depressing or potentiating certain processes or inducing differentiation events, mast cells themselves can be cytolytic for certain targets (e.g. fibrosarcoma [31, 43]). The in vivo significance of this cytotoxicity remains to be established.

Summary

Taken together, the potential activities of mast cells on a wide range of targets, and the diversity of cells and products, including those derived from local nerves, which modulate mast-cell function, it is obvious that in any working model of inflammatory diseases, mast cells must have a prominent position. This is complicated by the heterogeneity expressed by many cell types including mast cells, and our present ignorance of the nature and extent of this heterogeneity.

A more holistic and therefore realistic overview of the complex cellular interactions in inflammatory bowel disease and other diseases is needed. We must continue to identify the diversity of possible cellular interactions and direct research towards the many unexplored, but probably fundamentally important, aspects of gastrointestinal disease encompassing, for example, not only lymphocytes and mast cells, but also eosinophils, macrophages, epithelial cells, goblet cells and even nerves.

REFERENCES

1 Andre F, Andre C, Vialard JL: Role of homocytotropic antibodies in pathogenesis of gastric ulcer. Digestion 1979; 19:175–9.
2 Askenase PW: Immunopathology of parasitic diseases: involvement of basophils and mast cells. Springer Semin Immunopathol 1980; 2:417–42.
3 Askenase PW, Van Loveren H: Delayed-type hypersensitivity: activation of mast cells by antigen-specific T-cell factors initiates the cascade of cellular interactions. Immunol Today 1983; 4:259–64.
4 Askenase PW, Rosenstein RW, Ptak W: T cells produce an antigen-binding factor with in vivo activity analogous to IgE antibody. J Exp Med 1983; 157:862–73.
5 Azizkhan RG, Azizkhan JC, Zetter BR, Folkman J: Mast cell heparin stimulates migration of capillary endothelial cells in vitro. J Exp Med 1980; 152:931–44.
6 Barrett KE, Metcalfe DD: The mucosal mast cell and its role in gastrointestinal allergic diseases. Clin Rev Allergy 1984; 2:39–53.
7 Beaven MA: Histamine: its role in physiological and pathological processes. Monogr Allergy 1978; 13:1–113.
8 Beer DJ, Rocklin RE: Histamine-induced suppressor-cell activity. J Allergy Clin Immunol 1984; 73:439–52.
9 Befus AD, Bienenstock J: Factors involved in symbiosis and host resistance at the mucosa–parasite interface. Prog Allergy 1982; 31:76–177.
10 Befus D, Goodacre R, Dyck N, Bienenstock J: Isolation and characterization of human intestinal mast cells. Fed Proc 1984; 43:1973.

11 Befus AD, Johnston N, Berman L, Bienenstock J: Relationship between tissue sensitization and IgE antibody production in rats infected with the nematode, *Nippostrongylus brasiliensis*. Int Arch Allergy Appl Immunol 1982; 67:213–8.
12 Befus AD, Lee T, Denburg J, Bienenstock J: 'Mucosal'? mast cells. Immunol Today 1984; 5:218–9.
13 Befus AD, Pearce FL, Gauldie J et al: Mucosal mast cells. I. Isolation and functional characteristics of rat intestinal mast cells. J Immunol 1982; 128:2475–80.
14 Berman BA, Ross RN: Cromolyn. Clin Rev Allergy 1983; 1:105–21.
15 Bienenstock J, Befus AD, Pearce F et al: Mast cell heterogeneity: derivation and function with emphasis on the intestine. J Allergy Clin Immunol 1982; 70:407–12.
16 Busse WW, Sosman J: Histamine inhibition of neutrophil lysosomal enzyme release: an H_2 histamine receptor response. Science 1976; 194:737–8.
17 Butterworth AE, Wassom DL, Gleich GL et al: Damage to schistosomula of *Schistosoma mansoni* induced directly by eosinophil major basic protein. J Immunol 1979; 122:221–9.
18 Capron M, Rousseaux J, Mazingue E et al: Rat mast cell–eosinophil interaction in antibody dependent eosinophil cytotoxicity to *Schistosoma mansoni* schistosomula. J Immunol 1978; 121:2518–25.
19 Chensue SW, Boros DL, David CS: Regulation of granulomatous inflammation in murine schistosomiasis. II. T suppressor cell-derived, I-C subregion-encoded soluble suppressor factor mediates regulation of lymphokine production. J Exp Med 1983; 157:219–30.

20 Combs JW, Lagunoff D, Benditt EP: Differentiation and proliferation of embryonic mast cells of the rat. J Cell Biol 1965; 25:577–92.

21 Conscience JF, Conscience-Egli M, Fischer F et al: Rat monoclonal antibodies against differentiation and transformation markers in murine basophil/mast cells. Experientia 1984; 40:621.

22 Czarnetzki BM, Figdor CG, Kolde G et al: Development of human connective tissue mast cells from purified blood monocytes. Immunology 1984; 51:549–54.

23 Dannaeus A, Foucard T, Johansson SGO: The effect of orally administered sodium cromoglycate on symptoms of food allergy. Clin Allergy 1977; 7:109–15.

24 Denburg JA, Befus AD, Bienenstock J: Growth and differentiation in vitro of mast cells from mesenteric lymph nodes of *Nippostrongylus brasiliensis* infected rats. Immunology 1980; 41:195–202.

25 Donowitz M, Charney AN, Heffernan JM: Effect of serotonin treatment on intestinal transport in the rabbit. Am J Physiol 1976; 232:E85–E94.

26 Douch PGC, Harrison GBL, Buchanan LL, Greer KS: In vitro bioassay of sheep gastrointestinal mucus for nematode paralysing activity mediated by substances with some properties characteristic of SRS-A. Int J Parasitol 1983; 13:207–12.

27 Dullens HFJ, den Otter W: A small molecular weight peptide from P815 mastocytoma cells induces macrophage cytotoxicity. Immunopharmacology 1981; 3:309–16.

28 Enerback L: The gut mucosal mast cell. Monogr Allergy 1981; 17:222–32.

29 Ernst P, Befus AD, Bienenstock J: Leukocytes in the intestinal epithelium: a unique and heterogeneous compartment. Immunol Today 1985; 6:40–5.

30 Ernst PB, Petit A, Befus AD et al: Murine intestinal intraepithelial lymphocytes. II. Comparison of freshly isolated and cultured intraepithelial lymphocytes. Eur J Immunol 1985; 15:216–221.

31 Farram E, Nelson DS: Mouse mast cells as antitumor effector cells. Cell Immunol 1980; 55:294–301.

32 Foreman JC, Piotrowski W: Peptides and histamine release. J Allergy Clin Immunol 1984; 74:127–31.

33 Fox CF, Dvorak AM, Lichtenstein LM: The histamine-containing cells of the human peritoneum and gastrointestinal mucosa. J Allergy Clin Immunol 1984; 73:167.

34 Frieri M, Metcalfe DD: Analysis of the effect of mast cell granules on lymphocyte blastogenesis in the absence and presence of mitogens: identification of heparin as a granule-associated suppressor factor. J Immunol 1983; 131:1942–8.

35 Fromm D, Halpern N: Effects of histamine receptor antagonists on ion transport by isolated ileum of the rabbit. Gastroenterology 1979; 77:1034–8.

36 Ginsburg H, Sachs L: Formation of pure suspensions of mast cells in tissue culture by differentiation of lymphoid cells from the mouse thymus. J Natl Cancer Inst 1963; 31:1–39.

37 Gleich GJ, Frigas E, Loegerin DA et al: Cytotoxic properties of the eosinophil major basic protein. J Immunol 1979; 123:2925–7.

38 Goetzl EJ, Payan DG, Goldman DW: Immunopathogenetic roles of leukotrienes in human diseases. J Clin Immunol 1984; 4:79–84.

39 Goto T, Befus D, Low R, Bienenstock J: Mast cell heterogeneity and hyperplasia in bleomycin-induced pulmonary fibrosis of rats. Am Rev Respir Dis 1984; 130:797–802.

40 Guy-Grand D, Dy M, Luffau G, Vassalli P: Gut mucosal mast cells: origin, traffic and differentiation. J Exp Med 1984; 160:12–28.

41 Haig DM, McKee TA, Jarrett EEE et al: Generation of mucosal mast cells is stimulated in vitro by factors derived from T cells of helminth-infected rats. Nature 1982; 300:188–90.

42 Haslam PL, Cronwell O, Dewar A, Turner-Warwick M: Evidence of increased histamine levels in lung lavage fluids from patients with cryptogenic fibrosing alveolitis. Clin Exp Immunol 1981; 44:587–93.

43 Henderson WR, Chi EY, Jong EC, Klebanoff SJ: Mast cell-mediated tumor-cell cytotoxicity. Role of the peroxidase system. J Exp Med 1981; 153:520–33.

44 Horton MA, O'Brien HA: Characterization of human mast cells in long-term culture. Blood 1983; 62:1251–60.

45 Hunninghake GW, Moseley PL: Immunological abnormalities of chronic noninfectious pulmonary diseases. In: Bienenstock J, ed. Immunology of the lung and upper respiratory tract. New York: McGraw-Hill, 1984; 345–64.

46 Huntley JF, Newlands G, Miller HRP: The isolation and characterization of globule leukocytes: their derivation from mucosal mast cells in parasitized sheep. Parasite Immunol 1984; 6:371–90.

47 Ihle JN, Rebar L, Keller J et al: Interleukin 3: possible roles in the regulation of lymphocyte differentiation and growth. Immunol Rev 1982; 63:5–32.

48 Ishizaka T, Ishizaka K: Activation of mast cells for mediator release through IgE receptors. Prog Allergy 1984; 34:188–235.

49 Ishizaka T, Okudaira H, Mauser LE, Ishizaka K: Development of rat mast cells in vitro. I. Differentiation of mast cells from thymus cells. J Immunol 1976; 116:747–54.

50 Jarrett EEE, Haig DM: Mucosal mast cells in vivo and in vitro. Immunol Today 1984; 5:115–9.

51 Johnson AR, Erdos EG: Release of histamine from mast cells by vasoactive peptides. Proc Soc Exp Biol Med 1973; 142:1252–6.

52 Johnson HG, Chinn RA, Morton DR et al: Diphenhydramine blocks the leukotriene-C4 enhanced mucus secretion in canine trachea in vivo. Agents Actions 1983; 13:1–4.

53 Kaliner M: Hypotheses on the contribution of late-phase allergic responses to the understanding and treatment of allergic diseases. J Allergy Clin Immunol 1984; 73-3:311–5.

54 Kaliner M, Lemanske R: Inflammatory responses to mast cell granules. Fed Proc 1984; 43:2846–51.

55 Katz HR, LeBlanc PA, Russell SW: An antigenic determinant shared by mononuclear phagocytes and mast cells, as defined by monoclonal antibody. J Reticuloendothel Soc 1981; 30:439–43.

56 Katz HR, LeBlanc PA, Russell SW: Two classes of mouse mast cells delineated by monoclonal antibodies. Proc Natl Acad Sci USA 1983; 80:5916–8.

57 Kawanami O, Forram VJ, Fulmer JD, Crystal RG: Ultrastructure of pulmonary mast cells in patients with fibrotic lung disorders. Lab Invest 1979; 40:717–34.

58 Kenyon AJ, Ramos P, Michaels EB: Histamine-induced suppressor macrophage inhibits fibroblast growth and wound healing. Am J Vet Res 1983; 44:2164–6.

59 Kierszenbaum F, Ackerman SJ, Gleich GJ: Inhibition of antibody-dependent eosinophil-mediated cytotoxicity by heparin. J Immunol 1982; 128:515–7.

60 King SJ, Miller HRP: Anaphylactic release of mu-

cosal mast cell protease and its relationship to gut permeability in *Nippostrongylus*-primed rats. Immunology 1984; 51:653–60.

61 Kisloff B, Moore EW: Effect of serotonin on water and electrolyte transport in the in vivo rabbit small intestine. Gastroenterology 1976; 71:1033–8.

62 Lagunoff D, Martin TW, Read G: Agents that release histamine from mast cells. Annu Rev Pharmacol Toxicol 1983; 23:331–51.

63 Lee TDG, Shanahan F, Miller HRP et al: Intestinal mucosal mast cells: isolation from rat lamina propria and purification using unit gravity velocity sedimentation. Immunology 1985; 55:721–8.

64 Lee TDG, Sterk A, Ishizaka T, et al: Number and affinity of receptors for IgE on enriched populations of isolated rat intestinal mast cells. Immunology 1985; 55:363–6.

65 Leung KBP, Barrett KE, Pearce FL: Differential effects of anti-allergic compounds on peritoneal mast cells of the rat, mouse and hamster. Agents Actions 1984; 14:461–7.

66 Lewis RA, Austen F: The biologically active leukotrienes—biosynthesis metabolism, receptors, functions and pharmacology. J Clin Invest 1984; 73:889–97.

67 Lloyd G, Green FHY, Fox H et al: Mast cells and immunoglobulin E in inflammatory bowel disease. Gut 1975; 16:861–6.

68 McLean J, Fox JET: Mechanisms of action of neurotensin on motility of canine gastric corpus in vitro. Can J Physiol Pharmacol 1982; 61:29–34.

69 Maron Z, Shelhamer JH, Kaliner M: Effects of arachidonic acid, monohydroxyeicosatetraenoic acid and prostaglandins on the release of mucous glycoproteins from human airways in vitro. J Clin Invest 1981; 67:1695–702.

70 Marquardt DL: Histamine. Clin Rev Allergy 1983; 1:343–51.

71 Mazurek N, Berger G, Pecht I: A binding site on mast cells and basophils for the anti-allergic drug cromolyn. Nature 1980; 286:722–3.

72 Mazurek N, Bashkin P, Petran A, Pecht I: Basophil variants with impaired cromoglycate binding do not respond to an immunological degranulation stimulus. Nature 1983; 303:528–30.

73 Mazurek N, Schindler H, Schurholz TH, Pecht I: The cromolyn binding protein constitutes the Ca^{2+} channel of basophils opening upon immunological stimulus. Proc Natl Acad Sci USA 1984; 81:6841–5.

74 Metcalfe DD: Effector cell heterogeneity in immediate hypersensitivity reactions. Clin Rev Allergy 1983; 1:311–25.

75 Miller HRP: The structure, origin and function of mucosal mast cells: a brief review. Biol Cell 1980; 39:229–32.

76 Miller HRP: The protective mucosal response against gastrointestinal nematodes in ruminants and laboratory animals. Vet Immunol Immunopathol 1984; 6:176–259.

77 Mowat AM, Ferguson A: Intraepithelial lymphocyte count and crypt hyperplasia measure the mucosal component of the graft-versus-host reaction in the mouse small intestine. Gastroenterology 1982; 83:417–23.

78 Murray M, Miller HRP, Jarrett WFH: The globule leukocyte and its derivation from the subepithelial mast cell. Lab Invest 1968; 19:222–34.

79 Nabel G, Galli SJ, Dvorak AM et al: Inducer T lymphocytes synthesize a factor that stimulates proliferation of cloned mast cells. Nature 1981; 291:332–4.

80 Newson B, Dahlstrom A, Enerback L, Ahlman H: Suggestive evidence for a direct innervation of mucosal mast cells. Neuroscience 1983; 10:565–70.

81 Ninneman JL: Prostaglandins in inflammation and disease. Immunol Today 1984; 5:173–8.

82 Oertel HL, Kaliner M: The biologic activity of mast cell granules. III. Purification of inflammatory factors of anaphylaxis (IF-A) responsible for causing late-phase reactions. J Immunol 1981; 127:1398–402.

83 O'Flaherty JT, Wykle RL: Biology and biochemistry of platelet-activating factor. Clin Rev Allergy 1983; 1:353–67.

84 Palacios R, Garland J: Distinct mechanisms may account for the growth-promoting activity of interleukin 3 on cells of lymphoid and myeloid origin. Proc Natl Acad Sci USA 1984; 81:1208–11.

85 Payan DG, Levine JD, Goetzl EJ: Modulation of immunity and hypersensitivity by sensory neuropeptides. J Immunol 1984; 132:1324–601.

86 Pearce FL: Functional heterogeneity of mast cells from different species and tissues. Klin Wochenschr 1982; 60:954–7.

87 Pearce FL: Mast cell heterogeneity. Trends Pharm Sci 1983; 4:165–7.

88 Pearce FL, Befus AD, Bienenstock J: Mucosal mast cells. III. Effect of quercetin and other flavonoids on antigen-induced histamine secretion from rat intestinal mast cells. J Allergy Clin Immunol 1984; 73:819–23.

89 Pearce FL, Befus AD, Gauldie J, Bienenstock J: Mucosal mast cells. II. Effects of anti-allergic compounds on histamine secretion by isolated intestinal mast cells. J Immunol 1982; 128:2481–6.

90 Pearsall AD, Echt R, Ross LM et al: Morphologic and cytochemical characteristics of amine-containing globule leukocytes in rat tracheal epithelium. Am J Anat 1984; 170:83–99.

91 Perdue M, Gall DG: Intestinal dysfunction during IgE-mediated reactions: role of mast cell mediators. Gastroenterology 1983; 84:1272.

92 Perdue MH, Chung M, Gall DG: Effect of intestinal anaphylaxis on gut function in the rat. Gastroenterology 1984; 86:391–7.

93 Persinger MA: Handling factors not body marking influence thalamic mast cell numbers in the preweaned albino rat. Behav Neural Biol 1980; 30:448–59.

95 Persinger MA: Developmental alteration in mast cell numbers and distributions within the thalamus of the albino rat. Dev Neurosci 1981; 4:220–4.

95 Poole TJ, Zetter BR: Stimulation of rat peritoneal mast cell migration by tumor-derived peptides. Cancer Res 1983; 43:5857–61.

96 Ranadive NS, Cochrane CG: Mechanism of histamine release from mast cells by cationic protein (band 2) from neutrophil lysosomes. J Immunol 1971; 106:506–16.

97 Rao PVS, Friedman MM, Atkins FM, Metcalfe DD: Phagocytosis of mast cell granules by cultured fibroblasts. J Immunol 1983; 130:341–9.

98 Razin E, Mencia-Huerta JM, Lewis RA et al: Generation of leukotriene C_4 from a subclass of mast cells differentiated in vitro from mouse bone marrow. Proc Natl Acad Sci USA 1982; 79:4665–7.

99 Razin E, Stevens RL, Akiyama F et al: Culture from mouse bone marrow of a subclass of mast cell possessing a distinct chondroitin sulfate proteoglycan with glycosaminoglycans rich in *N*-

acetylgalactosamine-4,6-disulfate. J Biol Chem 1982; 257:7229-36.

100 Razin E, Stevens RL, Austen KF et al: Cloned mouse mast cells derived from immunized lymph node cells and from foetal liver cells exhibit characteristics of bone marrow-derived mast cells containing chondroitin sulphate E proteoglycan. Immunology 1984; 52:563-75.

101 Ruitenberg EJ, Elgersma A: Response of intestinal globule leukocytes in the mouse during a *Trichinella spiralis* infection and its independence of intestinal mast cells. Br J Exp Pathol 1979; 60:246-51.

102 Russell M, Dark KA, Cummins RW et al: Learned histamine release. Science 1984; 225:733-4.

103 Saavedra-Delgado AM, Metcalfe DD: The gastrointestinal mast cell in food allergy. Ann Allergy 1983; 51:185-9.

104 Samuelsson B: Leukotrienes: mediators of immediate hypersensitivity reactions and inflammation. Science 1983; 220:568-75.

105 Sandusky CB, Johnson AR, Moram NC: Effect of endotoxin and anaphylatoxin on rat mast cells and chopped rat lung. Proc Soc Exp Biol Med 1973; 143:764-8.

106 Schleimer RP, MacGlashan DW, Schulman ES et al: Human mast cells and basophils—structure, function, pharmacology, and biochemistry. Clin Rev Allergy 1983; 1:327-41.

107 Schrader DW, Scollay R, Battye F: Intramucosal lymphocytes of the gut: Lyt 2 and Thy 1 phenotype of the granulated cells and evidence for the presence of both T cells and mast cell precursors. J Immunol 1983; 130:558-64.

108 Schrader J: The ontogeny and differentiation of mast cells. In: Befus AD, Bienenstock J, Denburg JA, eds. Mast cell differentiation and heterogeneity. New York: Raven Press, 1986; 27-43.

109 Schulman ES, Kagey-Sobotka A, MacGlashan DW Jr et al: Heterogeneity of human mast cells. J Immunol 1983; 131:1936-41.

110 Schwartz LB, Austen KF: Structure and function of the chemical mediators of mast cells. Prog Allergy 1984; 34:271-321.

111 Selbekk BH: Neurotensin-induced mast cell degranulation in human jejunal mucosa. Scand J Gastroenterol 1983; 19:596-602.

112 Selbekk BH, Flaten O, Hanssen LE: The in vitro effect of neurotensin on human jejunal mast cells. Scand J Gastroenterol 1980; 15:457-60.

113 Shanahan F, Denburg JA, Bienenstock J, Befus AD: Mast cell heterogeneity. Can J Physiol Pharmacol 1984; 62:734-7.

114 Shanahan F, Lee TDG, Bienenstock J, Befus AD: The influence of endorphins on peritoneal and mucosal mast cell secretion. J Allergy Clin Immunol 1984; 74:499-504.

115 Shanahan F, Befus AD, Fox J et al: Mast cell subpopulations and their response to substance P. In: Skrabanek P, Powell D, eds. Substance P. Dublin: Book Press, 1983; 145-6.

116 Shelhamer JG, Maron Z, Kaliner M: Immunologic and neuropharmacologic stimulation of mucous glycoprotein release from human airways in vitro. J Clin Invest 1980; 66:1400:8.

117 Sher A, McIntyre SL: Receptors for C3 on rat peritoneal mast cells. J Immunol 1977; 119:722-5.

118 Siegel JN, Schwartz A, Askenase PW, Gershon RK: T-cell suppression and contrasuppression induced by histamine H_2 and H_1 receptor agonists, respectively. Proc Natl Acad Sci USA 1982; 79:5052-6.

119 Slauson DO, Walker C, Kristensen F et al: Mechanisms of serotonin-induced lymphocyte proliferation inhibition. Cell Immunol 1983; 84:240-52.

120 Sonoda T, Ohno T, Kitamura Y: Concentration of mast-cell progenitors in bone marrow, spleen and blood of mice determined by limiting dilution analysis. J Cell Physiol 1982; 112:136-40.

121 Sonoda T, Kanayama Y, Hara H et al: Proliferation of peritoneal mast cells in the skin of W/W^v mice that genetically lack mast cells. J Exp Med 1984; 160:138-51.

122 Sredni B, Friedman MM, Bland CE, Metcalfe DD: Ultrastructural, biochemical, and functional characteristics of histamine-containing cells cloned from mouse bone marrow: tentative identification as mucosal mast cells. J Immunol 1983; 131:915-22.

123 Stanworth DR: Immunochemical aspects of human IgG. Clin Rev Allergy 1983; 1:183-95.

124 Stenson WF, Parker CW: Metabolites of arachidonic acid. Clin Rev Allergy 1983; 1:369-84.

125 Strobel S, Busuttil A, Ferguson A: Human intestinal mucosal mast cells: expanded population in untreated coeliac disease. Gut 1983; 24:222-7.

126 Sugiyama K, Furuta H: Histamine release induced by dynorphin-(1-13) from rat mast cells. Jpn J Pharmacol 1984; 35:247-52.

127 Szewczuk MR, Campbell RJ, Smith JW: Evidence for histamine-induced auto-anti-idiotypic antibody immunoregulation in vivo. Cell Immunol 1981; 65:152-65.

128 Tanooka H, Kitamura Y, Sado T et al: Evidence for involvement of mast cells in tumor suppression in mice. J Natl Cancer Inst 1982; 69:1305-9.

129 Theoharides TC, Sieghart W, Greengard P, Douglas WW: Antiallergic drug cromolyn may inhibit histamine secretion by regulating phosphorylation of a mast cell protein. Science 1979; 207:80-2.

130 Van Loveren H, Kraiuter-Kops S, Askenase PW: Different mechanisms of release of vasoactive amines by mast cells occur in T cell-dependent compared to IgE-dependent cutaneous hypersensitivity responses. Eur J Immunol 1984; 14:40-7.

131 Van Loveren H, Meade R, Askenase PW: An early component of delayed-type hypersensitivity mediated by T cells and mast cells. J Exp Med 1983; 157:1604-17.

132 Victor M, Weiss J, Elsbach E: Heparin inhibits phagocytosis by polymorphonuclear leukocytes. Infect Immun 1981; 32:295-9.

133 Watkins SG, Dearin JL, Yong LC, Wilhelm DL: Association of mastopoiesis with haemopoietic tissues in the neonatal rat. Experientia 1976; 32:1339-40.

134 Weiner RI, Ganong WF: Role of brain monoamines and histamine in regulation of anterior pituitary secretion. Physiol Rev 1978; 58:905-76.

135 Weinstock JV, Boros DL: Heterogeneity of the granulomatous response in the liver, colon, ileum and ileal Peyer's patches to schistosome eggs in murine *Schistosomiasis mansoni*. J Immunol 1981; 127:1906-9.

136 Weinstock JV, Chensue SW, Boros DL: Modulation of granulomatous hypersensitivity. V. Participation of histamine receptor positive and negative lymphocytes in the granulomatous response of *Schistosomiasis mansoni*-infected mice. J Immunol 1983; 130:423-9.

137 Wells E, Mann J: Phosphorylation of a mast cell protein in response to treatment with anti-allergic compounds. Implication for the mode of action of sodium cromoglycate. Biochem Pharmacol 1983; 32:837-42.

138 West BC, Dunphy CH, Moore CA: Human neutrophil *N*-acetyl-glucosaminidase: heparin inhibition. Biochem Med 1983; 29:1–13.

139 Wiesner-Menzel L, Schulz B, Vakilzadeh F, Czarnetzki BM: Electron microscopical evidence for a direct contact between nerve fibres and mast cells. Acta Derm Venereol 1981; 61:465–9.

140 Wilson JG, Fearon DT, Stevens RL et al: Inhibition of the function of activated properdin by squid chondroitin sulfate E glycosaminoglycan and murine bone marrow-derived mast cell chondroitin sulfate E proteoglycan. J Immunol 1984; 132:3058–63.

141 Woodbury RG, Neurath H: Purification of an atypical mast cell protease and its levels in developing rats. Biochemistry 1978; 17:4298–304.

142 Woodbury RG, Gruzenski GM, Lagunoff D: Immunofluorescent localization of a serine protease in rat small intestine. Proc Natl Acad Sci USA 1978; 75:2785–9.

143 Woodbury RG, Miller HRP, Huntley JF et al: Mucosal mast cells are functionally active during spontaneous expulsion of nematode infections in rat. Nature 1984; 312:450–2.

144 Zifroni A, Treves AJ, Sachar DB, Rachmilewitz D: Prostanoid synthesis by cultured intestinal epithelial and mononuclear cells in inflammatory bowel disease. Gut 1983; 24:659–64.

145 Zweiman B: Mast cells in human disease. Clin Rev Allergy 1983; 1:417–26.

Chapter 6
The Mucosal T Cell

Stephan Strobel and John G. Shields

Introduction

The intestinal mucosa is a major barrier limiting foreign antigen access to the body. The means by which the body protects itself from the huge antigenic load presented at the intestinal mucosae have been studied for a long time. Being the first line of defence, the epithelium has been particularly well investigated and it has been realized for many years that non-epithelial cells are common within the epithelium [12, 22, 65, 83]. The cellular infiltrate consists of granular and non-granular lymphocytes, eosinophils, macrophages, mast cells (globule leukocytes) and the occasional neutrophil. All these cell types can be demonstrated both in the epithelium and the lamina propria; plasma cells, however, are restricted to the latter. Relatively little is known about the specific cellular immune functions of these non-epithelial cells and their role within the gut-associated lymphoid tissues (GALT). Of those cells residing within the mucosal epithelium, the intraepithelial lymphocytes (IEL) have attracted most attention (Fig. 6.1).

Intraepithelial 'lymphocytes'. These have the ultrastructural appearance of lymphocytes although some features distinguish them from the classical blood-borne lymphocytes [12, 22]. Their unique intraepithelial and interenterocytic location—only separated from the huge antigenic load of the gastrointestinal lumen by the epithelial cell tight junctions—makes them a likely candidate for an immunoregulatory role within the gut-associated lymphoid tissues.

Despite their early description in 1847 (Weber, cited in [83]) the lineage, function and fate of intraepithelial lymphocytes are still poorly understood. Some of the various hypotheses put forward are that these cells are effete lymphocytes undergoing degradation within the epithelium [82], being in transit to the gut lumen, or that they are presenting nutrients to the surrounding enterocytes [41]

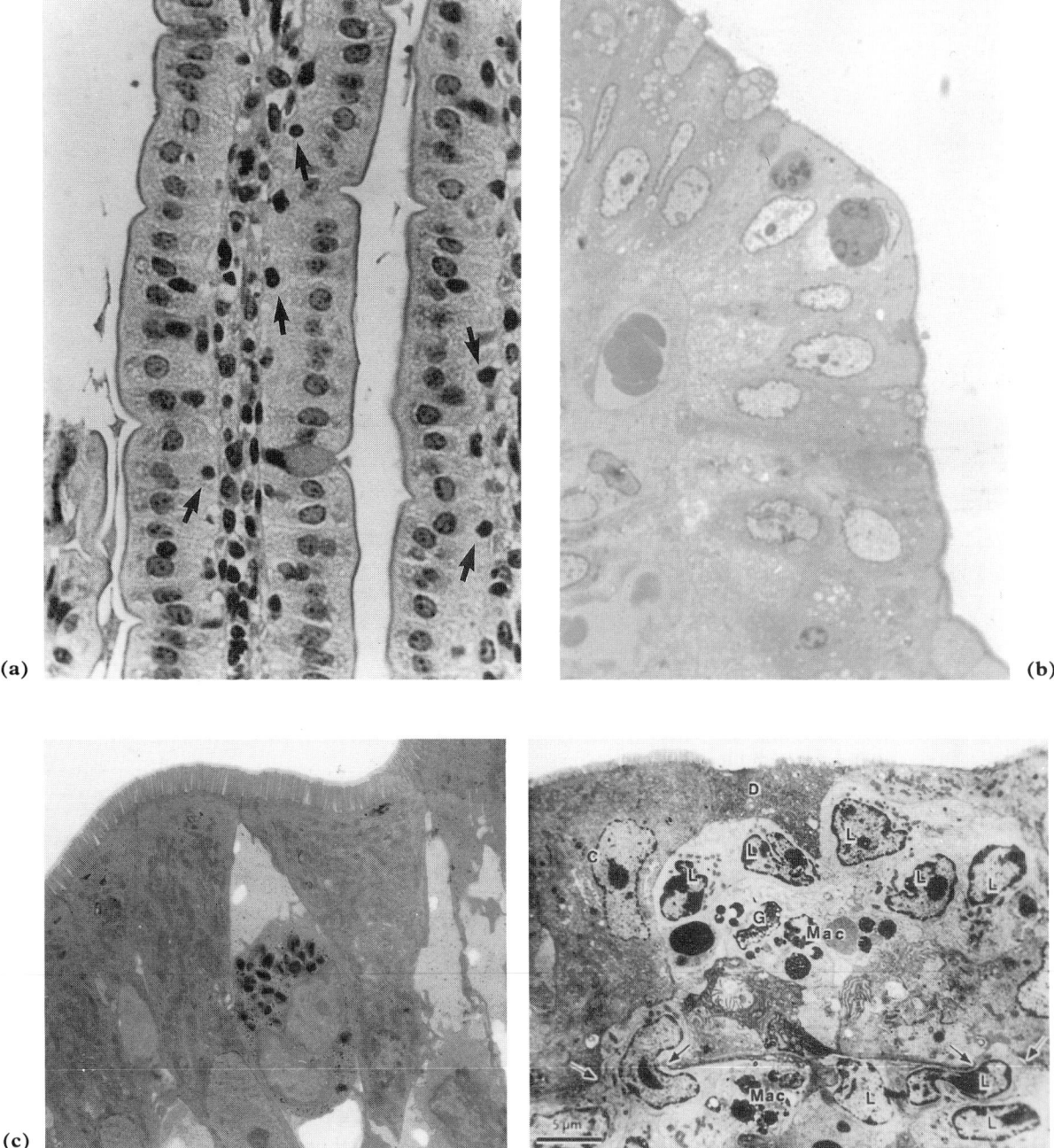

Fig. 6.1 (a) Section of normal mouse (BDF1) small intestinal villi demonstrating numerous intraepithelial lymphocytes which are clearly visible (arrows) above the basement membrane between the enterocytes. Fixative: formalin. Stain: haematoxylin–eosin. This staining technique is not suitable for distinguishing granulated from non-granulated intraepithelial lymphocytes. Original magnification × 500. (b) Semi-thin section of colonic mucosa of a child with Crohn's disease demonstrating intraepithelial granulocytes. Resin embedded, basic fuchsin-toluidine blue–polychrome stain. Original magnification × 1000. (c) Transmission electron microscopic picture of an intraepithelial eosinophil in a child with persistent diarrhoea. Original magnification × 3500. (Figs (b) and (c) kindly provided by Alan Phillips, Electron Microscopy, Queen Elizabeth Hospital for Sick Children, London.) (d) A giardia microorganism (G) within a macrophage (Mac) in the epithelium over the lymphoid follicle. Migrating lymphoblasts (L) in the epithelium are in direct contact with the macrophage. Two lymphocytes migrating through the basal laminia (arrows). (By courtesy of R. Owen and reproduced with permission from Owen RL et al, *Infection and Immunity*, 1981; 33:591–601.)

or forming a part of the (disputed) bursa equivalent in man [29, 30]. None of these hypotheses have been substantiated.

Lymphocyte diversity. The demonstration of functional and lineage-specific cell surface markers, and in particular the use of monoclonal antibodies, has broadened our views and understanding of the role(s) of mucosal T lymphocytes. Though our knowledge of the basic principles in gastrointestinal immunoregulation is still rudimentary, it is now possible to study the cell populations of the mucosa and to dissect the intestinal immune response in vivo and in vitro.

In this chapter we shall discuss intraepithelial and lamina propria T lymphocytes in humans and in selected laboratory rodents with reference to their heterogeneity and their role in food-related hypersensitivity reactions (food allergies) in the broadest sense.

ONTOGENY AND LIFESPAN OF MUCOSAL LYMPHOCYTES

Ontogeny of mucosal lymphocytes

The origin and fate of intraepithelial lymphocytes are still a matter of controversy and lymphoid as well as non-lymphoid origins have been proposed [26, 32, 33, 55]. In man they appear as early as the 20th gestational week and increase in numbers of up to 6–40 per 100 epithelial cells in the normal human small intestine [see 22, 65 for review]. In mice there is a steady increase after birth from 0.3 to 0.5 per 100 epithelial cells two days after birth to about 2/100 epithelial cells at one week of age, to around 11/100 epithelial cells in adult mice, although this can vary depending on animal house conditions (infections) and strains of mice studied [25, 84].

Site of first detection of granulated mucosal lymphocytes

Preliminary observations in BALB/c mice aged 1–14 days (Strobel, 1983, unpublished observations) have demonstrated that sparsely granulated mucosal cells (morphologically lymphocytes) are first detected in the lamina propria at the crypt level. These granulated lymphocytes appear in the villus lamina propria before they can be demonstrated in the epithelium. These observations however do not necessarily imply that these cells migrate from the lamina propria into the epithelium. Further radioactive labelling studies and the identification of their precursor cells are needed to answer these questions.

Thymus dependency and migration

Antigen-deprived mice or ectopic fetal gut grafts transplanted under the kidney capsule [25] exhibit smaller numbers of intraepithelial lymphocytes. Thymic aplasia, as in nude mice (nu/nu), also reduces, but does not totally abolish, the seeding of intraepithelial lymphocytes into the intestinal mucosa. This deficit involves mainly the non-granulated cell population. It seems likely that the non-granulated population of intraepithelial lymphocytes is thymus-dependent whereas the granulated cell population is not under thymus control [55, 56]. The balance of evidence supports the hypothesis that intraepithelial lymphocytes arise from precursor cells within the Peyer's patches and migrate via the mesenteric lymph nodes and thoracic duct lymph back to the mucosal epithelium through the normal routes of lymphoblast migration (see Chapters 1 and 2).

Lifespan

In a series of elegant studies, Röpke and Everett have shown by means of DNA synthesis that 70% of intraepithelial lymphocytes are short-lived ($T_{1/2}$ around three weeks), although a small proportion of long-lived small lymphocytes can also be demonstrated [71]. They are capable of local division within the epithelium and as an indicator, mitotic figures can be seen in man [28, 51] and in laboratory rodents [28, 71]. An increase in mitotic activity seems to be a marker of a raised cell turnover and has been reported during a graft-versus-host reaction in mice [28, 33] and in man with untreated coeliac disease [28, 52]. Intraepithelial lymphocytes are capable of active migration and have been identified crossing the basement membrane. The question of whether they migrate up the villus together with the epithelial cells [70, 71] or remain stationary against the upward movement of epithelial cells has not been conclusively answered [50].

MORPHOLOGY AND HISTOCHEMISTRY

Tissue sections from different species show that the majority of intraepithelial lympho-

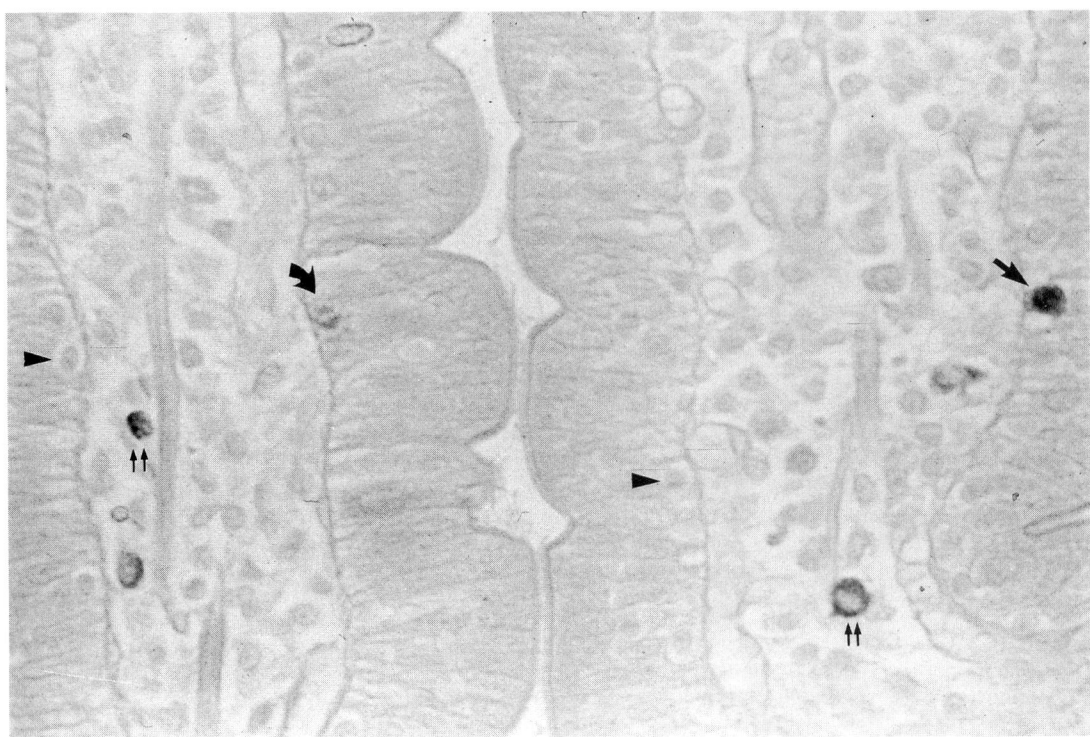

Fig. 6.2 Section of normal human (adult) small intestinal mucosa. Three different granulated mucosal cell populations are clearly distinguishable in this section: (a) a granulated intraepithelial lymphocyte (↘), (b) an intraepithelial mast cell (globule leukocyte) (↘), (c) lamina propria mast cells (↑↑) and (d) the non-granulated intraepithelial lymphocytes (▶). The granulated intraepithelial lymphocyte exhibits a polar distribution of its granule(s), whereas the lamina propria and intraepithelial mast cells demonstrate a non-polar distribution of their many granules which occasionally occlude the nucleus. Fixative: Carnoy's. Stain: astra blue/safranin, pH 0.3. Original magnification × 160.

cytes are medium sized [22, 71, 74]. When stained with Giemsa, they have abundant pale blue cytoplasm and a densely stained nucleus, thus demonstrating staining patterns typical of blood lymphocytes. Some intraepithelial lymphocytes have the features of basophilic lymphoblasts [32], one of the most distinctive features being polar distributed basophilic granules (range approximately 1–10, usually 1–4) within their cytoplasm. Histochemical and ultrastructural studies [33, 37, 62, 88] have led to the identification of various subpopulations (Table 6.1, Fig. 6.2).

In man 25–50% of intraepithelial lymphocytes are granulated [9]. In mice, up to 60% are granulated [66] reaching over 90% [84] in some inbred strains. Over 30% of the intraepithelial lymphocytes in rats and rabbits are granulated [55, 74]. Attempts to identify granulated intraepithelial lymphocytes in tissue sections of different species have yielded widely divergent results and are most likely due to differences in their fixation and staining properties [18, 54, 88].

Fixation and staining properties of granulated mucosal lymphocytes

The choice of the correct fixative for staining intraepithelial and mucosal granulated lymphocytes and mast cells is of great importance as has been shown in rodents and in man (see

Table 6.1 Monoclonal antibodies used in identifying T cell subsets in various species.

Species	Pan T cells	Helper/inducer T cell subset	Cytotoxic/suppressor T cell subset
Man	HuTLA; OKT 3	OKT 4	OKT 8
Mouse	anti-Thy 1	anti-Lyt 1	anti-Lyt 2, 3
Rat	W3/13	W3/25	MRC–OX8

below). A fixative with low formalin concentration (below 4%) or without formalin (Carnoy's fluid) gives best results. Varying reports on the existence and numbers of granulated intraepithelial lymphocytes and mucosal mast cells seem to be related to their sensitivity towards formalin containing fixatives.

Cytochemistry

Cytochemical studies of the basic contents of these granules have revealed glycosylaminoglycans in granulated intraepithelial lymphocytes, intraepithelial mast cells (globule leukocytes) and mucosal mast cells. After correct fixation, all granules stain with phthalodiazo dyes (astra blue, alcian blue, toluidine blue) in acid conditions (pH 0.5) (Fig. 2) [18, 37, 54, 88]. Granules of rodent cells con-

T LYMPHOCYTE SUBSETS WITHIN THE INTESTINAL MUCOSA

In studies using lymphocytes isolated from the mucosal epithelium it has been shown that intraepithelial lymphocytes have neither intracytoplasmic nor cell surface immunoglobulins (Ig^-), and that immunoglobulin positive (Ig^+) cells are confined to the lamina propria. This has led to the assumption that intraepithelial lymphocytes are a more or less homogeneous population of lymphocytes. However, the use of monoclonal antibodies (Table 6.2) and functional assays have yielded new insights into the cells taking part in host defence at the mucosal level and their immunoregulatory role within the gut-associated lymphoid tissues.

Table 6.2 Lymphocyte subsets found in cell suspensions isolated from small intestinal tissue.

		Staining: percentage positive		
Species	Lymphocyte subset	Intraepithelial lymphocytes	Lamina propria lymphocytes	Reference
Man	T cells (OKT 3)*	84	ND†	[9, 79]
	Th/ind (OKT 4)*	10	ND	
	Ts/c (OKT 8)*	68	ND	
Mouse	T cells (anti-Thy 1)	18	24	[66]
	Th/ind (anti-Lyt 1)	16	14	
	Ts/c (anti-Lyt 2)	60	12	
Rat	T cells (W3/13)	29	33	[47]
	Th/ind (W3/25)	13	15	
	Ts/c (MRC–OX 8)	73	26	

* Cell surface antigens detected with the above mentioned monoclonal antibodies have recently been designated as cluster determinant (CD) antigens CD3, CD4, CD8 according to the recommendations of the First International Workshop on Human Leukocyte Differentiation Antigens, Paris, 1982.
† ND = not done; Th/ind = helper or inducer T cell; Ts/c = suppressor or cytotoxic T cell.

tain histamine and serotonin [37]. Recent reports suggest that human granulated intraepithelial lymphocytes do not stain positively (with *o*-phthaldialdehyde) for histamine [9]. In rats it has been demonstrated that granulated intraepithelial lymphocytes lack a specific protease which is present in mucosal mast cells [37]. This is further evidence that granulated intraepithelial lymphocytes are of different lineage from mucosal mast cells or intraepithelial mast cells (see Chapter 5).

Similarities between granulated intraepithelial lymphocytes and large granular lymphocytes obtained from spleen and from the circulation in man have also been demonstrated. Both cell populations show alcian blue positive granules which contain a non-specific esterase and acid phosphatase [31] (see also Chapter 8).

Animal studies

T lymphocyte phenotypes

The subset profile of intraepithelial lymphocytes differs markedly from that of the lamina propria lymphocyte population. In mice, using the Lyt antisera, Parrott et al [66] found that, while most of the intraepithelial lymphocytes expressed antigens associated with T cell subsets, very few expressed the Thy 1$^+$ marker, an antigen usually found on all T cells in the mouse (Table 6.3). Almost 70% of the lymphocytes isolated from the epithelium of the small intestine had the Lyt 2$^+$ marker, normally associated with suppressor/cytotoxic cells in the mouse, yet did not have the Thy 1$^+$ marker present. Of the remaining 30% of

Table 6.3   Intraepithelial lymphocytes (IEL) in food-allergic and in inflammatory gastrointestinal disease.

Disease	IEL	Histology	Reference
Coeliac disease			
Untreated	+ +	A	[22, 24, 35]
On gluten-free diet	N	N	
Challenge after diet	+ +	A	
Transient gluten intolerance			
Untreated	+ +	A	[91]
Treated	N	N	
Gluten challenge after cessation of intolerance	N	N	
Cows' milk protein allergy			
Untreated	+(+)	(N)A	[34, 43, 69, 76]
On milk-free diet	N	N	
On milk challenge	+(+)	(N)A	
Soya protein allergy			
Untreated	+(+)	A	[67]
On soya-free diet	N	N	
On soya challenge		Data not available	
Crohn's disease			
Small intestinal focal lesion	+ +	A	[19]
Without focal small intestinal lesion	N	N	
Autoimmune gut disease	N(+)★	N(A)★	Milla and Walker-Smith (1985, personal communication)

Normal values: adults: 6–40, mean 21 IEL per 100 epithelial cells; children: 11–36, mean 23 IEL per 100 epithelial cells [22, 69].
N: normal values and normal histology; A: abnormal histology.
+ +: marked increase, +(+) slight to moderate increase of IEL.
★ Only single cases reported without formal IEL counts. Observations of P Milla and J Walker-Smith (1985) ($n=5$) suggest that IEL counts are within the normal range or slightly raised.
Formal studies of IEL numbers in other food-related enteropathies have not yet been reported.

lymphocytes most were Thy 1$^+$, Lyt 1$^+$, Lyt 2$^-$, a profile typical of the helper/inducer population.

This finding has been confirmed by two other groups who also found a large proportion of murine intraepithelial lymphocytes to be Thy 1$^-$, Lyt 2$^+$ [68, 77], although Leventon et al [45] found only 32% of intraepithelial lymphocytes expressing T cell markers. However, as pointed out by Ernst et al [20], the latter study was probably examining a mixed population of lamina propria and intraepithelial lymphocytes as judged by the presence of 30% surface immunoglobulin positive (sIg$^+$) cells in their cell preparation.

The unusual cell surface marker profile of murine intraepithelial lymphocytes has also been shown to be present in the rat [47]. Using the anti-T cell monoclonal antibody W3/13 and anti-T cell subset monoclonal antibody OX8, Lyscom and Brueton have found a similar proportion of isolated rat intraepithelial lymphocytes to be W3/13$^-$OX8$^+$ (see Table 6.3).

Pan T cell marker

The lack, or at least very low expression, of a pan T cell marker on these cells raises doubts as to whether they are true T cells. Their presence in the mucosa of congenitally athymic nude mice [66] and in thymectomized, irradiated and bone-marrow reconstituted rats [55] would argue that they are not T cells. However, both these animal models may not be as 'T cell free' as was originally believed and so the exact lineage of these cells remains controversial.

Lamina propria cells

The picture in the lamina propria is completely different: the cells exhibiting T cell subset markers also have Thy 1 (mouse) or W3/13 (rat) on their surface and thus are comparable in cell surface phenotype to T cells found in other lymphoid organs. Lamina propria lymphocytes contain a more heterogeneous population of lymphocytes including B cells, plasma cells and null cells with about 35% T cells present in both mice [66] and rats [47]. The T cells found in the murine lamina propria contain more Lyt 1^+ than Lyt 2^+ cells.

Human studies

T cell origin of intraepithelial lymphocytes

Lymphocyte subsets found in the mucosa of the human small intestine vary in cell surface marker profile from those found in small rodents. After isolation, most human intraepithelial lymphocytes will form spontaneous rosettes with sheep erythrocytes, as do mature T cells from other lymphoid organs [9]. Examinations of intraepithelial lymphocytes either in situ [39, 79] or after isolation [9] indicate that 80-99% of the cells stain with antibodies directed against the common T cell antigen. Most of these cells, 65-85%, exhibit the T8 marker, usually associated with cytotoxic/suppressor T cells, while a minority, <10%, show the T4 marker, normally found on helper/inducer T cells (see Table 6.3). Lamina propria T cells, on the other hand, are predominantly T8$^-$, further emphasizing the difference between intraepithelial and lamina propria populations.

Summary

Both rodents and humans have almost exclusively T cells in their intraepithelial lymphocyte population, while only 30-40% of the lamina propria lymphocytes are T cells. The majority of T cells in the intraepithelial lymphocyte pool are of the suppressor/cytotoxic phenotype (T8$^+$ in man, Lyt 2^+ in mouse and OX8$^+$ in rat) but in the lamina propria more of the T cells carry the helper/inducer marker (T4$^+$ in man, Lyt 1^+ in mouse and W3/25$^+$ in rat). These cell surface marker studies emphasize the fact that intraepithelial and lamina propria populations must be investigated separately in order to elucidate the role of each in gastrointestinal immune responses.

FUNCTIONAL ROLE OF MUCOSAL T CELLS

Effector functions

The effector function of mucosal T cells can be examined by using two basic approaches: firstly, one can extract the lymphocytes from the gut and study their functional potential in vitro or, upon transfer, in vivo. Alternatively, one can look for methods of measuring cell-mediated immune reactions in situ.

T cell mediated cytotoxicity

Using the former approach, several groups have investigated the potential of mucosal T cells to mediate cytotoxic reactions in vitro. Arnaud-Battandier et al [3] demonstrated that guinea-pig mucosal lymphocytes could, after mitogen stimulation, lyse target cells in vitro, a function known to be mediated by T cells. Mitogen-induced cellular cytotoxicity has also been observed using intraepithelial and lamina propria lymphocytes from human colon [11] and intraepithelial lymphocytes from human small intestine [48].

An interesting series of experiments undertaken by Davies and Parrott [13, 14] showed that intraperitoneal injection of a mastocytoma cell line, P815, into mice resulted in the rapid appearance of large numbers of cytotoxic T cells amongst the intraepithelial lymphocytes and, particularly, the lamina propria lymphocytes of the small intestine. These antigen-specific, Thy 1^+ cells persisted for several weeks in the lamina propria, longer than in any of the other organs studied. This work has been confirmed by a recent report from Klein and Kagnoff [42] using a different tumour cell line, EL-4.

Persistence of cytotoxic T cells

Why these cytotoxic cells appear and persist in the small intestine is still a mystery: it could be that the gut mucosa, with its constant antigenic stimulus, is a particularly suitable site to which activated T cells will localize. Microenvironmental conditions may have an important influence on the appearance and persistence of effector T cells in the mucosa.

Functional potential in vivo

Alternatively, one can examine the function of isolated mucosal lymphocytes in vivo upon transfer to naive syngeneic recipients. We have recently reported that oral immunization of mice with a protein antigen can lead to the presence of delayed hypersensitivity effector cells in the intraepithelial lymphocyte population which are capable of transferring a classical delayed hypersensitivity reaction to unimmunized recipient mice [81] (Fig. 6.3).

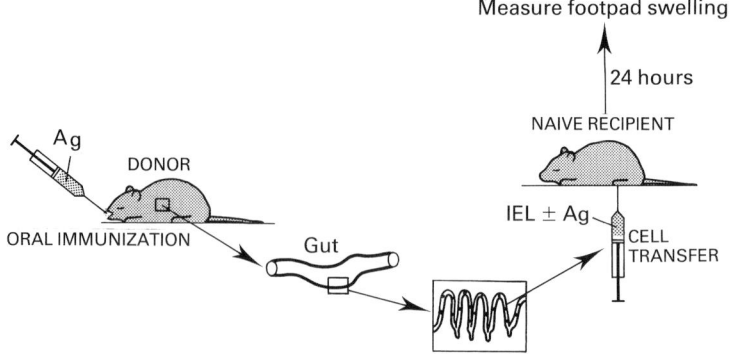

Fig. 6.3 Transfer of antigen (Ag) specific delayed-type hypersensitivity (DTH) with intraepithelial lymphocytes into naive recipients. Systemic DTH response of donor mice is negative. DTH in recipient mice is positive due to the presence of sensitized donor IELs and specific antigen; use of an unrelated antigen at the time of challenge produced no DTH reaction.

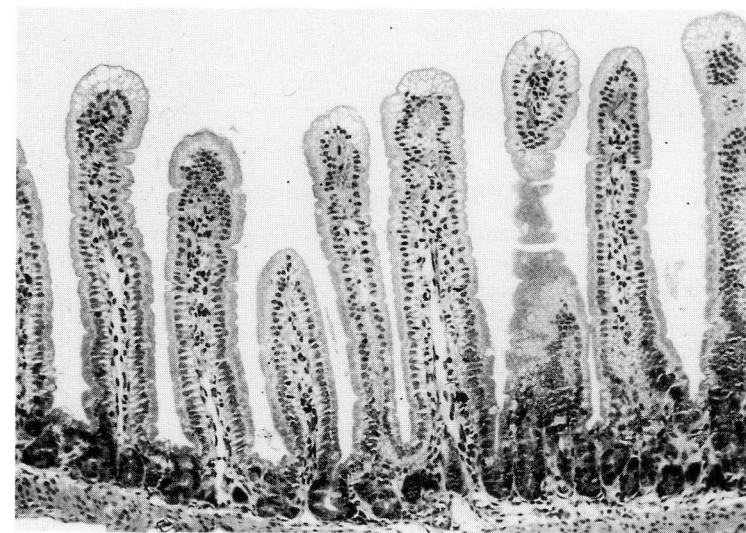

(a)

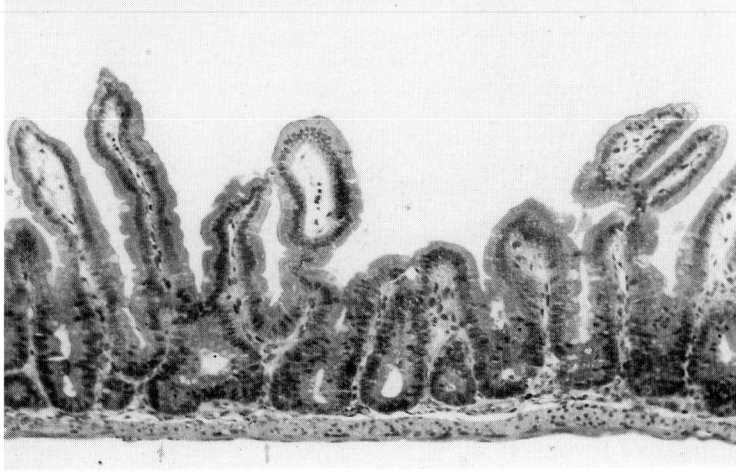

Fig. 6.4 Intestinal damage due to a cell mediated immune response: graft versus host disease. (a) Jejunum of a 15-day-old mouse (original magnification ×160) 14 days after intraperitoneal injection of syngeneic spleen cells (control). Note long fingershaped villi and short crypts. Villus/crypt ratio 5:1. (b) Jejunum of a 15-day-old mouse (original magnification ×160) 14 days after intraperitoneal injection of parental spleen cells (graft versus host disease). Note the irregular villus pattern with elongated crypts, shortened villi, mucosal oedema, and the only sparsely populated lamina propria. Villus/crypt ratio reduced to 1.8:1.

(b)

Although there was no evidence to suggest that oral immunization per se caused a gastrointestinal lesion in these animals, it would be interesting to examine those situations where oral immunization and challenge did lead to small intestinal pathology [59] to determine whether specific delayed hypersensitivity effector cells could be found in the intraepithelial lymphocyte population. Improved in vitro tests for identifying delayed hypersensitivity effector cells will be needed before it is possible to assess the relevance of these results to human disease.

Problems with isolated lymphocyte populations

The use of lymphocyte populations isolated from the mucosa leads to difficulties in the interpretation of results if the correct controls are not included. Lack of reactivity of mucosal cells may be due to a selective depletion and/or inactivation of responding cells by the preparative procedure. Control tissue or blood lymphocytes should be treated in an identical manner to assess the extent of altered reactivity caused by the procedure. Several groups have noted that cell-mediated cytotoxic function can be altered by the isolation protocol [7, 11]. Likewise, it is important to ascertain whether the reactivity of cells in mucosal lymphocyte preparations is due simply to activation of the cells during preparation.

Mucosal delayed hypersensitivity reactions

The alternative line of investigation, that of looking for in situ changes in the gut during mucosal cell-mediated immune (CMI) reactions, has been described by Ferguson and her co-workers. They hypothesized that the immunopathological findings in gastrointestinal diseases such as coeliac disease can be explained by local delayed hypersensitivity reactions occurring within the mucosa. This was based on the observation that classical cell-mediated immune reactions such as allograft rejection and graft-versus-host disease

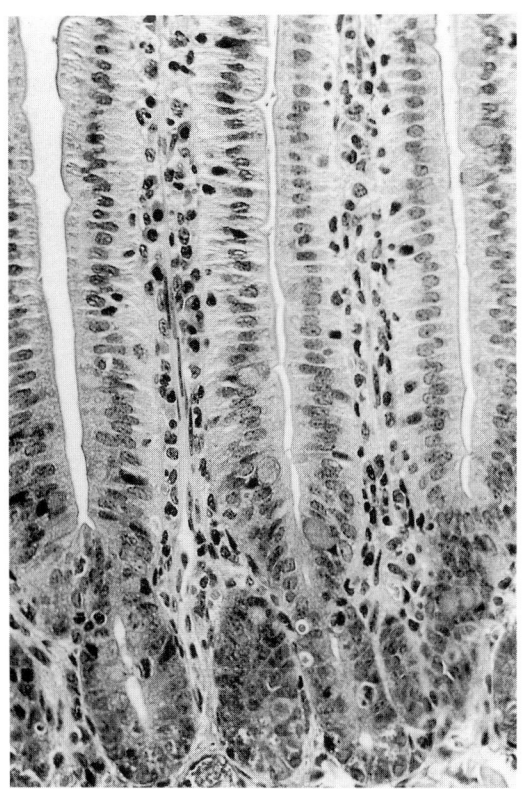 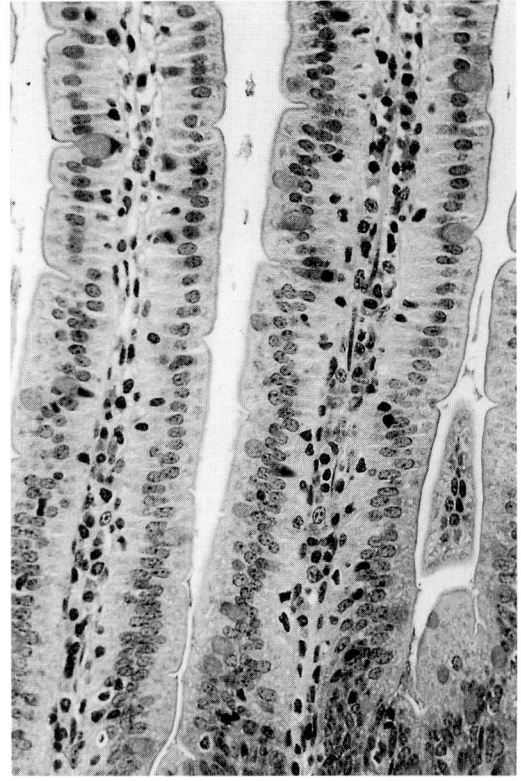

(a)   (b)

Fig. 6.5 Intraepithelial lymphocyte numbers during a cell mediated immune response to ovalbumin in the mouse. Original magnification ×320, haematoxylin–eosin. (a) Normal morphology and normal crypt cell kinetics in controls. Intraepithelial lymphocyte count: 11:1 per 100 epithelial cells. (b) Jejunum after induction of a cell mediated immune reaction to oral ovalbumin administration after injection of *N*-acetylmuramyl-dipeptide. (For full experimental details see [86].) Increased number of intraepithelial lymphocytes: 18.6 per 100 epithelial cells; otherwise normal morphology.

produced characteristic alterations in gut morphology (e.g. raised numbers of intraepithelial lymphocytes, increase in crypt length, villus atrophy) (Fig. 6.4) which were also seen, for example, in coeliac disease and cow's milk protein allergy.

Animal models. Three animal models have been studied by Ferguson et al: allograft rejection of fetal gut grafts [49], graft-versus-host disease induced in inbred mice by injecting parental spleen cells into F1 offspring [49, 60] and local hypersensitivity reactions produced by oral immunization and challenge using a soluble protein antigen [59, 84, 85]. In all three models there were comparable alterations in gut morphology and cell kinetics: increased numbers of intraepithelial lymphocytes (Fig. 6.5), increased crypt cell proliferation rates and increase in crypt length. The authors have proposed that these changes are indicative of a cell-mediated immune reaction taking place within the gut (Fig. 6.6). Based on these observations, the infiltration of the epithelium by lymphocytes has been examined in a number of clinical situations and their relevance to the pathogenesis will be discussed below.

Regulatory functions

Helper and suppressor T cells

T cells in the mucosa can operate not only as effector cells but also as regulatory cells influencing the appearance or activity of other cell types. Helper cells, specific for IgA, have been shown to be present in the Peyer's patches of mice [17] and it is likely that these are also to be found in the gut mucosa itself. Oral immunization with soluble or particulate antigen can lead to the production of specific IgA antibodies in a variety of mucosal tissues [10, 57]. Suppressor T cells can also be found in the gut-associated lymphoid tissues after oral immunization [4, 53] and this phenomenon of oral tolerance has been extensively studied in a variety of animal models (Chapter 14).

T cell requirement in response to parasites. A further regulatory role for mucosal T cells has been highlighted in experiments designed to investigate the immune response to gastrointestinal parasites. The crypt hyperplasia and villous atrophy associated with intestinal nematode infection are not seen in rats which have been rendered T cell depleted [23]. Both goblet cell hyperplasia [58] and mast cell hyperplasia [63, 75] found in the gut during helminth infestation were shown, by means of passive transfer experiments, to be controlled by T cells.

GASTROINTESTINAL T LYMPHOCYTES AND CLINICAL DISEASE

There are considerable problems in identifying and/or enumerating T cells or T cell subsets within the gastrointestinal mucosa and re-

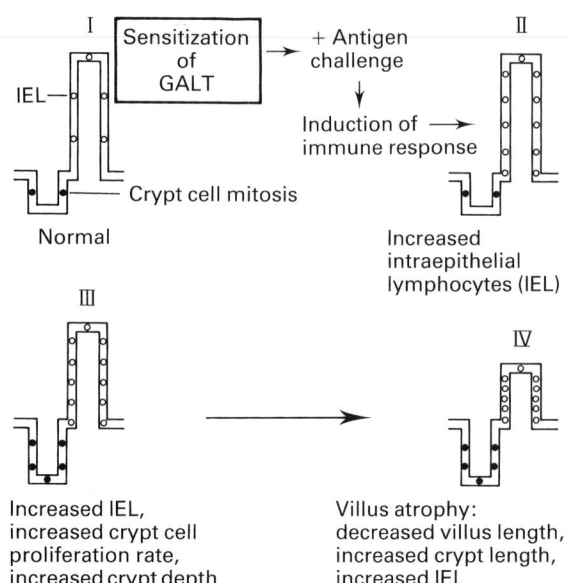

Fig. 6.6 Hypothetical chain of events in the generation of mucosal damage in intestinal cell-mediated immunity (hypertrophic villus atrophy). This model is derived from a series of observations and formal studies in human food-related enteropathies and experimentally induced cell-mediated immunity in animals. Still unresolved are the influences of genetic and environmental features involved in the pathogenesis of mucosal damage. Steps II and III can occur independently and need not necessarily progress to a more severe state of mucosal injury.

lating their presence or absence to disease. One major drawback is the difficulty in obtaining reasonably clean preparations without affecting their cell surface markers and/or functional properties in vitro. Another problem is that the functions of T cell subpopulations, as defined by their cell surface markers, do not necessarily correlate with their in vivo activity [46, 93].

An attempt will be made to summarize studies of cell numbers and cell surface markers of the gastrointestinal mucosa in food-related hypersensitivities and in inflammatory bowel disease.

Food-related enteropathy

Hypersensitivity reactions to foods have been implicated in a wide spectrum of clinical diseases including eczema, asthma, migraine, rheumatoid arthritis, behavioural disorders and others (for review see [16, 44]). In a considerable number of these conditions, a clear immunological pathogenesis has not yet been established. It is conceivable that some of these diseases represent direct toxic effects of the offending foods (for example due to histamine and/or tyramine content) or their contaminants (hormones, antibiotics), preservatives (salicylates, benzoates) or colourings (tartrazine, carnosine). We will concentrate on food-related hypersensitivities which cause gastroenteropathies with mucosal pathology.

Coeliac disease with its persistent intolerance to gluten has been studied most intensively [5, 21] (see Chapter 30). Similar mucosal abnormalities, although usually not as severe, have been reported in hypersensitivity reactions to milk, soya, rice, fish, egg and chicken [2, 38, 90, 91]. From an immunological point of view, however, any food antigen could cause a similar hypersensitivity reaction and careful evaluation of enteropathies in the future will most likely demonstrate clinical syndromes caused by a wide variety of foods and other antigens.

Gastrointestinal pathology

Increased numbers of intraepithelial lymphocytes have been demonstrated in patients with coeliac disease and cow's milk protein allergy when the intraepithelial infiltration of lymphocytes has been expressed in relation to the numbers of epithelial cells (see Table 6.3 for reference). This method has been criticized on the grounds that the apparent increase of in-

traepithelial lymphocytes is due to the 'cramming' of a normal number of lymphocytes into a reduced surface area [51].

Mucosal surface area and IEL infiltration. Observations in humans and in animal experiments [28, 33, 49, 87] suggest that an increased number of intraepithelial lymphocytes per 100 epithelial cells can be found even in a morphologically normal mucosa and there seems to be no consistent relationship between reduction of mucosal surface area and the infiltration with intraepithelial lymphocytes.

Cell surface markers in coeliac disease

In coeliac disease and other food-sensitive enteropathies, the number of intraepithelial lymphocytes returns to normal on an elimination diet and rises on subsequent challenge. Careful cell surface marker studies of the small intestinal epithelium in coeliac disease have not revealed a shift in OKT8$^+$, OKT4$^+$ and common T cell antigen (HuTLA)-positive cells when compared to normals (see Table 6.3). All intraepithelial lymphocytes were also HLA-DR$^-$, Tac$^-$ (present on activated T cells) and C3b receptor negative. A subset of intraepithelial lymphocytes (OKT8$^+$ and Leu 1$^+$) seems to be marginally increased in untreated coeliac disease. Slightly raised numbers of OKT8$^+$ were also found within the lamina propria lymphocyte population [79].

All abnormalities returned to normal on a gluten-free diet and these temporary abnormalities do not represent the underlying disorder of immunoregulation in coeliac disease.

A gluten responsive T cell? The higher percentage of OKT8$^+$, Leu 1$^+$ intraepithelial lymphocytes has been attributed to an increased cell traffic [79]. It is tempting to speculate that these cells indicate the arrival of a functionally distinct (gluten-responsive) cell population. It would be of particular interest to know which subpopulation of intraepithelial lymphocytes is changed, either quantitatively or qualitatively, during disease. Innate limitations of biopsy histopathology and of functional assays after complicated separation procedures have so far prevented unequivocal answers regarding the pathogenesis of food-related hypersensitivities [59].

Inflammatory bowel disease (IBD)

Although a role for food proteins in the pathogenesis of inflammatory bowel diseases (ulcerative colitis, Crohn's disease) has been suggested [1] this is still controversial and only a short discussion will be included here. Beneficial effects of oligoantigenic diets in the management of the acute phase of inflammatory bowel disease in adults and children have been published [36, 64]. Conclusive studies, however, as to the long-term benefits of these diets and their effects on the natural course of the disease are still needed (see Chaps. 31 and 32). A well-controlled study on colitis in infants under the age of two years has demonstrated the longer term curative effects of milk withdrawal on clinical symptoms and on mucosal morphology [40].

Intraepithelial lymphocytes in colonic tissue

Analysis of colonic tissue sections from patients with ulcerative colitis and Crohn's disease by Selby et al [78, 80] revealed that the majority of intraepithelial lymphocytes were T cells (HuTLA$^+$, UCHT1$^+$) and over 80% were of the suppressor/cytotoxic phenotype (OKT8$^+$) with a small population of helper/inducer type (OKT4$^+$) lymphocytes. Only about 30% of OKT8$^+$ cells reacted with a common T cell antibody (Leu 1). These cells were not activated (Tac$^-$) and were C3b receptor and surface immunoglobulin negative. Within the lamina propria OKT4$^+$ cells predominated (64%). There was no difference observed for normal or diseased intestinal mucosae.

Studies on venous blood lymphocytes

Several groups have reported changes in cell surface markers and functions of venous blood lymphocytes in inflammatory bowel disease. However since mucosal and systemic immune reactions are under separate cellular control [10, 89], these studies are potentially misleading. If one hypothesizes that the above mentioned diseases are due to an abnormal immune reaction, then investigations using venous blood lymphocytes may have little or no relevance to the disease process in the intestinal mucosa.

THE ROLE OF MUCOSAL T CELLS IN FOOD ANTIGEN-INDUCED ENTEROPATHY

Mechanisms of hypersensitivity

Evidence from studies of human diseases, clinical experience and animal studies point to an immunologically, cell-mediated mechanism for gluten and other food protein sensitive enteropathies [8, 23, 27, 59, 85, 86].

Humoral aspects

Immune reactions of the reaginic type (Type 1, IgE-mediated) do certainly play a role in immediate reactions to foods; however, enteropathies are not a feature of this immune response. Raised serum antibody titres to common food proteins can be found in diseased and healthy individuals with and without any gut damage [7, 21, 72, 73] and antibody titres are mainly a marker of active systemic immunity. A further important piece of evidence against the solitary role of antibodies in the pathogenesis of intestinal damage in coeliac disease is the well-documented case of a patient who had both coeliac disease and severe hypogammaglobulinaemia [92].

Cell-mediated mucosal reactions cause malabsorption

We believe there is persuasive evidence that cell-mediated mucosal reactions to foods and other enteric antigens cause or contribute to malabsorption syndromes in man. In all these conditions the normal patterns of immune responses to enteric antigens have been disturbed. A disturbance of immunoregulatory T cell function (reduction of T suppressor cell functions) allows sensitization within the gut-associated lymphoid tissues (see Fig. 6.7). This event would consequently lead to the activation of specific food-related memory and/ or effector T cells.

Seeding of effector cells for delayed hypersensitivity. Sensitized effector cells seed to the lamina propria via the established routes of lymphocyte recirculation. On contact with antigen these primed cells would then secrete enteropathic lymphokines. Damage of the gastrointestinal mucosa would be caused by altered crypt cell proliferation kinetics and/or by recruitment of delayed hypersensitivity effector cells. Animal studies have demonstrated that an increased crypt cell turnover is the first sign of intestinal damage caused by a cell-mediated immune response [60]. Thus the underlying pathogenesis can be envisaged as a failure of the immunoregulatory suppressor functions within the intestine and its associated lymphoid tissues.

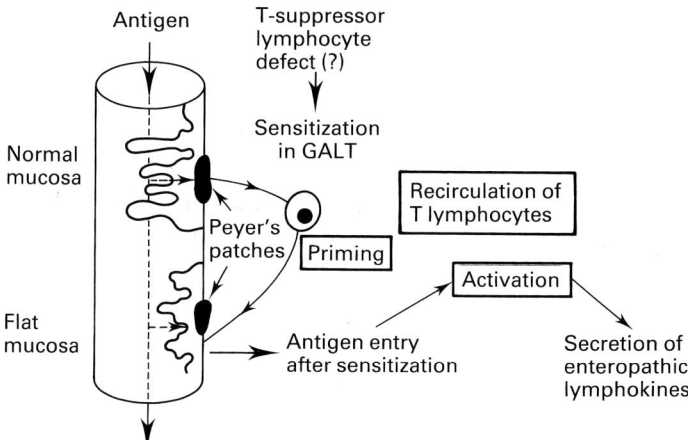

Fig. 6.7 Hypothetical chain of events in the generation of mucosal atrophy due to a cell-mediated immune reaction in the gut. (For further explanation please refer to the text.)

Prevention of food hypersensitivity

If this hypothesis proves to be correct, prevention or even reversal of food-related hypersensitivities should be feasible and become the ultimate goal of clinical management in sensitized patients. This could be achieved by antigen avoidance, by pharmacological manipulation of immuno-regulatory T cells and/or by the administration of tolerogenic antigen moieties to mucosa-associated lymphoid tissues. The existence of such immunosuppressive protein fragments has recently been demonstrated for the IgE system [15, 61].

More research into the pathogenesis of cell-mediated intestinal hypersensitivities, however, has to be carried out before the working hypothesis outlined above can be generally accepted—or dismissed—in the light of new findings.

REFERENCES

1 Acheson ED, Truelove SC: Early weaning in the aetiology of ulcerative colitis. Br Med J 1961; 2: 929–35.

2 Ament ME, Rubin CE: Soy protein—another cause of the flat intestinal lesion. Gastroenterology 1972; 62:227–34.

3 Arnaud-Battandier F, Bundy BM, O'Neill M et al: Cytotoxic activities of gut mucosal lymphoid cells in guinea pigs. J Immunol 1978; 121:1959–65.

4 Asherson GL, Zembala M, Perera MACC et al: Production of immunity and unresponsiveness in the mouse by feeding contact sensitizing agents and the role of suppressor cells in the Peyer's patches, mesenteric lymph nodes and other lymphoid tissue. Cell Immunol 1977; 33:145–55.

5 Asquith P, Haeney MR: Coeliac disease. In: Asquith P, ed. Immunology of the gastrointestinal tract. Edinburgh: Churchill-Livingstone, 1979; 66–92.

6 Bahna SL, Heiner DC: Allergies to milk. New York: Grune and Stratton, 1980.

7 Bland PW, Richens ER, Britton DC, Lloyd JV: Isolation and purification of human large bowel mucosal lymphoid cells; effect of separation technique on functional characteristics. Gut 1979; 20:1037–46.

8 Bullen AW, Losowsky MS: Cell mediated immunity to gluten fraction III in adult coeliac disease. Gut 1978; 19:126–31.

9 Cerf-Bensussan N, Guy-Grand D, Griscelli C: Intra-epithelial lymphocytes of human gut: isolation, characterization and study of natural killer activity. Gut 1985; 26:81–8.

10 Challacombe SJ, Tomasi TB: Systemic tolerance and secretory immunity after oral immunisation. J Exp Med 1980; 152:1459–72.

11 Chiba M, Bartnik W, ReMine SG et al: Human colonic intraepithelial and lamina propria lymphocytes: cytotoxicity in vitro and the potential effects of the isolation method on their functional properties. Gut 1981; 22:177–86.

12 Collan Y: Characteristics of non-epithelial cells in the epithelium of normal rat ileum. A light and electron microscopical study. Scand J Gastroenterol 1972; 7 [Suppl 18]: 1–66.

13 Davies MDJ, Parrott DMV: The early appearance of specific cytotoxic T cells in murine gut mucosa. Clin Exp Immunol 1980; 42:273–9.

14 Davies MDJ, Parrott DMV: Cytotoxic T cell in small intestine epithelial, lamina propria and lung lymphocytes. Immunology 1981; 44:367–71.

15 Dosa S, Pesce AJ, Ford DJ et al: Immunological properties of peptide fragments of bovine serum albumin. Immunology 1979; 38:509–17.

16 Egger J, Carter CM, Wilson J et al: Is migraine food allergy? A double-blind controlled trial of oligoantigenic diet treatment. Lancet 1983; ii:865–8.

17 Elson CO, Heck JA, Strober W: T cell regulation of murine IgA synthesis. J Exp Med 1979; 149:632–43.

18 Enerbäck L: Mast cells in rat gastrointestinal mucosa. II. Dye-binding and metachromatic properties. Acta Pathol Microbiol Immunol Scand 1966; 66:303–12.

19 Entrican JH, Busuttil A, Ferguson A: Histopathological features of lesions in the jejunal mucosa in Crohn's

disease are consistent with a cell mediated immune response. Gut 1984; 25:A1145-6.

20 Ernst PB, Befus AD, Bienenstock J: Leukocytes in the intestinal epithelium: an unusual immunological compartment. Immunol Today 1985; 6:50-5.

21 Ferguson A: Coeliac disease and gastrointestinal food allergy. In: Ferguson A, MacSween RNM, eds. Immunological aspects of the liver and gastrointestinal tract. Lancaster: MTP Press, 1976; 153-202.

22 Ferguson A: Intraepithelial lymphocytes of the small intestine. Gut 1977; 18:921-37.

23 Ferguson A, Jarrett EEE: Hypersensitivity reactions in the small intestine. I. Thymus dependence of experimental 'partial villus atrophy'. Gut 1975; 16:114-7.

24 Ferguson A, Murray D: Quantitation of intraepithelial lymphocytes in human jejunum. Gut 1971; 12:988-94.

25 Ferguson A, Parrott DMV: Growth and development of antigen-free grafts of fetal mouse intestine. J Pathol 1972; 106:95-101.

26 Ferguson A, Parrott DMV: The effect of antigen deprivation on thymus dependent and thymus independent lymphocytes in the small intestine of the mouse. Clin Exp Immunol 1972; 12:477-88.

27 Ferguson A, Parrott DMV: Histopathology and time course of rejection of allografts of mouse small intestine. Transplantation 1973; 15:516-24.

28 Ferguson A, Ziegler K, Strobel S: Gluten intolerance (Coeliac disease). Ann Allergy 1984; 53:637-42.

29 Fichtelius KE, Finstad J, Good RA: The phylogenetic occurrence of lymphocytes within the gut epithelium. Int Arch Allergy Appl Immunol 1969; 35:119-33.

30 Fichtelius KE, Yunis EJ, Good RA: Occurrence of lymphocytes within the gut epithelium of normal and neonatally thymectomised mice. Proc Soc Exp Biol 1968; 128:185-8.

31 Grossi CE, Cadoni A, Zizza A et al: Large granular lymphocytes in human peripheral blood: ultrastructural and cytochemical characterization of the granules. Blood 1982;59:277-83.

32 Guy-Grand D, Griscelli G, Vassalli P: The gut associated lymphoid system: nature and properties of the large dividing cells. Eur J Immunol 1974; 4:435-43.

33 Guy-Grand D, Griscelli C, Vassalli P: The mouse gut T lymphocyte, a novel type of T cell. Nature, origin and traffic in mice in normal and graft-versus-host conditions. J Exp Med 1978; 148:1661-77.

34 Harrison BM, Kilby A, Walker-Smith JA et al: Cow's milk protein intolerance: a possible association with gastroenteritis, lactose intolerance and IgA deficiency. Br Med J 1976; 1:1501-4.

35 Holmes GKT, Asquith P, Stokes PL, Cooke WT: Cellular infiltrate of jejunal biopsies in adult coeliac disease in relation to gluten withdrawal. Gut 1974; 15:278-93.

36 Hunter JO, Jones A, Freeman AH et al: Food intolerance in gastrointestinal disorders. In: Proceedings of Second Food Allergy Workshop. Oxford: Medicine Publishing Foundation, 1983:69-70.

37 Huntley JF, McGorum B, Newlands GFJ, Miller HRP: Granulated intraepithelial lymphocytes: their relationship to mucosal mast cells and globule leukocytes in the rat. Immunology 1984; 53:525-35.

38 Iyngkaran N, Abidin Z, Meng LL, Yadav M: Egg protein-induced villous atrophy. J Pediatr Gastroenterol Nutr 1982; 1:29-33.

39 Janossy G, Tidman N, Selby WS et al: Human T lymphocytes of inducer and suppressor type occupy different microenvironments. Nature 1980; 288:81-4.

40 Jenkins HR, Pincott JR, Soothill JF et al: Food allergy: the major cause of infantile colitis. Arch Dis Child 1984; 59:326-9.

41 Kelsall MA, Crabb ED: Lymphocytes and plasmacytes in nucleoprotein metabolism. Ann NY Acad Sci 1958; 72:293-317.

42 Klein JR, Kagnoff MF: Nonspecific recruitment of cytotoxic effector cells in the intestinal mucosa of antigen-primed mice. J Exp Med 1984; 160:1931-6.

43 Kuitunen P, Visakorpi J, Savilhati E, Pelkonen P: Malabsorption syndrome with cow's milk intolerance. Clinical findings and course in 54 cases. Arch Dis Child 1975; 50:351-6.

44 Lessof M, ed: Clinical reactions to food. Chichester: John Wiley and Sons, 1983.

45 Leventon GS, Kulkarni SS, Meistrich ML et al: Isolation of murine small bowel intraepithelial lymphocytes. J Immunol Methods 1983; 63:35-44.

46 Lin YL, Askonas BA: Biological properties of an influenza-A virus specific T cell clone. J Exp Med 1981; 154:225-34.

47 Lyscom N, Brueton MJ: Intraepithelial, lamina propria and Peyer's patch lymphocytes of the rat small intestine: isolation and characterisation in terms of immunoglobulin markers and receptors for monoclonal antibodies. Immunology 1982; 45:775-83.

48 McDermott RP, Franklin GO, Jenkins KM et al: Human intestinal mononuclear cells. I. Investigation of antibody-dependent, lectin-induced and spontaneous cell mediated cytotoxic capabilities. Gastroenterology 1980; 78:47-56.

49 MacDonald TT, Ferguson A: Hypersensitivity reactions in the small intestine. III. The effects of allograft rejection and of GvHD on epithelial cell kinetics. Cell Tissue Kinet 1977; 10:301-12.

50 Marsh MN: Studies of intestinal lymphoid tissue. II. Aspects of proliferation and migration of epithelial lymphocytes in the small intestine of mice. Gut 1975; 16:674-82.

51 Marsh MN: Studies of the intestinal lymphoid tissue. III. Quantitative analyses of epithelial lymphocytes in the small intestine of human control subjects and patients with coeliac sprue. Gastroenterology 1980; 79:481-92.

52 Marsh MN: Studies of intestinal lymphoid tissue. IV. The predictive value of raised mitotic indices among jejunal epithelial lymphocytes in the diagnosis of gluten-sensitive enteropathy. J Clin Pathol 1982; 35:517-27.

53 Mattingly JA, Waksman BH: Immunologic suppression after oral administration of antigen. J Immunol 1978; 121:1878-83.

54 Mayrhofer G: Fixation and staining of granules in mucosal mast cells and intraepithelial lymphocytes in the rat jejunum, with special reference to the relationship between acid glycosaminoglycans in the two cell types. Histochem J 1980; 12:513-26.

55 Mayrhofer G: Thymus-dependent and thymus-independent subpopulations of intestinal intraepithelial lymphocytes: a granular subpopulation of probable bone marrow origin and relationship to mucosal mast cells. Blood 1980; 55:532-5.

56 Mayrhofer G, Whately RJ: Granular intraepithelial lymphocytes of the rat small intestine. I. Isolation, presence in T lymphocyte-deficient rats and bone marrow origin. Int Arch Allergy Appl Immunol 1983; 71:317-27.

57 Mestecky J, McGhee JR, Arnold RR et al: Selective induction of an immune response in human external secretions by ingestion of bacterial antigen. J Clin Invest 1978; 61:731-7

58 Miller HRP, Nawa Y: *Nippostrongylus brasiliensis*: intestinal goblet cell response in adoptively immunised rats. Exp Parasitol 1979; 47:81–90.

59 Mowat AMcI, Ferguson A: Hypersensitivity in the small intestinal mucosa. V. Induction of cell mediated immunity to a dietary antigen. Clin Exp Immunol 1981; 43:574–82.

60 Mowat AMcI, Ferguson A: Intraepithelial lymphocyte count and crypt hyperplasia measure the mucosal component of the graft-versus-host reaction in mouse small intestine. Gastroenterology 1982; 83:417–23.

61 Muckerheide A, Pesce AJ, Michael JG: Modulation of the IgE immune response to BSA by fragments of the antigen. I. Suppression by free fragments and by fragments conjugated to homologous gamma-globulin. Cell Immunol 1981; 59:392–8.

62 Murray M, Miller HRP, Jarrett WFH: The globule leukocyte and its derivation from the subepithelial mast cell. Lab Invest 1968; 19:222–34.

63 Nawa Y, Miller HRP: Adoptive transfer of the intestinal mast cell response in rats infected with *Nippostrongylus brasiliensis*. Cell Immunol 1979; 42:225–39.

64 O'Morain C, Segal AM, Levi AJ, Valman HB: Elemental diet in Crohn's disease. Arch Dis Child 1983; 58:44–7.

65 Otto HF: The interepithelial lymphocytes of the intestine: morphological observations and immunological aspects of intestinal enteropathy. Curr Top Pathol 1973; 57:81–121.

66 Parrott DMV, Tait C, Mowat AMcI et al: Analysis of the effector functions of different populations of mucosal lymphocytes. Ann NY Acad Sci 1983; 409:307–20.

67 Perkkio M, Savilahti E, Kuitunen P: Morphometric and immunohistochemical study of jejunal biopsies from children with intestinal soy allergy. Eur J Pediatr 1981; 137:63–9.

68 Petit A, Ernst PB, Befus AD et al: Murine intestinal intraepithelial lymphocytes. I. Relationship of a novel Thy-1$^-$, Lyt-1$^-$, Lyt-2$^+$ granulated subpopulation to natural killer cells and mast cells. Eur J Immunol 1985; 15:211–5.

69 Phillips AD, Rice SJ, France NE, Walker-Smith JA: Small intestinal lymphocyte levels in cow's milk protein intolerance. Gut 1979; 20:509–12.

70 Röpke C, Everett NB: Kinetics of intraepithelial lymphocytes in the small intestine of thymus deprived mice and antigen deprived mice. Anat Rec 1976; 185:101–8.

71 Röpke C, Everett NB: Proliferative kinetics of large and small intraepithelial lymphocytes in the small intestine of the mouse. Am J Anat 1976; 145:395–408.

72 Rothberg RM, Farr RS: Anti-bovine serum albumin and anti-alpha lactalbumin in the sera of children and adults. Pediatrics 1965; 35:571–5.

73 Rothberg RM, Rieger CHL, Silverman GA, Peri BA: Antigen uptake and antibody production in the human newborn. In: Ogra PL, Bienenstock J, eds. The mucosal immune system in health and disease. Report of the 81st Ross conference on paediatric research, Columbus, Ohio: Ross Laboratories 1981: 57–62.

74 Rudzik O, Bienenstock J: Isolation and characteristics of gut mucosal lymphocytes. Lab Invest 1974; 30: 260–6.

75 Ruitenberg EJ, Elgersma A: Absence of intestinal mast

cell response in congenitally athymic mice during *Trichinella spiralis* infection. Nature 1976; 264:258–60.

76 Savilhati E, Kuitunen P, Visakorpi JK: Cow's milk allergy. In: Lebenthal E, ed. Textbook of gastroenterology and nutrition in infancy. Vol. 2. New York: Raven Press, 1981;689–708.

77 Schrader JW, Scollay R, Battye F: Intramucosal lymphocytes of the gut: Lyt-2 and Thy-1 phenotype of the granulated cells and evidence for the presence of both T cell and mast cell precursors. J Immunol 1983: 130:558–64.

78 Selby WS, Janossy G, Jewell DP: Intestinal lymphocyte subpopulations in inflammatory bowel disease: an analysis by immunohistological and cell isolation studies. Gut 1984; 25:32–40.

79 Selby WS, Janossy G, Bofill M, Jewell DP: Lymphocyte subpopulations in human small intestine. The findings in normal mucosa and in the mucosa of patients with adult coeliac disease. Clin Exp Immunol 1983; 52:219–28.

80 Selby WS, Janossy G, Goldstein G, Jewell DP: T-lymphocyte subsets in normal intestinal mucosa: the distribution and relationship to MHC-derived antigens. Clin Exp Immunol 1981; 44:453–8.

81 Shields JG, Parrott DMV: Appearance of delayed-type hypersensitivity effector cells in murine gut mucosa. Immunology 1985; 54:771–6.

82 Shields JW, Touchon RC, Dickson DR: Quantitative studies on small lymphocyte disposition in epithelial cells. Am J Pathol 1969;54:129–44.

83 Stenqvist H: Die 'Zellenwanderung' durch das Darmepithel. Anat Anz 1934; 78:68–79.

84 Strobel S: Modulation of the immune response to fed antigen in mice. Edinburgh: University of Edinburgh, 1983. 269 pp. PhD thesis.

85 Strobel S, Ferguson A: Effects of neonatal antigen feeding on subsequent systemic and local CMI responses. Gut 1982; 23:A895.

86 Strobel S, Ferguson A: Modulation of intestinal and systemic immune response to a fed protein antigen in mice. Gut 1986, in press.

87 Strobel S, Brydon WG, Ferguson A: Cellobiose/mannitol sugar permeability test complements biopsy histopathology in clinical investigation of the jejunum. Gut 1984; 25:1241–6.

88 Strobel S, Miller HRP, Ferguson A: Human intestinal mucosal mast cells: evaluation of fixation and staining techniques. J Clin Pathol 1981; 34:851–8.

89 Swarbrick ET, Stokes CR, Soothill JF: Absorption of antigens after oral immunisation and the simultaneous induction of specific systemic tolerance. Gut 1979; 20:121–5.

90 Vitoria JC, Camarero C, Sojo A et al: Enteropathy related to fish, rice and chicken. Arch Dis Child 1982; 57:44–8.

91 Walker-Smith JA: Dietary protein intolerance. In: Diseases of the small intestine in childhood, 2nd ed. Tunbridge Wells: Pitman Medical, 1979: 139–70.

92 Webster ADB, Slavin G, Shiner M et al: Coeliac disease with severe hypogammaglobulinaemia. Gut 1981; 22:153–7.

93 Weiss S, Dennert G: T cell lines active in the delayed-type hypersensitivity reaction. J Immunol 1981; 126:2031–5.

Chapter 7
The B Cell System

Per Brandtzaeg

Introduction

Secretory IgA. The interest in local humoral immunity was significantly boosted in the 1960s when it was reported by Tomasi and co-workers [233] that the predominant immunoglobulin (Ig) in external body fluids was IgA rather than IgG. This secretory IgA (SIgA) was shown to have unique immuno-chemical and physicochemical properties because of its dimeric nature and association with the secretory component (SC), which is

118

an epithelial glycoprotein of molecular weight (M_r) of approximately 80 000 [94, 232]. Shortly afterwards, Crabbé et al [57] demonstrated an isotype distribution of intestinal Ig-producing immunocytes strikingly different from that found for B cells in other lymphoid tissues; in mucosa IgA immunocytes were predominant—being more than 20 times as numerous as IgG-producing cells. This distribution has been repeatedly verified [34] although how it is regulated remains obscure. The first direct evidence indicating that the IgA immunocytes of the gut and other secretory tissues were peculiar in producing dimers rather than monomers was obtained in 1973 [21], but again the mechanism regulating this production is unknown.

Secretory IgM. In 1970 it was pointed out by our laboratory that IgM appears in exocrine fluids in addition to IgA and both because of selective transport [41]. Secretory IgM (SIgM) was later shown to be associated with SC and to follow the same intracellular route through glandular epithelia as SIgA [25, 46], and in 1974 a common epithelial transport model was proposed for dimeric IgA and pentameric IgM [22, 23].

J chain. The 'joining' (J) chain had been identified a few years earlier as a unique polypeptide ($M_r \sim 15\,000$) shared by these two Ig polymers [92, 159]. Our original suggestion that the J chain and epithelial SC represent the 'lock and key' in the selective external translocation of IgA and IgM has recently been firmly established [38] and it has been shown that prominent production of J chain is a common feature of B cells subjected to terminal differentiation at secretory sites [30, 37]. In teleological terms one would like to think that this complex cooperation between the B cell system and the glandular epithelium has been preserved in mammals because secretory antibodies are necessary for survival.

The latter view is challenged by the fact that patients totally lacking SIgA and SIgM sometimes have a perfectly functioning gut. At least in countries with good hygiene, therefore, the non-specific innate defence mechanisms may afford sufficient mucosal protection [148]. It is, moreover, difficult to evaluate the clinical role of secretory antibodies, even in subjects with a normal immune system, because a superimposed protective effect of concurrent systemic cellular and humoral immunity must always be considered.

GALT. The so-called gut-associated lymphoid tissue (GALT) is of central importance in the induction of secretory immunity. GALT includes lymphoepithelial structures such as Peyer's patches and solitary lymphoid follicles scattered throughout the gastrointestinal tract. Some authors also consider the mesenteric lymph nodes to be part of GALT. This chapter will focus on the functional characteristics of B cells in gastrointestinal mucosa and on their generation in GALT and other mucosa-associated lymphoid tissues (MALT). Emphasis will be placed on the human secretory immune system and on B cell alterations that take place in gut diseases. Initially a brief outline of the complex interactions between the various components of the gastrointestinal humoral defence system will be given as background information for subsequent discussions.

HUMORAL DEFENCE OF THE GUT

Immune exclusion

This term is coined for surface protection mediated by antibodies in cooperation with innate non-specific factors and thus refers to the 'first line' of defence (Fig. 7.1). Antibodies in gastrointestinal juice are mainly carried by actively secreted dimeric IgA and pentameric IgM, but there may be some contribution by serum-derived or locally produced IgG which reaches the surface by intercellular diffusion.

Immune regulation

Regulation of secretory immunity takes place both in organized parts of MALT (on the right in Fig. 7.1) and in glandular parts of the mucosa (on the left). Antigen is primarily taken up by MALT through follicle-associated epithelium (FAE) which contains 'membrane' (M) cells particularly designed for sampling and inward transport of luminal material (see Chapter 4).

Antigen presentation. Antigen is next either presented to sub- and intraepithelial T lymphocytes by dendritic antigen-presenting cells (APC) after initial processing in subepithelial macrophages, or it is subjected to direct presentation by epithelial cells. In man both APC and FAE express surface determinants encoded by HLA-DR and other loci [19] present in the class II region of the major histocom-

Fig. 7.1 Schematic representation of the three main components of mucosal immune defence: immune exclusion, immune regulation and immune elimination. Antigen stimulation in mucosa-associated lymphoid tissue provides 'first signals' to B cells which migrate to glandular parts of the mucosa via lymph and peripheral blood. 'Second signals' (dashed heavy arrow) induce local proliferation and terminal differentiation of the extravasated B cells. Most plasma cells generated in this way produce J-chain-containing dimeric IgA which is translocated to the lumen as stabilized SIgA. Also some IgM is actively transported by the crypt cells whereas small amounts of IgG normally reach the lumen by passive diffusion (dashed thin arrow).

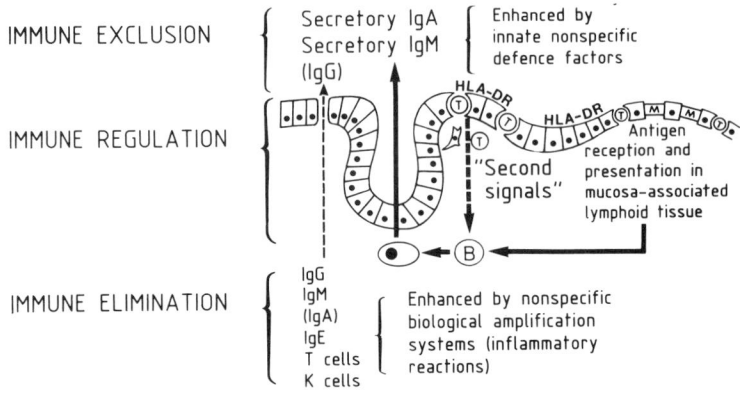

patibility complex (MHC). These gene products (human counterparts to Ia molecules) are required for appropriate antigen-presenting function. T cells thus subjected to MHC-restricted stimulation release immunoregulatory substances which act on other lymphocytes in the microenvironment.

B cells that become stimulated by 'first signals' in MALT migrate through lymph and peripheral blood and are finally seeded into distant sites of the lamina propria where they develop to Ig-producing plasma cells. This terminal differentiation is caused by 'second signals' which are modulated by various local cells expressing class II MHC molecules and by regulatory T lymphocytes (Fig. 7.1). Most of the B cells included in this traffic from MALT to glandular parts of the mucosa apparently belong to memory clones of an early maturation stage; this is indicated by their proneness to express cytoplasmic J chain regardless of concomitant isotype production (IgA normally being predominant). J-chain-containing dimeric IgA and pentameric IgM are finally transported to the gut lumen as SIgA and SIgM.

Immune elimination

This term refers to mechanisms involved in removal of foreign material which has penetrated the mucosal barrier; it represents a 'second line' of defence that depends partially on locally produced antibodies of various isotypes, probably often operating in combination with T cells and K ('killer') cells (Fig. 7.1). Immune elimination is enhanced by non-specific amplification mechanisms which,

however, may evolve into immunopathology and give rise to overt mucosal disease if satisfactory removal of antigen is not achieved. Such mechanisms are apparently involved in the pathogenesis of various gut disorders such as coeliac disease and inflammatory bowel disease.

B CELLS IN GUT MUCOSA

Ig-producing cells in normal mucosa

All normal secretory tissue sites in adults contain a remarkable preponderance of IgA-producing immunocytes (plasma cells and their immediate precursors). This is particularly true for the intestinal mucosa (Fig. 7.2) as first reported on the basis of immunohistochemical studies by Crabbé et al [57] and Rubin et al [198]. There are approximately 10^{10} such cells per metre of adult bowel [34]. Absolute figures are difficult to obtain for other secretory tissues where the cells are more heterogeneously distributed throughout the stroma than they are in the intestinal lamina propria, but it seems indisputable that most gland-associated IgA cells are located in the gut. Moreover, the size of this cell population is quite impressive compared with the figure of 2.5×10^{10} estimated for the total number of Ig-producing cells present in bone marrow, spleen and lymph nodes altogether [236].

B cells in intestinal mucosa. Analyses of B cells isolated from gut lamina propria of mice indicate a fairly similar content of Ig-producing immunocytes and B lymphocytes (22% versus

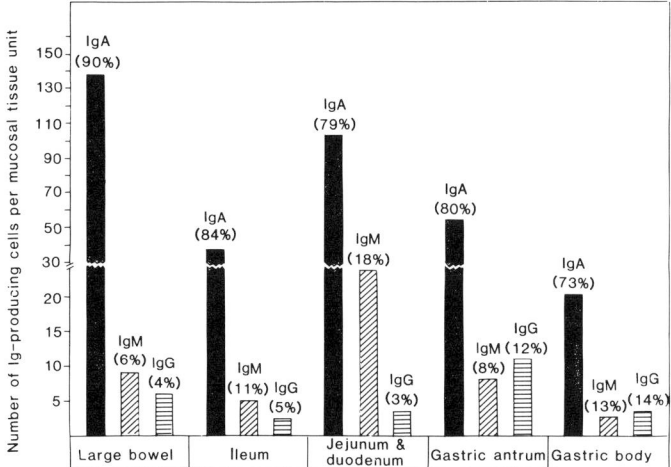

Fig. 7.2 Number of IgA-, IgM- and IgG-producing cells in various segments of normal human gastrointestinal mucosa. The counts are related to a 'tissue unit' which constitutes a 6 μm thick and a 500 μm wide mucosal block extending from the muscularis mucosae to the lumen (Fig. 7.6). The percentage isotype distribution of the immunocytes is indicated above the columns. Based on published data from the author's laboratory.

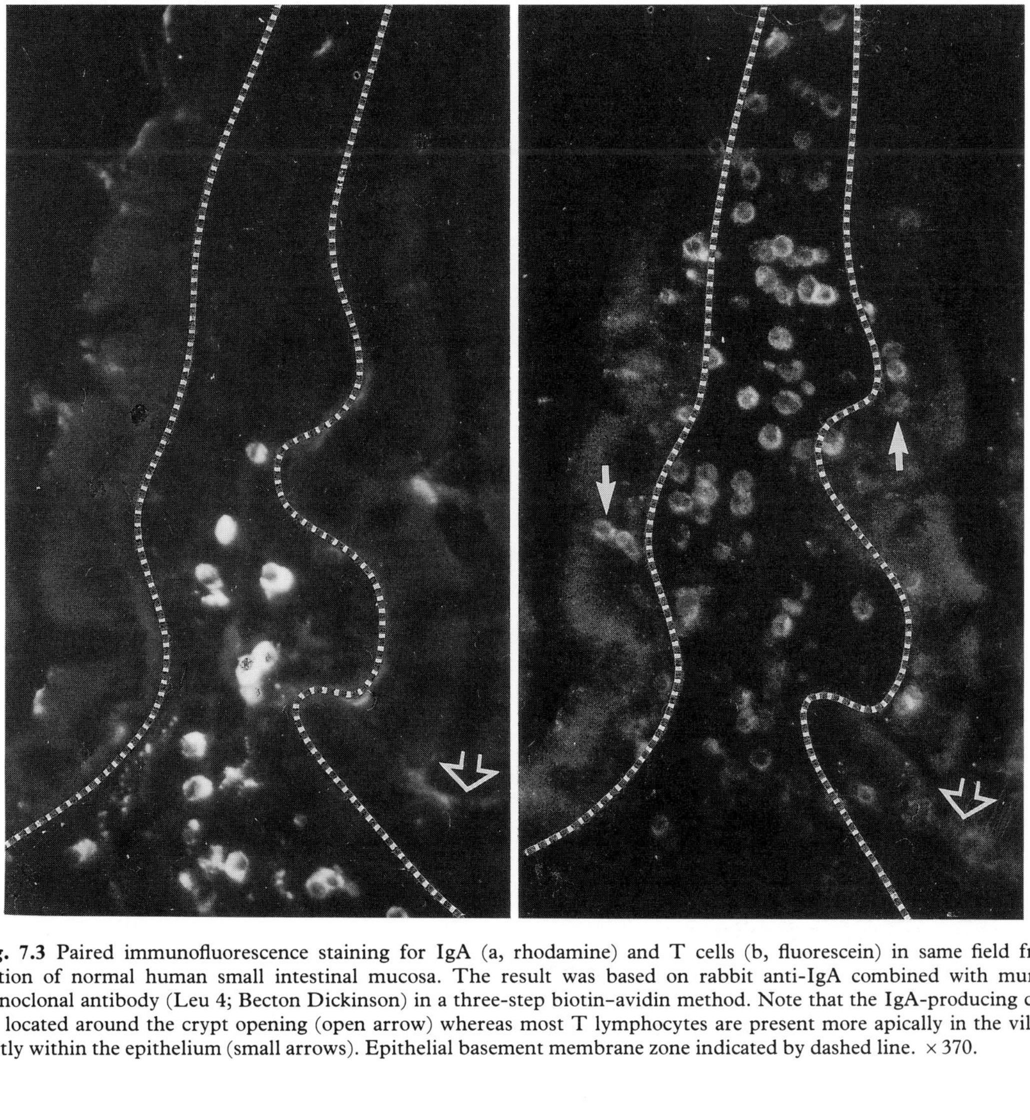

(b)

Fig. 7.3 Paired immunofluorescence staining for IgA (a, rhodamine) and T cells (b, fluorescein) in same field from section of normal human small intestinal mucosa. The result was based on rabbit anti-IgA combined with murine monoclonal antibody (Leu 4; Becton Dickinson) in a three-step biotin–avidin method. Note that the IgA-producing cells are located around the crypt opening (open arrow) whereas most T lymphocytes are present more apically in the villus, partly within the epithelium (small arrows). Epithelial basement membrane zone indicated by dashed line. $\times 370$.

18%). Most of the latter bear IgM or IgM + IgD on their surface [234]. The total fraction of B cells was found to equal that of T lymphocytes [234]. However, such studies probably underestimate the relative number of Ig-producing cells as it is difficult to exclude circulating lymphocytes from the tissue suspensions and because there may also be a selective loss of stimulated lymphoid cells during the isolation steps [80]. Analyses of B cells isolated from human intestinal mucosa have provided highly discrepant results and are inconclusive in quantitative terms [155].

Distribution of B cells. Preparation of mucosal suspensions does not take into account the fact that various lymphoid cells have different distributions in the lamina propria. Animal experiments have indicated that T cells become preferentially localized in the villi [16] whereas Ig-producing cells accumulate mainly around the crypt regions [104]. In the human jejunal mucosa, about 65% of all Ig-producing cells are normally located in a zone including the luminal 100 μm of the crypt layer and the basal 100 μm of the villi [6]. In this zone, which constitutes less than one-third of the total mucosal height, Ig-producing cells are intermingled with relatively few T lymphocytes, whereas the latter often abound more apically in the villi (Fig. 7.3).

Relative proportions of IgA1 and IgA2 cells. A relatively large contribution of the IgA2 subclass (35–60%) has been reported for the IgA immunocytes in gastrointestinal mucosa compared with that (13–24%) found in tonsils and peripheral lymph nodes [2, 60, 112]. A similarly high proportion of IgA2 (30–40%) is found in SIgA of intestinal fluid [112]; this may be important for the stability of SIgA because IgA2, in contrast to IgA1 is resistant to several IgA-specific proteases which are produced by a variety of bacterial species [117, 184].

IgM cells. IgM-producing cells constitute a substantial but variable fraction of the normal gastrointestinal immunocyte population in adults (Fig. 7.2). The reason for the relatively high proportion of this isotype in the proximal small intestine is unknown.

IgG, IgD and IgE cells. IgG-producing cells constitute 3–5% of the immunocytes in normal adult intestinal mucosa, but a considerably larger contribution is found in gastric mucosa (Fig. 7.2) which often is affected by low-grade gastritis even in healthy subjects [237]. Only occasional IgD and IgE immunocytes are encountered in the gastrointestinal mucosa, whereas IgD-producing cells constitute a significant fraction (2–10%) of the glandular immunocytes in the upper aeroalimentary tract (AAT) which includes nasal mucosa and salivary and lacrimal glands [44, 120].

J chain and nature of locally produced IgA and IgM

Demonstration of J chain and cytoplasmic SC affinity

The gastrointestinal IgA immunocytes differ from those found in tonsils, lymph nodes, spleen and bone marrow by showing a more prominent synthesis of dimers than of monomers. The presence of dimeric IgA in their cytoplasm can be immunohistochemically demonstrated by incubating tissue sections with purified free SC [21, 30]. The SC-binding site of dimeric IgA and pentameric IgM is generated at the cytoplasmic level by incorporation of J chain, and both IgA and IgM immunocytes in the gut produce abundant amounts of this polypeptide [24, 30].

Immunohistochemical staining of IgA-associated J chain is largely dependent on unmasking of antigenic determinants by acid urea treatment (Fig. 7.4). Conversely, intestinal IgM immunocytes seem to contain a substantial excess of free cytoplasmic J chain as indicated by 100% positivity even in untreated tissue sections (Fig. 7.4). Studies of murine plasmacytomas showed that J-chain production was excessive in IgM cells compared with that in IgA cells [176]. Moreover, a five-fold molar excess of cytoplasmic over secreted J chain was found in IgM-producing rabbit spleen cells after mitogen stimulation [196].

Local IgM production

SC-binding capacity of IgM immunocytes in various secretory tissues was 17–23% lower than the J-chain positivity [30]; in some intestinal specimens the proportion of SC-binding IgM cells was below 40% (Fig. 7.4). Such disparity between J-chain-expressing and SC-binding capacity was much smaller for the IgA immunocytes (Fig. 7.4). Perhaps J chain is often added to pentameric IgM during its secretion. Intracellular polymerization of IgM can take place without initial incorporation of

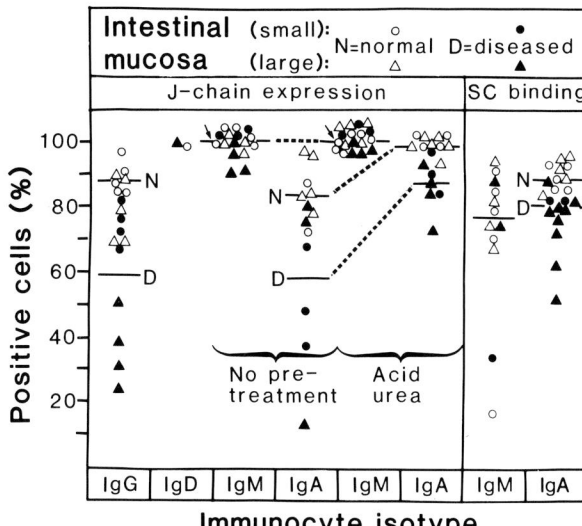

Fig. 7.4 Percentage of Ig-producing immunocytes showing J-chain positivity and cytoplasmic SC-binding properties in normal and diseased human intestinal mucosa as indicated. For IgM and IgA cells, J-chain data are based on both untreated and acid urea-treated tissue sections (medians connected by dashed lines). Adapted from Brandtzaeg and Korsrud [37].

J chain [227]. This may explain a lack of cytoplasmic SC affinity. A substantial fraction of cultured peripheral blood IgM immunocytes and some IgM-producing lymphoid cell lines have likewise been reported to lack SC-binding capacity [59, 73].

Dimeric and monomeric IgA production

About 90% of the intestinal IgA immunocytes are normally engaged in dimer production, but this does not exclude concurrent output of monomers [30, 37]. This was indicated by the finding that the venous effluent of perfused segments of human gut contained 20–30% monomeric IgA [47]. However, physicochemical analyses of the IgA spontaneously secreted by cultured mononuclear cells obtained from human gut mucosa have provided discrepant information: MacDermott et al [146] reported 31–37% monomers whereas Kutteh et al [123] concluded that about equal proportions of monomeric and dimeric IgA were produced. Contamination with epithelial cells, which release preformed SIgA, is an inherent problem in such experiments [123]. It is also possible that free SC, released from epithelial cells, may complex with dimeric IgA in the culture fluid and thereby partially mask the in vitro production of dimers. There is, on the other hand, evidence indicating that the proportion of secreted dimeric IgA may increase after prolonged incubation of lymphoid cells [161]. Altogether, therefore, no conclusive information is available as to the proportion of monomers actually produced by human intestinal IgA immunocytes.

Nature of intracellular IgA

There are likewise discrepant opinions with regard to the nature of intracellular IgA in dimer-producing immunocytes. We have maintained that the diffuse cellular binding of SC, along with the immunohistochemical requirement for unmasking of cytoplasmic J chain, constitutes direct evidence of a substantial intracellular dimerization in intestinal IgA immunocytes [30]. Our ultrastructural localizations of J chain in such normal cells have in fact suggested that the polymerization process begins in the endoplasmic reticulum [168]. Conversely, studies of pokeweed mitogen-stimulated human peripheral blood lymphoid cells, and of an Epstein Barr virus-transformed lymphoblastoid cell line, showed that most intracellular IgA occurred in a monomeric form even when the cells secreted mainly IgA dimers [161]. These results are in agreement with previous studies on murine tumour cells [69].

It is difficult to know to what extent such in vitro results reflect the normal situation in the gut. After B cell stimulation, there is increased intracellular expression of J chain [160, 196], and also induction of a sulphydryl oxidase catalysing the assembly of Ig polymer subunits [195]. The amount and subcellular distribution of this enzyme may influence the Ig polymerization process [68]. Direct analyses of normal intestinal IgA immunocytes are required before their content of monomers and dimers can be defined in quantitative terms.

J-chain expression unrelated to IgA and IgM

Almost 90% of the IgG immunocytes in normal intestinal mucosa express J chain (Fig. 7.4). However, J chain does not combine with IgG and is therefore not secreted from IgG-producing cells but becomes degraded intracellularly [166]. The same is probably true for J chain in IgD immunocytes which are almost 100% positive for this polypeptide in secretory tissues [37, 44]. J-chain-positive IgG and IgD immunocytes may represent 'spin-off' from the differentiation of relatively immature B cell memory clones on their way to IgA expression (Fig. 7.5).

In striking contrast to the situation in secretory tissues, IgA immunocytes show less than 50% and IgG immunocytes less than 10% J-chain positivity in non-glandular tissues [37]. Such down-regulation of J-chain synthesis seems to be a sign of clonal maturation (Fig. 7.5) as indicated by the fact that intrafollicular tonsillar IgG immunocytes show much more prominent J-chain expression than the extrafollicular counterparts [121]. It is possible that a negative feedback of cytoplasmic free J chain in IgG- (or IgD-) expressing precursor cells may be involved in the clonal differentiation process.

J chain and the B cell differentiation

Differentiation of B cells is an extremely complex process in both morphological and molecular terms. The mechanisms of isotype switching and the sequence of events involved in activation of resting B lymphocytes to clonal proliferation and terminal differentiation of Ig-producing immunocytes are only partly understood [49]. No direct role for the J chain in this process has yet been defined [122]. The J chain seems to be encoded by a single gene unlinked to other Ig genes, at least in the mouse [250].

J-chain expression. J-chain expression is an early event in B cell differentiation [122, 125] and may precede the appearance of cytoplasmic IgM [90, 168]. Recent studies of human cell lines [90, 142] have indicated that traces of J chain may be expressed even at the pre-B and 'null'-cell stage (Fig. 7.5); but, as mentioned above, the amounts produced increase markedly after mitogen or antigen stimulation, apparently with a slight delay in relation to activation of cytoplasmic IgM expression [126]. In murine B cells no evidence for J-chain expression before this activated stage has been obtained [126]. A recent study of human cell lines with a cloned gene

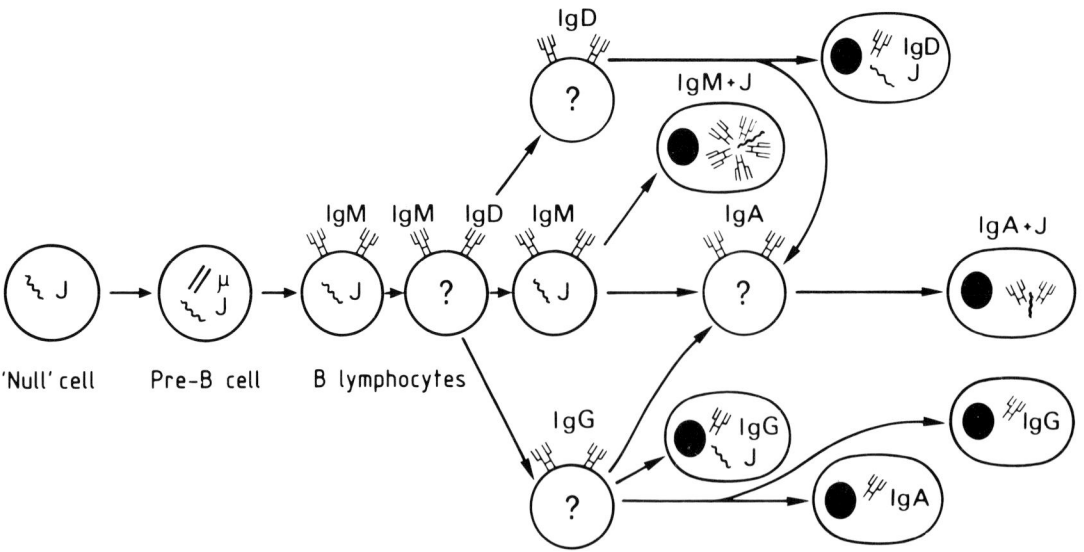

Fig. 7.5 Schematic representation of B cell development stages including various putative pathways to terminal differentiation of Ig-producing immunocytes, with or without concomitant cytoplasmic J-chain expression. It is postulated that J-chain-positive cells regardless of isotype, belong to relatively early memory clones which tend to seed preferentially secretory tissues, whereas J-chain-negative cells represent mature memory clones which terminate mainly in peripheral lymphoid tissues and inflammatory foci. Note that although J chain has been found in human lymphocytes expressing only surface IgM, the observed amounts are much smaller than in activated B cells. Unexplored cells are indicated by a question mark. Note also that there is discrepant information as to J-chain expression in 'null' cells (see text for details).

probe has, moreover, questioned whether the J chain can be expressed before the μ chain [154]. In any case, it is likely that substantial cytoplasmic J-chain expression is a marker of B cells belonging to relatively immature memory clones [26, 37, 44, 121].

Ig-producing cells in diseased mucosa

General comments. Immunohistochemical data on the major isotypes of Ig-producing cells in diseased gastrointestinal mucosae show striking discrepancies [31, 34]. In addition to general methodological difficulties, the selection of tissue samples poses a great problem in inflammatory bowel disease which may show highly varying histopathological features, even in the same specimen. In our laboratory, immunocyte counts have been based on a defined 'tissue unit' (Fig. 7.6) made up of a 6 μm thick and 500 μm wide mucosal block at full height from the muscularis mucosae to the lumen [34]; the aim has been to sample the total mucosal mass of Ig-producing cells in a representative manner.

Immunohistochemical findings. Our immunohistochemical results for various diseases in adult patients are schematically depicted in Fig. 7.7. A common feature is the relative increase in IgG immunocytes, although the IgA isotype remains predominant except adjacent to fissure-like ulcers in Crohn's disease. Both IgG and IgA cells in diseased mucosae show decreased expression of J chain, particularly in inflammatory bowel disease [37]; reduced SC-binding capacity likewise indicates a change towards production of monomeric IgA (Fig. 7.4). This finding is supported by observations on cultured cells obtained from lesions of ulcerative colitis and Crohn's disease [146]. Since production of dimeric IgA is of paramount importance in secretory immunity, its repression may contribute to persistence of mucosal disease. However, because of the substantial disease-associated expansion of the local IgA immunocyte population, decreased J-chain synthesis is probably of marginal pathogenic importance.

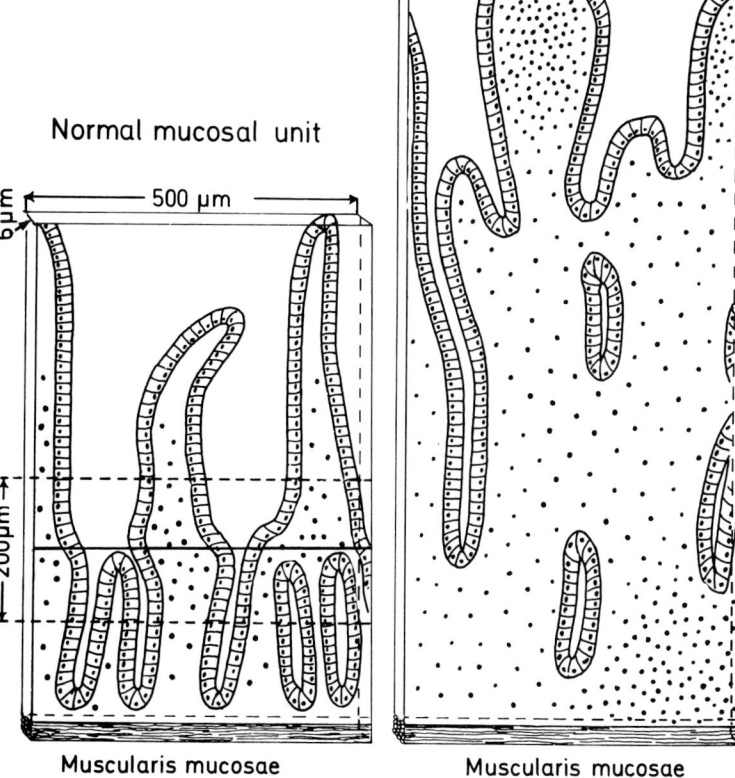

Crohn mucosal unit

Normal mucosal unit

Fig. 7.6 Schematic representation of mucosal 'tissue unit' from ileum of healthy individual (left) or from patient with Crohn's disease (right). The unit area of lamina propria will vary among different specimens; the total number of Ig-producing cells per tissue unit depends both on this variable and on cell density. The distribution of dots indicates arbitrarily heterogeneity in cell density. The highest density is normally found in the 200 μm zone around the crypt openings.

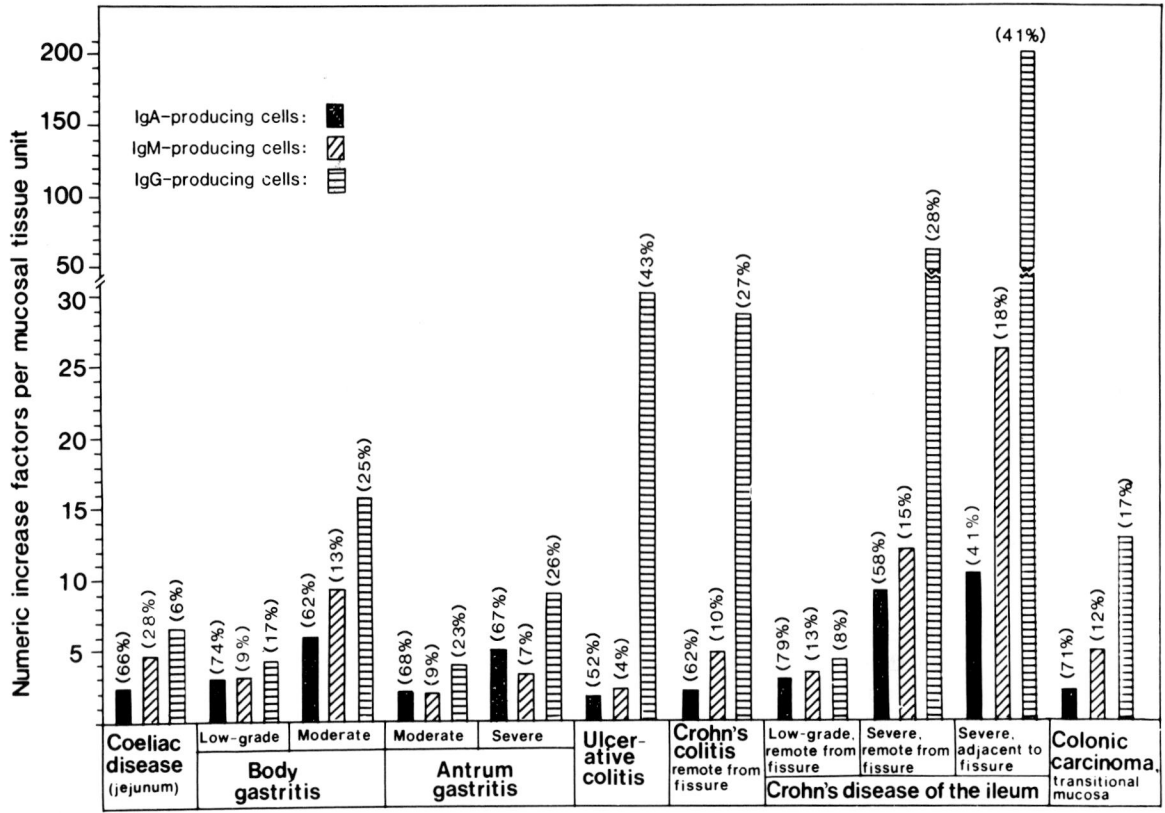

Fig. 7.7 Alterations in local immunocyte populations as indicated by numeric increase per mucosal 'tissue unit' (Fig. 7.6) in lesions of various gut diseases compared with normal counterparts. Immunocyte isotype distributions are indicated above the columns. Based on published data from the author's laboratory.

Coeliac disease

In untreated adult coeliac disease the average numbers of jejunal IgA, IgM and IgG immunocytes per mucosal 'tissue unit' were raised 2.4, 4.6 and 6.5 times, respectively [6]. Our results in children were comparable (Fig. 7.8) except that some of the young controls had a relatively high IgG-cell number [207]. Similar data have recently been published by others [194, 225], although a less prominent IgG-cell response was seen in diseased tissue specimens subjected to cross-linking fixatives [194]. The ethanol-fixation method is superior for immunohistochemical demonstration of IgG-producing cells [39].

In agreement with earlier observations [6], no increase of jejunal IgD- and IgE-producing cells has been found in recent investigations of coeliac disease [194, 225]. A highly discrepant report, indicating more IgE- than IgG-producing jejunal plasma cells both in coeliac disease and in normal control mucosa, remains unexplained [204].

Local B cell response to gluten. Immunohistochemical findings (Fig. 7.8) agree with studies of mucosal protein synthesis in tissue cultures; when jejunal biopsy specimens from patients with coeliac disease were compared with normal control specimens, incorporation of [^{14}C]leucine was highly elevated for both IgA and IgM [76, 136]. This emphasizes the importance of gluten as a stimulating antigen; when symptoms occurred after 8–12 days of gluten challenge in treated patients, the total IgA and IgM synthesis was increased two- to five-fold [76, 136].

Changes in B cell numbers with diet. We and others [194, 225] have found that a gluten-free diet reversed the changes of the jejunal immunocyte population in children with coeliac disease; after treatment for 1.2–9 years it was quite normal (Fig. 7.8) as was the mucosal morphology with the exception of minor villus changes [207]. Conversely, in treated adult patients both immunocyte numbers (Fig. 7.8) and isotype ratios fell between those of un-

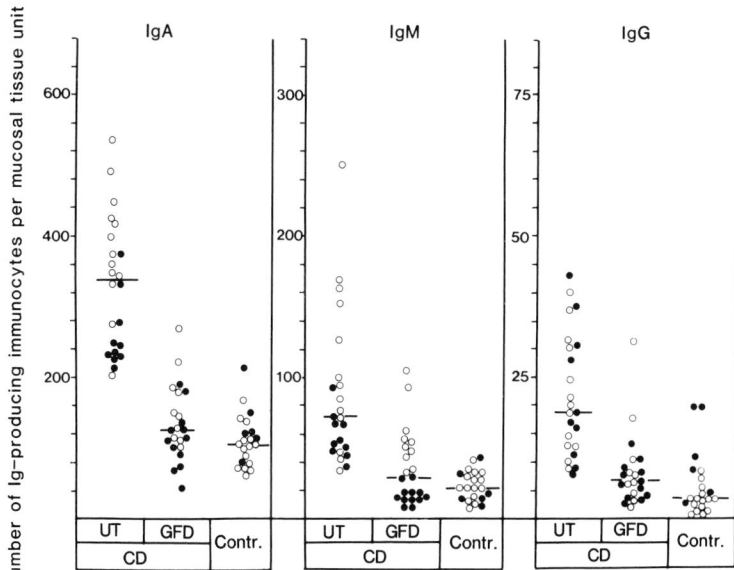

Fig. 7.8 Number of IgA-, IgM- and IgG-producing immunocytes in an individually defined mucosal 'tissue unit' (Fig. 7.6) of jejunal mucosa. Results from untreated patients with coeliac disease (UT), patients on a gluten-free diet (GFD) and controls (Contr.) are indicated for children (●) and adults (o). In untreated patients the absolute numerical increase was largest for IgA cells, but the relative increase was more pronounced for IgG cells (4.7-fold) than for IgA (3.0-fold) and IgM cells (3.3-fold). Note different scales on ordinates. Adapted from Baklien et al [6] and Scott et al [207].

treated patients and controls [6]. This difference indicates either that the adult jejunal mucosa does not have the same potential for improvement or that a strict gluten-free diet is more difficult to achieve in adults than in children.

Isotype of gluten antibodies. The increased mucosal Ig synthesis in tissue culture after gluten challenge was apparently largely due to gluten antibodies (29–75%); the isotype of these antibodies was not stated but experiments in one patient indicated that only 60% was accounted for by IgA + IgM [77]. In a preliminary study of an untreated adult with coeliac disease we found a small fraction of jejunal immunocytes with specificity for gluten and about 60% of these were of the IgA isotype [34]. However, a much larger proportion of the total IgG- than of the total IgA-cell population was positive (5.7% versus 1.6%). Another preliminary report based on children with coeliac disease indicated gluten specificity for 11%, 10.5% and 6.5% of the jejunal IgG, IgM and IgA immunocytes, respectively [224]. Moreover, in treated patients who were challenged with gluten, a significant inverse correlation appeared between the time to clinical relapse and the number of jejunal IgG immunocytes found after challenge (Fig. 7.9). This suggests that an imbalanced local immune response to gluten (and probably also to

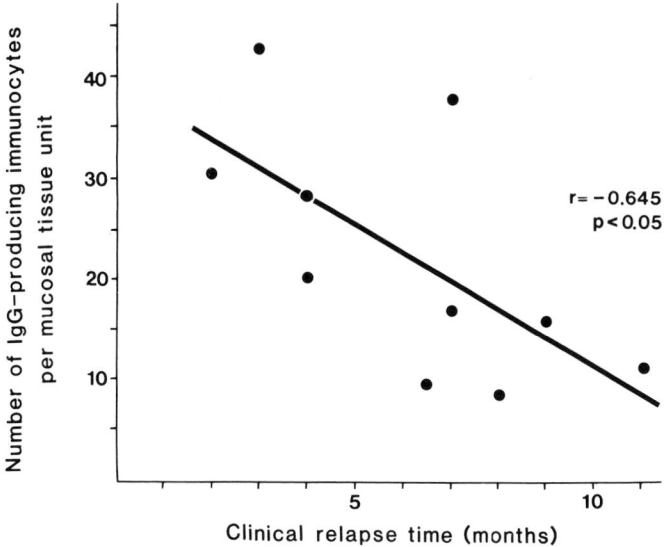

$r = -0.645$
$p < 0.05$

Fig. 7.9 Scatter diagram of relation in 10 children with coeliac disease between time to clinical relapse and number of IgG-producing immunocytes per jejunal mucosal 'tissue unit' (Fig. 7.6) as revealed by biopsy after completed gluten challenge. Relapse time was significantly shorter in patients with the brisker mucosal IgG response. Adapted from Scott et al [207].

other dietary antigens) with a shift towards IgG is involved in the pathogenesis of coeliac disease.

Cow's milk intolerance and other gastrointestinal diseases. In contrast to the strikingly disproportionate increase of IgG and IgM cells observed in the coeliac lesion (Fig. 7.7), a more proportionate and less pronounced increase of all major immunocyte isotypes has been reported for cow's milk intolerance [201, 225]. A selective mucosal IgA and IgM response was seen in patients with acute enteritis a few days after the diarrhoea ceased [222]. Acute gastrointestinal infection with the 'Norwalk agent' was found to induce a marked mucosal IgA response after 2 weeks in volunteers who became ill, whereas the initial response seemed to be brisker in those who did not [1]. Local IgM and IgG responses were not studied. In dermatitis herpetiformis, however, IgM and IgG cell numbers were found to be disproportionately raised as in coeliac disease when jejunal lesions of similar severity were compared [7].

Chronic gastritis

Relatively few immunohistochemical studies have been carried out on inflamed gastric mucosa; the results have been inconsistent and not related to the histopathological grade of gastritis. In a recent study, however, we showed that the number of Ig-producing cells rose strikingly with an increasing degree of inflammation (Fig. 7.7). IgG immunocytes showed the largest relative increase (4- to 16-fold), particularly in the basal part of the mucosa [237]. IgD and IgE immunocytes were only rarely found, although other authors have reported that some plasma cells of the latter isotype usually appear in gastric inflammatory infiltrates [170].

Locally produced IgG may be of protective value in the gastric mucosa in terms of 'second line' defence, but it may, at the same time, be involved in immunopathological mechanisms contributing to the chronicity of the disease. Virtually nothing is known about the antigens involved in the gastric immune responses. It is of interest, though, that local IgG-pro-

| (a) | (b) | (c) |

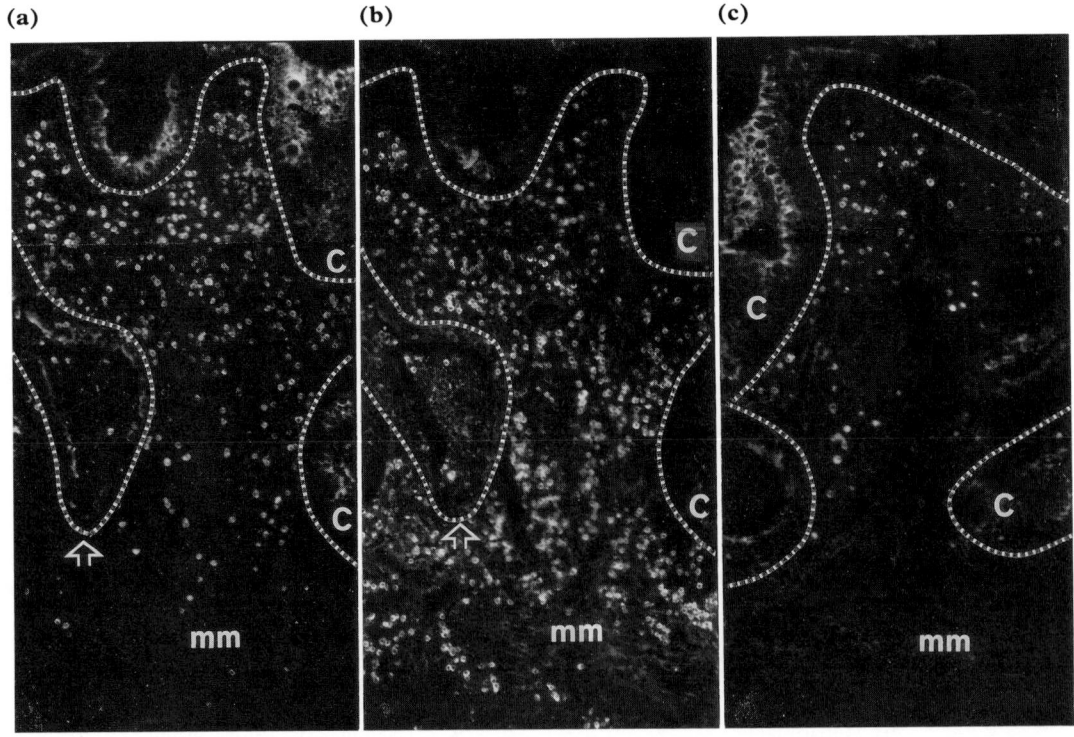

Fig. 7.10 Immunofluorescence staining for IgA (a), IgG (b) and IgM (c) in comparable fields from three serial sections of colonic mucosa from a patient with Crohn's disease. The epithelium (indicated by dashed lines) is preserved and shows secretory activity as signified by apical staining for IgA and IgM in crypts (C) with the exception of one in which an abscess has formed (arrow). Note that IgA-producing immunocytes abound mainly adjacent to well-preserved crypts (at the top), whereas IgG-producing immunocytes are predominant in the depths of the mucosa and below the muscularis mucosae (mm). Relatively few IgM immunocytes are present. × 135.

ducing cells with specificity for intrinsic factor have been found in pernicious anaemia [11].

Inflammatory bowel disease

Dramatic changes in the intestinal Ig-producing cell populations are found in ulcerative colitis and Crohn's disease (Fig. 7.10), depending on the histopathological features of the actual tissue unit examined [4, 5, 43]. In the severely affected tissue adjacent to fissure-like ulcers in Crohn's disease, the numbers of IgA, IgM and IgG immunocytes were raised 10, 26 and 201 times, respectively (Fig. 7.7). Compared with severely inflamed tissue remote from ulcers, this represented a doubling of the immunocyte population; IgG cells were responsible for about 75% of this increase.

Immunohistochemical studies of inflammatory bowel disease have provided highly discrepant results which partly remain unexplained [31], but a striking increase in IgG cells has also been found by others [116, 174]. Moreover, in vitro studies of lymphoid cells or mucosal tissue obtained from lesions of Crohn's disease and ulcerative colitis have confirmed that an enhanced local synthesis of IgG is a striking feature in both diseases [66, 79].

IgD and IgE cells. There is general agreement that no consistent increase of IgD-producing cells takes place in inflammatory bowel disease. Conversely, much confusion exists concerning IgE-producing cells. As discussed elsewhere [31], this can probably be ascribed to the inclusion of IgE-positive mucosal mast cells in the immunocyte counts.

Antibody specificities. Little is known about the antibody specificities of the local Ig-producing cells in these diseases. Monteiro et al [162] provided evidence indicating that immune responses against faecal anaerobic bacteria take place in the large bowel mucosa; these responses were especially enhanced in the IgG class when the mucosa was affected by ulcerative colitis. No local response was detected against faecal aerobic bacteria although corresponding antibodies were present in serum. Heddle et al [100] found that isolated intestinal mononuclear cells produced antibodies to common faecal *Escherichia coli* strains and that the IgG responses were particularly enhanced in Crohn's disease.

Miscellaneous large bowel disorders

The total number of Ig-producing cells in the transitional mucosa adjacent to large-bowel carcinomas is increased three-fold [190]. Again, this rise is disproportionate for the IgG isotype (Fig. 7.7). It is not known whether the local immune response is truly tumour-associated or reflects stimulation by microbial or dietary antigens passing through the tumour lesion.

A similar disproportionate increase of mucosal IgG-producing cells has been noted in the obstructed colon of children with Hirschsprung's disease [248]; this finding probably reflected a response to bacterial invasion resulting from faecal retention in the distended colon segment.

It was recently reported that a prominent IgG-cell response also takes place in the rectal mucosa of patients with ankylosing spondylitis, even when no inflammatory changes can be seen [226]. The authors speculated that the local immune response might reflect stimulation by an as yet unidentified agent involved in the pathogenesis of this disease.

DEVELOPMENTAL ASPECTS OF THE INTESTINAL B CELL SYSTEM

Perinatal immunity

Human exocrine fluids contain only occasional traces of IgA and IgM the first days after birth, whereas some IgG is usually present [82, 216]. Its immediate source is interstitial tissue fluid which after a gestational age of 18 weeks contains maternal IgG in substantial amounts [173]. Thus, immunohistochemistry of fetal intestinal mucosa shows bright diffuse staining for IgG in the lamina propria whereas IgA is totally lacking (Fig. 7.11).

Maternal IgG in the neonate's mucosa is unquestionably of value in protecting against infections, but IgG antibodies to dietary antigens may, in theory, adversely affect mucosal penetrability for macromolecules [40]. Mucosal integrity may be damaged by lysosomal enzymes released from polymorphonuclear granulocytes which are known to be attracted when complement (C)-activating immune complexes are formed locally [13]. This phlogistic mechanism may contribute to a greater influx of dietary antigens in newborn than in older infants, although the evidence for such a difference is rather circumstantial [189, 243].

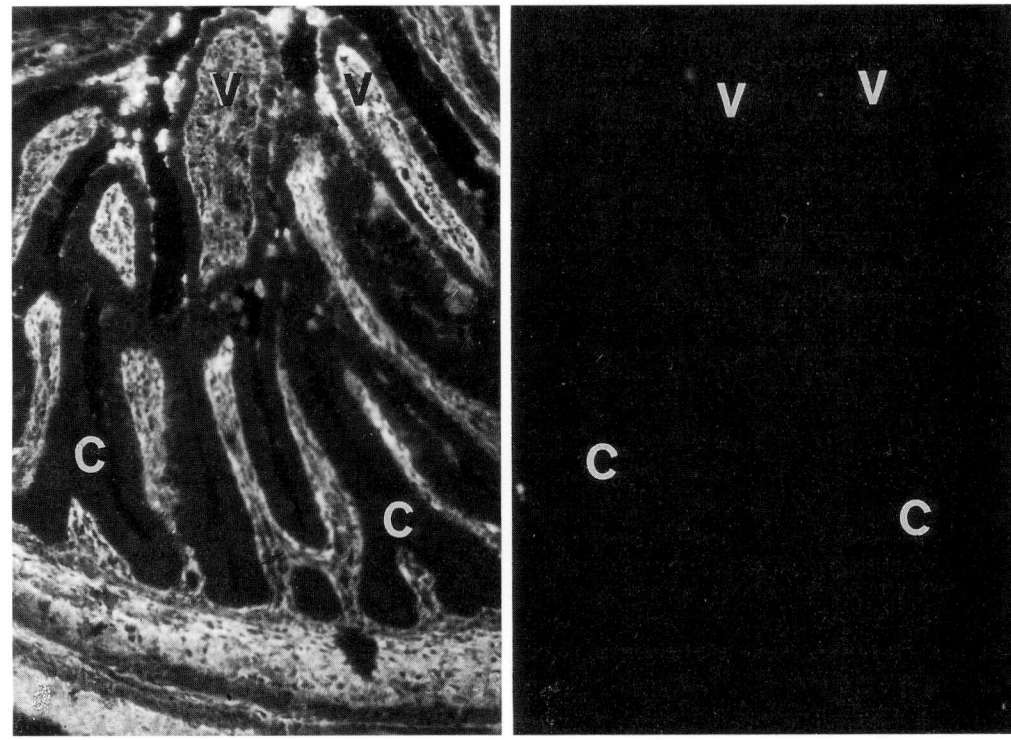

(a)

Fig. 7.11 Immunofluorescence staining for IgG (a) and IgA (b) in comparable fields from adjacent sections of proximal small intestinal mucosa from a 26-week-old fetus. The tissue was directly fixed in ethanol to retain diffusible proteins [23]. IgG abounds in connective tissue but is absent from crypt epithelium (C). The epithelium covering the villi (V) contains some intercellular IgG, indicating leakage of interstitial fluid to gut lumen where IgG is associated with mucous layer. Note complete lack of IgA. × 150.

Postnatal development

The literature contains highly discrepant information about the postnatal development of the human secretory immune system. This may be explained by methodological problems in quantifying SIgA [95], differences among various secretory sites, and large individual variations. In fact, re-evaluation of 19 children (1- to 5-year-olds) who at an earlier age had been diagnosed as IgA-deficient showed normalization of both serum and lacrimal IgA in almost half of them [111].

Ig-producing cells are not normally present in human intestinal mucosa before 10 days of age [178, 248]. Thereafter a rapid increase takes place, particularly of IgM immunocytes which usually dominate up to 1 month [178]. SIgM responses have been found to be relatively predominant early in infancy [82, 132, 158] and prominent development of IgM cells in the early phase of gut immune responses has been shown also in animal experiments [231].

Blanco et al [18] observed no significant increase of small intestinal IgA immunocytes in children after 1 year although IgM-producing cells decreased. A similarly decreasing trend for IgM immunocytes with age has been reported by others, but at the same time a continuing increase of IgA cells has been indicated, even after 2 years [149].

Role of antigen challenge in development of IgA

The antigenic and mitogenic load on the mucosa seems to be a decisive factor for the postnatal development of the secretory immune system. The indigenous microbial flora is probably of utmost importance, as indicated by the fact that the intestinal IgA system of germ-free or specific pathogen-free mice is normalized after about 4 weeks of conventionalization [58, 102]. *Bacteroides* and *E. coli* strains seem to be particularly stimulatory for the development of intestinal IgA immunocytes [135, 164]. Antigenic constituents of food may exert an additional stimulatory effect [200].

Reduced antigen load. Reduced amounts of microbial and dietary antigens obviously explain why the colonic numbers of IgA- and

IgM-producing cells are decreased by about 50% after 2–11 months in children who have been subjected to defunctioning colostomies [247]. Postnatal and prolonged observations on defunctioned ileal segments in lambs have even more strikingly revealed a scarcity of immunocytes in the lamina propria; this result was explained by reduced local accumulation of B cell blasts and might involve both hampered migration of such precursors into the mucosa and their subsequently decreased local proliferation and differentiation [188]. Also the number of intraepithelial lymphocytes was substantially decreased in the defunctioned ileum [188].

Development of the colonic and rectal secretory immune system

The observation that adult faecal levels of IgA were attained after 1–2 months [93a] is at variance with the fact that the average rectal number of IgA-producing cells in 1–3-month-old children is only about 20% of that seen after 2 years [178]. This discrepancy probably reflects how difficult it is to obtain a reliable measure for actual IgA secretion. In whole saliva adult levels were seldom seen before 12 months [158]. All in all, it seems that the human intestinal B cell system is usually poorly developed for several months after birth in countries with good hygiene (Fig. 7.12), although early IgM responses may afford some protective compensation.

Secretory component development

SC has been reported to appear in columnar crypt cells as early as the 18th gestational week [173]. This finding shows that its synthesis can take place in the absence of an activated B cell system, a fact that is also observed in immunodeficient patients [34].

Nutrition and intestinal immunity

Production of SIgA seems to depend more on the nutritional state of the child than does that of the various serum Ig classes. Thus, definitely decreased IgA concentrations in duo-

(a)

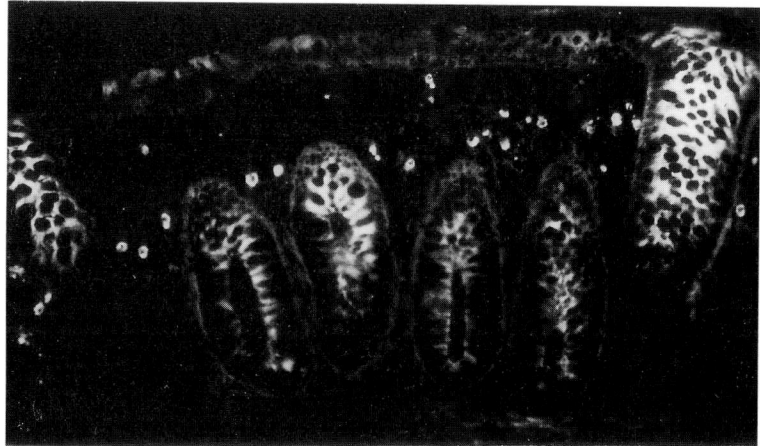

(b)

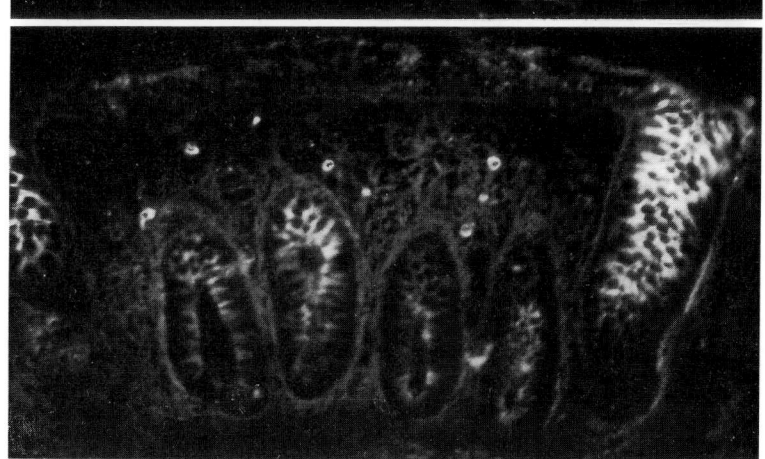

Fig. 7.12 Immunofluorescence staining for IgA (a) and IgM (b) in comparable fields from adjacent sections of histologically normal rectal mucosa from a 2-month-old girl (gut lumen at the top). Compared with normal adult mucosa the number of Ig-producing cells is small; the ratio of IgA to IgM immunocytes is about 2.5:1 compared with the adult colonic isotype ratio of 15:1 (Fig. 7.2). Despite relatively few local immunocytes, large amounts of IgA and IgM are taken up by columnar crypt cells—signifying external transport. Virtual absence of interstitial IgA staining reflects low serum level of IgA. × 150.

denal, nasal and salivary secretions have been reported for children with severe protein-calorie malnutrition [53, 186]. An immunohistochemical study of similar children reported selective reduction of IgA-producing cells in jejunal mucosa—indicating retarded maturation of the secretory immune system [83]. Animal experiments have suggested that hampered migration of IgA precursor cells to the secretory tissues may be involved in such an adverse development [144]. Also impairment of both T cell functions and innate defence factors probably contribute to the decreased resistance seen in malnutrition [245].

It should be noted that measurements of SIgA have not distinguished between decreased production and reduced external transport of IgA; the latter might be caused by adverse effects of vitamin A deficiency or infection on the secretory epithelium. Experiments in mice have in fact shown that only prolonged and severe malnutrition will lead to reduction of IgA immunocytes in the gut [241]. The intestinal immune system of undernourished children may respond to bacterial overgrowth with enhanced IgA synthesis and secretion [12]. Moreover, impaired secretory immunity can be restored by renourishment, both in experimental animals [10] and in children [186, 245].

Deficiency of IgA-producing cells

Selective lack of IgA is the most frequent immunodeficiency but obviously signifies a heterogeneous syndrome [96]. The activity of the secretory immune system in IgA-deficient subjects is fairly unpredictable on the basis of individual serum levels of IgA (see Chapter 12). Decreased intestinal IgA- to IgM-cell ratio reflects immaturity of the secretory immune system, and also seems to be a good indicator of a significant IgA deficiency after infancy. Thus, the intestinal IgA-cell population is commonly intact when serum IgA concentrations are above 18% of the normal average, whereas between 18% and 5% the number of jejunal IgA cells is usually decreased but that of IgM cells increased [202]. A dichotomy between the immunocyte patterns in jejunal and rectal mucosa is seen in some subjects [42, 203].

IgA cells in IgA-deficient subjects

In a group of IgA-deficient patients subjected to studies of their jejunal mucosa in this laboratory, all of the children presented with malabsorption and various degrees of villus atrophy. They seemed to have gluten-induced coeliac disease except one boy who after the age of 2.5 years has been well on a normal diet; his jejunal mucosa notably contained a considerable number of IgA-producing cells despite a low serum IgA level. The two adults likewise had no coeliac disease but showed a tendency to respiratory tract infections. In one of them both the rectal and jejunal IgA-cell populations were quantitatively fully developed, but an increased proportion of jejunal IgM cells, and an excess of free J chain in his intestinal IgA immunocytes, indicated some imbalance of the secretory immune system [42]. Nevertheless, this case demonstrated that a general defect of the IgA system does not necessarily prevent the development of intestinal IgA-producing cells. The reason for such a dichotomy between systemic and local IgA is probably the heavy stimulatory antigen and mitogen load on the mucosa.

It is interesting that the total number of jejunal Ig-producing cells was normal in the adult who completely lacked IgA immunocytes. The IgA-deficient children with diseased mucosae contained numerous jejunal immunocytes although in most of them the total number was only about half of that found in children with untreated coeliac disease [207].

Replacement of IgA-producing cells. These observations show that B cells can home to the intestinal lamina propria and become locally expanded and differentiated there even without possessing IgA-producing capacity. This has also been found in other secretory tissues [44]. But an important discrepancy appears when it comes to replacement of the lacking IgA immunocytes: in the upper aeroalimentary tract (AAT) numerous gland-associated IgD-producing cells (50-80%) are often found, whereas in the gastrointestinal tract such immunocytes usually make up less than 1% along with a regular predominance of IgM- and a varying fraction of IgG-producing cells. Regardless of isotype, however, the IgA-replacing immunocytes show prominent J-chain expression—attesting to their association with the secretory immune system [37].

Compensation with SIgM. Enhanced intestinal production and secretion of IgM in IgA deficiency may explain the fact that most subjects with this disorder have no gastro-intestinal symptoms; their problems are rather related to the upper AAT where compensation with IgM is often lacking [29]. However, immune exclusion in the intestine is clearly sub-optimal in IgA-deficient individuals as more than half of them have raised levels of IgG antibodies to bovine milk proteins and circulating immune complexes containing such antigens [61,63]. It seems that these phenomena, which obviously reflect increased gastrointestinal permeability, may explain the relatively high incidence of autoimmunity seen in selective IgA deficiency [64]. Moreover, the incidence of this deficiency is about 10 times higher among patients with coeliac disease than in the general population.

It is intriguing, however, that up to 50% of the jejunal immunocytes may produce IgG without causing clinical evidence of disturbed local homeostasis. At least in countries with good hygiene, therefore, SIgM may afford satisfactory surface protection of the gut in most IgA-deficient subjects as long as the non-specific defence mechanisms are functioning adequately [148]. However, associated T cell defects and genetic factors influencing the health of IgA-deficient individuals are poorly understood [93].

Generalized B cell deficiency

Still more intriguing is the fact that gastro-intestinal disorders are quite rare in patients with infantile X-linked (Bruton-type) B cell deficiency leading to agammaglobulinaemia [74, 171]. Conversely, 20–50% of the patients with common variable hypogammaglobulin-aemia develop diarrhoea and malabsorption. The intestinal lesions may vary over a wide range, from showing more or less villus atrophy to mimicking Crohn's disease. The common diagnoses of intestinal diseases should probably not be used in these cases because immunodeficiency apparently by 'imitation' may result in a variety of lesions.

The intestinal mucosa of patients with generalized B cell deficiency contains no or only very little extravascular IgG unless substitution therapy has been given [34]. However, some mucosal plasma cells (mainly of the IgM isotype) are often seen, particularly in hypo-gammaglobulinaemia [34,45]. SC occurs in a normal epithelial distribution so the small amounts of locally produced IgM can probably contribute to external defence. It may seem paradoxical, therefore, that the hypo-gammaglobulinaemic patients were usually found to have strikingly raised levels of bovine milk proteins in their blood whereas the agammaglobulinaemic ones apparently did not have more than normal [62] (see Chapter 12).

Solitary lymphoid follicles

Some patients with hypogammaglobulinaemia who present with diarrhoea show a markedly increased number of solitary lymphoid follicles in their gastrointestinal mucosa, mainly in the small intestine [74]. These follicles contain a distinct mantle zone of B lymphocytes which express surface IgM and IgD. The B cell maturation defect is only to a small extent overcome under the influence of antigens from the lumen as indicated by the development of a few IgM-producing immunocytes between the follicles and the surface epithelium. It is possible that nodular lymphoid hyperplasia reflects stimulation due to an excessive influx of antigens from the lumen [62], but there is no apparent relationship between this mode of reaction and development of intestinal lymphoma.

PROLIFERATION AND DIFFERENTIATION OF B CELLS IN GUT MUCOSA

Local development of IgA immunocytes

The B cells entering secretory tissues from peripheral blood are heterogeneous, comprising IgM-, IgD-, IgA- or IgG-bearing lymphocytes (or double-expressing ones) and IgA-producing blasts [147, 234, 235]. Since there is normally a prominent accumulation of IgA-positive cells at such sites, one can postulate that further B cell proliferation and differentiation takes place locally—including clonal expansion, isotype switching and terminal maturation to plasma cells (Fig. 7.13). The renewal rate of IgA immunocytes in the murine intestinal mucosa has been estimated at about 5 days [153].

Antigen-driven proliferation. Substantial antigen-driven proliferation of IgA-precursor cells has been revealed in the intestinal lamina propria of various experimental animals [105, 128, 181], especially in the crypt regions [104] where most IgA immunocytes are also found in the human jejunal mucosa [6]. Moreover, in the human secretory immune system, the role of topical antigens outside the Peyer's patches has been clearly demonstrated in terms of localization, magnitude and persistence of SIgA antibody responses [172].

Switching phenomenon. As discussed earlier, it seems that B cells triggered by 'second signals' in the mucosa belong to relatively early memory clones because they collectively show a striking J-chain-expressing potential [37]. Such an early clonal stage may also explain the fact that terminal differentiation gives rise to a remarkable predominance of IgA immunocytes. The J-chain-positive IgM-, IgG- and IgD-producing cells normally appearing in different secretory tissues probably reflect 'spin-off' from the clonal differentiation process, and their numbers may vary according to the pathway of switching followed to IgA expression (Fig. 7.13). Cebra et al [51] have proposed that this takes place in a vectorial

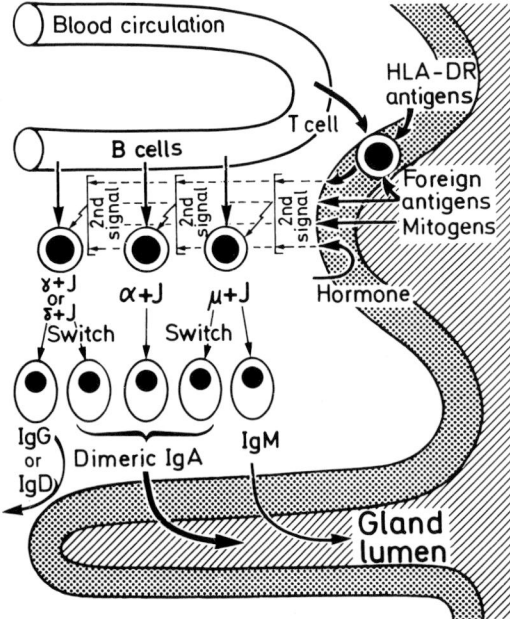

Fig. 7.13 Hypothetical scheme for maintenance and terminal differentiation of immunocytes at secretory sites. Circulating memory B cells of early clonal stage show high potential for J-chain expression and are receptive for 'second signals' after extravasation. After resulting proliferation and differentiation, most immunocytes normally end up as IgA-dimer producers owing to 'switching' of heavy-chain phenotype from μ to γ to α or directly from μ or δ to α in those cells that did not already express IgA at extravasation. A varying number of J-chain-positive immunocytes of the three other isotypes develop as 'spin-off' from the differentiation process. The 'second signals' that influence local B cells are largely mediated by T cells which are stimulated by HLA-DR and foreign antigens in or adjacent to the epithelium. Other putative factors may be mitogens or hormones.

manner (IgM→IgG→IgA), but direct switching from IgM to each of the other isotypes also seems to be possible [49].

It has been proposed that B cells may follow various differentiation pathways according to their place of origin (e.g. BALT and tonsils versus GALT) as indicated by the described dichotomy with regard to IgD-expressing potential [44]. However, it is also possible that the virtual lack of IgD-producing cells in the gut is a result of regional disparity in terms of 'second signals' which influence terminal B cell differentiation. For example, it has been indicated that lipopolysaccharide (LPS) may inhibit the expression of IgD [175].

Second signals for proliferation and terminal differentiation

With the exception of antigen-induced stimulation in gut mucosa, little is known about factors triggering terminal B cell differentiation at various secretory sites (Fig. 7.13). The immediate availability of antigens (and mitogens?) seems to be reflected by a density of Ig-producing cells that is about seven times higher in colonic mucosa than in parotid and lactating mammary glands [33]. It is indeed not obvious that foreign material, live or dead, gains access to the two latter organs—particularly not gut-related antigens. Perhaps secretory tissues remote from mucosae depend more on other types of stimulation.

Role of 'self' antigens

One possibility is epithelial expression of HLA-DR molecules, which are normally present on parotid intercalated duct cells [32] and on alveolar cells of lactating mammary glands [169]. Since the magnitude of immune responses may be related to the density of such 'self' antigens [108, 152], one may assume that their abundant epithelial expression—in combination with only trace amounts of foreign antigens or anti-idiotypic antibodies—may elicit sufficient 'second signals' for some terminal B cell differentiation to take place. It is also possible that hormones or unidentified epithelial factors contribute locally to specific or polyclonal B cell stimulation. Interestingly it has been reported that a factor from bursal epithelial cells can stimulate IgA production [72].

In the small intestine, HLA-DR expression on enterocytes (Figs. 7.14 and 7.15) may likewise contribute to the generation of 'second

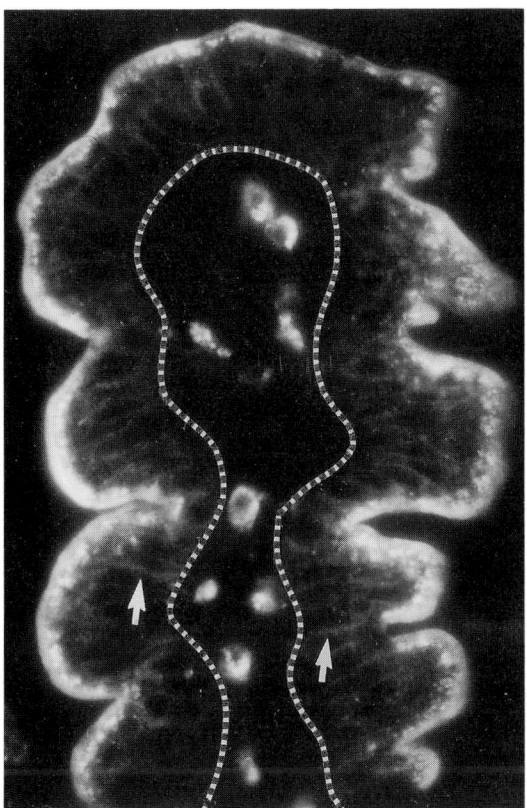

Fig. 7.14 Immunofluorescence staining with monoclonal antibody to HLA-DR as described in Fig. 7.15. Field from section of normal jejunal mucosa demonstrates characteristic distribution of DR determinants in epithelium of villus (gut lumen at the top). Note that, in addition to granular apical intensification, staining for DR appears diffusely in the cytoplasm of the enterocytes and along their basolateral membranes (arrows). Some DR-positive histiocytic cells are seen in the lamina propria. Epithelial basement membrane zone indicated by dashed line. × 530.

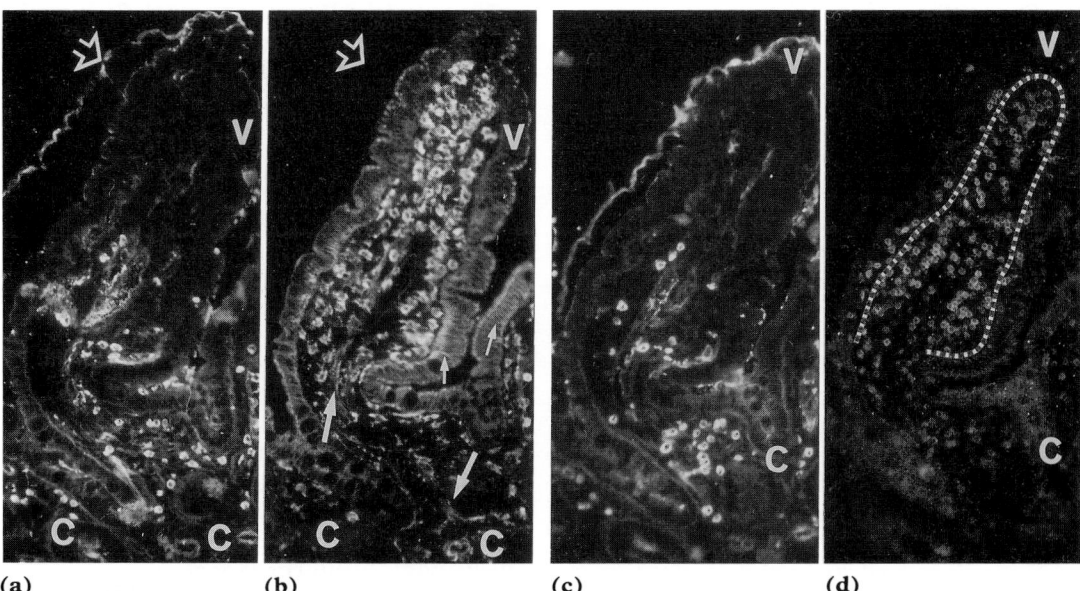

(a)   **(b)**   **(c)**   **(d)**

Fig. 7.15 Paired immunofluorescence staining for IgA (left panels, rhodamine) and (a) HLA-DR or (b) T cells (right panels, fluorescein) in two comparable fields from normal ileal mucosa. Murine monoclonal antibody to a non-polymorphic HLA-DR determinant or Leu 4 (Becton Dickinson) combined with rabbit anti-IgA in a three-step biotin-avidin method. (a) Note striking apical distribution of HLA-DR in villus epithelium (V) contrasting with crypt epithelium (C) that contains mainly IgA. Enterocytes show additional diffuse cytoplasmic DR staining with intensification along basolateral membranes (small arrows). Note that IgA-positive mucus layer (open arrows) has become detached from villus, thereby demonstrating that DR is epithelium-associated. Numerous DR-positive histiocytic cells occur in luminal part of villus whereas only few are intermingled with IgA immunocytes in the crypt region. In addition, there are a few DR-positive vessel walls (large arrows) and some intravascular IgA. (b) Few T lymphocytes are intermingled with IgA immunocytes in the crypt (C) region whereas numerous occur in villus (V), partly within the epithelium (basement membrane zone indicated by dashed line). × 80.

signals'. Perhaps DR determinants are involved in the presentation of foreign antigens to intraepithelial T cells, which can to some extent return to the lamina propria (Fig. 7.13). Whether the resulting immunoregulatory effects on mucosal B cells would be inductive or suppressive is unknown; the phenotypic characterization of the intraepithelial lymphocytes as mainly belonging to the putative T_S subset [211] is difficult to translate directly into functional terms (see Chapter 8).

Traffic of T cells from GALT to gut lamina propria

Since it has been shown that there is a traffic of T cells from GALT to the gut lamina propria [16, 88], one might expect transfer of the putative IgA-specific functional subsets apparently present in Peyer's patches (see Ch. 3); but support for this possibility has not been obtained in experimental animals [234]. Coculturing of B and T cells isolated from human gut mucosa has likewise provided inconclusive results with respect to enhancement of IgA production [56]. The reason for this may be that the IgA cells recovered from the lamina propria represent an activated population which apparently has received the 'second signals' required for terminal differentiation in vivo [70, 145].

Local terminal differentiation versus emigration of B cells

IgA-producing cells are usually present in the dome areas of Peyer's patches but rarely in the lymphoid follicles (Fig. 7.16). Most of the germinal-centre cells with a positive cytoplasm are of the IgM or IgG isotype, both in rat [219] and man [17], and a remarkably high proportion (38%) of the plasma cells found in the dome areas of normal human patches produce IgG [17]. These IgG immunocytes show much poorer J-chain expression than their counterparts in distant lamina propria (37% versus 82%), and a similar trend is seen for the IgA-producing cells present at these two sites (85% versus 97% J-chain positivity). Relatively decreased expression of J chain is likewise a characteristic of the IgG-producing cells that accumulate preferentially adjacent to solitary follicles elsewhere in the gut and particularly in the appendix (Fig. 7.17).

On the basis of these observations [17], it would seem that stimulated B cells with down-regulated J-chain-expressing potential

tend to remain in the lymphoepithelial structures and give rise to local Ig-producing immunocytes. These B cells apparently belong to mature memory clones, whereas most members of relatively early memory clones probably emigrate after stimulation and differentiate to J-chain-positive immunocytes at distant mucosal sites.

Production of antibodies in Peyer's patches

Local production of IgG along with IgA and IgM [58, 141, 219, 221], and specific antibodies of all three isotypes [139] have been observed in Peyer's patches of rats and mice. These and other studies [129, 220] contradict earlier observations which indicated that Peyer's patches do not generate local antibody-producing cells after topical stimulation [15, 114]. It has also been shown that antigens administered orally (but not by the parenteral route) induce germinal-centre formation [50] and elicit specific functional activation of both T and B cells [113]. The morphological evidence indicates that GALT contains all the accessory cells required for appropriate immune responsiveness (see Ch. 4).

The explanation for the relatively small number of Ig-producing immunocytes normally found in Peyer's patches [17] is probably that most stimulated lymphoid cells emigrate rapidly. This possibility was recently suggested for the behaviour of T cells after enteric immunization of rats with vaccinia virus [106]. As mentioned above, B cells subjected to such rapid emigration are largely of a clonal maturation stage compatible with J-chain expression since this is a common feature of immunocytes in secretory tissues—regardless of the isotype produced after terminal differentiation [37].

RELATIONSHIP OF GUT EPITHELIUM TO THE LOCAL B CELL SYSTEM

Secretory component-mediated immunoglobulin transport

Normal mucosa

Epithelial SC is a key factor in the secretory immune system. It is expressed on the basolateral surface of normal columnar epithelial cells [27] as part of a transmembrane protein [167]. In the small intestine, it is produced by

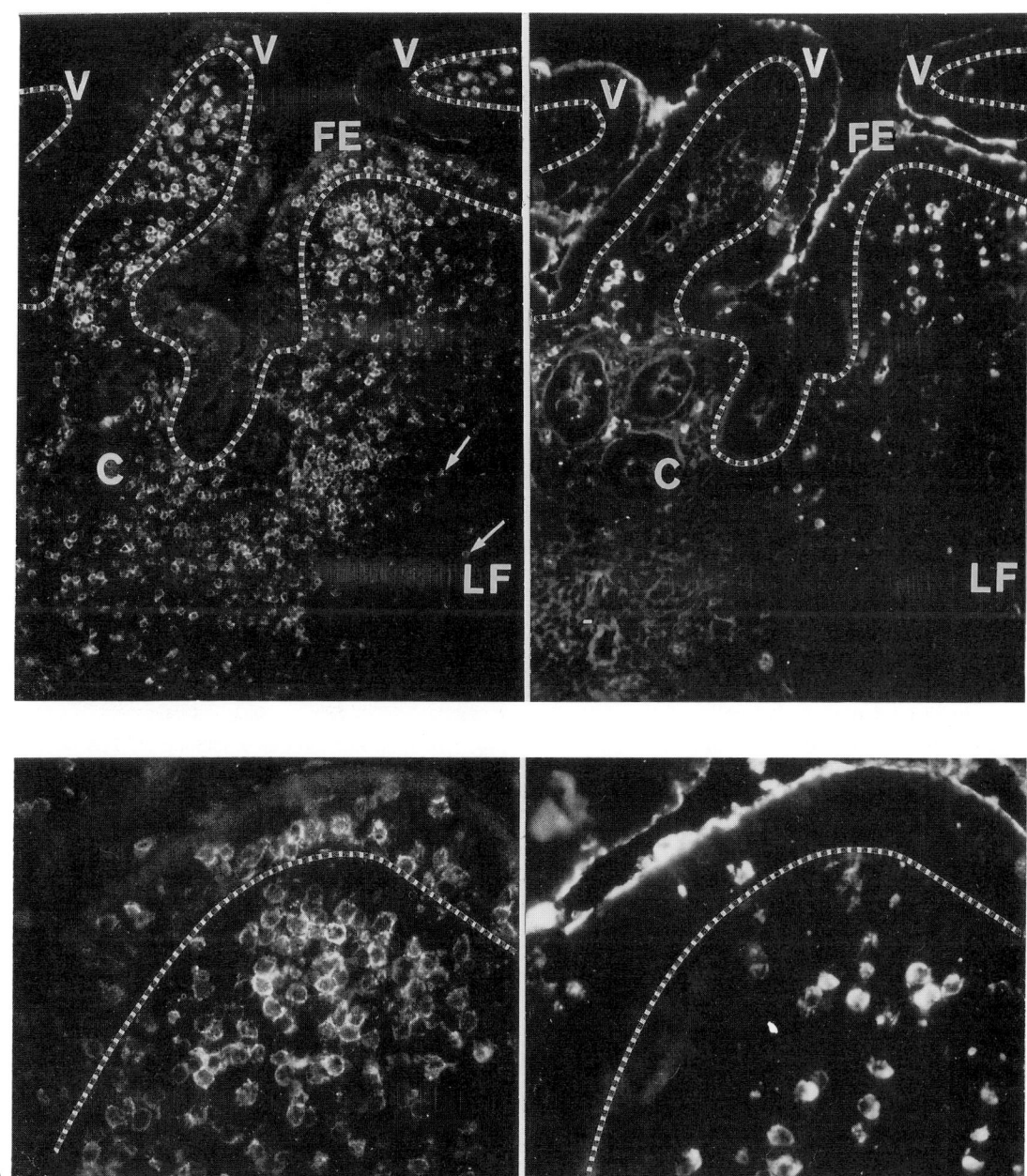

Fig. 7.16 Paired immunofluorescence staining of T cells (left panels, fluorescein) and IgA (right panels, rhodamine) in same field from section of normal human Peyer's patch. The result was based on monoclonal antibody to Leu 1 (Becton Dickinson) combined with rabbit anti-IgA in a three-step biotin–avidin method. (a) Numerous T lymphocytes are present in dome area beneath follicle-associated epithelium (FE), in T cell area alongside lymphoid follicle (LF), and in adjacent crypt (C) areas and villi (V). Note that more intraepithelial T lymphocytes are found in FE than in villi (epithelial basement membrane zone indicated by dashed line). Note also that some T cells (arrows) appear within LF. IgA-producing cells are found in dome area and at base of villi. Crypt epithelium shows uptake of IgA and surface mucus layer is IgA-positive. (b) Larger magnification of dome area. (a) ×150; (b) ×340.

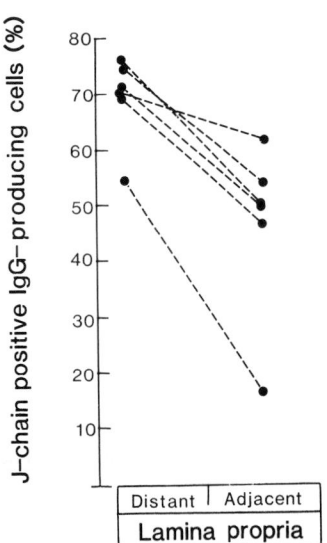

Fig. 7.17 Comparison of J-chain expression shown by IgG-producing cells in lamina propria of normal appendix mucosa distant from and adjacent to lymphoid follicles. Adapted from Bjerke and Brandtzaeg [17].

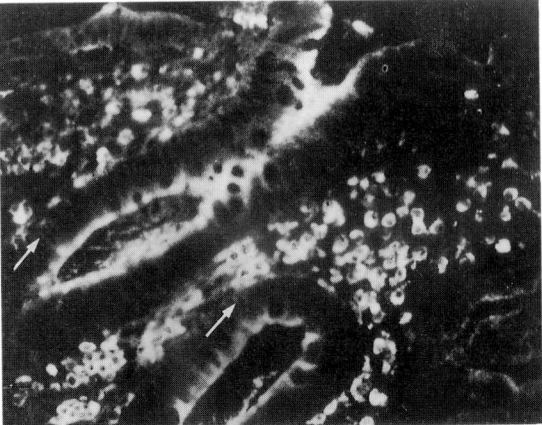

(a)

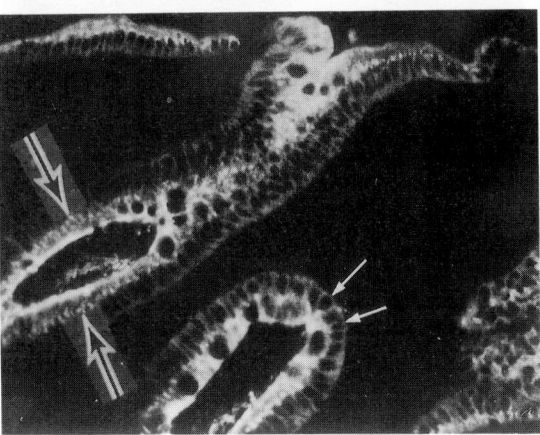

(b)

Fig. 7.18 Immunofluorescence staining for IgA (a) and SC (b) in comparable fields from adjacent sections of human colonic mucosa (lumen at the top) from a patient with ulcerative colitis. There is intense staining for IgA in columnar cells of glands, while surface epithelium contains less IgA. Note that SC is present in the Golgi regions (large arrows) which, by contrast, are devoid of IgA. Both SC and IgA are associated with the epithelial cell membranes (small arrows). Goblet cells are negative. ×250.

columnar cells of the crypts of Lieberkühn and decreases in concentration in the epithelium covering the villi [36]. In the large bowel it is generally present also in the surface epithelium (Fig. 7.18). In the normal gastric mucosa, SC is produced mainly by cells of the antral glands and their isthmus zones [238].

As reviewed elsewhere [28], several lines of evidence indicate that SC acts as a receptor in the selective external transport of J-chain-containing dimeric IgA and pentameric IgM [38]. After being formed on the basolateral surface of the epithelial cell, the Ig–SC complexes are translocated by endocytosis to the lumen (Fig. 7.19). As a consequence, the cytoplasmic distribution of SC and these two Ig classes is congruent except in the Golgi region (Fig. 7.18) where free SC is selectively accumulated [22]. The epithelial staining for IgA is normally stronger than that for IgM [25].

Diseased mucosa

A primary defect in epithelial immunoglobulin transport has not been convincingly identified as a cause of intestinal disease [36]. SC expression in jejunal mucosa from patients with coeliac disease mimics that in normal colon, and signs of epithelial IgA and IgM transport are seen along the entire hyperplastic crypts and surface epithelium [36]. It has been claimed that there is a marked 'backflow' of SIgA into the lamina propria in coeliac disease [217], but

we have been unable to confirm this observation.

Altered distribution of SC. Altered distribution of SC has also been reported in Crohn's disease and idiopathic proctitis [67, 84]. These findings can probably be ascribed to localized secondary events; no significant overall reduction of SC synthesis was shown when mucosal specimens from various intestinal diseases were cultured in vitro [141a]. Our studies of localized epithelial changes in longstanding ulcerative colitis showed reduced expression of both SC and IgA—progressively so from hyperplastic to dysplastic lesions [191]. The former type of lesion is considered to be caused by inflammation whereas the latter may

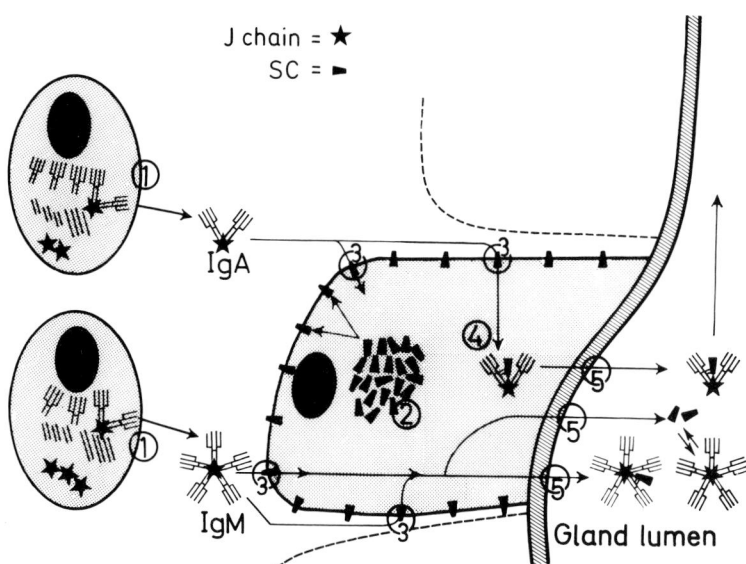

J chain = ★
SC = ►

IgA

IgM

Gland lumen

Fig. 7.19 Schematic representation of the various steps involved in local formation and selective glandular transport of dimeric IgA and pentameric IgM. (1) The two isotypes are produced along with J chain in local immunocytes. (2) SC is produced by serous-type secretory epithelial cells, accumulates in the Golgi complex and migrates to the basolateral plasma membrane. (3) Ig–SC complexes formed in the membrane are taken up by endocytosis and transported to the luminal face of the epithelial cell. (4) During this transport, covalent stabilization of the IgA–SC complexes takes place by disulphide-exchange reactions. (5) The Ig–SC complexes are extruded to the gland lumen along with an excess of free SC that serves to stabilize SIgM in which SC is mainly non-covalently bound. Modified from Brandtzaeg [22, 23].

represent an initial neoplastic alteration. Thus, there are probably different ways of repressing the production of SC and thereby the epithelial transport of dimeric IgA. Conversely, epithelial expression of SC and IgA was not reduced but rather enhanced in chronic gastritis [238]. We interpreted this finding as a reflection of augmented epithelial immaturity of the glandular isthmus zone where increased proliferation takes place in gastritis.

Epithelial HLA-DR expression

Normal mucosa

Another feature of great interest for epithelial interaction with the immune system is the expression of HLA-DR determinants on normal intestinal villi. This was first shown for the human small intestine in our laboratory [209] and has been confirmed by Selby et al [213]. Immunofluorescence for DR characteristically reveals a patchy apical distribution in the epithelium (Fig. 7.14). The staining is not associated with the mucous layer (Fig. 7.15a) but truly reflects apical DR expression by the enterocyte which also shows some faint diffuse cytoplasmic fluorescence and expression related to the basolateral plasma membrane (Fig. 7.14). It has been shown in the rat that enterocytes do not commence their production of class II MHC molecules until after weaning; normal Ia expression seemed to be independent of activated T cells but might, nevertheless, have been induced by microenvironmen-

tal influences [157]. Information on this point is apparently lacking in man.

The biological significance of the prominent HLA-DR expression shown by human intestinal villus epithelium is unknown, but a possible role in the presentation of luminal antigens to lymphocytes deserves consideration (Fig. 7.13).

Endothelial and histiocytic cells. In addition to their epithelial expression, HLA-DR determinants are also present on a varying number of endothelial and histiocytic cells in the lamina propria, mainly in the villi (Figs. 7.14 and 7.15a). In the gastric and large bowel mucosa there are also positive histiocytic cells of various morphology beneath the epithelium [215], but normally both glandular and surface epithelia are DR negative [209]. Studies in rats have indicated that the heterogeneous population of histiocytic cells in the intestinal mucosa is constitutively positive with regard to class II MHC determinants—that is, no stimulation was found to be required for Ia expression [157].

Antigen-presenting cells. Macrophages can take up foreign material, process it by poorly defined mechanisms and probably to some extent present it in a degraded form to T_h cells in the context of class II MHC molecules which they generally express [87]. However, dendritic histiocytic cells with such surface determinants are apparently functioning even better as accessory antigen-presenting cells (APC) (Fig.

Fig. 7.20 Schematic representation of HLA-DR-positive antigen-presenting cells which may be involved in immune regulation both in lymphoepithelial tissues and at glandular sites. Most soluble antigens must be presented to helper T (T_h) cells along with HLA-DR or other class II MHC determinants to elicit efficient B cell responses. Antigens presented by macrophages are first taken up by these cells (small arrows), processed by undefined mechanisms (?), and then presented on the cell surface in a modified form. A secretory IgA response may depend on release from activated T_h cells of immunoregulatory factors particularly enhancing IgA expression, but may in addition depend on stimulation of suppressor T (T_s) cells inhibiting the expression of other B cell isotypes.

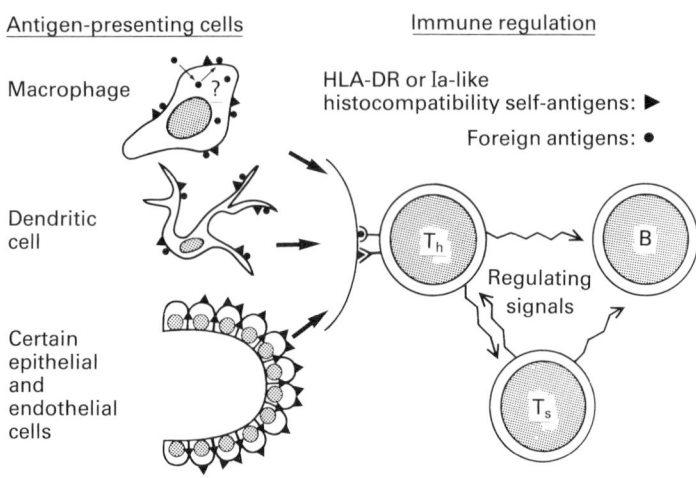

7.20). Recent evidence has indicated that also DR-positive human vascular endothelium [101] and thyroid epithelial cells [137] may present antigen which needs no prior processing. It is therefore tempting to believe that the enterocytes of the villi participate in presentation of degraded antigens from the intestinal lumen along with the subepithelial DR-positive histiocytic cells.

Diseased mucosa

Enhanced epithelial expression of HLA-DR in human intestinal mucosa was first reported in coeliac disease and dermatitis herpetiformis [206]; we found that bright immunohistochemical staining extended from the surface epithelium and deep into the hyperplastic crypts (Fig. 7.21). Selby et al [214] sub-

(a)

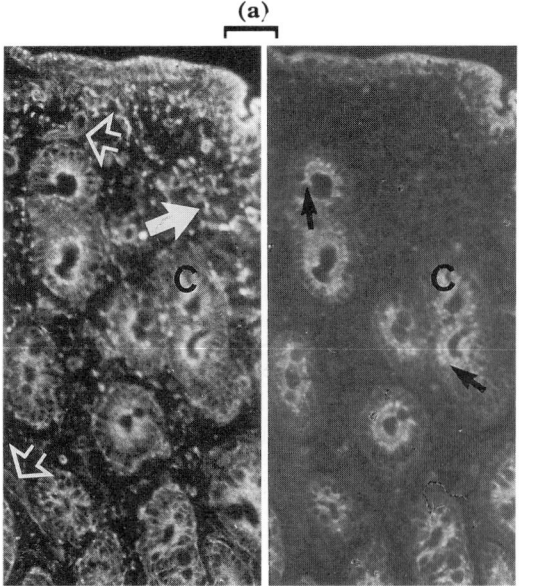

(b)

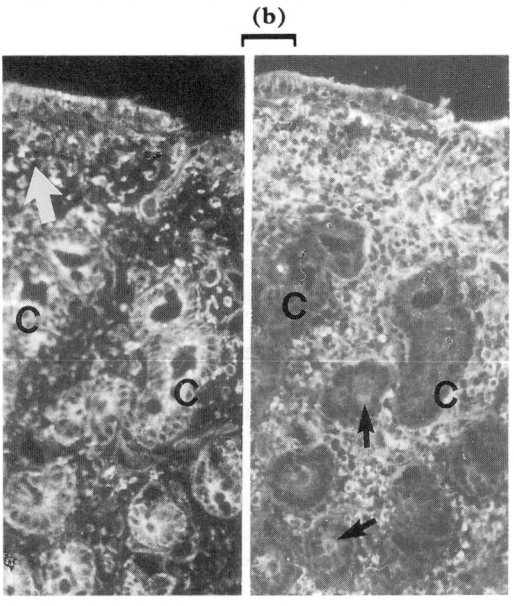

Fig. 7.21 Paired immunofluorescence staining for HLA-DR (left panels, fluorescein) and (a) SC or (b) IgA (right panels, rhodamine) in two comparable fields from adjacent sections of jejunal mucosa from a patient with untreated coeliac disease. Both surface epithelium (at the top) and hyperplastic crypts (C) show bright apical and membrane-related DR staining and there are DR-positive histiocytic cells (solid arrows) and endothelium (open arrows) in lamina propria. (a) In contrast to the normal situation DR is expressed along with SC by both surface and crypt epithelium, but the distribution of the two markers is not completely congruent; e.g. note selective accumulation of SC in Golgi zones (small arrow). (b) Numerous IgA immunocytes are present between DR-positive crypts and there is much extracellular IgA in lamine propria. Epithelial IgA staining signifies external transport (small arrows). × 150.

sequently observed epithelial expression of DR in about 70% of cases with active ulcerative colitis and in about 90% of those with active Crohn's disease. We have confirmed this observation [31] and have noted similarly enhanced epithelial DR expression in chronic gastritis (Valnes and Brandtzaeg, unpublished observations). In all four diseases there is, in addition, an increased number of DR-positive subepithelial histiocytic cells of various morphology [215].

Aberrant DR expression. It is currently unknown how the strikingly increased mucosal expression of HLA-DR in gastrointestinal diseases may influence local immune regulation, but augmented antigen presentation is one possibility. Experimental evidence indicates that the density of class II MHC molecules on APC is important for the magnitude of immune responsiveness [108, 152]. Enhanced epithelial DR expression may thus contribute to both food and microbial hypersensitivity and probably also to autoimmune phenomena [8, 20]. MHC molecules may, in addition, be directly involved in the binding of luminal substances to the epithelial cells [71].

The mechanisms underlying the increased mucosal DR expression are obviously complex but may primarily depend on stimulation of T cells. In the rat, gut epithelial cells can be induced to produce Ia molecules both by graft-versus-host reaction and by intestinal *Trichinella spiralis* infection [9]. Activated T cells produce γ-interferon which is a potent inducer of DR—not only on histiocytes but also on a variety of epithelial cells [103]. Synthesis of γ-interferon is regulated by interleukin 2 (IL-2) which acts as an amplifying signal [187]. Paradoxically, it has been reported that mucosal T cells isolated from Crohn lesions show decreased capacity for IL-2 synthesis [78]. It has, moreover, been reported that T cells from such lesions respond relatively poorly to this lymphokine [246]. However, factors derived from other as yet unidentified non-T cells participating in immune responses [48] and certain substances with lectin properties [185] may likewise induce epithelial Ia (or HLA-DR) expression.

Intraepithelial T cells. The finding that intraepithelial T lymphocytes isolated from rat gut can mediate epithelial Ia expression [52] is of great interest since a similar possibility exists in man. Although the total number of intraepithelial lymphocytes is decreased in coeliac disease (apparently because of excessive luminal loss), the flux of lymphocytes into the epithelium may be increased [151] in a dose-dependent response to gluten [130, 194]. As fewer circulating gluten-responding T cells are found in untreated than in treated patients [205], it is possible that the intraepithelial lymphocytes reflect sequestration of gluten-specific cells from blood. They are relatively large and highly mitotic [151], and small alterations of their phenotypic characteristics have been reported [212]. However, the possible contribution of intraepithelial lymphocytes to the augmented epithelial DR expression in coeliac disease remains uncertain.

IMMUNOLOGICAL HOMEOSTASIS IN GUT MUCOSA

Normal homeostasis

One may visualize that a humoral immunological homeostasis is maintained locally by a critical balance among available antibodies. This concept is schematically depicted in Fig. 7.22a, taking into account only the IgA and IgG isotypes. Dimeric IgA (and to some extent pentameric IgM) antibodies act in a 'first line' of defence by antigen exclusion on the mucosal surface. However, antigens bypassing the epithelial barrier will, within the mucosa, have the chance of meeting corresponding serum-derived or locally produced antibodies belonging to any of the three major isotypes. Since IgG (and IgM) can activate complement (C), which also permeates the lamina propria [3], inflammatory mediators of this enzyme system may regularly be generated to a limited extent.

Antiphlogistic activities of IgA. The phlogistic potential in the mucosa does not cause clinical symptoms as long as the local immunological homeostasis remains in control (Fig. 7.22a). Firstly, both within the mucosa and in the secretions, serum-derived monomeric and particularly locally produced dimeric IgA antibodies may reduce IgG-promoted phagocytosis [150, 249] and inhibit the C-activating properties of IgG antibodies and IgG-containing immune complexes by competition for the same antigenic determinants [86, 91, 199]. Secondly, IgA antibodies may prepare monocytes and lymphocytes for antibody-dependent cytotoxicity and thereby limit bacterial multiplication without inducing

Fig. 7.22 (a) It is postulated that normal immunological homeostasis is maintained in gut mucosa through critical balance between available immunoglobulins (for simplicity, only IgA and IgG are depicted). Dimeric IgA acts in a 'first line' of defence by antigen exclusion at the epithelial surface (to the right). Antigens bypassing this trapping mechanism may meet corresponding serum-derived IgG antibodies in lamina propria. Formed immune complexes will activate complement and inflammatory mediators are generated in mucosa. Such a development is moderated by 'blocking' antibody activities exerted in lamina propria by serum-derived or locally produced monomeric or dimeric IgA. (b) This homeostasis is altered when there is distorted immunological stimulation because of increased mucosal permeability and/or excessive antigen exposure. To limit dissemination of foreign substances a 'second line' of defence is then set up in the mucosa, including local production of IgG. Due to phlogistic properties of IgG antibodies, a vicious circle may develop with further increase of mucosal antigen penetrability, intensified complement activation and cytotoxic reactions, massive attraction of phagocytic cells, and release of lysosomal enzymes from phagocytes. Such a development will result in aggravation and perpetuation of inflammation and may lead to clinically overt gut disease.

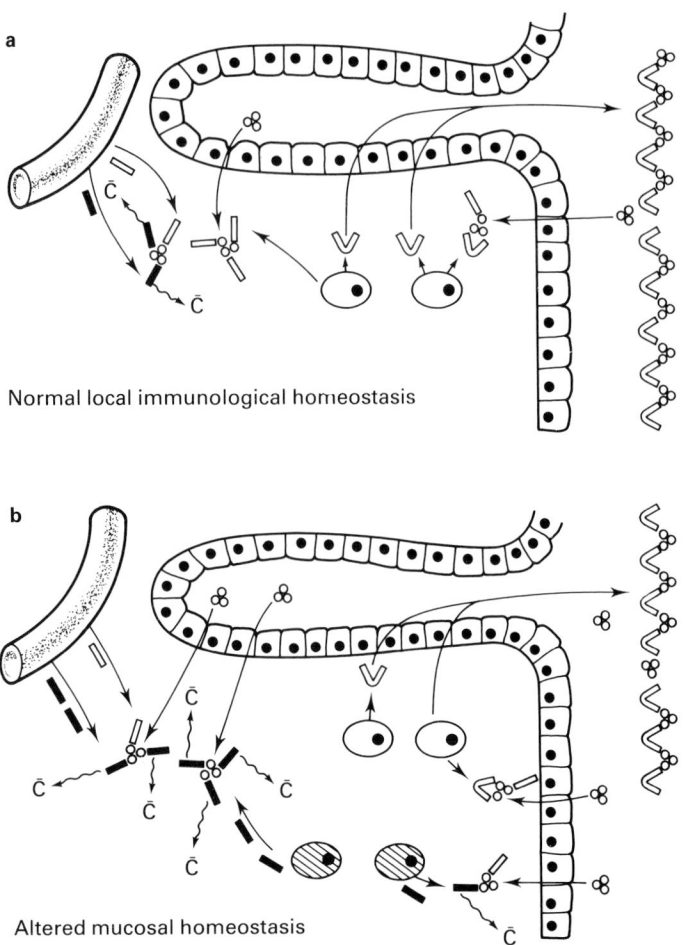

Normal local immunological homeostasis

Altered mucosal homeostasis

Antigen   IgG   IgA   Complement activation → C̄

C activation [138, 229]. Thirdly, and regardless of antibody specificity, locally produced dimeric IgA or soluble IgA-containing immune complexes may be able to suppress chemotaxis of neutrophils, eosinophils and monocytes [107, 115, 239].

IgA may thus in several ways dampen down potentially untoward inflammatory and cytotoxic reactions elicited indirectly by IgG antibodies. It is conceivable that IgA antibodies are likewise antagonistic to the phlogistic effect of IgE-mediated degranulation of local mast cells.

Altered homeostasis

Serum-derived and locally produced IgG antibodies (and mast cells armed with IgE antibodies) may be considered a 'second line' of humoral defence in the mucosa. IgG has a potent capacity for immune elimination, both through enhanced phagocytosis and antibody-dependent cytotoxicity involving activated C factors or K cells. It may be further visualized, however, that if immune elimination is unsuccessful due to continuous penetration of antigen, C-activating immune complexes will prevail locally. Mucosal penetrability may in that case increase for a variety of bystander antigens [40, 133]. Thus, a vicious circle could develop, perhaps also including arming of mast cells with IgE antibodies in individuals genetically susceptible to atopy. The result of such persistent phlogistic mechanisms will be overt clinical disease.

When noxious influences on the gastrointestinal mucosa are fairly well counterbalanced by a pronounced SIgA (and SIgM) response, only minor and reversible disturbances of the local immunological homeostasis take place and a normal condition may be established after removal of the aetiological agent. This is exemplified by successful treatment of coeliac disease when patients adhere strictly to a gluten-free diet and by the spontaneous recovery usually seen after acute gastroenteritis.

Crohn's disease and ulcerative colitis. Conversely, in Crohn's disease and ulcerative colitis, severe alterations of the mucosal homeostasis take place (Fig. 7.22b). In these disorders the pathogenetic antigens (and mitogens) have not been identified, and it is not known how they initially gain undue access to the lamina propria. Perhaps the first break in the epithelial barrier is caused by viral or bacterial infection, possibly combined with nutritional factors and genetic predisposition. Although enhanced local IgG responses may be regarded as an attempt to reinforce the 'second line' of defence against a battery of foreign substances and microbial agents, immune elimination is obviously unsuccessful in these severe disorders. Continued overproduction of IgG is probably at least in part responsible for the conversion of a self-limiting process into a chronic disease on the basis of immunopathological mechanisms.

Conclusions

These humoral aspects of mucosal homeostasis are obviously only part of a complex local immunological interplay. Much less is known about direct and indirect beneficial or detrimental effects exerted by T cells in the gastrointestinal mucosa. It should be re-emphasized that secretory antibodies are not always decisive for maintenance of immunological homeostasis.

RELATION OF INTESTINAL ALLERGY TO LOCAL IMMUNITY

Intestinal production of IgE

Several studies have been made to relate socalled 'IgE-containing' cells to gastrointestinal diseases [98]. Some workers have taken an increase of such cells to indicate ongoing local Type 1 hypersensitivity (atopy), whereas others have based the same conclusion on a reduced number—implying IgE consumption by the atopic reaction [35]. However, the contradictory views are difficult to evaluate because a distinction has not usually been made between IgE-positive mast cells and IgE-producing immunocytes [31]. This is also

true for the disease entities called allergic proctitis [99, 192] and infantile allergic colitis [109], which both are characterized by a high number of 'IgE-containing' cells in the mucosal lesions. The concomitant presence of numerous eosinophilic granulocytes, particularly in the latter disease, indicated mast-cell degranulation which results in release of socalled ECF-A or 'eosinophil chemotactic factor of anaphylaxis' [244].

IgE immunocytes or IgE-positive mast cells

Reported observations on jejunal mucosa of patients with food allergy are likewise difficult to interpret. Rosekrans et al [193] found a high number of 'IgE-containing' cells (up to 100 per mm² lamina propria area). In our opinion most of these were probably mast cells as we and others [201, 225] have been unable to find a consistent increase of IgE-producing cells associated with cow's milk protein intolerance, although we often see numerous IgE-positive mast cells. These cells are mainly located at the base of the crypts but are also found among the IgA-producing immunocytes around the level of the crypt openings (Fig. 7.23). They may be quite numerous, even in the complete absence of local IgE-producing cells. Such immunocytes are in our opinion just as sparse in the intestinal mucosa of patients with atopy as in non-specific chronic inflammatory lesions of various other origins [240]. An inconsistent and low number of jejunal and rectal IgE immunocytes has likewise been reported in children with food allergy and atopic eczema [177] and in children with soya protein allergy [179]. However, a recent study indicated that inflammatory lesions of the gastric mucosa often contain both plasma cells and mast cells positive for IgE [170].

It seems justifiable to conclude that IgE-positive mast cells may be involved in the pathogenesis of certain gastrointestinal diseases, whereas local synthesis of IgE in the lesions generally is small and inconsistent. This view accords with experimental investigations in infected rats which, on the basis of immunohistochemistry, have shown that IgE is produced chiefly in the regional lymph nodes and spleen rather than in the diseased intestinal mucosa [134, 156]. Direct evidence for a major clonal expansion of IgE-producing cells in mesenteric lymph nodes of rats after infestation with a gut-dwelling helminth parasite (*Nippostrongylus brasiliensis*) was recently obtained by an immunoplaque assay [210].

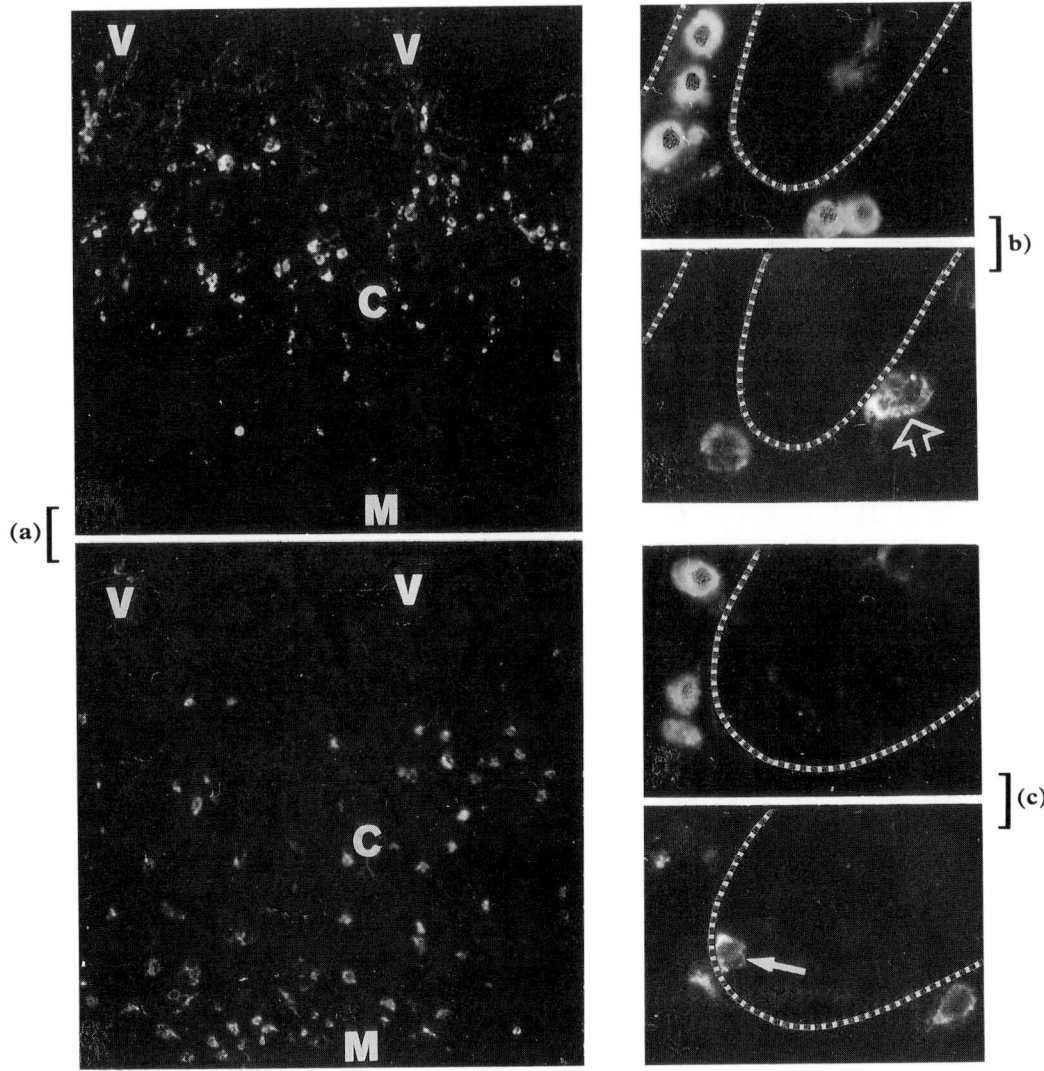

Fig. 7.23 Paired immunofluorescence staining for IgA (top panels, rhodamine) and IgE (bottom panels, fluorescein) in partly transverse section of jejunal mucosa from patient with food allergy. (a) IgA-producing immunocytes are found in normal distribution, mainly in the upper crypt (C) region and at the base of some villi (V); IgE-positive mast cells are found mainly between crypts and muscularis mucosae (M), but some are intermingled with IgA immunocytes. (b, c) Two fields adjacent to crypts (indicated by dashed lines) illustrate that IgA immunocytes and IgE-positive mast cells have different immunofluorescence appearance; the former show intense cytoplasmic staining whereas the latter show mainly plasma membrane-related granular staining (open arrow). Exposure times for mast cells were much longer than for immunocytes. Note that mast cells in crypt region are often juxtaposed to epithelium and sometimes intraepithelial (arrow in c). (a) × 150; (b, c) × 600.

Arming of intestinal mast cells with IgE

The balance of evidence indicates that intestinal mast cells acquire their IgE mainly in the regional lymph nodes (Fig. 7.24) as first proposed by Gillon [81]. In the mouse, when mucosal T cells are stimulated by topical antigen, they release IL-3 which induces local proliferation of mast-cell precursors; both stimulated T blasts and these precursors undergo cyclic traffic. They leave the regional lymph nodes and enter peripheral blood via thoracic duct lymph and then seed the whole length of the gut [89]. Under persistent antigen-induced IL-3 release from T blasts, the IgE-sensitized early mast cells will finally be transformed locally to mature mast cells (Fig. 7.24).

The excess of free IgE reaching the blood from the production site probably reflects rather poorly the extent of regional mast-cell sensitization, which depends not only on the availability of IgE but also on proliferation

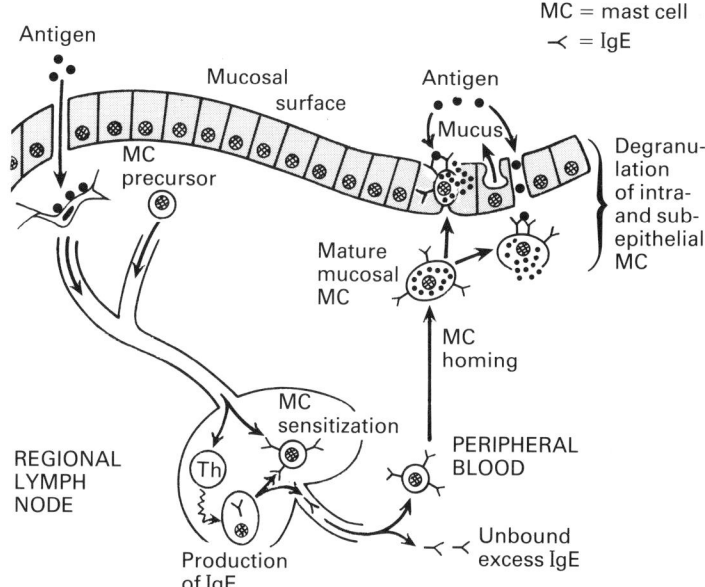

MC = mast cell
⤙ = IgE

Fig. 7.24 Hypothetical scheme for cyclic traffic and differentiation of mucosal mast cells. Bone-marrow-derived mast-cell precursors proliferate locally under the influence of IL-3 released from antigen-stimulated T cells. The precursors migrate to regional lymph nodes where they acquire surface IgE which is produced by immunocytes under regulation of helper T (T_h) cells. 'Armed' early mast cells home back to mucosa where they mature and are subjected to degranulation after exposure to antigen. Modified from Gillon [81].

and traffic of mast-cell precursors. Preferential regional sensitization would harmonize with the observation that distinctly IgE-positive mast cells are more often encountered in bronchial mucosa than in skin of allergic patients with recurrent pulmonary complaints [242]. The armed mast cells probably release their IgE both within the mucosa and, after entering the epithelium (Fig. 7.24), also directly into the lumen. This may be how IgE is carried by mast cells from regional lymph nodes to mucosal sites and exocrine secretions. This also explains the significantly raised levels of IgE (or rather IgE fragments) found in intestinal juice of patients with atopic food allergy, although the authors interpreted their observation to indicate mucosal synthesis of IgE [14]. As expected according to the model depicted in Fig. 7.24, there was no consistent relationship between IgE concentrations in serum and intestinal juice.

Production of IgA in atopy

The primary events in the development of atopic disease are poorly understood. On the basis of measurements of IgA in serum, it has been suggested that infants and children at hereditary risk of atopy have a relatively slow postnatal development of their IgA system [223, 230]. SIgA-mediated immunological exclusion may therefore be transiently deficient in these individuals. This notion has recently been supported by quantification of jejunal immunocytes, which indicated reduced IgA responses to luminal antigens without any IgM compensation in the mucosa of atopic children [218].

A recent study of T cell subsets in peripheral blood, moreover, suggested that such children have altered immune regulation; their T8 (putative 'suppressor') phenotype was numerically decreased, a finding that might explain their enhanced IgE-producing capacity [54]. Another recent study showed an inverse relationship between the serum IgE concentration and the number of IgA-producing cells in jejunal mucosa of food-allergic children [177]. A combination of reduced mucosal barrier function and brisk IgE responses may thus underlie the pathogenesis of gastrointestinal allergy, but there are most likely also other predisposing factors [131].

INTEGRATION OF MUCOSAL AND SYSTEMIC B CELL SYSTEMS

Implications for vaccination methods

There is normally a relatively high proportion of J-chain-positive IgA immunocytes ($\sim 50\%$) among the scarce Ig-producing cells found in normal human peripheral blood [26]. After mitogen stimulation, these cells secrete predominantly dimeric IgA with a subclass composition that matches the percentages of intestinal IgA1 and IgA2 immunocytes [124]. Moreover, when obtained from orally immunized volunteers, they have been found to pro-

duce specific IgA antibodies [85]. Such circulating B cells, therefore, may be representative
of those migrating from MALT to secretory
sites. However, other researchers were unable
to demonstrate memory B cells for an IgA response to influenza A virus in human peripheral blood, although this infectious agent
should have primed MALT; instead, specific
IgA precursors were found within peripheral
lymphoid tissue—indicating that IgA-memory
cells only temporarily circulate after priming
and do settle beyond secretory sites [140].

Relationship between systemic and secretory immune systems

Systemic dissemination of both IgG and IgA
responses has likewise been shown in man
after administration of a live mucosal immunogen such as Sabin attenuated poliomyelitis
vaccine [172]; the same is true in mice after
peroral immunization with cholera toxin [139].
There is direct experimental evidence indicating that the secretory and the systemic B cell

systems are not totally segregated [51, 143].
We have argued elsewhere that—rather than
depending on separate cell populations—the
two immune systems are integrated but preferentially retain memory B cells of different
clonal maturation stages [42]. In view of such
a putative integration, one would also expect
parenteral immunization to affect secretory
immunity; and there is increasing evidence
that this is the case, both with regard to induction and suppression (see below).

A considerable proportion of the Ig-producing cells generated in the follicular germinal centres of tonsils are J-chain-positive
regardless of isotype [121], and this is so also
in activated peripheral lymph nodes (unpublished observations). It is conceivable that B
cells of a clonal maturation stage compatible
with J-chain expression may migrate from
tonsils and lymph nodes to secretory sites and
settle there along with comparable GALT-
and BALT-derived cells (Fig. 7.25). This may
be the basis for several experimental observations showing that it is possible to prime for

Fig. 7.25 Schematic representation
of B cell traffic in the secretory
immune system. B lymphocytes
receive antigen-induced stimulatory
'first signals' in Peyer's patches,
other mucosa-associated lymphoid
structures (such as tonsils),
mesenteric lymph nodes and perhaps
to some extent in peripheral lymph
nodes. Most stimulated B cells
migrate from Peyer's patches
through lymph and peripheral blood
to various secretory tissues including
gut lamina propria. Such migrating
cells were previously thought to be
blasts but recent studies have
indicated that they are mainly
lymphocytes. They may receive
signals for further differentiation in
mesenteric lymph nodes and spleen.
Terminal differentiation to plasma
cells at secretory sites is induced by
'second signals' that are only partly
defined but largely antigen-
dependent, at least in the gut (cf.
Fig. 7.13).

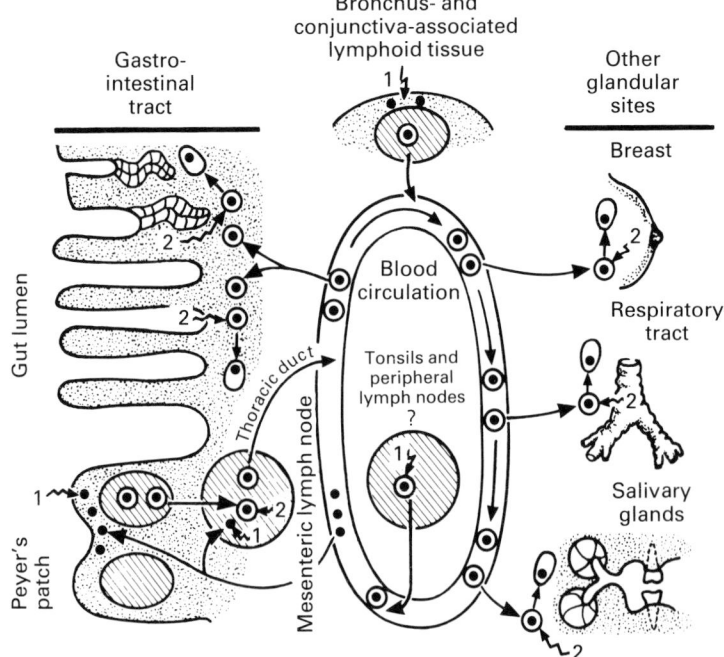

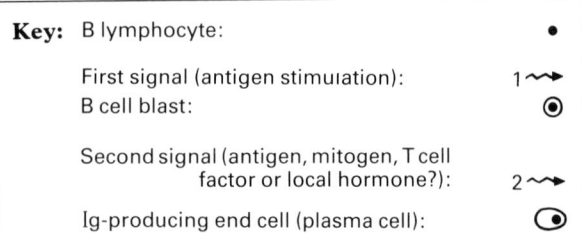

Key:	B lymphocyte:	●
	First signal (antigen stimulation):	1 ↝
	B cell blast:	◉
	Second signal (antigen, mitogen, T cell factor or local hormone?):	2 ↝
	Ig-producing end cell (plasma cell):	◉

an intestinal immune response by parenteral immunization [51, 118, 182], although it may be dependent on the antigen. In some combinations parenteral priming and subsequent topical boosting by the oral route have been more efficient than topical priming and boosting for the induction of secretory immunity, but the efficiency has depended on variables such as adjuvant, type of antigen (live versus dead; particulate versus soluble) and its dosage, routes and timing of administration [180] (see Chapter 15).

Cholera vaccination. Exciting vaccination results have been obtained with cholera toxin which is an exceptionally potent protein antigen, apparently because it binds to receptors on intestinal epithelial cells. Feeding this antigen does not induce oral tolerance, but stimulates both local and systemic immunity [139]. Its immunogenic properties are retained by the non-toxic B subunit, which has been administered successfully by both the intramuscular and oral routes for boosting of intestinal IgA antitoxin responses in naturally primed Bangladeshi adults [228]. An oral vaccine consisting of the B subunit and killed whole bacterial cells has likewise been shown to induce intestinal immunity in previously unprimed Swedish volunteers [110]. It may be difficult to evaluate the clinical effect of such vaccination in terms of SIgA antibodies, however, because it has recently been reported that other mechanisms may also be involved in acquired protection against cholera [127].

Experimental vaccinations. Other promising avenues of vaccination currently being explored in relation to secretory immunity are administration of oral adjuvant compounds and epithelial targeting of immunogens by cloning them into bacteria that are able to colonize GALT [65, 165].

Meanwhile much confusion prevails as to the long-term effect of enteric immunization. Both animal experiments [163] and human studies [97] have indicated that, with most antigens persistent topical stimulation may eventually result in a decreased IgA response, perhaps reflecting local induction of T_S cells. On the other hand, stimulation of a convincing secondary type of mucosal immune response seems to require the antigen to be applied to the site to be protected [183]. It is possible, therefore, that a combination of parenteral and enteric stimulation will turn out to be preferable.

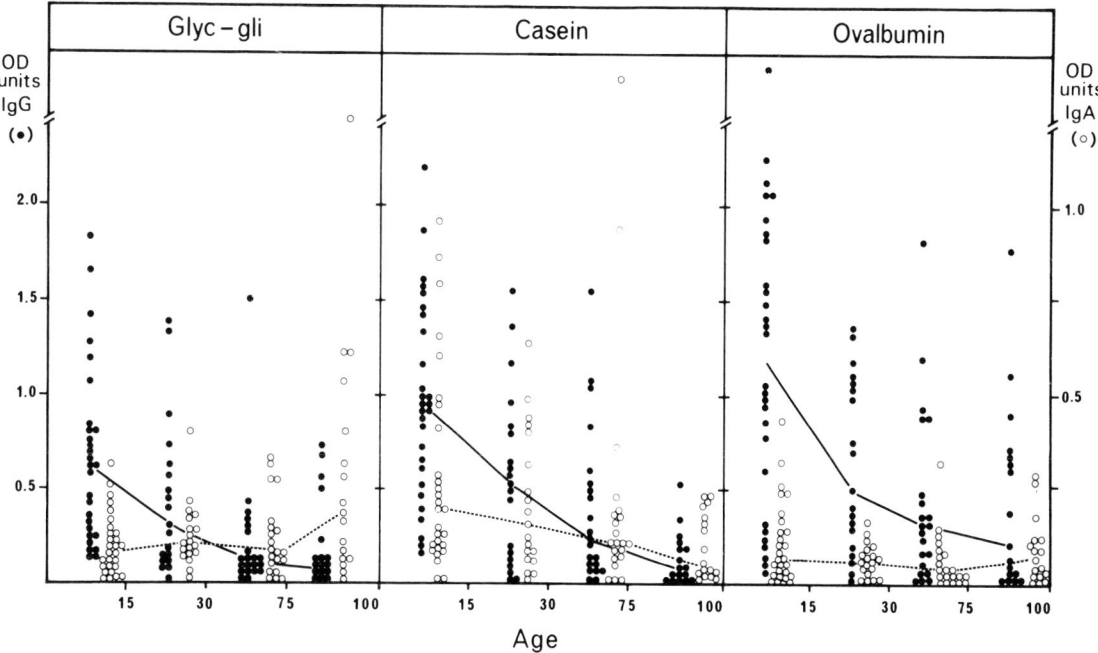

Fig. 7.26 Optical density (OD) measurements by enzyme-linked immunosorbent assay of serum IgG (●) and IgA (o) activities to gluten fraction glyc-gli, casein and ovalbumin in healthy children (5-15 years), young adults (16-30 years), adults (31-75 years) and old people (76-100 years). Medians connected by solid (IgG) and dotted (IgA) lines. Adapted from Scott et al [208].

Enterically induced hyporesponsiveness in man

In the light of the variable hyporesponsiveness obtained for systemic IgG-, IgE- and T cell-mediated (delayed-type) immunity in experimental animals [75], one may question the significance of oral tolerance as a general biological phenomenon (see Chapter 14). Nevertheless, the fact that human IgG (and IgM) serum antibody levels to most common dietary antigens decrease with increasing age (Fig. 7.26), is compatible with development of orally induced hyporesponsiveness with time [197, 208]. Direct evidence for a hyporesponsive state to bovine serum albumin was in fact shown by intradermal testing with this antigen in adults [119].

In contrast, persistence in the human gut of microbial antigens—including LPS—may lead to systemic hyporesponsiveness limited to IgM [55]. We found that serum IgM titres to several intestinal bacteria decreased selectively with age [208]. These findings in man may indicate a disparity between responses to dietary proteins and microbial antigens as suggested by animal experiments [75].

CONCLUSIONS

1 Humoral immunity in the gut depends on intimate cooperation between the B cell system and the secretory epithelium. The obvious biological significance of the striking J-chain expression shown by gut immunocytes is that SC-binding IgA and IgM polymers are generated locally and become readily available for external transport through SC-producing gut epithelium. This important functional goal, in terms of clonal differentiation, is sufficient justification for the J chain also to be expressed by B cells terminating locally with IgG or IgD production; these immunocytes may be considered as 'spin-off' from immature memory clones that through isotype switching are on their way to IgA expression.

2 It seems to be well established that gut immunocytes are largely derived from B cells generated in GALT. There is insufficient knowledge concerning the relative importance of M cells, HLA-DR-expressing epithelial and dendritic cells and macrophages in the transport, processing and presentation of luminal antigen that takes place in GALT to accomplish this extensive B cell generation. It is not known to what extent the germinal-centre ac-

tivity of the lymphoepithelial structures gives rise directly to the IgA precursors that seed the gut mucosa.

3 The regulatory T cells that participate in stimulation or suppression of B cells in GALT and mesenteric lymph nodes are still poorly defined. It is not known whether unique 'switch' T_h cells are necessary for generation of IgA precursors or whether IgA expression is a reflection of an early stage of expanded B cell clones.

4 Although B cell migration to the gut lamina propria may be guided by receptors for endothelial determinants, recent studies have indicated that a heterogeneous B cell population in terms of differentiation and origin extravasates largely at random but with some regional preferences.

5 Accumulation of B cells in gut mucosa seems to depend mainly on local proliferation and differentiation, which are largely antigen-driven. The role of HLA-DR-positive epithelial and dendritic cells, macrophages and T cells in mediating the necessary stimulatory signals to the extravasated B cells is unknown. The receptive B cell population seems to consist of relatively early memory clones with a high J-chain-expressing potential, which in part may explain why terminal differentiation chiefly gives rise to IgA immunocytes.

6 The mucosal barrier normally allows some uptake of antigens so there is probably always a need for immune elimination within the mucosa. If immune exclusion is insufficient (e.g. IgA deficiency), or if there is too large an antigen load on the mucosa (e.g. infection), non-specific amplication mechanisms involved in immune elimination may cause hypersensitivity which is observed clinically as gut disease. Such an immunopathological development is mainly precipitated by IgG and IgE antibodies. Although the phlogistic mechanisms induced by such antibodies may be pathogenetic in several types of gut disease, the reason for initial deterioration of the mucosal barrier is often unexplained.

7 Clinical observations of immunodeficient patients have shown that SIgA and SIgM are not the only important components of the humoral intestinal defence system, which is reinforced by a number of non-immunological factors.

Acknowledgements

This work was supported by the Norwegian Cancer Society, the Norwegian Research

Council for Science and the Humanities, and Anders Jahre's Foundation.

The following figures have been reproduced with kind permission of Universitetsforlaget, Oslo: Figures 7.1, 7.2, 7.7, 7.20 and 7.22 from Brandtzaeg P, Valnes K, Scott H, et al: The human gastrointestinal secretory immune system in health and disease. Scand J Gastroenterol 1985; 20 (suppl 114): 17–38; Fig 7.6 from Brandtzaeg and Baklien [34]; and Figures 7.13 and 7.24 from Brandtzaeg P: Research in gastrointestinal immunology—state of the art. Scand J Gastroenterol 1985; 20 (suppl 114): 137–56.

REFERENCES

1 Agus SG, Falchuk ZM, Sessoms CS, et al: Increased jejunal IgA synthesis in vitro during acute infectious non-bacterial gastroenteritis. Am J Dig Dis 1974; 19:127–31.

2 André C, André F, Fargier MC: Distribution of IgA1 and IgA2 plasma cells in various normal human tissues and in the jejunum of plasma IgA-deficient patients. Clin Exp Immunol 1978; 33:327–31.

3 Baklien K, Brandtzaeg P: Immunohistochemical localization of complement in intestinal mucosa. Lancet 1974; ii:1087–8.

4 Baklien K, Brandtzaeg P: Comparative mapping of the local distribution of immunoglobulin-containing cells in ulcerative colitis and Crohn's disease of the colon. Clin Exp Immunol 1975; 22:197–209.

5 Baklien K, Brandtzaeg P: Immunohistochemical characterisation of local immunoglobulin formation in Crohn's disease of the ileum. Scand J Gastroenterol 1976; 11:447–57.

6 Baklien K, Brandtzaeg P, Fausa O: Immunoglobulins in jejunal mucosa and serum from patients with adult coeliac disease. Scand J Gastroenterol 1977; 12:149–59.

7 Baklien K, Fausa O, Thune PO, Gjone E: Immunoglobulins in jejunal mucosa and serum from patients with dermatitis herpetiformis. Scand J Gastroenterol 1977; 12:161–8.

8 Ballardini G, Mirakian R, Bianchi FB, et al: Aberrant expression of HLA-DR antigens on bile duct epithelium in primary biliary cirrhosis: relevance to pathogenesis. Lancet 1984; ii:1009–13.

9 Barclay AN, Mason DW: Induction of Ia antigen in rat epidermal cells and gut epithelium by immunological stimuli. J Exp Med 1982; 156:1665–76.

10 Barry WS, Pierce NF: Protein deprivation causes reversible impairment of mucosal immune response to cholera toxoid/toxin in rat gut. Nature 1979; 281:64–5.

11 Baur S, Koo N, Taylor KB: The immunoglobulin class of autoantibody-containing cells in the gastric mucosa in pernicious anaemia. Immunology 1970; 19:891–4.

12 Beatty DW, Napier B, Sinclair-Smith CC: Secretory IgA synthesis in Kwashiorkor. J Clin Lab Immunol 1983; 12:31–6.

13 Bellamy JEC, Nielsen NO: Immune-mediated emigration of neutrophils into the lumen of the small intestine. Infect Immun 1974; 9:615–9.

14 Belut D, Moneret-Vautrin DA, Nicolas JP, Grilliat JP: IgE levels in intestinal juice. Dig Dis Sci 1980; 25:323–32.

15 Bienenstock J, Dolezel J: Peyer's patches: lack of specific antibody-containing cells after oral and parrenteral immunization. Immunology 1971; 106:938–45.

16 Bienenstock J, Befus D, McDermott M, et al: Regulation of lymphoblast traffic and localization in mucosal tissues, with emphasis on IgA. Fed Proc 1983; 41:3213–7.

17 Bjerke K, Brandtzaeg P: Immunoglobulin- and J-chain-producing cells associated with lymphoid follicles in human appendix, colon and ileum, including Peyer's patches. Clin Exp Immunol 1986; 64 (in press).

18 Blanco A, Linares P, Andión R, et al: Development of humoral immunity system of the small bowel. Allergol Immunopathol 1976; 4:235–40.

19 Bodmer J, Bodmer W: Histocompatibility 1984. Immunol Today 1984; 5:251–4.

20 Bottazzo GF, Pujol-Borrell R, Hanafusa T: Role of aberrant HLA-DR expression and antigen presentation in induction of endocrine autoimmunity. Lancet 1983; ii:1115–9.

21 Brandtzaeg P: Two types of IgA immunocytes in man. Nature, New Biol 1973; 243:142–3.

22 Brandtzaeg P: Mucosal and glandular distribution of immunoglobulin components. Differential localization of free and bound SC in secretory epithelial cells. J Immunol 1974; 112:1553–9.

23 Brandtzaeg P: Mucosal and glandular distribution of immunoglobulin components. Immunohistochemistry with a cold ethanol-fixation technique. Immunology 1974; 26:1101–14.

24 Brandtzaeg P: Presence of J chain in human immunocytes containing various immunoglobulin classes. Nature 1974; 252:418–20.

25 Brandtzaeg P: Human secretory immunoglobulin M. An immunochemical and immunohistochemical study. Immunology 1975; 29:559–70.

26 Brandtzaeg P: Studies on J chain and binding site for secretory component in circulating human B cells. II. The cytoplasm. Clin Exp Immunol 1976; 25:59–66.

27 Brandtzaeg P: Polymeric IgA is complexed with secretory component (SC) on the surface of human intestinal epithelial cells. Scand J Immunol 1978; 8:39–52.

28 Brandtzaeg P: Role of J chain and secretory component in receptor-mediated glandular and hepatic transport of immunoglobulins in man. Scand J Immunol 1985; 22:111–46.

29 Brandtzaeg P: Immune functions of human nasal mucosa and tonsils in health and disease. In: Bienenstock J, ed. Immunology of the lung and upper and respiratory tract. New York: McGraw-Hill, 1984;28–95.

30 Brandtzaeg P: Immunohistochemical characterization of intracellular J-chain and binding site for secretory component (SC) in human immunoglobulin (Ig)-producing cells. Mol Immunol 1983; 20:941–66.

31 Brandtzaeg P: Immunopathology of Crohn's disease. Ann Gastroentérol Hépatol 1985; 21:201–20.

32 Brandtzaeg P: The oral secretory immune system

with special emphasis on its relation to dental caries. Proc Finn Dent Soc 1983; 79:71-84.

33 Brandtzaeg P: The secretory immune system of lactating human mammary glands compared with other exocrine organs. Ann NY Acad Sci 1983; 409: 353-81.

34 Brandtzaeg P, Baklien K: Immunohistochemical studies of the formation and epithelial transport of immunoglobulins in normal and diseased human intestinal mucosa. Scand J Gastroenterol [Suppl 36] 1976; 11:1-45.

35 Brandtzaeg P, Baklien K: Inconclusive immunohistochemistry of human IgE in mucosal pathology. Lancet 1976; i:1297-8.

36 Brandtzaeg P, Baklien K: Intestinal secretion of IgA and IgM: a hypothetical model. Ciba Found Symp 1977; 46:77-108.

37 Brandtzaeg P, Korsrud FR: Significance of different J chain profiles in human tissues: generation of IgA and IgM with binding site for secretory component is related to the J chain expressing capacity of the total local immunocyte population, including IgG and IgD producing cells, and depends on the clinical state of the tissue. Clin Exp Immunol 1984; 58:709-18.

38 Brandtzaeg P, Prydz H: Direct evidence for an integrated function of J chain and secretory component in epithelial transport of immunoglobulins. Nature 1984; 311:71-3.

39 Brandtzaeg P, Rognum TO: Evaluation of nine different fixatives. 1. Preservation of immunoglobulin isotypes, J chain, and secretory component in human tissues. Pathol Res Pract 1984; 179:250-66.

40 Brandtzaeg P, Tolo K; Mucosal penetrability enhanced by serum-derived antibodies. Nature 1977; 266:262-3.

41 Brandtzaeg P, Fjellanger I, Gjeruldsen ST; Human secretory immunoglobulins. I. Salivary secretions from individuals with normal or low levels of serum immunoglobulins. Scand J Haematol [Suppl 12] 1970; 1-83.

42 Brandtzaeg P, Guy-Grand D, Griscelli C: Intestinal, salivary, and tonsillar IgA and J-chain production in a patient with severe deficiency of serum IgA. Scand J Immunol 1981; 13:313-25.

43 Brandtzaeg P, Baklien K, Fausa O, Hoel PS: Immunohistochemical characterization of local immunoglobulin formation in ulcerative colitis. Gastroenterology 1974; 66:1123-36.

44 Brandtzaeg P, Gjeruldsen ST, Korsrud F, et al: The human secretory immune system shows striking heterogeneity with regard to involvement of J chain-positive IgD immunocytes. J Immunol 1979; 122: 503-10.

45 Broom BC, de la Concha EG, Webster ADB, et al: Dichotomy between immunoglobulin synthesis by cells in gut and blood of patients with hypogammaglobulinaemia. Lancet 1975; ii:253-6.

46 Brown WR, Isobe Y, Nakane PK: Studies on translocation of immunoglobulins across intestinal epithelium. II. Immunoelectron-microscopic localization of immunoglobulins and secretory component in human intestinal mucosa. Gastroenterology 1976; 71:985-95.

47 Bull DM, Bienenstock J, Tomasi TB: Studies on human intestinal immunoglobulin A. Gastroenterology 1971; 60:370-80.

48 Callahan GN; Soluble factors produced during an immune response regulate Ia antigen expression by murine adenocarcinoma and fibrosarcoma cells. J Immunol 1984; 132:2649-57.

49 Calvert JE, Maruyama S, Tedder TF, et al: Cellular

50 Carter PB, Collins FM: Peyer's patch responsiveness to *Salmonella* in mice. J Reticuloendothel Soc 1975; 17:38-46.

51 Cebra JJ, Fuhrman JA, Horsfall DJ, Shahin RD: Natural and deliberate priming of IgA responses to bacterial antigens by the mucosal route. In: Weinstein L, Fields B, eds. Seminars in infectious disease, vol. 4: Robbins JB, Hill JC, Sadoff JC eds. Bacterial vaccines. New York: Thieme-Stratton, 1982; 6-12.

52 Cerf-Bensussan N, Quaroni A, Kurnick JT, Bhan AK: Intraepithelial lymphocytes modulate Ia expression by intestinal epithelial cells. J Immunol 1984; 132:2244-52.

53 Chandra RK: Reduced secretory antibody response to live attenuated measles and poliovirus vaccines in malnourished children. Br Med J 1975; 2:583-5.

54 Chandra RK, Baker M: Numerical and functional deficiency of suppressor T cells precedes development of atopic eczema. Lancet 1983; ii:1393-4.

55 Cižnár I, Farbakyova G, Draškovičová M, Karolcek J: Typhoid γG, γM and γA antibodies in persons with different relation to the typhoid infection. Zentralbl Bakteriol Hyg 1975; 231:108-15.

56 Clancy R, Cripps A, Chipchase H: Regulation of human gut B lymphocytes by T lymphocytes. Gut 1984; 25:47-51.

57 Crabbé PA, Carbonara AO, Heremans JF: The normal human intestinal mucosa as a major source of plasma cells containing $_{\gamma}$A-immunoglobulin. Lab Invest 1965; 14:235-48.

58 Crabbé PA, Nash DR, Bazin H, et al: Immunohistochemical observations on lymphoid tissues from conventional and germ-free mice. Lab Invest 1970; 22:448-57.

59 Crago SS, Mestecky J: Secretory component: interactions with intracellular and surface immunoglobulins of human lymphoid cells. J Immunol 1979; 122:906-11.

60 Crago SS, Kutteh WH, Moro I, et al: Distribution of IgA1-, IgA2-, and J chain-containing cells in human tissues. J Immunol 1984; 132:16-8.

61 Cunningham-Rundles C: The identification of specific antigens in circulating immune complexes by an enzyme-linked immunosorbent assay: detection of bovine κ-casein IgG complexes in human sera. Eur J Immunol 1981; 11:504-9.

62 Cunningham-Rundles C, Carr RI, Good RA: Dietary protein antigenemia in humoral immunodeficiency. Correlation with splenomegaly. Am J Med 1984; 76:181-5.

63 Cunningham-Rundles C, Brandeis WE, Good RA, Day NK: Bovine antigens and the formation of circulating immune complexes in selective immunoglobulin A deficiency. J Clin Invest 1979; 64:272-9.

64 Cunningham-Rundles C, Brandeis WE, Pudifin DJ, et al: Autoimmunity in selective IgA deficiency: relationship to anti-bovine protein antibodies, circulating immune complexes and clinical disease. Clin Exp Immunol 1981; 45:299-304.

65 Curtiss R, Holt RG, Barletta RG: *Escherichia coli* strains producing *Streptococcus mutans* proteins responsible for colonization and virulence. Ann NY Acad Sci 1983; 409:688-95.

66 Danis VA, Harries AD, Heatley RV: In vitro immunoglobulin secretion by normal human gastrointestinal mucosal tissues, and alterations in patients with inflammatory bowel disease. Clin Exp Immunol 1984; 56:159-66.

67 Das KM, Erber WF, Rubinstein A: Immunohisto-

events in the differentiation process of antibody-secreting cells. Semin Hematol 1984; 21:226-43.

chemical changes in morphologically involved and uninvolved colonic mucosa of patients with idiopathic proctitis. J Clin Invest 1977; 59:379-85.

68 Delamette F, Marty MC, Panijel J: In vitro study of IgM polymerization. Cell Immunol 1975; 19:262-75.

69 Della Corte E, Parkhouse RME: Biosynthesis of immunoglobulin A (IgA) and immunoglobulin M (IgM). Requirement for J-chain and a disulphide-exchange enzyme for polymerization. Biochem J 1973; 136: 597-606.

70 Drew PA, La Brooy JT, Shearman DJC: In vitro immunoglobulin synthesis by human intestinal lamina propria lymphocytes. Gut 1984; 25:649-55.

71 Edidin M: MHC antigens and non-immune functions. Immunol Today 1983; 4:269-70.

72 Eerola E, Jalkanen S, Granfors K, Toivanen A: Immune capacity of the chicken bursectomized at 60 h of incubation. Effect of bursal epithelial cells and bursal epithelium-conditioned medium on the production of immunoglobulins and specific antibodies in vitro. Scand J Immunol 1984; 19:493-500.

73 Egido J, Blasco R, Sancho J, et al: Increased rate of polymeric IgA synthesis by circulating cells in mesangial glomerulonephritis. Clin Exp Immunol 1982; 47:309-16.

74 Eidelman S: Intestinal lesions in immune deficiency. Hum Pathol 1976; 7:427-34.

75 Elson CO: Induction and control of the gastrointestinal immune system. Scand J Gastroenterol [Suppl] 1985; 114:1-15.

76 Falchuk ZM, Strober W: Increased jejunal immunoglobulin synthesis in patients with nontropical sprue as measured by a solid phase immunoadsorption technique. J Lab Clin Med 1972; 6:1004-13.

77 Falchuk ZM, Strober W: Gluten-sensitive enteropathy: synthesis of antigliadin antibody in vitro. Gut 1974; 15: 947-52.

78 Fiocchi C, Hilfiker ML, Youngman KR, et al: Interleukin 2 activity of human intestinal mucosa mononuclear cells. Decreased levels in inflammatory bowel disease. Gastroenterology 1984; 86:734-42.

79 Fiorilli M, Luzi G, Aiuti F: Immunoglobulin production by the rectal mucosa in subjects with ulcerative colitis. Rend Gastroenterol 1975; 7:1-4.

80 Fossum S, Rolstad B, Tjernshaugen H: Selective loss of S-phase cells when making cell suspensions from lymphoid tissue. Cell Immunol 1979; 48:149-54.

81 Gillon J: Where do mucosal mast cells acquire IgE? Immunol Today 1981; 2:80-1.

82 Gleeson M, Cripps AW, Clancy RL, et al: Ontogeny of the secretory immune system in man. Aust NZ J Med 1982; 12:255-8.

83 Green F, Heyworth B: Immunoglobulin-containing cells in jejunal mucosa of children with protein-energy malnutrition and gastroenteritis. Arch Dis Child 1980; 55:380-3.

84 Green FH, Fox H: The distribution of mucosal antibodies in the bowel of patients with Crohn's disease. Gut 1975; 16:125-31.

85 Gregory RL, Schöller M, Filler SJ, et al: IgA antibodies to oral and ocular bacteria in human external secretions. Protides Biol Fluids 1985; 32:53-6.

86 Griffiss JM, Goroff DK: IgA blocks IgM and IgG-initiated immune lysis by separate molecular mechanisms. J Immunol 1983; 130:2882-3.

87 Guidos C, Wong M, Lee K-C: A comparison of the stimulatory activities of lymphoid dendritic cells and macrophages in T proliferative responses to various antigens. J Immunol 1984; 133:1179-84.

88 Guy-Grand D, Griscelli C, Vassalli P: The mouse gut T lymphocyte, a novel type of T cell. Nature,

origin, and traffic in mice in normal and graft-versus-host conditions. J Exp Med 1978; 148:1661-77.

89 Guy-Grand D, Dy M, Luffau G, Vassalli P: Gut mucosal mast cells. Origin, traffic, and differentiation. J Exp Med 1984; 160:12-28.

90 Hadju I, Moldoveanu Z, Cooper M, Mestecky J: Ultrastructural studies of human lymphoid cells. μ and J chain expression as a function of B cell differentiation. J Exp Med 1983; 158:1993-2006.

91 Hall WH, Manion RE, Zinneman HH: Blocking serum lysis of *Brucella abortus* by hyperimmune rabbit immunoglobulin A. J Immunol 1971; 107:41-6.

92 Halpern MS, Koshland ME: Novel subunit in secretory IgA. Nature 1970; 228:1276-8.

93 Hammarström L, Axelsson U, Björkander J, et al: HLA antigens in selective IgA deficiency: distribution in healthy donors and patients with recurrent respiratory tract infections. Tissue Antigens 1984; 24:35-9.

93a Haneberg B, Aarskog D: Human faecal immunoglobulins in healthy infants and children, and in some with diseases affecting the intestinal tract or the immune system. Clin Exp Immunol 1975; 22:210-22.

94 Hanson LÅ: Comparative immunological studies of the immune globulins of human milk and of blood serum. Int Arch Allergy Appl Immunol 1961; 18:241-67.

95 Hanson LÅ, Brandtzaeg P: The mucosal defense system. In: Stiehem ER, Fulginiti WA, eds. Immunological disorders in infants and children. Philadelphia: WB Saunders 1980; 137-62.

96 Hanson LÅ, Björkander J, Oxelius V-A: Selective IgA deficiency. In: Chandra RK, ed. Primary and secondary immunodeficiency disorders. New York: Churchill Livingstone, 1983; 62-84.

97 Hanson LÅ, Carlsson B, Jalil F, et al: Different secretory IgA antibody responses after immunization with inactivated and live poliovirus vaccines. Rev Infect Dis [Suppl 2] 1984; 6:S356-S360.

98 Heatley RV: The gastrointestinal mast cell. Scand J Gastroenterol 1983; 18:449-53.

99 Heatley RV, Rhodes J, Calcraft BJ, et al: Immunoglobulin E in rectal mucosa of patients with proctitis. Lancet 1975; ii:1010-12.

100 Heddle RJ, La Brooy JT, Shearman DJC: *Escherichia coli* antibody-secreting cells in the human intestine. Clin Exp Immunol 1982; 48:469-76.

101 Hirschberg H, Braathen LR, Thorsby E: Antigen presentation by vascular endothelial cells and epidermal Langerhans cells: the role of HLA-DR. Immunol Rev 1982; 66:57-77.

102 Horsfall DJ, Cooper JM, Rowley D: Changes in the immunoglobulin levels of the mouse gut and serum during conventionalisation and following administration of *Salmonella typhimurium*. Aust J Exp Biol Med Sci 1978; 56:727-35.

103 Houghton AN, Thomson TM, Gross D, et al: Surface antigens of melanoma and melanocytes. Specificity of induction of Ia antigens by human γ-interferon, J Exp Med 1984; 160:255-69.

104 Husband AJ: Kinetics of extravasation and redistribution of IgA-specific antibody-containing cells in the intestine. J Immunol 1982; 128:1355-9.

105 Husband AJ, Monié HJ, Gowans JL: The natural history of cells producing IgA in the gut. Ciba Found Symp 1977; 46:29-42.

106 Issekutz TB: The response of gut-associated T lymphocytes to intestinal viral immunization. J Immunol 1984; 133:2955-60.

107 Ito S, Mikawa H, Shinomiya K, Yoshida T: Suppressive effect of IgA soluble immune complexes on

neutrophil chemotaxis. Clin Exp Immunol 1979; 37:436–40.

108 Janeway CA, Bottomly K, Babich J, et al: Quantitative variation in Ia antigen expression plays a central role in immune regulation. Immunol Today 1984; 5:99–105.

109 Jenkins HR, Pincott JR, Soothill JF, et al: Food allergy: the major cause of infantile colitis. Arch Dis Child 1984; 59:326–9.

110 Jertborn M, Svennerholm A-M, Holmgren J: Gut mucosal, salivary and serum antitoxic and antibacterial antibody responses in Swedes after oral immunization with B subunit-whole cell cholera vaccine. Int Arch Allergy Appl Immunol 1984; 75:38–43.

111 Joller PW, Buhler AK, Hitzig WH: Transitory and persistent IgA deficiency. Reevaluation of 19 pediatric patients once found to be deficient in serum IgA. J Clin Lab Immunol 1981; 6:97–101.

112 Jonard PP, Rambaud JC, Dive C, et al: Secretion of immunoglobulins and plasma proteins from the jejunal mucosa. Transport rate and origin of polymeric immunoglobulin A. J Clin Invest 1984; 74:525–35.

113 Kagnoff MF: Functional characteristics of intestinal Peyer's patch lymphoid cells. Ann NY Acad Sci 1976; 278:539–45.

114 Kagnoff MF, Campbell S: Functional characteristics of Peyer's patch lymphoid cells. I. Induction of humoral antibody and cell-mediated allograft reactions. J Exp Med 1974; 139:398–406.

115 Kemp AS, Cripps AW, Brown S: Suppression of leucocyte chemokinesis and chemotaxis by human IgA. Clin Exp Immunol 1980; 40:388–95.

116 Keren DF, Appelman HD, Dobbins WO, et al: Correlation of histopathologic evidence of disease activity with the presence of immunoglobulin-containing cells in the colons of patients with inflammatory bowel disease. Hum Pathol 1984; 15:757–63.

117 Kilian M, Thomsen B, Petersen TE, Bleeg HS: Occurrence and nature of bacterial IgA proteases. Ann NY Acad Sci 1983; 409:612–23.

118 Klipstein FA, Engert RF, Clements JD: Arousal of mucosal secretory immunoglobulin A antitoxin in rats immunized with *Escherichia coli* heat-labile enterotoxin. Infect Immun 1982; 37:1086–92.

119 Korenblat PE, Rothberg RM, Minden P, Farr RS: Immune responses of human adults after oral and parenteral exposure to bovine serum albumin. J Allergy Clin Immunol 1968; 41:226–35.

120 Korsrud FR, Brandtzaeg P: Quantitative immunohistochemistry of immunoglobulin- and J-chain-producing cells in human parotid and submandibular glands. Immunology 1980; 39:129–40.

121 Korsrud FR, Brandtzaeg P: Immunohistochemical evaluation of J-chain expression by intra- and extra-follicular immunoglobulin-producing human tonsillar cells. Scand J Immunol 1981; 13:271–80.

122 Koshland ME: Presidential address: molecular aspects of B cell differentiation. J Immunol 1983; 131:I–IX.

123 Kutteh WH, Prince SJ, Mestecky J: Tissue origins of human polymeric and monomeric IgA. J Immunol 1982; 128:990–5.

124 Kutteh WH, Koopman WJ, Conley ME, et al: Production of predominantly polymeric IgA by human peripheral blood lymphocytes stimulated in vitro with mitogens. J Exp Med 1980; 152:1424–9.

125 Kutteh WH, Moldoveanu Z, Prince SJ, et al: Biosynthesis of J-chain in human lymphoid cells producing immunoglobulins of various isotypes. Mol Immunol 1983; 20:967–76.

126 Lamson G, Koshland ME: Changes in J chain and μ

chain RNA expression as a function of B cell differentiation. J Exp Med 1984; 160:877–92.

127 Lange S, Lönnroth I, Nygren H: Protection against experimental cholera in the rat. A study on the formation of antibodies against cholera toxin and desensitization of adenylate cyclase after immunization with cholera toxin. Int Arch Allergy Appl Immunol 1984; 75:143–8.

128 Lange S, Nygren H, Svennerholm A-M, Holmgren J: Antitoxic cholera immunity in mice: influence of antigen deposition on antitoxin-containing cells and protective immunity in different parts of the intestine. Infect Immun 1980; 28:17–23.

129 Layton GT, Smithyman AM: The optimum conditions for antibody production in vitro by Peyer's patch lymphocytes and a comparison between total immunoglobulins and antigen (TNP)-specific antibody synthesis following mitogen stimulation. Int Arch Allergy Appl Immunol 1983; 72:158–63.

130 Leigh RJ, Marsh MN, Crowe P, et al: Studies of intestinal lymphoid tissue. IX. Dose-dependent, gluten-induced lymphoid infiltration of coeliac jejunal epithelium. Scand J Gastroenterol 1985; 20:715–9.

131 Levinsky RJ; Natural resistance of the gastrointestinal tract. Clin Immunol Allergy 1983; 3:441–56.

132 Lie SO, Fröland S, Brandtzaeg P, et al: Transient B cell immaturity with intractable diarrhoea: a possible new immunodeficiency syndrome. J Inherit Metab Dis 1978; 1:137–43.

133 Lim PL, Rowley D: The effect of antibody on the intestinal absorption of macromolecules and on intestinal permeability in adult mice. Int Arch Allergy Appl Immunol 1982; 68:41–6.

134 Lindsay MC, Blaies DB, Williams JF: *Taenia taeniaeformis*: immunoglobulin E-containing cells in the intestinal and lymphatic tissues of infected rats. Int J Parasitol 1983; 13:91–9.

135 Lodinova R, Jouja V, Wagner V: Serum immunoglobulins and coproantibody formation in infants after artificial intestinal colonization with *Escherichia coli* 083 and oral lysozyme administration. Pediatr Res 1973; 7:659–69.

136 Loeb PM, Strober W, Falchuk ZM, Laster I: Incorporation of L-Leucine-¹⁴C into immunoglobulins by jejunal biopsies of patients with celiac sprue and other gastrointestinal disease. J Clin Invest 1971; 50:559–69.

137 Londei M, Lamb JR, Bottazzo GF, Feldmann M: Epithelial cells expressing aberrant MHC class II determinants can present antigen to cloned human T cells. Nature 1984; 312:639–41.

138 Lowell GH, Smith LF, Griffiss JM, Brandt BL: IgA-dependent, monocyte-mediated, antibacterial activity. J Exp Med 1980; 152:452–7.

139 Lycke N, Lindholm L, Holmgren J: IgA isotype restriction of the mucosal but not in the extramucosal immune response after oral immunizations with cholera toxin or cholera B subunit. Int Arch Allergy Appl Immunol 1983; 72:119–27.

140 McCaughan GW, Adams E, Basten A: Human antigen-specific IgA responses in blood and secondary lymphoid tissue: an analysis of help and suppression. J Immunol 1984; 132:1190–6.

141 McClelland DBL: Peyer's-patch-associated synthesis of immunoglobulin in germ-free, specific-pathogen-free, and conventional mice. Scand J Immunol 1976; 5:909–15.

141a McClelland DBL, Shearman DJC, Lai a Fat RFM, van Furth R: In vitro synthesis of immunoglobulins, secretory component, complement and lysozyme by human gastrointestinal tissues—II. Pathological tissues. Clin Exp Immunol 1976; 23:20-7.

142 McCune JM, Fu SM, Kunkel HG: J chain biosynthesis in pre-B cells and other possible precursor B cells. J Exp Med 1981; 154; 138-45.

143 McDermott MR, Bienenstock J: Evidence for a common mucosal immunologic system. I. Migration of B immunoblasts into intestinal, respiratory, and genital tissues. J Immunol 1979; 122:1892-8.

144 McDermott MR, Mark DA, Befus AD, et al: Impaired intestinal localization of mesenteric lymphoblasts associated with vitamin A deficiency and protein-calorie malnutrition. Immunology 1982; 45:1-5.

145 MacDermott RP, Nash GS, Bertovich MJ: Alterations of IgM, IgG, and IgA synthesis and secretion by peripheral blood and intestinal mononuclear cells from patients with ulcerative colitis and Crohn's disease. Gastroenterology 1981; 81:844-52.

146 MacDermott RP, Beale MG, Alley CD, et al: Synthesis and secretion of IgA, IgM, and IgG by peripheral blood mononuclear cells in human disease states, by isolated human intestinal mononuclear cells, and by human bone marrow mononuclear cells from ribs. Ann NY Acad Sci 1983; 409:498-508.

147 McGee DW, Franklin RM: Lymphocyte migration into the lacrimal gland is random. Cell Immunol 1984; 86:75-82.

148 McLoughlin GA, Hede JE, Temple JG, et al: The role of IgA in the prevention of bacterial colonization of the jejunum in the vagotomized subject. Br J Surg 1978; 65:435-7.

149 Maffei HVL, Kingston D, Hill ID, Shiner M: Histopathologic changes and the immune response within the jejunal mucosa in infants and children. Pediat Res 1979; 13:733-6.

150 Magnusson KE, Stjernström I: Mucosal barrier mechanisms. Interplay between secretory IgA (SIgA), IgG and mucins on the surface properties and association of salmonellae with intestine and granulocytes. Immunology 1982; 45:239-48.

151 Marsh MN: Studies of intestinal lymphoid tissue. III. Quantitative analyses of epithelial lymphocytes in the small intestine of human control subjects and of patients with celiac sprue. Gastroenterology 1980; 79:481-92.

152 Matis LA, Glimcher LH, Paul WE, Schwartz RH: Magnitude of response of histocompatibility-restricted T-cell clones is a function of the product of the concentrations of antigen and Ia molecules. Proc Natl Acad Sci USA 1983; 80:6019-23.

153 Mattioli CA, Tomasi TB: The life span of IgA plasma cells from the mouse intestine. J Exp Med 1973; 138:452-60.

154 Max EE, Korsmeyer SJ: Human J chain gene. Structure and expression in B lymphoid cells. J Exp Med 1985; 161:832-49.

155 Mayrhofer G: Physiology of the intestinal immune system. In: Newby TJ, Stokes CR, eds. Local immune responses of the gut. Boca Raton, Florida: CRC Press, 1984: 1-96.

156 Mayrhofer G, Bazin H, Gowans JL: Nature of cells binding anti-IgE in rats immunized with *Nippostrongylus brasiliensis*: IgE synthesis in regional nodes and concentration in mucosal mast cells. Eur J Immunol 1976; 6:537-45.

157 Mayrhofer G, Pugh CW, Barclay AN: The distribution, ontogeny and origin in the rat of Ia-positive cells with dendritic morphology and of Ia antigen in epithelia, with special reference to the intestine. Eur J Immunol 1983; 13:112-22.

158 Mellander L, Carlsson B, Hanson LÅ: Appearance of secretory IgM and IgA antibodies to *Escherichia coli* in saliva during early infancy and childhood. J Pediatr 1984: 104:564-8.

159 Mestecky J, Zikan J, Butler W: Immunoglobulin M and secretory immunoglobulin A: evidence for a common polypeptide chain different from light chains. Science 1971; 171:1163-5.

160 Mestecky J, Winchester RJ, Hoffman T, Kunkel HG: Parallel synthesis of immunoglobulins and J-chain in pokeweed mitogen-stimulated normal cells and in lymphoblastoid cell lines. J Exp Med 1977; 145:760-5.

161 Moldoveanu Z, Egan ML, Mestecky J; Cellular origins of human polymeric and monomeric IgA: intracellular and secreted forms of IgA. J Immunol 1984; 133:3156-62.

162 Monteiro E, Fossey J, Shiner M: Antibacterial antibodies in rectal and colonic mucosa in ulcerative colitis. Lancet 1971; i:249-51.

163 Montgomery PC, Majumdar AS, Shandera CA, Rockey JH: The effect of immunization route and sequence of stimulation on the induction of IgA antibodies in tears. Curr Eye Res 1984; 3:861-5.

164 Moreau MC, Ducluzeau R, Guy-Grand D, Muller MC: Increase in the population of duodenal immunoglobulin A plasmocytes in axenic mice associated with different living or dead bacterial strains of intestinal origin. Infect Immun 1978; 121:532-9.

165 Morisaki I, Michalek SM, Harmon CC, et al: Effective immunity to dental caries: enhancement of salivary anti-*Streptococcus mutans* antibody responses with oral adjuvants. Infect Immun 1983; 40:577-91.

166 Mosmann TR, Gravel Y, Williamson AR, Baumal R: Modification and fate of J chain in myeloma cells in the presence and absence of immunoglobulin secretion. Eur J Immunol 1978; 8:94-101.

167 Mostov KE, Blobel G: A transmembrane precursor of secretory component. The receptor for transcellular transport of polymeric immunoglobulins. J Biol Chem 1982; 157:11816-21.

168 Nagura H, Brandtzaeg P, Nakane PK, Brown WR: Ultrastructural localization of J chain in human intestinal mucosa. J Immunol 1979; 123:1044-50.

169 Newman RA, Ormerod MG, Greaves MF: The presence of HLA-DR antigens on lactating human breast epithelium and milk fat globule membranes. Clin Exp Immunol 1980; 41:478-86.

170 Niedobitek F, Volkheimer G, Dumke K, Schlecht M: Zur Häufigheit und Verteilung IgE-haltiget Zellen in der Magenschleimhaut. Pathologe 1984; 5:212-5.

171 Ochs HD, Ament ME: Gastrointestinal tract and immunodeficiency. In: Ferguson A, MacSween RNM, eds. Immunological aspects of the liver and gastrointestinal tract. Lancaster: MTP Press, 1976; 82-120.

172 Ogra PL, Karzon DT: The role of immunoglobulins in the mechanism of mucosal immunity to virus infection. Pediat Clin North Am 1970; 17:385-400.

173 Ogra SS, Ogra PL, Lippes J, Tomasi TB: Immunohistologic localization of immunoglobulins, secretory component, and lactoferrin in the developing human fetus. Proc Soc Exp Biol Med 1972; 139: 570-2.

174 Otto HF, Gebbers J-O: Electron microscopic, ultracytochemical and immunohistological observations in Crohn's disease of the ileum and colon. Virchows Arch [Pathol Anat] 1981; 391:189-205.

175 Parkhouse RME, Cooper MD: A model for the dif-

ferentiation of B lymphocytes with implications for the biological role of IgD. Immunol Rev 1977; 37:105-26.

176 Parkhouse RMF, Della Corte E: Control of IgA biosynthesis. In: Beers RF, Bassett EG, eds. The role of immunological factors in infections, allergic, and autoimmune processes. New York: Raven Press, 1976; 389-401.

177 Perkkiö M: Immunohistochemical study of intestinal biopsies from children with atopic eczema due to food allergy. Allergy 1980; 35:573-80.

178 Perkkiö M, Svailahti E: Time of appearance of immunoglobulin-containing cells in the mucosa of the neonatal intestine. Pediatr Res 1980; 14:953-5.

179 Perkkiö M, Savilahti E, Kuitunen P: Morphometric and immunohistochemical study of jejunal biopsies from children with intestinal soy allergy. Eur J. Pediatr 1981; 137:63-9.

180 Pierce NF: The role of antigen form and function in the primary and secondary intestinal immune responses to cholera toxin and toxoid in rats. J Exp Med 1978; 148:195-206.

181 Pierce NF, Cray WC: Determinants of the localization, magnitude, and duration of a specific mucosal IgA plasma cell response in enterically immunized rats. J Immunol 1982; 128:1311-5.

182 Pierce NF, Gowans JL: Cellular kinetics of the intestinal immune response to cholera toxoid in rats. J Exp Med 1975; 142:1550-63.

183 Pierce NF, Koster FT: Specific immunologic memory in the secretory mucosal immune system. In: Weinstein L, Fields B, eds. Seminars in infectious disease, vol. 4: Robbins JB, Hill JC, Sadoff JC, eds. Bacterial vaccines, New York: Thieme-Stratton, 1982; 19-23.

184 Plaut AG: The IgA1 proteases of pathogenic bacteria. Ann Rev Microbiol 1983; 37:603-22.

185 Pujol-Borrell R, Hanafusa T, Chiovato L, Bottazzo GF: Lectin-induced expression of DR antigen on human cultured follicular thyroid cells. Nature 1983; 304:71-3.

186 Reddy V, Raghuramulu N, Bhaskaram C: Secretory IgA in protein-calorie malnutrition. Arch Dis Child 1976; 51:871-4.

187 Reem GH, Yeh N-H: Interleukin 2 regulates expression of its receptor and synthesis of gamma interferon by human T lymphocytes. Science 1984; 225:429-30.

188 Reynolds JD, Morris B: The influence of gut function on lymphoid cell populations in the intestinal mucosa of lambs. Immunology 1983; 49:501-9.

189 Roberton DM, Paganelli R, Dinwiddie R, Levinsky RJ: Milk antigen absorption in the preterm and term neonate. Arch Dis Child 1982; 57:369-72.

190 Rognum TO, Brandtzaeg P, Baklien K, Hognestad J: Immunoglobulin-producing cells in the 'transitional' mucosa adjacent to adenocarcinomas of the human large bowel. Int J Cancer 1979; 23:165-73.

191 Rognum TO, Elgjo K, Fausa O, Brandtzaeg P: Immunohistochemical evaluation of carcinoembryonic antigen, secretory component, and epithelial IgA in ulcerative colitis with dysplasia. Gut 1982; 23:123-33.

192 Rosekrans PCM, Meijer CJLM, van der Wal AM, Lindeman J: Allergic proctitis, a clinical and immunopathological entity. Gut 1980; 21:1017-23.

193 Rosekrans PCM, Meijer CJLM, Cornelisse CJ, et al: Use of morphometry and immunohistochemistry of small intestinal biopsy specimens in the diagnosis of food allergy. J Clin Pathol 1980; 33:125-30.

194 Rosekrans PCM, Meijer CJLM, Polanco I, et al: Long-term morphological and immunohistochemical observations on biopsy specimens of small intestine from children with gluten-sensitive enteropathy. J Clin Pathol 1981; 34:138-44.

195 Roth R, Koshland ME: Identification of a lymphocyte enzyme that catalyzes pentamer immunoglobulin M assembly. J Biol Chem 1981; 256:4633-9.

196 Roth R, Mather EL, Koshland ME: Intracellular events in the differentiation of B lymphocytes to pentamer IgM synthesis. In: Pernis B, Vogel HJ, eds. Cells of immunoglobulin synthesis. London: Academic Press, 1979; 141-51.

197 Rothberg RM, Farr RS: Anti-bovine serum albumin and anti-alpha lactalbumin in the serum of children and adults. Pediatrics 1965; 35:571-88.

198 Rubin W, Fauci AS, Sleisenger MH, Jeffries GH: Immunofluorescent studies in adult celiac disease. J Clin Invest 1965; 44:475-85.

199 Russell-Jones GJ, Ey PL, Reynolds BL: The ability of IgA to inhibit complement consumption by complement-fixing antigens and antigen-antibody complexes. Aust J Exp Biol Med Sci 1984; 62:1-10.

200 Sagie E, Tarabulus J, Maeir DM, Freier S: Diet and development of intestinal IgA in the mouse. Isr J Med Sci 1974; 10:532-4.

201 Savilahti E: Immunochemical study of the malabsorption syndrome with cow's milk intolerance. Gut 1973; 14:491-501.

202 Savilahti E: Workshop on secretory immunoglobulins. In: Brent L, Holborow J, eds. Progress in immunology. Amsterdam: North-Holland Publishing, 1974; 2:238-43.

203 Savilahti E, Pelkonen P: Clinical findings and intestinal immunoglobulins in children with partial IgA deficiency. Acta Paediat Scand 1979; 68:513-9.

204 Scott BB, Goodall A, Stephenson P, Jenkins D: Small intestinal plasma cells in coeliac disease. Gut 1984; 25:41-7.

205 Scott H, Fausa O, Thorsby E: T-lymphocyte activation by a gluten fraction, glyc-gli. Scand J Immunol 1983; 18:185-91.

206 Scott H, Brandtzaeg P, Solheim BG, Thorsby E: Relation between HLA-DR-like antigens and secretory component (SC) in jejunal epithelium of patients with coeliac disease or dermatitis herpetiformis. Clin Exp Immunol 1981; 44:233-8.

207 Scott H, Ek J, Baklien K, Brandtzaeg P: Immunoglobulin-producing cells in jejunal mucosa of children with coeliac disease on a gluten-free diet and after gluten challenge. Scand J Gastroenterol 1980; 15:81-8.

208 Scott H, Rognum TO, Midtvedt T, Brandtzaeg P: Age-related changes of human serum antibodies to dietary and colonic bacterial antigens measured by an enzyme-linked immunosorbent assay. Acta Pathol Microbiol Immunol Scand [C] 1985; 93:65-70.

209 Scott H, Solheim BG, Brandtzaeg P, Thorsby E: HLA-DR-like antigens in the epithelium of the human small intestine. Scand J Immunol 1980; 12:77-82.

210 Sedgwick JD, Holt PG: Kinetics and distribution of antigen-specific IgE-secreting cells during the primary antibody response in the rat. J Exp Med 1983; 157:2178-83.

211 Selby WS, Janossy G, Jewell DP: Immunohistological characterization of intraepithelial lymphocytes of the human gastrointestinal tract. Gut 1981; 22:169-76.

212 Selby WS, Janossy G, Bofill M, Jewell DP: Lymphocyte subpopulations in the human small intestine.

The findings in normal mucosa and in the mucosa of patients with coeliac disease. Clin Exp Immunol 1983; 52:219–28.

213 Selby WS, Janossy G, Goldstein G, Jewell DP: T lymphocyte subsets in human intestinal mucosa: the distribution and relationship to MHC-derived antigens. Clin Exp Immunol 1981; 44:453–8.

214 Selby WS, Janossy G, Mason DY, Jewell DP: Expression of HLA-DR antigens by colonic epithelium in inflammatory bowel disease. Clin Exp Immunol 1983; 53:614–8.

215 Selby WS, Poulter LW, Hobbs S, et al: Heterogeneity of HLA-DR-positive histiocytes in human intestinal lamina propria: a combined histochemical and immunohistological analysis. J Clin Pathol 1983; 36:379–84.

216 Selner JC, Merrill DA, Claman HN: Salivary immunoglobulin and albumin: development during the newborn period. J Pediat 1968; 72:685–9.

217 Shiner RJ, Ballard J: Mucosal secretory IgA and secretory piece in adult coeliac disease. Gut 1973; 14:778–83.

218 Sloper KS, Brook CGD, Kingston D, et al: Eczema and atopy in early childhood: low IgA plasma cell counts in the jejunal mucosa. Arch Dis Child 1981; 56:939–42.

219 Sminia T, Plesch BEC: An immunohistochemical study of cells with surface and cytoplasmic immunoglobulins in situ in Peyer's patches and lamina propria of rat small intestine. Virchows Arch [Cell Pathol] 1982; 40:181–9.

220 Sminia T, Delemarre F, Janse EM: Histological observations on the intestinal immune response towards horseradish peroxidase in rats. Immunology 1983; 50:53–6.

221 Sminia T, Janse EM, Plesch BEC: Ontogeny of Peyer's patches of the rat. Anat Rec 1983; 207:309–16.

222 Söltoft J, Söeberg B: Immunoglobulin-containing cells in the small intestine during acute enteritis. Gut 1972; 13:535–8.

223 Soothill JF: Some intrinsic and extrinsic factors predisposing to allergy. Proc R Soc Med 1976; 69:439–42.

224 Stern M, Dietrich R, Grüttner R: Gliadin-binding immunocytes in small intestinal lamina propria of children with coeliac disease. Pediatr Res 1981; 15:1196.

225 Stern M, Dietrich R, Müller J: Small intestinal mucosa in coeliac disease and cow's milk protein intolerance: morphometric and immunofluorescent studies. Eur J Pediatr 1982; 139:101–5.

226 Stodell MA, Butler RC, Zemelman VA, et al: Increased numbers of IgG-containing cells in rectal lamina propria of patients with ankylosing spondylitis. Ann Rheum Dis 1984; 43:172–6.

227 Stott SI: Biosynthesis and assembly of IgM. Addition of J-chain to intracellular pools of 8S and 19S IgM. Immunochemistry 1976; 13:157–61.

228 Svennerholm A-M, Sach DA, Holmgren J, Bardhan PK: Intestinal antibody responses after immunisation with colera B subunit. Lancet 1982; i,305–8.

229 Tagliabue A, Boraschi D, Villa L, et al: IgA-dependent cell-mediated activity against enteropathogenic bacteria: distribution, specificity, and characterization of the effector cells. J Immunol 1984; 133:988–92.

230 Taylor B, Norman AP, Orgel HA, et al: Transient IgA deficiency and pathogenesis of infantile atopy. Lancet 1973; ii:111–3.

231 Tlaskalová H, Mandel L, Cerná J: Kinetics of cellular

and humoral IgM, IgG and IgA antibody formation in germfree piglets after peroral immunization. Folia Microbiol (Praha) 1979; 24:82.

232 Tomasi TB, Tan EM, Solomon A, Prendergast RA: Characteristics of an immune system common to certain external secretions. J Exp Med 1965; 121:101–24.

233 Tomasi TB, Zigelbaum S: The selective occurrence of γ_{1A} globulins in certain body fluids. J Clin Invest 1963; 42:1552–60.

234 Tseng J: Expression of immunoglobulin isotypes by lymphoid cells of mouse intestinal lamina propria. Cell Immunol 1982; 73:324–36.

235 Tseng J: Population of resting IgM-IgD double-bearing lymphocytes in Peyer's patches: the major precursor cells for IgA plasma cells in the gut lamina propria. J Immunol 1984; 132:2730–5.

236 Turesson I: Distribution of immunoglobulin-containing cells in human bone marrow and lymphoid tissues. Acta Med Scand 1976; 199:293–304.

237 Valnes K, Brandtzaeg P: Localization of cells producing immunoglobulins and other immune factors in human gastric mucosa. Protides Biol Fluids 1985; 32:315–8.

238 Valnes K, Brandtzaeg P, Elgjo L, Stave R: Specific and nonspecific humoral defense factors in the epithelium of normal and inflamed gastric mucosa. Immunohistochemical localization of immunoglobulins, secretory component, lysozyme, and lactoferrin. Gastroenterology 1984; 86:402–12.

239 Van Epps DE, William RC: Suppression of leucocyte chemotaxis by human IgA myeloma components. J Exp Med 1976; 144:1227–42.

240 Van Spreeuwel JP, Lindeman J, van Maanen J, Meyer CJLM: Increased numbers of IgE containing cells in gastric and duodenal biopsies. An expression of food allergy secondary to chronic inflammation? J Clin Pathol 1984; 37:601–6.

241 Wade S, Lemonnier D, Alexiu A, Bocquet L: Effect of early postnatal under- and overnutrition on the development of IgA plasma cells in mouse gut. J Nutr 1982; 112:1047–51.

242 Wagenaar SS, Peters A, Westermann CJJ, Oosting J: IgE bound to mast cells in bronchial mucosa and skin in atopic subjects. Respiration 1981; 41:258–63.

243 Walker WA: Mechanisms of antigen handling by the gut. In: Brostoff J, Challacombe SJ, eds. Clinics in immunology and allergy, vol. 2, Food Allergy. London: WB Saunders, 1982;15–40.

244 Warren SL: A new look at type I immediate hypersensitivity immune reactions. Ann Allergy 1976; 36:337–41.

245 Watson RR, McMurray DN: The effects of malnutrition on secretory and cellular immune processes. CRC Crit Rev Food Sci Nutr 1979; 12:113–59.

246 Weiserbs DB, Elson CO: Abnormal T cell–T cell communication in the lesions of active Crohn's disease. Gastroenterology 1983; 84:1348.

247 Wijesinha SS, Steer HW: Studies of the immunoglobulin-producing cells of the human intestine: the defunctioned bowel. Gut 1982; 23:211–4.

248 Wijesinha SS, Steer HW: Observations on the immunocytes and macrophages in megacolon. Dis Colon Rectum 1982; 25:312–20.

249 Wilton JMA: Suppression by IgA of IgG-mediated phagocytosis by human polymorphonuclear leucocytes. Clin Exp Immunol 1978; 34:423–8.

250 Yagi M, D'Eustachio P, Ruddle FH, Koshland ME: J chain is encoded by a single gene unlinked to other immunoglobulin structural genes. J Exp Med 1982; 155:647–54.

Chapter 8
Natural Killer Cells and Intestinal Immunity

A. Mowat

Introduction

It is clear that the intestine is equipped with a large array of specific immunological mechanisms which may be of potential importance both in local defence and in conditions of immunopathological origin. In addition, the gut and its lymphoid tissues contain large numbers of non-specific effector cells, including macrophages, mast cells, eosinophils and other leukocytes. In view of the necessity for the gut to handle rapidly large amounts of antigen, the complexity of the intestinal immune apparatus is perhaps not surprising and it follows that there is also a wide range of regulatory factors involved in its control.

Natural killer (NK) cells are one population of non-specific effector cells which may also have immunoregulatory properties and it is the purpose of this chapter to outline the characteristics and possible roles of NK cells in the intestine.

Definition of NK cells

Natural killer cells may be defined as a population of lymphocytes which will rapidly lyse certain susceptible target cells in a non-antigen-specific manner and without the need for prior immunization. They are therefore well suited to the purpose of effective immune surveillance in an organ with a large, constantly changing antigen load, such as the gut.

Characteristics of NK cells

NK cells belong to the subset of large granular lymphocytes (LGL) which are characterized by the presence of azurophilic cytoplasmic granules. They comprise approximately 15% of human peripheral blood lymphocytes (PBL) and can be identified by the specific markers Leu 7 (HNK-1) and Leu 11 in humans [1, 40] or asialo GM_1 and NK1 in mice [4, 38]. In addition, NK cells have receptors for the Fc portion of IgG (Fcγr) [32] and in most species may carry T cell markers, including those of the suppressor/cytotoxic subset [1, 8, 10,

Table 8.1 Phenotypic characteristics of human NK cells in comparison with T cells and macrophages/monocytes.

Marker	NK	T	Macrophage/monocyte
sIg	−	−	−
FcγR	+	−(+)	+
T3	+/−	+ + +	−
T4	−	+ +/−	−
T8	+/−	+/−	−
Mac 1	+	−	+ +
Leu 7/Leu 11	+ + +	−	−
HLA–ABC	+	+	+
HLA–DR	−	−(+)	+/−
Phagocytosis	−	−	+ +
PBL (%)	10–15	70–80	10–20
Granules	+ + +	−	+ +
Esterase	−	+/−	+ + +

Symbols (+ or −) denote the presence or absence of the marker. +/− denotes markers present only on certain subpopulations and −(+) represents results which are doubtful.

59, 61]. For these reasons, NK cells are frequently assigned to the Tγ subset of lymphocytes, but the exact relationship to the T cell lineage is unclear. It is possible that NK cells represent an unusual or parallel line of T cell differentiation [23]. NK cells are most numerous in blood and spleen, less so in lymph nodes, and NK activity in bone marrow and thymus is low or undetectable. Within organized lymphoid tissues, NK cells are found predominantly within germinal centres, raising the possibility that they are involved in immunoregulation [33, 61]. These and other characteristics are summarized in Table 8.1.

Functions of NK cells

Cell lysis

NK cells will bind to and kill a wide range of susceptible tumour cell targets in vitro and, unlike conventional cytotoxic T lymphocytes (CTL), are not antigen-specific. In addition, products of the major histocompatibility complex (MHC) are not involved in target cell recognition. NK cells will also lyse virally infected cells [63], certain normal cell types such as bone marrow cells and thymocytes [53, 60] and even some parasites [49] (Table 8.2). The target structures are unknown, but may be a group of closely related differentiation markers expressed on immature or activated cells [35]. Target cell lysis occurs rapidly (<four hours) after binding to a susceptible target and may involve secretion of a granule-associated lymphotoxin with a serine protease activity [11, 57]. NK cell activity is markedly enhanced by interferons (IFN) and T cell growth factor (IL-2) [15, 20, 28] and shows a marked age pendency in many species, with maximal

Table 8.2 Functional characteristics of NK cells.

In vitro
Rapid lysis (<four hours) of selected tumour cells,
   virally infected cells, bone marrow cells, thymocytes
No antigenic specificity or MHC restriction
Enhanced by IFN, IL-2
Inhibited by macrophages, neutrophils, T lymphocytes
Suppress colony formation by bone marrow cells and Ig
   synthesis

In vivo
Can prevent tumour induction and metastasis
Mediate resistance to viral infections (especially herpes
   viruses) and parasites
Reject allogeneic haemopoietic cells
Augmented by IL-2, IFN, GvHR, allograft responses
Under genetic control (MHC and non-MHC)

levels appearing in early adult life and declining thereafter.

Human NK cell activity, however, is more stable and is present from birth onwards [56, 74]. There is also a strong genetic basis for NK cell levels, and this may be determined by the MHC [37]. Genetic defects in lysosome function as seen in beige mice and humans with Chédiak–Higashi syndrome are associated with low or absent NK activity.

Anti-tumour activity

The ability of NK cells to kill tumour cells in vitro has led to the concept that NK cells are the principal non-specific immune surveillance mechanism in the defence against tumours. This is supported by the accelerated growth and metastasis of tumours in NK-cell-depleted animals and by the ability of NK-cell-enriched populations to mediate tumour resistance in vivo [35]. In addition, NK cells have been implicated in resistance to several virus infections and certain parasitic infestations, including babesiosis and cryptococcosis [30].

Immune effector cells

A further role for NK cells as immune effector cells is in T cell-mediated immune responses, where NK cell activation has been described during allograft rejection [67], graft-versus-host reactions (GvHR) [7, 39, 62], in skin delayed type hypersensitivity reactions [71] and in the response to allogeneic cells [13]. Thus NK cells may play an important role as non-specific effector cells in cell-mediated immune (CMI) responses. While it is probable that cytotoxicity is the principal feature of NK cell activation in CMI, it should be noted that NK cells have also been shown to secrete soluble immune mediators, thus increasing the possible effects of NK cells in immune reactions [29].

Immunoregulation

A final property ascribed to NK cells is that of immunoregulation [29]. As noted above, bone marrow cells and thymocytes are susceptible to NK cell activity in vitro as is the colony-forming potential of bone marrow stem cells [25]. Furthermore, NK cells are probably responsible for the natural resistance which irradiated animals show to allogeneic haemotopoietic cells [36]. There are also several reports which indicate that lymphocytes with an NK phenotype can suppress antibody production [50, 72], supporting their presence within germinal centres in vivo (see above). These findings suggest that NK cells may represent a population of 'natural' regulatory cells which are important in maintaining homeostasis of lymphoid cell production and function.

Thus, NK cells are a rapidly acting population of cells which do not require immunological priming and which may combine effector and regulatory functions in the immune response. In theory, these properties make NK cells ideally suited as important components of the immune apparatus in tissues encountering large amounts of antigen and the next sections will consider the evidence that NK cells are involved in local intestinal immunity.

INTESTINAL NATURAL KILLER ACTIVITY

Introduction

The antigenic load which the intestine encounters makes it likely that the mucosa should contain a wide range of effector lymphocytes, including NK cells. For many years the study of intestinal NK cells was limited by difficulties in obtaining pure populations of mucosal lymphoid cells and by early assumptions that NK cells were relevant only to tumour immunology. In recent years, several workers have turned their interests to the role of non-specific effector cells in intestinal immunity and this section will deal with those studies addressing intestinal NK cells.

Mucosal NK cells

It has long been known that the intraepithelial lymphocytes (IEL) of the small intestine contain a large proportion of medium-large lymphocytes with azurophilic cytoplasmic granules [14, 24] (Fig. 8.1). This similarity to the large granular lymphocytes (LGL) responsible for NK activity in other tissues was the observation which first focused attention on mucosal NK cells and on IEL in particular.

Animal studies

In an early study of guinea pig small intestine, Arnaud-Battandier et al [2] showed that IEL had equivalent spontaneous cytotoxicity to spleen cells, when assayed over 18 hours in

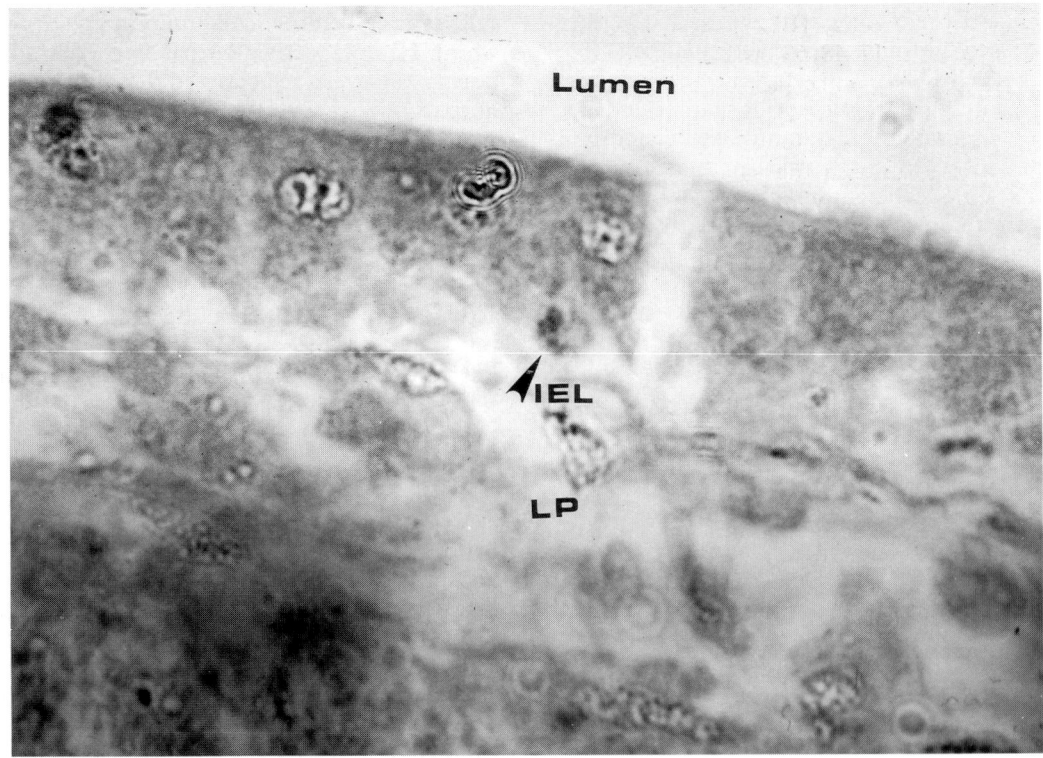

Fig. 8.1 Granulated intraepithelial lymphocyte in mouse small intestine (arrow). Astra blue × 1000.

vitro, but this was not confirmed as true NK activity. These experiments employed preparations of IEL which had not been purified, and subsequently it was shown in humans that colonic mucosal cells [45] and colonic IEL [12] had little or no NK activity against defined NK cell targets. More recently, studies of highly purified IEL from rat and mouse intestine have indicated the presence of significant NK activity, although there is some disagreement over the exact characteristics of the NK cells responsible (Table 8.3). As with

Table 8.3 Summary of the comparison between peripheral and intraepithelial NK cells in mice.

	Peripheral	Intraepithelial
LGL	+ + +	(+ + +)
Thy 1	+/−	(+/−)
Lyt 2	−/(+)	−
NK1/asialo GM$_1$	+ + +	+
4 hour lysis	+ + +	+
18 hour lysis	+ + +	+ + +
Induced by IFN	+ + +	+
Activity in beige mice	↓↓	↓↓
Activity in athymic mice	↑	↑
Activity in aged mice	↓	↓↓
Target selectivity	+	+

+ or − indicate the presence or absence of a given characteristic. (+) denotes the result requires confirmation.

peripheral NK cells, IEL lyse only defined NK cell targets [7, 48, 69] while their activity is absent in beige mice [48, 68] but enhanced in athymic mice [48, 54]. In addition, large numbers of LGL are found in the intestine of athymic rats, with the small intestine and stomach having many more than the colon. Interestingly, the intestine is the major non-lymphoid source of LGL in these animals [75].

The studies of Tagliabue et al also indicate that mouse IEL have NK activity in conventional four-hour assays which is equal to the high levels of activity found in spleen. IE NK activity was further similar to its peripheral counterpart in its enhancement by interferon, in its age-related decline and in its enrichment in low-density fractions of Percoll gradients where LGL are found [7, 68, 69]. However, Tagliabue et al also showed that the IE NK cells carried more Thy 1 than spleen NK cells, but fewer NK cell-specific markers such as asialo GM$_1$ and NK1. Significantly, the NK cells appeared to belong to the small proportion of IEL which are Lyt 2$^-$ [55, 68].

Comparison with humans

In contrast to these findings, others have shown that few IEL in humans have the Leu 7$^+$ phenotype [22, 64]; also it has been reported that rat and mouse IEL have deficient NK activity and require prolonged contact (18–20 hours) with the target cells to produce full lysis [17, 48]. In these latter studies, IE NK cells were Thy 1$^-$ [48] and responded poorly to interferon [17]. Similarly conflicting results have been obtained in studies of purified colonic IEL, where in humans few Leu 7$^+$ cells and little short-term NK activity were found [12, 19]. In contrast, rat colonic IEL had high NK levels (as measured in longer assays) with identical target cell specificity to peripheral NK cells [51].

The reasons for these discrepancies are not clear, but several groups have suggested that the isolation procedures used to obtain IEL may inhibit cytotoxicity [6, 12]. In the studies described above these factors were controlled for, but it is possible that different isolation techniques induce different inhibitory variables. In addition, it has been suggested that the lytic activity and characteristics of IE NK cells may depend on the level of endogenous interferon [17] and this may of course vary from laboratory to laboratory.

Together these studies suggest that a significant proportion of IEL have the potential for considerable NK activity, but it remains an open question whether this is normally expressed by IEL in situ. In vitro studies have suggested that IEL have a defective lytic mechanism [17, 48] (MacKenzie and Mowat, unpublished) and their NK activity is less than would be anticipated from the numbers of IEL with an NK cell phenotype [19]. Most workers agree that artefacts of isolation do not account for these findings and it may be that the full expression of natural cytotoxicity requires activation of IEL by a local immune response (see below).

Lamina propria lymphocytes and NK activity

The position with the NK activity of lamina propria lymphocytes (LPL) is less complex. In all species in which isolated LPL have been examined, little or no NK cell activity has been detected, irrespective of the systems used to detect this [2, 12, 19, 51, 54, 68, 70]. Of particular note is the consistent finding that, when compared directly, LPL have always been shown to have considerably lower NK activity than the equivalent population of IEL. This correlates with a lower proportion of LGL in the lamina propria [54, 68] but whether it reflects differential localization of NK cells within the mucosa or differentiation of cells after entering the epithelium is unclear.

NK cell activity in the gut-associated lymphoid tissues

It is paradoxical that NK cells in the organized tissues of the GALT have received less attention than those distributed throughout the mucosa despite the relative ease of obtaining GALT cells. In those studies which have been reported, however, there is a general agreement that both Peyer's patches and mesenteric lymph nodes (MLN) have little or no NK activity [2, 7, 17, 48, 69] although LGL of NK phenotype have been found in the T cell areas of the GALT in nude rats [75]. Furthermore, MLN have few Leu 7$^+$ cells in humans, indicating that the absence of cytotoxic activity reflects a lack of NK cells rather than a deficient lytic ability, as may be the case with mucosal NK cells [18]. As NK precursor cells are also Leu 7$^+$ [1], this observation indicates that mucosal NK cells do not originate from the GALT in the same way as other intestinal lymphocytes, and are presumably derived directly from the bone marrow.

The reasons for this compartmentalization of NK cells within the intestine and GALT are unclear, but it should be noted that NK cells are also rarely found in peripheral lymph nodes [58]. Thus, it is likely that NK effector cells are distributed to tissues such as the mucosa, where contact with antigen is most likely and where their rapid functional activity is most required.

Regulation of intestinal NK cell activity

Systemic NK cells are subject to positive and negative regulation by several components of the lymphoid system. Thus, T cell products such as interleukin 2 (IL-2) and γ-interferon (γ-IFN) enhance NK cell activity as does endotoxin [65], while suppression by T cells, macrophages, prostaglandins and granulocytes has been described [56]. If intestinal NK cells are important in mucosal immunity it would be anticipated that their activity will also be regulated by local cells and mediators.

Augmented NK activity

Augmented NK activity has been described in the IEL of mice rejecting allogeneic tumour cells (Fig. 8.2) [47] and also during GvHR [7]. In the latter case, the enhanced NK activity paralleled the increased number of IEL which characterizes the intestinal phase of GvHR and was preceded by a delayed type hypersensitivity reaction in the host animal [7, 48a]. Tagliabue et al [68] have also cited an increased NK activity by IEL from mice with giardiasis or with a helminth infection, but these findings remain to be confirmed. Thus it seems likely that intestinal NK cells can be recruited and activated during local immune reactions and that T lymphocytes may be the critical factors involved in this phenomenon.

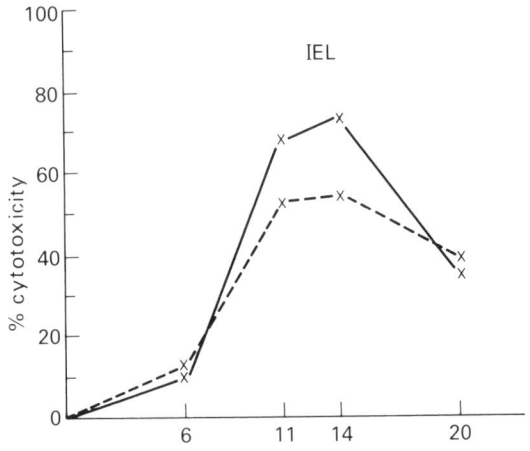

Fig. 8.2 Activation of IE NK cells in CBA mice injected intraperitoneally with allogeneic tumour cells (P815). The NK activity of IEL against YAC-1 target cells rises in exact parallel with the specific cytotoxic T cell activity against P815 target cells. Cytotoxic activity assayed at 50:1 effector target cell ratio for four hours.

Suppression of NK activity

Suppression of mucosal NK cells by other lymphoid cells has not been described, but it has been shown that IEL themselves can regulate the NK activity of spleen cells (Fig. 8.3) [48]. Despite their apparent suppressor T cell phenotype, IEL do not suppress specific immune responses in vivo or in vitro [44] and the suppression of NK cell activity has not been characterized. However, these results raise the intriguing possibility that the mucosal lymphoid system may regulate its own natural cytotoxicity.

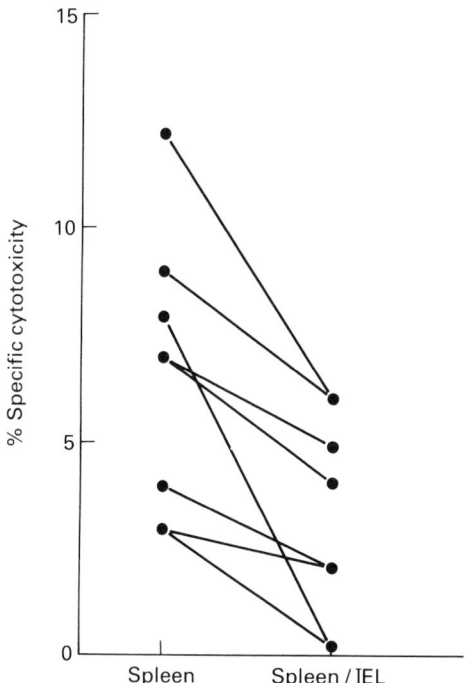

Fig. 8.3 Suppression of spleen NK activity by syngeneic IEL. Spleen cells were assayed against YAC-1 target cells, either alone, or mixed with an equal number of IEL, for four hours at 25:1 effector target ratio.

Table 8.4 Relationship of NK cells to intestinal disease/pathology.

Disease	Behaviour of NK cells
Colonic tumour	Intestinal NK activity normal
Ulcerative colitis	PBL NK activity normal
Crohn's disease	PBL NK activity normal, but NK cells have suppressor activity. Mesenteric plasma highly inhibitory to NK cells
Coeliac disease	Normal numbers of IE NK cells
GvHR (mice)	Enhanced NK activity by IEL, MLN

selves. However, animal studies do indicate that NK cells are important in preventing the progress of neoplasia [31] and thus it might be anticipated that NK cells are involved in local responses to intestinal tumours. Indeed, colonic cancer cells may be sensitive to NK cells [27] and it has been suggested that the low incidence of small intestinal neoplasia is related to the higher number of LGL found in the upper gut than in the colon [75].

Unfortunately, studies of intestinal NK cells in tumour-bearing intestine do not shed light on this hypothesis—only low NK cell activity has been found, which is identical to that in normal intestine [5]. Assays of systemic NK cells are similarly unhelpful and prospective studies of NK cell activity in patients at risk of malignant disease are required to resolve the issue.

Inflammatory bowel disease

The non-specific cytotoxic activity of NK cells makes them ideal candidates for effector cells in the pathogenesis of inflammatory bowel disease, but there are several reports of low NK activity in the blood of patients with both Crohn's disease [3, 21, 34] and ulcerative colitis [21]. Clearly these findings could reflect secondary effects of the diseases, and indeed, it has been shown that mesenteric vein plasma from patients with inflamed intestine is usually inhibitory to NK cells [18]. Nevertheless, the possibility that the low NK levels in blood could be due to sequestration of effector cells in the mucosa has not been excluded. A recent interesting finding is that patients with Crohn's disease have very high levels of circulating suppressor cells with an NK cell phenotype despite normal levels of NK activity [34]. If confirmed, this would suggest a possible regulatory role for NK cells which have differentiated unusually in Crohn's disease.

A further mechanism of suppression which has been demonstrated is an inhibitory effect of mesenteric vein plasma on NK cell activity in vitro, and this was markedly increased in patients with inflammatory bowel disease [18]. The authors suggest that inhibitory mediators are released from the intestinal mucosa and that these account for the low levels of unstimulated NK activity in intestinal sites. These mediators have not been characterized and it remains to be proved that they have any role in regulating NK cells in situ and whether this is altered in disease states.

NK cells and intestinal disease

Neoplastic disease

The association of NK cells with immuno-surveillance against neoplastic disease has led to a large number of clinical studies of NK cell activity in tumour-bearing individuals. In many cases, clear-cut results have not been obtained, because it is difficult to determine whether abnormalities in NK activity precede the development of the tumour or are merely secondary to the disease (Table 8.4). Furthermore, assays of peripheral NK activity may not reflect events in the affected tissues them-

Food-sensitive enteropathies

There are no studies of PBL NK cells in food-sensitive enteropathies, but normal numbers of IE NK cells are found in coeliac mucosa, despite the large increase in IEL count [19, 64]. As discussed in later chapters, many patients with atopic eczema also have evidence of food hypersensitivity and recently it was shown that such patients have low PBL NK cell activity [41]. As yet, the phenomenon has not been correlated directly with the presence of food allergy or with suppressor cell function, but it is tempting to speculate that the low NK cell activity is associated with the deficient level of suppression which is found in atopic eczema [9].

Infections

Finally, in this section, it should be noted that there are no studies of NK cell activity in intestinal infections, despite the evidence from animal experiments that NK cells may be involved in local defence.

Functional relevance of intestinal NK cells

The evidence discussed in the preceding sections indicates that significant numbers of NK cells may be present only within the epithelial compartment of the intestine. This observation is compatible with local NK cells having a role in the surface defence of the mucosa itself as the epithelium is the layer which is in direct contact with antigen (Fig. 8.4).

This concept is supported by studies which have implicated NK cells in the defence against systemic infections due to herpes virus [42], trypanosomiasis [26], babesiosis and cryptococcosis [30]. Furthermore, local NK cells are the major defence mechanism against pulmonary infection by cytomegalovirus in mice [66] and, as noted above, may be activated by intestinal parasitic infestations. NK cells are also found in increased numbers in the intestine of nude rats with enteritis [75].

Antibacterial activity

Recently, it has been shown that mouse IEL may have a direct natural antibacterial activity which is effective against *Salmonella typhimurium* in vitro [52]. Although there are certain properties of these antibacterial effector cells which are unlike conventional NK cells and the findings require confirmation and extension, this work does raise the possibility that IEL may possess natural antibacterial properties. As this suggests that they are the first line of protection against pathogenic organ-

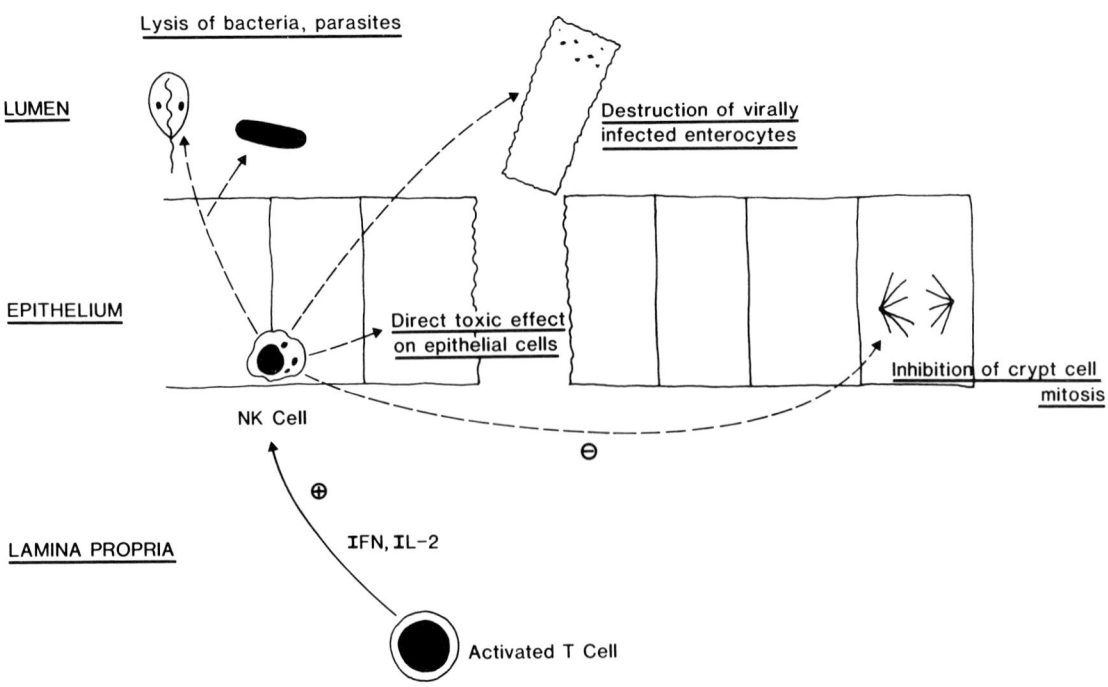

Fig. 8.4 Possible roles for mucosal NK cells.

isms, it will be important in future to assess the sensitivity of different intestinal pathogens to the lytic activity of peripheral and mucosal NK cells.

Epithelial cell damage

An additional potential effector role for intestinal NK cells is that of causing epithelial cell damage in intestinal disease. There has been considerable research into the possibility that specific autoimmunity may be involved in inflammatory bowel disease but non-specific mechanisms have received less attention. In a recent report, it has been shown that lymphoid cells isolated from human colonic mucosa showed spontaneous cytotoxicity against autologous colonic epithelial cells. The effector cells had the characteristics of NK cells and target cell lysis was enhanced by IFN [51]. This study supports the hypothesis that in intestinal disease NK cells may be recruited locally by a specific immune response and may contribute to the intestinal damage.

NK activity in cell-mediated immune reactions

As noted above, experimental CMI in the intestine activates local NK cells and it would be of interest to investigate whether these NK cells are also activated to lyse intestinal epithelial cells. Furthermore, intestinal CMI may be the mechanism underlying entropathies due to food hypersensitivity [16], and thus it would also be important to demonstrate similar enhanced NK activity in the intestine of animals with experimentally induced CMI to a dietary protein [46]. Such experiments might help elucidate the pathogenesis of inflammatory bowel disease and enteropathy due to food hypersensitivity.

Immunoregulatory role

In addition to their effector cell function, NK cells may have an immunoregulatory role in vivo [29], and it has been shown that patients with Crohn's disease have increased numbers of suppressor cells of NK cell phenotype [34]. The possibility then arises that these recruited NK cells may play an important role in regulating disease activity in the intestinal wall. Alternatively, this accumulation of peripheral NK cells may be due to defective entry of cells into the intestine [18] and thus the mucosal pathology may reflect a local deficiency of NK cells.

If NK cells have a regulatory function in intestinal disease, this is likely to operate on the immune system itself. However, it is also believed that NK cells may be able to recognize target structures on all dividing cells and it is possible that NK cell inhibition of epithelial cell renewal may reflect a further level of local regulation. Detailed studies of local and peripheral NK cells and their target cell specificity in intestinal disease are required to define their role in the evolution of intestinal pathology.

Conclusions

NK cells represent a population of rapidly acting effector lymphocytes which function in the absence of specific immunization and without clear antigenic specificity. They are effective against target cells infected by intracellular parasites and are thus particularly suited to mount a rapid defence of a mucosal surface. The evidence presented here indicates that the intestinal epithelium is rich in cells with a considerable potential for NK cell activity and that IE NK cells can be recruited by local T lymphocyte-mediated immune responses. These findings are especially interesting in view of the increased IEL count found in diseases associated with hypersensitivity to dietary antigens, including coeliac disease and cow's milk protein intolerance. The lamina propria and GALT, however, are deficient in NK cell activity, suggesting that local factors in the epithelium are responsible for activating these cells. Thus, the intestinal immune system has evolved in such a way that its non-specific cytotoxic effector lymphocytes are concentrated in the most superficial layer of the mucosa, where antigenic contact is most frequent and where rapid elimination of infected cells is most required.

There is some evidence that intestinal NK cells may be involved in local infections but no firm relationship between NK cell function and other intestinal diseases has been established. Nevertheless, the enhanced activity of intestinal NK cells in local CMI suggests this may be an important pathogenic mechanism in diseases associated with mucosal CMI, such as coeliac disease and graft-versus-host disease. In addition, NK cells can regulate cellular proliferation and lymphocyte function and this immunosuppressive activity is increased in Crohn's disease. Thus, abnormal NK cell activity may be one of the immune abnormalities which are important in the pathogenesis of inflammatory bowel disease.

NK cell activity can be measured rapidly and reproducibly, the cells identified and purified and IE NK cells can now be propagated in vitro [55]. Thus, there is considerable scope for examining mucosal NK cells in detail and their combined effector and regulatory roles makes their study a potentially fascinating area for the future.

REFERENCES

1 Abo T, Cooper MD, Balch CM: Characterisation of HNK-1$^+$ (Leu 7) human lymphocytes. I. Two distinct phenotypes of human NK cells with different cytotoxic capability. J Immunol 1982; 129:1752–7.

2 Arnaud-Battandier F, Bundy BM, O'Neill M et al: Cytotoxic activities of gut mucosal lymphoid cells in guinea pigs. J Immunol 1978; 121:1059.

3 Auer IO, Ziemer E, Sommer H: Immune status in Crohn's disease. V. Decreased in vitro natural killer activity in peripheral blood. Clin Exp Immunol 1980; 42:41–9.

4 Beck BN, Gillis S, Henney CS: Display of the neutral glycolipid ganglio-N-tetraosylceramide (asialo GM$_1$) on cells of the natural killer and T lineages. Transplantation 1982; 33:118–22.

5 Bland PW, Britton DC, Richens ER, Pledger JV: Peripheral, mucosal and tumour-infiltrating components of cellular immunity in cancer of the large bowel. Gut 1981; 22:744–51.

6 Bland PW, Richens ER, Britton DC, Lloyd JV: Isolation and purification of human large bowel mucosal lymphoid cells: effect of separation technique on functional characteristics. Gut 1979; 20:1037–46.

7 Borland A, Mowat AMcI, Parrott DMV: Augmentation of intestinal and peripheral natural killer activity during the graft-versus-host reaction in mice. Transplantation 1983; 36:513–9.

8 Brooks CG, Kuribayashi K, Sale GE, Henney CS: Characterisation of five cloned murine cell lines showing high cytolytic activity against YAC-1 cells. J Immunol 1982; 128:2326–35.

9 Butler M, Atherton D, Levinsky RJ: Quantitative and functional deficit of suppressor T cells in children with atopic eczema. Clin Exp Immunol 1982; 50:92.

10 Cantrell DA, Robins RA, Brooks CG, Baldwin RW: Phenotype of rat natural killer cells defined by monoclonal antibodies marking rat lymphocyte subsets. Immunology 1982; 45:97–103.

11 Carpen O, Virtanen I, Saksela E: Ultrastructure of human natural killer cells: nature of the cytolytic contacts in relation to cellular secretion. J Immunol 1982; 128:2691–7.

12 Chiba M, Bartnik W, Remine SG et al: Human colonic intraepithelial and lamina proprial lymphocytes: cytotoxicity in vitro and the potential effects of the isolation method on their functional properties. Gut 1981; 22:177–86.

13 Clark EA, Holly RD: Activation of natural killer (NK) cells in vivo with H-2 and non-H-2 alloantigens. Immunogenetics 1981; 12:221–35.

14 Collan Y: Characteristics of non-epithelial cells in the epithelium of normal rat ileum: a light and electron microscopical study. Scand J Gastroenterol [Suppl 18] 1972; 7.

15 Domzig W, Stadler BM, Herberman RB: Interleukin 2 dependence of human natural killer (NK) cell activity. J Immunol 1983; 130:1970–3.

16 Ferguson A, Mowat AMcI: Immunological mechanisms in the small intestine. In: Wright R, ed. Recent advances in gastrointestinal pathology. Philadelphia: WB Saunders 1980; 93–103.

17 Flexman JP, Shellam GR, Mayrhofer G: Natural cytotoxicity, responsiveness to interferon and morphology of intra-epithelial lymphocytes from the small intestine of the rat. Immunology 1983; 48:733–41.

18 Gibson PR, Verhaar HJJ, Selby WS, Jewell DP: The mononuclear cells of human mesenteric blood, intestinal mucosa and mesenteric lymph nodes: compartmentalisation of NK cells. Clin Exp Immunol 1984; 56:445–52.

19 Gibson PR, Dow EL, Selby WS et al: Natural killer cells and spontaneous cell-mediated cytotoxicity in the human intestine. Clin Exp Immunol 1984; 56:438–44.

20 Gidlund M, Orn A, Wigzell H et al: Enhanced NK cell activity in mice injected with interferon and interferon inducers. Nature 1978; 273:759–61.

21 Ginsburg CH, Dambrauskas JT, Ault KA, Falchuk ZM: Impaired natural killer cell activity in patients with inflammatory bowel disease: evidence for a qualitative defect. Gastroenterology 1983; 85:846–51.

22 Greenwood JH, Austin LL, Dobbins WO: In vitro characterisation of human intestinal intraepithelial lymphocytes. Gastroenterology 1983; 85:1023–35.

23 Grossman Z, Herberman RB: Hypothesis on the development of natural killer cells and their relationship to T cells. In: Heberman RB, ed. NK cells and natural effector cells. New York: Academic Press, 1982; 229–38.

24 Guy-Grand D, Griscelli C, Vassalli P: The mouse gut T-lymphocyte, a novel type of T-cell: nature, origin and traffic in mice in normal and graft-versus-host conditions. J Exp Med 1978; 148:1661–77.

25 Hansson M, Beran M, Andersson B, Kiessling R: Inhibition of in vitro granulopoiesis by autologous allogeneic human NK cells. J Immunol 1982; 129:126–32.

26 Hatcher FM, Kuhn RE: Destruction of *Trypanosoma cruzi* by natural killer cells. Science 1982; 218:295–6.

27 Helms RA, Bull DM: Natural killer activity of human lymphocytes against colon cancer cells. Gastroenterology 1980; 78:738–44.

28 Henney CS, Kuribayashi K, Kern DE, Gillis S: Interleukin-2 augments natural killer cell activity. Nature 1981; 291:335–8.

29 Herberman RB: Immunoregulation and natural killer cells. Mol Immunol 1982; 19:1313–21.

30 Herberman RB: Natural resistance mechanisms. Adv Exp Med Biol 1982; 155:799–808.

31 Herberman RB, Ortaldo JR: Natural killer cells: their role in defenses against disease. Science 1981; 214:24–31.

32 Herberman RB, Bartram S, Haskill JS et al: Fc receptors on mouse effector cells mediating natural cytotoxicity against tumour cells. J Immunol 1977; 19:322.

33 Itoh K, Suzuki R, Umezu Y et al: Studies of murine large granular lymphocytes. II. Tissue, strain and age distributions of LGL and LAL. J Immunol 1982; 129:395–400.

34 James SP, Neckers LM, Graeff AS et al: Suppression of immunoglobulin synthesis by lymphocyte subpopulations in patient with Crohn's disease. Gastroenterology 1984; 86:1510–8.

35 Kiessling R, Hansson M, Gromberg A: Natural killer cells as regulators of malignant and normal cell growth. Prog Immunol 1983; 5:1181–94.

36 Keissling R, Hochman PS, Haller O et al: Evidence for a similar or common mechanism for natural killer activity and resistance to haemopoietic grafts. Eur J Immunol 1977; 7:655–63.

37 Klein GO: NK-activity against YAC-1 is regulated by two H-2 associated genes. In: Herberman RB, ed. NK cells and other natural effector cells. New York: Academic Press, 1982; 275–80.

38 Koo GC, Peppard JR, Hatzfeld A, Cayre Y: Ontogeny of NK-1$^+$ natural killer cells. In: Herberman RB, ed. NK cells and other natural effector cells. New York: Academic Press, 1982; 325–8.

39 Kubota E, Ishikawa H, Saito K: Modulation of F$_1$ cytotoxic potentials by GvHR. Host and donor-derived cytotoxic lymphocytes arise in the unirradiated F$_1$ host spleens under the condition of GvHR-associated immunosupression. J Immunol 1983; 131:1142–8.

40 Lanier LL, Loken MR: Human lymphocyte subpopulations identified by using three-colour immunofluorescence and flow cytometry analysis. Correlation of Leu-2, Leu-3, Leu-7, Leu-8 and Leu-11 cell surface antigen expression. J Immunol 1984; 132:151–6.

41 Lever RS, Lesko MJ, MacKie RM, Parrott DMV: Natural killer cell activity in atopic dermatitis. Clin Allergy 1984; 14:483–90.

42 Lopez C: Resistance to herpes simplex virus-Type 1 (HSV-1). Curr Top Microbiol Immunol 1981; 92:15–24.

43 Luini W, Boraschi D, Alberti S et al: Morphological characterisation of a cell population responsible for natural killer activity. Immunology 1981; 43:663–8.

44 Lyscom N, Brueton MJ: Study of the transfer of tolerance by mucosal intraepithelial and Peyer's patch lymphocytes. Gut 1983; 24:A473.

45 MacDermott RP, Franklin GO, Jenkins KM et al: Human intestinal mononuclear cells. I. Investigation of antibody-dependent, lectin-induced and spontaneous cell-mediated cytotoxic capabilities. Gastroenterology 1980; 78:47.

46 Mowat AMcI, Ferguson A: Hypersensitivity in the small intestinal mucosa. V. Induction of cell mediated immunity to a dietary antigen. Clin Exp Immunol 1981; 43:574–82.

47 Mowat AMcI, Borland A, Tait RC, Parrott DMV: Natural killer cells and small intestinal immunity. In: Mechanisms of gastrointestinal immunity. Welwyn Garden City: Smith, Kline & French Laboratories, 1984; 5–9.

48 Mowat AMcI, Tait RC, MacKenzie S et al: Analysis of natural killer effector and suppressor activity by intraepithelial lymphocytes from mouse small intestine. Clin Exp Immunol 1983; 52:191–8.

48a Mowat AMcI, Borland A, Parrott DMV: Augmentation of natural killer cell activity by anti-host delayed-type hypersensitivity during the graft-versus-host reaction in mice. Scand J Immunol 1985; 22:389–99.

49 Murphy JW, McDaniel DO: In vitro reactivity of natural killer (NK) cells against *Cryptococcus neoformans*. J Immunol 1982; 128:1577–83.

50 Nabel G, Allard WJ, Cantor H: A cloned cell line mediating natural killer cell function inhibits immunoglobulin secretion. J Exp Med 1982; 156:658–63.

51 Nauss KM, Pavlina TM, Kumar V, Newberne PM: Functional characteristics of lymphocytes isolated from the rat large intestine. Gastroenterology 1984; 86:468–75.

52 Nencioni L, Villa L, Boraschi D et al: Natural and antibody-dependent cell-mediated activity against *Salmonella typhimurium* by peripheral and intestinal lymphoid cells in mice. J Immunol 1983; 130:903–7.

53 Nunn ME, Herberman RB, Holden HT: Natural cell-mediated cytotoxicity in mice against non-lymphoid tumour cells and some normal cells. Int J Cancer 1977; 20:381–7.

54 Parrott DMV, Tait C, Mackenzie S et al: Analysis of the effector functions of different populations of mucosal lymphocytes. Ann NY Acad Sci 1982; 409:307–20.

55 Petit A, Ernst P, Rosenthal K et al: Murine intestinal intraepithelial lymphocytes (IEL) and their relationship to T-cells, NK cells and mast cells. Fed Proc 1983; 42:1218.

56 Petranyi GyG, Benczur M, Laskai T et al: Natural killer cells in man: genetic and other factors regulating their activity. Prog Immunol 1983; 5:1169–80.

57 Quan P-C, Ishizaka T, Bloom BR: Studies on the mechanism of NK cell lysis. J Immunol 1982; 128:1786–91.

58 Reynolds CW, Timonen T, Herberman RB: Natural killer (NK) cell activity in the rat. I. Isolation and characterisation of the effector cells. J Immunol 1981; 127:282–8.

59 Reynolds CW, Sharrow SO, Ortaldo JR, Herberman RB: Natural killer activity in the rat. II. Analysis of surface antigens on LGL by flow cytometry. J Immunol 1981; 127:2204–8.

60 Riccardi C, Santoni A, Barlozzari T, Herberman RB: In vivo reactivity of mouse natural killer (NK) cells against normal bone marrow cells. Cell Immunol 1981; 60:136–43.

61 Ritchie AWS, James K, Micklem HS: The distribution and possible significance of cells identified in human lymphoid tissue by the monoclonal antibody HNK-1. Clin Exp Immunol 1983; 51:439–47.

62 Roy C, Ghayur T, Kongshavn PAL, Lapp WS: Natural killer activity by spleen, lymph node and thymus cells during the graft-versus-host reaction. Transplantation 1982; 34:144–6.

63 Santoli D, Trinchieri G, Leif FS: Cell-mediated cytotoxicity against virus-infected target cells in humans. I. Characterisation of effector lymphocytes. J Immunol 1978; 121:526–31.

64 Selby WS, Janossy G, Bofill M, Jewell DP: Lymphocyte subpopulations in the human small intestine. The findings in normal mucosa and in the mucosa of patients with adult coeliac disease. Clin Exp Immunol 1983; 52:219–28.

65 Shacter B, Kleinherz ME, Edmonds K, Ellner JJ: Spontaneous cytotoxicity of human peripheral blood mononuclear cells for the lymphoblastoid cell line CCRF-CEM: augmentation by bacterial lipopolysaccharide. Clin Exp Immunol 1981; 46:640–8.

66 Shellam GR, Allan JE, Papadimitrious JM, Bancroft GJ: Increased susceptibility to cytomegalovirus infection in beige mutant mice. Proc Natl Acad Sci USA 1981; 78:5104–8.

67 Soulillou JP, Vie H, Moreau JF et al: Increased NK cell activity in rats rejecting heart allografts. Transplantation 1983; 36:726–7.

68 Tagliabue A, Befus AD, Clark DA, Bienenstock J: Characteristics of natural killer cells in the murine intestinal epithelium and lamina propria. J Exp Med 1982; 155:1785–96.

69 Tagliabue A, Luini W, Soldateschi D, Boraschi D: Natural killer activity of gut mucosal lymphoid cells in mice. Eur J Immunol 1981; 11:919–22.

70 Targan S, Britvan L, Kendal R et al: Isolation of spontaneous and interferon inducible natural killer-like cells from human colonic mucosa: lysis of lymphoid and autologous epithelial target cells. Clin Exp Immunol 1983; 54:14–22.

71 Tartof D, Curran JD, Yung C, Livingston C: Mononuclear cells (MNC) mediating natural killer cell-like cell mediated cytolysis (NK-like CMC) are present in the delayed type hypersensitivity (DTH) response in man. Fed Proc 1983; 42:1219.

72 Tilden AB, Abo T, Balch CM: Suppressor cell function of human granular lymphocytes identified by the HNK-1 (Leu 7) monoclonal antibody. J Immunol 1983; 130:1171–5.

73 Timonen T, Ortaldo JR, Herberman RB: Characteristics of human large granular lymphocytes and relationship to natural killer and K-cells. J Exp Med 1981; 153:569–82.

74 Uksila J, Lassila O, Hirvonen T, Toivanen P: Development of natural killer cell function in the human foetus. J Immunol 1983; 130:153–6.

75 Ward JM, Argilan F, Reynolds CW: Immunoperoxidase localisation of large granular lymphocytes in normal tissues and lesions of athymic nude rats. J Immunol 1983; 131:132–9.

SECTION C
SPECIALIZED SECRETIONS OF THE GUT

Chapter 9
Mucosal Antibodies

S.S. Crago and T.B.Tomasi

Introduction

The mucosal surfaces of the body, including those associated with the gastrointestinal tract, respiratory tract, lacrimal glands, salivary glands and mammary glands, provide an extensive protective barrier to the entry of foreign substances. A variety of immune and non-immune factors have developed which prevent the colonization, invasion and subsequent pathologies associated with contact between a vast array of potential pathogens and the secretory mucosae. The most important of the immune factors, and the subject of this chapter, are the secretory antibodies found in external secretions bathing mucosal surfaces. These antibodies function to inhibit bacterial adherence, to neutralize viruses and toxins, to prevent the absorption of antigens (immune exclusion) and to regulate mucus secretion. In addition to these important biological functions, secretory antibodies elicited

167

by active immunization could provide protection against a variety of pathogens for which vaccines are not currently available. (For a detailed review of the secretory immune system, the reader is referred to refs. 8, 16, 111, 117, 144, 189, 195, 197.)

The predominant immunoglobulin found in external secretions such as saliva, tears and milk is IgA, locally produced by IgA-containing plasma cells distributed throughout glandular tissue [203]. Low levels of IgG [12, 73], IgM [14] and traces of IgD [179] and IgE [207] have also been detected in milk and other secretions. Secretory IgA (SIgA) differs from serum IgA in physical and immunochemical properties; IgA found in secretions exists mainly in the polymeric form (11S and 19S), while serum IgA is mainly monomeric [203] (see Table 9.1). In addition, IgA (and IgM) in

Table 9.1 Properties of secretory and serum IgA.

	Secretory	Serum
Form	Polymer	Monomer
Sedimentation	11S (90%)	7S (90%)
Size	390 000	165 000
Secretory component	+	−
J chain	+	−
IgA1	50–75%	80–90%
IgA2	25–50%	10–20%

secretions have been found to be associated with two additional polypeptides, secretory component (SC) [203] and J chain [69, 122]. Polymeric IgA and IgM containing J chain are selectively transported into external secretions by binding to SC which is expressed on the basolateral membrane of epithelial cells lining mucosal surfaces, and which serves as a receptor [16]. The mechanisms by which IgG,

IgD and IgE reach external secretions are not known.

Defects in the secretory immune system such as those seen in patients with a selective deficiency of IgA (if not compensated for by the presence of SIgM) can lead both to recurrent infections and to 'leaky' mucous membranes which will allow the absorption of a variety of ingested and inhaled antigens. These antigens may elicit the formation of immune complexes and/or the development of hypersensitivities and autoimmune syndromes. More subtle defects in the secretory immune system may also occur in a variety of diseases, including other immune deficiencies, autoimmune syndromes and inflammatory bowel disease. Studies on the role of the secretory system in these diseases is just beginning.

PHYSICOCHEMICAL PROPERTIES OF SECRETORY IMMUNOGLOBULINS

SIgA (and SIgM) is the product of two cell types: plasma cells underlying mucosal surfaces produce the heavy (H), light (L) and joining (J) chain components of the immunoglobulin molecule, while epithelial cells lining the mucosae produce the SC. SIgA usually occurs as an 11S molecule (MW 390 000) consisting of two IgA monomers covalently bonded to the J chain and complexed to one molecule of SC (Fig. 9.1).

Characteristics of J chain

J chain has a molecular weight of 15 600 and is covalently associated with polymeric IgA

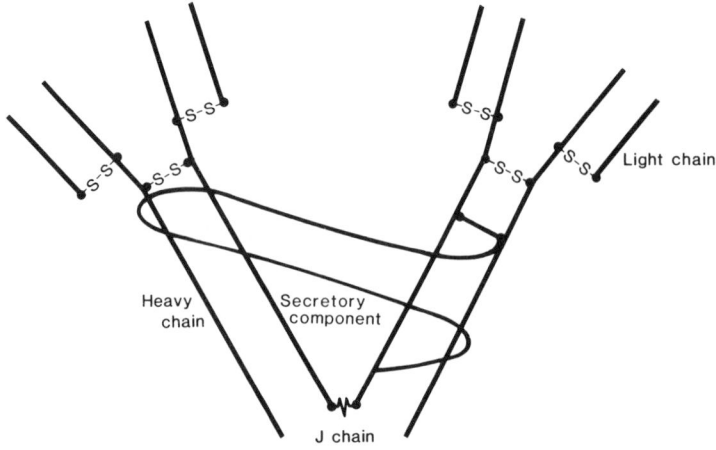

Fig. 9.1 Model of the secretory IgA molecule. Dimeric IgA is depicted, joined by the J chain molecule. SC covalently binds to one monomeric subunit and interacts with the second, perhaps affording protection to the hinge region. Heavy and light chains are shown covalently bound (-S-S-) although in some species and allotypes, these subunits are not connected by disulphide bonds.

and IgM [218, 220]. A single J chain is present per mole of polymeric immunoglobulin, regardless of the polymer size [102]. The carbohydrate portion of J chain consists of a single asparagine-linked oligosaccharide comprising about 7.5% of its molecular weight. The primary structure of the polypeptide portion of the J chain has been elucidated [130] and the complete structure of the carbohydrate moiety has recently been established [4]. In IgM and polymers of IgA, J chain binds, via a disulphide linkage, to the penultimate cysteine residue of the two heavy chains of the monomer. Apparently this association with J chain results in a dimeric conformation which tends to promote interaction with additional monomeric subunits, giving rise to higher order IgA polymers and to the pentameric IgM molecule [76, 102]. Little J chain is present in unstimulated B cells, but following exposure to mitogen or antigen, there is a marked increase (100–200 fold) in intracellular J chain [103]. The presence of J chain has also been described (by immunoelectron microscopy and radioimmunoassay) in pre-B cells and in HLA-DR$^+$ null cell leukaemias [68, 116], suggesting that J chain expression precedes antigen-induced events. Thus, J chain expression may be one of the earliest markers for differentiation along the B cell pathway, since it is not detectable in malignant cells of the T or myeloid lineages.

Detection in cells

J chain has been detected in cells containing all classes of monomeric as well as polymeric immunoglobulins [19, 123], but is incorporated into immunoglobulin and secreted only by cells producing polymeric IgA or IgM. J chain has also been demonstrated within the cytoplasm of a number of human lymphoid neoplasms, including myeloma, Waldenström's macroglobulinaemia, heavy chain disease and non-Hodgkin's lymphoma [18, 85, 125, 225]. It has been suggested that the presence of J chain in these lymphoid disorders is a marker of immaturity and may be used to distinguish malignant from non-malignant proliferations [6, 85]. The production of J chain appears to decrease as the cell matures [15], and the protein may be rapidly degraded in mature plasma cells which produce monomeric immunoglobulins [131].

Role of J chain

Because of its association with polymeric immunoglobulins, it has been proposed that J chain plays a role in the polymerization process [32, 76]. However, studies have shown that polymeric immunoglobulins can be assembled both in vitro and in vivo without the incorporation of J chain [49, 50, 104, 199]. It appears that binding of J chain during immunoglobulin assembly confers a conformation on the protein which enhances subsequent polymer formation. In addition to J chain, there is recent evidence that an enzyme present in stimulated but not unstimulated B lymphocytes catalyses polymer assembly [174]. Analysis of the polymerization reactions suggests that the enzyme is a sulphydryl oxidase, directly catalysing the oxidation of disulphide bonds, rather than an interchange enzyme as previously postulated.

It has also been suggested that J chain is necessary in order for polymeric molecules to bind SC. It should be emphasized that although polymers lacking J chain are capable of binding SC, they do so in smaller amounts and with less affinity than those containing J chain [199]. Thus the conformation induced by J chain may be optimal for the subsequent binding of SC.

Genetic analysis

Genetic analysis [223] indicates that there is a single J chain gene located on chromosome 5 in the mouse haploid genome, which is unlinked to any of the immunoglobulin genes. The same gene product must therefore be used for polymerization in both IgM and IgA. The localization of the genes for J chain, H and L chains on different chromosomes suggests that activation of polymeric immunoglobulin production in B cells is mediated by mechanisms which can either generate three separate signals or one signal that subsequently affects loci on the other chromosomes. The presence of J chain in cells containing immunoglobulins other than IgM and IgA suggests that once the J chain gene is activated, it continues to be expressed during the subsequent H chain class switches.

Secretory component

Secretory component is a glycoprotein with a molecular weight of approximately 80 000, which is synthesized by epithelial cells of mucous membranes [203]. SC isolated from human milk contains 23.4% carbohydrate [167], and the precise structure of the carbohydrate moieties has recently been reported [129, 159]. In addition to the bound form (in IgA and IgM), SC also occurs in a free or unbound form in secretions from the digestive, respiratory and other exocrine glands [200]. A glycoprotein analogous to human SC has been detected in secretions from several mammalian and avian species [156, 210]. SC has been localized by immunohistochemistry and immunoelectron microscopy to the basolateral membrane of epithelial cells lining exocrine glands [16, 23, 35, 138], to ductal epithelial cells in salivary, bile, pancreatic and lacrimal ducts and on hepatocyte membranes of certain species, where it allows for the transport of IgA and immune complexes involving IgA through the liver cells into the biliary system.

In human IgA and IgM, the majority of SC is complexed by disulphide bonds (not directly involving J chain) to a single monomer subunit [206], but in the rabbit a significant portion of the SC is non-covalently bound [28]. Free SC has been shown to complex in vitro with polymeric IgA and IgM, and this does not require the formation of a covalent bond [13, 197, 217]. The reaction is not species-restricted: human SC complexes with IgA from a variety of species including the chicken. The affinity constant for the binding of free SC to the intact IgA dimer in solution is approximately 10^8 M^{-1} [105] but the apparent affinity constant for SC binding to mammary gland and liver membranes is significantly higher ($K_A = 10^9$ M^{-1}).

Binding sites

The binding of ^{125}I-labelled IgA dimer to SC-bearing membranes is saturable, reversible, and is a time- and temperature-dependent process. The number of measureable IgA dimer binding sites per epithelial cell varies (260 to 7000 sites per mammary cell), and is directly related to the number of unoccupied SC receptor molecules in the membrane [106].

IgE as a secretory antibody

The initial observations that the majority of IgE-producing cells in the body are associated with the respiratory and gastrointestinal mucosa [192] prompted the theory that IgE might be a locally produced secretory antibody. Subsequently, it was shown that IgE/IgG ratios were higher in sputum [82, 141], nasal washings [46, 77] and urine [5] than in serum, again indicating a local production. In addition, following chronic lung infections the number of IgA- and IgE-containing cells rises disproportionately to other immunoglobulin classes in the bronchial lamina propria [25]. However, significant differences are found between secretory IgA and IgE. SIgA exists in a molecular form (polymer plus SC) different from that observed in its serum counterpart (monomer with no SC), while IgE from secretions lacks SC and has a sedimentation coefficient similar to that seen in serum [141]. The ratio of IgE to total protein is greater in serum than in secretions, although the ratio of IgE to non-secretory proteins such as albumin indicates local production rather than a passive diffusion [140]. In contrast to IgA produced at mucosal surfaces (which is primarily transported into secretions), the major part of locally produced IgE goes into the serum [140]. In concordance with this finding, after either intraperitoneal or intratracheal priming, neither the kinetics nor distribution of the IgE responses in various lymphoid tissues followed those seen with mucosal IgA responses [58]. Finally, while IgE has been detected in sputum and nasal washings, it appears to be absent from other secretions such as milk or parotid fluids [140, 207].

Features of IgE antibody responses

The IgE antibody response also has some characteristic regulatory features; IgE is regulated by antigen-specific helper and suppressor cells, and also by isotype-specific IgE binding factors (for review see ref. 84). These binding factors act on surface IgE$^+$ (sIgE$^+$) B cells and by themselves do not induce differentiation, but rather enhance the effects of antigen and T cells. These factors are released by T cells with receptors for the Fc portion of IgE (FcϵR$^+$), and can serve to potentiate or suppress the IgE response. Potentiating and suppressive factors are derived from the same T cell subset and have similar molecular weights, but differ in their carbohydrate composition. Failure to glycosylate the core protein results in IgE suppressive factor; the ability of T cells to glycosylate the parent structure is controlled by accessory cells and glycosylation-enhancing factors released by other T cells.

ORIGIN OF SECRETORY ANTIBODIES

Because of the preponderance of IgA-containing cells associated with secretory tissues (for review see [111, 195]), it is assumed that the majority of IgA found in a particular secretion is produced locally. Investigations have indicated that under normal conditions, little serum IgA is transported into secretions [24, 29, 188, 189, 203]. Recent studies [43] suggest that less than 2% of the total salivary polymeric IgA originated from plasma, which is consistent with older [203] as well as recent work [7] indicating that only a small portion of the salivary IgA of patients with myeloma of the IgA class is derived from the circulating monoclonal protein. Following the original description of the predominance of IgA plasma cells at mucosal sites, a variety of studies have quantitated the classes of the immunoglobulin-containing cells in various secretory as well as peripheral lymphoid tissues (for review see [111, 195]).

IgA antibodies of local origin

Recently, Kutteh et al [108] found that intestinal lamina propria cells secrete the largest amount of polymeric IgA (although these cells also produce monomeric IgA), while cultured spleen and bone marrow cells produce predominantly monomeric (7S) IgA. There is also a positive correlation between the amount of polymeric IgA produced and the presence of cytoplasmic J chain. The authors suggested that the bone marrow may be a major source of serum 7S IgA. In humans, there is not only a difference in molecular form between secretory and serum IgA, but also a difference in subclass distribution. Serum contains 10-20% IgA2, while in external secretions 25-50% of total IgA belongs to the IgA2 class [43, 64, 209]. Crago et al [36] showed that human spleen, tonsils, bone marrow and peripheral lymphoid tissues contain predominantly IgA1-staining cells (75-90%) while the small and large intestine, and salivary and lacrimal glands exhibit approximately equal numbers of IgA1 and IgA2 plasma cells. A larger number of cells staining for J chain were found in the mucosal tissues and a higher percentage of the IgA2 cells contained J chain than IgA1 positive cells. Thus it appears that the proportion of IgA1 and IgA2 molecules in serum and secretions is similar to the tissue

distribution of the cells containing the two subclasses. These studies on the cellular content of tissues strengthens the evidence for the local production of SIgA.

IgA antibodies of distant origin

It has been proposed that the IgA in a particular secretion may originate in distant mucosal tissues, enter the circulation and be selectively transported from the blood into exocrine secretions. Recent evidence has indicated that in several species, dimeric IgA is indeed rapidly transported from serum through the liver into bile and hence into intestinal fluids (for review see [149]). Halsey et al [70-72] also reported significant transport of IgA from serum into the mammary secretions of mice. Similarly, Sheldrake et al [180] found that the bulk of IgA in sheep milk was derived from serum during early and mid-lactation, while during mammary involution, IgA was locally produced; concomitant studies on sheep *intestinal* IgA production suggested that the vast majority was locally produced. Brandtzaeg [17] has carefully studied human mammary glands and concluded that the IgA in human milk is synthesized in cells intrinsic to the lactating gland; the density of IgA-producing cells and the daily output of IgA per kilogram of wet weight of tissue is similar for salivary and lactating mammary tissues.

Transport and synthesis

These apparently conflicting data can be rationalized on the following basis: transport of IgA from serum depends on (a) the concentration of dimeric IgA in serum, (b) the ability of dimeric IgA to permeate the capillaries of a particular tissue and (c) the availability of SC locally to mediate transport across the epithelial cells of a particular tissue. In ruminants such as the sheep, serum IgA is primarily dimeric (derived largely from the gut) while in humans 90% of the serum IgA is monomeric. Therefore, the interstitial regions of the sheep mammary glands would contain large amounts of potentially transportable dimeric IgA derived from serum. Thus an inverse correlation might be expected between the extent of local production and serum transport; i.e. in tissues such as the gastrointestinal tract where IgA-producing cells (and therefore dimeric IgA) are abundant, the SC is unavailable for transporting molecules derived from serum since it is 'pre-empted' or occupied by locally pro-

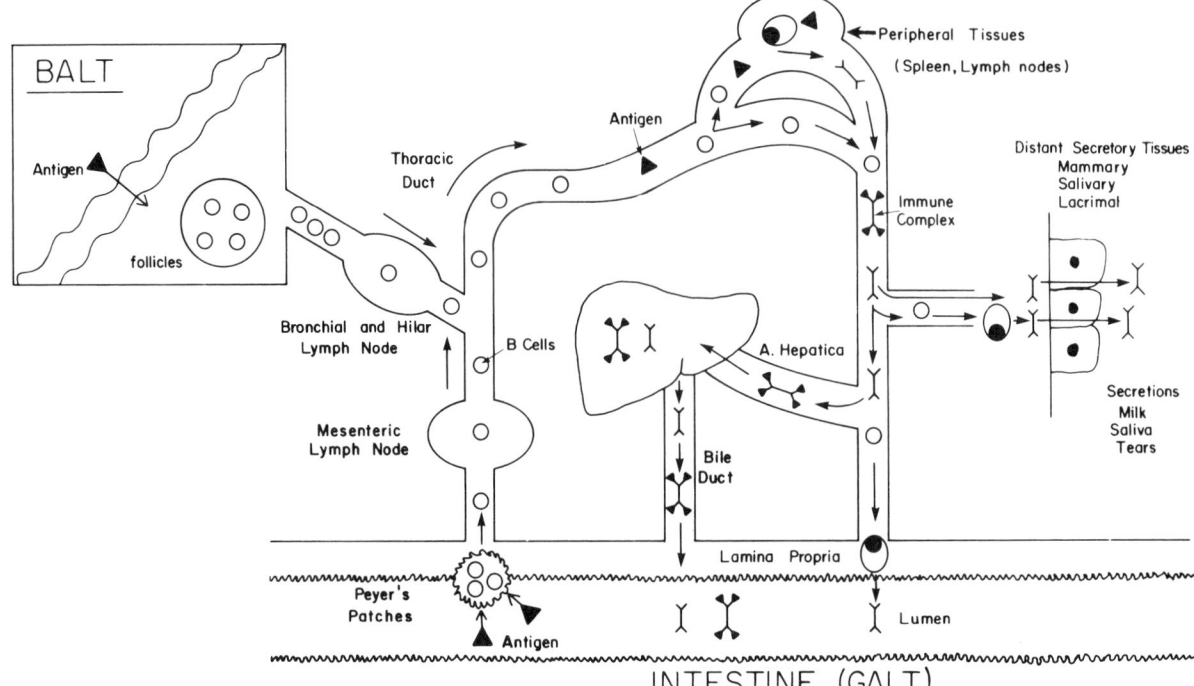

Fig. 9.2 Origin of secretory antibodies. Antigen impinging on mucosal surfaces is taken up through the GALT (or BALT) and sensitizes IgA precursor B cells which migrate out of the lymphoid follicles and enter the circulation through the thoracic duct. These cells begin maturation and may leave the circulation to selectively populate other mucosal tissues or may travel back to the lamina propria of the gut. After settling at mucosal surfaces, B cells complete differentiation into mature plasma cells and secrete antibodies specific for the immunizing agent which are selectively transported into external secretions. This pathway represents local synthesis. B cells may also encounter antigen in peripheral lymphoid tissues and mature into plasma cells which secrete antibodies into the circulation. Circulating dimeric IgA antibodies and immune complexes may then be selectively transported into gut secretions by the liver or into distant exocrine secretions by secretory mucosae.

duced IgA. Since the liver does not produce IgA, the hepatic cell plasma membrane receptor (SC on the sinusoidal surface) would be freely available to transport serum IgA without competition from any locally produced dimer. Few plasma cells are present in the mammary gland during early lactation [219], allowing transport of serum IgA. As lactation progresses, the number of IgA-containing cells in the mammary tissues increases and transport from serum ceases. However, in the rat very few cells are found even in the lactating breast and yet dimeric IgA is reportedly not transferred to milk [41]. Here one could evoke a particularly active 'competitive' biliary transport (known to occur in this species) which rapidly removes serum dimeric IgA, and/or the relative impermeability of the mammary capillaries of this species to dimeric IgA. Hormonal fluctuations appear to affect the levels of SC available to transport immunoglobulins into secretions [222]. Obviously, additional studies are needed to evalu-

ate how much of a given antibody is produced in cells indigenous to the tissues versus the amount derived from serum (see Fig. 9.2).

Cell traffic to secretory tissues

The origin of cells residing at mucous membranes will be reviewed in more detail in Chapter 3 and will be briefly touched on here in order to set the stage for a discussion of antibody production, secretion and function. It should be emphasized that the mucosal system, particularly the gut, contains more lymphoid tissue than the spleen and peripheral lymph nodes. Of the mucosal tissues the gut has been most extensively studied and the lamina propria has been shown to contain B cells, plasma cells, macrophages and T cells; the latter mediate help, alloreactivity and cytotoxicity. In intraepithelial locations, large granular lymphocytes predominate and have been shown to be involved in antibody-dependent, cell-mediated cytotoxicity (ADCC) and natural killer (NK) activity (for review see [10]). Key components of the lymphoid tissues of the gut are focal collections of lymphoid cells scattered throughout the small intestine (gut-associated lymphoid tissue, GALT) of which the Peyer's patches are the most prominent. Similar lymphoid follicles are present in the lungs (bronchial associated lymphoid tissues, BALT) and perhaps the eye and tonsils. Although lymphoid cells are first sensitized in Peyer's patches, production of antibody does not begin until the B cells leave the patches and migrate to other sites. Sensitized cells undergo a remarkable journey which involves migration to the mesenteric lymph nodes and then, via the thoracic duct, to the circulation. These cells subsequently seed not only the whole length of the gut lamina propria but other mucosal tissues as well [9, 38, 219]. Such migratory phenomena have important implications, since deposition of antigens in the gastrointestinal tract (and possibly the respiratory tract) can elicit specific antibodies at distant mucosal sites. A similar migratory pattern has been described for T cells, but localization in this case occurs predominantly in the intraepithelial regions of the mucosal membranes [67]. Work in several laboratories is currently attempting to devise a means of immunization via the gut and respiratory tract that takes advantage of these migratory patterns.

TRANSPORT OF SECRETORY IMMUNOGLOBULINS

Mucosal transport

The transport of polymeric IgA (and IgM) into secretions is a highly specific mechanism which results in the accumulation of secretory immunoglobulins in exocrine fluids against a concentration gradient. In order to reach those fluids, IgA must be transported through epithelial cells lining mucosal surfaces, as tight junctional complexes preclude movement of the large IgA molecule through intercellular spaces. This intracellular passage involves SC, a glycoprotein synthesized by mucosal epithelial cells and expressed on the basolateral surfaces. The association of IgA with SC not only results in the transport of IgA, but also serves to protect and stabilize the IgA molecule [87, 114, 198], allowing it to function in an enzyme-filled environment.

This dual role of SC both as a secretory protein and as a receptor prompted investigations into the biosynthesis and function of the molecule. It was postulated [105] that SC might serve as a 'linker', forming a complex with polymeric immunoglobulins and then attaching to a surface receptor on epithelial cells which would function as the effector in transcytosis. Subsequent studies, however, showed that in the rabbit SC was synthesized as a large transmembrane protein which was proteolytically cleaved to form the smaller, secreted form [135]. Analyses of SC isolated from deoxycholate-solubilized plasma membranes from rabbit liver and mammary glands reveal a heterogeneous population of larger molecules which show extensive structural homology to the smaller, secreted forms [107]. High molecular weight SC precursors have also been noted in rat hepatocyte golgi membranes [191].

Studies on the structure of SC have been extended by the analysis of a human adenocarcinoma cell line (HT-29) which synthesizes SC [82], has polarity [138] and is capable of binding dimeric IgA at the basal and lateral plasma membranes and translocating it across the cell to the luminal membrane. mRNA extracted from HT-29E.10 cells (a subclone of HT-29 which produces significantly more SC than the parent line) and translated in a cell-free system produced proteins which, when precipitated with anti-SC and analysed by sodium dodecyl sulphate polyacrylamide gel electrophoresis, gave a primary product with a molecular weight of 80 000 [132, 133]. Moreover, when microsomal vesicles from the dog pancreas were added to the translation reaction, the primary product had a molecular weight of 95 000 (converted to MW 100 000 by addition of peripheral sugars). The presence of trypsin post-translationally resulted in a reduction in size of the 95 000 molecule suggesting that the precursor molecule contained trypsin-sensitive domain as well as membrane-protected portions. The undigested precursor (MW 95 000–100 000), free SC (MW 80 000) as well as the intracellular cleavage product of the precursor form (MW 80 000) all have the same N-terminal amino acid sequence. This result suggests that the 80 000 MW form of SC (free SC and that complexed with IgA and IgM) is proteolytically cleaved from the N-terminal (ectoplasmic) domain of the transmembrane precursor molecule.

Model of secretory IgA transport

Fig. 9.3 represents a hypothetical model for
the transport pathway of IgA across the epithelial cell. SC is synthesized and undergoes
core glycosylation on polysomes as a transmembrane protein which is integrated into the
rough endoplasmic reticulum (RER) with its
ectoplasmic domain projecting into the lumen
of the RER. After transport to the golgi

(where terminal saccharide units are added)
SC is inserted into the basolateral region of
the epithelial cell membrane. The ectoplasmic
domain of the transmembrane protein projects
from the cell surface and acts as a receptor for
polymeric IgA and IgM. After complexing
with J chain-containing polymers, endocytosis
is initiated and immunoglobulins are transported across the cell within vesicles that
ultimately fuse with the apical plasma

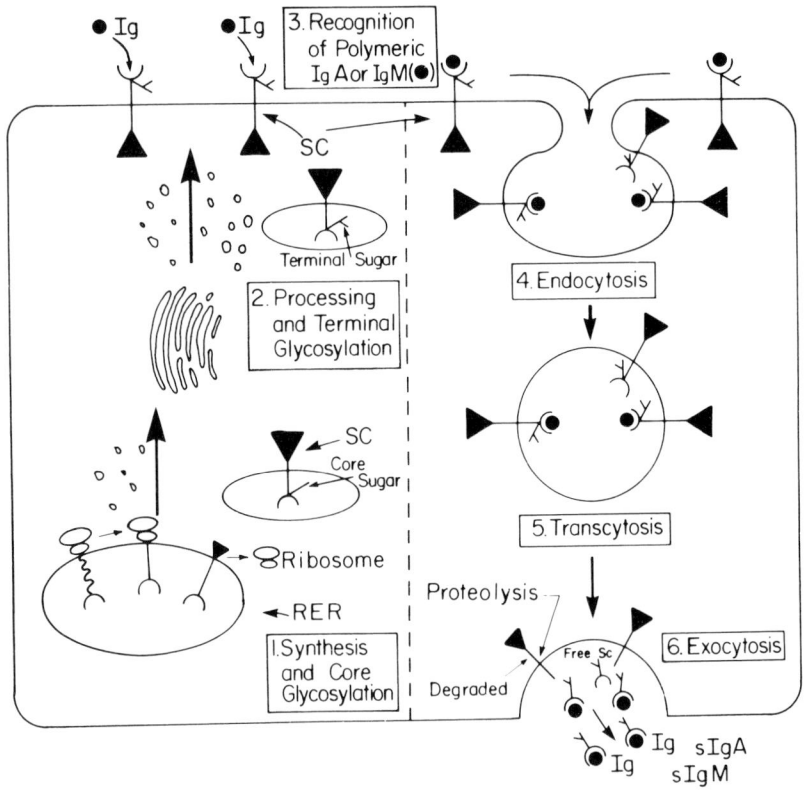

Fig. 9.3 Model for transport of IgA and IgM across the mucosal epithelial cell or hepatocyte. The synthesis of secretory
component (SC) (left side) and the steps in the transport of Ig across the cell (right side) are graphically represented. SC
is synthesized and core glycosylated on membrane-bound polysomes [rough endoplasmic reticulum (RER)] as an approximately 95 000 molecular weight transmembrane protein and is cotranslationally inserted into the RER. Further processing
may occur in the golgi (including the addition of terminal sugars). SC then becomes integrated into the basal (and lateral)
plasma membranes of the mucosal epithelial cell or the sinusoidal membrane of the hepatocyte. The transmembrane SC
(∪) consists of three domains: (a) cytoplasmic (⊥), (b) membrane-spanning (|) and (c) ectoplasmic (Y). The ectoplasmic
domain acts as the external receptor for J chain-containing polymeric Igs, such as IgA and IgM (● = Ig). Endocytosis
of the receptor is probably occurring continuously. Transcytosis of the complexes and of SC not associated with Ig
occurs in vesicles (endosomes) which probably do not fuse with lysosomes but do fuse with the plasma membrane thus
carrying the Ig–receptor complex to the luminal surface. Proteolysis occurs at an unknown stage leaving behind the
cytoplasmic and membrane-spanning portions (MW ~ 20 000). The Ig is secreted covalently attached to the ectoplasmic
domain (MW ~ 80 000).

membrane. Since colchicine has little effect on binding and internalization of IgA [62], but does effect translocation, it has been suggested that microtubules are involved in vesicular movement across the cell. There are no data suggesting fusion of these vesicles with lysosomes but this has not been excluded.

At some point in this transcytotic process, the transmembrane–immunoglobulin complex is proteolytically cleaved, releasing soluble SIgA and leaving behind the protected residual membrane and cytoplasmic domains. The location and characteristics of the proteolytic enzyme that is responsible for this cleavage are unknown, but the cleavage site may be highly specific (similar to that of IgA protease, see below). The SC attached to IgA (and IgM) as well as free SC has a molecular weight of 80 000, and therefore the portion remaining in the cell has a molecular weight of approximately 20 000. Most of the residual SC represents an intracytoplasmic domain that is unusually large compared to other transmembrane proteins. This transport scheme is consistent with previous immunofluorescence studies localizing SC and IgA to the same regions of the basolateral plasma membrane of intestinal cells, and with the concurrent presence of IgA and SC in membrane-bound intracytoplasmic vesicles [16, 23, 35, 138]. Similar transport mechanisms may be operative in the transfer of dimeric IgA from serum to bile (see below) in which the sinusoidal plasma membrane is equivalent to the basolateral membrane of the intestinal epithelial cell and the bile caniculus corresponds to the apical (luminal) membrane. The various historical models suggested for the transport of IgA and IgM have been reviewed by Brandtzaeg [16].

Structure of secretory component

A very recent study [134] reports the complete amino acid sequence of the polymeric immunoglobulin receptor derived from rabbit liver and lactating mammary glands as deduced from its gene sequence. The entire SC molecule consists of 773 amino acids (aa) and includes: an 18 aa signal peptide, a 629 aa ectoplasmic domain, a 23 aa (largely hydrophobic) membrane-spanning segment and a 103 aa cytoplasmic tail. The extracellular portion consists of five highly conserved domains of 100–115 aa. A sixth domain is somewhat more distantly related and includes the membrane-spanning portion. When the domains were compared with each other and with other proteins using the Dayhoff Protein Data Bank, homologies were found with immunoglobulins as well as related proteins such as Thy 1. The most significant homologies were found between kappa variable (V) regions with an average of 28% identical aa; when comparisons were based on the similarities of side chains, homology increased to 56%. A striking feature was a highly conserved 18 residue consensus sequence which is found in each of the five domains and which closely resembles a segment which has been reported to represent the primordial building block of immunoglobulin heavy chain variable regions [146]. The similarity of the receptor to its ligand is not unique to immunoglobulins and could indicate that domains on the receptor and ligand interact via a mechanism similar to the interaction between immunoglobulin domains in polymeric molecules [76].

Receptor specificity

Alternatively, the receptor may have antibody V region-like specificity with a site on polymeric IgA and IgM. In any case, these homologies, if biologically relevant, could have implications for other receptors, particularly those involved in transport of immunoglobulins across the neonatal intestine and placenta. Recent studies [224] have cloned and sequenced mRNA specific for mammalian T cells which may correspond to a message for part of the T cell antigen receptor. This protein also shows homology with immunoglobulin light chains, suggesting a 'superfamily' of receptor-like molecules including Thy 1, β_2 microglobulin, Ia, SC, immunoglobulins and possibly the Fc receptors on T cells (Fig. 9.4).

The role of SC in transport of immunoglobulins differs from that of other receptors which are degraded in lysosomes or recycled for use again [59, 90, 152–155, 173] SC is proteolytically altered but not destroyed, and remains associated with its ligand so that it can not be used in subsequent translocations. For this reason SC has been termed a 'sacrificial receptor'. The fate of the intracytoplasmic and transmembrane portions of the molecules are not known, but they are probably rapidly degraded.

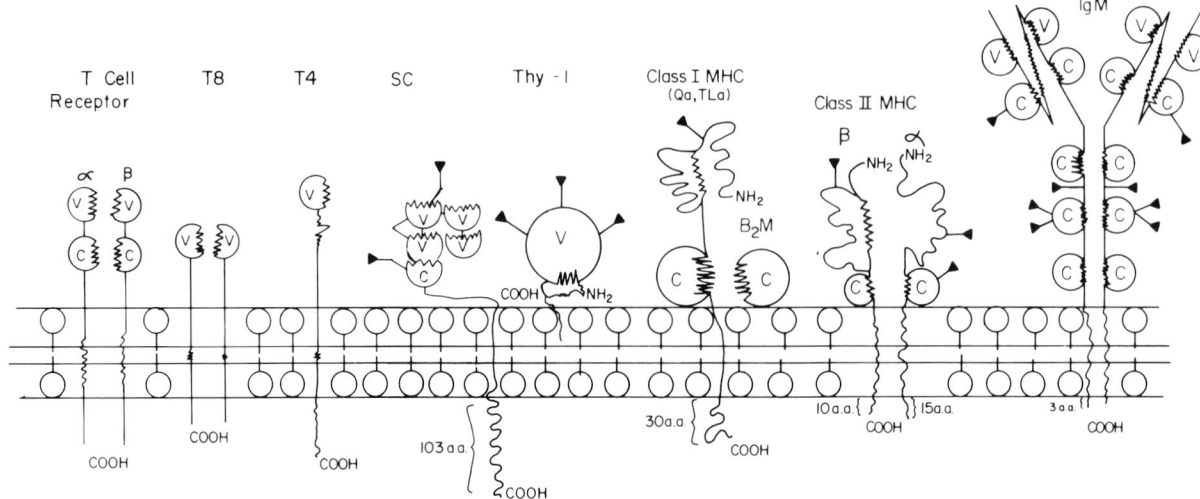

Fig. 9.4 Structural homology among cell surface receptor-like molecules. IgM is shown as a model for the antigen receptor on B cells. Immunoglobulin domains and homologous sequences in other molecules are depicted by circles designated V or C to indicate homology with variable or constant regions. The ⌁ symbols show interchain or intrachain disulphide bonds, while ◄ designates N-linked carbohydrate chains. Covalent bond and carbohydrate chain positions on SC are predicted by the sequence but not determined analytically. The number of residues in the intracytoplasmic portion of each molecule is indicated.

Hepatobiliary transport

Transport in animals

Mucosal surfaces are not the only sites at which polymeric IgA is selectively transported; studies in several laboratories have shown that IgA is transported across rat hepatocytes from serum into bile by receptor-mediated endocytosis [86, 147]. IgA is bound to SC on the sinusoidal surface of the hepatocyte, transferred across the cell in vesicles and released into the bile at the canicular membrane [54, 148, 183]. The ability to transport IgA from serum to bile and eventually into the proximal small intestine shows great species variation (for review see [149]), but there is no obvious phylogenetic relationship involved in transport of one species' IgA by another. Biliary transport mechanisms appear to be mediated by the cross-linking of the SC receptor, since IgG class anti-SC antibodies (but not univalent Fab fragments) also initiate the transcellular movement of endocytic vesicles [54]. SC-mediated vesicular transport appears to differ from lysosomal degradation of proteins [208]; in isolated, perfused rat livers, interruption of the lysosomal pathway with chloroquine inhibits the uptake processing of asialoorosomucoid but has no effect on uptake and transport of IgA. However, poly-

meric human IgA has been shown to compete for the asialo-receptor on rat hepatocytes, presumably through interaction with terminal galactose residues [187]. These studies indicate that mechanisms other than SC may also mediate interaction of IgA with rat liver membranes.

Although several unresolved issues related to the hepatobiliary transport of IgA remain, this pathway in rodents is apparently an efficient route for antigen disposal into the gut [157, 175, 184]. Russell et al [175] have demonstrated that trinitrophenyl- (TNP)-human serum albumin complexed with TNP-specific mouse IgA myeloma protein MOPC 315 was efficiently transported into mouse bile from the blood, but similar complexes involving IgG and IgM antibodies were not. Pneumococcal type III capsular antigens are similarly transported when complexed with polymeric IgA myeloma proteins or hybridoma antibody [177]. Little radioactivity was recovered in other secretions or tissues which would indicate other secretory pathways [176]. The transport process could not be inhibited by blockade of the mononuclear-phagocytic system or depletion of C3 by cobra venom factor, but was sensitive to large excesses of IgA of a different antibody specificity [22]. The size of circulating complexes is important in the biliary transport mechanism because exceptionally large complexes exceeding a molecular weight of 10^6 are inefficiently cleared and may be degraded by the reticuloendothelial system of the liver [158, 172, 182]. In some species the liver–bile pathway may be a major route for the elimination of foreign proteins that gain access to the body. Disease of the hepatobiliary system may significantly disrupt this pathway, leading to an accumulation of antigens and immune complexes in the circulation.

Transport in man

Hepatobiliary transport of IgA in man is less well defined; human hepatocytes apparently do not synthesize or express SC, at least not in amounts detectable utilizing the methods applied to date [42, 81, 139]. However, studies of biliary transport of IgA in patients with indwelling bile duct T-tubes indicate that 160–400 mg of IgA enter the bile in a 24–hour period [109] and transport of polymeric IgA from serum to bile is approximately 10 times greater than that of monomeric IgA. In addition, serum polymeric IgA levels are high in parenchymal liver disease [109, 124, 142] although the significance of this with respect to IgA transport is unclear because common bile duct obstruction does not result in elevated serum IgA in man [44]. The source of biliary IgA in man is unclear; some may be locally synthesized by plasma cells in the bile ducts or gall bladder, but indirect evidence such as the high fractional catabolic rate of polymeric versus monomeric IgA [42] suggests that plasma clearance through some undefined transport mechanism probably exists. Although the existence of SC in bile ducts suggests that these epithelial cells may play a key role in transport, several workers [31, 40] have suggested a dual role of the liver and bile duct in transporting serum IgA. The possibility that hepatic receptors other than SC may be involved in transport in the human has also been suggested [109].

Animal models

Because of the considerable difference detailed above between rodent hepatobiliary transport and that seen in man, it has been difficult to find a suitable animal model. However, it has recently been shown that the dog may be a candidate for such a model [45]. Like the human, dogs secrete polymeric IgA into bile across a concentration gradient. The coefficient of biliary excretion of polymeric IgA re-

lative to albumin is 9.2 for the dog compared to 4.9 for man and 1060 and 320 for rat and rabbit, respectively [43]. In addition, similarities exist in the fractional catabolic rate for polymeric IgA (26–36% per day) while the catabolic rate for rats is 100% per hour [44, 45]. Mechanisms of transport may be similar in dogs and man, as neither express SC on hepatocytes and may utilize a transbiliary ductal route [139].

REGULATION OF MUCOSAL ANTIBODIES

In the adult, most macromolecular absorption across the intestinal epithelium probably occurs via the microfold (M) cells of the Peyer's patches (PP) [11, 27, 150, 151]. PP contain macrophages, regulatory T lymphocytes and B lymphocytes, but, following contact with antigen, they do not exhibit local immune responses. It has been proposed that the relative absence of antibody-containing cells in PP is secondary to a lack of, or defect in, accessory cells [89], particularly adherent, antigen-presenting cells and classical dendritic cells [202]. While PP appear to contain cells capable of presenting antigen [170, 185, 202] the nature of those cells remains to be defined. It is possible that several cell types may be involved in presentation, including Ia-positive macrophages [205], dendritic cells [214] and B cells [33]. In recent work the population derived from PP which displayed the greatest antigen-presenting activity was enriched for B blasts. In this regard, lipopolysaccharide (LPS), which is present in the gut of conventionally fed mice, has a dramatic effect on the activation of B cells for presentation of antigen [33].

Following oral immunization, antigen-sensitive cells leave the PP and migrate through the thoracic duct, into the circulation and eventually lodge at mucosal surfaces resulting in an antigen-specific IgA response in secretions. In parallel, oral immunization and stimulation of PP may result in a state of *systemic* unresponsiveness termed oral tolerance (see Chapter 14). The mechanisms regulating these events (isotypic expression, suppressor mechanisms, localization of IgA precursor cells and terminal differentiation of IgA precursors to IgA plasma cells) are unknown. Previous studies have indicated that the IgA response is highly T cell dependent and may be regulated by isotope-specific T cells of both helper

(Th) and suppressor (Ts) phenotypes. It appears that the oral administration of antigen results in the simultaneous appearance of IgA-specific Th cells which remain in the secretory tissues and IgG- and IgE-specific Ts cells [119, 120, 143, 171] which migrate to the spleen and peripheral lymphoid tissues. The result is a concomitant induction of local immunity and systemic tolerance.

Role of T helper cells

The concept that mucosal tissues may be enriched for IgA-specific Th cells [47] has been tested directly using T cells cloned from PP which have been shown to stimulate the appearance of cells bearing IgA on their surface (sIgA$^+$) [91, 92] or of IgA plaque-forming cells (PFC) [96, 127]. These cells appear to operate at different levels of B cell maturation. The regulatory cell described by Kawanishi et al is termed a 'switch T cell' which is purported to drive B cells to 3' DNA rearrangements resulting in cells committed to the production of IgA. The PP appear to be enriched in these cells, as cloned T cells from spleen

did not induce the appearance of IgA B cells. Furthermore, only sIgM$^+$ cells could be induced to switch, suggesting that the regulation is at the level of DNA rearrangement, rather than the result of proliferation of preexisting cells committed to IgA production. Final differentiation into IgA-secreting cells is presumably governed by other Th cells or macrophages or by factors derived from these cells [93].

Kiyono et al [96] report the generation of IgA Th cells and their clones from PP after gut stimulation with erythrocyte antigens. These clones fall into two functional groups; one set allows development of only IgA and IgM PFC while the other set results in development of IgM, IgG and IgG$_2$ in addition to IgA. The target of these Th cells is an sIgA$^+$ B cell [97].

The PP T cell clones described by Kawanishi et al [92] and Kiyono et al [96] bear Fc receptors for IgA, which suggests that they recognize antigen and IgA simultaneously, making them good candidates for IgA regulators [48, 78].

It has also been postulated that IgA cells

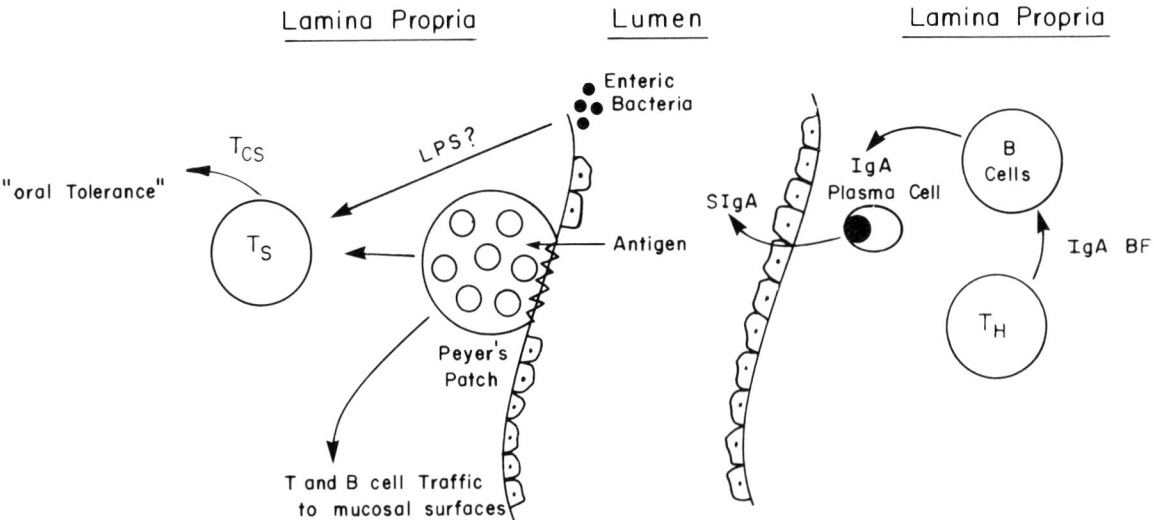

Intestine

Fig. 9.5 Regulation of mucosal antibodies. Antigens encountered at mucosal surfaces such as those associated with the gastrointestinal tract stimulate T lymphocytes of both helper (Th) and suppressor (Ts) phenotype. Th cells with receptors for the Fc portion of IgA (FcαR) remain in the mucosa and enhance the expression of IgA by B cells selectively lodging at these sites. This enhancement is possibly through IgA binding factors (IgA BF) released from FcαR$^+$ Th cells. The exact point at which IgA Th cells interact with B cells is not defined. FcαR$^+$ Ts cells generated by antigenic stimulation leave mucosal tissues and migrate to peripheral tissues such as spleen or lymph nodes where they suppress production of circulating antibodies of other isotypes (oral tolerance). Suppression may also be mediated by IgA BF. Immunomodulatory agents such as LPS present at external mucosae may induce regulatory cells. The contrasuppressor circuit also functions at mucosal surfaces, although the exact point at which it interacts with secretory immune responses is unclear.

arise in PP as a result of multiple divisions following exposure to a particular kind and pattern of antigenic or mitogenic stimuli [57]. These divisions are accompanied by successive switches to more 3′ sites in the heavy chain DNA, with eventual isotype restriction to IgA which is the most 3′ of the heavy chain genes.

The production of mucosal antibodies is also influenced by contact with immunomodulatory substances present in the gastrointestinal tract; central among these agents is LPS. It has been suggested that precursors of Ts present in the GALT are sensitive to LPS, and are stimulated by this substance [127]. Experiments by this group have shown that germ-free mice (LPS-free) and LPS-non-responsive C3H/HEJ mice demonstrated high IgA responses to enteric immunizations due to the absence of Ts activation by LPS.

Oral tolerance: mechanisms

Systemic suppression after oral feeding has been demonstrated with a variety of thymic-dependent antigens including heterologous erythrocytes and haptens as well as various soluble proteins [196]. Some workers ascribe suppression to soluble serum factors, particularly antigen–IgA antibody complexes [2, 88], some report antigen-specific suppressor cells [120] and other investigators have implicated at least two distinct T cell-derived soluble suppressive factors [121]. Another type of regulatory cell, the contrasuppressor cell, has been identified in PP [63]. This is a cell which inhibits the function of suppressor cells, thereby enhancing the immune response. The IgA response thus also appears to be influenced by contrasuppressor regulatory circuits. Many (or all) of these cells may have different migratory patterns to various lymphoid tissues at different times following immunization and thus a detailed analysis is

necessary to dissect out the relative roles of each cell type (Fig. 9.5). (See also Chap. 14.)

EFFECTOR FUNCTIONS OF MUCOSAL ANTIBODIES

The effector functions of mucosal antibodies, particularly IgA, have been debated for many years (for review see [26, 98, 201, 221]. Both IgA and IgM have properties that ensure efficient translocation across epithelial membranes, and these properties are central to their action (Table 9.2).

When compared with IgG and IgM antibodies of similar specificities, IgA antibodies are silent as mediators of inflammatory reactions such as complement activation, neutrophil chemotaxis and phagocytosis [98, 201, 221]. Although the failure of IgA to participate in inflammatory events was originally regarded as puzzling (some reports questioned the biological value of IgA) it is now recognized that IgA mediates an 'escort' function involving efficient disposal of antigens. As reviewed below, the mucosal immune system is part of a comprehensive local and systemic defence mechanism in which IgA plays a major role by disposing of microbial and dietary antigens locally and/or preventing them from entering the blood. The fact that continuous encounters with antigen at mucosal surfaces do not trigger vigorous inflammatory responses can be regarded as advantageous.

Complement activation

Neither secretory IgA nor serum IgA monomers or dimers activate complement by the classical pathway in vivo. There is experimental and theoretical evidence showing that circulating IgA blocks complement-mediated lysis or opsonization by serum IgG and IgM antibodies in cases of infection with *Neisseria*

Table 9.2 Effector functions of mucosal antibodies.

Functional activities	Blocking activities
Immune exclusion	Blocking of chemotaxis
Viral neutralization	Blocking of chemiluminescence
Toxin neutralization	Blocking of opsonization
Mucus regulation	Blocking of ADCC in meningococcal infections
Inhibition of bacterial colonization	
Opsonization by mucosal macrophages expressing FcαR	
Collaboration with IgG in ADCC	
Mediation of ADCC by mucosal effector cells	
Plasmid elimination	

meningitidis [65,66] *Streptococcus pneumoniae* [21], *Haemophilus influenzae* [137] and *Pseudomonas aeruginosa* [178]. The ability of serum IgA to block complement-mediated immune effector functions has prompted the hypothesis that it functions as an anti-inflammatory agent [211]. The significance of the components of the alternative pathway (properdin, etc.) which are seen in association with IgA deposits in certain diseases [166] is unclear, but at present there is no definitive evidence that IgA antibodies can mediate immunological tissue damage through a complement-dependent mechanism.

IgA and phagocytosis

In addition to lack of activity (or inhibition) in complement-mediated interactions, IgA appears to play little role in opsonization for phagocytosis by polymorphonuclear leukocytes (PMN). While receptors for IgA of both subclasses have been detected on PMN [53,113], the role of these receptors in promoting phagocytosis is unclear. On the contrary, Van Epps and colleagues reported that polymeric IgA paraproteins inhibited chemotaxis of neutrophils [212] and eosinophils [168]. These proteins also suppressed the bactericidal activity of neutrophils without interfering with cell metabolism, membrane fluidity or the ability of the neutrophils to participate in the lysis of IgG-coated avian erythrocytes in an antibody-dependent cytotoxicity system [213].

However, it appears that the anatomical source of phagocytic cells is important in their ability to ingest particles opsonized by secretory antibodies. Fanger et al [52] reported that although circulating human neutrophils were unable to phagocytose erythrocytes sensitized by specific rabbit IgA antibodies, neutrophils recovered from mucosal sites, such as the gingival crevice of teeth, were able to phagocytose such cells. They also demonstrated that: (a) more gingival neutrophils (62%) than peripheral blood neutrophils (35%) had IgA receptors; (b) the presence of IgA evoked both an increase in the number of IgA receptors per neutrophil and the overall number of receptor-positive cells; and (c) that the simultaneous sensitization of erythrocytes with IgA and IgG lowered the level of IgG needed to promote phagocytosis. SIgA from milk has also been reported to increase phagocytosis of human erythrocytes. Further examination of these issues is clearly needed because of the

obvious importance of the neutrophil in the host response to diverse bacterial infections of mucosal tissues.

This anatomical compartmentalization also appears to function for monocytes and macrophages. Earlier studies had failed to show cytophilic attachment of IgA to spleen macrophages [200]. However, using as a model mice infected with the parasite *Nippostrongylus brasiliensis*, Gauldie et al [56] found that on the second day of infection, when parasites were passing through the lung, resident macrophages having IgA receptors increased their numbers from 14% to 29%. Such cells were activated, and had an enhanced ability to ingest TNP-coated erythrocytes sensitized by the mouse IgA myeloma protein MOPC 315. Other studies, however, have shown that IgG is more efficient in enhancing phagocytosis by alveolar macrophages [169]. The failure to detect Fc receptors for IgA on peripheral macrophages may also have been due to lack of sensitivity of the assay system. Recently, Fanger et al [51] were able to demonstrate IgA binding to human circulating monocytes employing a sensitive assay involving cytofluorographic analysis of the binding of fluorescein isothiocyanate-labelled human myeloma IgA. These investigators also showed that proteins of IgA2 isotype bound to peripheral mononuclear cells, but IgA1 proteins did not. The explanation for this differential binding of the two human IgA subclasses is not clear.

Cell receptors for IgA

Receptors for the Fc portion of IgA have also been detected on lymphoid cells, but their expression appears to be a function of circulating levels of IgA. The twice-daily injection of BALB/c mice with the murine myeloma protein MOPC 315 was shown by Hoover et al [79] to induce expansion of a pool of Ts lymphocytes that have IgA receptors (FcαR$^+$). They also showed that FcαR$^+$T cells could be expanded in a pool of BALB/c spleen cells incubated with MOPC 315 in vitro, a phenomenon that was dependent on both DNA and protein synthesis. FcR$^+$ cells are increased in patients with IgA and IgG myeloma [80], and cells with IgE receptors are elevated in rats having high circulating levels of IgE, indicating that increased expression of immunoglobulin receptors as a result of elevated levels of circulating antibody is neither species- nor isotype-specific [186,226]. In patients with IgA nephropathy, characterized by higher levels of serum polymeric IgA [204], increased numbers of T cells bearing IgA receptors were found. The expression of IgA receptors apparently represents an unusual example of 'upregulation' of receptor expression by ligand leading to suppression. Although the significance of these findings for the function of IgA antibodies and effector cells of both the lymphocytic and monocytic macrophage system is not completely clear, it has been suggested that $Fc\alpha R^+$ cells are involved in isotype-specific helper activity [48] as well as suppressor functions [79]. Thus, the observed changes in $Fc\alpha R$ may represent regulatory factors for IgA.

Antibody-dependent cellular cytotoxicity

IgA has also been shown to participate in antibody-dependent cell-mediated cytotoxicity (ADCC). Lowell et al [115] demonstrated that circulating, non-adherent mononuclear cells in patients recovering from type C meningococcal infections were bactericidal for the infecting organism in the presence of serum IgA antibodies. This activity was complement-independent and was not found after immunization of normal individuals with type C polysaccharide vaccine. Shen and Fanger [181] reported that IgA could synergize with IgG to mediate ADCC. Recent studies [193, 194] demonstrated that murine lymphocytes from GALT but not other tissues (thymus or popliteal lymph nodes) exerted natural antibacterial activity, specifically enhanced by SIgA (but not IgG or IgM). The type of cell involved was not defined but some evidence was presented that a null or K lymphocyte and not a macrophage was mediating the ADCC by SIgA. If this work is verified it represents an important new role for SIgA in protection of the host against infectious agents at the mucosal level.

Other effector functions of IgA

IgA antibodies have been shown to have several effector functions that are not dependent on phagocytic cells, lymphocytes or complement which may be crucial in defence against mucosal pathogens and the undesirable gastrointestinal absorption of ingested antigenic materials. Most of these are well known and have been extensively reviewed (see [118]). Mucosal IgA neutralizes viruses as exemplified by the extensive studies of Ogra and co-

workers on poliovirus immunization by the oral route [145]. In the case of bacterial infections, IgA blocks the attachment of pathogens to relevant mucosal tissues and cells [55, 60, 190].

Porter and Lingood [165] have reported that mucosal antibodies may eliminate ('cure') plasmids coding for K88 adhesive determinants in *Escherichia coli* strains that are common intestinal pathogens of pigs. The phenomenon of sustained plasmid elimination represents a potentially important function of mucosal antibody because it may reduce the virulence of bacterial strains in the environment. The mechanisms involved in plasmid exclusion are, however, unknown.

Another biologically relevant function of mucosal antibodies is the binding and subsequent inhibition of absorption of soluble macromolecular antigens (immune exclusion) as shown in extensive studies by Walker and colleagues [215]. These investigators also showed that intestinal inflammation in the rat (by *Nippostrongylus brasiliensis* infection) or intestinal anaphylaxis caused enhanced uptake into the systemic circulation of intestinal 'bystander' macromolecules. It has been postulated that immune exclusion is mediated by antibodies bound to the surface of the mucosal epithelium, although other ultrastructural studies suggest that IgA does not bind to the apical plasma membrane of normal or neoplastic colon cells [23, 138].

An important function of mucosal antibodies might be associated with the IgA found in milk and milk cells. Previous studies have shown that phagocytic cells in human milk (which constitute 90% of the cell population) contain IgA antibodies which they acquire from the external environment and subsequently release [37, 112, 160, 216]. These studies suggest that milk phagocytes function as vehicles for the transport and release of secretory antibodies, and may continue to serve this function in the intestine of the nursing infant. Recent studies have shown the presence of antibodies to food antigens in human colostrum [1, 34, 39, 74] and colostral cells [34]. The potential value of such antibodies in preventing the entry of food antigens through the infant's gut is evident, but not proven.

It has been well established that in infants who have been formula-fed, antibodies to cow's milk proteins may be found [99]. The effect of these IgA antibodies present in colostrum and milk on the uptake of antigens present in cow's milk is not clear. Infants on mixed feedings of human milk and cow's milk for less than one week had higher levels of antibodies to the cow's milk than those on mixed feeding for three weeks or longer [75]. These findings suggest that colostral and milk antibodies to cow's milk prevented the uptake of those antigens through the infant's gut. Antibodies present in milk seem to affect the appearance of atopic diseases [3, 30] and children with atopic conditions may have decreased levels of SIgA [164]. It has also been reported that IgA class antibodies to allergens block the release of histamine by IgE antibodies [161].

IgA1 PROTEASES

A medically important group of bacterial pathogens produce IgA1 proteases, highly substrate-specific extracellular enzymes that cleave human IgA1 proteins [126, 136, 163]. The enzymes are metal dependent (Mg^{2+}) and some evidence has been presented [110] that specificity may depend on the combination of a protease and a dextran sucrase. Bacteria releasing these proteases include the two pathogenic *Neisseria* (*N. meningitidis* and *N. gonorrhoeae*), *Haemophilus influenzae*, *Streptococcus pneumoniae* and bacteria involved in dental caries and periodontal infections (*Streptococcus sanguis* and *Bacterioides melaninogenicus* [162]. In addition, IgA1 protease activity has recently been found among fresh clinical isolates of *E. coli* and certain other urinary tract pathogens [128]. Among *Neisseria* and *Haemophilus* species, IgA1 protease activity is confined to the human pathogens; non-pathogens within these two genera are not only enzyme-negative, but they also lack the gene specifying the enzyme in their chromosomal DNA [20]. Because IgA1 proteases are found only among bacteria capable of causing human infections, and because they are present in infected secretions and exhibit substrate specificity for human IgA1, it is likely that they take part in the infectious process, although the precise mechanisms have not been defined.

Variation in proteases

The IgA1 proteases are variably antigenic in man and experimental animals; high titres of antibodies that inhibit the proteolytic function of the IgA1 proteases from *Neisseria* are found in the SIgA purified from normal human colostrum [61], and serum antibody titres (of the IgG class) rise markedly in patients convalescing from meningococcal meningitis. Inhibiting

antibodies are present in low titre in all normal sera, but the role these play in normal resistance is unknown. In marked contrast, the IgA1 proteases of *Streptococcus sanguis* are not antigenic for man. These variations in antigenicity reflect the pronounced differences among the enzymes [95] that is also apparent at the genetic level (see below). Enzyme-neutralizing antibodies have been used to examine the relationships between IgA1 proteases. Within the *Haemophilus* species, 15 patterns of protease activity were detected which were correlated to capsular serotype [94]. A similar pattern of complexity may exist within other species of IgA1 protease-producing bacteria.

Each IgA1 protease identified to date cleaves a single peptide bond in the hinge region of the IgA1 H chain, and proline residues invariably contribute the carboxyl group to the bond cleaved. There are multiple such Pro-R bonds in the hinge region of IgA1 because of the unique proline-rich stretch of 16 amino acids that represents the duplication of an octapeptide having the composition Thr-Pro-Pro-Thr-Pro-Ser-Pro-Ser. IgA2 proteins have a deletion of 13 hinge residues and are therefore resistant to such proteolytic hydrolysis (Fig. 9.6).

Gene coding

Production of active IgA1 protease is encoded by a single gene on the chromosomal DNA of both *Neisseria gonorrhoeae* [101] and *Haemophilus influenzae* [20]. DNA probes prepared from the cloned genes of both strains showed strong homology with DNA restriction fragments of bacterial species from within the respective genera, but homology was marginal with DNA of other protease-positive bacteria. This suggests that the IgA1 proteases from various bacteria will have structural differences, a result consistent with the biochemical diversity discussed above. The genetic studies of these enzymes has not as yet revealed their function. A *Neisseria gonorrhoeae* mutant produced by the reintroduction of a physically modified (deleted) gene failed to produce the active enzyme but was found to be phenotypically indistinguishable from its protease-positive but otherwise isogenic counterpart [100]. The participation of IgA1 protease function in virulence could be tested with a protease-negative strain transfected with the protease gene, but the paucity of animal models of infection by these strictly human pathogens is a continuing impediment to such studies.

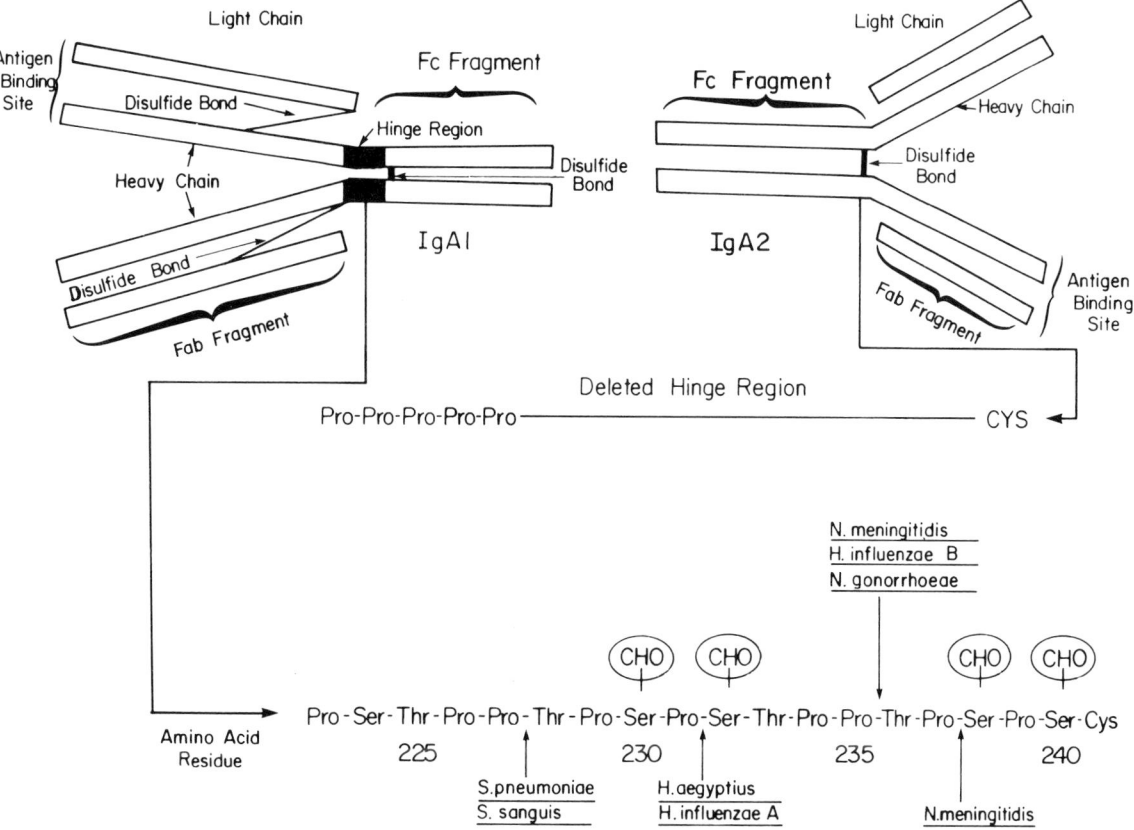

Fig. 9.6 Cleavage of the IgA1 molecule by IgA1 proteases. The diagram shows the structure of the two subclasses of human IgA, showing Fab and Fc regions, placement of disulphide bonds and the differences in hinge region structure. The lower half of the diagram outlines the amino acid structure of the IgA1 hinge region and the cleavage points for various proteases. The IgA2 molecule lacks the bonds cleaved by the various IgA1 proteases and is resistant to hydrolysis.

REFERENCES

1 Ahlstedt S, Carlsson B, Fällstrom SP et al: Antibodies in human serum and milk induced by enterobacteria and food proteins. Ciba Found Symp 1977; 46:115–34.

2 André C, Heremans JF, Vaerman JP, Cambiaso CL: A mechanism for the induction of immunological tolerance by antigen feeding: antigen–antibody complexes. J Exp Med 1975; 142:1509–19.

3 Atherton DJ: Breast feeding and atopic eczema. Br Med J 1983; 287:775–6.

4 Baenziger JU: Structure of the oligosaccharide of human J chain. J Biol Chem 1979; 254:4063–71.

5 Barratt TM, Turner MW, Johansson SG: Urinary excretion of immunoglobulin E in the nephrotic syndrome and atopic eczema. Lancet 1970; ii:402–3.

6 Bast EJE, Vancamp B, Boom SE et al: Differentiation between benign and malignant monoclonal gammopathy by the presence of the J chain. Clin Exp Immunol 1981; 44:375–82.

7 Bertolli LF, Kubagawa H, Koopman WF et al: Presence of monoclonal immunoglobulins in saliva of myeloma patients. Fed Proc 1983; 42:840.

8 Bienenstock J, Befus AD: Mucosal immunity. Immunology 1980; 41:249–70.

9 Bienenstock J, Dolezel J: Peyer's patches: lack of specific antibody-containing cells after oral and parenteral immunization. J Immunol 1971; 106:938–45.

10 Bienenstock J, Befus AD, McDermott M et al: The mucosal immunological network: compartmentalization of lymphocytes, natural killer cells, and mast cells. Ann NY Acad Sci 1983; 409:164–70.

11 Bockman DE, Cooper MD: Pinocytosis by epithelium associated with lymphoid follicles in the bursa of Fabricius, appendix, and Peyer's patches. An electron microscopic study. Am J Anat 1973; 136:455–78.

12 Brandtzaeg P: Human secretory immunoglobulins. II. Salivary secretions from individuals with selectively excessive or defective synthesis of serum immunoglobulins. Clin Exp Immunol 1971; 8:69–85.

13 Brandtzaeg P: Characteristics of SC-Ig complexes found in vitro. Adv Exp Med Biol 1974; 45:87–97.

14 Brandtzaeg P: Human secretory immunoglobulin M. An immunochemical and immunohistochemical study. Immunology 1975; 29:559–70.

15 Brandtzaeg P: Studies on J chain and binding site for secretory component in circulating B cells. II. The cytoplasm. Clin Exp Immunol 1976; 25:59–66.

16 Brandtzaeg P: Transport models for secretory IgA and secretory IgM. Clin Exp Immunol 1981; 44:221-32.

17 Brandtzaeg P: The secretory immune system of lactating human mammary glands compared with other exocrine organs. Ann NY Acad Sci 1983; 409:353-81.

18 Brandtzaeg P, Berdal P: J-chain in malignant human IgG immunocytes. Scand J Immunol 1975; 4:403-7.

19 Brandtzaeg P, Gjeruldsen ST, Korsrud F et al: The human secretory immune system shows striking heterogeneity with regard to involvement of J-chain-positive IgD immunocytes. J Immunol 1979; 122:503-10.

20 Bricker J, Mulks MH, Plaut AG et al: IgAl proteases of *Haemophilus influenzae*: Cloning and characterization in *E. coli* K-12. Proc Natl Acad Sci USA 1983; 80:2681-5.

21 Briles DE, Forman C, Hudak S, Claflin L: Blocking effect of IgA in infections with *Streptococcus pneumoniae*. Am Soc Microbiol 1983; abstract:E40:83.

22 Brown TA, Russell MW, Mestecky J: Hepatobiliary transport of IgA immune complexes: molecular and cellular aspects. J Immunol 1982; 128:2183-6.

23 Brown WR, Isobe Y, Nakane PK: Studies on translocation of immunoglobulins across intestinal epithelium. II. Immunoelectron microscopic localization of immunoglobulins and secretory component in human intestinal mucosa. Gastroenterology 1976; 71:985-95.

24 Butler WT, Rossen RD, Waldman TA: The mechanism of appearance of immunoglobulin A in nasal secretions in man. J Clin Invest 1967; 46:1813-93.

25 Callerame ML, Condemi JJ, Ishizaka K et al: Immunoglobulins in bronchial tissues from patients with asthma with special reference to immunoglobulin E. J Allergy 1971; 47:187-97.

26 Calvanico NJ, Tomasi TB: Effector sites on antibodies. In: Immunochemistry of proteins. New York: Plenum Press, 1979.

27 Carter PB, Collins FM: The route of enteric infection in normal mice. J Exp Med 1974; 139:1189-203.

28 Cebra JJ, Small PA: Polypeptide chain structure of rabbit immunoglobulin. III. Secretory αA-immunoglobulin from colostrum. Biochemistry 1967; 6:503-12.

29 Challacombe SJ, Russell MW, Hawkes JE et al: Passage of immunoglobulins from plasma to the oral cavity in rhesus monkeys. Immunology 1978; 35:923-31.

30 Chandra RK: Prospective studies of the effect of breast feeding on incidence of infection and allergy. Acta Paediatr Scand 1979; 68:691-4.

31 Chandy KG, Hübscher SG, Elias E et al: Dual role of the liver in regulating circulating polymeric IgA in man: studies on patients with liver disease. Clin Exp Immunol 1983; 53:207-18.

32 Chapius RM, Koshland ME: Mechanism of IgM polymerization. Proc Nat Acad Sci 1974; 71:657-61.

33 Chesnut RW, Colon SM, Grey HM: Antigen presentation by normal B cells, B cell tumors amd macrophages: functional and biochemical comparison. J Immunol 1982; 128:1764-8.

34 Crago SS, Mestecky J: Presence of antibodies to food antigens in human milk and milk cells. Protides of the Biological Fluids XXXII Colloquium 32:277-30.

35 Crago SS, Kulhavy R, Prince SJ, Mestecky J: Secretory component on epithelial cells is a surface receptor for polymeric immunoglobulins. J Exp Med 1978; 147:1832-6.

36 Crago SS, Kutteh WH, Moro I et al: Distribution of

37 Crago SS, Prince SJ, Pretlow TG et al: Human colostral cells. I. Separation and characterization. Clin Exp Immunol 1979; 38:585-97.

38 Craig SW, Cebra JJ: Rabbit Peyer's patches, appendix and popliteal lymph node B lymphocytes: a comparative analysis of their membrane immunoglobulin components and plasma cell precursor potential. J Immunol 1975; 114:492-502.

39 Cruz JR, Garcia B, Urrutia JJ et al: Food antibodies in milk from Guatemalan women. J Pediatr 1981; 99:600-2.

40 Cuadrado E, Arenas JI, Echaniz P et al: Rapid decrease of secretory IgA serum levels in extrahepatic obstructive jaundice after surgical relief of the bile duct obstruction. Gastroenterology 1983; 84:203-4.

41 Dahlgren U, Ahlstedt S, Hedman L et al: Dimeric IgA in the rat is transferred from serum into bile but not into milk. Scand J Immunol 1981; 14:95-8.

42 Delacroix DL, Vaerman JP: Function of the human liver in IgA homeostasis in plasma. Ann NY Acad Sci 1983; 409:383-401.

43 Delacroix DL, Dive C, Rambaud JC, Vaerman JP: IgA subclasses in various secretions and in serum. Immunology 1982; 47:282-5.

44 Delacroix DL, Elkom KB, Geubel AP et al: Changes in size, subclass, and metabolic properties of serum immunoglobulin A in liver diseases and in other diseases with high serum immunoglobulin A. J Clin Invest 1983; 71:358-67.

45 Delacroix DL, Furtado-Barreira G, de Hemptinne B et al: The liver in the IgA secretory immune system. Dogs, but not rats and rabbits, are suitable models for human studies. Hepatology 1983; 3:980-2.

46 Deuschl H, Johansson SGO: Immunoglobulins in tracheo-bronchial secretion with special reference to IgE. Clin Exp Immunol 1974; 16:401-6.

47 Elson CO, Weiserbs DB, Ealding E, Machelski E: T helper cell activity in intestinal lamina propria. Ann NY Acad Sci 1983; 409:230-7.

48 Endoh M, Sakai H, Nomoto Y et al: IgA-specific helper activity of Tα cells in human peripheral blood. J Immunol 1981; 127:2612-3.

49 Eskeland T: IgM reassociation in vitro: no influence of J chain on the amount of polymers. Scand J Immunol 1974; 3:757-68.

50 Eskeland T, Brandtzaeg P: Does J chain mediate the conformation of 19s IgM and dimeric IgA with the secretory component rather than being necessary for its polymerization? Immunochemistry 1974; 11:161-3.

51 Fanger MW, Goldstine SN, Shen L: Cytofluorographic analysis of receptors for IgA on human polymorphonuclear cells and monocytes and the correlation of receptor expression with phagocytes. Mol Immunol 1983; 20:1019-27.

52 Fanger MW, Goldstine SN, Shen L: The properties and role of receptors for IgA on human leukocytes. Ann NY Acad Sci 1983; 409:552-63.

53 Fanger MW, Shen L, Pugh L, Bernier GM: Subpopulations of human peripheral granulocytes and monocytes express receptors for IgA. Proc Natl Acad Sci USA 1980; 77:340-4.

54 Fisher MM, Nagy B, Bazin H, Underdown BJ: Biliary transport of IgA: role of secretory component. Proc Natl Acad Sci USA 1979; 76:2008-12.

55 Freter R, Jones GW: Models for studying the role of bacterial attachment in virulence and pathogenesis. Rev Infect Dis 1983; 5:5647-58.

IgA1-, IgA2- and J chain-containing cells in human tissues. J Immunol 1984; 132:16-18.

56 Gauldie J, Richards C, Lamontagne L: Fc receptors for IgA and other immunoglobulins on resident and activated alveolar macrophages. Mol Immunol 1983; 20:1029-37.

57 Gearheart PJ, Cebra JJ: Differentiated B lymphocytes. Potential to express particular antibody variable and constant regions depends on site of lymphoid tissue and antigen load. J Exp Med 1979; 149:216-27.

58 Gerbrandy JLF, Bienenstock J: Kinetics and localization of IgE tetanus antibody response in mice immunized by the intratracheal, intraperitoneal and subcutaneous routes. Immunology 1976; 31:913-9.

59 Geuze HJ, Slot JW, Strous GJ: Intracellular site of asialoglycoprotein receptor–ligand uncoupling: double-label immunoelectron microscopy during receptor-mediated endocytosis. Cell 1983; 32:277-87.

60 Gibbons RJ, van Houte J: Bacterial adherence in oral microbial ecology. Ann Rev Microbiol 1975; 29:19-44.

61 Gilbert JV, Plaut AG, Longmaid B, Lamm ME: Inhibition of microbial IgA proteases by secretory IgA and serum. Mol Immunol 1983; 20:1039-49.

62 Goldman IS, Jones AL, Hradek GT, Huling S: Hepatocyte handling of immunoglobulin A in the rat: the role of microtubules. Gastroenterology 1983; 85:130-40.

63 Green DR, Gold J, St Martin S et al: Microenvironmental immunoregulation: possible role of contrasuppressor cells in maintaining immune response in gut-associated lymphoid tissues. Proc Natl Acad Sci USA 1982; 79:889-92.

64 Grey HM, Abel CA, Yount WJ, Kunkel HG: A subclass of human αA-globulins (αA2) which lacks the disulfide bonds linking heavy and light chains. J Exp Med 1968; 128:1223-36.

65 Griffiss J McL: Epidemic meningococcal disease: synthesis of a hypothetical immunoepidemiologic model. Rev Infect Dis 1982; 4:159-72.

66 Griffiss J McL: Biologic function of the serum IgA system: modulation of complement-mediated effector mechanisms and conservation of antigenic mass. Ann NY Acad Sci 1983; 409:698-707.

67 Guy-Grand D, Griscilli C, Vassali P: The mouse gut T lymphocyte—a novel type of T cell. J Exp Med 1978; 148:1661-77.

68 Hajdu I, Moldoveanu Z, Cooper MD, Mestecky J: Ultrastructural studies of human lymphoid cells. J Exp Med 1983; 158:1193-2006.

69 Halpern MS, Koshland ME: A novel subunit in secretory IgA. Nature 1970; 228:1276-78.

70 Halsey JF, Johnson BF, Ceba JJ: Transport of immunoglobulins from serum into colostrum. J Exp Med 1980; 151:767-72.

71 Halsey JF, Mitchell CS, McKenzie SJ: The origins of secretory IgA in milk: a shift during lactation from a serum origin to a local synthesis in the mammary gland. Ann NY Acad Sci 1983; 409:452-9.

72 Halsey JF, Mitchell CS, Meyer R, Ceba JJ: Metabolism of immunoglobulin A in lactating mice: origins of immunoglobublin A in milk. Eur J Immunol 1982; 12:107-12.

73 Hanson LÅ: Comparative immunological studies of the immunoglobulins of human milk and blood serum. Int Arch Allergy Appl Immunol 1961; 18:241-67.

74 Hanson LÅ, Ahlstedt S, Carlsson B, Fällstrom SP: Secretory IgA antibodies against milk proteins in human milk and their possible effect in mixed feeding. Int Arch Allergy 1977; 54:457-62.

75 Hanson LÅ, Ahlstedt S, Carlsson B et al: Secretory IgA antibodies to enterobacterial virulence antigens: their induction and possible relevance. Adv Exp Med Biol 1977; 107:165-76.

76 Hauptman SP, Tomasi TB: Mechanism of immunoglobulin A polymerization. J Biol Chem 1975; 250:3891-6.

77 Hobday JD, Cake M, Turner KJ: A comparison of the immunoglobulins IgA, IgG and IgE in nasal secretions from normal and asthmatic children. Clin Exp Immunol 1971; 9:577-83.

78 Hoover RG, Lynch RG: Isotype-specific suppression of IgA: suppression of IgA responses in Balb/c mice by Tα cells. J Immunol 1983; 130:521-3.

79 Hoover RG, Dieckgraefe BK, Lynch RG: T cells with Fc receptors for IgA: induction of tα cells in vivo and in vitro by purified IgA. J Immunol 1981; 127:1560-3.

80 Hoover RG, Hickman S, Gebel HM et al: Expansion of Fc receptor-bearing T lymphocytes in patients with immunoglobulin G and immunoglobulin A myeloma. J Clin Invest 1981; 67:308-11.

81 Hopf U, Brandtzaeg P, Hutteroth Th, Meyer Zum Buschenfelde KH: In vivo and in vitro binding of IgA to the plasma membrane of hepatocytes. Scand J Immunol 1978; 8:543-9.

82 Huang SW, Fogh J, Hong R: Synthesis of secretory component by colon cancer cells. Scand J Immunol 1976; 5:263-8.

83 Ishizaka K, Newcomb RW: Presence of γE in nasal washings and sputum from asthmatic patients. J Allergy 1970; 46:197-202.

84 Ishizaka K, Yodoi J, Seremura M, Hirashima M: Isotype-specific regulation of the IgE response of IgE-binding factors. Immunol Today 1983; 4:192-6.

85 Issacson P: Immunochemical demonstration of J chain. A marker of B-cell malignancy. J Clin Pathol 1979; 32:802-7.

86 Jackson GDF, Lamaitre-Coelho I, Vaerman JP et al: Rapid disappearance from serum of intravenously injected rat myeloma IgA and its secretion into bile. Eur J Immunol 1978; 18:123-6.

87 Jerry LM, Kunkel HG, Adams L: Stabilization of dissociable IgA2 proteins by secretory component. J Immunol 1972; 109:275-83.

88 Kagnoff MF: Effects of antigen-feeding on intestinal and systemic immune responses. III. Antigen-specific serum-mediated suppression of humoral antibody responses after antigen feeding. Cell Immunol 1978; 40:186-203.

89 Kagnoff MF, Campbell S: Functional characteristics of Peyer's patch lymphoid cells. I. Induction of humoral antibody and cell-mediated allograft reactions. J Exp Med 1974; 139:398-406.

90 Kaplan J: Polypeptide-binding membrane receptors: analysis and classification. Science 1981; 212:14-20.

91 Kawanishi H, Strober W: T cell regulation of IgA immunoglobulin production in gut-associated lymphoid tissues. Mol Immunol 1983; 20:917-30.

92 Kawanishi H, Saltzman L, Strober W: Mechanisms regulating IgA class-specific immunoglobulin production in murine gut-associated lymphoid tissues I. J Exp Med 1983; 157:433-50.

93 Kawanishi H, Saltzman L, Strober W: Mechanisms regulating IgA class-specific immunoglobulin production in murine gut-associated lymphoid tissues II. J Exp Med 1983; 158:649-69.

94 Kilian M, Thomsen B, Petersen TE, Bleeg H: Molecular biology of *Haemophilus influenzae* IgA1 proteases. Mol Immunol 1983; 20:1051-9.

95 Kilian M, Thomsen B, Peterson TE, Bleeg HS:

Occurrence and nature of bacterial IgA proteases. Ann NY Acad Sci 1983; 409:612-24.

96 Kiyono H, McGhee JR, Mosteller LM et al: Murine Peyer's patch T cell clones. Characterization of antigen-specific helper T cells for immunoglobulin A responses. J Exp Med 1982; 156:1115-30.

97 Kiyono H, Phillips JO, Colwell DE et al: Murine Peyer's patch T cell clones: Fcα receptors regulate T and B cell collaboration for IgA responses. J Immunol 1984; 133:1087-9.

98 Klein M, Haeffner-Cavaillon N, Isenman DE et al: Expression of biological effector functions by immunoglobulin G molecules lacking the hinge region. Proc Natl Acad Sci USA 1981; 78:524-8.

99 Kletter B, Gery I, Freier S, Davies AM: Immune responses of normal infants to cows milk. II. Decreased immune reaction in initially breast-fed infants. Int Arch Allergy Appl Immunol 1971; 40:667-74.

100 Koomey JM, Falkow S: Nucleotide sequence homology between the immunoglobulin A1 protease genes of *Neisseria gonorrhoeae*, *Neisseria meningitidis*, and *Haemophilus influenzae*. Infect Immun 1984; 43:101-7.

101 Koomey JM, Gill RE, Falkow S: Genetic and biochemical analysis of gonococcal IgA1 protease: cloning in *Escherichia coli* and construction of mutants of gonococci which fail to produce the activity. Proc Natl Acad Sci USA 1982; 79:7881-5.

102 Koshland ME: Structure and function of the J chain. Adv Immunol 1975; 20:41-69.

103 Koshland ME: Presidential address: molecular aspects of B cell differentiation. J Immunol 1983; 131:i-ii.

104 Kownatzki E: Reassociation of IgM subunits in presence and absence of J chain. Immunol Commun 1973; 2:105-13.

105 Kuhn LC, Kraehenbuhl JP: Interaction of rabbit secretory component with rabbit IgA dimer. J Biol Chem 1979; 254:11066-71.

106 Kuhn LC, Kraehenbuhl JP: Role of secretory component, a secreted glycoprotein in the specific uptake of IgA dimer by epithelial cells. J Biol Chem 1979; 254:11072-81.

107 Kuhn LC, Kraehenbuhl JP: The membrane receptor for polymeric immunoglobulins is structurally related to secretory component. J Biol Chem 1981; 256:12490-5.

108 Kutteh WH, Prince SJ, Mestecky J: Tissue origins of human polymeric and monomeric IgA. J Immunol 1982; 128:990-5.

109 Kutteh WH, Prince SJ, Phillips JO et al: Properties of immunoglobulin A in serum of individuals with liver diseases and in hepatic bile. Gastroenterology 1982; 82:184-93.

110 Labib RS, Calvanico C, Tomasi TB: Studies on extracellular proteases of *Streptococcus sanguis*: purification and characterization of human IgA1 specific protease. Biochim Biophys Acta 1978; 526:547-59.

111 Lamm ME: Cellular aspects of immunoglobulins. Adv Immunol 1976; 22:223-90.

112 Laven GT, Crago SS, Kutteh WH, Mestecky J: Hemolytic plaque formation by cellular and noncellular elements of human colostrum. J Immunol 1981; 127:1967-72.

113 Lawrence DA, Weigle WO, Spiegelberg HL: Immunoglobulins cytophilic for human lymphocytes, monocytes and neutrophils. J Clin Invest 1975; 55:368-87.

114 Lindh E: Increased resistance of immunoglobulin A

dimers to proteolytic degradation after binding of secretory component. J Immunol 1975; 114:284-6.

115 Lowell GH, Smith LF, Griffiss J McL, Brandt BL: IgA-dependent monocyte-mediated, antibacterial activity. J Exp Med 1980; 152:452-7.

116 McCune JM, Fu SM, Kunkel HG: J chain biosynthesis in pre-B cells and other possible precursor B cells. J Exp Med 1981; 154:138-45.

117 McGhee JR, Mestecky J: Ann NY Acad Sci 1983; 409:

118 McNabb P, Tomasi TB: Host defense mechanisms at mucosal surfaces. Ann Rev Microbiol 1981; 35:477-96.

119 Mattingly JA: Cellular circuitry involved in orally induced systemic tolerance and local antibody production. Ann NY Acad Sci 1983; 409:204-13.

120 Mattingly JA, Waksman BH: Immunologic suppression after oral administration of antigen I. Specific suppressor cells formed in rat Peyer's patches after oral administration of sheep erythrocytes and their systemic migration. J. Immunol 1978; 121:1878-83.

121 Mattingly JA, Kaplan JM, Janeway CA Jr: Two distinct antigen-specific suppressor factors induced by the oral administration of antigen. J Exp Med 1980; 152:545-54.

122 Mestecky J, Zikan J, Butler WT: Immunoglobulin M and secretory immunoglobulin A: presence of a common polypeptide chain different from light chains. Science 1971; 171:1163-5.

123 Mestecky J, Winchester RJ, Hoffman T, Kunkel HG: Parallel synthesis of immunoglobulins and J chain in pokeweed mitogen-stimulated normal cells and in lymphoblastoid cell lines. J Exp Med 1977; 145:760-5.

124 Mestecky J, Kutteh WH, Brown TA et al: Function and biosynthesis of polymeric IgA. Ann NY Acad Sci 1983; 409:292-305.

125 Mestecky J, Preud'Homme J-L, Crago SS et al: Presence of J chain in human lymphoid cells. Clin Exp Immunol 1980; 39:371-85.

126 Metha SK, Plaut AG, Calvanico NJ, Tomasi TB: Human immunoglobulin A: production of an Fc fragment by an enteric microbial proteolytic enzyme. J Immunol 1973; 111:1274-6.

127 Michalek SM, McGhee JR, Kiyono H et al: The IgA response: inductive aspects, regulatory cells, and effector functions. Ann NY Acad Sci 1983; 409:448-69.

128 Miluzzo FH, Delisle GJ: Immunoglobulin A proteases in gram-negative bacteria isolated from human urinary tract infections. Infect Immun 1984; 43:11-13.

129 Mizoguchi A, Mizoguchi T, Kobata A: Structures of the carbohydrate moieties of secretory component purified from human milk. J Biol Chem 1982; 257:9612-21.

130 Mole JE, Bhown AS, Bennett JC: Primary structure of human J chain: alignment of peptides from chemical and enzymatic hydrolyses. Biochemistry 1977; 16:3507-13.

131 Mossman TR, Gravel Y, Williamson AR: Modification and fate of J chain in myeloma cells in the presence and absence of polymeric immunoglobulin secretion. Eur J Immunol 1978; 8:94-101.

132 Mostov KE, Blobel G: A transmembrane precursor of secretory component. The receptor for transcellular transport of polymeric immunoglobulins. J Biol Chem 1982; 257:11816-21.

133 Mostov KE, Blobel G: Transcellular transport of polymeric immunoglobulin by secretory component:

a model system for studying intracellular protein sorting. Ann NY Acad Sci 1983; 409:441–51.

134 Mostov KE, Friedlander M, Blobel G: The receptor for transepithelial transport of IgA and IgM contains multiple immunoglobulin-like domains. Nature 1984; 308:37–43.

135 Mostov KE, Kraehenbuhl JP, Blobel G: Receptor-mediated transcellular transport of immunoglobulin: synthesis of secretory component as multiple and larger transmembrane forms. Proc Natl Acad Sci USA 1980; 77:7257–61.

136 Mulks MH, Plaut AG: IgA protease production as a characteristic distinguishing pathogenic from harmless Neisseriaceae. N Engl J Med 1978; 299:973–6.

137 Musher DM, Goree A, Baughn RE, Birdsall HH: Immunoglobulin A from bronchopulmonary secretions blocks bactericidal and opsonizing effects of antibody to nontypable *Haemophilus influenzae*. Infect Immun 1984; 45:36–40.

138 Nagura H, Nakane P, Brown WR: Translocation of dimeric IgA through neoplastic colon cells in vitro. J Immunol 1979; 123:2359–68.

139 Nagura J, Smith PD, Nakane PK, Brown WR: IgA in human bile and liver. J Immunol 1981; 126:587–95.

140 Nakajima S, Gillespie DN, Gleich GJ: Differences between IgA and IgE as secretory proteins. Clin Exp Immunol 1975; 21:306–17.

141 Newcomb R, Ishazaka K: Physiochemical and antigenic studies in human αE respiratory fluids. J Immunol 1970; 105:85–9.

142 Newkirk MM, Klien MH, Katz A et al: Estimation of polymeric IgA in human serum: an essay based on binding of radiolabeled human secretory component with applications in the study of IgA nephropathy, IgA monoclonal gammapathy and liver disease. J Immunol 1983; 130:1176–81.

143 Ngan J, Kind LS: Suppressor T cells for IgE and IgG in Peyer's patches of mice made tolerant by the oral administration of ovalbumin. J Immunol 1978; 120:861–5.

144 Ogra PL, Dayton DH: Immunology of breast milk. New York: Plenum Press, 1979.

145 Ogra PL, Karzon DT, Righthand F, McGillivray M: Immunoglobulin response in serum and secretions after immunization with live and inactivated poliovaccine and natural infection. N Engl J Med 1968; 279:894–900.

146 Ohno S, Matsunaga T, Wallace RB: Identification of the 48-base-long primordial building block sequence of mouse immunoglobulin variable region genes. Proc Natl Acad Sci USA 1982; 79:1999–2002.

147 Orlans E, Peppard J, Reynolds J: Rapid active transport of immunoglobulin A from blood to bile. J Exp Med 1978; 147:588–92.

148 Orlans E, Peppard J, Fry JR et al: Secretory component as the receptor for polymeric IgA on rat hepatocytes. J Exp Med 1979; 150:1577–81.

149 Orlans E, Peppard JV, Payne AWR et al: Comparative aspects of the hepatobiliary transport of IgA. Ann NY Acad Sci 1983; 409:411–26.

150 Owen RL: Sequential uptake of horseradish peroxidase by lymphoid follicle epithelium of Peyer's patches in the normal unobstructed mouse intestine: an ultrastructural study. Gastroenterology 1977; 72:440–51.

151 Owen RL, Jones AL: Epithelial cell specialization within human Peyer's patches: an ultrastructural study of intestinal lymphoid follicles. Gastroenterology 1974; 66:189–90.

152 Palade G: Intracellular aspects of the process of protein synthesis. Science 1975; 189:347–58.

153 Pastan IH, Willingham MC: Journey to the center of the cell: role of the receptosomes. Science 1981; 214:504–9.

154 Pearse BM: Clathrin: a unique protein associated with intracellular transfer of membrane by coated vesicles. Proc Natl Acad Sci USA 1976; 73:1255–9.

155 Pearse BM: On the structural and functional components of coated vesicles. J Mol Biol 1978; 126:803–12.

156 Peppard JV, Rose ME, Hesketh P: A functional homologue of mammalian secretory component exists in chickens. Eur J Immunol 1983; 13:566–70.

157 Peppard J, Orlans E, Payne AWR, Andrew E: The elimination of circulating complexes containing polymeric IgA by excretion into the bile. Immunology 1981; 42:83–9.

158 Phillips JO, Russell MW, Brown TA, Mestecky J: Selective hepatobiliary transport of monoclonal IgA but not IgM anti-idiotypic antibodies by IgA. Ann NY Acad Sci 1983; 409:859–60.

159 Pierce-Cretal A, Pamblanco M, Strecker G et al: Primary structure of the N-glycosidically linked sialoglycans of secretory immunoglobulins A from human milk. Eur J Biochem 1982; 125:383–8.

160 Pittard WB, Polmar SH, Fanaroff AA: The breast milk macrophage: a potential vehicle for immunoglobulin transport. J Reticuloendothel Soc 1977; 22:597–603.

161 Platts-Mills TAE, van Maur RK, Ishizaka K et al: IgA and IgG anti-ragweed antibodies in nasal secretions. Quantitative measurements of antibodies and correlation with inhibition of histamine release. J Clin Invest 1976; 57:1041–50.

162 Plaut AG: The IgA1 proteases of pathogenic bacteria. Ann Rev Microbiol 1983; 37:603–22.

163 Plaut AG, Gilbert JV, Artenstein MD, Capra JD: *Neisseria gonorrhoeae* and *Neisseria meningitidis*: extracellular enzyme cleaves human immunoglobulin A. Science 1978; 190:1103–5.

164 Plebani U, Monato M, Giannetti A, Uqazio AG: Different role of secretory IgA in the pathogenesis of RAST-positive and RAST-negative atopic dermatitis. Clin Allergy 1982; 12:403–7.

165 Porter P, Lingood MA: Novel mucosal antimicrobial functions interfering with the plasmid-mediated virulence determinants of adherence and drug resistance. Ann NY Acad Sci USA 1983; 409: 564–79.

166 Provost TT, Tomasi TB: Evidence for the activation of complement via the alternate pathway in skin diseases. II. Dermatitis herpetiformis. Clin Immunol Immunopathol 1974; 3:178–86.

167 Purkayastha S, Rav CVN, Lamm ME: Structure of the carbohydrate chain of free secretory component from human milk. J Biol Chem 1979; 254:6583–7.

168 Reed KJ, van Epps DE, Williams RC Jr: Inhibition of human eosinophil chemotaxis by IgA paraproteins. Inflammation 1979; 3:405–16.

169 Reynolds HY, Kazmierowski JA, Newball HA: Specificity of opsonic antibodies to enhance phagocytosis of *Pseudomonas aeruginosa* by human alveolar macrophages. J Clin Invest 1975; 56:376–85.

170 Richman LK, Graeff AS, Strober W: Antigen presentation by macrophage-enriched cells from the mouse Peyer's patch. Cell Immunol 1981; 62:110–18.

171 Richman LK, Graeff AS, Yarchoan R, Strober W: Simultaneous induction of antigen-specific IgA helper T cells and IgG suppressor T cells in the murine

Peyer's patch after protein feeding. J Immunol 1981; 126:2079–82.

172 Rifai A, Mannik M: Clearance, kinetics and fate of mouse IgA immune complexes prepared with monomeric or dimeric IgA. J Immunol 1983; 130:1826–32.

173 Rodewald R: Distribution of immunoglobulin G receptors in the small intestine of the young rat. J Cell Biol 1980; 85:18–32.

174 Roth RA, Koshland ME: Identification of a lymphocyte enzyme that catalyzes pentamer immunoglobulin M assembly. J Biol Chem 1983; 256:4633–9.

175 Russell MW, Brown TA, Mestecky J: Role of serum IgA: hepatobiliary transport of circulating antigen. J Exp Med 1981; 153:968–76.

176 Russell MW, Brown TA, Mestecky J: Preferential transport of IgA and IgA immune complexes to bile compared with other external secretions. Mol Immunol 1982; 19:677–82.

177 Russell, MW, Brown TA, Claflin JL et al: Immunoglobulin A-mediated hepatobiliary transport constitutes a natural pathway for disposing of bacterial antigens. Infect Immun 1983; 42:1041–8.

178 Schiller NL, Millard RL: *Pseudomonas*-infected cystic fibrosis patient sputum inhibits the bactericidal activity of normal human serum. Pediatr Res 1983; 17:747–52.

179 Sewell HF, Matthews JB, Flack V, Jeffrees R: Human immunoglobulin D in colostrum, saliva and amniotic fluid. Clin Exp Immunol 1979; 36:183–8.

180 Sheldrake RF, Husband AJ, Watson PL, Cripps AW: Selective transport of serum-derived IgA into mucosal secretions. J Immunol 1984; 132:363–8.

181 Shen L, Fanger MW: Secretory IgA antibodies synergize with IgG in promoting ADCC by human polymorphonuclear cells, monocytes and lymphocytes. Cell Immunol 1981; 59:75–81.

182 Skogh T: Tissue distribution of intravenously injected dinitrophenylated human serum albumin (DNP-HSA) preparations. Effects of specific IgG and IgA antibodies. Scand J Immunol 1982; 16:465–75.

183 Socken DJ, Jeejeebhoy KN, Bazin H, Underdown BJ: Identification of secretory component as an IgA receptor on rat hepatocytes. J Exp Med 1979; 150:1538–48.

184 Socken DJ, Sims ES, Nagy B et al: Transport of IgA antibody-antigen complexes by the rat liver. Mol Immunol 1981; 18:345–8.

185 Spalding DM, Koopman WJ, McGhee JR: Identification of a nonadherent accessory cell in murine Peyer's patches. Ann NY Acad Sci USA 1983; 409:880–1.

186 Spiegelberg HL, O'Connor RD, Simon RA, Mathison DA: Lymphocytes with immunoglobulin E Fc receptors in patients with atopic disorders. J Clin Invest 1979; 64:714–8.

187 Stockert RJ, Kressner MS, Collins JC et al: IgA interaction with asialoglycoprotein receptor. Proc Natl Acad Sci USA 1982; 79:6229–31.

188 Strober W, Blaese RM, Waldman TA: The origin of salivary IgA. J Lab Clin Med 1970; 75:856–62.

189 Strober W, Hanson LÅ, Sel KW: Recent advances in mucosal immunity. New York: Raven Press, 1982.

190 Svanborg-Éden C, Freter CR, Hagbert R et al: Inhibition of experimental ascending urinary tract infection by receptor analogue. Nature 1982; 298:560–2.

191 Sztul ES, Howell KE, Palade GE: Intracellular and transcellular transport of secretory component and albumin in rat hepatocytes. J Cell Biol 1983; 97:1582–91.

192 Tada T, Ishizaka K: Distribution of αE-forming cells in lymphoid tissues of the human and monkey. J Immunol 1970; 104:377–87.

193 Taqliabue A, Boraschi D, Villa L et al: IgA-dependent cell-mediated activity against enteropathogenic bacteria: distribution specificity and characterization of the effector cells. J Immunol 1984; 133:988–92.

194 Taqliabue A, Nencioni L, Villa L et al: Antibody-dependent cell-mediated antibacterial activity of intestinal lymphocytes with secretory IgA. Nature 1983; 306:184–6.

195 Tomasi TB: The immune system of secretions. Englewood Cliffs, New Jersey: Prentice Hall, 1976.

196 Tomasi TB: Oral tolerance. Transplantation 1980; 29:353–73.

197 Tomasi TB, Bienenstock J: Secretory immunoglobulins. Adv Immunol 1968; 9:2–96.

198 Tomasi TB, Czerwinski DS: The secretory IgA system. In: Immunologic deficiency diseases in man, Vol. IV, New York: The National Foundation-March of Dimes, 1968.

199 Tomasi TB, Czerwinski DS: Naturally occurring polymers of IgA lacking J chain. Scand J Immunol 1976; 5:647–53.

200 Tomasi TB, Grey HM: Structure and function of Immunoglobulin A. Prog Allergy 1972; 16:81–213.

201 Tomasi TB, Plaut AG: Humoral aspects of mucosal immunity. Adv Host Defense Mech (in press).

202 Tomasi TB, Barr WG, Challacombe SJ, Curran G: Oral tolerance and accessory cell function of Peyer's patches. Ann NY Acad Sci 1983; 409:145–63.

203 Tomasi TB, Tan EM, Soloman A, Prendergast RA: Characteristics of an immune system common to certain external secretions. J Exp Med 1965; 121:101–24.

204 Trascasa ML, Egido J, Sancho J, Hernando L: IgA glomerulonephritis (Berger's disease): evidence of high serum levels of polymeric IgA. Clin Exp Immunol 1980; 142:247–54.

205 Unanue ER, Beller DI, Lu CY, Allen PM: Antigen presentation: comments on its regulation and mechanism. J Immunol 1984; 132:15.

206 Underdown BJ, Derose J, Plaut AG: Disulfide bonding of secretory component to a single monomer subunit in human secretory IgA. J Immunol 1977; 118:1816–21.

207 Underdown BJ, Knight A, Paspin FR: The relative paucity of IgE in human milk. J Immunol 1976; 116:1435–8.

208 Underdown BJ, Schiff JM, Nagy B, Fisher MM: Differences in processing of polymeric IgA and asialoglycoproteins by the rat liver. Ann NY Acad Sci 1983; 409:402–10.

209 Vaerman JP, Heremans JF, Laurell CB: Distribution of α chain subclasses in normal and pathological IgA-globulins. Immunology 1968; 14:425–32.

210 Vaerman JP, Heremans JF, Bazin H, Beckers A: Identification and some properties of rat secretory component. J Immunol 1975; 114:265–9.

211 Van Epps DE, Brown SL: Inhibition of formyl-methionyl-leucyl-phenylalanine-stimulated neutrophil chemiluminescence by human immunoglobulin A paraproteins. Infect Immun 1981; 34:864–70.

212 Van Epps DE, Williams RC: Suppression of leukocyte chemotaxis by human IgA myeloma components. J Exp Med 1976; 144:1227–42.

213 Van Epps DE, Reed K, Williams RC Jr: Suppression of human PMN bacterial activity by human IgA para-proteins. Cell Immunol 1978; 36:363–76.

214 Van Voorhis WC, Witmer MD, Steinman RM: The

phenotype of dendritic cells and macrophages. Fed Proc 1983; 42:3114.

215 Walker WA, Bloch KJ: Intestinal uptake of macromolecules: in vitro and in vivo studies. Ann NY Acad Sci 1983; 409:593-601.

216 Weaver EA, Tsuda H, Goldblum RM et al: Relationship between phagocytosis and immunoglobulin A release from human colostral macrophages. Infect Immun 1982; 38:1073-7.

217 Weicker J, Underdown BJ: A study on the association of human secretory component with IgA and IgM proteins. J Immunol 1975; 114:1137-344.

218 Weinheimer PF, Mestecky J, Acton RT: Species distribution of J chain. J Immunol 1971; 107:1211-12.

219 Weisz-Carrington P, Roux ME, McWilliams M et al: Hormonal induction of the secretory immune system in the mammary gland. Proc Natl Acad Sci USA 1978; 75:2928-32.

220 Wilde CE, Koshland ME: Molecular size and shape of the J chain from polymeric immunoglobulins. Biochemistry 1973; 12:3218-24.

221 Winkelhake JL: Immunoglobulin structure and effector functions. Immunochemistry 1978; 14:695-714.

222 Wira CR, Sullivan DA, Sandoe CP: Estrogen-mediated control of the secretory immune system in the uterus of the rat. Ann NY Acad Sci 1983; 409:534-51.

223 Yagi M, D'Eustachio P, Ruddle FH, Koshland ME: J chain is encoded by a single gene unlinked to other immunoglobulin structural genes. J Exp Med 1982; 155:647-52.

224 Yangi Y, Yoshikai Y, Leggett K et al: A human T cell specific cDNA clone encodes a protein having extensive homology to immunoglobulin chains. Nature 1984; 308:145-9.

225 Yasuda N, Kanoh T, Uchino H: J chain synthesis in human myeloma cells: light and electron microscopic studies. Clin Exp Immunol 1980; 40:573-80.

226 Yodoi J, Ishizaka K: Lymphocytes bearing receptors for IgE. Presence of human and rat T lymphocytes with FcE receptors. J Immunol 1979; 122:2577-81.

Chapter 10
The Properties of the Mucus Gel Layer in the Gastrointestinal Tract

J. R. Clamp

Introduction

Humans are most vulnerable where they come into contact with the environment, and the body deals with this problem in different ways. The external surface of the body is protected by a thick layer of keratinized epithelium. However, the 'internal' epithelial surfaces tend of necessity to be only a few cells thick or to be composed of a single cell layer. Virtually all these internal surfaces are protected by an adherent layer of mucus. This is true not only of the gastrointestinal tract but also of the conjunctiva [53, 93], urogenital system [18], respiratory system [105] and so on. The nature of this mucus layer and the way in which it protects the underlying mucosa form the basis of this chapter. Any chapter on mucus must be selective and include studies on species other than man. Fortunately differences in the properties of mucus between species, for example rat and man [58], are relatively minor and are greatly outweighed by the similarities.

Nomenclature. The nomenclature followed in this chapter is that suggested by Reid and Clamp [112]. The only extension to that nomenclature is to acknowledge that the histochemical term 'mucin' is now being increasingly used by biochemists as a convenient term for the rather cumbersome phrase 'mucus glycoprotein'. The two terms 'mucin' and 'mucus glycoprotein' will therefore be used interchangeably and 'mucus' will be used for the whole secretion.

MUCUS-SECRETING CELLS

Origin

Unlike the respiratory tract where most of the secretions arise from submucosal glands, the only true submucosal glands in the gut are in the duodenum, namely Brunner's glands [61]. Thus most of the mucus in the gastrointestinal tract arises from cells in the surface epithelium. These cells have a characteristic shape and are known as goblet cells, although the term is often used for all mucus-secreting cells, of whatever shape and wherever they occur. Other authors however distinguish between typical goblet cells and 'mucus-secreting non-goblet cells' [4].

Migration of crypt epithelial cells

All crypt epithelial cells, including goblet cells, arise from single progenitor stem cells [104]. For example, in the duodenum cell division takes place in the base of a crypt and the cells then migrate upwards. After division the cells take about 15 hours to mature, emerge from the crypt and spend about 4 days migrating up the villus [135]. The migration pattern is more complicated in the stomach. Here the proliferative zone is in the neck of the gastric glands and cells migrate from this zone in both upward and downward directions. The colon also appears to have a zone of mitotic activity in mid-crypt [4]. Interestingly the number of secretory cells in the deep crypts varies from ascending to descending colon. About one-third of the cells in the former are mucus-secreting cells and this number drops to 5% in the descending colon. Possibly this reflects the harsher conditions in the ascending colon which are due to the discharge of small intestinal contents.

Types of mucus-secreting cell

Two types of acidic group are present in mucins. The first is a sugar acid, namely sialic acid, which will be discussed below. The other is a sulphate ester, i.e. sulphate linked through one of its acid groups to the hydroxyl group of sugar. There is a difference in the strength (pK) of these two acids and this can be exploited by the differential binding of cationic dyes such as Alcian blue. Thus mucins in general, including those in the gastrointestinal tract, are divided by histochemists into three main types, namely neutral mucins, sialomucins and sulphomucins (see Table 10.1) [39, 74]. Stomach and duodenum possess neutral mucins and little or no acidic mucin. The remaining small intestine shows in addition to neutral mucin a gradual increase in the

amount of sialomucin from the duodenum to the terminal ileum [40]. In addition to this regional variation in the intestines, the crypts and villi themselves show a variation in mucin type in that the amount of sialomucin increases towards the top of the villus [40].

Sulphomucins on the other hand are largely confined to the colon [27, 40], and as with sialomucins in the small intestine, there is regional variation with most of the sulphomucin being present in the distal colon [113, 117].

Relationship of mucus-secreting cell to surrounding epithelium

As mentioned above, the main function of the mucus layer is to protect the underlying mucosa. The character of this layer must depend to a considerable extent on the number and type of mucus-secreting cells in the epithelium. The mucus is released from these cells and must then flow over and form a layer upon the epithelium. Another factor that may be important in the development of a protective layer may therefore be the relationship of the goblet cell orifices to the surrounding epithelial cells. Toad bladder is ideal for the visualization of such goblet cell patterns. It can be distended and prepared for electron microscopy in this state. Any folds are thereby largely eliminated and the cell junctions which do not collapse so much during dehydration stand out in relief. Fig. 10.1 shows firstly that cell boundaries radiate from goblet cell orifices and secondly that every epithelial cell is in contact with a goblet cell. This pattern may be fortuitous and result from the way cells are packed together. However the pattern is dependent on the small size of the goblet cell orifice in comparison to the size of the epithelial cells and this must be a consequence of the goblet shape. Human tissue is difficult to visualize in quite the same way, but a pattern does appear to be discernible in the intestines (Fig. 10.2).

SECRETION

Mechanism of mucus secretion

The goblet cell arises in the proliferative zone and matures as it migrates up the crypt and villus. During this process the mucus-filled vesicles fuse to form large vacuoles or granules [68]. Those granules formed early in the life of the cell occupy the central zone whereas the

Table 10.1 Histochemical types of gastrointestinal mucus

Type	Characteristic sites
Neutral mucins	Stomach and duodenum
Sialomucin	Jejunum and ileum
Sulphomucins	Colon and rectum

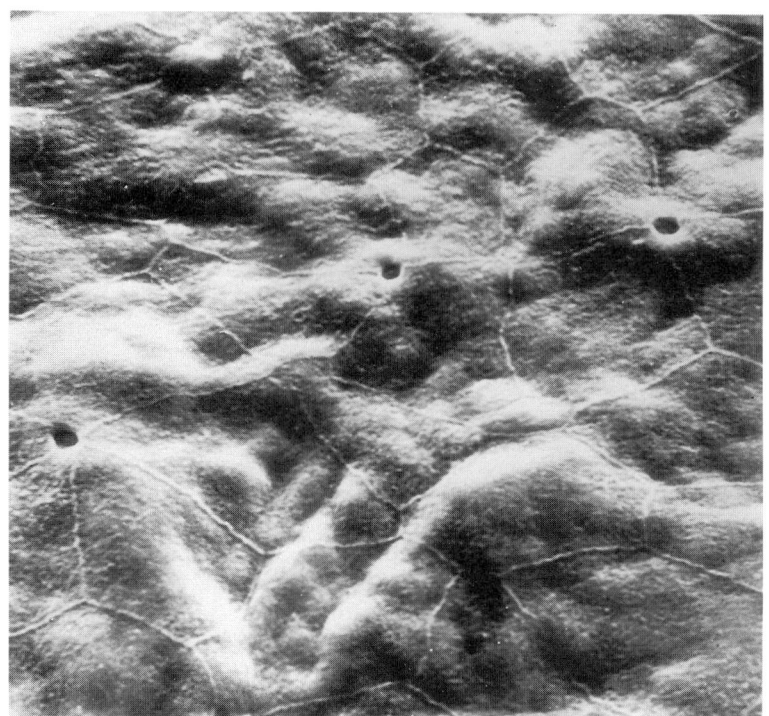

Fig. 10.1 Scanning electron microscopy of toad bladder epithelium. Epithelial cell boundaries are seen radiating from goblet cell orifices.

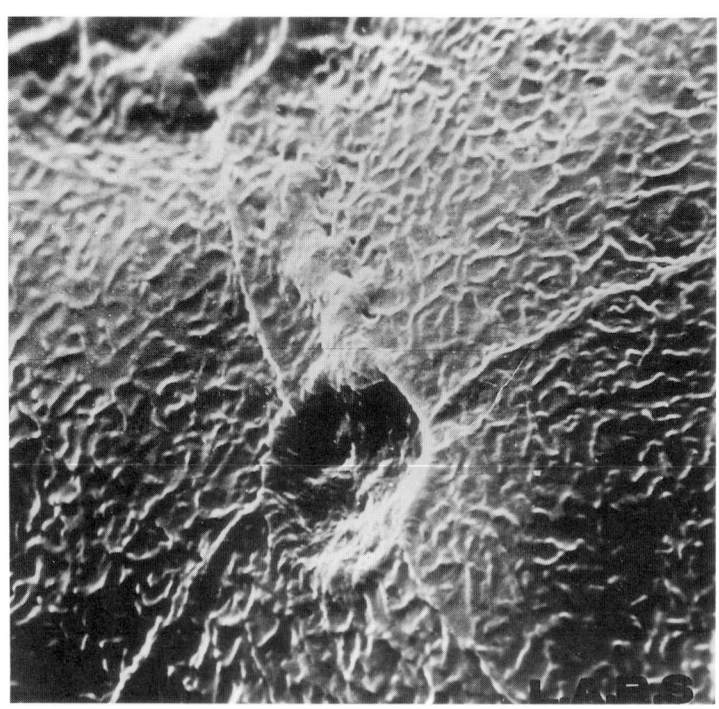

Fig. 10.2 Scanning electron microscopy of large bowel mucosa. A goblet cell orifice is seen in contact with four epithelial cells.

newly formed granules move along the periphery and do not mix freely with the central mucus granules [97]. The goblet cell only secretes mucus in substantial amounts during the later part of its life span [29] and the central mucus granules are released before the peripheral granules [97].

Mechanisms of mucus release

Three mechanisms of mucus release have been described [137] (Table 10.2). A slow baseline secretion is achieved by the process of exocytosis in which a single granule [121] or a few granules are released intermittently. Apical expulsion is the term used for the explosive release of an entire mucus package often followed by degeneration of the cell [137]. This may be the process of accelerated secretion by compound exocytosis described by Specian and Neutra [121]. Finally goblet cell exfoliation is a rare event in which the entire cell with its contained mucus is extruded from the epithelium [137].

Table 10.2 Mucus release from goblet cells.

Mechanisms of release	Effect
Intermittent exocytosis of single granules	Slow release
Apical expulsion of entire mucus contents	Explosive release
Goblet cell exfoliation	Cell and mucus

Factors affecting mucus secretion

The thickness of the mucus gel layer is the result of a steady-state situation where the rate of loss of mucus at the luminal surface is balanced by the rate of mucus production by the mucosa. The thickness varies at different levels of the gastrointestinal tract, being thickest in the stomach. The actual thickness in human stomach is controversial, one measurement indicating a layer nearly 600 μm thick [8] whereas other workers [62] suggest that the value is less than 200 μm. However, the mucus gel layer is extremely variable and the thickness may vary 10-fold in the same specimen [81]. Fewer studies have been carried out on other regions of the gastrointestinal tract. However, it would appear that in a number of species the mucus gel layer of the proximal colon is thicker than that of the distal colon [113] and this would be in keeping with the

different environment found in that part of the large intestine.

Endogenous control of mucus secretion

Mucus secretion in the intestines appears to be influenced by the parasympathetic system as indicated by the effect of acetylcholine [96, 121, 138] but it is not affected by adrenergic substances.

Acetylcholine. The action of acetylcholine in stimulating mucus release is predominantly an effect on goblet cells of the crypts with little effect on those at the mucosal surface [121]. Possibly the mature goblet cells characteristic of the surface are more susceptible to local factors.

Prostaglandins. Prostaglandins stimulate the output of gastric mucus and this may be one mechanism whereby they protect the stomach from ulcerogenic agents. Most prostaglandins seem to have this property [83] although those of the E [10] and F [30] series have the greatest effect.

Somatostatin. The action of somatostatin in stimulating gastric mucus output in man is probably mediated through its effect on prostaglandin synthesis since the activity is abolished by prior administration of indomethacin [59].

Serotonin. Other substances may also act endogenously to stimulate mucus secretion. For example, the neurotransmitter 5-hydroxytryptamine (serotonin) has a prolonged action on mucus output [11] which is not abolished by atropine [12]. The authors suggest that there may be two mechanisms for stimulating mucus release, one cholinergic and the other involving 5-hydroxytryptamine.

Externally acting secretagogues

It has been known for many years that irritants cause the discharge of mucus from goblet cells, for example the action of alcohol on the stomach [44] or of mustard oil on the colon [45]. No doubt food contains a range of substances that have a direct irritant effect upon the stomach or small intestine. Physiological substances may act in a similar way. Acid will cause mucus release in the stomach [57] and most of the bile acids induce mucus secretion in the colon [76] although it is not clear whether this is a direct effect or mediated through the cholinergic system [15].

Bacterial products. Certain bacterial products appear to stimulate mucus secretion directly. Proteinases, for example from *Pseudomonas aeruginosa*, will cause mucus release from tracheal epithelium [65]. This is a general effect of most proteinases, including trypsin, acting directly upon goblet cells [9] and for this reason it is likely to be a feature of the gastrointestinal tract as well.

Bacterial toxins will also cause mucus hypersecretion in the gut. The classical example is cholera toxin [118, 136] but other toxins have this property including those from *Shigella* [124] and *Escherichia coli* [92].

Lectins. Of more interest from the point of view of food allergy and intolerance is the effect of certain food constituents upon mucus release. A great many foods contain lectins and these are discussed more fully elsewhere in this book (see Chapter 21). However, one important aspect of certain lectins, for example concanavalin A from jack bean, that is relevant to this chapter is that they act directly upon goblet cells to cause mucus release [47]. In addition to lectins, foods no doubt contain other toxins and irritants that may have similar actions.

Food as antigen. Food proteins, by acting as antigens, may also elicit an effect on the goblet cell in the immunized animal. However, in this case the animal must be orally immunized. Thus rats that were immunized by the intraperitoneal route did not show mucus discharge when antigen was introduced into the duodenum [69]. Presumably in this mechanism the lymphoid aggregates of the intestine must be involved in the development of the immune response. Possibly this is mediated through the production of secretory IgA (SIgA) antibodies since immune complexes introduced into the duodenum of a normal rat will induce mucus release.

Immune complexes. The action of immune complexes is quite specific: it occurs in non-immunized animals and neither antigen nor antibody alone has any effect [130]. Thus the immune complex is another agent that appears to act directly upon the goblet cell. This study [130] used serum antibody which would be of less significance in the gut, but so far no studies have been carried out to test the effect of complexes containing SIgA antibodies.

Anaphylactic mucus release. An alternative explanation for the effect of antigen upon mucus release may be that some antigen reaches the submucosa to trigger the anaphylactic response [70]. The various mast cell-derived factors may then act upon the goblet cell. Other cell-derived secretagogues are known. For example, activated pulmonary macrophages secrete a factor that causes mucus release from cultured human airways [86].

CONSTITUENTS OF MUCUS

Mucus glycoprotein (mucin)

The component that is present in mucus in the greatest amount and which confers upon the secretion its characteristic physicochemical properties is a high molecular mass glycoprotein [21]. The actual molecular mass varies somewhat depending upon the source but is always in the region of several million. Mucins from whatever origin have a similar subunit structure consisting of a long polypeptide chain to which are attached many hundreds of oligosaccharide units. These subunits are conveniently termed glycopolypeptides [112]. The way in which the subunits or glycopolypeptides are linked together to form the glycoprotein is still a matter of some controversy and will be discussed later.

The polypeptide chain has a characteristic and rather unusual amino acid content. About half of the total amino acids consist of serine, threonine and proline. Glycine and alanine are the next most common amino acids and these five together account for about two-thirds of the polypeptide chain. There are only small amounts of basic, aromatic and sulphur-containing amino acids.

Carbohydrate constituents of mucus glycoprotein

The carbohydrate content of mucus glycoprotein accounts for about three-quarters of the total weight of the molecule. Most of this carbohydrate is present in units containing less than 10 monosaccharide residues. These may therefore be correctly called oligosaccharide units and the term is usually extended to include all units, even those containing more than 10 residues. When one considers the fact that the large mucus glycoprotein molecule contains over 70% carbohydrate and that this carbohydrate is present in relatively small oligosaccharide units, it is obvious that the molecule must possess a very large number of units. Indeed every third or fourth amino acid residue carries an oligosaccharide unit so that the carbohydrate is tightly packed along and around the chain.

Types of monosaccharide

There are five different types of sugar (monosaccharide) that may be present in the oligosaccharide units of mucin, namely galactose, fucose, *N*-acetylglucosamine, *N*-acetylgalactosamine and sialic acid. These are usually abbreviated to Gal, Fuc, GlcNAc, GaINAc and SA, respectively. The monosaccharides are shown in Fig. 10.3 as the Haworth representation on the left-hand side and the more correct chair-like conformational representation on the right-hand side of the figure. Fucose is a derivative of L-galactose in which a methyl group replaces the primary alcohol group at C-6. Sialic acid is a general name for all substituted neuraminic acids. Neuraminic acid is a nine-carbon ketose sugar with a carboxyl group at C-1 and an amino group at C-5 [115]. The amino group is always substituted with either an acetyl group (*N*-acetylneuraminic acid) or a glycolyl group (*N*-glycolylneuraminic acid). Although *N*-glycolylneuraminic acid is found widely amongst mammals only the *N*-acetyl derivative is found in man. There may be additional substitutions in the molecule. Thre are, for example, hydroxyl groups at C-4, C-7, C-8 and C-9 that may be substituted with acetyl groups (*O*-acetyl derivatives). The subsequent sialic acids tend to be characteristic of the species. Thus horses and donkeys have a 4-*O*-acetylsialic acid but this particular derivative is never found in man. However, the C-7, C-8 or C-9 derivatives are found, particularly in the colon, and resistance to the action of sialidase is correlated with the degree of substitution so that the 7,8,9-tri-*O*-acetylsialic acid is most resistant.

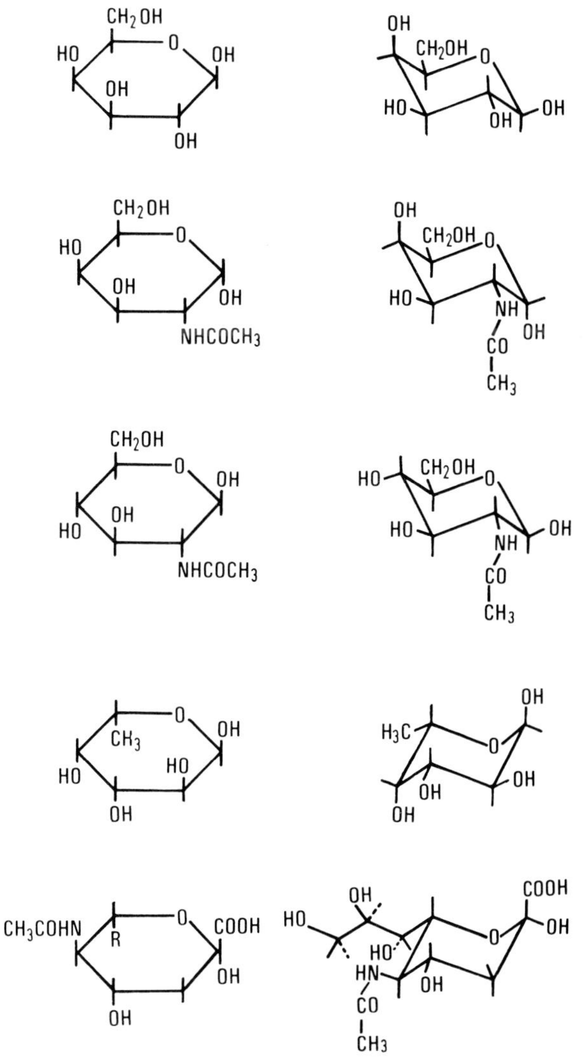

Fig. 10.3 Structure of the monosaccharides found in mucus glycoproteins. The monosaccharides are, from above downwards: galactose; *N*-acetylgalactosamine; *N*-acetylglucosamine; fucose; *N*-acetylneuraminic acid (sialic acid). On the left-hand side the Haworth representation is used and on the right is the corresponding chair conformation.

Hexosamines

The oligosaccharide units also contain two hexosamines, namely *N*-acetylglucosamine and *N*-acetylgalactosamine. *N*-Acetylglucosamine may be present in the core or in the backbone region of the oligosaccharide unit [56]. *N*-Acetylgalactosamine on the other hand is present in only two positions. It is the monosaccharide that links the oligosaccharide unit to the protein. This link is from C-1 (the potential reducing group) of the sugar to the hydroxyl group of either serine or threonine. As the link is through an oxygen atom, this type of bond is called an *O*-glycosidic linkage. The other position that *N*-acetylgalactosamine may occupy is as a non-reducing terminal sugar in the mucin of blood group A secretors.

Oligosaccharide regions

For ease of description Hounsell and Feizi [56] and others have divided the oligosaccharide unit into three regions, namely the core region, the backbone region and the peripheral region (Fig. 10.4).

Core region. The core region consists of the linkage N-acetylgalactosamine together with the monosaccharides immediately attached to it. There are five possible core structures ranging from the unsubstituted N-acetylgalactosamine (structure 1) to a structure where the linkage sugar carries N-acetylglucosamine at positions 3 and 6 (structure 5). Probably the commonest core is structure 2 consisting of the following attached to protein:

$$Gal(\beta 1\text{-}3)GalNAc(\alpha 1\text{-})Ser/Thr$$

The core structures described by Hounsell and Feizi [56] for gastrointestinal mucins are identical to those described by Lamblin et al [71] for bronchial mucins and may therefore be a common feature of all mucus glyco-proteins.

Backbone region. The backbone region is attached to the core region, that is to the substituents of N-acetylgalactosamine, and consists of alternating galactose and N-acetylglucosamine. There are two types of backbone differing in the position of attachment of galactose to the N-acetylglucosamine residue. In type 1, galactose is attached to the 3 position whereas in type 2 it is attached to the 4 position.

Peripheral region. The peripheral region consists of the terminal non-reducing sugars that are attached to the backbone region and which often carry known antigenic activities. There are a large number of these, for example blood groups A, B, H, Lewis[a] and Lewis[b], I, SSEA-1, C14 [37, 56], Sd[a] [31] and so on. The expression of the A, B, H blood group activities in mucus secretions is unusual in that it is controlled by a separate gene.

Secretor status. This 'secretor' gene is present in about three-quarters of the population and those that possess it have a particular glycosyltransferase in their epithelial tissue. They are thereby able to synthesize the H structure which is an absolute substrate requirement for the glycosyltransferases that synthesize A and B blood group structures. Thus 'non-secretors' lack A, B and H activities in their secretions although of course they are able to synthesize these structures in membrane glycolipids, for example of red cells.

As can be seen from the above discussion, the striking property of all mucins is the

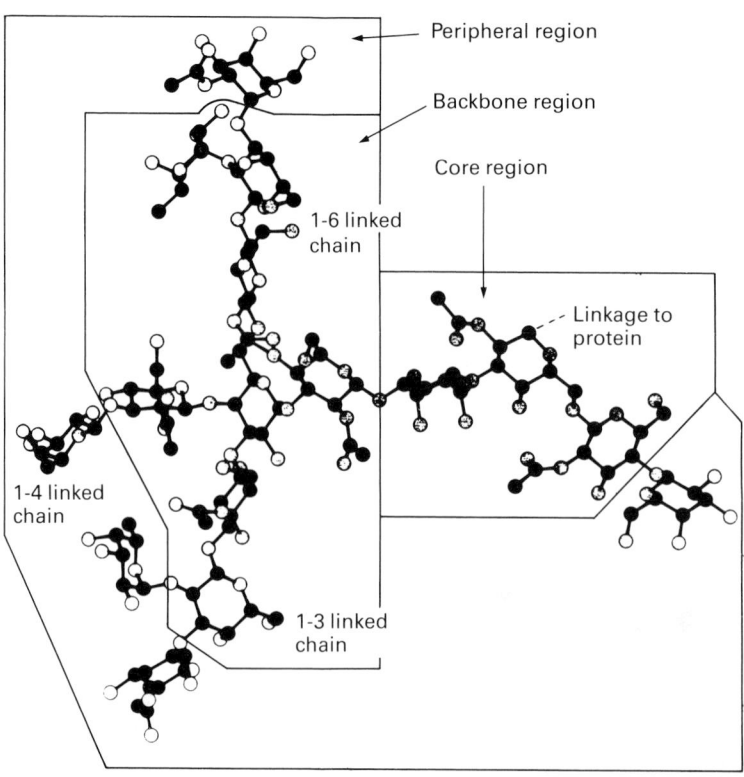

Fig. 10.4 The subdivision of oligosaccharide units into three regions for descriptive purposes. As discussed in the text, oligosaccharides may be divided into three regions. The core region consists of the linkage N-acetylgalactosamine and the monosaccharides directly attached to it; the peripheral region consists of the terminal monosaccharides and the backbone region is the remaining carbohydrate. The oligosaccharide used for illustration is the computational model shown in Fig. 10.7.

Peripheral region

Backbone region

Core region

1-6 linked chain

Linkage to protein

1-4 linked chain

1-3 linked chain

tremendous heterogeneity of their oligosaccharide units. For example, 26 different oligosaccharides were found in just two fractions from bronchial mucin [71] and at least 10 were present in the neutral oligosaccharides of human gastric mucin [119].

Models of mucus glycoprotein structure

The fundamental aspects of the mucus glycoprotein molecule are clear. It is an extremely large molecule with a molecular mass ranging from 10 to 20 million [16, 23, 87]. It is both polydisperse and heterogeneous, and thus shows variability with respect to size and charge [123]. It can be broken down to smaller fragments by either proteolysis or reduction of disulphide bridges [49] to give glycopolypeptides with a mass which for many mucins is about 500 000 [103]. Often the two techniques used sequentially [84, 87] will reduce the size of the glycopolypeptide more than either used alone, indicating the presence of two kinds of disulphide bridges, namely those between glycopolypeptide subunits (interchain) and those within a subunit (intrachain).

Structure of glycopeptide

The glycopolypeptide therefore is a polypeptide chain studded with oligosaccharide units but with sections that are devoid of carbohydrate namely the 'naked peptide' regions. These regions possess disulphide bonds, both intrachain and more importantly linking one glycopolypeptide to another to form the glycoprotein molecule. The polypeptide chain would be shielded by carbohydrate from proteolysis except in the naked peptide region. Thus proteolysis or disulphide reduction of the overall glycoprotein molecule will give rise to similar but not identical subunits.

Glycoprotein structure (1). Two kinds of model have been proposed for the mucus glycoprotein molecule (Fig. 10.5). The first is that proposed for pig gastric mucin where four glycopolypeptide subunits are assembled into a windmill-like structure [85]. This model has been criticized on two grounds: firstly, that the molecular mass proposed for pig gastric mucin of approximately 2×10^6 is too low [16, 23], and secondly that the model cannot accommodate the degree of polydispersity that is found in mucins.

Glycoprotein structure (2). An alternative model is what might be termed the 'necklace' or 'string-bead' structure. Here the polypeptide subunits are joined end-to-end to form a long, linear flexible chain [16]. It is possible that the structure of mucin is somewhat more

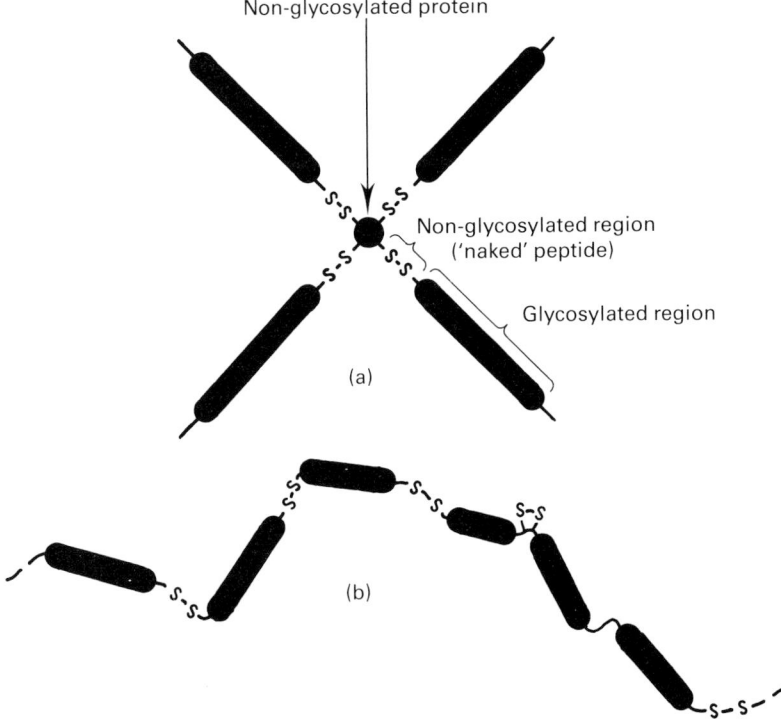

Non-glycosylated protein

Non-glycosylated region ('naked' peptide)

Glycosylated region

(a)

(b)

Fig. 10.5 Models proposed for the structure of human gastric mucus glycoprotein. The figure shows a diagrammatic representation of the two models proposed for gastric mucin as discussed in the text. The thick sausage-shaped regions are glycosylated protein and the thinner lines are non-glycosylated protein ('naked' peptide) as indicated in (a). The windmill-like structure [85] is shown in (a). The necklace-like structure [16] is shown in (b). The non-glycosylated regions show both interchain and intrachain disulphide bonds. A necklace-like structure is shown as an expanding view in Fig. 10.6.

complicated than either of these models would suggest. For example, non-mucin protein has been found covalently attached to both gastric [85] and small intestinal [102] mucus glycoprotein. Obviously with such a large molecule, protein may be trapped within the structure and not removed by the usual dissociative techniques. Alternatively, disulphide interchange might have occurred at some stage between mucin and protein. Nevertheless it would be a mistake to assume that the nature of the gel has been fully explained.

An attempt has been made to show the relationship between mucus gel, glycoprotein, glycopolypeptide and the oligosaccharide units in Fig. 10.6. This is an expanding view of mucus gel, assuming that it consists of tangled

and interacting glycoprotein molecules of the string-bead or necklace type. The final expansion in the figure is to show a typical oligosaccharide unit. This has a core region of the structure 2 type that is

$$\text{Gal}(\beta1\text{-}3)\text{GalNAc}(\alpha1\text{-})O\text{-Ser/Thr}$$

To this is attached a branched backbone structure of the type 1 sequence, that is

$$\text{Gal}(\beta1\text{-}3)\text{GlcNAc}(\beta1\text{-})$$

where the branch is present at C-6 of galactose.

Oligosaccharide structure. A composite structure has been published [79] which attempts to incorporate into one theoretical

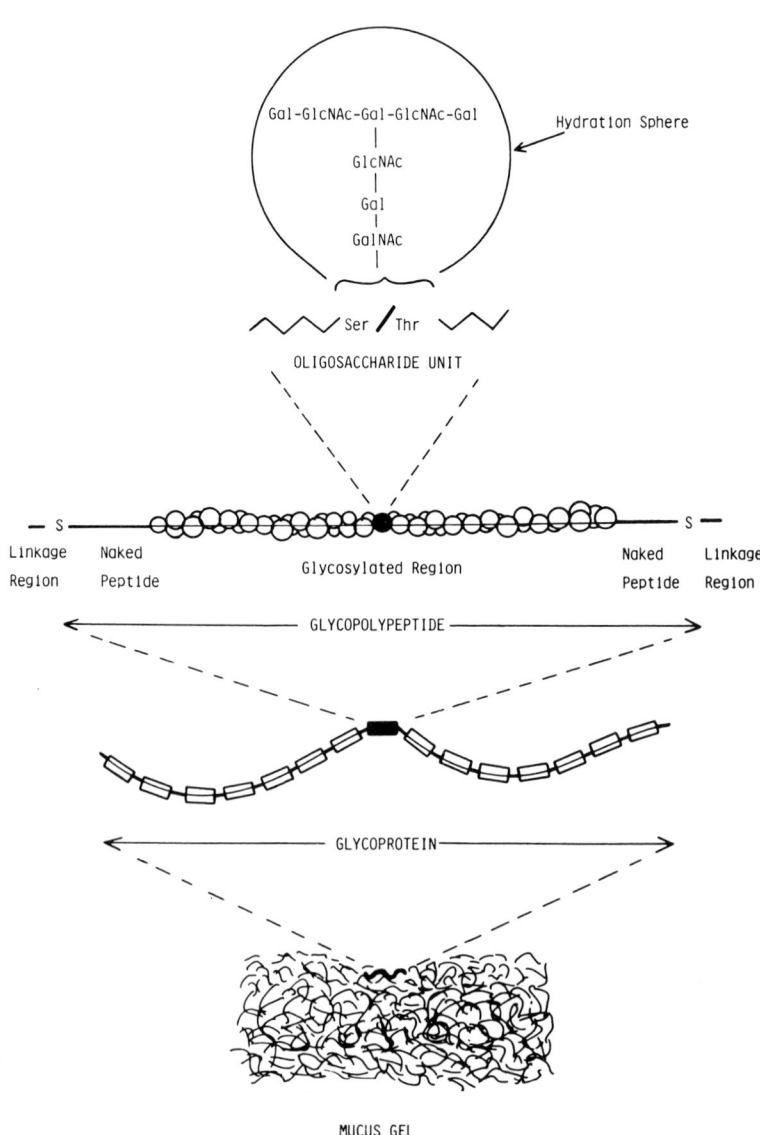

Fig. 10.6 An expanding view of the mucus gel structure. The structures are expanded from below upwards. Each component to be enlarged is shown in black with dotted lines indicating the expansion. The model assumes that the mucus glycoprotein is a long linear chain, corresponding to the string-bead or necklace model.

oligosaccharide all the possible side-chains and branches. Thus Fig. 10.7 is a computational model which tries to show the actual relationship of the monosaccharides in such an oligosaccharide. It is evident that the main backbone sequence is more or less at right angles to the polypeptide chain. The main backbone galactose carries three substituent chains namely at C-3, C-4 and C-6. The C-4 chain carries on in the line of the backbone but the C-3 and C-6 branches are at right-angles to

Non-mucin components of mucus

In addition to the mucus glycoprotein, mucus contains a large number of other substances as well as the products of epithelial cell breakdown such as membrane components [72] and DNA. Obviously substances such as inorganic material and plasma proteins may arise by transudation but this discussion will be confined to those constituents that appear to be specifically added to mucus secretions.

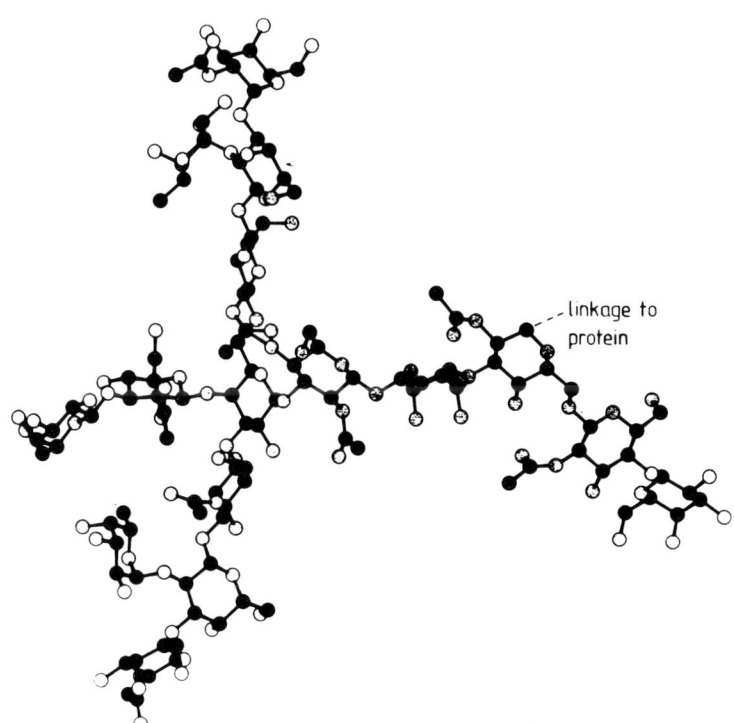

-- linkage to protein

Fig. 10.7 Computational model of an oligosaccharide unit. The monosaccharides are shown in a skeletal representation for clarity with carbon atoms in black, other atoms shaded and with hydrogen atoms omitted. Reproduced with permission from Professor E. Atkins, University of Bristol.

the backbone and at 180° to each other. Thus they resemble two arms embracing the polypeptide chain. If this structure were to be present in a substantial number of oligosaccharide units one can see how effective the carbohydrate would be at surrounding and protecting the protein. Another important prediction of the model concerns any substituent at C-6 of the linkage *N*-acetylgalactosamine. A branch at this position appears to lie along the polypeptide chain and would therefore hinder the attachment of adjacent oligosaccharide units. The degree of hindrance would be related to the size of the branch and this may be a way of controlling the number or possibly types of oligosaccharide units in particular areas of the mucus glycoprotein.

Bicarbonate

The surface epithelial cells of both the stomach and the duodenum actively secrete bicarbonate into the lumen [42]. The factors which cause acid secretion in the stomach appear to cause a simultaneous secretion of bicarbonate in both stomach and duodenum. In addition, when the stomach contents empty into the duodenum the resulting acid in the lumen stimulates the duodenal mucosa to secrete bicarbonate [43].

Lipid

Lipid appears to be associated with gastric mucus [120]. Mucus glycoproteins were prepared from human gastric secretions and exhaustively extracted with lipid solvents. A small amount of covalently bound lipid remained consisting principally of C_{16} and C_{18} fatty acids. These were attached by ester linkages to the glycoprotein though whether these bonds were to the hydroxyl groups of sugars or of amino acids was not clear. The total amount of fatty acid amounted to 2.9 nmol/mg and this corresponds to about one or two fatty acid residues in a glycopolypeptide subunit. This is a very small amount and is indeed two or three orders of magnitude less than the amount of carbohydrate. This probably explains why the presence of lipid has been overlooked for so long.

Polysaccharide

Human gastric mucus also contains polysaccharide [22]. This polysaccharide has a molecular mass of about 300 000 and is unusual in containing a large amount of galactose. It is a not insignificant component of mucus because about a quarter of the total galactose in gastric secretions is present in the polysaccharide. Other monosaccharides that have been found in the polysaccharide include glucose and glucuronic acid. The function of this polysaccharide is not clear and will therefore not be discussed in the final section of this chapter. Possibly it is a renewable cell-surface component that interacts with and thereby 'anchors' the gel layer [22].

Lysozyme

A number of proteins are added to mucus secretions. The best known of these is perhaps lysozyme. Lysozyme cleaves muramic acid linkages in the cell walls of susceptible bacteria causing lysis of the organism and it was this activity that was discovered in a number of bodily secretions by Fleming in 1922 [41] and led to its name. The enzyme has a number of interesting properties. It is a small protein with a mass of only 14 500 [60] and it strongly interacts with mucus glycoproteins [24]. It is present in many secretions in relatively high concentrations which may amount to 0.5 mg/ml. Lysozyme is synthesized by epithelial cells, but a subpopulation of epithelial cells has been described [91] in the small intestine which appears to synthesize both lysozyme and mucin. Such cells would certainly ensure that lysozyme and mucin are intimately mixed in the mucus layer.

Lactoferrin

Lactoferrin is another important protein component of mucus secretions. It is a larger protein than lysozyme with a mass of 76 400 [107]. Although similar to plasma transferrin in many ways, there are important differences between the two iron-binding proteins, no doubt reflecting the requirements of their different environments. For example lactoferrin binds iron 200 times more avidly than transferrin [1] and therefore the amount of free iron in equilibrium with lactoferrin would be virtually zero [20]. In addition, lactoferrin remains iron-binding under acidic conditions that would dissociate the transferrin–iron complex. Obviously this could be an important property in the upper gastrointestinal tract. Lactoferrin is secreted by epithelial cells for example in duodenum, but in stomach the mucus neck cells appear to have this function [88]. The relationship between iron, lactoferrin, mucus and the epithelium is a complex one, particularly as goblet cells of the small intestine appear to be involved in iron excretion [111].

Epidermal growth factor–urogastrone

Mucus secretions may contain a number of other interesting proteins or polypeptides. For example, epidermal growth factor has been found in two regions of the human digestive tract, namely the submandibular glands and Brunner's glands [33]. It has a powerful inhibitory effect on gastric acid secretion both unstimulated and stimulated and irrespective of whether the stimulant is pentagastrin, histamine or insulin [34]. Epidermal growth factor is almost certainly identical to the acid-inhibiting factor found in the urine of pregnant women and called 'urogastrone'. Indeed the polypeptide is often given the conjoint name 'epidermal growth factor–urogastrone' [52]. It is a 53 amino acid polypeptide that is derived from a much larger precursor [108] and, in addition to its effect on gastric acidity, it is an epithelial mitogen. Consequently it has been implicated in the control of secretions and of mucosal cell renewal in the gastrointestinal tract [33]. In view of these properties it is not surprising that the growth factor exhibits cytoprotective action in both the stomach [66] and the duodenum [63].

Control of epidermal growth factor. The secretion of epidermal growth factor itself appears to be under hormonal control. Vasoactive intestinal polypeptide increases the secretion of the factor and this is inhibited by somatostatin [64]. Two further intriguing observations have been made recently about epidermal growth factor and its receptor. Intestinal goblet cells have been shown to contain a novel proteolytic enzyme [98] that cleaves the growth factor. This would have the effect of shortening it to a 48 amino acid polypeptide which has lost its mitogenic activity but still retains its acid-inhibitory activity [98]. Cell-surface receptors for epidermal growth factor have been characterized [100] and some of these have been shown to have blood group A activity. This implies a high density of non-reducing terminal *N*-acetylgalactosamine residues as would also be present for example in mucus glycoproteins of A secretors. The relationship between epidermal growth factor and its receptor, mucus, and goblet cells is obviously complex but likely to be important in understanding the mechanism of cytoprotection.

Secretory IgA

A further important protein component that is present in mucus secretion is secretory IgA (SIgA). This immunoglobulin exists in two subclasses, namely IgA1 and IgA2. An important difference between them is that the putative hinge region of IgA1 is deleted in IgA2. This is an interesting region in that the polypeptide chain is largely composed of serine, threonine and proline to which is attached a number of *O*-glycosidically linked oligosaccharide units. It must be of significance therefore that one of the immunoglobulin subclasses charged with the protection of mucous membrane itself contains a mucus-like stretch [19].

BIOLOGICAL FUNCTIONS OF MUCUS

The mucus gel layer has evolved to protect the underlying epithelial surface very efficiently. Indeed, so effective is the mucus layer together with its non-immune components in this respect, that the relatively common condition of IgA deficiency [5] is not accompanied in most patients by a marked increase in mucosal infections.

Antidesiccant properties

The overall structure of the gel is determined by the properties of the mucus glycoproteins. These, because of their high carbohydrate content, are very hydrophilic and as a consequence the gel consists of more than 95% water. This means that the mucosal cells are virtually covered by a continuous water layer and this constitutes an important moisturizing or antidesiccant activity on the part of the gel.

Mucus as a physical barrier

Molecular sieve. The long glycoprotein molecules, interacting at intervals, form a mesh-like structure and it is not surprising therefore that mucus has properties that are similar in many ways to those of a gel-permeation or molecular sieve resin. The size of the molecules excluded from the gel has been studied [3] and appears to be quite low, namely in the region of 17 000. In the gut this would have the effect of keeping the various proteolytic enzymes away from the mucosa and also of excluding intact food proteins. However, smaller molecules or those that have been partially digested would be able to enter the gel as would the final products of digestion.

Phase partition. An additional barrier property that the mucus layer may possess, but which is so far largely theoretical, is that of phase partition. This is the tendency for chemically different polymers to segregate into separate aqueous phases [2]. This would have the effect of keeping dissimilar macromolecules out of the mucus phase and such molecules would once again be food proteins and proteolytic enzymes [32]. These properties, namely gel-permeation and phase partition, explain the concept put forward 25 years ago that the mucus layer acts as a diffusion barrier or an unstirred layer [51].

pH gradient

The unstirred layer is exploited by the body in a number of ways, for example by the establishment of a pH gradient across the mucus gel of stomach and duodenum. Both gastric and duodenal epithelium secrete bicarbonate ions which by diffusing through the mucus layer ensure that the fluid in contact with the mucosa is kept at or near neutrality [132, 133]. The mucus glycoproteins of stomach and duodenum may have modified properties to allow bicarbonate diffusion and to enable a pH gradient to be established. Firstly both gastric and duodenal mucus glycoproteins are unusual in that they are largely neutral mucins. Presumably the presence of a large amount of negatively charged sialic acid would interfere with the diffusion of the negatively charged ions and therefore with the establishment of a bicarbonate concentration gradient across the gel. Also the association of lipid with mucus glycoproteins retards in some way the diffusion of hydrogen ions through gastric mucus [114].

Penetration of the mucus layer

The barrier properties of the mucus layer are of course not absolute. Proteolytic enzymes degrade the glycoproteins at the surface and almost certainly penetrate the layer by disrupting the gel structure. However, the layer is renewed from below and the result is a steady movement of the gel from epithelium to lumen counteracting to some extent any penetration by food and other proteins. Indeed, where there is any interaction between proteins and the mucus coat [126] the process will be even more efficient. There is one level in the gut where it is necessary for macromolecules to come into contact with the mucosal surface and that is the epithelium, and in particular the M cells, overlying Peyer's patches [99]. Here the epithelium has reduced numbers of mucus-secreting cells as one would expect from the foregoing discussion.

Trapping of molecules

An important property of the mucus layer therefore is to act as a physical barrier to molecules and particles. However, an equally important function is to actually 'trap' them. This process implies an interaction between the molecules or particles on the one hand and mucin on the other. This interaction can be non-specific or specific. The non-specific interactions are a consequence of the general 'stickiness' of mucus, which can be explained by physicochemical forces such as multiple hydrogen bonding, charged residues and hydrophobic interactions involving the associated lipid.

Bacterial adhesion

The specific associations between microorganisms and mucins are an extension of such interactions at the cell surface. Both viruses and bacteria adhere to structures at the epithelial cell surface as a feature of their pathogenicity [35]. These structures are usually the carbohydrate moieties of glycoproteins or glycolipids. The terminal carbohydrate sequences of these two types of glycoconjugate are structurally similar [110] and are likely therefore to be equally acceptable to a compatible microorganism. Attachment to carbohydrate has been shown for a range of microorganisms including *Escherichia coli* [67, 77, 78], *Mycoplasma pneumoniae* [80], streptococci [94] and many others [35]. Viruses appear to share the same requirement as has been shown with influenza [17], polyoma [48], myxovirus [101] and so on.

The oligosaccharide units of mucus glycoproteins show considerable heterogeneity as has been discussed earlier. Many of the carbohydrate antigens detected at epithelial cell surfaces are also present in mucus glycoproteins. Thus mucin is a mirror of the epithelial surface and so offers spurious carbohydrate attachment sites for microorganisms. Attachment to mucin has been shown for streptococci [75, 131], *Pseudomonas aeruginosa* [109, 129], *Vibrio cholerae* [116] and its toxin [127] and so on. Actually one of the first to observe a specific interaction of this kind was Burnet who in 1951 [14] showed the relationship between influenza virus and 'mucoprotein'. A way that microorganisms could overcome this trapping mechanism is by degrading the mucin structure in their immediate environment. Pathogenic *Shigella flexneri* carries this out by producing glycosidases [106] which attack the oligosaccharide units. An even more effective way would be the production of extracellular proteinases and it may be to compensate for this possibility that proteinases are very effective at increasing the rate of mucus release [9].

Expulsion of intestinal parasites

The role of mucus in the expulsion of intestinal parasites is probably a non-specific mechanism in which immunity plays a part. In previously primed rats, worms are rapidly expelled in a copious secretion of thick mucus (Fig. 10.8). This has been shown with *Nippostrongylus brasiliensis* [89] and *Trichinella spiralis* [6, 73]. Mast cells are active in this process [134] and some of their products may be responsible for mucus secretion.

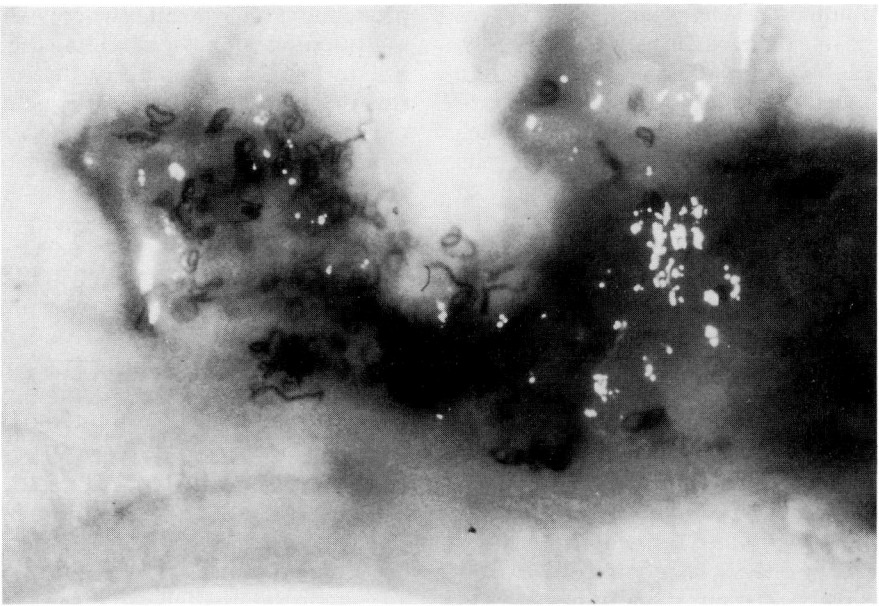

Fig. 10.8 Worms enveloped in thick mucus in the intestine of an immune rat. *Nippostrongylus brasiliensis* caught up in thick viscous mucus 2 hours after challenge in an immune rat. Reproduced with permission from Dr HRP Miller, Moredun Institute, Edinburgh.

Lectins

Lectins have been identified as an important class of food protein that may have toxic effects upon the gastrointestinal tract [46, 95]. Lectins are, by definition, proteins (of non-immune origin) that have a specific binding affinity for monosaccharide residues. They would be expected therefore to bind to the corresponding groupings in mucus glycoproteins. As discussed above, the oligosaccharide units of mucins are very heterogeneous and may have terminal residues of fucose, galactose, N-acetylglucosamine, sialic acid and often N-acetylgalactosamine. Thus mucus glycoproteins present many of the known affinities of lectins.

Peristalsis (the 'waterfall' effect)

The interaction of microorganisms with mucin or indeed of toxins or lectins with mucin would not be a satisfactory protective mechanism unless mucus with its trapped material was being continually removed. This of course is carried out by peristalsis and this process alone, without the assistance of any immune mechanism, appears to be sufficient to prevent colonization by bacteria artificially introduced into the small intestine [28].

Non-mucin components and protection

So far the role of mucus glycoproteins in gastrointestinal protection has been discussed without reference to the other proteins that are present in the secretions. However, these non-mucin components greatly enhance the properties of mucus.

Lysozyme

Lysozyme, for example, is a small protein and can therefore readily enter the mucus gel structure. To retain it within the gel, lysozyme binds to the mucin molecule. Thus susceptible organisms, that is those organisms that have muramic acid-containing cell walls, if they are not trapped during their journey through the mucus gel, are likely to be attacked by lysozyme.

Lactoferrin

Lactoferrin probably plays a complicated role in mucus secretions. Its avidity for iron is such that little free iron remains in solution with the non-saturated protein. Thus at one level lactoferrin is a very effective bacteriostatic agent for iron-requiring microorganisms [13, 36] and this action is enhanced in the presence of SIgA [125]. However, the relationship between mucus, iron, lactoferrin and oxygen radicals may be more complicated. Lactoferrin is secreted by epithelial cells, probably as the apoprotein, and is too large to enter the mucus gel freely. Thus it is likely to remain in the vicinity of the epithelium together with leukocytes such as polymorphs and macrophages [38]. Goblet cells appear to be involved in iron secretion [111] and mucins themselves bind iron [7]. It is possible that a function of lactoferrin is to mop up any free iron in the fluid adjacent to the epithelium, not only for bacteriostasis but also to prevent the catalytic production of hydroxyl radicals [50].

Superoxide

Leukocytes such as polymorphs and macrophages probably produce some active oxygen species non-specifically in contact with particles but this is greatly increased in the presence of triggering microorganisms. Superoxide (or peroxide) diffuses from the site of release but will only produce the powerful oxidizing species, the hydroxyl radical, in the presence of iron. The mucosa is therefore protected, but hydroxyl radicals can be produced within the mucus gel for microbial killing. Excess radicals may be mopped up by the mucus layer itself [26]. In addition the mucus glyco-

protein is cleaved within the polypeptide chain at histidine residues [25]. Thus the mucus gel is liquefied very effectively in the region of superoxide release and subsequent hydroxyl radical production, thereby facilitating the rapid clearance of any contaminated mucus.

Subclasses of IgA

The relationship of the two subclasses of IgA to the mucus gel is not known in detail. IgA does seem to be non-covalently associated with for example, gastric mucus [122] but in that study the subclass of the immunoglobulin fraction was not determined. It is tempting to speculate that SIgA1 with its mucus-like stretch would be the subclass associated with the mucus gel. SIgA2, on the other hand, one would expect to be excluded from the gel and, therefore, to some extent confined to the vicinity of the epithelium. This subdivision of function would be very useful in dealing with pathogenic organisms or toxins by sterically interfering with attachment. In addition there is evidence that SIgA renders bacteria 'mucophilic' [82], and so impedes their progress through the gel. Again this could be a property of SIgA1. A similar process might occur with food proteins where SIgA1 antibodies would render the proteins 'mucophilic' retaining

Table 10.3   A summary of the biological functions of the mucus gel layer in the gut.

1. Lubrication
   To facilitate passage of food in the gut
2. Antidesiccant action
   To retain an aqueous environment at the mucosal surface
3. Protection
   (a) Physical barrier
      (i) Unstirred layer
         To maintain a pH gradient in the stomach and duodenum
      (ii) Gel-permeation or molecular sieve properties
         Molecules larger than about 17 000 tend to be excluded from the gel
      (iii) Phase-partition properties
         Non-mucin-type molecules tend to be excluded from the gel phase
   (b) Biological barrier
      (i) Non-specific trapping
         Particles trapped by general 'stickiness'
      (ii) Specific trapping
         Mucin oligosaccharides mirror the epithelial cell surface and therefore offer spurious attachment sites to lectins, toxins and pathogens etc
      (iii) Lysozyme
         A small bacteriolytic enzyme that can enter the gel and is retained there by interacting with mucin
      (iv) Lactoferrin
         Maintains an iron-free environment at the mucosal surface for bacteriostasis and to prevent catalytic production of hydroxyl radicals
      (v) Secretory IgA
         SIgA1 with its mucus-like stretch associates with gel whereas SIgA2 is excluded
4. Mucus release and clearance
   Triggered by irritants, toxins, lectins, immune complexes, proteolytic enzymes etc. Net flow from epithelium to lumen is therefore increased
5. Food source for colonic microflora

them in the mucus gel to be returned eventually to the lumen.

Summary

All these aspects of the mucus gel layer work in a synergistic fashion to enhance the overall protection of mucosal surfaces. In addition, many of the harmful influences in the gut act as mucus secretagogues. The net flow of mucus from epithelium to lumen is thereby increased counteracting any diffusion of toxic substances through the gel. It must also be remembered that many substances which act as secretagogues appear to stimulate peristalsis. These two processes therefore complement each other to remove the irritant from the vicinity of the mucosa and clear it from the gut.

One important function principally of colonic mucus should be mentioned. The amount of undigested food, particularly nitrogen-containing material, that reaches the colon must be small and variable. Colonic mucus is therefore an important food source for the symbiotic and commensal bacteria that exist in the colon [54, 55, 90, 128].

The various biological functions of the mucus gel layer are summarized in Table 10.3.

REFERENCES

1 Aisen P, Leibman A: Lactoferrin and transferrin: a comparative study. Biochim Biophys Acta 1972; 257: 314–23.

2 Albertson PA: Separation of particles and macromolecules by phase partition. Endeavour 1977; 1 (2): 69–74.

3 Allen A, Bell A, Mantle M, Pearson JP: The structure and physiology of gastrointestinal mucus. Adv Exp Med Biol 1981; 144: 115–33.

4 Altmann GG: Morphological observations on mucus-secreting non-goblet cells in the deep crypts of the rat ascending colon. Am J Anat 1983; 167: 95–117.

5 Bachmann R: Studies on the serum γA-globulin levels. III. The frequency of A-γ A-globulinemia. Scand J Clin Lab Invest 1965; 17: 316–20.

6 Bell RG, Adams LS, Ogden RW: Intestinal mucus trapping in the rapid expulsion of *Trichinella spiralis* by rats. Induction and expression analyzed by quantitative worm recovery. Infect Immun 1984; 45: 267–72.

7 Bella A, Kim YS: Iron binding of gastric mucins. Biochim Biophys Acta 1973; 304: 580–5.

8 Bickel M: Effect of 16,16-dimethyl-prostaglandin E_2 on gastric mucus gel thickness. Prostaglandins 1981; 21: 63–5.

9 Boat TF, Cheng PW, Klinger JD et al: Proteinases release mucin from airways goblet cells. Ciba Found Symp 1984; 109: 72–88.

10 Bolton JP, Palmer D, Cohen MM: Stimulation of mucus and non-parietal cell secretion by the E_2 prostaglandins. Am J Dig Dis 1978; 23: 359–64.

11 Bradbury JE, Black JW, Wyllie JH: Stimulation of colonic mucus output. Gut 1979; 20: A444–5.

12 Bradbury JE, Black JW, Wyllie JH: Stimulation of mucus output from rat colon in vivo. Eur J Pharmacol 1980; 68: 417–25.

13 Bullen JJ, Rogers HJ, Leigh L: Iron-binding proteins in milk and resistance to *Escherichia coli* infection in infants. Br Med J 1972; i: 69–75.

14 Burnet FM: Mucoproteins in relation to virus action. Physiol Rev 1951; 31: 131–50.

15 Camilleri M, Murphy R, Chadwick VS: Pharmacological inhibition of chenodeoxycholate-induced fluid and mucus secretion and mucosal injury in the rat colon. Dig Dis Sci 1982; 27: 865–9.

16 Carlstedt I, Sheehan JK: Is the macromolecular architecture of cervical, respiratory and gastric mucins the same? Biochem Soc Trans 1984; 12: 615–17.

17 Carroll SM, Higa HH, Paulson JC: Different cell-surface receptor determinants of antigenically similar influenza virus haemagglutinins. J Biol Chem 1981; 256: 8357–63.

18 Chantler E: Structure and function of cervical mucus. Adv Exp Med Biol 1982; 144: 251–63.

19 Clamp JR: The relationship between secretory immunoglobublin A and mucus. Biochem Soc Trans 1977; 5: 1579–81.

20 Clamp JR, Creeth JM: Some non-mucin components of mucus and their possible biological roles. Ciba Found Symp 1984; 109: 121–136.

21 Clamp JR, Allan A, Gibbons RA, Roberts GP: Chemical aspects of mucus. Br Med Bull 1978; 34 (1): 25–41.

22 Clamp JR, Cooper B, Creeth JM et al: The presence of polysaccharide in normal human gastric mucus. Biochem J 1983; 215: 421–3.

23 Creeth JM, Cooper B: Studies on the molecular weight distributions of two mucins. Biochem Soc Trans 1984; 12: 618–21.

24 Creeth JM, Bridge JL, Horton JR: An interaction between lysozyme and mucus glycoproteins. Implications for density-gradient separations. Biochem J 1979; 181: 717–24.

25 Creeth JM, Cooper B, Donald ASR, Clamp JR: Studies on the limited degradation of mucus glycoproteins. The effect of dilute hydrogen peroxide. Biochem J 1983; 211: 323–32.

26 Cross CE, Halliwell B, Allen A: Antioxidant protection: a function of tracheobronchial and gastrointestinal mucus. Lancet 1984; i: 1328–30.

27 Culling CF, Reid PE, Dunn WL, Clay MG: Histochemical comparison of the epithelial mucins in the ileum in Crohn's disease and in normal controls. J Clin Pathol 1977; 30: 1063–7.

28 Dixon JMS: The fate of bacteria in the small intestine. J Pathol Bacteriol 1960; 79: 131–40.

29 Doidge JM, Millar SJ, Yeomans ND: Changes in volume of stored mucus in pit and surface cells during their maturation and migration in the antral mucosa of the mouse. Cell Tissue Res 1982; 227: 459–63.

30 Domschke W, Domschke S, Hornig D, Demling L:

Prostaglandin-stimulated gastric mucus secretion in man. Acta Hepatogastroenterol 1978; 25: 292-4.

31 Donald ASR, Yates AD, Soh CPC et al: The human blood-group-Sd^a determinant: a terminal non-reducing carbohydrate structure in N-linked and mucin-type glycoproteins. Biochem Soc Trans 1984; 12: 596-9.

32 Edwards PAW: Is mucus a selective barrier to macromolecules? Br Med Bull 1978; 34 (1): 55-6.

33 Elder JB, Williams G, Lacey E, Gregory H: Cellular localisation of human urogastrone/epidermal growth factor. Nature 1978; 271: 466-7.

34 Elder JB, Ganguli PC, Gillespie IE et al: Effect of urogastrone on gastric secretion and plasma gastrin levels in normal subjects. Gut 1975; 16: 887-93.

35 Elliott K, O'Connor M, Whelan J, eds: Adhesion and microorganism pathogenicity. Ciba Found Symp 1981: 80: 1-346.

36 Emery T: Iron deprivation as a biological defence mechanism. Nature 1980; 287: 776-7.

37 Feizi T, Gooi HC, Childs RA et al: Tumour-associated and differentiation antigens on the carbohydrate moieties of mucin-type glycoproteins. Biochem Soc Trans 1984; 12: 591-6.

38 Ferguson A: Mast cells and other reactive cells in the gut. Hosp Update 1984; 10: 371-83.

39 Filipe MI: Mucins in the human gastrointestinal epithelium: a review. Invest Cell Pathol 1979; 2: 195-216.

40 Filipe MI, Fenger C: Histochemical characteristics of mucins in the small intestine. A comparative study of normal mucosa, benign epithelial tumours and carcinoma. Histochem J 1979; 11: 277-87.

41 Fleming A: On a remarkable bacteriolytic element found in tissues and secretions. Proc R Soc Lond B 1922; 93: 306-17.

42 Flemstron G, Garner A: Gastroduodenal HCO$_3$-transport: characteristics and proposed role in acidity regulation and mucosal protection. Am J Physiol 1982; 242: G183-93.

43 Flemstron G, Garner A, Nylander O et al: Surface epithelial HCO$_3^-$ transport by mammalian duodenum in vivo. Am J Physiol 1982; 243: G348-58.

44 Florey HW: Mucin and the protection of the body. Proc R Soc Lond B 1955; 143: 147-58.

45 Florey HW: Electron microscopic observations on goblet cells of the rat colon. Q J Exp Physiol 1960; 45: 329-36.

46 Freed DLJ: Lectins. Br Med J 1985; 290: 584-5.

47 Freed DLJ, Buckley CH: Mucotractive effect of lectin. Lancet 1978; i: 585-6.

48 Fried H, Cahan LD, Paulson JC: Polyoma virus recognises specific sialyloligosaccharide receptors on host cells. Virology 1981; 109: 188-92.

49 Gibbons RA: Mucus of the mammalian genital tract. Br Med Bull 1978; 34 (1): 34-8.

50 Gutteridge JMC, Rowley DA, Halliwell B: Superoxide-dependent formation of hydroxyl radicals in the presence of iron salts. Detection of 'free' iron in biological systems by using bleomycin-dependent degradation of DNA. Biochem J 1981; 199: 263-5.

51 Heatley NG: Mucosubstance as a barrier to diffusion. Gastroenterology 1959; 37: 313-7.

52 Hollenberg MD: Epidermal growth factor-urogastrone, a polypeptide acquiring hormonal status. Vitam Horm Adv Res Applic 1979; 37: 69-110.

53 Holy FJ, Lemp MA: Tear physiology and dry eyes. Surv Ophthalmol 1977; 22: 69-87.

54 Hoskins LC: Human enteric population ecology and degradation of gut mucins. Dig Dis Sci 1981; 26: 769-72.

55 Hoskins LC, Boulding ET: Mucin degradation in human colon ecosystems—evidence for the existence and role of bacterial subpopulations producing glycosidases and extracellular enzymes. J Clin Invest 1981; 67: 163-72.

56 Hounsell EF, Feizi T: Gastrointestinal mucins: structures and antigenicities of their carbohydrate chains in health and disease. Med Biol 1952; 60: 227-36.

57 Ivy AC, Oyama Y: Studies on the secretion of the pars pylorica gastri. Am J Physiol 1921; 57: 51-60.

58 Jabball I, Kells DI, Forstner G, Forstner J: Human intestinal goblet cell mucin. Can J Biochem 1976; 54: 707-16.

59 Johansson C, Aly A: Stimulation of gastric mucus output by somatostatin in man. Eur J Clin Invest 1982; 12: 37-9.

60 Jolles P: Lysozyme: a chapter of molecular biology. Angew Chem Int Edn 1969; 8: 227-94.

61 Jones R, Reid L: Secretory cells and their glycoproteins in health and disease. Br Med Bull 1978; 34 (1): 9-16.

62 Kerss S, Allen A, Garner A: A simple method for measuring thickness of the mucus gel layer adherent to rat, frog and human gastric mucosa: influences of feeding, prostaglandin, N-acetylcysteine and other agents. Clin Sci 1982; 63: 187-95.

63 Kirkegaard P, Olsen PS, Poulsen SS, Nexo E: Epidermal growth factor inhibits cysteamine-induced duodenal ulcer. Gastroenterology 1983; 85: 1277-83.

64 Kirkegaard P, Olsen PS, Nexo E et al: Effect of vasoactive intestinal polypeptide and somatostatin on secretion of epidermal growth factor and bicarbonate from Brunner's glands. Gut 1984; 25: 1225-9.

65 Klinger JD, Tandler B, Liedtke CM, Boat TF: Proteinases of *Pseudomonas aeruginosa* evoke mucin release by tracheal epithelium. J Clin Invest 1984; 74: 1669-78.

66 Konturek SJ, Radecki T, Brzozowski T et al: Gastric cytoprotection by epidermal growth factor. Gastroenterology 1981; 81: 438-43.

67 Korhonen TK, Vaisanen-Rhen V, Rhen M et al: *Escherichia coli* fimbriae recognising sialyl galactosides. J Bacteriol 1984; 159: 762-6.

68 Kurasumi K, Shibuichi I, Tosaka H: Ultrastructural studies on the secretory mechanism of goblet cells in the rat jejunal epithelium. Arch Histol Jpn 1981; 44: 263-84.

69 Lake AM, Bloch KJ, Neutra MR, Walker WA: Intestinal goblet cell mucus release. II. In vivo stimulation by antigen in the immunized rat. J Immunol 1979; 122: 834-7.

70 Lake AM, Bloch KJ, Sinclair KJ, Walker WA: Anaphylactic release of intestinal goblet cell mucus. Immunology 1980; 39: 173-8.

71 Lamblin G, Lhermitte M, Klein A et al: Carbohydrate chains from human bronchial mucus glycoproteins: a wide spectrum of oligosaccharide structures. Biochem Soc Trans 1984; 12: 599-600.

72 LaMont JT, Ventola A: Synthesis and secretion of colonic glycoproteins. Evidence for shedding in vivo of low molecular weight membrane components. Biochim Biophys Acta 1980; 629: 553-65.

73 Lee GB, Ogilvie BM: The intestinal mucus barrier to parasites and bacteria. Adv Exp Med Biol 1982; 144: 247-8.

74 Lev R: The histochemistry of mucus-producing cells

in the normal and diseased gastrointestinal mucosa. Prog Gastroenterol 1970; 2: 13–41.

75 Levine MJ, Carese JM, Prakobphol A et al: Adherence of *Streptococcus sanguis* to salivary mucin bound to glass. J Dent Res 1982; 61: 1390–3.

76 Lewin MR, El Masri SH, Clark CG: Effects of bile acids on mucus secretion in the dog colon. Eur Surg Res 1979; 11: 392–9.

77 Lindahl M, Wadstrom T: Terminal *N*-acetylgalactosamine and sialic acid residues are recognised by the K99 surface haemagglutinin of enterotoxigenic *E. coli*. IRCS Med Sci Biochem 1983; 11: 790–1.

78 Lindahl M, Wadstrom T: K99 surface haemagglutinin of enterotoxigenic *E. coli* recognise terminal *N*-acetylgalactosamine and sialic acid residues of glycophorin and other complex glycoconjugates. Vet Microbiol 1984; 9: 249–58.

79 Lloyd KO, Kabat EA: Immunochemical studies on blood groups. XLI. Proposed structures for the carbohydrate portions of blood groups A, B, H, Lewis[a] and Lewis[b] substances. Proc Natl Acad Sci USA 1968; 61: 1470–7.

80 Loomes LM, Uemura K, Childs RA et al: Erythrocyte receptors for *Mycoplasma pneumoniae* are sialylated oligosaccharides of Ii antigen type. Nature 1984; 307: 560–3.

81 McQueen S, Allen A, Garner A: Measurement of gastric and duodenal mucus gel thickness. In: Allen A, Flemstron G, Garner A et al, eds. Mechanisms of mucosal protection in the upper gastrointestinal tract. New York: Raven Press, 1984; 215–21.

82 Magnusson KE, Stjernstrom I: Mucosal barrier mechanisms. Interplay between secretory IgA (SIgA), IgG and mucins on the surface properties and association of *Salmonellae* with intestine and granulocytes. Immunology 1982; 45: 239–48.

83 Mahoney JM, Waterbury LD: The effect of orally administered prostaglandins on gastric mucus secretion in the rat. Prostaglandins Med 1981; 7: 101–7.

84 Mantle M, Mantle D, Allen A: Polymeric structure of pig small intestinal mucus glycoprotein. Dissociation by proteolysis or by reduction of disulphide bridges. Biochem J 1981; 195: 277–85.

85 Mantle M, Pearson J, Allen A: Pig gastric and small-intestinal mucus glycoproteins: proposed role in polymeric structure for protein joined by disulphide bridges. Biochem Soc Trans 1980; 8: 715–6.

86 Marom Z, Shelhamer JH, Kaliner M: Human pulmonary macrophage-derived mucus secretagogue. J Exp Med 1984; 159: 844–60.

87 Marshall T, Allen A: The isolation and characterisation of the high molecular glycoprotein from pig colonic mucus. Biochem J 1978; 173: 569–78.

88 Mason DY, Taylor CR: Distribution of transferrin, ferritin and lactoferrin in human tissues. J Clin Pathol 1978; 32: 316–27.

89 Miller HRP, Huntley JF, Wallace GR: Immune exclusion and mucus trapping during the rapid expulsion of *Nippostrongylus brasiliensis* from primed rats. Immunology 1981; 44: 419–29.

90 Miller RS, Hoskins LC: Mucin degradation in human colonic ecosystems. Fecal population densities of mucin-degrading bacteria estimated by a 'most probable number' method. Gastroenterology 1981; 81: 759–65.

91 Montero C, Erlandsen SL: Immunocytochemical and histochemical studies on intestinal epithelial cells producing both lysozyme and mucosubstance. Anat Rec 1978; 190: 127–41.

92 Moon HW, Whipp SC, Baetz AL: Comparative effects of enterotoxins from *Escherichia coli* and *Vibrio cholerae* on rabbit and swine small intestine. Lab Invest 1971; 25: 133–40.

93 Moore JC, Tiffany JM: Human ocular mucus. Origins and preliminary characterization. Exp Eye Res 1979; 29: 291–301.

94 Murray PA, Levine MJ, Tabak LA, Reddy MS: Specificity of salivary-bacterial interactions. II. Evidence for a lectin on *Streptococcus sanguis* with specificity for a NeuAcα2,3Galβ1,3GalNAc sequence. Biochem Biophys Res Commun 1982; 106: 390–6.

95 Nachbar MS, Oppenheim JD: Lectins in the US diet: a survey of lectins in commonly consumed foods and a review of the literature. Am J Clin Nutr 1980; 33: 2338–45.

96 Neutra MR, O'Malley LJ, Specian RD: Regulation of intestinal goblet cell secretion. II. A survey of potential secretagogues. Am J Physiol 1982; 242: G380–7.

97 Neutra MR, Phillips TL, Phillips TE: Regulation of intestinal goblet cells in situ, in mucosal explants and in the isolated epithelium. Ciba Found Symp 1984; 109: 20–39.

98 Nexo E, Poulsen SS, Hansen SN et al: Characterisation of a novel proteolytic enzyme localised to goblet cells in rat and man. Gut 1984; 24: 656–64.

99 Owen RL: And now pathophysiology of M cells—good news and bad news from Peyer's patches. Gastroenterology 1983; 85: 468–70.

100 Parker PJ, Young S, Gullick WJ et al: Monoclonal antibodies against the human epidermal growth factor receptor from A431 cells. Isolation, characterization and use in the purification of active epidermal growth factor receptor. J Biol Chem 1984; 259: 9906–12.

101 Paulson JC, Sadler JE, Hill RL: Restoration of specific myxovirus receptors to asialo-erythrocytes by incorporation of sialic acid with pure sialotransferases. J Biol Chem 1979; 254: 2120–4.

102 Pearson JP, Allen A, Parry S: A 70 000-molecular weight protein isolated from purified pig gastric mucus glycoprotein by reduction of disulphide bridges and its implication in the polymeric structure. Biochem J 1981; 197: 155–62.

103 Pearson J, Allen A, Venables C: Gastric mucus: isolation and polymeric structure of the undegraded glycoprotein: its breakdown by pepsin. Gastroenterology 1980; 78: 709–15.

104 Ponder BAJ, Schmidt GH, Wilkinson MM et al: Derivation of mouse intestinal crypts from single progenitor cells. Nature 1985; 313: 689–91.

105 Porter R, Rivers J, O'Connor M, eds: Respiratory tract mucus 1978. Ciba Found Symp 1978; 54: 1–334.

106 Prizont R: Degradation of intestinal glycoproteins by pathogenic *Shigella flexneri*. Infect Immun 1982; 36: 615–20.

107 Querinjean P, Masson PL, Heremans JF: Molecular weight, single-chain structure and amino acid composition of human lactoferrin. Eur J Biochem 1971; 20: 420–5.

108 Rall LB, Scott J, Bell GI et al: Mouse prepro-epidermal growth factor synthesis by the kidney and other tissues. Nature 1985; 313: 228–31.

109 Ramphal R, Pyle M: Evidence for mucins and sialic acid as receptors for *Pseudomonas aeruginosa* in the lower respiratory tract. Infect Immun 1983; 41: 339–44.

110 Rauvala H, Finne J: Structural similarity of the terminal carbohydrate sequences of glycoproteins and glycolipids. FEBS Lett 1979; 97: 1–8.

111 Refsum SB, Schreiner B: Iron excretion from the goblet cells of the small intestine in man. An additional regulatory mechanism in iron homeostasis? Scand J Gastroenterol 1980; 15: 1013-20.

112 Reid L, Clamp JR: The biochemical and histochemical nomenclature of mucus. Br Med Bull 1978; 34 (1): 5-8.

113 Sakata T, Von Engelhardt W: Luminal mucin in the large intestine of mice, rats and guinea pigs. Cell Tissue Res 1981; 219: 629-35.

114 Sarosiek J, Slomiany A, Takagi A, Slomiany BL: Hydrogen ion diffusion in dog gastric mucus glycoprotein. Effect of associated lipids and covalently bound fatty acids. Biochem Biophys Res Commun 1984; 118: 523-31.

115 Schauer R: Chemistry, metabolism and biological function of sialic acids. Adv Carbohydr Chem Biochem 1982; 40: 131-234.

116 Schrank GD, Verwey WF: Distribution of cholera organisms in experimental *Vibrio cholerae* infections: proposed mechanisms of pathogenesis and antibacterial immunity. Infect Immun 1976; 13: 195-203.

117 Sheahan DC, Jervis HR: Comparative histochemistry of gastrointestinal mucosubstances. Am J Anat 1976; 146: 103-32.

118 Sherr HP, Mertens RB, Broock R: Cholera toxin-induced glycoprotein secretion in rabbit small intestine. Gastroenterology 1979; 77: 18-25.

119 Slomiany BL, Zdebska E, Slomiany A: Structural characterization of neutral oligosaccharides of human H^+Le^{b+} gastric mucin. J Biol Chem 1984; 259: 2863-9.

120 Slomiany A, Slomiany BL, Witas H et al: Isolation of fatty acids covalently bound to the gastric mucus glycoprotein of normal and cystic fibrosis patients. *Biochem Biophys Res Commun* 1983; 113: 286-93.

121 Specian RD, Neutra MR: Mechanism of rapid mucus secretion in goblet cells stimulated by acetylcholine. J Cell Biol 1980; 85: 626-40.

122 Spohn M, McColl I: Studies on gastric mucosal IgA: separation of immunoglobulin rich fraction from gastric mucoproteins. Biochem Biophys Res Commun 1977; 79: 837-42.

123 Stanley RA, Lee SP, Robertson AM: Heterogeneity in gastrointestinal mucins. Biochim Biophys Acta 1983; 760: 262-9.

124 Steinberg SE, Banwell JG, Yardley JH et al: Comparison of secretory and histological effects of *Shigella* and *Cholera* enterotoxins in rabbit jejunum. Gastroenterology 1975; 68: 309.

125 Stephens S, Dolby JM, Montreuil J, Spik G: Differences in inhibition of the growth of commensal and enteropathogenic strains of *Escherichia coli* by lacto-ferrin and secretory immunoglubulin A isolated from human milk. Immunology 1980; 41: 597-603.

126 Stern M, Pang KY, Walker WA: Food proteins and gut mucosal barrier. Differential interaction of cows milk proteins with the mucous coat and the surface membrane of adult and immature rat jejunum. Pediatr Res 1984; 18: 1252-6.

127 Strombeck DR, Harrold D: Binding of cholera toxin to mucins and inhibition by gastric mucin. Infect Immun 1974; 10: 1266-72.

128 Variyam EP, Hoskins LC: Mucin degradation in human colon ecosystems. Degradation of hog gastric mucin by fecal extracts and fecal cultures. Gastroenterology 1981; 81: 751-8.

129 Vishwanath S, Ramphal R: Adherence of *Pseudomonas aeruginosa* to human tracheobronchial mucin. Infect Immun 1984; 45: 197-202.

130 Walker WA, Wu M, Bloch KJ: Simulation by immune complexes of mucus release from goblet cells of the rat small intestine. Science 1977; 197: 370-2.

131 Williams RC, Gibbons WJ: Inhibition of streptococcal attachment to receptors on human buccal epithelial cells by antigenically similar salivary glycoproteins. Infect Immun 1975; 11: 711-8.

132 Williams SE, Turnberg LA: Retardation of acid diffusion by pig gastric mucus: a potential role in mucosal protection. Gastroenterology 1980; 79: 299-304.

133 Williams SE, Turnberg LA: Demonstration of a pH gradient across mucus adherent to rabbit gastric mucosa—evidence for a mucus-bicarbonate barrier. Gut 1981; 22: 94-6.

134 Woodbury RG, Miller HRP, Huntley JF, et al: Mucosal mast cells are functionally active during spontaneous expulsion of intestinal nematode infections in rat. Nature 1984; 312: 450-2.

135 Wright NA: Role of mucosal cell renewal in mucosal protection in the gastrointestinal tract. In: Allen A, Flemstrom G, Garner A et al eds. Mechanisms of mucosal protection in the upper gastrointestinal tract. New York: Raven Press, 1984; 15-20.

136 Yardley JH, Bayless TM, Leubbers EH et al: Goblet cell mucus in the small intestine. Findings after net fluid production due to cholera toxin and hypertonic solutions. Johns Hopkins Med J 1972; 131: 1-10.

137 Zalewsky CA, Moody FG: Mechanisms of mucus release in exposed canine gastric mucosa. Gastroenterology 1979; 77: 719-29.

138 Zalewsky CA, Moody FG, Allen M, Davis EK: Stimulation of canine gastric mucus secretion with intra-arterial acetylcholine chloride. Gastroenterology 1983; 85: 1067-75.

SECTION D
ANTIGEN HANDLING

Chapter 11
Role of the Mucosal Barrier in Antigen Handling by the Gut

W. Allan Walker

Introduction

Since the principal function of the gastro-intestinal tract is digestion and absorption of nutrients, it is assumed that intraluminal protein antigens are completely digested, thus preventing their appreciable transport across the epithelium into the lamina propria or systemic circulation. Despite this notion, there is increasing experimental and clinical evidence to suggest that large antigenically active molecules can penetrate the intestinal epithelial surface, not in sufficient quantities to be of nutritional importance, but in quantities that may be of immunological importance [31, 49, 72, 77]. This observation could mean that the intestinal tract represents a potential site for the absorption of bacterial breakdown products such as endotoxins and enterotoxins, of proteolytic and hydrolytic enzymes or of ingested food antigens that normally exist in the intestinal lumen, and therefore might be of considerable importance in the pathogenesis of a number of immunologically mediated gastrointestinal disease states.

This topic is reviewed in an attempt to bring the immunologist and allergist up to date on our current understanding of small intestinal permeability to antigens and to underscore the potential importance of excessive large molecular absorption in mechanisms of clinical disease. Since the vast majority of mammals show no ill-effects from a limited intestinal permeability to large molecules, it seems likely that some additional alteration must take place in intraluminal or membrane factors controlling permeability of macromolecules before the process results in clinical disease. Therefore, factors (immunological, mucosal and intraluminal) which contribute to the physiological control of antigen uptake will be reviewed and the circumstances in which pathological (excessive) penetration of antigens occur will be considered. The scope of this topic will focus on available human studies. However, when pertinent, studies on experimental animals will be cited but details can be obtained from additional comprehensive reviews in the references (see also Chapter 16).

CONCEPT OF THE MUCOSAL BARRIER

As a result of a variety of recent observations [75], it is now apparent that non-immunological processes working independently and in concert with the local mucosal immune system collectively comprise an effective barrier, 'the mucosal barrier', to the attachment and penetration of antigens, microorganisms and toxins present in the intraluminal environment. Table 11.1 lists some of these processes which comprise the mucosal barrier.

Table 11.1 Representative components of the mucosal barrier to microorganisms/toxins.

Non-immunological
  Intraluminal
    gastric barrier
    proteolysis
    peristalsis
  Mucosal surface
    mucous coat
    microvillus membrane

Immunological
  Secretory IgA system

Combination of immunological and non-immunological
  Immune complex-mediated goblet cell mucus release
  Immune complex-facilitated mucosal surface
    proteolysis
  Kupffer cell phagocytosis of immune complexes

Non-immunological components of the mucosal barrier

Gastric function

Gastric acidity represents an important deterrent to the colonization of the upper small in-

testine by gram-positive organisms present in the oral cavity. Kraft et al reported increasing amounts of bovine serum albumin (BSA) antibodies in adults with achlorhydria and suggested that these individuals do not adequately hydrolyse the common food antigen BSA in the stomach [43]; the BSA may therefore be present in greater concentrations for absorption by the small intestine. Bloch et al [7] demonstrated increased macromolecular transport when bicarbonate was administered with antigen (BSA) to neutralize gastric acidity. Presumably, the neutralization of gastric pH retarded the initiation of protein digestion by pepsin and so increased amounts of antigen were available for release into the small intestine.

Intestinal proteolysis

Proteolytic activity in the small intestine also determines to an extent the composition of microbial surface factors, enterotoxins and antigens and may contribute to their capacity to attach to and penetrate the microvillus surface. Walker et al have shown that the breakdown of ^{125}I-labelled BSA by jejunal gut sacs from pancreatic duct-ligated rats is significantly decreased in comparison to sham-operated controls [80]. In addition, feeding of pancreatic extracts to rats with pancreatic duct ligations prior to removal of the small intestine for gut-sac experiments leads to an increase in digestion of ^{125}I-labelled BSA by in vitro gut sacs. These findings suggest that pancreatic enzymes absorbed onto the surface of the intestine contribute to the proteolysis of antigens.

More recently, Saffron et al [64] administered lysine vasopressin (LVP) by gavage to rats simultaneously with the trypsin inhibitor aprotinin and noted an increased physiological effect of the hormone (antidiuretic effect) in these animals compared to control animals given LVP alone. This finding extends the earlier in vitro studies of Walker et al [80] and demonstrates that in vivo inhibition of pancreatic enzymes leads to increased amounts of vasopressin being transported across the intestine and into the bloodstream. Similar processes may be controlling bacterial entero- and endotoxin penetration.

Peristalsis

In order for microorganisms to adhere to appropriate receptors on the microvillus surface, they must come in direct contact with the receptor. The longer the time taken for diffusion through the mucous coat and for attachment to carbohydrate receptors on the microvillus membrane, the more likely it is that microorganisms will attach and colonize the gastrointestinal tract. Rhythmic movement of the small and large intestine in the form of smooth muscle contraction (peristalsis) acts to regulate bacterial attachment and colonization. In the presence of antibodies attached to the mucous coat forming complexes with bacteria the process is further enhanced. In an elegant study to demonstrate the phenomenon, Pang et al [57] provided evidence that antigen–antibody formation in the mucous coat coupled with peristalsis resulted in rapid expulsion of antigens from the small intestine.

Mucous coat

The thickness and composition of the mucous coat overlying the microvillus surface contributes to the defence of mucosal surfaces against toxins and bacterial attachment and penetration. With an increase of goblet cell mucus discharge into the mucosal surface the physical thickness of the mucous coat can increase providing a more extensive barrier to diffusion of microorganisms from the lumen to the microvillus surface. This enhanced thickness of the mucous coat may be a contributing factor in the expulsion phenomenon for parasites described by Miller and Nawa [50].

Another protective property of mucus is related to the observation that microorganisms can attach to carbohydrate moieties (receptors) of glycoprotein components of the microvillus surface. Examples of this phenomenon are the mannose receptor [10] for *Escherichia coli* and the fucose receptor for *Vibrio cholera* [38]. Recent studies from our laboratories (Snyder and Walker, unpublished results) and other studies [30] suggest that mucus may contain carbohydrate moieties which can act as receptor inhibitors thereby specifically interfering with the attachment of microorganisms to the microvillus surface. Interference of bacterial attachment by carbohydrate mucus inhibitors provides evidence for a specific protection against bacterial penetration. Additional studies in this are are needed to further delineate this process.

Membrane composition

The composition of the intestinal cell membrane changes as the epithelial cell migrates up the villus [26, 59, 61] and as the animal ages [26, 47, 70]. Changes in membrane composition may determine whether bacteria or toxins bind to the cell. Bresson et al [13] have studied isolated microvillus membranes from the intestine of newborn and adult rabbits. They have shown that the membrane protein/phospholipid ratio is dramatically decreased in newborn membranes compared with those of adults. In addition, they noted increased cholera enterotoxin binding to newborn microvillus membranes compared with those of adults. These studies of the development of the intestinal surface may help us to understand better why antigen transport is greater early in life and why newborn infants have a high incidence of infectious diarrhoea. In recent studies, a direct association between maturity of the microvillus membrane and antigen attachment has been demonstrated (Fig. 11.1) [68].

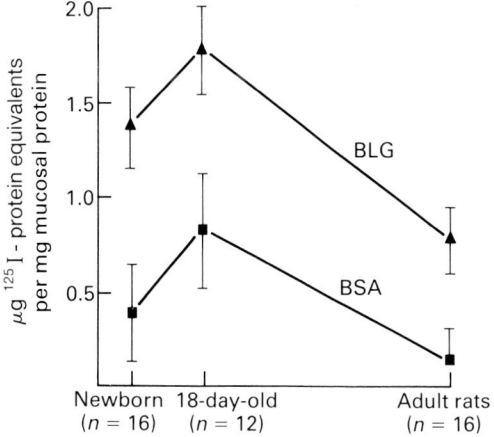

Fig. 11.1 Binding of ^{125}I-labelled BSA and β-lactoglobulin (BLG) by the jejunal microvillus membrane in the rat, showing the effect of maturity. Numbers of experiments are given in parentheses. Means $\pm$ 1 SD are shown. Protein concentration of BSA and BLG 0.1 mg/ml; microvillus membrane protein concentration 1.5 mg/ml. Differences in binding between immature and adult groups are statistically highly significant ($P < 0.001$) for both proteins. Reproduced from [68], with kind permission of the editor of *Pediatric Research*.

Immunological components of the mucosal barrier

IgA

The adequacy of immune function in the gastrointestinal tract affects the attachment and penetration of bacteria and toxins. IgA is the immunoglublulin present in highest concentration in intestinal secretions [16,54]. It has been postulated that this immunoglobulin prevents the transport of microbes, antigens and toxins by complexing with them in the lumen or within the mucous coat, thereby impeding absorption [75,78]. The concentration of IgA in saliva, stool and serum of newborn animals and humans [1,14,30,65] is decreased, and it has been hypothesized that this transient deficiency in part accounts for the increased transport of antigens, and presumably bacteria attachment, in newborn animals.

Selective IgA deficiency. This hypothesis is supported by studies of patients with selective IgA deficiency. These patients have circulating immune complexes and precipitating antibodies to adsorbed bovine milk proteins [21] (see Chapter 12). Again, when the serum of IgA-deficient individuals was studied for the appearance of complexes after milk ingestion, three of seven subjects had increases in anti-

body–antigen complexes, which peaked at 120–150 minutes [22]. In another three subjects, there was a tendency towards the formation of two peak concentrations of complexes, the first at 30–60 minutes and the second at 120–150 minutes after drinking milk. Additionally, the circulating immune complexes found in some patients contained bovine milk proteins. Presumably the same process occurs in the transient IgA deficiency of the newborn as a contributing factor in the increased incidence of necrotizing enterocolitis, a bacterial invasive disease occurring during infancy and in the increased incidence of microbial infections (giardiasis, toxigenic diarrhoea) occurring in selective IgA-deficient patients.

Antigen access to lymphoid tissue

Another important component of mucosal immunity is the access of intestinal antigens to

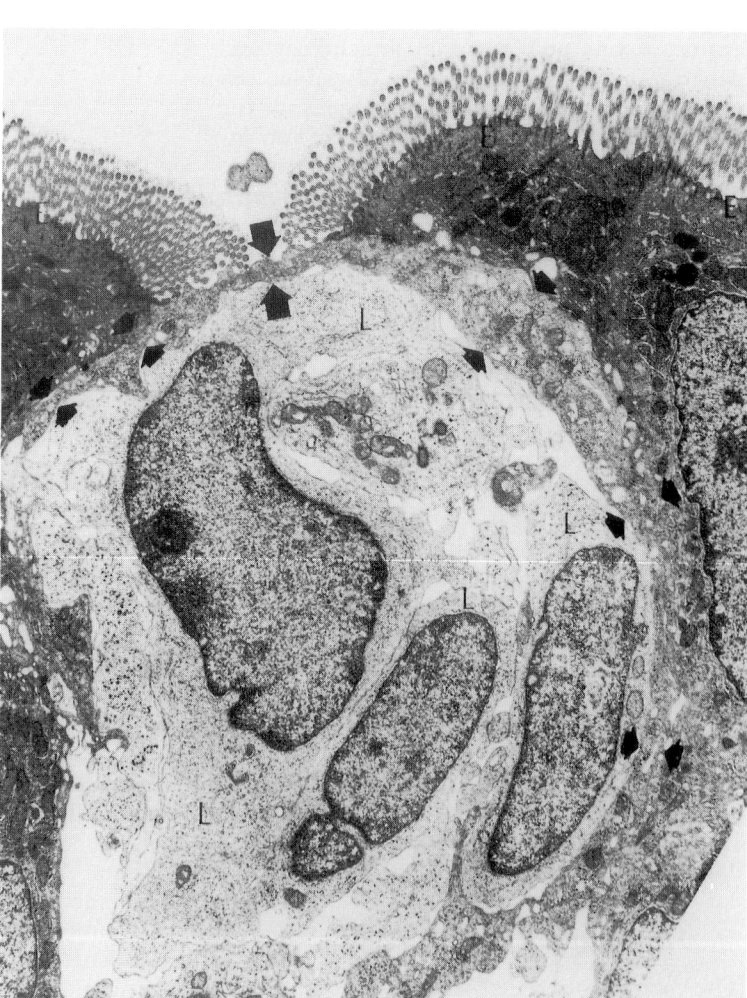

Fig. 11.2 Transmission electron micrograph from the non-columnar region of the Peyer's patch epithelium of the small intestine showing a cross-sectional view of the apex of an M cell, associated microvillus-covered epithelial cells (E) and at least three lymphoid cells (L). Note the attenuated cytoplasm of the M cells (between arrows) that bridges the surface between microvillus-covered cells, forming tight junctions with them and producing a barrier between the lymphoid cells and the intestinal lumen. Reproduced from [55], with kind permission of Elsevier Science Publishing Co., Inc. Copyright 1977 by The American Gastroenterological Association.

lymphoid elements in Peyer's patches, a necessary first step in the secretory IgA cycle [78] (see Chapter 9). Owen and Jones [56] and Owen [55] have demonstrated that macromolecular protein antigens can also traverse the epithelial barrier of the intestine. This occurs in the distal small intestine via specialized M cells overlying Peyer's patches. Electron microscopical studies of these cells indicate that they have few microvilli, a poorly developed glycocalyx and an absence of lysosomal organelles (Fig. 11.2) [55, 56] (see Chapter 4). Using electron microscopy, Owen has observed uptake and processing of horseradish peroxidase by M cells. The marker is first taken up by these specialized cells and then extruded into an extracellular space, where it is phagocytosed by lymphoid cells circulating through Peyer's patches [55, 56].

This type of antigen absorption in the gut has not yet been shown to occur via receptors, but nonetheless appears to represent an important access route for ingested antigen, bacteria and viruses [85] to reach lymphoid tissues and thereby stimulate the local and distant immune system. More research is needed to define the composition of the M cell membrane surface and to determine if composition is important in microbial attachment.

Combined effect of immunological and non-immunological components of the mucosal barrier

Several recent observations have suggested that the local immune process can augment the protective capacity of the previously mentioned non-immunological protective components of the mucosal barrier. Representative examples can be used to illustrate this phenomenon.

Enhanced proteolysis

In previous work Walker et al [79, 80] reported that proteolysis of intestinal antigens was considerably greater in immunized animals than in non-immunized controls and that enhanced proteolysis most likely resulted from the interaction of immune complexes present in the mucous coat with pancreatic enzymes adsorbed onto the surface of the intestine after secretion into the lumen. Fig. 11.3 illustrates our concept of this augmented protective process.

Mucin release

Another example of combined protection is the enhanced discharge of goblet cell mucin occurring in intestinal anaphylaxis as reported by Lake et al [44]. Using radiolabelled goblet cell mucus to quantitate release, he showed that IgE-mediated mast cell discharge of histamine resulted in enhanced goblet cell mucus release into the intestinal tract. This observation probably explains the mucous coat expulsion phenomenon of parasites described by Miller and Nawa [50] as discussed earlier and may represent an important factor in host protection against parasitic infestation of the intestine. Fig. 11.4 illustrates the possible mech-

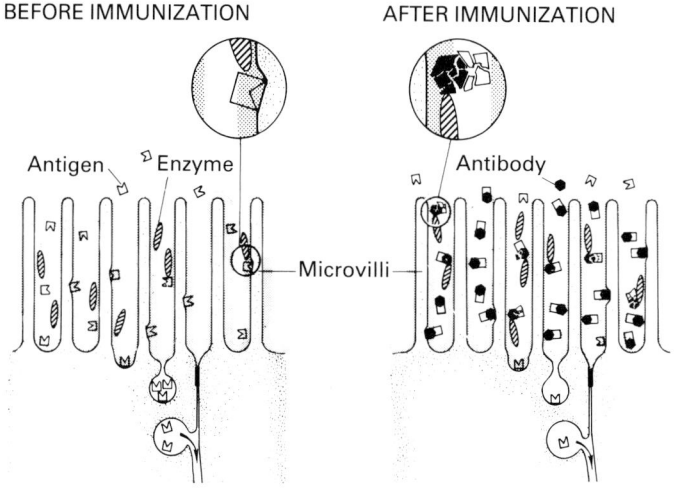

BEFORE IMMUNIZATION   AFTER IMMUNIZATION

Antigen   Enzyme   Antibody

Microvilli

Fig. 11.3 Schmatic representation of the processing of protein antigen at the surface of the gut. Prior to immunization, a small portion of ingested protein escapes intraluminal digestion and is taken up by the enterocyte and transported to the intercellular spaces. After immunization, antibodies present on the gut surface interact with antigen to form complexes thereby preventing or decreasing the binding of antigen to, and subsequent pinocytosis of antigen by, intestinal epithelial cells. Antigens complexed with antibodies in the mucous coat (glycocalyx) may be degraded by pancreatic enzymes adsorbed to the gut surface; consequently, there is less antigen available by intestinal epithelial cells. Reproduced from [80], by permission of Elsevier Science Publishing Co., Inc. Copyright 1975 by The American Gastroenterological Association.

Fig. 11.4 Possible mechanism(s) of immune-complex-mediated goblet cell mucus release on the intestinal surface. (a) Formation of IgA or IgE immune complexes with intestinal antigens within the intestinal lumen or the intestinal surface can possibly cause direct release of goblet cell mucus after interaction of the complex with the goblet cell surface. (b) Alternatively, formations of immune complexes may be absorbed across the intestinal surface and trigger a mediator (histamine/lymphokine) release of mucus after interaction with cells (mast cell/T cell) within the intestinal interstitium.

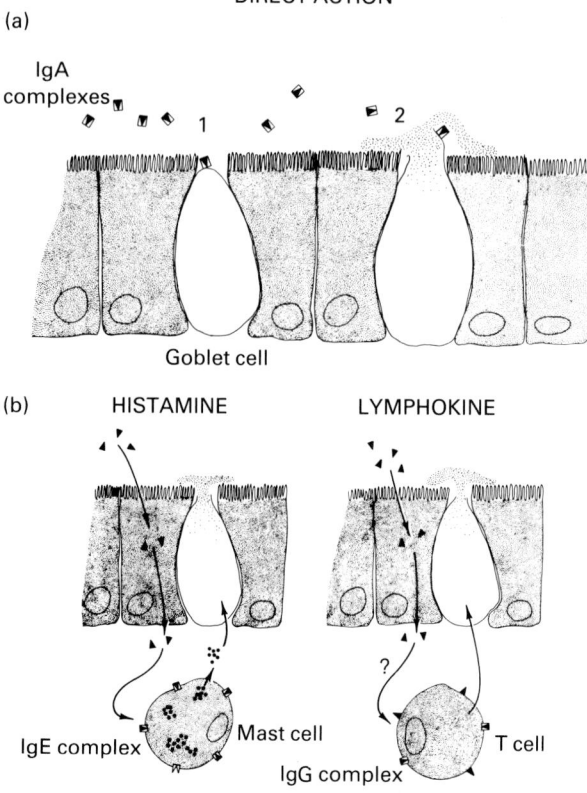

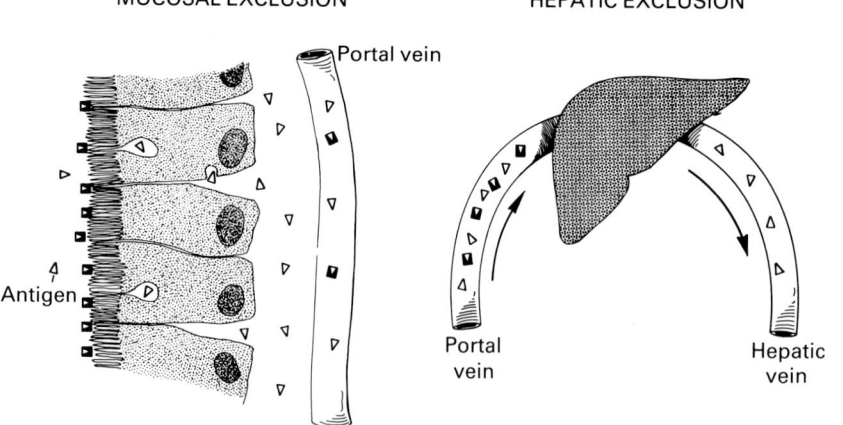

Fig. 11.5 Hepatic filtration of immune complexes from the portal circulation. Immune complexes form within the intestinal lumen or on the intestinal surface and may be excluded from the systemic circulation at the mucosal surface (mucosal exclusion) or if absorbed by a secondary defence mechanism, within the Kupffer cells of the liver (hepatic exclusion).

anism(s) of immune complex-mediated goblet cell mucus release on the intestinal surface.

Clearance of absorbed immune complexes

A final example of the combined effect of immunological and non-immunological processes in controlling host defence at the mucosal surface is the role of cells in clearing immune complexes absorbed from the gastrointestinal tract. Several years ago in an animal model, Walker et al demonstrated that immune complexes to intestinal antigens formed on the intestinal surface or within the intestinal interstitium were cleared more readily by Kupffer cells within the liver than were antigens alone [76]. This second line of mucosal defence may be important in preventing gram-negative microorganisms gaining access to the portal circulation and in the clearance of endotoxins known to be taken up into the portal circulation. Fig. 11.5 illustrates the concept of hepatic filtration of intestinal immune complexes.

ANTIGEN TRANSPORT IN THE IMMATURE INTESTINE

Endocytosis of large molecules

The neonatal mammalian small intestine, like the reticuloendothelial system in humans, has a capacity to ingest macromolecules by an endocytotic mechanism. The initial event in this process is an interaction between large molecules within the intestinal lumen and components of the microvillus membrane of intestinal absorptive cells (adsorption). When a sufficient concentration of molecules comes into contact with the cell membrane, invagination occurs and small vesicles are formed. In studies of endocytosis using macrophages, the invagination process can be induced by antibodies (opsonins) which combine with antigens on the cell surface to facilitate their membrane attachment. In the neonatal intestine a similar induction process may occur, but so far no specific factors have been isolated. However, the uptake process is energy dependent, since invagination can be inhibited with metabolic inhibitors of both glycolysis and oxidative phosphorylation. Energy is presumably

required for the resynthesis of cell membrane to replace that utilized as a result of invagination.

After invagination, macromolecules migrate within membrane-bound vesicles (phagosomes) to the supranuclear region of the cell where the vesicles coalesce with lysosomes to form large vacuoles (phagolysosomes). Within these structures intracellular digestion occurs. However, small quantities of ingested macromolecules escape breakdown and migrate to the basal-lateral surface of the cell to be deposited in the intercellular space by reverse endocytosis (exocytosis) (Fig. 11.6). Very little is known about those conditions of adsorption that can inhibit or facilitate invagination, nor is the mechanism of lysosomal migration to the site of vesicle formation clearly understood.

The concept of 'closure'

During the perinatal period in all mammalian species studied, the operational mucosal barrier to antigen uptake and transport remains immature for varying time periods. During this time, excessive quantities of antigen may be transported across the intestinal epithelium into the systemic circulation. At the time when intestinal immunological and non-immunological host defences develop and intestinal epithelial cells mature functionally and morphologically, the uptake of macro-

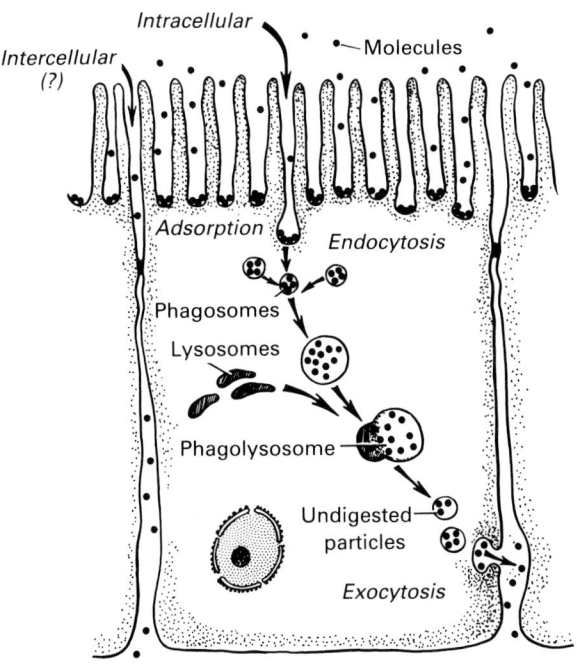

Fig. 11.6 General mechanisms for the uptake and transport of macromolecules by the intestine. Intracellular uptake—after adsorption and endocytosis by the microvillus membrane, macromolecules are transported in small vesicles and larger phagosomes. Intracellular digestion occurs when lysosomes combine to form phagolysosomes. Intact molecules that remain after digestion are deposited in the intercellular space by reverse endocytosis (exocytosis). Intercellular uptake— alternatively, macromolecules may cross the 'tight junction' barrier between cells and diffuse into the intercellular space. Reproduced from [77] by permission of Elsevier Science Publishing Co., Inc. Copyright 1974 by The American Gastroenterological Association.

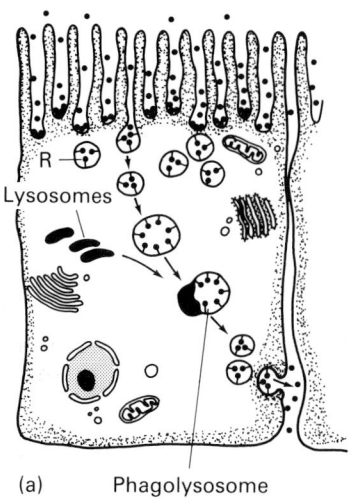 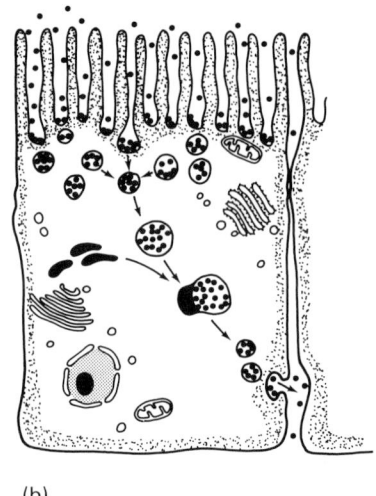

(a)   Phagolysosome   (b)

Fig. 11.7 Mechanisms of macromolecular absorption in the neonatal mammalian intestine. (a) Selective transport of maternal γ-globulins in colostrum occurs in the jejunum of newborn rats via a specific receptor site (R) present on the microvillous membrane. γ-Globulins are presumed to be protected from intracellular lysosomal digestion because of attachment to the receptor site and are transported in large quantities out of the cell. (b) A non-selective uptake and transport of other macromolecules occurs throughout the small intestine of most neonatal animals. Immature intestinal absorptive cells engulf large quantities of macromolecules. After intracellular digestion in phagolysosomes, very small quantities are deposited in the intercellular space. Reproduced from [77] by permission of Elsevier Science Publishing Co., Inc. Copyright 1974 by The American Gastroenterological Association.

molecules decreases. This phenomenon, known as 'closure', is the result of maturational events in gastrointestinal development. To illustrate this process, Fig. 11.7 depicts our current concept of the two different processes for the transport of maternal γ-globulins into the systemic circulation of newborn mammals prior to closure of the gastrointestinal tract [34, 41, 57, 62, 74].

'Closure' phenomenon in humans

The process of closure in humans is more subtle than in other animals. The bulk of the evidence to be presented suggests that excessive quantities of macromolecular antigens can cross the mucosal barrier of the underdeveloped intestine (newborn), compared with the mature intestinal epithelium (adult) [71]. Increased uptake appears to be related to a number of factors, including decreased breakdown of macromolecules, increased attachment of large molecules to the intestinal epithelial surface and less inhibition of uptake by ingested antibodies. These factors will be discussed in more detail later.

There is little evidence in humans to suggest that γ-globulins are either absorbed in bulk quantities with other colostral proteins (ruminants) or selectively transported by a specific transport system (rodents) (see Fig. 11.7). This observation is reasonable in the light of two facts. Since transplacental transmission of maternal γ-globulins represents the primary process for passive systemic immunity in the human newborn there is very little, if any, need for intestinal transport of systemic antibodies. In a similar fashion, the predominant class of antibody in human colostrum and milk is secretory IgA (SIgA), an antibody suited for functioning on epithelial surfaces and not in the circulation. Bierring et al [6] and Gitlin et al [3] have provided indirect evidence that the human small intestine in utero has the capacity to absorb macromolecules, particularly γ-globulins. However, Dancis et al [24] could not demonstrate a significant intestinal absorption of tetanus antibody injected into the amniotic fluid, suggesting that the intestinal route for antibody transport into the circulation was limited. Although specific antibodies can be detected in the serum of newborn infants fed human colostrum, as compared with those on formula feedings, the antibody levels detected suggest an unselective intestinal permeability to macromolecules rather than the selective transport of γ-globulin as shown in the newborn rat.

These studies demonstrate that γ-globulin absorption by the human intestine does not contribute significantly to the passively acquired serum antibody levels in the newborns. In recent studies, however, Ogra et al [54] have suggested that infants who are fed polio virus IgA antibody-rich human colostrum shortly after birth have appreciable levels of active antibody in their circulations shortly after. This study suggests that limited passive immunity may be passed from maternal colostrum to neonatal circulation. It is possible that factors in colostrum may facilitate this transport process.

Antigen transport in humans: effect of age

Several clinical studies suggest that macromolecules can cross the mucosal barrier under normal physiological conditions in humans [84]. Since pinocytosis represents a more primitive absorptive process in the alimentary canal, the capacity to absorb large molecules should be more extensive in an immature small intestine than in a well-differentiated mature intestine. In fact, this observation is supported by several clinical studies suggesting that premature and newborn infants can absorb greater quantities of ingested food antigens than older infants or adults are able to [35]. Rothberg [63], for example, has measured bovine serum albumin (BSA) in the serum of premature infants fed quantities of this protein, normally present in the daily milk requirement. In contrast, circulating BSA could not be detected in serum samples from older children fed equivalent quantities of protein. We have also reported a larger percentage of infants under three months with serum samples containing antibodies to food antigens than of infants exposed to antigen after three months, which suggests that food proteins are absorbed more readily into the circulation during the first three months than later on [27].

Animal studies. The implication of these studies is that the neonatal intestine may absorb antigenic quantities of ingested protein more readily than the more mature adult intestine. In support of this hypothesis, Lev and Orlic [46] in morphological studies with fetal monkeys, and Moxey and Trier [52] with human fetuses, have shown excessive uptake of large molecules by intestinal epithelial cells. They also described morphological features of epithelial cells suggesting structural immaturity. This same immaturity of gastrointestinal function and structure may persist beyond fetal life into the newborn period, at a time when the small intestine is exposed to increased quantities of both bacterial and food

antigens. In addition to increased macromolecular uptake, it is also possible that a greater quantity of protein ingested by intestinal epithelial cells escapes intracellular proteolysis as a result of immature lysosomal function, and therefore more protein becomes available for subsequent transport out of the cell and into the circulation.

The studies suggest that because of an immaturity of gastrointestinal function, uptake of intestinal macromolecules may be enhanced during infancy. The implications of this increased transport will be discussed later.

ANTIGEN TRANSPORT ACROSS MATURE INTESTINAL EPITHELIUM

As stated previously, the uptake and transport of γ-globulins markedly decreases when the neonatal small intestinal epithelial cell matures [14, 62]. At the time of closure, there is morphological and physiological evidence that the capacity of absorptive cells to endocytose other macromolecules decreases [15]. Based on these observations, it has been assumed that macromolecular absorption ceases entirely with epithelial cell maturation. However, reports have appeared indicating that small, nutritionally insignificant numbers of antigenically intact macromolecules may be transmitted across the mature mammalian gut [5, 15, 17]. For example, Danforth and Moore [25] noted that insulin injected into isolated loops of adult rat small intestine causes hypoglycaemia, suggesting that this protein was absorbed in biologically active quantities. Furthermore, Bernstein and Ovary [35] demonstrated that haptens and larger antigens were absorbed from guinea pig small intestine in quantities that could produce passive cutaneous anaphylaxis.

Animal studies. In the laboratory, direct morphological and physiological evidence has been provided for macromolecular transport with an enzyme marker, horseradish peroxidase (HRP) [18–20, 77]. This enzyme is an especially useful marker since it can be detected histochemically at both light- and electron-microscopical levels [31]; it can also be measured quantitatively in very small concentrations [48]. After intraluminal injection of HRP into ligated segments of jejunum and ileum in the rat, the marker was found absorbed to the apical surface membranes and within membrane-bound cytoplasmic canalicular vesicular and vacuolar structures. Also, extracellular, absorbed HRP was noted in the intercellular spaces between adjacent absorptive cells, traversing the basement membranes and in the spaces of the lamina propria [20].

These studies indicated that an intraluminal antigen can be taken up by a characteristic pinocytotic mechanism within rat small intestine absorptive cells, and the larger molecules can be transmitted by these cells to the extracellular space of the lamina propria. Furthermore, the mechanism of uptake is similar to that described previously for γ-globulin absorption in the neonatal mammalian intestine (Fig. 11.7). In a parallel physiological experiment, the ability of the rat small intestinal mucosa to transmit macromolecules from its lumen to mesenteric lymph and portal venous blood was determined by means of a quantitative study of HRP absorption [82]. After infusion of HRP into jejunum through an indwelling catheter, small but significant amounts of protein tracer were consistently transmitted across the gut into intestinal lymph and portal blood. The uptake of HRP into absorptive cells and HRP transport into intercellular spaces and the lamina propria was the same as that which had been reported in the ligated loop experiments.

Human studies. In humans, several studies suggest that macromolecules can cross the mature mucosal barrier under normal physio-logical conditions [23, 25]. Korenblat et al [40] showed that a considerable proportion (15–30%) of normal adults developed milk precipitins after ingestion of a physiological amount of milk protein. In earlier studies, Wilson and Walzer [84] reported uptake and transport of undigested protein using a passive cutaneous anaphylaxis technique to measure circulating food proteins; they also demonstrated precipitins to these proteins in the serum of adults fed these proteins in physiological quantities. Absorption appears to be related to the concentration of ingested protein. In order for uptake to occur, sufficient protein must escape intraluminal proteolysis. In turn, protein taken up into cells must exceed the lysosomal digestive capacity to permit intact molecules to be transported out of the cell into the circulation.

Specialized mechanisms for antigen transport

Membranous epithelial cell

Recent studies have demonstrated that a specialized epithelial cell (membranous epithelial cell or 'M' cell) exists within the gut to facilitate the access of antigens to intestinal lymphoid tissue [8, 55, 56] (see Chapter 4). This specialized macromolecular transport process may be important in the IgA-producing plasma cell cycle and may facilitate the

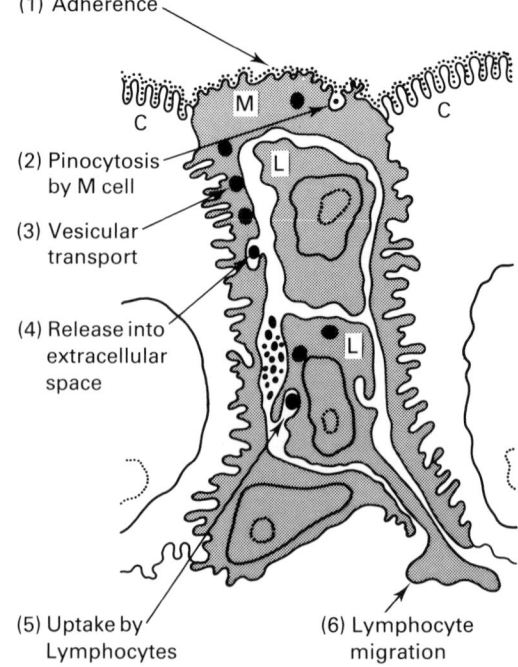

(1) Adherence

(2) Pinocytosis by M cell

(3) Vesicular transport

(4) Release into extracellular space

(5) Uptake by Lymphocytes

(6) Lymphocyte migration

Fig. 11.8 Diagram summarizing the stages observed in the transport of horseradish peroxidase by the M cell from the intestinal lumen to the intraepithelial lymphocyte. C, columnar cells; L, lymphocytes. Reproduced from [55] by permission of Elsevier Science Publishing Co., Inc. Copyright 1977 by The American Gastroenterological Association.

local immune response. These clusters of specialized epithelial cells ('M' cells) have been recognized overlying gut-associated lymphoepithelial tissue (GALT) in the ileum of several species, including humans, and may represent an important pathway for the direct access of intestinal antigens to lymphoid tissue [73].

Morphological features of M cells, including a paucity of microvilli, a poorly developed glycocalyx and an absence of lysosomal organelles, support the view that these cells are especially adapted for antigen transport (Fig. 11.8). Histochemical studies have demonstrated a preferential uptake of HRP into M cells after exposure of the gut to small quantities of that antigen. After exposure to larger amounts of the enzyme, uptake of HRP was noted, not only in M cells, but in all epithelial cells, suggesting that the mode of antigen access to GALT may be dependent on the concentration of antigens in the intestinal lumen. At physiological or lower levels of luminal antigen, the specialized uptake pathway is preferred; at increased antigen levels, a more generalized uptake of antigen takes place. After uptake into M cells, HRP is rapidly released into the interstitial space and processed by lymphoid cells circulating through Peyer's patches. This mechanism of antigen handling by the gut appears to represent an important specialized access route for intestinal macromolecules to reach lymphoid tissues and thereby stimulate the local immune system.

Uptake of antigen–antibody complexes

Another physiological event occurring within the small intestine which may facilitate uptake of intestinal macromolecules is the formation of immune complexes and the specialized uptake of large molecules as complexes. Bockman and Winborn [9] originally reported that ferritin absorption was greater in sensitized animals than in unsensitized controls. They hypothesized that systemic immunization somehow facilitated intestinal epithelial handling of intraluminal antigens. Subsequent studies have shown that facilitated uptake of macromolecules require serum-derived (IgG) antibodies [8, 12]. It was assumed that formation of IgG immune complexes might trigger a chemotactic-mediated response resulting in enhanced penetration of all intraluminal macromolecules. Recent reports, however, have suggested that receptors exist for IgG antibody and IgG complexes on the epithelial

surface and may represent a facilitated transport process for antigens, just as facilitated IgG transport has been reported in newborn rodents [11, 37].

This immunologically mediated facilitated uptake of macromolecules may have an important influence on the development of mucosal immune competence in young infants. Alternatively it may represent an important mechanism whereby excessive uptake of large molecules contributes to adverse reactions which are manifested as clinical disease states (see below).

CLINICAL CONDITIONS POSSIBLY ASSOCIATED WITH PATHOLOGICAL (EXCESSIVE) ANTIGEN TRANSPORT

Table 11.2 lists clinical conditions known to be associated with pathological uptake of antigens. The pathophysiological mechanism(s) of representative conditions will be discussed in this section to illustrate the association between antigen transport and clinical disease. A comprehensive review of all clinical conditions is beyond the scope of this chapter.

Table 11.2 Clinical conditions possibly associated with pathological transport of macromolecules.

Newborn and early childhood (immediate clinical response)
  Necrotizing enterocolitis
  Gastrointestinal allergy
  Sudden infant death syndrome
  Dermatitis
  Toxigenic diarrhoea
  Malabsorption

Later childhood and adulthood (delayed clinical response)
  Inflammatory bowel disease
  Chronic active hepatitis
  Nephritis
  Autoimmune (immune-complex-mediated) diseases

As a result of the pathological transport of antigens across the small intestine, ingested antigens may traverse the mucosal barrier and predispose to allergic and toxic reactions leading to a number of gastrointestinal diseases. The gastrointestinal diseases possibly associated with antigen absorption are gastrointestinal allergy [7, 39, 42, 45, 64] inflammatory bowel disease [29, 39, 83], coeliac disease [66], toxigenic diarrhoea [53, 58], chronic hepatitis [60, 81], necrotizing enterocolitis [71, 72] and autoimmune disease [67, 72]. Since the evidence cited to support the hypothesis that intestinal permeability to antigens is involved in the pathogenesis of human disease is largely indirect, one should realize that these comments are somewhat speculative and still remain to be proved by more direct evidence [71, 72]. For purposes of this report only gastrointestinal allergy will be discussed in detail as a prototype condition.

Gastrointestinal allergy

Probably the most striking association between antigen handling and clinical disease is shown with gastrointestinal allergy. Several clinical symptoms of such allergy have been described which appear to relate specifically to the ingestion of certain foods (particularly cow's milk). These conditions may be localized to the gastrointestinal tract and present with diarrhoea, gastrointestinal bleeding or protein-losing enteropathy, or they may be represented by systemic manifestations of allergy ranging in severity from exanthema to anaphylaxis. The clinical expression of allergy may relate to the transport of antigens into (a) the lamina propria alone (local allergic reactions), or (b) into both the lamina propria and the systemic circulation (systemic allergic response). Factors which determine the nature of the allergic response are not entirely understood, but they undoubtedly relate to the degree of sensitivity of the allergic patient and/ or the concentration of allergen ingested.

Although the mechanism(s) of gastrointestinal allergy is at present obscure, it would appear that the intestinal transport of allergens is a necessary initial step in the process. In fact, it has been suggested that during the neonatal period when increased antigen permeability exists, susceptible infants may become sensitized to specific ingested proteins. With re-exposure at a time when much less macromolecular absorption is

occurring, minute quantities of allergen may be absorbed and result in allergic symptoms. These symptoms can then be propagated by further uptake of allergens across a disrupted mucosal surface [7]. In recent experimental studies Walker et al [79, 80] have reported that intestinal anaphylaxis can lead to increased uptake of non-specific intestinal allergens which in turn can evoke an IgG-mediated reaction leading to further propagation of disease. This secondary process occurring with classic IgE-mediated disease may be very important in converting a self-limiting process into a chronic disease state.

CONCLUSIONS

In this review, I have attempted to summarize the research done in a poorly understood area of gastroenterology, namely the role of the intestine in controlling uptake of ingested antigens (i.e., macromolecules). The mature gut retains the capacity to absorb antigens by an energy-dependent, pinocytotic mechanism similar to that described for the transport of γ-globulins in certain mammalian species in the neonatal state. The vast majority of adults show no ill-effects as a result of this physiological phenomenon due to mucosal barrier function. However, when the barrier is disturbed and increased (pathological) quantities of toxic or antigenic macromolecules gain access to the body because of a derangement in the intraluminal digestive process or a defect in the mucosal barrier, macromolecular absorption may be altered and result in either local intestinal or systemic disorders. The speculative concepts suggesting that clinical disease states may be associated with altered mucosal permeability have been discussed.

REFERENCES

1 Abrahamson DR, Powers A, Rodewald R: Intestinal absorption of immune complexes by neonatal rats: a route of antigen transfer from mother to young. Science 1979; 206:567-9.

2 Allansmith M, McClellan BH, Butterworth M, Maloney JR: The development of immunoglobulin levels in man. J Pediatr 1968; 72:276.

3 Alpers DH, Isselbacher KJ: Protein synthesis by the rat intestinal mucosa: the role of ribonuclease. J Biol Chem 1967; 242:5617-20.

4 Bamford DR: Studies in vitro of passage of serum proteins across the intestinal wall of young rats. Proc R Soc Lond [B] 1966; 166:30-47.

5 Bernstein ID, Ovary Z: Absorption of antigens from the gastrointestinal tract. Int Arch Allergy Appl Immunol 1968; 33:521-9.

6 Bierring F, Anderson H, Eveberg J: On the nature of the meconium corpuscles in human foetal intestinal epithelium. I. Electron microscopic studies. Acta Pathol Microbiol Scand 1964; 61:363-76.

7 Bloch KJ, Bloch KB, Sterns M, Walker WA: Intestinal uptake of macromolecules. VI. Uptake of protein antigen in vivo in normal rats and rats infected with Nippostronglyus brasiliensis or subjected to mild systemic anaphylaxis. Gastroenterology 1968; 77:1039.

8 Bockman DE, Cooper MD: Pinocytosis by epithelium

associated with lymphoid follicles in the bursa of Fabricius, appendix and Peyer's patches. An electron microscopy study. Am J Anat 1973; 136:455-77.

9 Bockman DE, Winborn WB: Light and electron microscopy of intestinal ferritin absorption. Observations in sensitized and non-sensitized hamsters (*Mesocricetus auratus*). Anat Rec 1966; 155:603-22.

10 Boedeker EC: Enterocyte adherence of *Escherichia coli*: its relation to diarrheal disease. Gastroenterology 1982; 83:489.

11 Borthisle B, Dubo RT, Brown WR, Gray HM: Studies on receptors for IgG on epithelial cells of the rat intestine. J Immunol 1977; 119:471-6.

12 Brandtzaeg P: Mucosal penetrability enhanced by serum-derived antibodies. Nature 1977; 266:262-3.

13 Bresson JL, Pang K, Udall J, Walker WA: Evidence for increased enterotoxin binding to newborn microvillus membranes: possible explanation for enhanced toxigenic diarrhea in infancy. Gastroenterology 1980; 78:1145.

14 Burgio GR, Lanzavecchia A, Plebani A et al: Ontogeny of secretory immunity: levels of secretory IgA and natural antibodies in saliva. Pediatr Res 1980; 14:1111.

15 Casley-Smith JR: The passage of ferritin into jejunal epithelial cells. Experientia 1967; 23:370-1.

16 Chandra RK: Food antibodies in malnutrition. Arch Dis Child 1975; 50:532-4.

17 Chisiu N St: Morphological aspects suggesting the transfer procedure absorption of some proteins in intestine of adult rats. Med Interne 1968; 5:65-71.

18 Clarke RM, Hardy RN: Factors influencing the uptake of (^{125}I) polyvinyl pyrrolidine by the intestine of the young rat. J Physiol (Lond) 1971; 212:801-7.

19 Cooper M, Teichberg S, Lifshitz F: Alterations in rat jejunal permeability to a macromolecular tracer during a hyperosmotic load. Lab Invest 1978; 38:447-51.

20 Cornell R, Walker WA, Isselbacher KJ: Intestinal absorption of horseradish peroxidase. A cytochemical study. Lab Invest 1971; 25:42-8.

21 Cunningham-Rundles C, Brandeis WE, Good RA, Day NK: Milk precipitins, circulating immune complexes and IgA deficiency. Proc Natl Acad Sci USA 1978; 75:3387.

22 Cunningham-Rundles C, Brandeis WE, Good RA, Day NK: Bovine antigens and the formation of circulating immune complexes in selective immunoglubulin A deficiency. J Clin Invest 1979; 64:272.

23 Dack GM, Petran E: Bacterial activity in different levels of intestine and in isolated segments of small and large bowel in monkeys and in dogs. J Infect Dis 1934; 54:204-7.

24 Dancis J, Lind J, Oratz M: Placental transfer of proteins in human gestation. Am J Obstet Gynecol 1961; 82:167-71.

25 Danforth E, Moore RD: Intestinal absorption of insulin in the rat. Endocrinology 65:118-26.

26 DeBoth NJ, Van Der Kamp AW, Van Dongen JM: The influence of changing crypt cell kinetics on functional differentiation in the small intestine of the rat. Nucleotide and protein synthesis. Differentiation 1975; 4:175.

27 Eastham EJ, Lichauco T, Grady MI, Walker WA: Antigenicity of infant formulas: role of immature intestine in protein permeability. J Pediatr 1978; 93:561-4.

28 Etzler ME, Branstrator ML: Cell surface components of intestinal epithelial cells and their relationship to cellular differentiation. In: Ciba Foundation Symposium 70, Development of mammalian absorptive processes. Amsterdam: Excerpta Medica, 1979; 51-68.

29 Ferguson A: Intraepithelial lymphocytes of the small intestine. Gut 1977; 18:921-37.

30 Forstner G, Sturgess J, Forstner J: Malfunction of intestinal mucus and mucus production. Adv Exp Med Biol 1976; 89:349.

31 Galant SP: Biological and clinical significance of the gut as a barrier to penetration of macromolecules. Clin Pediatr (Phila) 1976; 15:731-4.

32 Gitlin D, Kumate J, Morales C: The turnover of amniotic fluid protein in the human conceptus. Am J Obstet Gynecol 1972; 113:632-45.

33 Graham RC, Karnovsky ML: The early stage of absorption of ingested horseradish peroxidase in the proximal tubule of the mouse kidney: ultrastructural cytochemistry by a new technique. J Histochem Cytochem 1966; 14:291-302.

34 Graney D: The uptake of ferritin by ileal absorptive cells in suckling rats. An electron microscopic study. J Anat 1968; 123:227-54.

35 Grusky FL, Cooke RE: The gastrointestinal absorption of unaltered protein in normal infants and in infants recovering from diarrhea. Pediatrics 1955; 16:763-8.

36 Haneberg B, Aarskog D: Human fecal immunoglobulins in healthy infants and children and in some diseases affecting the intestinal tract or the immune system. Clin Exp Immunol 1975; 22:210.

37 Jones EA, Waldmann TA: The mechanism of intestinal uptake and transcellular transport of IgG in the newborn rat. J Clin Invest 1972; 51:2916-27.

38 Jones GW, Freter R: Adhesive properties of *Vibrio cholera*: nature of the interaction with isolated rabbit brush border membranes and human erythrocytes. Infect Immun 1976; 14:240.

39 Kjellman NIM, Johansson SGO: Soy versus cow's milk in infants with a biparental history of atopic disease: development of atopic disease and immunoglobulins from birth to 4 years of age. Clin Allergy 1979; 9:347-58.

40 Korenblat RE, Rothberg RM, Minden P: Immune response of human adults after oral and parenteral exposure to bovine serum albumin. J Allergy 1968; 41:226-35.

41 Krachenbuhl JP, Campiche MA: Early stages of intestinal absorption of specific antibodies in the newborn. An ultrastructural, cytochemical and immunological study in the pig, rat and rabbit. J Cell Biol 1969; 42:345-65.

42 Kraft S, Kirsner JB: Immunological apparatus of the gut and inflammatory bowel disease. Gastroenterology 1971; 60:922-5.

43 Kraft SC, Rothberg RM, Knauer CM et al: Gastric acid output and circulating antibovine serum albumin in adults. Clin Exp Immunol 1967; 2:231.

44 Lake AM, Bloch KJ, Leuter MR, Walker WA: Intestinal goblet cell mucus release. J Immunol 1979; 122:834.

45 Lake AM, Bloch KJ, Sinclair KJ, Walker WA: Anaphylactic release of intestinal goblet cell mucus. Immunology 1980; 39:1-6.

46 Lev R, Orlic D: Uptake of proteins in swallowed amniotic fluid by monkey fetal intestine in utero. Gastroenterology 1973; 65:60-8.

47 Lojda Z: Cytochemistry of enterocytes and of other cells in the mucosal membrane of the small intestine. In: Smyth DH, ed. Biomembranes, Vol.4A, Intestinal absorption. London: Plenum Press, 1974; 43-122.

48 Maehly AC, Chance B: The assay of catalases and

peroxidases. In: Glick D, ed. Methods of biochemical analysis, Vol. 1. New York: John Wiley, 1954; 357–64.

49 McClelland DBL, Sampson RR, Parkin DM: Bacterial agglutination studies with secretory IgA prepared from human gastrointestinal secretions and colostrum. Gut 1972; 13:450–5.

50 Miller HRP, Nawa Y: Immune regulation of intestinal goblet cell differentiation: specific induction of nonspecific protection against helminths? Nouv Rev Fr Hematol 1979; 21:31.

51 Morris IG: Gamma globulin absorption in the newborn. In: Cole CF, Heidel W, eds. Handbook of physiology. Baltimore: Williams and Wilkins, 1968; 1491–512.

52 Moxey PC, Trier JS: Structural features of the mucosa of human fetal small intestine. Gastroenterology 1975; 68:1002–9.

53 Ogra PL, Karzon DT: The role of immunoglobulins in the mechanisms of mucosal immunity to viral infection. Pediatr Clin North Am 1970; 17:385–9.

54 Ogra SS, Weintraub D, Ogra PL: Immunologic aspects of human colostrum and milk. III. Fate of absorption of cellular and soluble components in the gastrointestinal tract of the newborn. J Immunol 1979; 119:245–8.

55 Owen RL: Sequential uptake of horseradish peroxidase by lymphoid follicle epithelium of Peyer's patches in the neonatal unobstructed mouse intestine: an ultrastructural study. Gastroenterology 1977; 72:440–51.

56 Owen RL, Jones AI: Epithelial cell specialization within human Peyer's patches: an ultrastructural study of intestinal lymphoid follicles. Gastroenterology 1974; 66:189–203.

57 Pang KY, Walker WA, Bloch KJ: Intestinal uptake of macromolecules: difference in distribution and degradation of protein antigen in control and immunized rats. Gut 1981; 22:1018.

58 Payne LC, Marsh CL: Gamma globulin absorption in the baby pig: the nonselective absorption of heterologous globulins and factors influencing absorption time. J Nutr 1962; 76:151–8.

59 Quaroni A, Kirsch K, Herscovics A, Isselbacher KJ: Surface-membrane biogenesis in rat intestinal epithelial cells at different stages of maturation. Biochem J 1980; 192:133.

60 Quinton PM, Philpott CW; A role of anionic sites in epithelial architecture. Effects of cationic polymers on cell membrane structure. J Cell Biol 1973; 56:878–96.

61 Raul F, Simon P, Kedinger M, Haffer K: Intestinal enzymes activities in isolated villus and crypt cells during postnatal development of the rat. Cell Tissue Res 1977; 172:167.

62 Rodewald R: Intestinal transport of antibodies in the newborn rat. J Cell Biol 1973; 58:189–211.

63 Rothberg RM: Immunoglobulin and specific antibody synthesis during the first weeks of life of premature infants. J Pediatr 1969; 75:391–9.

64 Saffron M, Franco Saenz R, Kong A et al: A model for the study of the oral administration of peptide hormones. Can J Biochem 1979; 57:548.

65 Selner JC, Merrill DA, Claman NH: Salivary immunoglobulins and albumin: development during the newborn period. J Pediatr 1968; 72:685.

66 Shiner VM, Ballard J: Antibody–antigen reactions in jejunal mucosa in childhood coeliac disease after gluten challenge. Lancet 1972; i:1202–5.

67 Smith CB, Purcell RH, Bellanti JA, Chanock RM: Protective effect of antibody to parainfluenza type I virus. N Engl J Med 1966; 275:1145–50.

68 Stern MS, Pang KY, Walker WA: Food proteins and gut mucosal barrier. II. Differential interaction of cow's milk proteins with the mucous coat and the surface membrane of adult and immature rat jejunum. Pediat Res 1984; 18:1252–7.

69 Taylor B, Normal AP, Orgel HA, Stoken CR: Transient IgA deficiency and pathogenesis of infantile atopy. Lancet 1973; ii:111–13.

70 Toofanian F, Kidder DE, Hill FW: The postnatal development of intestinal disaccharidases in the calf. Res Vet Sci 1975; 16:382.

71 Walker WA: Antigen absorption from the small intestine and gastrointestinal disease. Pediatr Clin North Am 1975; 22:731–46.

72 Walker WA: Host defense mechanisms in the gastrointestinal tract. Pediatrics 1976; 57:901–6.

73 Walker WA: Antigen handling by the gut. Arch Dis Child 1978; 53:527–31.

74 Walker WA: Gastrointestinal host defense: importance of gut closure in control of macromolecular transport. In: Ciba Foundation Symposium 70. Development of mammalian absorptive processes. Amsterdam: Excerpta Medica, 1979; 201–16.

75 Walker WA: Intestinal transport of macromolecules. In: Johnson J, Christensen J, Grossman M et al, eds. Physiology of the gastrointestinal tract. New York: Raven Press, 1981; Chapter 51:1271.

76 Walker WA, Bloch KJ: Uptake of antigen–antibody complexes prepared in antibody or antigen excess by normal rat intestine in vitro. Gastroenterology 1976; 70:948.

77 Walker WA, Isselbacher KJ: Uptake and transport of macromolecules by the intestine: possible role in clinical disorders. Gastroenterology 1974; 67:531–50.

78 Walker WA, Isselbacher KJ: Intestinal antibodies. N Engl J Med 1977; 297:767–73.

79 Walker WA, Wu M, Isselbacher KJ, Bloch KJ: Intestinal uptake of macromolecules. III. Studies on the mechanism by which immunization interferes with antigen uptake. J Immunol 1975; 115:854–861.

80 Walker WA, Wu M, Isselbacher KJ, Bloch KJ: Intestinal uptake of macromolecules. IV. The effect of pancreatic duct ligation on the breakdown of antigen and antigen–antibody complexes on the intestinal surface. Gastroenterology 1975; 69:1223–9.

81 Walzer M: Studies in absorption of undigested proteins in human beings. I. A simple direct method of studying the absorption of undigested proteins. J Immunol 1927; 14:143–9.

82 Warshaw AL, Walker WA, Cornell R, Isselbacher KJ: Small intestinal permeability to macromolecules: transmission of horseradish peroxidase into mesenteric lymph and portal blood. Lab Invest 1971; 25:675–84.

83 Wilson ID, Onstad GR, Williams RC Jr, Carey JB Jr: Selective immunoglobulin A deficiency in two patients with alcoholic cirrhosis. Gastroenterology 1968; 54:253–9.

84 Wilson SJ, Walzer M: Absorption of undigested proteins in human beings. Am J Dis Child 1935; 50:49–57.

85 Wolfe JL, Rubin DH, Finberg R et al: Intestinal M cells: a pathway for entry of reovirus into the host. Science 1981; 212:471.

Chapter 12
Failure of Antigen Exclusion

Charlotte Cunningham-Rundles

Introduction

Despite the large number of mechanisms present in the gastrointestinal tract which provide for the exclusion of undigested macromolecules from systemic compartments, dietary and other antigens normally confined to the intestinal tract do indeed enter the systemic circulation. Since all healthy, non-immunocompromised humans develop and maintain serum antibodies to specific dietary antigens one must assume that the continual absorption of small amounts of such molecules is a normal event. Exactly what amounts and what types of intestinal antigens are normally absorbed into the circulation are largely unknown. However, in order to decide how much mucosal permeation could be considered abnormal, it is useful to recall that in animal studies, Block et al [7] showed that feeding bovine serum albumin 4 g/kg body weight to rats resulted in serum levels of this antigen of 170 ng/ml after 6 hours, and that in humans, Paganelli and Levinsky [56] showed that three adults had a maximum of 3 ng of α-lactoglobulin in their serum after ingesting 1.2 litres of milk. Similarly, Husby et al [40] showed that

seven of eight individuals had a maximum of 10.5 ng of ovalbumin in their serum 2 to 3 hours after a test meal containing 3 g of ovalbumin. While the exact amounts of each antigen differ in various studies according to dose, antigen and means of measurement, it appears that small but significant amounts of at least some intact antigen are continually absorbed from the intestinal tract in normal subjects.

Using these studies as background, there are numerous reports in the literature which tend to show that in certain disease states and other conditions, gastrointestinal absorption of luminal antigens may exceed that which is considered normal. In some cases, this phenomenon has been linked to a specific pathological outcome; in many other instances, the relationship between cause and effect is much more obscure. For example, both non-specific inflammatory processes and specific lesions such as a lack of secretory IgA (SIgA), can lead to excess absorption. In other instances, specific and non-specific lesions can exist simultaneously, as for example in IgE-mediated intestinal permeability which is initiated by a specific allergen, but then permits other bystander antigens to gain systemic access. In this chapter, the mechanism of failure of antigen exclusion and the known or suspected results will be discussed. While animal experiments will be cited where appropriate, the major intent of this chapter is to examine the evidence in human systems. The instances to be discussed in this chapter are listed in Table 12.1. For each of these situations, the mechanisms of failure and the possible results are described.

Table 12.1 Mechanisms of failure of antigen exclusion.

1. Immaturity

2. Congenital immune deficiency
   IgA deficiency
   Common varied immunodeficiency

3. Allergic

4. Gastrointestinal disease
   Inflammatory bowel diseases
   Gluten-sensitive enteropathy
   Other gastrointestinal diseases

5. Miscellaneous
   Protein malnutrition
   Surgery
   Drugs
   Radiation

IMMATURITY

Physiology of closure

The mucosal cells of the immature gastrointestinal tract have the ability to ingest directly macromolecules by an endocytic mechanism. This occurs by a direct invagination of the cell surface, and the subsequent formation of an intracytoplasmic vesicle. The ingested molecules are transported in an undigested state into the systemic circulation. At the time when this process ceases, the immature gut is said to have undergone 'closure'. Although this process of maturing has not been as extensively studied in humans as in animals, it appears that prior to 3 months of age, much more extensive absorption of food proteins occurs than after 3 months of age [28, 37, 75]. In animals, this mechanism may provide for an enhanced absorption of maternal antibodies present in amniotic fluid and milk, but in humans the evidence for this has been harder to demonstrate, although Ogra et al [55] have shown that infants fed human colostrum rich in IgA antibodies to poliovirus have high titres of anti-polio antibody in their serum.

Absorption of dietary proteins: serum antibodies in children

With regard to specific dietary proteins presented by the gastrointestinal tract, it has been known since the early part of this century that the intestinal tract of infants can be permeable to proteins of egg [49, 65, 77] and milk [5, 48, 65]. Moro [54] first showed that precipitating antibodies (or antibodies with a titre sufficiently increased to permit detection in an agar diffusion assay) to bovine milk proteins were often present in the sera of marasmic infants. Because of the antigens present, these sera were later found to be capable of producing anaphylaxis in sensitized guinea-pigs and of producing a positive reaction in the Schultz-Dale test, in which smooth muscle contraction occurs even if very minute amounts of the specific antigen are present [2]. Somewhat later, precipitating antibodies to bovine milk were found in the sera of many apparently healthy infants up to 15 months of age. Precipitins have, however, rarely been observed in the sera of healthy children between the ages of 2 and 5, and in most studies have not been found in the sera of normal children over the age of 5 [39, 58, 64]. Using haemagglutination or ELISA (enzyme-linked immunosorbent assay) antibody titre determinations to milk proteins, it has been shown that a gradual decline in antibodies to bovine proteins occurs not only in childhood but ac-

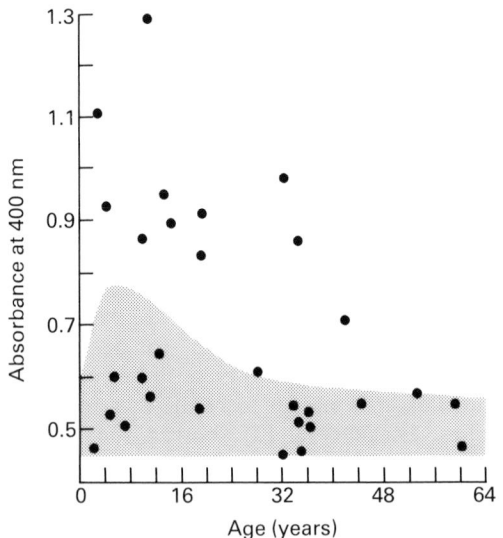

Fig. 12.1 Antibody to bovine milk proteins (absorbance 400 nm) by patient age for 30 IgA-deficient subjects. The values for the 45 healthy controls are within the hatched area. Reproduced from [21], with permission.

tually over about four to five decades, reaching for healthy adults, a stable but still detectable low level at about age 45 [46, 61, 62] (see Fig. 12.1).

Consequences of serum antibodies

Immune complex formation

Since it is clear from the above discussion that the absorption of dietary antigen is a normal event, it is interesting to review the possible immunological effects of this absorption. If antibody titres are high in infancy and continued exposure occurs, one likely outcome would be the formation of circulating immune complexes. As an early indication of this, Matthews and Soothill reported that following milk ingestion in infants, the level of serum C3 fell, which suggested that antigen–antibody complexes had been formed [50]. Later it was reported that antigen–antibody complexes were present in the sera of newborns fed cow's milk 6 days after birth, while these were not detected in the sera of breast-fed infants [26]. Others have criticized this latter report because a relatively insensitive test (inhibition of latex IgG agglutination by polyclonal rheumatoid factor) was used and because a C1q–staphylococcus protein A method did not confirm the presence of complexes [24]. However, using the Raji cell radioimmunoassay and a Raji cell ELISA, we have also found circulating immune complexes in the sera of infants 3–12 months old fed cow's milk (Cunningham-Rundles and Fikrig, unpublished observations).

At present, it seems entirely probable that infants with sufficient antibody directed towards cow's milk proteins could transiently develop immune complexes in the serum after a milk feeding, although the biological significance of this is entirely unknown. Indeed, it may even be possible that these immune complexes present a stimulus for the formation of anti-idiotypic antibodies, or antibodies directed to the antigen-binding regions of previously formed antibodies to dietary proteins. Since antigen–antibody complexes can serve as an excellent immunogen in animals for anti-idiotype production [44] and anti-idiotypes can exert a powerful suppressive effect upon further production of the primary antibody [45] it is possible that the production of immune complexes in the sera of infants presents a mechanism whereby this immunological control is first established (see Fig. 12.2). Some precedent for this possibility exists for humans, since anti-idiotypic antibodies directed to anticasein have been found in IgA-deficient sera, as will be discussed below.

Oral tolerance

Another possible outcome for the early absorption of dietary proteins could be the first step in the production of oral tolerance. Tolerance is the inability to produce a specific antibody in response to a parenteral immunization; oral tolerance is induced by a prior feeding of the same antigen by mouth [3, 10, 13, 66]. Since antibody titres to numerous dietary substances decrease with age and reach a stable low level somewhere around the age of 40–50 for most individuals, it is possible that the development of oral tolerance could be an eventual result of continued antigen absorption [46, 62]. In line with this, some studies show that immune complexes may play a particular role in the production of tolerance [3] although the immunological mechanisms involved are not understood (see Chap. 14).

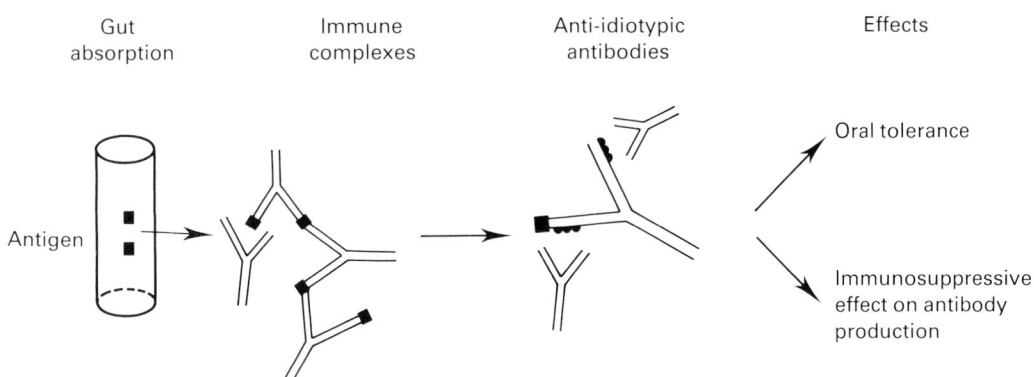

Fig. 12.2 Consequences of neonatal absorption of antigen.

Summary. In summary, the immature gastro-intestinal tract apparently permits the absorption of a wide range of antigens, many of which stimulate antibody production. With increasing age, this absorption diminishes in normal infants. While immune complexes may be detected in the sera of cow's milk-fed infants, the biological significance of this phenomenon is open to question.

CONGENITAL IMMUNE DEFICIENCY

In some ways, the immature gastrointestinal tract resembles the gastrointestinal tract of the congenitally immunodeficient patient. In each, the secretory mucosal immune system is defective. Specific analyses of the gastrointestinal absorption of dietary antigens in the immunodeficient patient have helped to define certain aspects of the secretory immune barrier.

IgA deficiency

Secretory IgA (SIgA) is the predominant immunoglobulin of exocrine secretions and it is abundant in the glycocalyx mucous coat of the intestinal tract [71]. It has been calculated that 3 g of SIgA are produced daily by lamina propria plasma cells [14]. The role of SIgA is not completely elucidated, but several important aspects are known: (a) SIgA contains antibody directed to bacteria, viruses and proteins which are normally restricted to the intestinal tract, and (b) SIgA can reduce the uptake of these substances from the intestinal lumen [15, 35, 38, 76, 81].

If secretory IgA constitutes an important barrier to the absorption of dietary substances, patients who are IgA deficient could be expected to have an excessive absorption of various antigens presented in the gastrointestinal tract. That this is a correct assumption is demonstrated by the observation that the sera of IgA-deficient patients is much more likely to contain precipitating antibodies to cow's milk than that of normal subjects [9]. In addition, it has been shown that circulating immune complexes, which have been demonstrated to contain bovine proteins, appear in the sera of IgA-deficient patients as early as 15-30 minutes after milk ingestion and often are present for at least 2-4 hours in the sera [19, 20, 22]. Fig. 12.3 shows the levels of circulating immune complexes found in the sera of six IgA-deficient individuals after milk ingestion.

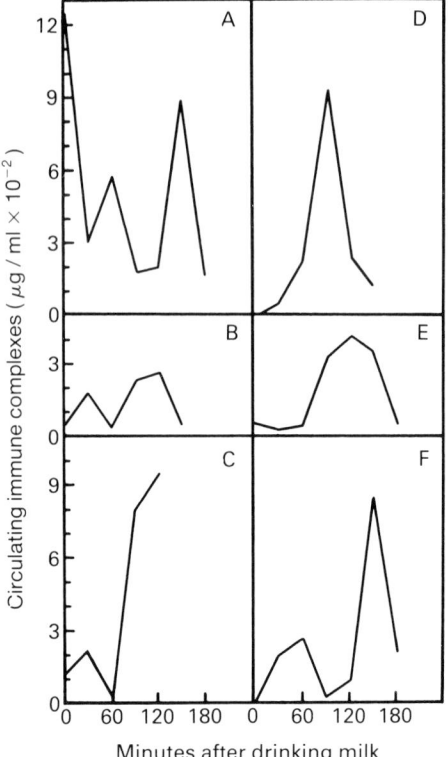

Fig. 12.3 The level of circulating immune complex was measured by the Raji cell radioimmunoassay in the sera of six IgA-deficient subjects for 2-3 hours after drinking 100 ml of milk.

Antigen absorption in IgA deficiency

In order to determine whether the amount of immune complex formed in IgA deficiency is in any way related to the levels of serum or salivary IgA, the data for 24 patients tested in this way have been collected (Table 12.2). Here, IgA-deficient patients are listed in order of the amount of serum IgA present. The levels for salivary IgA are included. From these data it is clear that a few patients having little or no serum or salivary IgA had no circulating immune complexes following milk ingestion (example, patient 12), while other patients with detectable serum and salivary IgA had large amounts of immune complex after drinking milk. In addition, some patients who had only a modest deficit of serum IgA, had large amounts of bovine antigens detectable in their sera after exposure to milk (patients 19 and 23). These data were surprising because no predictable association could be established between the amount of immune complex formation and the degree of the IgA deficit. In fact, these data show that a relatively leaky

Table 12.2 Antigen absorption in IgA deficiency.

Patient number	Serum immunoglobulins			Salivary IgA† (ng/dl)	Maximum CIC‡ (μg/ml)	Antigens detected by agar diffusions§		
	IgG	IgA	IgM			Casein	α-Lactalbumin	β-Lactoglobulin
1	1161	0	97	0	6400	+	0	+
2	1685	0	153	2	6400	+	0	+
3	664	0	103	0	6400	+	+	+
4	1489	0	33	0	1680	ND	ND	ND
5	2300	0	220	11	1700	+	0	0
6	1130	0	100	0	1280	+	0	0
7	1500	0	172	0	928	+	+	+
8	1550	0	78	0	500	+	+	+
9	1096	0	187	0	256	0	0	+
10	1213	0	425	ND¶	176	ND	ND	ND
11	1087	0	86	9	220	ND	ND	ND
12	1940	0	98	0	0	0	0	0
13	757	5	198	0	40	0	0	0
14	1420	10	105	ND	992	0	0	+
15	1340	12	98	ND	20	+	0	+
16	812	13	312	31	880	0	0	0
17	2940	19	165	6	6240	0	0	0
18	689	20	70	5	1360	ND	ND	ND
19	910	31	165	ND	250	0	0	+
20	775	32	55	13	400	0	0	0
21	766	33	96	0	1760	ND	ND	ND
22	675	44	222	0	0	ND	ND	ND
23	747	48	132	11	80	+	0	0
24	1098	83	122	2	528	ND	ND	ND

* Serum immunoglobulins: normal range for adults is IgG = 800–1800 mg/dl, IgA = 90–450 mg/dl; IgM = 90–300 mg/dl.
† Salivary IgA: normal range for adults is 5–30 mg/dl.
‡ Circulating immune complexes (CIC): normal serum contains < 16 μg/ml equivalent to heat-aggregated IgG/ml.
§ Antigens tested for were casein, α-lactalbumin, and β-lactoglobulin.
¶ Not done.

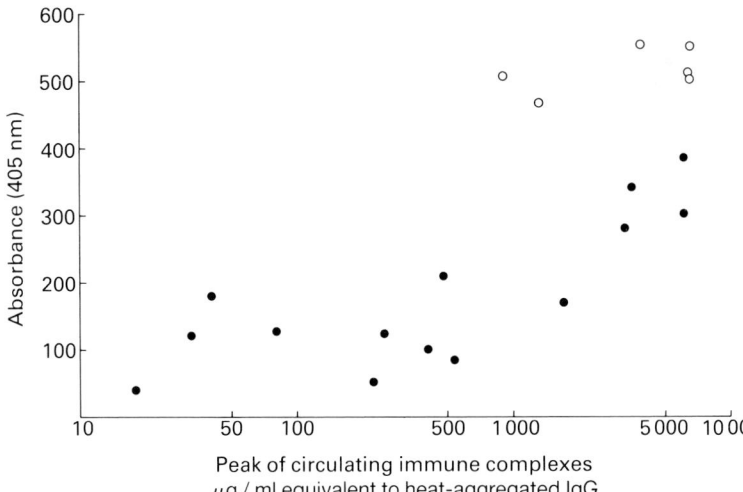

Fig. 12.4 The peak level of circulating immune complexes after ingestion of 100 ml of milk for 20 IgA-deficient patients is given on the abscissa (log scale) and for each patient's serum the corresponding amount of antibody (as determined by ELISA) to a mixture of milk proteins is given on the ordinate (absorbance 405 nm). Sera which contained precipitating antibodies (generally those with the highest titre of antibody) are shown as open circles. The relationship between the peak level of immune complexes and the amount of antibody is statistically significant ($P < 0.01$).

intestinal tract can be present in individuals who have only a modestly reduced level of serum IgA; many of these patients would not normally be classified as immune deficient. While the exact reasons for these findings are not established, we have determined that the level of immune complex which is formed is closely correlated ($P < 0.01$) with the amount of serum antibody which is present to bovine milk proteins (Fig. 12.4).

Absence of coexisting IgE-mediated antigen absorption

In an attempt to clarify these observations, and to identify an additional mechanism for antigen absorption, we considered the possibility of a coexisting IgE-mediated antigen absorption. However, this possibility was excluded by double-blind antigen feeding experiments, in which cromolyn sodium had no effect upon excess antigen absorption in IgA-deficient subjects (Cunningham-Rundles, unpublished observations).

Consequences of excessive antigen absorption

Autoimmunity. The pathological significance of excessive antigen absorption in the IgA-deficient patient population is unknown. However, in one study, increased amounts of antibody to bovine milk proteins were found to be associated with the presence of positive serological tests for autoimmunity (Fig. 12.5) [21].

Autologous anti-idiotypic antibodies. Another effect of the continually absorbed gastrointestinal antigens could be the potential formation of autologous anti-idiotypic antibodies, or antibodies directed at the variable regions of antibodies made to bind the absorbed antigens. A specific example of this has already been demonstrated, since antibodies to anti-bovine casein have been detected in the sera of several IgA-deficient donors with large amounts of anti-casein [16]. The regulatory effects of the autologous anti-idiotypes are not yet defined; however, these anti-idiotypes are likely candidates for participation in immune complex formation [17].

Delayed oral tolerance. As discussed above, the absorption of dietary antigens in infants could result in the production of oral tolerance.

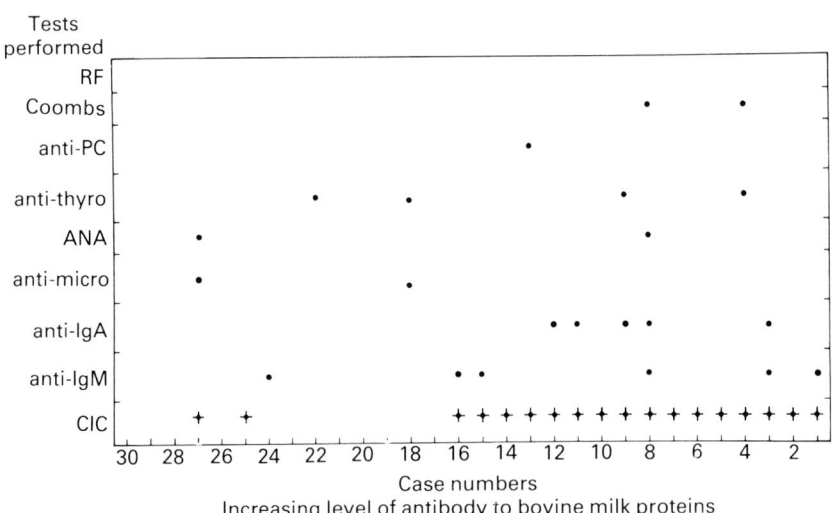

Fig. 12.5 IgA-deficient sera were studied for the amount of antibody to bovine milk proteins and for the presence of autoantibodies. The sera are ranked according to the level of antibody to milk proteins on the ordinate (with serum number 1 having the largest amount of antibody). The presence of circulating immune complex (CIC) is indicated as (+). Sera containing various autoantibodies are indicated as (●). The relationship between the amount of antibody to bovine proteins and the presence of an autoimmune reaction was statistically significant ($P < 0.05$). Reproduced from [21], with permission.

While a mechanism for this particular association is difficult to elucidate in precise terms, it has previously been proposed that the presence and degree of the intestinal permeability defect in IgA deficiency could permit the excessive absorption of numerous exogenous antigens to which a variety of antibodies could then be raised. Some of these antigens could share antigenic cross-reactivity with internal antigens and thus provide a basis for auto-antibody formation [1, 21].

Because of this, we were interested to determine if the IgA-deficient individual, who clearly absorbs more antigen from the gastro-intestinal tract, would develop tolerance more quickly than non-immunodeficient individuals. In determining the amount of antibody to two major dietary antigens, casein and ovalbumin, in sera of IgA-deficient and normal subjects age 3 months to 66 years old, we found that IgA-deficient subjects actually appear to become tolerant more slowly than normals, since the antibody titres were increased for IgA-deficient subjects of all ages and apparently began to reach a stable low level at an age somewhat later than that found for normals (Figs. 12.6 and 12.7) [59]. The development of oral tolerance in the IgA-deficient population is clearly a complex topic, the elucidation of which would require further analyses.

Common varied immunodeficiency

Increased circulating antigen levels

Since patients with common varied immuno-deficiency (adult onset or acquired hypogam-maglobulinaemia) also lack SIgA, one might expect that patients with this defect could have an equally excessive gastrointestinal permeability compared with the IgA-deficient patients. However, since hypogammaglobuli-naemic patients produce antibodies poorly, the ingested proteins could not engage in immune complex formation with endogenous immuno-globulin. For this reason, the absorbed antigens would not be eliminated via the mechanism of immune complex clearance, and could potentially accumulate in the blood. In analysing a recent series of such patients, it was shown that this prediction is true; very

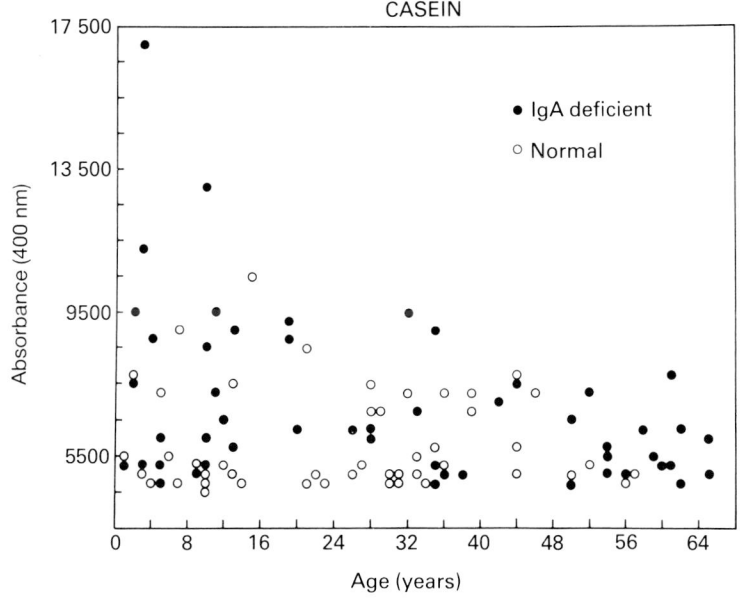

Fig. 12.6 The amount of antibody to casein was determined by ELISA for a large panel of IgA-deficient and normal sera obtained from individuals of various ages.

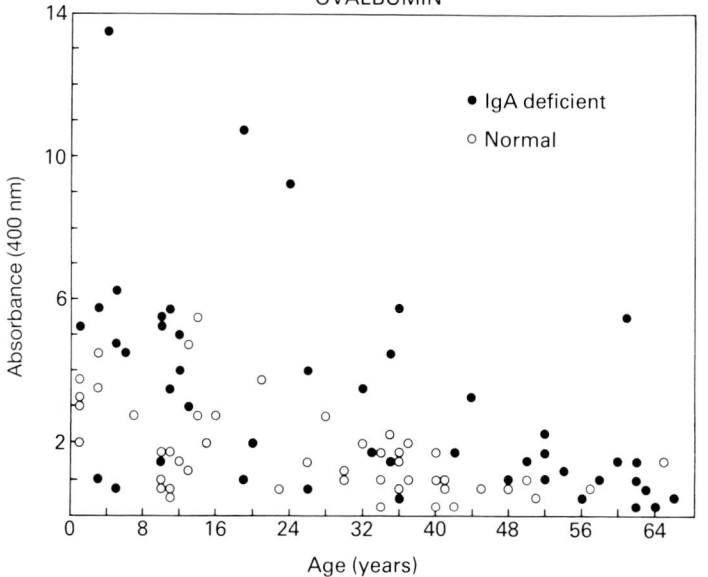

Fig. 12.7 The amount of antibody to ovalbumin was determined by ELISA for a large panel of IgA-deficient and normal sera obtained from individuals of various ages.

large amounts of bovine casein and bovine gamma globulin can be detected in the sera of most hypogammaglobulinaemic patients.

Splenomegaly and lymphadenopathy

The amount of foreign protein in the sera cannot be correlated with gastrointestinal disease nor to any specific immunological parameter; however, for still unknown reasons, the amounts of protein in the serum of each patient is closely associated with the presence of splenomegaly and/or lymphadenopathy (Table 12.3). The reasons for this association are not known but it seems possible that the continued absorption of external antigens, which cannot be readily eliminated by immune complex function, could serve to stimulate lymphoid tissue [18].

Apparently normal antigen exclusion in agammaglobulinaemia. The reason for the relative lack of these antigens in the sera of three agammaglobulinaemic patients is not known. While this could be due to the particular patients studied, it is also not impossible that

this form of immunodeficiency is not accompanied by excess antigen absorption. If this proves to be true, it will be quite interesting to determine why this is so, since patients with common varied immunodeficiency and X-linked agammaglobulinaemia have an equal deficit of SIgA.

Summary. In summary, the humoral immunodeficient patient who lacks SIgA often has an excessive absorption of numerous dietary antigens which results in immune complex formation. While the pathological result of immune complex formation is not clear, the titre of antibody to bovine milk is related to the presence of autoimmunity. For the hypogammaglobulinaemic patient who makes little or no antibody to gastrointestinal antigen, high levels of bovine antigens can be detected in the serum; these high levels of antigens are related to lymphoid hypertrophy.

ALLERGY

One of the most common mechanisms for the penetration of dietary antigens into the sys-

Table 12.3 Casein and bovine γ-globulin levels.

Patient number	Bovine casein (ng/ml)	Bovine gamma globulin (ng/ml)	Spleen*	Presence of lymphoid hypertrophy
Hypogamma-globulinaemia				
1	1600	650	+ + +	Cervical lymphadenopathy†, nodular lymphoid hyperplasia
2	1200	500	0	Lymphoid and pulmonary infiltration
3	1280	300	+ + +	
4	1080	250	+ +	
5	1000	<40	+ +	
6	980	700	+ +	Nodular lymphoid hyperplasia
7	980	<40	0	Cervical lymphadenopathy†
8	970	<40	0	
9	960	<40	0	
10	960	<40	+	
11	930	260	+	
12	900	<40	0	
13	900	800	+ +	Nodular lymphoid hyperplasia
14	400	<40	0	
15	400	<40	0	
16	300	<40	0	
Agamma-globulinaemia				
17	80	<40	0	
18	<40	<40	0	
19	Trace	<40	0	
20	<40	<40	0	

* Spleen: + + + = enlarged by 6 cm or more (to umbilicus or below); + + = enlarged by 2–6 cm; + = just palpable.
† On biopsy, benign lymphoid hyperplasia.
Reproduced from [22], with permission.

temic circulation is that associated with the mucosal alterations present in allergy. The usual effects that this can produce on the individual are well established and are described elsewhere in this volume. Aside from the urticaria, wheezing, vomiting, diarrhoea and abdominal pain, numerous other symptoms are very probably also allergic in nature. The appearance of the small bowel mucosa in allergy can vary from normal to villous atrophy [67]. There is a variable increase in the number of mucosal inflammatory cells such as polymorphonuclear leukocytes, eosinophils, macrophages and mast cells [47, 67].

Immunological mechanisms:
IgE-mediated reactions

The immunological mechanisms which are involved in the systemic reactions to specific food substances are not entirely clarified, but IgE, specific antibody and complement and T cell reactions are certainly involved [33, 34, 67]. The best studied of these are the IgE-mediated allergies. In the gastrointestinal tract, IgE is produced by plasma cells which lie in the lamina propria. The allergic potential of IgE is exerted through the degranulation of mast cells which also reside in the submucosa. The degranulation process is initiated by bridging of pairs of IgE surface receptors on mast cells by IgE immune complexes [41]. Degranulation results in the release of potent pharmacological agents such as histamine, leukotrienes, serotonin, platelet activation factor and arachidonic acid metabolites (for a review, see [78]). These agents cause smooth muscle contraction, vasodilation, bronchoconstriction and platelet aggregation. In an allergic subject, one must assume that the local hyperaemic effects permit the absorption of increased amounts of the specific allergen and as it has been shown, even other bystander antigens through the mucosal surface [6].

Systemic access of food allergens

Whatever the exact mechanism of entrance, in gastrointestinal allergy specific food allergens can be detected in the circulation after specific antigen challenge [8, 25, 57]. In atopic patients with sensitivity to eggs, IgG immune complexes and ovalbumin can be detected in the serum for 5 hours after a challenge consisting of two soft-boiled eggs. After pretreatment with cromolyn sodium, the quantities of both ovalbumin and immune complexes in the serum can be reduced [57]. Normal controls fed 1.2 litres of milk have also been shown to form immune complexes in the serum, but the clearance of these complexes is possibly more rapid than for atopic subjects [57].

Components of immune complexes

In further studies it has been shown that for normal subjects IgA containing immune complexes may actually predominate after specific food challenge [8] but for the atopic patient more IgG and IgE complexes are formed [57]. This is of interest because it may explain in part one reason why the atopic patient deviates from the normal methods of antigen handling, and thereby develops some of the specific allergic consequences. Skin biopsy samples of lesions in atopic eczema do not show lesions of Type I hypersensitivity, but have predominantly a mononuclear cell infiltrate closely resembling a Type IV reaction [53]. Possibly this is actually due to the deposition of immune complexes, which can produce this picture experimentally [8].

IgA deficiences and atopy

There are other aspects of gastrointestinal allergy which might be important in excessive absorption of antigens. One of these is the observation that a proportion of atopic individuals are IgA deficient, although most are not. When present, IgA deficiency (and as discussed above, possibly even partial IgA deficiency) can certainly contribute to excess antigen absorption. In addition, it has been found that some infants born to atopic parents may have transient IgA deficiency which could produce an early sensitizing effect [70]. Conclusive studies on this topic are still lacking.

Possible intestinal tract lesions

Aside from the immunological mechanisms discussed above, it is possible that allergic subjects may have specific structural lesions in the intestinal tract. Jackson et al [42] found, for example, that patients with eczema have an abnormally increased absorption of polyethyleneglycol (PEG) from the intestinal tract. Polyethyleneglycol is biologically inert, non-immunogenic and is excreted unchanged in the urine. Nine of 18 patients with eczema had increased excretion of PEG 4000 when compared to normal controls. These data appear to show that patients with eczema may have a distinct mucosal lesion. However, this may also be due to IgE-mediated mechanisms, as Falth-Magnussun et al [32] have shown that pre-medication with cromolyn sodium can also diminish the absorption of PEG.

Summary. In summary, one of the most common conditions in which excessive amounts of various antigens can enter the systemic circulation is by the mechanisms of gastrointestinal allergy. While the effects of allergy are described thoroughly elsewhere in this volume, IgE activation, specific antigenic absorption and immune complex formation are biological events which have been documented.

GASTROINTESTINAL DISEASE

Although failure of antigen exclusion is suggested in numerous gastrointestinal diseases, actual evidence for this is lacking in most of these conditions. In the following discussion, the available information is discussed.

Inflammatory bowel disease

Inflammation of the gastrointestinal mucosa, regardless of specific cause, could potentially permit luminal antigens to enter the general circulation. In acute ulcerative colitis for example, several immunological mechanisms for increased antigen absorption are possible. The presence of increased numbers of IgG-positive B cells [36] could mean the production of local immune complexes and subsequent complement activation. Eosinophils are also present which could produce increased local mediator release [36]. In addition, T cells cytotoxic to the intestinal wall, and circulating anti-colon antibodies [79] could further produce local damage. Through these immunological mechanisms of mediator release and mucosal damage, various dietary components could more readily gain entrance to the circulation, although whether any of these potential mechanisms actually do lead to increased absorption of luminal antigens is still unknown.

Gluten-sensitive enteropathy

Gluten-sensitive enteropathy (coeliac disease or non-tropical sprue) is a disease in which the intestinal mucosa is injured by the ingestion of glutens derived from wheat, rye, barley or oat flour [74]. The exact mechanisms of tissue damage are uncertain but individuals having major histocompatibility antigens HLA-1,

HLA-B8 and/or -DR3, and certain immunoglobulin allotype markers are at increased risk for this disease [31, 80]. HLA antigens appear to direct T cell proliferation responses to wheat gluten fractions [23]. In addition, patients with coeliac disease have increased amounts of antibodies to gluten in their serum [29,68] and synthesis of anti-gliadin antibody in vitro is known [30]. This implies that wheat fractions have been absorbed in an antigenically intact form, and have served as systemic immunogens. The sera of patients with coeliac disease also may have circulating immune complexes [27]. From these observations, it seems probable that mucosal perturbation, induced by various immunological and non-immunological mechanisms, does permit the excess absorption of various antigens into the circulation [68, 73]. This seems particularly possible since excess absorption of orally administered ovalbumin can be demonstrated in children with coeliac disease but not in healthy children [25].

Other gastrointestinal diseases

In other gastrointestinal diseases, excess antigen absorption could also occur. This would be true for diseases which do not have an immune basis as well as those which have. For example, excess antigen absorption is probably quite common in infants and children after gastroenteritis since the intestinal mucosa has sustained injury and the increased permeability which results may take 1–2 weeks to heal [4, 37, 82].

Liver diseases. In chronic liver disease, the serum may contain abnormally high titres of antibodies to intestinal microorganisms and dietary proteins [72]; these observations imply excess antigen absorption. In addition, increased levels of IgA-containing circulating immune complexes can be found in sera of cirrhotic patients, although the exact mechanism for these findings is still unknown [63]. Initially the phenomenon was considered to be due to extrahepatic or intrahepatic shunts, but subsequent analysis has shown that the increased antibody levels may be due to a combination of shunting and abnormal drainage through liver cells [51].

Investigating other mechanisms for antigen penetration, Block and Walker [6] have shown that intestinal inflammation resulting from an infection with the nematode *Nippostrongylus brasiliensis* resulted in the passage of increased

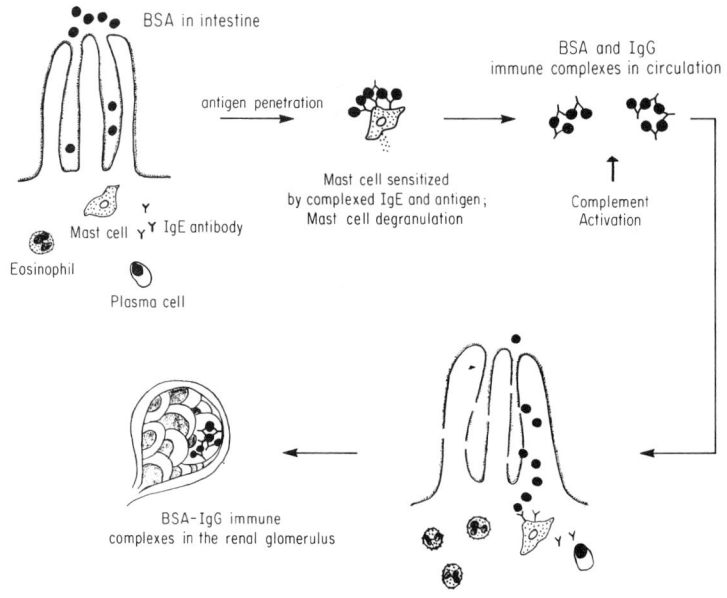

BSA in intestine

antigen penetration

Mast cell ᵧᵧ IgE antibody

Eosinophil

Plasma cell

Mast cell sensitized
by complexed IgE and antigen;
Mast cell degranulation

BSA and IgG
immune complexes in circulation

Complement
Activation

BSA-IgG immune
complexes in the renal glomerulus

Intestinal oedema and hyperpermeability
permit BSA to enter; further
accumulation of eosinophils

Fig. 12.8 A child who had eosinophilic gastroenteritis and a high level of IgE and a strongly positive RAST for beef. He also had a large amount of anti BSA in his serum, and circulating immune complexes containing BSA. A renal biopsy showed BSA-IgG complexes in his kidney. After removing beef from his diet, his recurrent nephrotic syndrome was eliminated.

amounts of bovine serum albumin into the blood stream.

Eosinophilic gastroenteritis. Another condition in which systemic absorption of excess dietary antigens is likely is eosinophilic gastro-enteritis. A dramatic example of this was recently presented by a child who had nephrotic syndrome due to renal disposition of immune complexes containing bovine serum albumin (BSA) of dietary origin. The boy had increased IgE, a strongly positive RAST (radio-allergosorbent test) to BSA and intestinal eosinophilia. Presumably, IgE released from mast cells due to BSA exposure resulted in enough local hyperaemia to permit BSA (and probably other antigens) to enter the systemic circulation, engage in immune complex formation and later to be deposited in the renal glomerulus [52]. (See Fig. 12.8.)

Summary. In summary, although there are numerous indications that the mucosal disruption which accompanies gastrointestinal disease can permit excessive antigen absorption, complete data for these conditions are not yet available.

MISCELLANEOUS MECHANISMS

Protein malnutrition

Malnutrition in infancy and failure to thrive were first associated with the presence of milk

precipitins by Schloss and Anderson in 1923. In animal studies, protein malnutrition has been found to promote an actual increase in the absorption of ingested proteins. This has been shown by various in vitro assays involving inverted intestinal sacs [43] and in studies using intact animals [83]. In the latter study, morphological evaluation of jejunal tissue showed an initial increase in pinocytotic activity with a later deterioration of apical junctions and movement of protein molecules directly between cells [83]. While the mechanisms for these changes are not known, a reduction of the concentration of both secretory IgA and mucosal antibody responses has been found in patients with protein energy malnutrition [11]. This reduction in responsiveness includes antibodies to several vaccines as well as to dietary macromolecules [11]. The effect that increased absorption and diminished immunological secretory responsiveness may have in humans is not clarified due to the complexities of the situation. Speculations about the possibility of Arthus-like reactions in malnourished subjects repeatedly exposed to the same substances have been put forward [12].

Surgery

After even rather minor surgical trauma to the intestinal tract, such as an open biopsy of the small intestine and placing of a suture, extensive gastrointestinal uptake of a luminal antigen (horseradish peroxidase) has been observed in animal studies. These effects were noted for at least 10 cm in either direction from the initial biopsy, and could not be found in control animals who had been anaesthetized and subjected to laparotomy [60]. While the exact localization of the created defect was not specifically demonstrated, the data suggest that disruption of the epithelial tight junctions might have occurred. Similar studies have not been reported in humans, and more information will be needed to clarify this relatively unexplored topic.

Summary and conclusions

This chapter discusses specific conditions in which antigens normally confined to the intestinal tract are able to gain access to the general circulation. Although there are numerous diseases in which such antigen exposure is considered possible, the actual situations in which excess absorption has been well documented are in immaturity, immunodeficiency and atopy. Suggestive, but less conclusive, evidence for excess antigen absorption has been obtained from studies of various gastrointestinal diseases, and of malnourished individuals. In almost all of these areas, the pathological results of excess absorption are still uncertain.

Acknowledgements

Supported by grants from the National Institute of Health AI-15809, CA-29502, the American Cancer Society 1M245, The National Foundation March of Dimes, the Beneficial Corporation and the Zelda Radow Weintraub Cancer Fund.

REFERENCES

1 Ammann AJ: Immunodeficiency disorders and autoimmunity. In: Talal N, ed. Genetic, immunologic, viral and clinical aspects of autoimmunity. New York: Academic Press, 1977;479.

2 Anderson AF, Schloss OM: Allergy to cow's milk in infants with nutritional disorders. Arch Dis Child 1923; 26:341–5.

3 André C, Heremans JF, Vaerman JP, Cambiaso CL: A mechanism for the induction of immunological tolerance by antigen feeding: antigen–antibody complexes. J Exp Med 1975; 142:1509–19.

4 Barnes GL, Townley RRW: Duodenal mucosal damage in 31 infants with gastroenteritis. Arch Dis Child 1973; 48:343–9.

5 Bauer J: Weber den Nachweis der pracipitablen. Substanz der Kuhmilch in Blute atrophescher Sanglige. Berl Klin Wochenschr 1906; 43:711–19.

6 Block FJ, Walker WA: Effect of locally induced intestinal anaphylaxis on the uptake of a bystander antigen. J Allergy Clin Immunol 1981; 67:312–16.

7 Block KJ, Block DB, Stearns M, Walker WA: Intestinal uptake of macromolecules. IV. Uptake of protein antigen in vivo in normal rats and rats infected with *Nippostrongylus brasiliensis* or subjected to mild systemic anaphylaxis. Gastroenterology 1979; 77:1039–44.

8 Brostoff J, Carini C, Wraith DG et al: Immune complexes in atopy. In: Pepys J, Edwards AM eds. The mast cell. London: Pitman, 1979; 380–93.

9 Buckley RH, Dees SC: Correlation of milk precipitins with IgA deficiency. N Engl J Med 1969; 281:465–7.

10 Challacombe SJ, Tomasi TB: Systemic tolerance and secretory immunity after oral immunization. J Exp Med 1980; 152:1459–72.

11 Chandra RK: Reduced secretory antibody responses to live attenuated measles and poliovirus vaccines in malnourished children. Br Med J 1975; 2:583–5.

12 Chandra RK: Malnutrition. In: Chandra RK, ed. Primary and secondary immunodeficiency disorders. Edinburgh: Churchill Livingstone, 1983; 187–203.

13 Chase MW: Inhibition of experimental drug allergy by prior feeding of the sensitizing agent. Proc Soc Exp Biol Med 1946; 61:257–9.

14 Clancy R, Bienenstock J: Secretion immunoglobulins. Clin Gastroenterol 1976; 5:229–49.

15 Crabbé PA, Bazin H, Eyssen H, Heremans JF: The normal microbial flora as a major stimulus for proliferation of plasma cells synthesizing IgA in the gut. Int Arch Allergy 1968; 34:362–75.

16 Cunningham-Rundles C: Naturally occurring autologous anti-idiotypic antibodies: participation in immune complex formation in selective IgA deficiency. J Exp Med 1982; 155:711–19.

17 Cunningham-Rundles C: Isolation and analysis of anti-idiotypic antibodies from IgA-deficient sera. Ann NY Acad Sci 1983; 409:469–77.

18 Cunningham-Rundles C, Carr RI, Good RA: Dietary protein antigenemia in humoral immunodeficiency disease: correlation with splenomegaly. Am J Med 1984; 76:181–5.

19 Cunningham-Rundles C, Brandeis WE, Good RA, Day NK: Milk precipitins, circulating immune complexes and IgA deficiency. Proc Nat Acad Sci USA 1978; 75:3387–9.

20 Cunningham-Rundles C, Brandeis WE, Good RA, Day NK: Bovine antigens and the formation of circulating immune complexes in selective IgA deficiency. J Clin Invest 1979; 64:270–2.

21 Cunningham-Rundles C, Brandeis WE, Pudifin DJ et al: Autoimmunity in selective IgA deficiency: relationship to anti-bovine protein antibodies, circulating immune complexes and clinical disease. Clin Exp Immunol 1981; 45:299–304.

22 Cunningham-Rundles C, Brandeis WE, Safai B et al: Selective IgA deficiency and circulating immune complexes containing bovine proteins in a child with chronic graft vs. host disease. Am J Med 1979; 67:883–9.

23 Cunningham-Rundles S, Cunningham-Rundles C, Pollack MS et al: Response to wheat antigen in an in vitro lymphocyte transformation among HLA-B8 positive normal donors. Trans Proc 1978; 10:977–9.

24 D'Amelio R, Seminara R, Galli E et al: Circulating immune complexes in infants fed on cow's milk. Nature 1982; 298:72-3.

25 Dannaeus A, Inganas M, Johansson SGO, Foucard T: Intestinal uptake of ovalbumin in malabsorption and food allergy in relation to serum IgG antibody and orally administered sodium cromoglycate. Clin Allergy 1979; 9:263-70.

26 Delire M, Cambiasco CL, Masson P: Circulating immune complexes in infants fed on cow's milk. Nature 1978; 272:632-8.

27 Doe WF, Brown D: Evidence for circulating immune complexes in inflammatory bowel disease and adult celiac disease. Gut 1973; 14:429.

28 Eastham FJ, Lichauco T, Grady MI, Walker WA: Antigenicity of infant formulas: role of immature intestine in protein permeability. J Pediatr 1978; 93: 561-4.

29 Eterman KP, Feltkamp TEW: Antibodies to gluten and reticulin in gastrointestinal disease. Clin Exp Immunol 1978; 31:92-9.

30 Falchuck ZM, Strober W: Gluten-sensitive enteropathy: synthesis of antigliadin antibody in vitro. Gut 1974; 15:947-52.

31 Falchuk ZM, Rogentine GM, Strober W: Predominance of histocompatibility antigen HLA-8 in patients with gluten-sensitive enteropathy. J Clin Invest 1972; 51:1602-5.

32 Falth-Magnusson K, Kjellman N-IM, Magnusson K-E, Sundqvist T: Intestinal permeability in healthy and allergic children before and after sodium-cromoglycate treatment assessed with differently-sized polyethyleneglycols (PEG 400-PEG 1000) Clin Allergy 1984; 14:277-86.

33 Ferguson A: Pathogenesis and mechanisms in the gastrointestinal tract. In: Proceedings of the first food allergy workshop (Chairman, Prof RRA Coombs). Oxford: Oxford Medical Education Services, 1980; 28-38.

34 Fontaine JL, Navarro J: Small intestinal biopsy in cow's milk protein allergy in infancy. Arch Dis Child 1975; 50:351-62.

35 Fubura ES, Freter R: Availability of locally synthesized and systemic antibodies in the intestine. Infect Immun 1973; 6:365-99.

36 Goldgraber MB, Kirsner JB, Palmer WL: The histopathology of chronic ulcerative colitis and its pathogenic implications. Gastroenterology 1960; 38:596-604.

37 Gruskay FL, Cooke RE: The gastrointestinal absorption of unaltered protein in normal infants and in infants recovering from diarrhea. Pediatrics 1955; 16:763-8.

38 Hanson LA, Ahlstedt S, Anderson B et al: The biologic properties of secretory IgA. J Recticuloendothel Soc 1980; 28:1.

39 Holland NH, Hong R, Davis NC, West CD: Significance of precipitating antibodies to milk proteins in the serum of infants and children. J Pediatr 1962; 61:181-95.

40 Husby S, Jensenius JC, Svehag SE: Passage of undegraded dietary antigen into the blood of healthy adults. Quantification, estimation of size, distribution and relations of uptake to levels of specific antibodies. Scand J Immunol (in press).

41 Ishizaka K, Ishizaka T: Immune mechanisms of reversed type reaginic hypersensitivity. J Immunol 1969; 103:588-95.

42 Jackson PG, Baka RWR, Lessof MH et al: Intestinal permeability in patients with eczema and food allergy. Lancet 1981; i:1285-6.

43 Kirsch RE, Saunders SJ, Brock JF: Animal models and human protein calorie malnutrition. Am J Clin Nutr 1968; 21:1225-8.

44 Klaus CGB: Antigen antibody complexes elicit anti-idiotypes. Nature 1978; 272:265-7.

45 Kohler H: The response to phosphorylcholine: dissecting an immune response. Transplant Rev 1975; 27:24-39.

46 Korenblat PE, Rothberg RM, Minden P, Farr RS: Immune responses of human adults after oral and parental exposure to bovine serum albumin. J Allergy 1969; 41:226-35.

47 Kuitunen P, Visakorpi JK, Savilahti E, Pelkonen P: Malabsorption syndrome with cow's milk intolerance. Arch Dis Child 1975; 50:351-6.

48 Lippard VW: Immunologic response to ingestion of foods by normal and eczematous infants. Am J Dis Child 1939; 57:524-40.

49 Lust F: Die Durchlassigkeet des Magendarmkanales fur heterologes Eiweiss bei ernal irungsgestortes Sauglengen. Jahrb Kinderheilk 1913; 77:244-50.

50 Matthews TS, Soothill JF: Complement activation after milk feeding in children with cow's milk allergy. Lancet 1970; ii:893-5.

51 McCoughan C, Basten A: Immune system of the gastrointestinal tract: In: Young JA, ed. Gastrointestinal physiology IV. International Review of Physiology, Vol. 28. Baltimore: University Park Press, 1983; 131-56.

52 McCrory WW, Becker CG, Cunningham-Rundles C et al: Milk protein immune complex glomerulonephritis in a child with eosinophilic gastroenteritis. (Submitted.)

53 Mihm MC, Soter NA, Dvorak HJ, Austen KF: The structure of normal skin and the morphology of atopic eczema. J Invest Dermatol 1976; 67:305-12.

54 Moro E: Kuhmilch Prazipitin im Blute. Eines $4\frac{1}{2}$ monate alten Atrophikers. Munch Med Wochenschr 1906; 51:214-20.

55 Ogra SS, Weintraub D, Ogra PL: Immunologic aspects of human colostrum and milk. III. Fate of absorption of cellular and soluble components in the gastrointestinal tract of the newborn. J Immunol 1979; 119:245-8.

56 Paganelli R, Levinsky RJ: Solid phase radioimmunoassay for detection of circulating food protein antigens in human sera. J Immunol Methods 1980; 37:333.

57 Paganelli R, Levinsky RJ, Brostoff J, Wraith DG: Immune complexes containing food proteins in normal and atopic subjects after oval challenge and effect of sodium cromoglycate on antigen absorption. Lancet 1979; i:1270-2.

58 Peterson RDA, Good RA: Antibodies to cow's milk proteins—their presence and significance. Pediatrics 1965; 31:209-21.

59 Pudifin DJ, Cunningham-Rundles C, Good RA: Circulating antibodies to chicken ovalbumin in IgA deficient subjects. Fed Proc 1979; 38:52-63.

60 Rhodes RS, Karnovsky MJ: Loss of macromolecular barrier function associated with surgical trauma to the intestine. Lab Invest 1971; 25:220-5.

61 Rothberg RM: Immunoglobulin and specific antibody synthesis during the first weeks of life of premature infants. J Pediatr 1969; 75: 391-9.

62 Rothberg RM, Farr RS: Anti-bovine serum albumin and anti-alpha lactalbumin in the serum of children and adults. Pediatrics 1965; 33:571-88.

63 Sancho J, Edigo J, Sanchez-Crespo M, Blasco R: Detection of monomeric and polymeric IgA containing immune complexes in serum and kidney from patients

with alcoholic liver disease. Clin Exp Immunol 1982; 47:327-35.

64 Saperstein S, Anderson DW, Gredman AS, Kinder WT: Immunologic studies with sera from allergic and normal children. Pediatrics 1963; 32:580-6.

65 Schloss OM, Worthen TW: The permeability of the gastroenteric tract of infants to undigested protein. Am J Dis Child 1916; 11:342-60.

66 Sewell HF, Gell PGH, Basu MK: Immune responsiveness and oral immunization. Int Arch Allergy Appl Immunol 1979; 58: 414-25.

67 Shiner M, Ballard J, Smith ME: The small intestine mucosa in cow's milk allergy. Lancet 1975; i:136-40.

68 Signer E, Burgin-Wolff A, Berger R et al: Antibodies to gliadin as a screening test for celiac disease. Helv Paediatr Acta 1979; 34:41-52.

69 Taylor KB, Truelove SC, Thompson DL, Wright R: An immunological study of celiac disease and idiopathic steatorrhea. Br Med J 1961; 2: 1727-31.

70 Taylor B, Norman AP, Orgel HA et al: Transient IgA deficiency and pathogenesis of infantile atopy. Lancet 1973; ii:111-13.

71 Tomasi TB Jr, Tan EM, Solomon A, Prendergast RA: Characteristics of an immune system common to certain external secretions. J Exp Med 1965; 121: 101-7.

72 Triger DR, Alp MH, Wright R: Bacterial and dietary antibodies in liver disease. Lancet 1972; i:60.

73 Unsworth DJ, Manuel PD, Walker-Smith JA et al: New immunofluorescent blood test for gluten sensitivity. Arch Dis Child 1981; 56:864-8.

74 Van der Kamer JH, Weisjers HA, Dicke WK: Celiac disease. IV. An investigation into the injurious constituents of wheat in connection with the action on patients with celiac disease. Acta Paediatr 1953; 42:223-6.

75 Walker WA, Isselbacher KJ: Uptake and transport of macromolecules by the intestine: possible role in clinical disorders. Gastroenterology 1974; 67:531-50.

76 Walker WA, Isselbacher KJ, Bloch KJ: Intestinal uptake of macromolecules: effect of oral immunization. Science 1972; 608-10.

77 Walzer M: Studies in absorption of undigested proteins in human beings. I. A simple direct method of studying the absorption of undigested proteins. J Immunol 1927; 14:143-9.

78 Wasserman SI: The mast cell—introduction. Clin Rev Allergy 1983; 1:309-10.

79 Watson DW, Quigley WA, Blot RJ: Effect of lymphocytes from patients with ulcerative colitis on human adult colon epithelial cells. Gastroenterology 1966; 51:985-93.

80 Weiss JB, Austin RK, Schanfield MS, Kognoff MF: Gluten-sensitive enteropathy. Immunoglobulin G—heavy chain allotypes and the immune response to wheat gliadin. J Clin Invest 1983; 72:96-101.

81 Williams RC, Gibbons RJ: Inhibition of bacterial adherence by secretory immunoglobulin A: a mechanism of antigen disposal. Science 1972; 177:697.

82 Wilson JJ, Walzer M: Absorption of undigested proteins in human beings. Am J Dis Child 1935; 50:49-57.

83 Worthington BS, Boatman ES, Kenny GE: Intestinal absorption of intact proteins in normal and protein-deficient rats. Am J Clin Nutr 1974; 27:276-86.

SECTION E
MECHANISMS OF DAMAGE

Chapter 13a
Immunologically Mediated Damage—
Local and Distant

R. Wright and D. Robertson

Introduction

The gastrointestinal tract is exposed to an enormous load of potentially antigenic foreign material, and it is a measure of the efficient exclusion and handling of these antigens that damaging immune reactions to food are so uncommon. However, adverse reactions to food do occur, and some of these are thought to have an allergic basis. In this chapter possible mechanisms of food allergy are discussed.

This is a controversial area and little is known for certain about the mechanisms of food-allergic reactions in man. For example, the best-studied and commonest food allergy in children is cow's milk allergy, yet the immunopathogenesis remains unclear. Similarly, in coeliac disease it is not clear whether the abnormal immunological phenomena demonstrated in this condition are of primary importance or secondary to a biochemical abnormality [33].

The normal systemic immune response

After systemic exposure to an antigenic stimulus, the individual responds by the primary immune reaction, which may involve the development of specific antibody, the development of cell-mediated immunity or both. Alternatively, the specific state of nonresponsiveness known as tolerance may be induced.

Humoral response. In the humoral response, B lymphocytes differentiate into plasma cells, producing specific antibody which combines with soluble antigen such as bacterial toxins to produce immune complexes. These are then phagocytosed by polymorphonuclear leukocytes or macrophages/monocytes with or without the fixation of complement. Complexes with excess antigen will not activate complement and will utilize the Fc receptor mechanism. Cellular antigens such as bacteria will

237

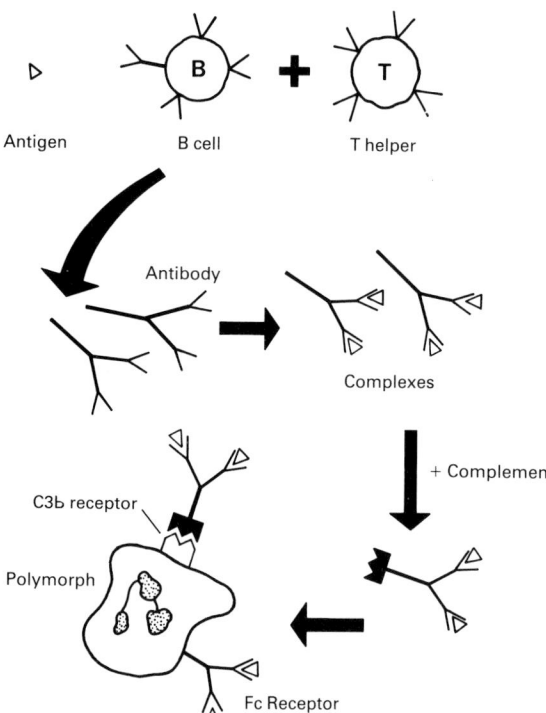

Fig. 13a.1 The humoral antigen elimination system. B lymphocytes differentiate into plasma cells, producing specific antibodies. T helper cells are important at this stage. Immune complexes are formed which fix complement if there is antibody excess, or are phagocytosed using the Fc receptor mechanism if there is antigen excess.

be coated with antibody (opsonized) to enhance phagocytosis (Fig. 13a.1).

Cell-mediated response. The cell-mediated response is directed primarily towards intracellular microorganisms, such as viruses and mycobacteria, and to foreign cells (allografts). Sensitized T cells proliferate and differentiate to produce two major effector mechanisms— cytotoxic cells and cells which release lymphokines (Table 13a.1). These polypeptides modulate the behaviour of other cells, enhancing phagocytosis non-specifically and activating macrophages with T cell antigen-specific factors (Fig. 13a.2).

After effective elimination of the antigen, the systemic immune system remains primed and able to respond promptly should the antigen be encountered once more.

Specific tolerance. The alternative to specific immunization is the development of specific tolerance, where further exposure to an antigen leads to a state of non-responsiveness. Activated T and B cells being rendered unresponsive by antigen-specific suppressor T cells

is thought to be one of the major mechanisms involved.

Control of the immune response

The magnitude and quality of the immune response is highly specific and under control at a variety of levels. Immune response genes are closely linked to the HLA genes and provide a genetic level of control, and high and low responders to a specific antigenic stimulus can be identified. The monocyte/macrophage series is important in processing of antigens and presenting them to the lymphocyte in such a way that an appropriate immune response is triggered. There are interactions between T cells and B cells, such that certain antibody responses are T cell-dependent. Helper and suppressor T cells regulate the immune response, helper cells amplifying the system, suppressor cells, which may be antigen-specific or non-specific, applying a brake to the system. Control is exerted by other factors, including the feedback inhibition of specific antibody.

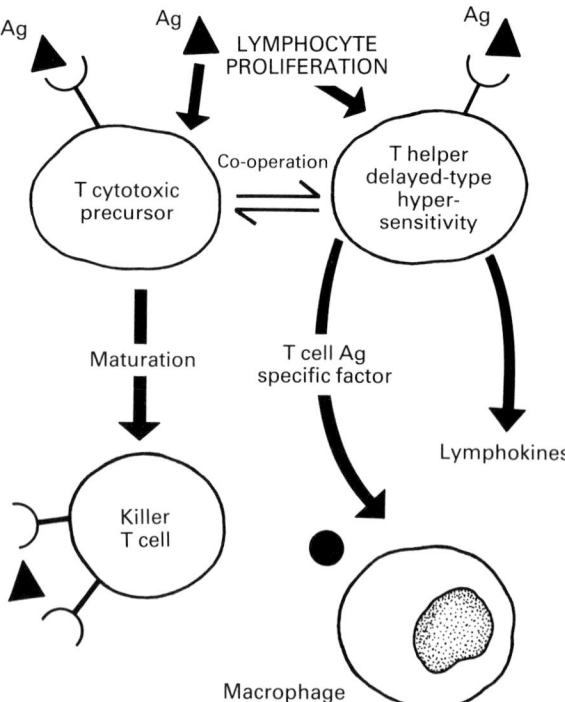

Fig. 13a.2 The cellular antigen (Ag) elimination system. Sensitized T cells differentiate into cytotoxic cells, or cells releasing lymphokines and antigen-specific factors which activate macrophages.

Table 13a.1 Lymphokines: polypeptides of molecular weight 20 000 to 80 000.

Mononuclear phagocyte chemotactic factor Migration inhibition factor (MIF)	Increase local macrophage population
Macrophage activating factor α-Interferon	Synonymous. Stimulates killing of intracellular organisms and inhibits viral replication
Interleukin 2	T cell proliferation
Lymphocyte inhibitory factor (LIF)	T suppressor function
Others, of uncertain function	

Antigenic exclusion

Despite the enormous antigenic load present in the gut, the systemic immune response is relatively small. This is because the majority of antigens are excluded by non-immune means (Chapter 11). Most of the antigens that do stimulate a response are effectively contained within the mucosa and the systemic response is more likely to involve the development of specific tolerance to the antigen [9]. However, under certain circumstances an immunizing reaction may occur, which normally leads to the effective elimination of the antigen without tissue damage. If the antigen is present in sufficiently large amounts or if the cellular or humoral response is excessive, then host tissue damage can occur. This is called hypersensitivity and forms the basis of food-allergic reactions.

HYPERSENSITIVITY REACTIONS

Coombs and Gell [10] describe four groups of hypersensitivity reactions. This remains a useful classification, but it is not clear whether all types of reaction are involved in the pathogenesis of food allergy, either in the gut itself or in remote organs. The four groups are not intended to be mutually exclusive and more than one mechanism may operate in any allergic reaction.

Type I. Anaphylactic sensitivity
(Fig. 13a.3)

Type I hypersensitivity occurs when antigen combines with reaginic antibody (usually IgE) bound by its Fc piece to the surface of tissue and blood mast cells or basophils. The bound antibodies are cross-linked by antigen, the basophil degranulates and releases large amounts of stored, pharmacologically active substances including histamine, 5-hydroxytryptamine and heparin; other substances are synthesized, such as leukotrienes, prostaglandins and thromboxanes. The combined effect of these

agents is to constrict smooth muscle and dilate capillaries (Table 13a.2). This mechanism underlies the common problem of atopic allergy, which affects approximately 10% of the population. Following intradermal injection of antigen in a sensitized subject, a local wheal and flare reaction occurs, and it is this that forms the basis of intradermal skin testing. In the nasal mucosa the reaction causes the rhinorrhoea and congestion typical of hay fever. In the bronchial tree, bronchial constriction and a clinical asthmatic attack may be precipitated. Rarely systemic anaphylaxis with bronchoconstriction, hypotension and death can occur following exposure to antigens such as a bee sting. Figure 13a.4(a) shows mucosal oedema in the ileum in a patient with urticaria

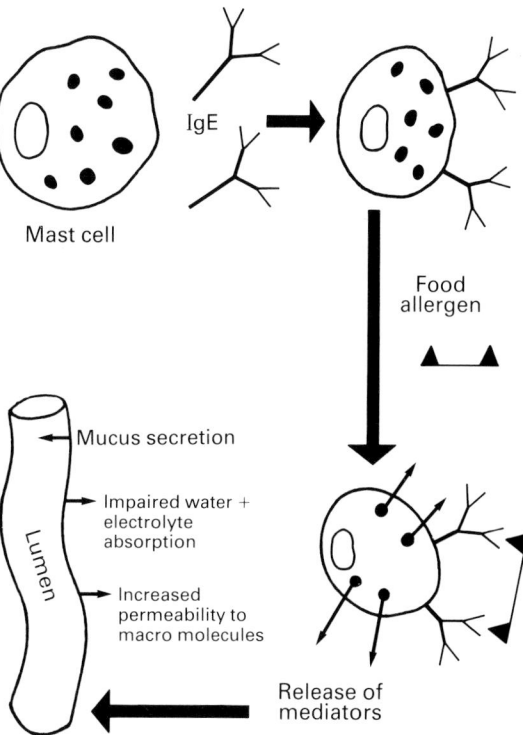

Fig. 13a.3 Type I hypersensitivity. A food allergen cross-links two mast-cell-bound IgE molecules, causing local release of mediators. These cause increased mucus secretion, impaired absorption and increased permeability.

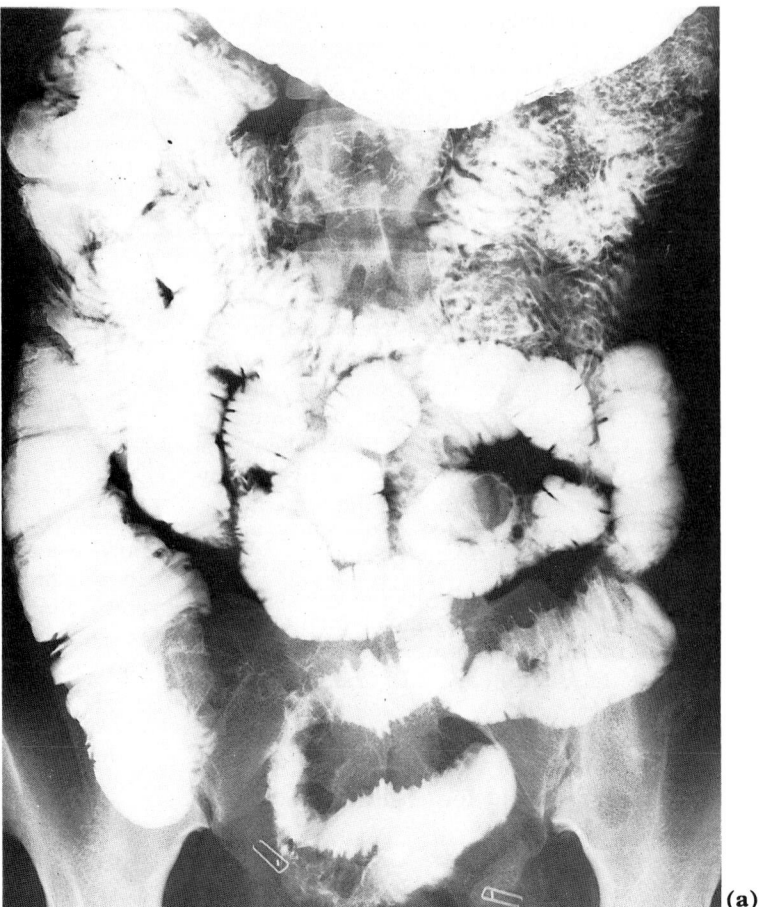

(a)

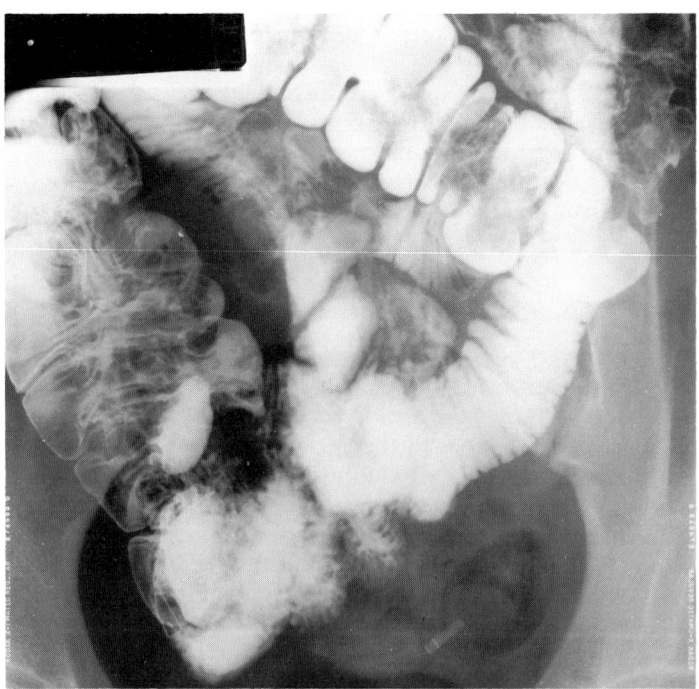

(b)

Fig. 13a.4 Barium followthrough examination in a patient with urticaria and abdominal pain. During an acute attack of abdominal pain there is gross mucosal oedema (a), which is not present between attacks (b).

Table 13a.2 Mediators released by mast-cell triggering.

Granule release (preformed)	
Histamine	Vasodilatation: increased permeability
	Chemotaxis: bronchoconstriction
Heparin	Anticoagulant
Tryptase	Activates complement
Eosinophil chemotactic factors	
Neutrophil chemotactic factors	
Platelet-activating factor	
Newly synthesized	
Lipoxygenase pathway	Leukotrienes B_4 C_4 D_4—histamine-like
Cyclooxygenase pathway	Prostaglandins Platelet aggregation
	Thromboxanes and vasodilatation

and abdominal pain. The ileum appears normal between attacks of pain (Fig. 13a.4(b)).

Atopic food sensitivity

In atopic food hypersensitivity, shortly after ingestion of the offending food the subject may develop a local reaction such as swelling of the tongue or oral mucosa. Diarrhoea and vomiting may occur within a few minutes or a more generalized reaction may occur, such as urticaria or, rarely, anaphylaxis. Such food allergies are well recognized. On the whole, the subject correctly identifies the offending foodstuff and avoids it thereafter. There is evidence that less obvious symptoms can be attributed to Type I reactions to food.

IgE-producing plasma cells are distributed throughout the gastrointestinal tract and are present in increased numbers in the jejunal mucosa of patients with food allergy [34]. Mast cells are also widely distributed throughout the gut [3] (Chapter 5), so the potential for Type I reactions is present in the gut in healthy individuals.

Type I-mediated damage: hypotheses

There are two main hypotheses to explain how certain predisposed individuals develop IgE antibodies and Type I hypersensitivity reactions. The first suggests that atopy is a consequence of overstimulation by antigens during early life. In infants there is a relative IgA deficiency in the gut resulting in an increased capacity to absorb macromolecules [41]. Events such as gastroenteritis can further disrupt intestinal integrity and lead to further antigen exposure and uptake.

The alternative hypothesis suggests that antigen stimulation results in T suppressor cell activation, which suppresses IgE synthesis and the atopic individual has a specific suppressor T cell deficiency [21].

Gut changes following Type I reactions

Important changes in gut physiology can be demonstrated in sensitized experimental animals undergoing exposure to antigen. Thus, large changes in water and electrolyte transport [31], goblet cell mucus release [24] and enterocyte turnover and differentiation [15] can be demonstrated following gut challenge, and it is proposed that IgE-mediated mast-cell release of chemical mediators, in particular histamine, accounts for the functional abnormalities demonstrated. A similar sequence of events in man may account for a variety of gastrointestinal symptoms, such as abdominal pain, distension and diarrhoea.

Type II. Antibody-dependent cytotoxic hypersensitivity

The best recognized example of a Type II reaction occurs when an antigen present on a cell surface combines with antibody, either IgG or IgM, to cause cellular destruction by one of a number of pathways.

1 Antibody-dependent cell-mediated cytotoxicity can occur. Non-sensitized lymphoreticular cells bind to the antibody by specific receptors. Polymorphs, macrophages and killer cells may be involved and killing occurs by an extracellular mechanism (Fig. 13a.5).

2 The antibody-coated (opsonized) cell will be phagocytosed, e.g. hyperimmune graft rejection reaction.

3 Complement is activated as far as C3: C3A has an anaphylotoxic activity causing mast-cell degranulation and release of chemotactic factors. There are specific receptors to C3B on polymorphs and macrophages, permitting immune adherence and facilitating phagocytosis.

4 Complement is activated through to C8, C9 and cell lysis occurs.

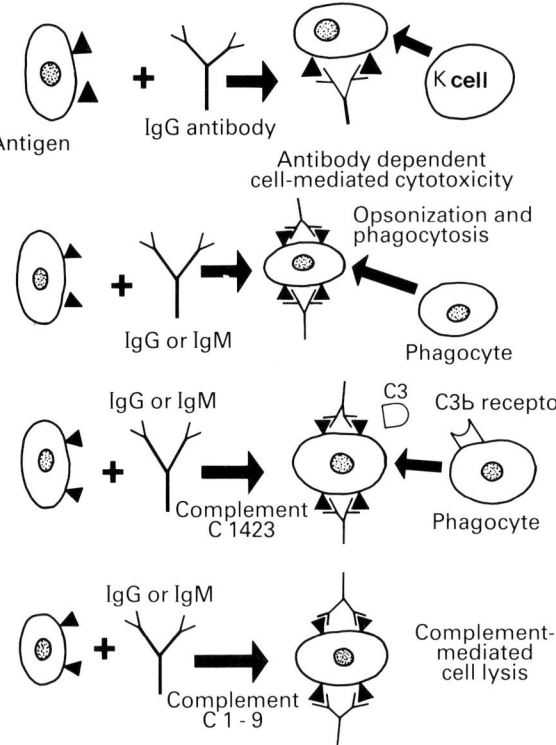

Fig. 13a.5 Type II hypersensitivity. Destruction of antigen-bearing cells may be accomplished by a number of mechanisms. Antibody-dependent cell-mediated cytotoxicity, opsonization and phagocytosis, or complement activation.

Type II reactions and autoimmunity

Type II reactions form the basis of auto-immune haemolytic anaemia and thrombocytopenia. In other autoimmune diseases, the mechanism is less clear. In Goodpasture's syndrome there is good evidence that anti-glomerular basement membrane antibodies fix complement and are directly responsible for the glomerulonephritis. In pernicious anaemia, gastric parietal cell antibodies are cytotoxic to isolated parietal cells [13], but in other conditions where autoantibodies are common, e.g. Hashimoto's thyroiditis, the evidence for a pathogenic role of the antibody is less clear, and it may represent an epiphenomenon.

Non-IgE antibodies to food

Circulating non-IgE antibodies to food can be readily demonstrated in low concentrations in health and in an increased prevalence and concentration in a variety of groups of individuals, such as normal infants and people with selective IgA deficiency, inflammatory bowel dis-

ease, coeliac disease and gastroenteritis. These antibodies do not appear to be of pathological significance and reflect the normal response to impaired exclusion of antigen. Antibody titres fall with appropriate treatment of the underlying condition [23]. Theoretically, tissue damage might occur if food antigens cross-react with host tissue antigens, initiating an autoimmune process. For example, there are reports of antibodies to *Escherichia coli* (a gut bacterial antigen but not a food antigen) cross-reacting with human colon in ulcerative colitis [32], and it has been suggested that these antibodies are cytotoxic, but it is now widely held that *E. coli* antibodies are not of pathogenic significance and may occur in a variety of other disease states [42].

There is therefore no evidence that Type II reactions are an important mechanism in food allergy.

Type III. Immune-complex mediated

Food antigens are often absorbed from the gut in small amounts and encounter specific antibodies in the circulation with the formation of

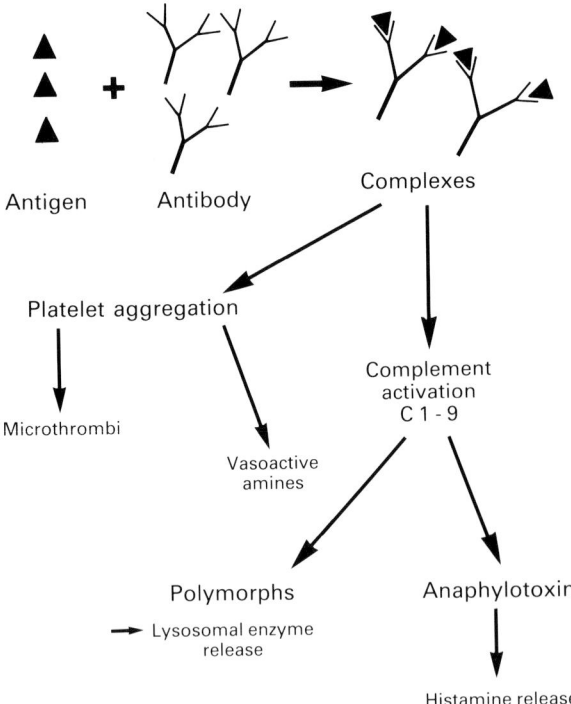

Fig. 13a.6 Type III hypersensitivity. Complexes formed in antigen excess are deposited in vessel walls with aggregation of platelets and local release of inflammatory mediators. In antibody excess there is local precipitation of complexes with fixation of complement and release of inflammatory mediators.

immune complexes. These are normally cleared rapidly by the reticuloendothelial system and they are of no pathological significance. Tissue damage will result, however, if there are high concentrations of complexes and the nature of the damage depends upon whether antigen or antibody is present in excess (Fig. 13a.6).

Antigen excess (serum sickness reaction)

These are usually generalized reactions associated with circulating complexes. When large doses of foreign antigens, e.g. horse serum, are given therapeutically, a specific antibody response is provoked with the formation of immune complexes in the presence of gross antigen excess. If the complexes are of an appropriate size, they are deposited in vessel walls and an inflammatory reaction is provoked in the endothelium with exposure of the basement membrane to which the complexes attach. Deposition in skin, kidney and joints leads to the clinical features of urticaria, albuminuria and arthritis, together with fever and lymphadenopathy.

Antibody excess (Arthus-type reaction)

These are usually local reactions. By injecting hyperimmune rabbits intradermally with the appropriate antigen, Arthus induced a characteristic skin lesion with erythema and induration. There is a local deposition of complexes with fixation of complement, anaphylotoxin release, mast-cell degranulation and local intravascular reactions. This type of reaction occurs in man in the lungs, in farmer's lung and aspergillosis, in the lymphatics in response to filarial worm infestation, and Type III reactions are implicated in the joints of patients with rheumatoid arthritis.

Immune complexes and food allergy. In food allergy, circulating immune complexes are demonstrable after ingestion of antigen, but are quantitatively and qualitatively different from the small amounts found in normal subjects [30]. In animal studies, the secondary development of immune complexes following increased absorption of antigen as the result of intestinal anaphylaxis (Type I) reaction may be important in the pathogenesis of the intestinal lesion [44].

Animal models of Type III reactions

In animal models, Type III reactions can cause gastrointestinal abnormalities. In immunized pigs, ingestion of high levels of antigen leads to polymorph migration to the epithelium but no tissue damage or functional derangement [4]. In hyperimmune animals, there is a deposition of immune complexes in the gut, with only minor histological damage [1]. Major histological damage can be induced in the colon by injecting immune complexes into an animal where the colon has previously been traumatized by exposure to formalin [19], and it has been suggested that the immune complexes found inconstantly in inflammatory bowel disease may be important in initiating a relapse of disease activity or perpetuating the disease.

Dermatitis herpetiformis

The skin lesions associated with dermatitis herpetiformis may be the result of a local Type III reaction. Patients with dermatitis herpetiformis have elevated antibody levels to gluten of IgA, IgG and IgM classes, and skin lesions and unaffected skin have linear deposits of IgA which bind gluten [43]. Gluten challenge in patients on a gluten-free diet produces elevated levels of gluten-containing immune complexes and clinical relapse [20]. It is not clear, however, whether the IgA deposits are directed against skin components, e.g. reticulin, where a Type II mechanism would be implicated, or whether they are deposited in the form of immune complexes (Type III reaction).

It seems probable that, if immune complexes are formed after ingestion of antigen, damage, if it occurs, will be in distant organs rather than in the gut.

Type IV. Delayed hypersensitivity
(Fig. 13a.7)

The classic reaction is the Mantoux reaction, where 1 to 3 days after injection of tuberculin into a sensitized subject (previously exposed to TB), an indurated erythematous lesion appears. Histologically, there is perivascular cuffing with mononuclear cells and later extensive exudation of monocytes and polymorphs. The predominant cell type is the macrophage/monocyte. If the reaction continues because of continuing antigen exposure (persistent infection), the macrophages differentiate to form

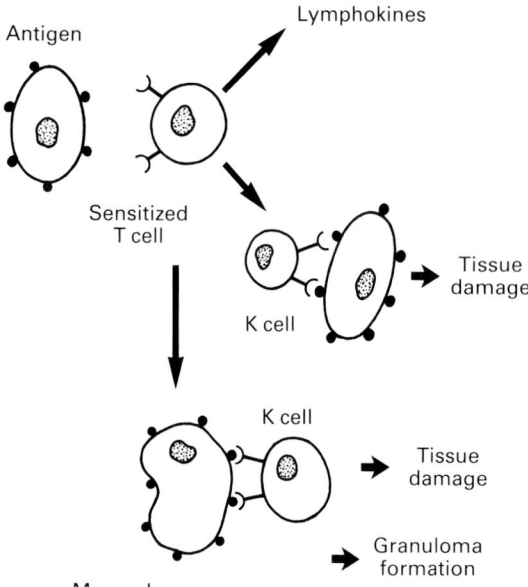

Fig. 13a.7 Type IV hypersensitivity. In response to a cellular antigen, sensitized T cells differentiate to produce lymphokines and cytotoxic cells. Antigens are expressed on the surface of macrophages, and tissue damage results from continued infection or autoimmunization.

epithelioid cells and fuse to form giant cells. This is a T cell-dependent mechanism. Some of the stimulated T cells produce soluble factors mediating the hypersensitivity reaction (Fig. 13a.7), while others develop cytotoxicity. Tissue damage occurs as a result of persisting antigenic stimulation, either because of continuing infection or because of autoimmunization. Macrophages with bacterial antigens on the surface will be destroyed by K cells and other cells are killed as innocent bystanders by non-specifically activated macrophages.

Type IV reactions and food antigens

There is evidence that Type IV reactions can cause intestinal damage, including villus atrophy, in a variety of animal models, including parasitic infections and graft-versus-host disease [16].

The importance of cell-mediated hypersensitivity reactions in the pathogenesis of food allergy is not clear. It is widely held that the enteropathy of coeliac disease is due to a local cell-mediated immune response to dietary gluten. Cell-mediated immunity to gluten in coeliac disease can be demonstrated by inhibition of leukocyte migration [7], which persists despite a gluten-free diet. However, cell-mediated immunity to food antigens other than gluten can be demonstrated in coeliac disease [39] and this may be the result rather than the cause of villus atrophy.

Assessment of cell-mediated reactions. One of the major problems encountered in the assessment of cell-mediated immunity to food allergens is the inadequacy of the immunological methods available. For example, the phenomenon of leukocyte migration inhibition is thought to be due to macrophage migration inhibitory factor (MIF) production, a lymphokine. Studies in patients with coeliac disease have shown that the marked migration inhibition that occurs in the presence of gluten is not due to lymphokine release but may reflect cytophilic antibody, implying an entirely different mechanism, probably unrelated to the pathogenesis of coeliac disease [40].

Mechanisms operating simultaneously

As emphasized previously, the hypersensitivity reactions Type I–IV of Gell and Coombs are not intended to be mutually exclusive and one might expect two or more mechanisms to operate simultaneously on occasion. Furthermore, these mechanisms were elucidated in the systemic immune response and have not been shown unequivocally to be operative in the gut. One might expect reactions to vary from tissue to tissue and indeed from time to time in the same tissue. The varied clinical features that can occur in cow's milk protein intolerance suggest different mechanisms in different patients [17]. It is not surprising, therefore, that clear immunogenic pathways of food allergy have not yet been defined. Even in the best-studied example, cow's milk protein intolerance, evidence is indirect and often conflicting and the distinction between primary pathogenic events and immunological phenomena secondary to mucosal damage is often difficult to assess.

Three of the best-understood examples of food allergy are described here to illustrate the mechanisms and are discussed in greater detail in other chapters.

The mechanisms of cow's milk intolerance (see also Chapter 18)

There is evidence to implicate all four types of reaction in cow's milk protein intolerance. In Type I reactions there is often a family or personal history of atopy. There are elevated titres of IgE specific for cow's milk protein, and skin testing may be positive [11]. There is an increase in IgE plasma cell numbers in the small bowel mucosa following challenge [38]. Type II reactions are considered to be rare, but may account for the occasional thrombocytopenia seen in cow's milk protein intolerance [22], particularly in association with the absent radius syndrome [45]. Type III reactions may well be important. Immune complexes of IgE, IgG and IgM with cow's milk proteins, such as β-lactalbumin, are present after feeding [5,18]. Reduced complement levels [27] may be the result of clearance of immune complexes after challenge. Type IV reactions are suggested by studies demonstrating in vitro milk-induced lymphoblast transformation [37] and reduced neutrophil chemotaxis [8,28]. However, none of the above phenomena are specific for cow's milk protein intolerance, and there are many false-positive and false-negative reactions.

MECHANISMS INVOLVED IN EXTRAINTESTINAL ABNORMALITIES

Hypersensitivity reactions to food can occur when the predominant clinical abnormality occurs outside the gastrointestinal tract. The development of extraintestinal phenomena implies that antigen is being absorbed and circulated in excess amounts, and that the usual state of tolerance to that antigen is not operating [9] (see Chapter 14). Here we will consider the mechanisms of two such phenomena—asthma and atopic eczema.

Asthma (see also Chapter 27)

Asthma is known to have a multifactorial aetiology and the overall contribution of allergic reactions to food in the pathogenesis is unknown. There are undoubtedly cases where wheezing follows quickly and reliably upon the ingestion of foods and in these cases the association is clear. However, there are many more cases of intrinsic asthma where unsuspected food allergy may be an important factor. Immune complexes containing food antigens may be detected in the blood of asthmatic subjects undergoing challenge, and these may trigger bronchoconstriction. The abnormal immune reaction starts in the gut, however, and it seems likely the local mast-cell degranulation which may or may not cause gastrointestinal symptoms leads to increased perme-

ability of mucosa and increased absorption of antigens [12,14] which are complexed with IgE or IgG. IgE complexes can lead to bronchial mast-cell degranulation and bronchoconstriction. Since mucosal permeability may remain altered for days after challenge and since immune complexes may persist for several days in the circulation, there may be no obvious temporal relationship to eating. If the antigenic food is frequently eaten, e.g. milk, symptoms are likely to be continuous.

Identification of such cases is difficult, and if other important factors are not operative, such as exercise or stress, then a provocation test may not lead to a clinical attack. However, more subtle changes such as an increase in bronchial reactivity to histamine may be noted [46].

The sensitizing dose of antigen need not necessarily enter the body through the gastrointestinal tract. Allergic reactions, including asthma and anaphylaxis, occur after eating where sensitization has occurred by inhalation, such as after exposure to ispaghula husk used in bulk laxatives [26].

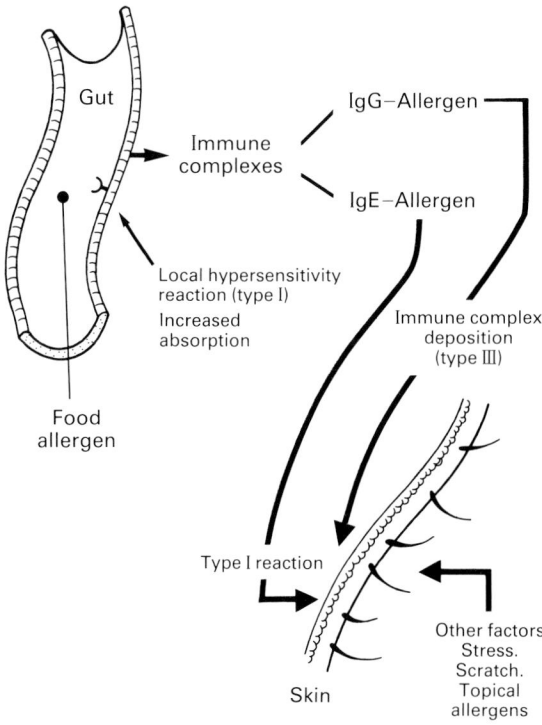

Fig. 13a.8 Suggested mechanism of food allergy in atopic eczema. A Type I reaction in the gut (which may or may not cause symptoms) causes increased permeability and antigen is absorbed. IgE complexes cause a secondary Type I reaction in the skin with further release of mediators, and IgG complexes are deposited in skin, causing a Type III reaction.

Asthma occurring as a result of food allergy appears to be an atopic phenomenon (Type I), mast-cell degranulation occurring in the gut and in the bronchial tree.

Atopic eczema (see also Chapter 34)

Children with atopic eczema demonstrate cutaneous reactions to food administered in a double-blind placebo-controlled manner [35]. Challenge is associated with marked increase in blood histamine levels [36], prostaglandins [25] and a decrease in complement levels [27]. Circulating immune complexes which bind to C1q [6] and contain food antigens [29] can be demonstrated. The increase in blood histamine demonstrated is not all attributable to release of histamine from gut-associated mast cells, as histamine is rapidly metabolized in the portal circulation [2].

The combination of Type I and Type III reactions appears to be involved and circulating IgE complexes may trigger cutaneous mast cells, allowing the secondary release of vasoactive substances and contributing, along with immune complex deposition, to the lesion of atopic eczema. Non-immune factors, such as scratching, may complete the clinical picture (Fig. 13a.8).

The mechanisms involved in food allergy are poorly understood and the traditional classification of sensitivity reactions into Types I–IV may be insufficient to explain all the abnormalities seen. As further research provides information about immune mechanisms in food allergy, a new classification may evolve.

REFERENCES

1 Accini L, Brentjens JR, Albini B, et al: Deposition of circulating antigen–antibody complexes in the gastrointestinal tract of rabbits with chronic serum sickness. Am J Dig Dis 1978; 23:1098–106.

2 Arnoldsson H, Melander C-G, Melander E: Elimination of C^{14} histamine from the blood of man. Scand J Clin Lab Invest 1962; 14:241–6.

3 Befus AD, Pearce FL, Gauldie J, et al: Mucosal mast cells. I. Isolation and functional characteristics of rat intestinal mast cells. J. Immunol 1982;128:2475–80.

4 Bellamy JEC, Nielsen NO: Immune mediated emigration of neutrophils into the lumen of the small intestine. Infect Immun 1974; 9:615.

5 Brostoff J, Carinii C, Wraith DG, Johns P: Production of IgE complexes by allergic challenge in atopic patients and the effect of sodium cromoglycate. Lancet 1979; ii:1268–9.

6 Brostoff J, Carini C, Wraith DG, et al: Immune complexes in atopy. In: Pepys J, Edwards AM, eds. The mast cell. Tunbridge Wells: Pitman Medical, 1979;380–93.

7 Bullen A, Losowsky MS: Cell-mediated immunity to gluten fraction III in adult coeliac disease. Gut 1978; 19:126–31.

8 Butler HL, Byrne WJ, Marmer DJ, et al: Depressed neutrophil chemotaxis in infants, with cow's milk intolerance and/or soy protein intolerance. Pediatrics 1981;67:264–8.

9 Challacombe SJ, Tomasi TB: Systemic tolerance and secretory immunity after oral immunisation. J. Exp Med 1980;152:1459–72.

10 Coombs RRA, Gell PGH, Lachmann PJ: Clinical aspects of immunology. 3rd edn. Oxford: Blackwell Scientific, 1974.

11 Dannaeus A, Johansson SGO: A follow-up study of infants with adverse reactions to cow's milk. I. Serum test, skin test reactions and RAST in relation to clinical course: Acta Paediatr Scand 1979; 68:377–82.

12 Danneus A, Inganäs M, Johansson SGO, Foucard T: Intestinal uptake of ovalbumin in malabsoption and food allergy in relation to serum IgG antibodies and orally administered sodium cromoglycate. Clin Allergy 1979; 9:263–70.

13 De Aizpurua JH, Cosgrove LJ, Ungar B, Toh B-H: Autoantibodies cytotoxic to gastric parietal cells in serum of patients with pernicious anaemia. N Engl J Med 1983; 309:625–9.

14 Du Mont GCL, Beach RC, Menzies IS: Gastrointestinal permeability in food allergic eczematous children. Clin Allergy 1984; 14:55–9.

15 Ferguson A, Jarrett EG: Hypersensitivity reactions in the small intestine. I. Thymus-dependent experimental partial villous atrophy. Gut 1975; 16:114–7.

16 Ferguson A, Macdonald TT: Effects of local delayed hypersensitivity on the small intestine. Immunology of the gut. Ciba Found Symp 46: 305.

17 Firer MA, Hosking CS, Hill DJ: Cow's milk allergy and eczema: patterns of the antibody response to cow's milk in allergic skin disease. Clin Allergy 1982; 12:385–90.

18 Frick OL: B-lactoglobulin in immune complexes in milk-sensitive children. J Allergy Clin Immunol [Suppl] 1982; 69:187.

19 Hodgson HJF, Potter BJ, Skinner J, Jewell DP: Immune complex mediated colitis in rabbits. An experimental model. Gut 1978; 19:225–31.

20 Induction of IgA circulating immune complexes after wheat feeding in dermatitis herpetiformis patients. J Dermatol Invest 1982; 78:375–80.

21 Jarrett E: Activation of IgE regulatory mechanisms by transmucosal absorption of antigen. Lancet 1977; ii:223–5.

22 Jones RHT: Milk induced thrombocytopenia. Arch Dis Child 1977; 52:744–5.

23 Kendrick KG, Walker-Smith JA: Immunoglubulins and dietary protein antibodies in childhood coeliac disease. Gut 1970; 11:635–40.

24 Lake AM, Bloch KJ, Walker WA: Anaphylactoid release of intestinal goblet cell mucus. Immunology 1980; 39:1–6.

25 Lessof MH, Buisseret PD, Merrett TG, et al: Mechanisms involving prostaglandins in food tolerance. In: Pepys J, Edwards AM, eds. The mast cell. Tunbridge Wells: Pitman Medical, 1979; 406–10.

26 Machado L, Fagerborg E, Zetterström D: Occupational allergy in nurses to a bulk laxative. Allergy 1979; 34:5.

27 Matthews TS, Soothill JE: Complement activation after milk feeding in children with cow's milk allergy. Lancet 1970; ii:893–5.

28 Minor JED, Tolber SG, Rick OKL: Leucocyte inhibition factor in delayed-onset food allergy. J Allergy Clin Immunol 1980; 66:314–21.

29 Paganelli R, Levinsky RJ, Brostoff J: Detection of specific antigen within circulating immune complexes. Validation of the assay and its application to food antigen-antibody complexes found in healthy and food allergic subjects. Clin Expl Immunol 1981; 46:44–53.

30 Paganelli R, Levinsky RJ, Brostoff J, Wraith DG: Immune complexes containing food proteins in normal and atopic subjects after oral challenge and effect of sodium cromoglycate on antigen absorption. Lancet 1979; ii:1270–2.

31 Perdue MH, Chung M, Grantgall D: Effect of intestinal anaphylaxis on gut function in the rat. Gastroenterology 1984; 86:391–7.

32 Perlmann P, Hammarstrom S, Lagercrantz R, Campbell D: Autoantibodies to colon in rats and human ulcerative colitis: cross-reactivity with *E. coli* 014 antigen. Proc Soc Expl Biol 1967; 125;975–80.

33 Peters TJ, Bjarnason I: Coeliac syndrome: biochemical mechanisms and the missing peptidase hypothesis revisited. Gut 1984; 28:913–8.

34 Rosekrans PCM, Meijer CJLM, Cornellise CJ, et al: Use of morphometry and immunohistochemistry of small intestinal biopsy specimens in the diagnosis of food allergy. J Clin Pathol 1980; 33:125–30.

35 Sampson HA: Role of immediate food hypersensitivity in the pathogenesis of atopic dermatitis. J Allergy Clin Immunol 1983; 71:473–80.

36 Sampson HA, Jolie PL: Increased plasma histamine concentrations after food challenge in children with atopic dermatitis. N Engl J Med 1984; 311:372–6.

37 Scheinmann P, Genorel D, Charlas J, Paupe J: Value of lymphoblast transformation test in cow's milk protein intolerance. Clin Allergy 1976; 6:515–21.

38 Shiner M, Ballard J, Smith ME: The small intestinal mucosa in cow's milk allergy. Lancet 1975; i:136–40.

39 Simpson FG, Robertson DAF, Howdle PD, Losowsky MS: Cell-mediated immunity to dietary antigens in coeliac disease. Scand J Gastroenterol 1982; 17:671–6.

40 Simpson FG, Field MP, Howdle PD, et al: Leucocyte migration inhibition test in coeliac disease—a reappraisal. Gut 1983; 24:311–7.

41 Taylor B, Norman AP, Orgel HA, et al: Transient IgA deficiency and pathogenesis of infantile atopy. Lancet 1973; ii: 111–3.

42 Triger DR, Alp MH, Wright R: Bacterial and dietary antibodies in liver disease. Lancet 1972; i:60–3.

43 Unsworth DJ, Johnson GD, Haffenden G, et al: Binding of wheat gliadin in vitro to reticulin in normal and dermatitis herpetiformis skin. J Dermatol Invest 1981; 76:88–93.

44 Walker WA, Wu M, Isselbacher KJ, Bloch KJ: Intestinal uptake of macromolecules. III. Studies on the mechanism by which immunisation interferes with antigen uptake. J Immunol 1975; 119: 854–61.

45 Whitfield MF, Barr DGD: Cow's milk allergy in the syndrome of thrombocytopenia with absent radius. Arch Dis Child 1976; 51:337–43.

46 Wilson N, Silverman M: Diagnosis of food sensitivity in childhood. J R Soc Med [Suppl 5] 1985; 78:11–6.

Chapter 13b
Non-immune Damage to the Gut

R. Wright and D. Robertson

Introduction

Adverse organic reactions to food which do not involve the immune system can be classified into three main groups (Table 13b.1). The first group involves predictable reactions to food where adverse effects would be expected to occur in any individual exposed to that food, although there may be individual variations in susceptibility. Examples include microbial contamination causing gastroenteritis, the pharmacological effects of foods containing, for example, caffeine or alcohol, or a direct toxic effect of non-nutrients contained in foods.

The second group of disorders is rather rare and is attributable to a specific inborn or acquired error of metabolism, and symptoms occur after ingestion of a food that in most people would not cause adverse effects.

The final group includes idiosyncratic reactions where the mechanism of intolerance may be obscure but does not involve allergic responses.

Table 13b.1 Classification of non-immunological mechanisms of damage.

Type	Example
1 Predictable reactions	Microbial contamination Alcohol
2 Errors of metabolism	Enzyme deficiencies Hypolactasia
3 Idiosyncratic reactions	Non-IgE mast-cell degranulation

Diagnosis

Some reactions, particularly the predictable ones, are readily recognized as being associated with the ingested food, but the nature of the illness does not suggest an allergic mechanism either to the patient or the physician. Other reactions may closely resemble an allergic response, indeed they may share a common pathway, such as anaphylactoid reactions where histamine release is brought about by foods such as shellfish, causing symptoms and signs of a Type I reaction without involving IgE.

There are a large number of chronic diseases where the diet is an important pathogenic factor. These include ingestion of sodium in the development of hypertension, of saturated fats in the pathogenesis of atherosclerosis, and of smoked foods in the development of gastric cancer. The important role of foods is not in doubt in these conditions and the mechanisms will not be considered here.

PREDICTABLE REACTIONS

Man's diet contains many thousands of chemical compounds, only a few of which are of nutritional significance [24]. Many of the other compounds are not characterized chemically and may be toxic under certain circumstances, although centuries of use suggest that these reactions are not common. However, changes in food production, storing and processing may uncover toxic effects of these food substances.

Lectins

Leguminous plants contain biologically active substances that can cause marked gastro-intestinal symptoms, particularly if ingested in a raw state. Substances such as phytohaemag-glutinins or lectins have a number of biological properties, including agglutination of red cells, intense stimulation of mitosis and inflammation. Examples of such substances are ricin from the castor bean, concanavalin A from the jack bean and phytohaemagglutinin from the red kidney bean [11] (see Chapter 21). Ingestion of these beans can cause intense epithelial inflammation, producing diarrhoea and abdominal pain.

Protease inhibitors

Protease inhibitors are widely found in vegetables and are present in raw soya beans, peanuts, lentils, rice, corn and potatoes, and in small concentrations in many other foods [20].

Whether their presence significantly inhibits digestion of the nutrients in food is not certain, but their presence may be important in cases of borderline nutrition as, for example, in patients with enzyme deficiency or protein calorie malnutrition. Further toxic effects of naturally occurring foods are listed in Table 13b.2.

Pharmacological effects

Caffeine

Caffeine (a methyl xanthine) is the most widely used stimulatory drug, pharmacologically active effects becoming apparent after ingestion of approximately 200 mg or two strong cups of coffee. The effects are predictable and include stimulation of the central nervous system, diuresis, gastric acid secretion and tachycardia. Some susceptible individuals develop severe symptoms such as abdominal pain, hypertension, supraventricular tachycardia and depression, which respond to withdrawal of the drug [8]. Such patients usually drink large amounts of coffee, and it is possible that all the effects are not due to caffeine but to

Table 13b.2 Some naturally occurring toxic substances contained within foods.

Toxic substance	Food source	Toxic effect
Proteases	Legumes	Impaired growth
Lectins	Seeds	Haemagglutination Stimulation of mitosis Inflammation
Aflatoxins	Fungal contamination of cereals	Hepatotoxic Carcinogenic
Saponins	Many plants	Haemolysis
Oxalates	Spinach Rhubarb	Oxalate renal stones
Hypoglycin	Akee plant	Hypoglycaemia
Cycads	Palm tree nuts	Amytrophic lateral sclerosis
Herb teas and tobacco	Thyme Rosemary Spearmint	Psychoactive, contains atropine and scopolamine
Cyclopeptides	Mushrooms *Amanita phalloides*	Vomiting, diarrhoea Liver and renal necrosis
Muscarin	Mushrooms *Amanita muscaria*	Salivation, vomiting Abdominal pain, diarrhoea
Methyl mercury	Fish	Minimata disease
Arsenic	Insecticides Water supply	Hepatotoxic Carcinogenic
Lead	Environmental contaminant	Neuropathy Encephalopathy
Cadmium	Environmental contaminant and shellfish	Vomiting, diarrhoea Nephrotoxic Osteomalacia

some of the many other organic substances contained in coffee. Caffeine is a drug of addiction: withdrawal symptoms such as irritability, lassitude and headache may be anticipated.

Salt

Ingestion of large amounts of salt may lead to symptoms of headache, thirst and bloating. These occur particularly after eating Chinese take-away meals which may contain up to 200 mmol of sodium and cause an elevation of serum sodium of approximately 5 mmol per litre [17]. Some of the sodium is in the form of monosodium glutamate and in the susceptible individual this can give rise to the 'Chinese restaurant syndrome' [28], where, 10 to 20 minutes after eating the food, the subject develops chest pain, facial flushing and headache. The mechanism of chest pain is uncertain, but it seems likely to be due to an oesophageal spasm. A high prevalence of vitamin B6 deficiency has been noted in sufferers, and this may increase sensitivity to monosodium glutamate [6].

Natural laxatives

Natural laxatives contained within foods or taken in the form of proprietary purgatives or tonics may cause gastrointestinal symptoms, usually cramp and diarrhoea. Magnesium, sulphate or phosphate, as naturally occurring laxatives, will cause osmotic diarrhoea. Senna and rhubarb increase intestinal secretions and motility. Castor oil, containing ricolinic acid, has a structure similar to that of bile acids and stimulates colonic secretion [4].

Vasoactive amines

Vasoactive amines are commonly found in small amounts in normal foods and can cause a wide variety of symptoms, particularly affecting the gastrointestinal tract and central nervous system (Table 13b.3). Adrenaline, noradrenaline, serotonin and histamine are all present in cheeses, cooked meats and sausages. Tyramine is produced by bacterial activity from tyrosine in fermented cheeses. Dihydroxyphenylalanine occurs in broad beans. Normally, ingested amines are rapidly metabolized by the monoamine oxidase enzymes, but if very large quantities of a food are eaten, then symptoms can result. These include erythema, headaches, hypotension and migraine. The food additive sodium nitrite causes similar symptoms in susceptible individuals [15, 25].

Bacterial effects

Enterotoxins

After ingestion of food or water contaminated by pathogenic bacteria or their enterotoxins, diarrhoea and vomiting is a common sequel and can involve a variety of mechanisms. One of the best-studied mechanisms is shared by the enterotoxins of cholera, *Staphylococcus aureus* and *Escherichia coli* (heat-labile enterotoxin). After penetrating the non-specific defences of the gastric acid barrier and the mucous coating of the small intestine, the protein subunit B of the enterotoxin adheres to a receptor on the epithelial cell of the small intestine and permits entry of subunit A, which is the active toxin. Subunit A binds irreversibly to the enzyme adenylate cyclase and stimulates production of cyclic adenosine monophosphate (AMP). This produces active secretion of chloride and bicarbonate ions and inhibits absorption of sodium and chloride. The colon is unaffected, but its absorptive

Table 13b.3 Vasoactive amines in foods.

Amine	Food source	Approximate concentration (μg/g)
Serotonin	Cheeses	
Histamine	Fermented cheese	up to 1300
	Smoked herring roe	350
	Tinned tuna	20
Tyramine	Cheddar cheese	1500
	Camembert	50
Octopamine	Citrus fruits	
Phenylethylamine	Chocolate	60
Dopamine	Chocolate	
Dopa (dihydroxyphenylalanine)	Broad beans	

capacity is exceeded by the massive small bowel secretion and copious diarrhoea results. Adenylate cyclase is permanently damaged by the toxin and recovery occurs only after replacement of the affected cell [30].

Toxic changes induced by bacteria

Other bacteria, such as *Shigella*, cause invasive bacterial infection of the epithelial mucosa. Bacteria can produce toxic changes in food, even though the bacteria themselves are not responsible for infection. Bacterial decarboxylation of histidine accounts for very high levels of histamine in certain cheeses and sausages, which can lead to diarrhoea and nausea, rashes, flushing and headaches. Scombrotoxic fish poisoning occurs after eating poorly preserved mackerel or tuna, the characteristic illness produced being due to bacterial generation of histamine from histidine [9]. Toxicity can occur because of toxins ingested by foodstuffs lower in the food chain. Nausea, vomiting, diarrhoea and, occasionally, paralysis are produced by ingestion of shellfish which have themselves ingested certain planktonic dinoflagellates which produce curare-like neurotoxins [5]. These reactions are predictable and would occur in many normal people exposed to the same food. There are considerable individual variations in the response. This variation may be accentuated by other factors, such as drug ingestion and bacterial flora of the gastrointestinal tract. The rapid hepatic metabolism of histamine is inhibited in patients taking isoniazid, and patients taking monoamine oxidase inhibitors develop headache and hypertensive crises after ingestion of foods containing tyramine, which can normally be ingested without ill-effects.

ADVERSE FOOD REACTIONS ASSOCIATED WITH METABOLIC DEFECTS

The majority of these rather rare disorders are inherited, systemic, single enzyme deficiencies, but the commonest cause of symptoms is hypolactasia, an acquired defect of lactose digestion confined to the gastrointestinal tract. In biological terms, lactose is an important foodstuff only during childhood and in adult life there is no advantage to maintaining an enzyme system with no substrate. It is not surprising, therefore, that lactase activity diminishes with age.

Hypolactasia

Hypolactasia is found in 5–10% of Caucasians and in up to 90% of some other races [7]. Most individuals are able to tolerate moderate quantities of lactose, such as 25 g contained within 1 pint of cow's milk daily, without symptoms, but the lactase-deficient subject may develop bloating, abdominal pain and diarrhoea. The mechanism is that of an osmotic diarrhoea: 25 g of lactose retain 250 ml of water in the small intestine to preserve isotonicity and bacterial metabolism in the colon leads to the formation of lactic acid, short-chain fatty acids, carbon dioxide and hydrogen, with further osmotic and cathartic effects. If bacteria containing β-galactosidase, such as the lactabacilli in yoghurt, are present, then this enzyme may substitute in part for the deficient brush border enzyme and permit lactase-deficient subjects to ingest lactose in the form of yoghurt without symptoms and with nutritional benefit [16].

Hypolactasia is not uncommon in inflammatory bowel disease and may contribute to the diarrhoea [23], but does not occur with increased frequency in patients with the irritable bowel syndrome [7].

Primary enzyme deficiencies
(Table 13b.4)

Primary deficiencies of sucrase-isomaltase can occur, causing symptoms in childhood which often improve in adult life [12]. In trehalase deficiency, exposure to trehalose contained in certain species of mushroom leads to severe symptoms which may be mistaken for toxic effects or food allergy [18]. Inherited disorders of protein digestion, such as trypsinogen deficiency, are rare and lead to failure to thrive in infancy. Fat malabsorption, leading to steatorrhoea, occurs rarely as a result of isolated deficiency of lipase or colipase or, more commonly, in cystic fibrosis or Swachmann's syndrome.

Food ingestion may precipitate symptoms in other metabolic disorders. A carbohydrate

Table 13b.4 Enzyme deficiencies giving gastrointestinal reactions to foods.

Hypolactasia
Sucrase–isomaltase deficiency
Trehalase deficiency
Trypsinogen deficiency
Lipase deficiency
Glucose-6-phosphate dehydrogenase deficiency

meal may precipitate symptoms in periodic familial hypokalaemic paralysis, where the insulin response to a meal leads to an intracellular shift of potassium and flaccid paralysis [21]. Ingestion of broad beans in glucose-6-phosphate dehydrogenase-deficient subjects may lead to haemolysis (favism) [3].

IDIOSYNCRATIC REACTIONS

Mast cells may be degranulated other than by antigen cross-linked IgE. Mediator release may follow contact with endogenous proteins on neutrophils and eosinophils or the anaphylatoxins generated by activation of the complement cascade. Exogenous polypeptides in foodstuffs which may bind to receptors for IgE include egg-white, lectins in legumes [14], nuts and cereals, proteolytic enzymes in pineapple and polypeptides present in shellfish, strawberries, tomatoes and fish [19] (Fig. 13b.1). Small amounts of naturally occurring salicylates in food can cause symptoms such as wheeze, urticaria or angioedema, and the response of aspirin-sensitive subjects to the tiny doses contained in foods might suggest an allergic reaction. However, sensitivity to aspirin and related substances usually occurs in otherwise non-atopic individuals and often in middle life, suggesting a non-atopic mechanism [27].

Food additives and dyes

The molecular structure of other agents capable of producing bronchoconstriction is varied, making immunological cross-reactivity unlikely. Similar reactions occur relatively frequently to food additives and dyes, such as tartrazine, sodium benzoate, butylated hydroxytoluene and butylated hydroxyanisole [31]. Sodium metabisulphite is a widely used food and drug preservative found in relatively high concentrations in alcoholic beverages, soft drinks, dried fruit and sausages. Exposure can produce bronchoconstriction, both after oral ingestion [29] and following inhalation of sulphur dioxide liberated by opening bottles and packages, suggesting a direct toxic effect of sulphur dioxide [13]. These are examples of common idiosyncratic reactions to foods or additives. The vast range of chemical substances contained in foods suggests an enormous

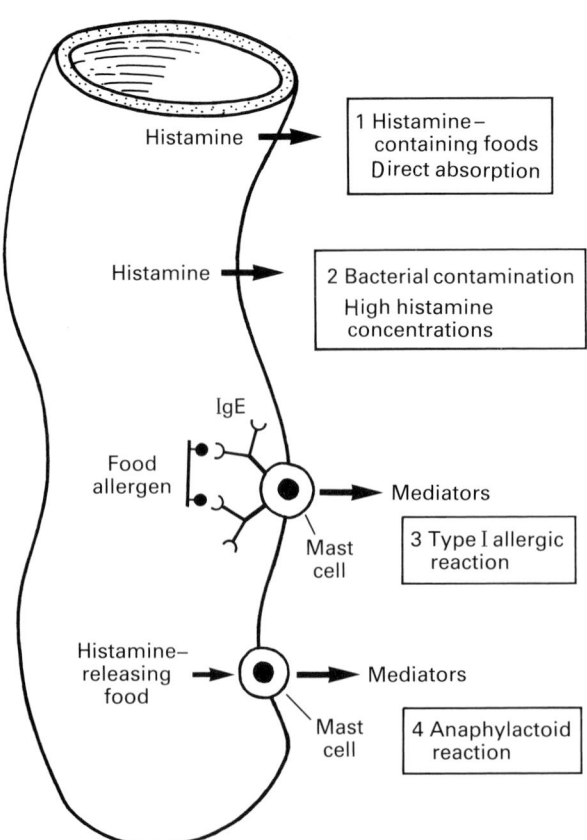

Fig. 13b.1 Histamine may be absorbed directly from foods that contain large quantities either naturally or as a result of bacterial contamination. Alternatively, histamine and other mediators may be absorbed as a result of mast-cell degranulation, either immunologically or non-immunologically mediated.

potential for reactions, although in practice they appear relatively uncommon.

Irritable bowel syndrome

The development of symptoms in the irritable bowel syndrome is often related by the patient to the ingestion of specific foods, including bran, widely used in the treatment of the condition. Evidence for food intolerance has been sought in patients with the irritable bowel syndrome, with conflicting results (see Chapter 32). Alun Jones et al [1] found that symptoms could be produced in 14 of 21 patients on double-blind reintroduction of foods, and that relapse was associated with an increase in rectal levels of prostaglandin E$_2$, suggesting that prostaglandins were implicated in the pathogenesis of diarrhoea in this condition. Bentley et al found evidence of food hypersensitivity in 3 of 27 patients, each of whom had a previous history of atopic disease. A high prevalence of minor psychiatric disorders was found in this group of subjects, and it seems likely that psychological factors are most important in the pathogenesis of the irritable bowel syndrome. Very real changes in gastrointestinal motility occur under stress, and diarrhoea, nausea and abdominal pain can be provoked by telling patients that they have been given a food to which they believe themselves allergic [10].

Pseudo-food allergy. Pseudo-food allergy [22], where the patient falsely believes he or she is allergic to a particular food, has become increasingly common in the last decade, and can lead to severe dietary restriction which should not be encouraged unless there is good evidence for intolerance to a specific food. Treatment of the underlying psychiatric problems, such as chronic hyperventilation or depression, is more appropriate [26]. (See Ch. 39.)

REFERENCES

1 Alun Jones V, Shorthouse M, McLaughlan P, et al: Food intolerance: a major factor in the pathogenesis of the irritable bowel syndrome. Lancet 1982; ii:1115–8.

2 Bentley SJ, Pearson DJ, Rix KJB: Food hypersensitivity in irritable bowel syndrome. Lancet 1983; ii:295–7.

3 Beuler E: Glucose-6-phosphate dehydrogenase deficiency. In: Stanbury JB, Wyngaarden JB, Fredrichson DS, et al., eds. The metabolic basis of inherited disease. 3rd edn. New York: McGraw-Hill, 1972; 1629–53.

4 Binder MJ: Pharmacology of laxatives. Annu Rev Pharmacol Toxicol 1977; 17:355–67.

5 Clarke RB: Biological causes and effects of paralytic shellfish poisoning. Lancet 1968; ii:770–1.

6 Editorial: Possible B6 deficiency uncovered in persons with the Chinese restaurant syndrome. Nutr Rev 1982; 40:15–6.

7 Ferguson A, Macdonald DM, Brydon WG: Prevalence of lactase deficiency in British adults. Gut 1984; 25:163–7.

8 Finn R, Cohen MN: 'Food allergy'. Fact or fiction? Lancet 1978; i:426–8.

9 Gilbert RJ, Hobbs G, Murray CK, et al: Scrombrotoxic fish poisoning; features of the first 50 incidents to be reported in Britain (1976–1979). Br Med J 1980; 281:71–3.

10 Graham DT, Wolf S, Wolff HG: Changes in tissue sensitivity associated with varying life situations and emotions: their relevance to allergy. J Allergy 1950; 21:478–86.

11 Grant G, More L, McKenzie NH, et al: A survey of the nutritional and haemagglutination properties of legume seeds generally available in the UK. Br J Nutr 1983; 50:207–14.

12 Gray GM: Intestinal disaccharidase deficiencies and glucose–galactase malabsorption. In: Stanbury JB, Wyngaarden JB, Fredrichson DS, et al, eds. The metabolic basis of inherited disease. 3rd edn. New York: McGraw-Hill, 1983; 1729–42.

13 Harries MG, Parkes PEG, Lessof MH, Orr TSC: Role of bronchial irritant receptors in asthma. Lancet 1981; i:5–9.

14 Helm RM, Froese A: Binding of the receptors for IgE by various lectins. Intern Arch Allergy, Suppl Immunol 1981; 65:81–4.

15 Henderson WR, Raskin NH: Hot dog headache; individual susceptibility to nitrite. Lancet 1972; i:1162–3.

16 Kolars JC, Levitt MD, Aouji M, Savaiano DA: Yoghurt—an autodigesting source of lactose. N Engl J Med 1984; 310:1–3.

17 MacGregor GA: New or old Chinese restaurant syndrome. Br Med J 1982; 285:1205.

18 Madrazarovova-Nohejlova J: Trehalase deficiency in a family. Gastroenterology 1973; 65:130–3.

19 Moneret-Vautrin DA: False food allergies: nonspecific reactions to foodstuffs. In: Lessof M, ed. Clinical reactions to food. Chichester: John Wiley, 1973.

20 Newberne PM: Naturally occurring food-borne toxicants. In: Goodhart RS, Shils ME, eds. Modern nutrition in health and disease. Philadelphia: Lea and Febiger, 1978; 463–96.

21 Pearson CM, Kalyanaraman K: The periodic paralyses. In: Stanbury JB, Wyngaarden JB, Fredrichson DS, et al, eds. The metabolic basis of inherited disease. 3rd edn. New York: McGraw-Hill, 1972; 1181–203.

22 Pearson DJ: Food allergy, hypersensitivity and intolerance. J R Coll Physicians Lond 1983; 19:154–62.

23 Pena AS, Truelove SC: Hypolactasia and ulcerative colitis. Gastroenterology 1973; 64:400–4.

24 Rampton RF, Charlesworth FA: Occurrence of natural toxins in food. Br Med Bull 1975; 31:209–13.

25 Rice SL, Eitenmiller RR, Koehler PE: Biologically ac-

tive amines in food: a review. J Milk Food Technol 1976; 39:353-8.

26 Rix KJB, Pearson DJ, Bentley SJ: A psychiatric study of patients with supposed food allergy. Br J Psychiatry 1984; 145:121-6.

27 Samter M, Beers RF: Intolerance to aspirin. Clinical studies and consideration of the pathogenesis. Ann Intern Med 1968; 68:975-82.

28 Schaumberg HH, Byck R, Gerstl R, Mashman JH: Monosodium glutamate; its pharmacology and role in the Chinese restaurant syndrome. Science 1969; 826-8.

29 Stevenson DD, Simon RA: Sensitivity to ingested metabisulfites in asthmatic subjects. J Allergy Clin Immunol 1981; 68:26-32.

30 Van Heyningen WE, Seal JR: The biochemistry of cholera. In: Cholera, the American Scientific Experience. Boulder, CO: Westview Press, 1983; 249-84.

31 Weber RW, Hoffmann M, Raine DA, Nelson HS: Incidence of bronchoconstriction due to aspirin, azodyes, non-azodyes and preservatives in a population of perennial asthmatics. J Allergy Clin Immunol 1979; 64:32-7.

SECTION F
MODEL SYSTEMS OF ANTIGEN HANDLING

Chapter 14
Oral Tolerance

S. J. Challacombe and T. B Tomasi

Introduction

It has been known since the work of Besredka in 1909 [6, 7] and H. G. Wells in 1911 [73] that animals fed soluble proteins lose their ability to respond to that specific antigen on subsequent systemic challenge. The elegant studies of Chase in 1946 [14] confirmed and extended these findings to show that guinea pigs fed a skin-sensitizing agent were rendered anergic to a normal sensitizing dose. Curiously the 'Chase phenomenon' was then little studied until the last 10 years when the importance of antigen handling by the gut in terms of both general and secretory immunity became realized.

Thus recently, many investigators have studied the systemic hyporesponsiveness after enteric antigen administration, as well as the induction of secretory responses [10,50]. The latter are discussed in detail in Chapter 15. Whilst in certain situations enteric immunization can result in priming (see below), there is an impressive degree of agreement that, despite marked differences in experimental design such as feeding protocols, species of the experimental animals used and the type of response measured, the ingestion of antigen will lead to systemic hyporesponsiveness. A common feature of all these studies has been the fact that the immunological unresponsiveness after such antigen feeding is to a remarkable degree antigen specific. This hyporesponsiveness has been shown in both humoral and

Fig. 14.1 Effect of sequence of intragastric and intraperitoneal immunizations on the subsequent serum IgG antibody response to ovalbumin. I/G = intragastric immunization (three daily doses of 10 mg of ovalbumin). I/P = intraperitoneal injection of 50 µg in Freund's incomplete adjuvant. Serum antibodies assayed by radioimmunoassay.

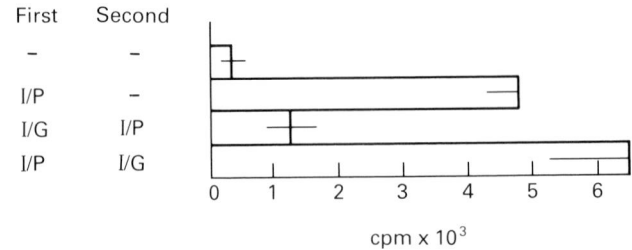

cellular arms of the systemic response, and has become known as oral tolerance [70].

Systemic immune responses after oral immunization

Deposition of antigen in the gut may lead either to immunization in the systemic system (enhancement) or to hyporesponsiveness (oral tolerance). Whether priming or tolerance occurs is dependent on a number of complex immunoregulatory mechanisms and also depends on the nature of the antigen and on whether the animals had prior exposure to the antigen. Although presentation of antigen by the enteric route appears to prime particularly well for local immune responses of the IgA class (see Chapter 15), this is not exclusive to this isotype [15].

In the dog, Pierce and Koster [52] have shown that if animals are given cholera toxoid intraperitoneally in adjuvant 2 weeks before oral immunization with cholera toxin, then this leads to an enhanced mucosal anticholera response and also to an augmented systemic response. In studies with mice we have been able to show that oral immunization with ovalbumin leads to systemic hyporesponsiveness; however, if the animals have been primed then the same immunization may give rise to enhanced systemic IgG antibody responses (Fig. 14.1). This concept has important implications for the responses to ingested material but it is unclear whether this is dependent on the nature of the antigen and whether this applies to both the humoral and cellular arms of the immune response. The importance of the nature of the antigen is discussed in more detail below.

Oral enhancement

In experiments comparing soluble with insoluble antigen on the humoral antibody responses in serum and secretions after intragastric immunization with streptococcal antigen

I/II, different serum antibody responses were found according to whether the antigen was soluble (Fig. 14.2) or insoluble (Fig. 14.3). When the antigen was given intragastrically in the soluble form in three daily doses of either 1, 10 or 50 µg, dose-dependent systemic hyporesponsiveness was found. If the same doses of antigen were given in the insoluble form then a dose-dependent enhancement of the subsequent systemic immune response of the IgG, IgA and IgM isotypes was found (Fig. 14.3). This is similar to that previously described with whole bacteria of *Streptococcus mutans* [10].

Oral enhancement has been reported with other antigens and animal models also. Serum antibody to the O antigen of *Escherichia coli* was found to be enhanced after feeding *E. coli* to pigs [48]. Similarly mice fed *E. coli* showed an increased serum antibody response to the somatic antigen [63]. With bacterial antigens, it is unclear whether the enhanced systemic

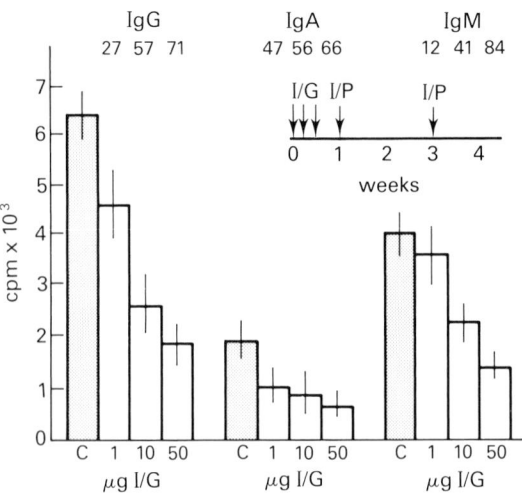

Fig. 14.2 Serum antibody responses after intragastric (I/G) immunization and intraperitoneal (I/P) challenge with streptococcal antigen (SA) I/II. Doses of 1, 10 or 50 µg of SA I/II given on 3 consecutive days, followed by I/P challenge of 2 µg of SA I/II in adjuvant at 1 and 3 weeks. Serum taken at 4 weeks and antibodies assayed by solid phase radioassay.

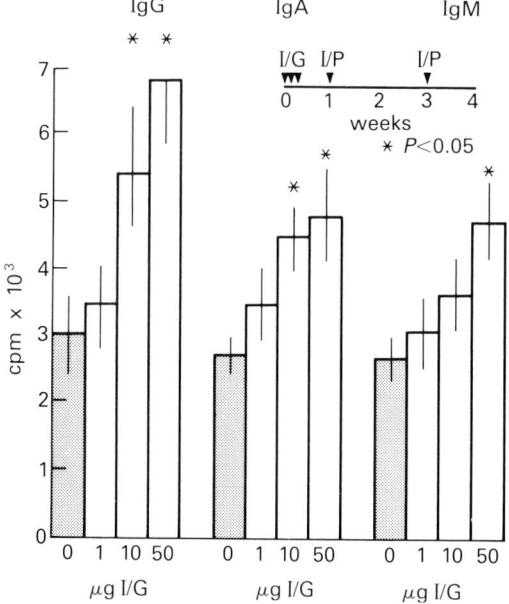

IgG IgA IgM

* P<0.05

Fig. 14.3 Serum antibody responses after intragastric (I/G) immunization and intraperitoneal (I/P) challenge with insolubilized streptococcal antigen (SA) I/II. Experimental protocol as in Fig. 14.2. SA I/II insolubilized on Sepharose beads.

response is due to the nature of the antigen itself or to prior exposure to similar or cross-reacting antigens. In the example shown in Fig. 14.3 with insolubilized streptococcal antigen, it seemed unlikely that prior exposure was the explanation since giving the same antigen in the soluble form resulted in dose-dependent suppression of the systemic humoral antibody response [11] (Fig. 14.2). Thus it seems that the nature of the antigen itself is one of the most important influences on whether systemic tolerance or enhancement occurs after the ingestion of antigen.

Animal models

A variety of animal models have been used in the study of oral tolerance. An impressive degree of concordance throughout the various experiments indicates that this is a response which may have wide biological relevance, and certainly is present with regard to the response to food antigens in man. Some examples of animal models are shown in Table 14.1. The guinea pig was the first animal model to be examined scientifically in this system and both Wells [73] and Chase [14] used this animal model to show depressed passive cutaneous anaphylaxis (PCA) and delayed-type hypersensitivity (DTH) respectively after feeding of antigen or hapten.

However, most investigators have used either mice or rats in attempts to understand and dissect some of the mechanisms underlying this phenomenon. Thus in mice, the various authors have assayed PCA, DTH and plaque-forming cells. Proliferative asays have been used to determine T cell responses [12,57] and serum antibody has been measured by others [22,60,67]. Few larger animals have been used, though diminished serum responses in pigs have been reported [48]. Some evidence exists in man that ingestion of antigenic material may result in systemic hyporesponsiveness [33]. There is some debate as to the exact mechanisms involved in the induction of oral tolerance in each of the different systems and this is discussed in more detail below.

Main features of oral tolerance

Oral tolerance can affect different aspects of the immune response, and split tolerance is sometimes found with normal or enhanced re-

Table 14.1 Some examples of oral tolerance.

Species	Antigens	Route	Assay	Author	Reference
Guinea pig	OVA	Oral feeding	PCA	Wells, 1911	73
Guinea pig	DNCB	Oral feeding	DTH	Chase, 1946	14
Mice	SRBC	Intragastric	PFC	Andre et al, 1975	1
Mice	OVA	Intragastric	PCA	Vaz et al, 1977	72
Mice	OVA	Intragastric	PA	Richman et al, 1978	57
Mice	Picryl chloride	Oral feeding	DTH	Asherson et al, 1977	3
Mice	Antigen I/II	Intragastric	Antibody	Challacombe, 1983	10
Rats	SRBC	Oral feeding	PFC	Mattingly et al, 1978	37
Pigs	BGG	Oral feeding	Antibody	Newby et al, 1981	48

Abbreviations: OVA = ovalbumin, DNCB = dinitrochlorobenzene, BGG = bovine gamma globulin, SRBC = sheep red blood cells, PCA = passive cutaneous anaphylaxis, DTH = delayed-type hypersensitivity, PFC = plaque-forming cells, PA = proliferative assay.

sponses in the humoral or cellular arm with hyporesponsiveness in the other.

Humoral tolerance

Hyporesponsiveness of systemic antibody production has been demonstrated in several studies after enteric immunization, though the majority of investigations have been concerned with cellular immunity (see below). Many authors have examined plaque-forming cells and have shown that animals given oral antigen have reduced numbers of splenic IgM and IgG plaque-forming cells, though few authors have examined IgA [1,27,29]. However, hyporesponsiveness does appear to extend to all three main isotypes where this has been examined [10], Fig. 14.2). The demonstration that systemic antibodies and passive cutaneous anaphylaxis can be inhibited in orally immunized animals [5,49] suggests that IgE responses are also depressed. In fact suppressor cells for IgE have been shown in Peyer's patches [49].

Cellular tolerance

Orally induced tolerance can certainly affect cell-mediated responses and several authors have examined delayed-type hypersensitivity reactions after such oral immunization [3,43,68]. The proliferation of antigen-sti-

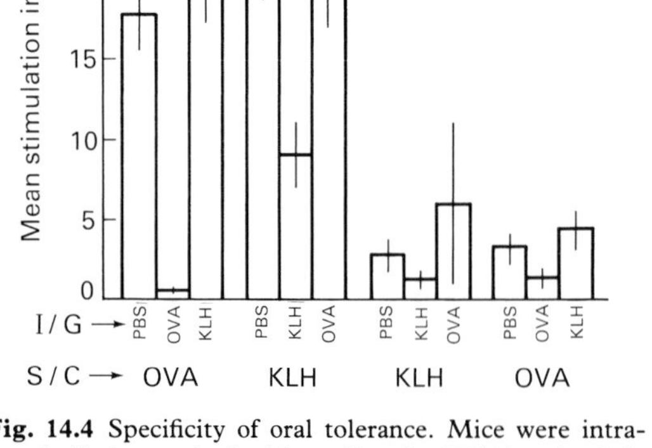

Fig. 14.4 Specificity of oral tolerance. Mice were intragastrically immunized with ovalbumin (OVA) or keyhole limpet haemocyanin (KLH). Subcutaneous challenge with the homologous antigen resulted in a very marked suppression of the proliferative responses of draining lymph nodes whereas a normal response was seen to heterologous antigen.

mulated lymphocytes in vitro is also reduced in animals given oral antigen [12]. A striking feature of oral tolerance is the degree of specificity. This applies to both the humoral and cellular arms of the systemic immune response. Thus many authors have shown that feeding of ovalbumin tolerizes animals to this protein but not to unrelated antigens such as human γ-globulin and serum albumin [12,22,68] (Fig. 14.4).

T cell-dependent antigens

It should be noted that oral tolerance applies primarily to T cell-dependent antigens and that the tolerance is maintained at the T cell level. It seems likely that in most instances the B cell itself is not tolerized [16,70]. Whilst tolerance is a very common feature in animal models following ingestion of antigenic material, this is not an absolutely consistent response. A number of factors will contribute to whether tolerance or immunization results as discussed above, and one of the most important of these appears to be the immune status of the animal. Thus it is difficult to detect the tolerizing effects of intragastric immunization feeding in animals which have already been primed systemically. There is also some evidence of species differences with regard to systemic responses to orally administered protein antigens, and there are also detectable genetic differences (see below).

Bronchial-associated lymphoid tissue (BALT) and tolerance

It should be noted that presentation of antigen by the enteric route is not the only way in which antigen present at mucosal surfaces can induce tolerance. Holt and his colleagues [24] have demonstrated that antigen presented in an aerosol to rats can lead to systemic hyporesponsiveness. In addition, antigen presentation by this route can result in the induction of secretory antibodies in bronchial secretions and also in secretions distant from the lung such as saliva ([44] and see Chapter 15). In these respects BALT seems to act in a manner analogous to gut-associated lymphoid tissue (GALT) (Fig. 14.5).

In general the doses reported for tolerance via inhalation seem to be lower than those needed via the enteric route. At certain doses split tolerance is seen in the humoral arm of the systemic immune response with IgE responses suppressed but IgG responses enhanced [24].

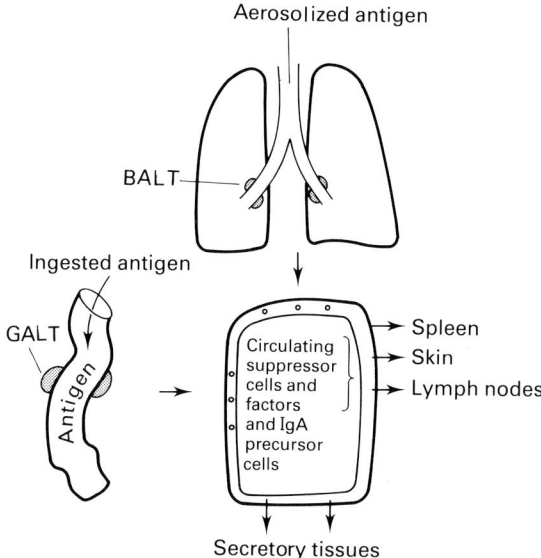

Fig. 14.5 Similarity of tolerance induction by bronchial-associated lymphoid tissue (BALT) and gut-associated lymphoid tissue (GALT).

FACTORS INFLUENCING ORAL TOLERANCE

Nature of the antigen

The tolerogenicity of an orally delivered antigen is determined by a number of factors including its degree of T cell dependence but also by other properties such as whether it is particulate or soluble, easily digested by proteases or resistant and whether it is easily aggregated or survives in the intestinal tract. There are differences between antigens in their ability to induce oral tolerance which may depend on their mechanical structure. For example soluble proteins can lead to a long-lasting systemic tolerance (and an active mucosal response) whereas tolerance to more complex antigens such as cell walls of bacteria may require larger amounts of antigen for tolerance induction and this tolerance may be relatively short lived [12,53]. With certain complex antigens such as *S. mutans*, a significant proliferative response may be found in Peyer's patches within 10 days following feeding whereas no proliferative response was detected with soluble proteins such as ovalbumin or keyhole limpet haemocyanin (KLH) [12].

Antigen structure

The importance of the role of the antigen structure is demonstrated by studies with cholera [53] where it seems that antigen combinations may be more effective than antigens given singly. Analysis of the mechanisms of oral tolerance after antigen feeding is made more challenging by the observation that with certain complex antigens like a bacterium, oral tolerance may be seen to one of the surface antigens and yet enhancement to another [63]. This presumably may be due to prior exposure to antigens which cross-react with one but not another of the surface antigens.

Polysaccharide antigens

Although most studies have been performed with protein antigens it has been demonstrated that humoral antibody responses to the polysaccharide dextran B1355 can be markedly diminished following oral feeding. Thus Kagnoff [29] showed that the IgM and IgA plaque-forming cell responses in spleens were markedly diminished following feeding. B1355 is thought to be a thymus-independent antigen. In contrast, Chiller et al [16] found that feeding lipopolysaccharide, polyvinyl pyrolidone or trinitrophenyl–ficoll did not suppress antibody responses when animals were subsequently challenged with the same antigen. It is possible though that these variances in results may reflect differences in the protocols rather than the effect of the different antigens since the dextran was fed daily for 6 days (10 mg per dose) before suppression was noted, whereas the other antigens were fed as single doses of 20 mg or as 20 mg divided over 3 days.

Skin-sensitizing agents. The ability of skin-sensitizing agents and haptens to induce oral tolerance has been noted above, and indeed is one of the best analysed systems following the work of Chase [14]. In a hapten-carrier system, the tolerance induced is carrier specific [26]. In other words, it requires challenge with the same carrier and hapten to demonstrate the oral tolerance.

Passive cutaneous anaphylaxis. Passive cutaneous anaphylaxis has been examined in the guinea pig [14] and more recently the mouse [72]. In both species enteric immunization appears to tolerize the animal.

Antigen dose and frequency of exposure to antigen

The dosage of antigen and the schedule of feeding seem to be important parameters in the induction of oral tolerance. It is dependent on both the antigen and the animal species examined. For example, with certain contact sensitizing agents (e.g. oxazolone) small doses such as 0.1–1 mg given intragastrically would tolerize the animal where higher doses (10 mg) would lead to sensitization [2]. With a well-studied antigen such as ovalbumin, varying responses have been reported according to antigen dose. Thus oral tolerance to ovalbumin could be achieved by feeding either very small or large doses. It has been reported that with small doses, delayed-type hypersensitivity (DTH) and IgE antibody formation might be diminished but higher doses of antigen were required for inhibition of IgG responses [46, 58, 59].

Low dose antigen. In contrast, it has been reported that feeding of ovalbumin in very small amounts in mice (1–100 μg) may prime rather than tolerize animals [40, 50]. In our own experiments in mice with ovalbumin, we have found a wide range of antigen doses capable of inducing oral tolerance. Thus with cell-mediated responses, single oral doses of between 1 and 20 mg would give rise to oral tolerance [12] and a similar range of antigen doses gave rise to suppression of the humoral antibody response in terms of the IgG, IgA and IgM isotypes [10]. This wide range of antigen doses giving rise to oral tolerance is in contrast to the narrow range of antigen doses which can give rise to the induction of secretory IgA antibodies (see Chapter 15).

Immune status and effect of prior antigen exposure

The immune status of the animal appears to be a critical determinant with respect to the type of systemic response to ingested antigen. Thus in mice it has been demonstrated that soluble antigen given to an immunologically virgin animal may result in oral tolerance, whereas if the same amount of antigen is given to a primed animal, then enhancement of the subsequent systemic response may be seen [11]. An example is shown in Fig. 14.1 where a comparison was made of the effect of the sequence of immunization on the serum IgG antibodies to ovalbumin. If an intraperitoneal immunization was preceded by intragastric immunization then tolerance occurred. However, if the intraperitoneal immunization was followed by an intragastric immunization then the IgG antibody response was greater than intraperitoneal alone. These observations suggest that prior sensitization may have profound effects on the nature of the systemic response.

Induction of oral tolerance in a sensitized host

The demonstrated importance of the state of the systemic immune system in the induction of oral tolerance also raises the question of which conditions might allow feeding of antigen to tolerize an already primed host. Recent studies [32] suggest that in mice, subsequent feeding abrogates the serum antibody response of parentally immunized mice and can modify the course of antigen-induced immune complex disease [17]. Partial systemic tolerance has been reported in primed rats after prolonged oral administration of antigen [9]. This however, is not a universal finding and it is a most important point in terms of the potential of treatment by the oral route of previously sensitized patients. Thus more work is needed in this area to determine the exact parameters which might result in enhancement or tolerance in already primed subjects.

Prolonged antigen feeding. One of these parameters seems to be prolonged antigen feeding. For example, Kagnoff [27] shows that whilst short-term feeding of sheep red blood cells (SRBC) boosted the IgA and IgG serum antibody titres in mice, if antigen feeding was continued over longer periods then the animals were tolerized. In a similar system oral tolerance to SRBC was induced in primed mice by prolonged feeding [28]. This rationale has already been applied in humans in attempts to tolerize allergic patients by oral immunization [8, 66].

Passive immunization. Prior passive immunization with specific antibodies may reduce the tolerogenic activity of fed ovalbumin [22, 23]. It is not clear whether this can be explained by the antigen being absorbed or bound by circulating antibodies or how this affects the induction of suppressor cells in the Peyer's patch, but it is an observation which may have biological relevance.

Duration of tolerance (see Fig. 14.6)

Oral tolerance to most protein antigens and to erythrocytes has been shown to be long lasting in most animal models, and in the mouse and rat persists for several months [12,27,71]. However, this observation is not universal to all antigens and in a system in mice when tolerance was induced to *S. mutans*, the tolerance lasted for relatively brief periods [12]. Since in most systems oral tolerance applies primarily to T cell-dependent antigens and the B cell is not tolerized [16,70], it is possible that active suppression may be present for much longer periods of time than the adoptive transfer studies have indicated. For example, suppressive factors have been found in extracts of spleen taken from HGG-tolerant animals as long as 4 months after induction of oral tolerance, whereas T suppressor cells could only be demonstrated for 3 months [71]. This raises the possibility that relatively low levels of suppressor activity are necessary to maintain T cell unresponsiveness late in tolerance. The mechanisms involved in tolerance are discussed in more detail below.

Effect of age

The age of the host at the time of oral immunization may affect both secretory and systemic responses [10]. With regard to secretory responses in the mouse, significant responses were not found in mice under 5 weeks of age nor in aged mice [11]. However, tolerance to ovalbumin assayed by plaque-forming cells could be induced in young animals though not to the same degree as in adults [10]. In other work in mice it was shown that systemic or primary tolerance resulted from enteric immunization and was related to the age at which antigen was first encountered [64].

Genetic influences

Several studies suggest that species differences may be important in the systemic responses to ingested antigen. Decreased DTH responses and decreased anttibody responses to parenteral challenge have been reported not only in the various animal models but in humans after mucosal exposure to reactive chemicals or protein antigens [30,33]. However, whilst results in humans seem to follow the results of most animal models, not all animals respond in the same way. For example, feeding of antigens such as bovine serum albumin (BSA) tolerizes both mice and rats [60,61] but the same antigen given to rabbits seems to have a priming effect [51].

Oral versus systemic tolerance. Initial studies have shown that oral tolerance may be different from systemic tolerance with regard to genetic control [71]. It seems that within strains bearing the same H-2K histocompatibility locus, there are significant differences in the ease of induction of oral tolerance to deaggregated human γ-globulin. This suggests that non-H2-linked genes are also important in oral tolerance. This would be similar to findings with systemic tolerance where Ranges and Azar [54] have shown that both H-2 and non-H-2 genes influence systemic tolerance.

Antigen handling by the gut. Stokes et al [62] examined genetic differences in tolerance and the ability to exclude ingested antigen in different strains of mice. Distinct differences were found in the capacity to absorb antigen between the four strains of mice examined and also differences were detected in the ability to develop oral tolerance.

Taken together these results clearly suggest

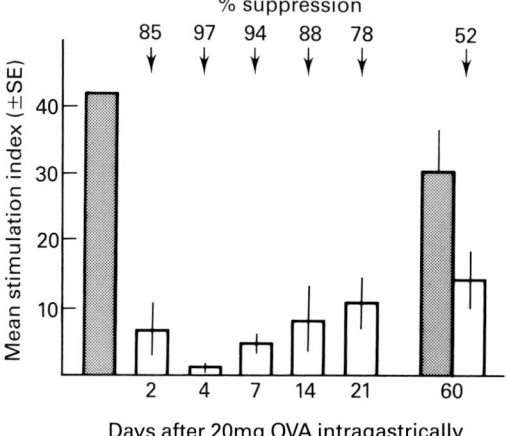

Fig. 14.6 Duration of oral tolerance. Mice were challenged at intervals after intragastric immunization with ovalbumin. Oral tolerance was still demonstrable after 2 months.

that genetic differences exist in the handling of antigen by the gut and are of obvious relevance in man with regard to differential susceptibility to food allergy. It was interesting to note that the ability to develop tolerance did not correlate with the ability to develop immune exclusion and thus suggests that these two functions are inherited independently [62].

Role of gut flora and lipopolysaccharide in oral tolerance

A number of substances within the lumen may have an effect upon the response to a particular antigen. It is known that the normal gut flora has a pronounced effect upon the immune system and a wide range of immune activities are modified including macrophage function [4] and the ability to mount DTH reactions [34]. Using the mouse model, McGhee et al [36] have shown that bacterial lipopolysaccharide (LPS) can profoundly influence the regulation of IgA responses and the generation of tolerance. Feeding with LPS enhances oral tolerance to antigens such as sheep red blood cells given at the same time. Thus oral tolerance to SRBC could not be induced in LPS-non-responsive mice or in germ-free mice, whilst in genetically related LPS-responsive mice and in germ-free mice pretreated with LPS, tolerance to SRBC could be induced [42].

Expansion of suppressor cells. It is possible that LPS derived from the normal microflora contributes to expansion of suppressor cells in the gut-associated lymphoid tissues. In the DTH model in mice, feeding of LPS has been shown to enhance oral tolerance to oxazolone and picryl chloride [47]. However, this might not apply to all antigens since oral tolerance to ovalbumin was induced equally well in LPS-responsive or non-responsive mice [58]. It also seems that oral tolerance to an antigen can be avoided if this is given within 48 hours of primary contact with a non-related antigen [62]. This suggests that a response to an ingested antigen may be modified if an immune response is already being generated to an unrelated antigen. This is clearly an interesting area which deserves further investigation.

Antigen-presenting cells

Another factor which may affect either immune regulation or tolerance is the nature of the antigen-presenting cell. It has not been ex-cluded that antigen presentation for the induction of IgA-producing cells is mediated by different cells from those responsible for suppression of the systemic immune responses. It is also possible that different structural forms of antigen might be handled differentially and account for differences in responses to ingestion of soluble or particulate antigens. Peyer's patches certainly contain cells capable of presenting antigen to induce immune responses. Both macrophages and Ia-positive cells have been found within Peyer's patches (Chapter 4 and [31].

Peyer's patch macrophages. In addition, Peyer's patch macrophages have been shown to be capable of supporting the induction of immune responses in vitro [55]. However, these functional cells may not be identical to antigen-presenting cells elsewhere since adherent Ia-positive cells from Peyer's patches do not seem to be so effective in antigen presentation [31, 71].

The absolute requirement for Peyer's patches and other gut-associated lymphoid tissue for the induction of human secretory immunity and oral tolerance has been subject to much investigation. This will not be reviewed here but whilst early studies indicated that Peyer's patches were essential, more recent studies have suggested that in addition to the special epithelium of Peyer's patches and lymphoid follicles, other areas of the intestine may be engaged in antigen presentation (see review by Mayrhofer [41].

MECHANISMS OF ORAL TOLERANCE

As can be seen from Table 14.2, in the various animal models a large number of mechanisms have been postulated as underlying oral tolerance. They can be broadly divided into humoral or cellular mechanisms though there is no reason to suppose that both types of mechanisms might not be operative simultaneously.

Humoral factors

In early studies in orally induced hyporesponsiveness in mice, Andre et al [1] showed that the hyporesponsiveness could be transferred with serum, and postulated the suppressive role of immune complexes containing IgA antibody. A number of other investigators, particularly those using the sheep red blood

Table 14.2 Mediators of oral tolerance.

Mediator	Species	Antigen	Assay	Author	Reference
IgA Ag/Ab	Mice	SRBC	PCA	Andre et al, 1975	1
B cell	Mice	Picryl chloride	DTH	Asherson et al, 1977	3
T cell	Rats	SRBC	PFC	Mattingly and Waksman, 1978	37
T cell	Mice	OVA	PCA	Ngan and Kind, 1978	49
T cell	Mice	OVA	DTH	Miller and Hanson, 1979	43
Serum factor	Mice	SRBC	PFC	Kagnoff, 1978	27
IgG1	Mice	SRBC	PFC	Chalon et al, 1979	13
Ts factor	Rats	SRBC	PFC	Mattingly and Waksman, 1980	38
T cell	Mice	OVA	PA	Challacombe and Tomasi, 1980	12
Ly 1$^+$ T cells	Mice	BSA	PA	Silverman et al, 1982	61
Ly 2$^+$ T cells	Mice	OVA	Ab	Challacombe, 1985	11

Abbreviations: see footnote to Table 14.1. Ag = antigen, Ab = antibody.

cell system, showed that the suppression could be transferred with mouse sera but that this activity was attributable to IgG or IgG1 antibodies and not IgA [13,27,28]. Adoptive transfer studies failed to show that T suppressor cells were responsible [27].

Serum suppressive factors

The factor in the serum was also suppressive for the induction of IgM anti-sheep red blood cell responses in normal spleen cultures, and both the in vivo and in vitro suppression was highly specific [27,28]. Characterization of the factor revealed that it was not H-2 restricted and did not block the expression of previously established spleen IgM and anti-SRBC responses. The suppressor factor had a molecular weight of 150 000, was heat stable and contained immunoglobulin determinants but not erythrocyte determinants. Interestingly, IgA and IgE secondary anti-SRBC responses in vitro were not inhibited by the factor.

Serum factors and protein antigens

With oral tolerance to protein antigens, the picture is less clear with regard to serum factors. Thus tolerance to HSA or ovalbumin could not be transferred with sera obtained at 7–14 days or 30–70 days after stopping feeding [21,22,60]. However, recently it has been reported that serum taken 4 days after oral immunization with ovalbumin can transfer suppression to syngeneic recipients [10]. Strobel et al [65] have described transfer of tolerance by serum taken 1 hour after ingestion. Activity in serum could be absorbed out with antibody to ovalbumin. Chromatographic analysis revealed this activity to be in areas of very low molecular weight suggesting that the

tolerogenic effect was due to low molecular weight antigen and quickly absorbed breakdown products of ovalbumin.

Anti-idiotypic antibodies

Jackson and Mestecky [25] have demonstrated IgG auto-anti-idiotypic cells to be induced by oral–parenteral immunization with HSA in rabbits. It is possible that such autoantibodies might contribute to oral tolerance, though it should be remembered that previous evidence suggests that rabbits may not respond in the same way as other animal species. However, these findings may offer an explanation for the results of Asherson et al [3] who showed in mice using picryl chloride that suppression of delayed hypersensitivity could be transferred with B cells.

Cellular factors

Suppressor cells. It is clear that, in many of the animal systems discussed, ingestion of antigenic material results in oral tolerance and the production of suppressor cells. These have been demonstrated in Peyer's patches [37], mesenteric lymph nodes [12] and spleens of animals orally tolerized to soluble proteins [43,49,56,57]. These cells have been shown to be of T cell phenotype by using fractionation on nylon wool columns or treatment of cells with anti-thy 1.2 [43,56,57]. These suppressor cells have also been shown to be radiosensitive [23].

Cyclophosphamide treatment

Further evidence for the T cell nature of the suppressor cells is indicated by the fact that pretreatment with cyclophosphamide will abrogate the induction of oral tolerance in the mouse model [45]. However, this has not been found in all models and Tomasi et al [71] report that in their system, the induction of tolerance was unaffected by pretreatment with cyclophosphamide. It has also been suggested that the phenomenon of oral tolerance could be manifested by a functional deletion of T helper cells [68]. These authors suggested that small doses of ovalbumin would activate T suppressor cells and that pretreatment with cyclophosphamide would prevent the development of tolerance but that large dosage resulted in alteration of other T cell functions including diminished carrier-dependent T helper cell activity.

Phenotype of T suppressor cells

Recent work with treatment with anti-Ly 1 and anti-Ly 2 antisera has attempted to elucidate further the phenotype of suppressor cells. Silverman et al [61] showed that although in vitro antigen-induced proliferation could not be detected in whole lymphocyte preparations from lymph nodes from orally tolerized animals, if cells from these nodes were treated with anti-Ly 1 plus complement then a significant proliferative response was found. This would seem to suggest that T suppressor cells elicited by oral immunization are of the Ly 1$^+$ phenotype.

Contrasuppressor cells

An alternative possibility is that treatment with anti-Ly 1 in this mouse system enriches for proliferating Ly 2$^+$ suppressor cells known to be induced by oral immunization [57] and would be part of the contrasuppressor system described by Gershon and his associates in Peyer's patches [20]. This would suggest that failure to observe T suppressor activity in adoptive transfer experiments may be due to the use of whole populations of cells in which suppressor activity is contraregulated.

Immunoregulatory networks: induction of both help and suppression

These findings suggest a complex immunoregulatory network within the Peyer's patch. A commonly suggested view is that oral immunization leads to isotype-specific T suppressor cells for IgG and IgM which then migrate to systemic lymphoid tissues while helper cells for IgA remain locally in the intestine [56]. However, these findings would not explain diminished serum IgA responses found in

some studies [10], especially when secretory IgA antibodies can be induced at the same time.

Streptococcus mutans. In recent studies with whole bacteria [11] it has been shown that intragastric immunization with *S. mutans* leads not only to the production of suppressor cells but also to the production of helper cells. Both enhancement and suppression could be transferred to syngeneic recipients by separation of the cell populations and this suggests that what is detected in vivo is the balance between the two systems.

Ovalbumin. With ovalbumin [11] (Fig. 14.7) no helper cells were detected and this suggests that in the case of soluble protein antigens, the dominant effect is of suppression due to the

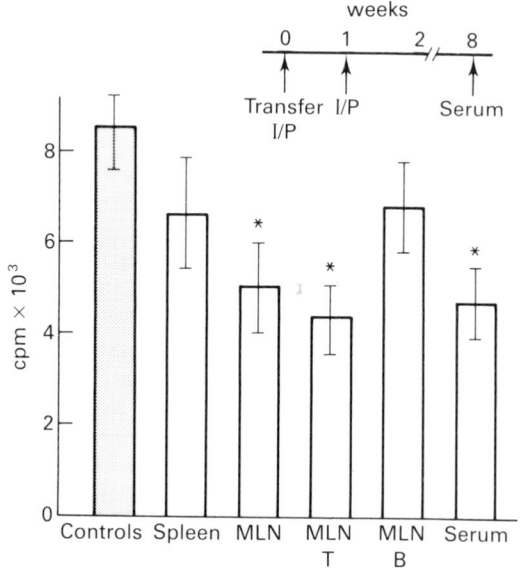

Fig. 14.7 Serum IgG antibodies to ovalbumin in recipients of 40×10^6 cells from mice immunized with ovalbumin intragastrically. Immunization schedule as indicated. Cells removed 4 days after intragastric immunization and transferred to syngeneic recipients. I/P = intraperitoneal, MLN = mesenteric lymph node.

induction of T suppressor cells. However, with ovalbumin, tolerance could be transferred with T cells and with serum suggesting that at least two mechanisms were operative simultaneously, though the duration of each is not known (Fig. 14.5).

T cell phenotype

Characterization of the phenotype of these T cells with antisera revealed that with *S. mutans*, the enhancement could be abolished by treatment with anti-Ly 1 antisera and suppression could be abolished by the pretreatment with anti-Ly 2 antisera. In addition, with ovalbumin, suppression could be transferred only by $Ly 2^+$ cells, and no enhancement was seen following the transfer of $Ly 1^+$ cells [11]. It appears therefore that with a complex antigen such as a bacterial cell both helper and suppressor cells are induced, whereas with a simpler antigen such as ovalbumin only suppressor cells were induced. However, the inability to detect enhancement may be due either to a lack of helper cells, or to inhibited helper cells. An interesting area of current research is into the immunoregulatory networks within the gut-associated lymphoid tissue.

Suppressor factors

Suppressor factors have been described which were produced in vitro from spleen cells from rats which had been fed sheep red blood cells [38]. These suppressor factors were antigen specific and suppressed the plaque-forming cells of three allogeneic strains. The factor had a molecular weight of about 65 000 and its production was unaffected if the animals had been thymectomized. Interestingly helper factors were produced in the same in vitro culture system, but suppression always showed dominance over help. Feeding of a single antigen may give rise to two different suppressor factors from T cells [39].

Maintenance of oral tolerance

Thus a number of different mechanisms may be operative in the induction of oral tolerance according to the animal model and system. However, it is possible that more than one mechanism is operative in any system, and it is also possible that mechanisms responsible for the maintenance of tolerance differ from those responsible for the induction of tolerance. It would be interesting for the transfer of oral tolerance to be more fully dissected to determine the duration of particular mechanisms.

The significance of findings in animal models to man

Vaccination. It is clear that the use of animal models has allowed major advances in the understanding of the physiology of the gastrointestinal tract. With regard to the secretory system, the use of animal models, particularly those in which genetic and dynamic studies can be performed, has allowed the cellular basis of the secretory system to be examined. The findings have obvious implications with regard to man in terms of vaccination against diseases particularly those affecting mucosal surfaces. One of the great difficulties of putting this into practice is the difficulty in prolonging secretory responses and currently many authors are examining the use of oral adjuvants. There seems to be no doubt that secretory IgA has the functional capabilities of antigenic exclusion, virus neutralization, inhibition of microbial adherence and enzyme modulation but these functions cannot be brought into useful practice unless the secretory response can be stimulated for greater duration than seems likely at present (see Chapter 15).

Coeliac disease. Understanding the physiology of the gut is an essential prerequisite for the understanding of pathology of the gut. Animal models have been less useful in the study of certain gut diseases such as coeliac disease because of the absence hitherto of suitable models. However, the interesting graft-versus-host model of local cell-mediated immunity [35, 46] seems to allow further possibilities of understanding the mechanisms of this and other diseases.

Oral desensitization. One practical application of the phenomenon of oral tolerance would appear to be in the field of oral desensitization. Although attempts have already been made to use desensitization therapy in allergic diseases, these have not been outstandingly successful and it can be anticipated that with more extensive knowledge about the immunology of the gastrointestinal tract and the systemic manifestations of the immune responses to ingested materials, that further attempts will be made in this field. The difficulty in inducing oral tolerance in primed animals (see above) militates against this as an easy option. However, as discussed, a number of studies have shown that tolerance or partial tolerance in primed animals can be achieved and clearly this is an area which is worthy of some detailed analysis because of its clinical implications.

Induction of secretory IgA antibodies. In the case of allergy, it is attractive to hypothesize that the dual response to ingested material would have a primary purpose of exclusion of unwanted antigens, allergens and cross-reacting antigens from the body and this state would be mediated by the induction of secretory IgA antibodies. The ingestion of antigen would allow the production of antibodies in most secretions but antibodies would continue to be secreted only at sites where antigen was still present. Oral tolerance would allow the negation of any damaging systemic reactions to ingested antigens, and this might be particularly pertinent with antigens cross-reacting with host tissue. It may be that the efficient delivery of dimeric IgA from serum into bile via the liver is an extension to this system whereby unwanted antigens and antigen–antibody complexes can be rapidly cleared from the body without any further damaging reactions.

CONCLUSIONS

Dual responses. Deposition of antigenic material in the gut may lead to the simultaneous induction of secretory antibodies and systemic hyporesponsiveness [12]. Under different circumstances such deposition may lead to the simultaneous induction of secretory antibodies and systemic enhancement. This raises intriguing questions as to the relationship between the two systems, and also concerning the conditions which determine which of the different types of response are triggered.

This dual response has hitherto only been demonstrated in the murine model, and it remains to be shown that this is a general phenomenon common to all species. However, this seems likely since the secretory responses and the systemic hyporesponsiveness have been shown separately in a number of different species.

Species similarity. Immunochemically and functionally the secretory systems of many if

not most species appear to be similar (Chapter 9). There seems no doubt that the gut has a role to play in the general induction of secretory responses, and also in the regulation of systemic immune responses. With regard to oral tolerance, there is a remarkable degree of unanimity in the results from all the different animal models. These results suggest that it is a widespread and general phenomenon for systemic hyporesponsiveness to arise after feeding of antigen. This appears at first sight to be difficult to reconcile with the large amount of antigen which is ingested and normally present. Several studies suggest that it is a change in normal antigenic exposure which results in the induction and stimulation of tolerance.

Maintenance of tolerance. The maintenance of tolerance to ingested antigens is an area of great importance which requires further investigation. It is clear that contrary to the earlier views, antigenic material does get through the stomach and is delivered to the duodenum. This appears to apply to man as well as to other species. The nature of the subsequent systemic immune response depends on the nature of the antigen which has survived, whether it is soluble or particulate and its molecular size as well as the species of animal, the genetic strains, the dosage of the antigen and prior antigen exposure. One of the intriguing challenges, now that understanding of the oral tolerance system is better, is to determine parameters by which previously sensitized individuals may become hyposensitized with antigens. It has great implications in respect of desensitization of humans and also in enhancing understanding of the relationship between the secretory and systemic immune systems.

REFERENCES

1 Andre C, Heremans JF, Vaerman JP, Cambiaso CL: A mechanism for the induction of immunological tolerance by antigen feeding: antigen–antibody complexes. J Exp Med 1975; 142:1509.

2 Asherson GL, Perera MACC, Thomas WR, Zembala M: Contact sensitizing agents and the intestinal tract: the production of immunity and unresponsiveness by feeding contact sensitizing agents and the role of suppressor cells. In: Immunology of breast milk. New York: Raven Press, 1979; 19.

3 Asherson GL, Zembala M, Perera MACC et al: Production of immunity and unresponsiveness in the mouse by feeding contact sensitizing agents and the role of suppressor cells in the Peyer's patches, mes-

enteric lymph nodes and other lymphoid tissues. Cell Immunol 1977; 33:145.

4 Bauer H, Paronetto F, Burns WA, Einherber A: The enhancing effect of microbial flora on macrophage function and the immune response. J Exp Med 1966; 123:1013.

5 Bazin H, Platteau B: Oral feeding of ovalbumin can make rats tolerant to an intraperitoneal injection of dinitrophenylated ovalbumin and *Bordetella pertussis* vaccine. Biochem Soc Trans 1977; 5:1571.

6 Besredka A: De l'anaphylaxie. Sixième mémoire de l'anaphylaxie lactique. Ann Inst Pasteur 1909; 23:166.

7 Besredka A: Local immunization. Baltimore, Maryland: Williams and Wilkins, 1927.

8 Bierme SJ, Blanc M, Abral M, Fournie A: Oral Rh treatment for severely immunized mothers. Lancet 1979; i:605.

9 Bloch KJ, Perry R, Bloch M, Walker A: Induction of (partial) systemic tolerance in primed rats subjected to prolonged oral administration of antigen. Ann NY Acad Sci 1983; 409:787.

10 Challacombe SJ: Salivary antibodies and systemic tolerance in mice after oral immunization with bacterial antigens. Ann NY Acad Sci 1983; 409:177.

11 Challacombe SJ: Systemic tolerance and salivary antibodies after oral immunization. In: Revillard J-P, Wierzbicki CN, eds. Mucosal immunity, IgA and polymorphonuclear neutrophils. Journées immunologiques. Fondation Franco-Allemande, 1985.

12 Challacombe SJ, Tomasi B: Systemic tolerance and secretory immunity after oral immunization. J Exp Med 1980; 152:1459.

13 Chalon MP, Milne RW, Vaerman JP: In vitro immunosuppressive effect of serum of orally immunised mice. Eur J Immunol 1979; 9:747.

14 Chase MW: Inhibition of experimental drug allergy by prior feeding of the sensitizing agent. Proc Soc Exp Biol Med 1946; 61:257.

15 Childow JW, Porter P: The role of oral immunization in stimulating *Escherichia coli* antibody of the IgM class in porcine colostrum. Res Vet Sci 1978; 24: 254.

16 Chiller JM, Titus RG, Etlinger HM: Cellular dissection of tolerant states induced by the oral route or in neonatal animals. Dev Immunol 1979; 4:195.

17 Devey ME, Bleasdale K: Antigen feeding modifies the course of antigen–induced immune complex disease. Clin Exp Immunol 1984; 53:637–44.

18 Fujita K, Finkelstein RA: Antitoxic immunity in experimental cholera: comparison of immunity induced perorally and parenterally in mice. J Infect Dis 1972; 125:647.

19 Gautam SC, Battisto JR: Suppression of contact sensitivity and cell-mediated lympholysis by oral administration of hapten is caused by different mechanisms. Cell Immunol 1983; 78:295–304.

20 Green DR, St Martin S: Suppression and contrasuppression in the regulation of gut-associated immune responses. Ann NY Acad Sci 1983; 409:284.

21 Hanson DG, Morimoto T: A role of digestion in orally induced tolerance to ovalbumin. J Allergy Clin Immunol 1980; 65:227.

22 Hanson DG, Vaz NM, Maia LCS, Lynch JM: Inhibition of specific immune responses by feeding protein antigens. III. Evidence against maintenance of tolerance to ovalbumin by orally induced antibodies. J Immunol 1979; 123:2337.

23 Hanson DG, Vaz NM, Rawlings LA, Lynch JM: Inhibition of specific immune responses by feeding protein antigens. II. Effects of prior passive and active immunization. J Immunol 1979; 122:2261.

24 Holt PG, Leivers S: Tolerance induction via antigen inhalation: isotype specificity, stability and involvement of suppressor T cells. Int Arch Allergy Appl Immunol 1982; 67:155–60.

25 Jackson DE, Lally ET, Nakamura MC, Montgomery PC: Migration of IgA-bearing lymphocytes into salivary glands. Cell Immunol 1981; 63:203.

26 Kagnoff MF: Functional characteristic of Peyer's patch cells. III. Carrier priming of T cells by antigen feeding. J Exp Med 1975; 142:1425.

27 Kagnoff MF: Effects of antigen feeding on intestinal and systemic immune responses. III. Antigen-specific serum mediated suppression of humoral antibody responses after antigen feeding. Cell Immunol 1978; 40:186.

28 Kagnoff MF: Effects of antigen feeding on intestinal and systemic immune responses. II. Similarity between the suppressor factor in mice after erythrocyte lysate injection and erythrocyte feeding. Gastroenterology 1980; 79:54.

29 Kagnoff MF: Immunological unresponsiveness after enteric antigen administration. In: Strober W, Hanson L, Sell K, eds. Recent advances in mucosal immunity. New York: Raven Press, 1982; 95.

30 Korenblat PE, Rothberg RM, Minden P, Farr RS: Immune responses of adults after oral and parenteral exposure to bovine serum albumin. J Allergy 1968; 411:226.

31 Krco CJ, Challacombe SJ, Lafuse WP et al: Expression of Ia antigens by mouse Peyer's patch cells. Cell Immunol 1981; 57:420.

32 Lafont S, Andre C, Andre F et al: Abrogation by subsequent feeding of antibody response, including IgE, in parenterally immunized mice. J Exp Med 1982; 155:1973.

33 Lowney ED: Immunological unresponsiveness to a contact sensitizer in man. J Invest Dermatol 1968; 512:411.

34 MacDonald TT, Carter PB: Requirement for a bacterial flora before mice generate cells capable of mediating the delayed hypersensitivity reaction to sheep red blood cells. J Immunol 1979; 122:2624.

35 MacDonald TT, Ferguson A: Hypersensitivity reactions in the small intestine. III. The effects of allograft rejection and of graft-versus-host disease on epithelial cell kinetics. Cell Tissue Kinet 1977; 10:301.

36 McGhee JR, Kiyono H, Michalek SM et al: Lipopolysaccharide regulation of the immune response: T lymphocytes from normal mice suppress mitogenic and immunogenic responses to LPS. J Immunol 1980; 124:1603.

37 Mattingly JA, Waksman BH: Immunologic suppression after oral administration of antigen. I. Specific suppressor cells formed in rat Peyer's patches after oral administration of sheep erythrocytes and their systemic migration. J Immunol 1978; 121:1878.

38 Mattingly JA, Waksman BH: Immunological suppression after oral administration of antigen. II. Antigen-specific helper and suppressor factors produced by spleen cells of rats fed sheep erythrocytes. J Immunol 1980; 125:1044.

39 Mattingly JA, Kaplan JM, Janeway CA Jr: Two distinct antigen-specific suppressor factors induced by the oral administration of antigen. J Exp Med 1980; 152:545–54.

40 Matuhasi T, Usui M, Iwata M: IgA and IgG enhancing but IgE suppressing characteristics of lipopolysaccharide or cholesterol-ovalbumin conjugate in intubated mice. Naturwissenschaften 1982; 69:397.

41 Mayrhofer G: Physiology of the intestinal immune system. In: Newby TJ, Stokes CR, eds. Local immune responses in the gut. Boca Raton: CRC Press, 1984.

42 Michalek SM, Kiyono H, Wannemuehler MJ et al: Lipopolysaccharide (LPS) regulation of the immune response: LPS influence in oral tolerance induction. J Immunol 1982; 128:1992.

43 Miller SD, Hanson DG: Inhibition of specific immune responses by feeding protein antigens. II. Evidence for tolerance and specific active suppression of cell-mediated immune response to ovalbumin. J Immunol 1979; 123:2344.

44 Montgomery PC, Connell KM, Cohn J, Skandera CA: Remote site stimulation of secretory IgA antibodies

following bronchial and gastric stimulation. Adv Exp Med Biol 1978; 107:113.

45 Mowat AM, Strobel S, Drummond HE, Ferguson A: Immunological responses to fed protein antigens in mice. I. Reversal of oral tolerance to ovalbumin by cyclophosphamide. Immunology 1982; 45:105.

46 Mowat A, Tait RC, Mackenzie S et al: Analysis of natural effector and suppressor activity by intraepithelial lymphocytes from mouse small intestine. Clin Exp Immunol 1983; 52:191.

47 Newby T J, Stokes CR, Bourne F J: Effect of feeding bacterial lipopolysaccharide and dextran sulphate on the development of oral tolerance to contact sensitizing agents. Immunology 1980; 41:617.

48 Newby T J, Stokes CR, Evans PA, Bourne F J: The immune response following oral vaccination with *E. coli*. Curr Top Vet Med Anim Sci 1981; 12:377.

49 Ngan J, Kind LS: Suppressor T cells for IgE and IgG in Peyer's patches of mice made tolerant by the oral administration of ovalbumin. J Immunol 1978; 120:861.

50 Nicklin S, Miller K: Local and systemic immune responses to intestinally presented antigen. Int Arch Allergy Appl Immunol 1983; 72:87-90.

51 Peri BA, Rothberg RM: Circulating antitoxin in rabbits after ingestion of diphtheria toxoid. Infect Immun 1981; 32:1148.

52 Pierce NF, Koster FT: Priming and suppression of the intestinal immune response to cholera toxoid/toxin by parenteral toxoid in rats. J Immunol 1980; 124:307.

53 Pierce NF, Cray WC Jr, Saccri JB Jr: Oral immunization against experimental cholera: the role of antigen form and antigen combinations in evoking protection. Ann NY Acad Sci 1983; 409:724.

54 Ranges GE, Azar MM: Inheritance of tolerance susceptibility to human γ-globulin in congenic mice. J Immunol 1979; 123:1151.

55 Richman LK, Graeff AS, Strober W: Antigen presentation by macrophage enriched cells from the mouse Peyer's patch. Cell Immunol 1981; 62:110.

56 Richman LK, Graeff AS, Yarchoan R, Strober W: Simultaneous induction of antigen–specific IgA helper T cells and IgG suppressor T cells in the murine Peyer's patch after protein feeding. J Immunol 1981; 126:2079.

57 Richman LK, Chiller JM, Brown, WR et al: Enterically induced immunologic tolerance. I. Induction of suppressor T lymphocytes by intragastric administration of soluble proteins. J. Immunol 1978; 121:2429.

58 Saklayen M, Pesce A J, Pollak VE, Michael JG: Induction of oral tolerance in mice unresponsive to bacterial lipopolysaccharide. Infect Immun 1983; 41:1383.

59 Saklayen M, Pesce A J, Pollak VE, Michael JG: Kinetics of oral tolerance: study of variables affecting tolerance induced by oral administration of antigen. Int Arch Allergy Appl Immunol 1984; 73:5.

60 Sewell HF, Gell PH, Bazu MK: Immune responsiveness and oral immunization. Int Arch Allergy Appl Immunol 1979; 58:414.

61 Silverman GA, Peri BA, Rothberg RM: Systemic antibody responses of different species following ingestion of soluble protein antigens. Dev Comp Immunol 1982; 6:747.

62 Stokes CR, Newby T J, Bourne F J: The influence of oral immunization on local and systemic immune responses to heterologous antigens. Clin Exp Immunol 1983; 52:399.

63 Stokes CR, Newby T J, Huntley JH et al: The immune response of mice to bacterial antigens given by mouth. Immunology 1979; 38:497.

64 Strobel S, Ferguson A: Immune responses to fed protein antigens in mice. III. Systemic tolerance or priming is related to age at which antigen is first encountered. Pediatr Res 1984; 18:588-94.

65 Strobel S, Mowat AM, Drummond HE et al: Immunological responses to fed protein antigens in mice. II. Oral tolerance for CMI is due to activation of cyclophosphamide sensitive cells by gut processed antigen. Immunology 1983; 49:451.

66 Sullivan T J, Wedner, J J, Parker, CHW: Densensitization of patients allergic to penicillin using oral penicillin. J Allergy Clin Immunol 1980; 65:195.

67 Swarbrick ET, Stokes CR, Soothill JF: Absorption of antigens after oral immunization and the simultaneous induction of specific systemic tolerance. Gut 1979; 20:121.

68 Titus RG, Chiller JM: Orally induced tolerance. Definition at the cellular level. Int Arch Allergy Appl Immunol 1981; 65:323.

69 Tomasi TB: The immune system of secretions. New Jersey: Prentice-Hall, 1976.

70 Tomasi TB: Oral tolerance (an overview). Transplantation 1980; 29:353.

71 Tomasi TB, Barr WG, Challacombe SJ, Curran G: Oral tolerance and accessory-cell function of Peyer's patches. Ann NY Acad Sci 1983; 409:145.

72 Vaz NM, Maia LCS, Hanson DG, Lynch JM: Inhibition of homocytotropic antibody responses in adult inbred mice by previous feeding of the specific antigen. J Allergy Clin Immunol 1977; 60:110.

73 Wells HG: Studies on the chemistry of anaphylaxis. III. Experiments with isolated proteins, especially those of the hen egg. J Infect Dis 1911; 9:147.

Chapter 15
The Induction of Secretory IgA Responses

Stephen J. Challacombe

Introduction

The discovery of IgA by Heremans [48] and of secretory IgA by Tomasi et al [100] led to the realization that there existed a secretory immune system which could be stimulated and act independently of the systemic immune system. Earlier Besredka [9] had recognized a dichotomy between antibodies in stools and serum, and Burrows [14] had shown that gut immunity could be stimulated separately from systemic immunity. During the last 20 years, significant advances have been made in understanding the secretory immune system. Much has been learned about the importance of humoral antibody responses at mucosal surfaces and their regulation. Rather less has been learned about the importance of cell-mediated immune responses at mucosal surfaces. Nevertheless there has been extensive characterization of the cells involved in the induction of secretory responses and the relationship between antigen-sensitive cells in the intestine and extraintestinal sites.

Normal antigenic challenge

The intestinal lymphoid cell populations participate in immune responses that are essential components of the host interaction with its environment. Food antigens, bacterial, parasitic and chemical antigens encountered in the gut present a normal and major antigenic challenge throughout the life of the host. These also appear to be important in the development and function of the host immune system. The mucosal immune system can be regarded as functioning to counteract and handle a major antigenic challenge which is present continuously. The nature of these interactions between the host immune system and environmental antigens on mucosal surfaces has been extensively studied and characterized in the last few years, and has led to the revision of concepts about the secretory system.

Properties of the mucosal immune system

The older concept that antibodies in secretions of the gut and other mucosal surfaces were derived from serum was shown to be incorrect, and it was established on the basis of a variety of criteria that antibodies in secretions were locally derived [97]. Secretory antibodies were mainly of the IgA class. The IgA in secretions was dimeric whereas serum IgA was monomeric. Antibodies could be induced by local immunization, and antibody levels in secretions did not correlate with those in serum. Early work on the mucosal responses of the gut to antigenic material concentrated almost entirely on analyses of localized responses to antigen, since at that time it had not been appreciated that there might be effects at sites quite distant from the gut.

Elsewhere in this book various components of the secretory immune system are discussed in some detail including the lymphoid tissue of the gut (Chapter 1), the specialized cells of the gut (Chapters 4–8) and the structure and function of mucosal antibodies (Chapter 9) as well as circulation of lymphocytes from the gut to secretory tissues (Chapter 3). This chapter is therefore limited to the induction of secretory responses.

Development of mucosal immunocompetence

The development of immunocompetency in mammals, including that of intestinal lymphoid tissue, occurs during fetal life [24, 89]. The lymphoid tissue of the intestine shows development during the first days after birth and this postnatal development is thought to be a response to antigenic challenge [57].

Role of normal flora

There is experimental evidence for this concept since the intestinal IgA system of germfree animals seems to be considerably reduced in comparison with normal mice [25]. However, if these germ-free mice are normalized there is an increase in IgA levels which reaches normal values after 4 weeks or so [49]. In infants, deliberate colonization with a nonpathogenic strain of *Escherichia coli* was shown to enhance the IgA concentration in the gut [55]. These observations suggest that antigenic

challenge plays a role in the development of enteric immunocompetence. On balance it seems that in the human, mucosal immunocompetence is not complete until between 1 and 2 years of age (see Chapter 7). Nevertheless, the secretory IgA system reaches adult values well before serum IgA [45]. Developmental aspects of the gut B cell system are covered in further detail in Chapter 7.

Local or central stimulation of secretory antibodies

It has become evident that secretory responses may be induced locally or centrally (Table 15.1). These two mechanisms may be synergistic in many circumstances with a primary signal in gut-associated lymphoid tissue (GALT) leading to release of IgA precursors destined for secretory tissues [16] (see Chapter 4) and a secondary signal in the local tissue leading to further differentiation and proliferation.

Table 15.1 Methods of induction of secretory responses.

Local	1	Topical application of antigen
	2	Injection of antigen near secretory glands
Central GALT	1	Enteric immunization
	2	Antigens given in diet
Central BALT	1	Bronchial or tracheal immunization
	2	Antigens aerosolized in environment

Concept of an enteromucosal system

It has become evident that the gut is closely associated with other mucosal surfaces and that IgA precursor cells originate in Peyer's patches and are stimulated by intestinal antigens to leave the Peyer's patch, migrate through the mesenteric lymph nodes, the thoracic duct and blood and return to the gut and a variety of other mucosal surfaces [99] (Fig. 15.1). This has been described as the common mucosal system [11]. A similar pathway appears to be true for T cells originating in the gut and these also migrate to other mucosal surfaces [75, 76]. Thus the gastrointestinal tract appears to be intimately associated with other mucosal surfaces.

The deposition of antigens in the gut has been shown to lead to the production of IgA antibodies in secretions at sites distant from the gut such as colostrum, lacrimal and salivary secretions in man [63] and salivary secretions in rhesus monkeys [20] and in rats [64].

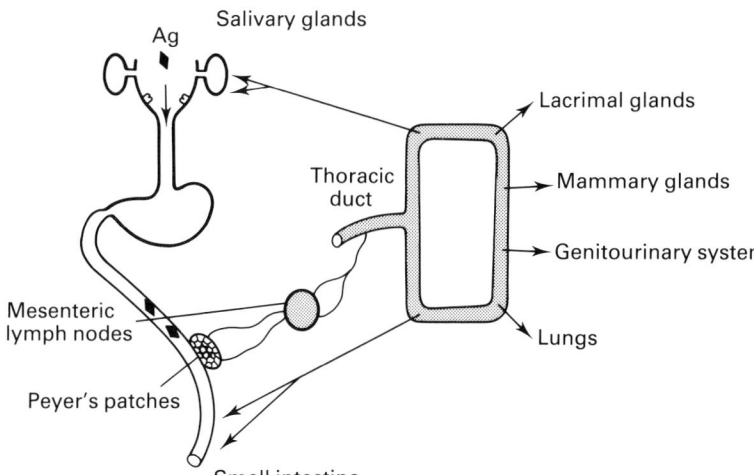

Fig. 15.1 Cellular migration in the secretory system after antigenic stimulation of gut-associated lymphoid tissue. Cells migrate from Peyer's patches to all secretory sites where further differentiation takes place. The resulting plasma cells secrete secretory IgA. Ag = antigen.

A general conclusion therefore is that the secretory immune system can be stimulated centrally and that precursors of IgA-producing cells migrate from the gut-associated lymphoid tissue to several secretory sites in addition to the lamina propria of the gut itself.

Common mucosal system

The evidence that cells migrate from the gut to various secretory tissues, and that immunization in the gut leads to antibodies at various secretory sites has led to the concept of a common mucosal system [10, 11]. However, this concept may be an oversimplification, since although immunization in the lung may lead to antibodies in distant secretory sites such as the salivary glands [66] and immunization in the lacrimal glands has also been shown to lead to the production of antibodies in saliva [66], it is not a general observation that immunization at one secretory site leads to antibodies at another.

Thus with firm evidence that antigen deposition in the gut may lead to antibodies not only in the gut but also in saliva [20, 21], lungs [11], lacrimal secretions [63] and genitourinary tract, it is probably more correct to designate the system as an enteromucosal system.

INDUCTION OF SECRETORY RESPONSES BY LOCAL IMMUNIZATION

Topical application of antigen has been the classical method of inducing antibodies in the secretory system (Fig. 15.2). The role of topically applied antigen in the localization and persistence of SIgA responses has been demonstrated in several secretory sites including the respiratory tract [73], oral cavity [31], gut [51, 78] and vagina [74].

Intestinal responses

It is now quite clear that antigen encountered by the enteric route can stimulate antibody responses in the intestine in the absence of any detectable systemic immune responses. Besredka [9] and Davies [28] recognized many years ago that the stools of patients with dysentery may contain a high titre of anti-*Shigella* antibodies whereas antibodies could not be detected in the serum. It has now been established with a variety of antigens that specific IgA antibody can be induced in the intestine which might mediate local protective immunity [16, 73, 81]. The production of secre-

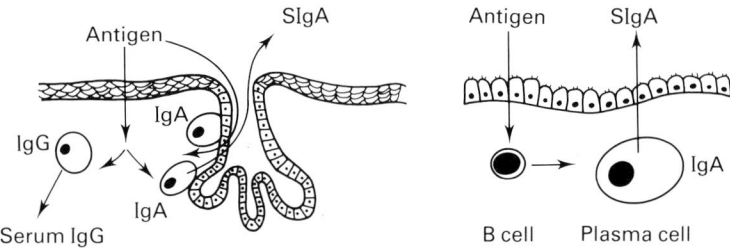

Fig. 15.2 Induction of secretory IgA (SIgA) antibodies by local immunization. Antigen can either be injected into submucosal tissues, where it is likely to induce serum IgG antibodies as well as secretory IgA antibodies, or applied topically where SIgA is the main product.

tory antibody may be very localized and in a number of experiments it has been shown that application of antigen to one segment of the gut may lead to antibodies in that section but not necessarily in other segments [73].

It should be noted that whilst local immunization may give rise to the local production of secretory antibodies, it may nevertheless, depending on the conditions used, have an effect systemically. Enteric antigen administration can result either in enhancement of a systemic immune response [18] or hyporesponsiveness of the systemic immune response [22,107]. The different types of systemic immune responses after oral immunization have now been studied in some detail using a variety of different antigens, test systems and animal models and are discussed in Chapter 14.

Saliva and other secretions (local immunization)

The major salivary glands are not immediately adjacent to the oral mucosa and are connected by ducts. Local immunization has taken the form of injecting the antigen near to the salivary glands [95] or instillation of antigen into the parotid duct [34,60]. The latter method has been shown to induce salivary IgA antibodies in rodents and primates [34,60]. These methods indicate that a local secretory response can be induced by local immunization. They do not, however, seem to be appropriate for human studies although injection of antigen around the salivary glands in man has been performed [67].

Minor salivary glands abound in the oral mucosa and may produce some 25% of the total salivary IgA [26] though only 10% of the volume. Repeated application of antigen to the lips may give rise to detectable IgA antibody in minor salivary gland secretions [53]. Topical application in the mouse with bacterial antigens may also give rise to serum antibodies as well as to salivary antibodies [31].

Mammary glands

Mammary glands will respond to the local application of antigen [65]. Thus Taubman some years ago demonstrated that intramammary deposition of antigen in rabbits led to a convincing secretory IgA response in mammary secretions [94]. In humans infections with microorganisms may lead not only to antibody in breast milk but also to the passage of the microorganisms involved [72].

INDUCTION OF SECRETORY ANTIBODIES BY CENTRAL (GALT) IMMUNIZATION

Intestinal responses

There is now convincing evidence to suggest that enteric immunization will lead to antibodies in the gastrointestinal tract which are derived from release of cells from Peyer's patches and subsequent migration to the gut rather than from direct local stimulation [51]. Indeed bronchial-associated lymphoid tissue (BALT) can also be stimulated and lead to the induction of antibodies in gut secretions. Thus Montgomery et al [66] using dinitrophenylated bovine γ-globulin (BGG), keyhole limpet haemocyanin and pneumococcus organisms showed that in rabbits intragastric or bronchial immunizations would give rise to IgA antibodies in milk, saliva, bronchial fluid as well as in intestinal fluid (Fig. 15.3).

Experiments in dogs and rats with Thiry-Vella loops and using cholera toxin as the antigen have shown the importance of Peyer's patches in the induction of secretory responses in the gut [79,81]. Interestingly immunization of a loop containing a Peyer's patch resulted in a detectable antibody response in a loop

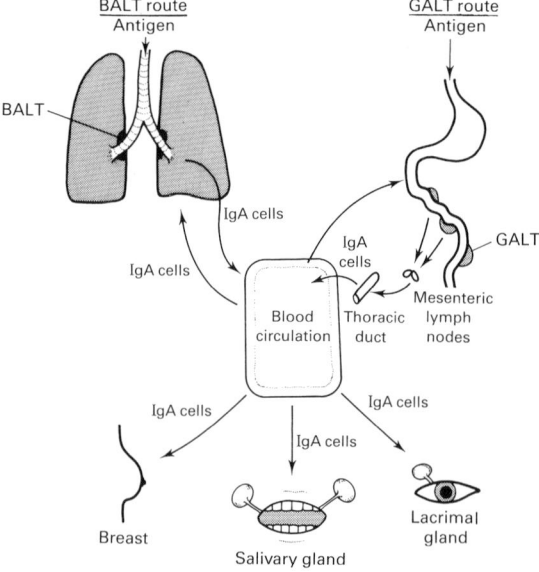

Fig. 15.3 Cellular traffic in the secretory system. Antigen stimulation of either bronchial-associated lymphoid tissue (BALT) or gut-associated lymphoid tissue (GALT) may lead to the release of IgA immunocytes which migrate to the general circulation and are retained in various secretory tissues where secretory IgA antibodies can be detected.

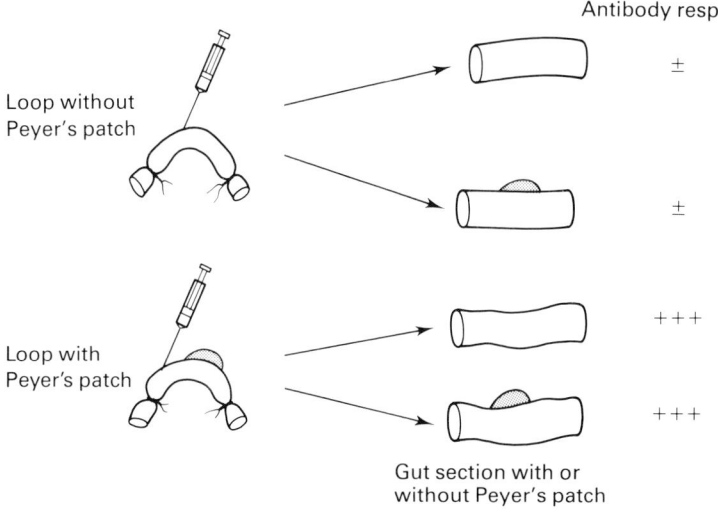

Antibody response

Loop without Peyer's patch

±

±

Loop with Peyer's patch

+++

+++

Gut section with or without Peyer's patch

Fig. 15.4 Importance of Peyer's patches in the induction of secretory antibodies in the intestine. Thiry-Vella loops have been prepared and segments isolated by ligation. Intestinal antibody responses are found only after immunization of loop containing Peyer's patches.

without patches, suggesting that cells had migrated to other segments of the gut (Fig. 15.4).

Salivary responses

Salivary antibody induction has been widely used as a model system to study secretory responses to ingested material, primarily because saliva is an easy secretion to collect and analyse. It seems to be a general feature that salivary IgA antibodies can be induced in a variety of species in the absence of serum antibodies (Table 15.2). This has been demonstrated after immunization with particulate bacterial antigens in the human [63], monkeys [20], rabbits [66], rats [64] and mice [21]. The appearance of salivary antibodies after immunization or intragastric deposition of soluble antigens has been less widely reported, though salivary antibodies after intragastric immunization with bovine gamma globulin (BGG) has been reported in rabbits by Montgomery et al [66] and in mice using ovalbumin [21] and antigen I/II, a soluble protein antigen derived from *Streptococcus mutans* [18].

Mammary glands

Whilst direct immunization of mammary glands in the rabbit led to the formation of antibodies in milk [65,94], it seems that in women who have been naturally primed with *Vibrio cholerae*, subcutaneous immunization would enhance the IgA antibody response in milk [92]. Also Goldblum et al [41] showed that after feeding of non-pathogenic *E. coli* to lactating females, specific IgA antibodies appeared in breast secretions (Table 15.3). These observations clearly suggest that antibodies in milk can be induced by central (GALT) stimulation, and that this route of immunization may have potential in terms of neonatal protection.

Central stimulation may also occur via bronchial-associated lymphoid tissue (BALT). Intragastric or intratracheal immunization with viruses or with bovine serum albumin (BSA) of pregnant rabbits led to antigen-specific IgA in colostrum and milk [77] (Table 15.3).

Table 15.2 Induction of salivary antibodies by stimulation of gut-associated lymphoid tissue.

Species	Antigen	Route	Salivary IgA antibodies	Serum antibodies	Author	Reference
Human	*Streptococcus mutans*	Oral	+ +	−	Mestecky et al, 1978	63
Monkeys	*Streptococcus mutans*	Intragastric	+ +	−	Challacombe and Lehner, 1980	20
Rabbits	*Pneumococcus/BGG*	Intragastric	+ +	−	Montgomery et al, 1978	66
Rats	*Streptococcus mutans*	Oral	+ +	−	Michalek et al, 1976	64
Mice	*Streptococcus mutans/ Ovalbumin*	Intragastric	+ +	−	Challacombe and Tomasi, 1980	21

NB Serum antibodies are not induced normally in unprimed animals. BGG = bovine gamma globulin.

Table 15.3 Immunological responses of mammary glands.

Species	Antigen	Route of immunization	Presence of serum antibodies	Antibody response in milk or colostrum	Reference
Human	Cholera toxin	Subcutaneous	−	−	91
Human	Cholera toxin	Subcutaneous	+	+ +	91
Human	*E. coli*	Feeding	ND	+ +	41
Rabbit	Streptococcal carbohydrate	Intramammary	−	+ +	94
Human	*Streptococcus mutans*	Feeding	+	+ +	63
Rabbit	Viruses, BSA	Intratracheal	−	+ +	77

ND = Not done. BSA = bovine serum albumin.

The relevance of animal models of humans

Several species have secretory systems analogous to that described in man. These include the monkey, rabbit, dog, guinea-pig, rat, mouse, hamster, cat and hedgehog [101]. In these species IgA is the predominant immunoglobulin in secretions including saliva and milk. In most of these species the physicochemical properties of the predominant form of IgA in secretions is similar to that of man, with a sedimentation coefficient of about 11 *s*. In monkey, dog, cow, rabbit and guinea-pig a polypeptide chain probably similar to the secretory component has been detected [97]. There appears to be antigenic cross-reactivity between the secretory component (SC) of man, monkey and cow, and the IgA of other species such as chicken, dolphin and seal will combine with human SC [97].

These various species have secretory systems which appear to be analogous to that described in man, on the basis of immunochemical studies. However, in several of these species the mechanisms involved in the actual induction of secretory antibodies has not been examined, particularly with regard to the stimulation of secretory responses by intragastric or intraduodenal immunization. In addition, there are quantitative differences between the species with regard to the IgG content of secretions such as saliva. For example in the rat, almost 50% of the total immunoglobulin in saliva appears to be IgG [32] whereas in primates IgG only accounts for about 2% of the total immunoglobulin [13].

FACTORS INFLUENCING SECRETORY RESPONSES TO INGESTED MATERIAL

The main secretions that have been examined with regard to the induction of secretory responses after ingested materials have been those in the gut and in saliva. Saliva has been selected not only because of its relevance in oral disease, but mainly because it is an accessible fluid, easy to collect and is thought to show representative responses in secretions after central or intragastric immunization. There are a number of factors which influence successful induction of secretory antibody by this route. Some of these are listed in Table 15.4.

Table 15.4 Factors which have been shown to influence the induction of secretory antibody by ingestion of antigen.

Frequency of antigenic challenge
Duration of antigenic challenge
Dosage of antigen
Nature of antigen—soluble or particulate
　　　　　　　　—viable or non-viable (vaccines)
　　　　　　　　—size of aerosol particles
Age of host
Use of adjuvants
Species of animal
Previous exposure of host to antigen (a) systemic
　　　　　　　　　　　　　　　　　(b) secretory
Nature of antigen-presenting cells
Site of immunization

Antigen dose

It has been a general finding from many studies in a variety of species that very large antigen doses are needed to induce a secretory response after deposition of antigen in the gut. Thus in mice, Michalek et al [64] delivered 10^{10} organisms daily for 10 days to get a salivary response, whilst in pigs Dziaba et al [30] gave greater than 10^{11}, and in man Dupont et al [29] found that 10^{12} was optimal. Interestingly, in the experiments involved with vaccination against disease, protection achieved was incomplete and usually inferior to that following natural infection or vaccination with living organisms.

Several studies have analysed dose responses with regard to the secretory system.

The results suggest that there may be a window of responsiveness in a wall of unresponsiveness. In the studies of Michalek et al [64] and Challacombe [18], non-responsiveness was found in the lowest and highest of three or four immunization doses (Fig. 15.5). Thus,

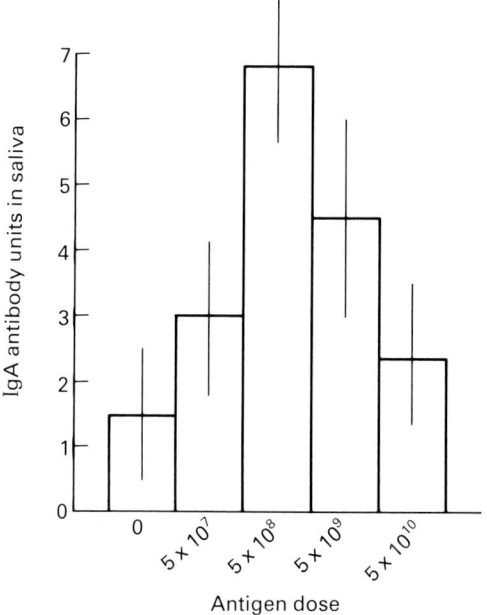

Fig. 15.5 Effect of antigen dose on salivary IgA antibody responses by distant (GALT) immunization. CBA mice were given three daily intragastric immunizations and the salivary antibody response at 14 days was assayed by solid-phase radioimmunoassay. Hyporesponsiveness is seen at high antigen doses.

giving mice either 5×10^8 or 5×10^{10} on 3 consecutive days did not result in a detectable salivary antibody response. However, salivary antibody titres were detected after administration of 5×10^9 [18]. The fact that in both these studies there was an upper limit of responsiveness suggests that the secretory system can be hyporesponsive if the antigen dose is large enough.

Frequency of immunization

The frequency of immunization is another factor which has been considered. In experiments in man, 12 daily intragastric immunizations with *Streptococcus mutans* resulted in successful induction of secretory antibodies in parotid and submandibular saliva and the lacrimal secretions [63]. A similar regime resulted in antibodies in secretions in monkeys [20] though failures have also been reported using similar regimes in the monkey model [54,105].

In rats, Taubman et al [95] have orally immunized up to 24 times to induce salivary antibodies. However, schedules at less frequent immunization were not examined.

In our work, we have examined the minimum immunization schedule that will give rise to salivary antibody responses after oral immunization. Although a single immunization can sometimes give rise to detectable antibody responses, a more consistent response is found with a minimum of three or four oral immunizations [19]. Weekly immunizations over several months in contrast did not give rise to a consistent response in saliva. Thus not only the antigen dose, but also the frequency of immunization seems to be critical in inducing secretory antibody responses.

Nature of antigen

Living or dead vaccines

It is a general finding that living organisms orally administered appear to have greater immunogenicity than inactivated oral vaccines. The greater response and functional capacity in terms of protection elicited by viable organisms has been reported by a large number of workers who have used a variety of organisms including *Vibrio cholerae*, *E. coli*, *Salmonella typhi* and *Shigella* [5, 37, 73, 108]. It seems probable that in order to elicit a strong response, colonization of the intestinal tract with the immunizing strain is necessary.

This is supported by work with poliovirus and by the observation from experiments in pigs with *E. coli* that local antibody production was detected only in animals in which the organisms could be cultured from the faeces [69]. Interestingly, animals lacking a binding receptor for the K88 antigen of *E. coli*, which is involved in adherence, did not give a satisfactory response to the *E. coli* [86].

Immunization with attenuated strains of bacteria, or mutants lacking virulence determinants, has been recently explored with the objective that these non-pathogenic organisms might colonize the gut and not only prevent the colonization of pathogenic strains by direct niche competition but also induce a secretory immune response. Non-pathogenic strains of *Salmonella typhimurium* have been used in cows and apparently do exert a protective effect [5]. However, the mechanism of protection is not clear.

Attenuated strains of *Salmonella typhi* substrain Ty[21a], which lacks an enzyme essential to the utilization of galactose and thus to its survival in the host, have also been examined as a possible vaccine in man [40]. Initial results suggest that it may offer protection.

Particulate versus soluble antigens

As the results in Table 15.2 indicate, particulate antigens whether viable or inactivated have been rather more effective in inducing secretory antibodies than have soluble antigens. This particular aspect has been examined in more detail recently [18, 19]. A comparison of salivary antibody responses after oral immunization in mice with ovalbumin and with inactivated *Streptococcus mutans* indicated that the responses with the streptococcus were always greater. In addition, an anamnestic response could be induced with whole cells of *Streptococcus mutans* but not with ovalbumin.

This result was confirmed in subsequent experiments comparing soluble antigen with that insolubilized on Sepharose beads. The antigen used was a soluble protein of 185 000 molecular weight derived from *Streptococcus mutans*. As seen in Fig. 15.6, when antigen was given intragastrically on three occasions into mice in the soluble or insoluble form, a similar response was detected in saliva. However, when animals were given a second series of immunizations intragastrically some weeks later, the antigen in the insoluble form gave a significantly greater response than in the soluble form.

This can be interpreted as evidence of an anamnestic response in secretions, though not classical of those described with systemic responses. The nature of antigens also has implications with regard to the systemic immune responses (see Chapter 14) since in general, soluble antigens give rise to oral tolerance whilst particulate antigens do not.

With regard to respiratory secretory responses, the particle size may be important. Waldman et al [104] have shown that the particle size of aerosolized influenza virus had a substantial effect on the development of the secretory IgA antibodies in the lung. Similar results were found with rubella as antigen [103].

Effect of age

There has been relatively little work in animal models on the effects of age on secretory antibody responses. In man the secretory system is thought to mature in advance of the systemic immune system in terms of IgA. Recent work suggests that the IgA levels in whole unstimulated saliva, which may be representative of the mucosal immune system, reach adult values at between 1 and 2 years of age [46]. It had been assumed previously that the secretory IgA system matured even faster [47]. It is not known whether the IgA response shows any decrease in old age.

In mice, the salivary IgA response does appear to be age dependent. The salivary response to either soluble protein antigens or to whole bacteria was greater in mature animals of 17 weeks of age or greater than in young animals [19]. Since no differences were found in the systemic IgA antibody responses in young or mature mice, it is possible that maturation of the secretory system is delayed in comparison with the systemic immune system in mice, even though this is the reverse of that found in man. In these experiments (Fig. 15.7) it was not possible to induce responses in aged animals, and it is therefore possible that the secretory immune system becomes less efficient with age. However, further work is needed in this area and in other animal models.

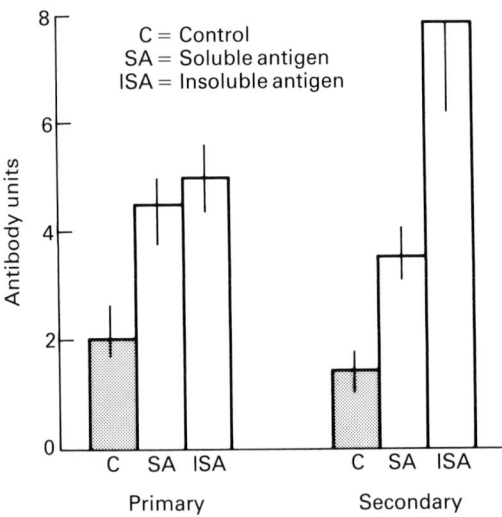

Fig. 15.6 Comparison of soluble and particulate antigens in the induction of secretory immune responses. Balb/c mice were given streptococcal antigen I/II in a soluble form or linked to Sepharose beads intragastrically on three consecutive days. After a first series of immunizations comparable salivary IgA antibody responses were found, but after a second series the insoluble form of antigen induced significantly greater responses.

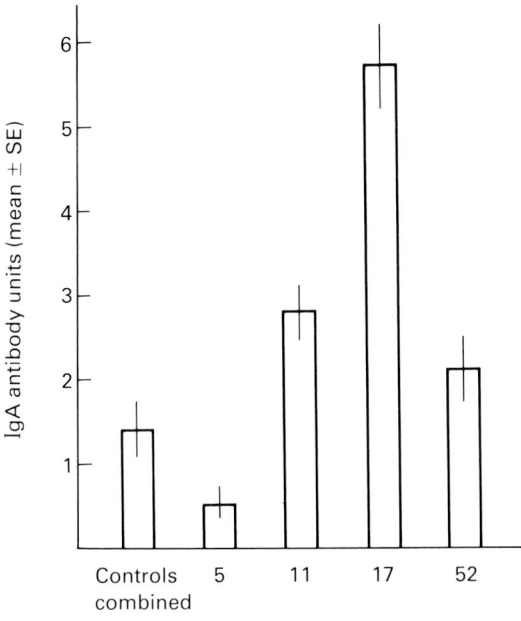

Fig. 15.7 Effect of age on the induction of salivary IgA antibodies to *Streptococcus mutans* by intragastric immunization. Neither young (5 weeks) nor aged mice (52 weeks) gave a significant antibody response. Optimal responses were found in young adult mice.

Effect of immune status on secretory responses

Effect of prior systemic exposure to antigen

In some studies it has been possible to stimulate the production of mucosal antibody by non-mucosal presentation of antigen. Svennerholm et al [92] showed that a subcutaneous vaccination with *Vibrio cholerae* led to an enhanced IgA antibody response in saliva and breast milk of women who had evidence of exposure to *V. cholerae*—in other words had serum IgG antibodies to this organism. Other studies have examined the concept of systemic priming with oral boosting and Pierce et al

[78, 81] found that, with cholera toxin, a single intraperitoneal injection in adjuvant followed 2 weeks later with intestinal immunization produced a maximal IgA antitoxin response which peaked 4 days after the boost. This regime was shown by the same authors to be protective in the dog.

Protection of lambs from *Salmonella typhimurium* infection has been shown also to be effectively induced by a combination of systemic priming and oral boost [50], and intravenous challenge of mice primed previously enterically with *V. cholerae* led to a good secondary response in the gut [78] (Table 15.5).

These results would seem to suggest that secretory responses are enhanced by prior systemic sensitization. Unfortunately, these observations do not seem to be universal for all antigens or systems. Intraperitoneal immunization can make an animal unresponsive to subsequent challenge in the gut [80] which suggests that such intraperitoneal immunization may have some direct effect on the Peyer's patches [56]. However, this may not be the only explanation since in other experiments subcutaneous priming of rabbits followed by oral dosing has been shown to suppress subsequent IgA antibody responses [43]. Similar results have been shown with sheep [7]. Thus it seems that the animal species and the nature of the antigen are as important as is whether the animals have had prior systemic exposure to the antigen (Table 15.4).

Cholera immunization

Cholera immunization has been extensively studied in both human and animal models. Using the subunit B vaccine, a number of workers have demonstrated that it is possible to prime for an intestinal immune response by parenteral immunization [38]. However, since this antigen binds to receptors on intestinal

Table 15.5 Effect of prior systemic exposure of antigen to secretory antibody responses.

	Species	Systemic immunization	Antigen	Secretory antibody	Effect	Reference
1	Man	Subcutaneous	*V. cholerae*	Milk, saliva	Enhanced	92
	Dogs, rabbit	Intraperitoneal	*V. cholerae*	Intestinal	Enhanced	81
	Lambs	Intraperitoneal	*S. typhimurium*	Intestinal	Protection enhanced	50
	Mice	Intravenous	*V. cholerae*	Intestinal	Enhanced	78
2	Mice	Intraperitoneal	*V. cholerae*	Intestinal	Suppressed	80
	Rats	Intraperitoneal	Ovalbumin	Intestinal	Suppressed	80
	Rabbits	Subcutaneous	Cholera toxin	Intestinal	Suppressed	43
	Sheep	Intraperitoneal	Toxin	Intestinal	Suppressed	7

epithelial cells the responses seen may not be typical of enterically applied antigens. In addition, intraperitoneal immunization may have a direct effect on Peyer's patches, and parenteral immunization elsewhere in the body may not prime for a secretory response in the same way. Indeed this antigen behaves differently in terms of oral tolerance, since feeding cholera toxin does not seem to induce oral tolerance, but instead both systemic and secretory immunity are stimulated [38, 71]. Pierce et al [79, 81] have shown that with this antigen, parenteral priming and subsequent oral immunization give a better response in the gut than the reverse sequence.

Effect of prior mucosal exposure to antigen: memory in the secretory system

With regard to previous exposure of the secretory system alone, or previous antigen exposure in the gut, the results from different animal models vary with respect to the evidence for immunological memory within the secretory immune system. Repeated oral immunization in man leads to a modified secondary response in secretions which is larger but of similar duration to the primary response [63]. In monkeys, a secondary series of intragastric immunizations gave rise to a similar response with no evidence of an anamnestic response [20].

It has been shown that orally immunized rabbits may show an anamnestic response in the mammary gland [65] and rats immunized by injection into the Peyer's patches with suboptimal doses of antigen produce a more rapid and greater biliary IgA response on challenge up to 1 year later [2]. Taken overall, the results suggest that the nature of the secretory response to ingested material may certainly depend on prior antigen exposure, but that this may vary according to the nature of the antigen.

Duration of secretory responses

It has been a general finding from animal models that the duration of secretory responses after gut immunization is short-lived. In experiments reported in mice [18, 31], secretory responses have been detectable 1–2 weeks after immunization but diminished by 3 or 4 weeks. In man, the secretory antibody responses in lacrimal and salivary secretions after intragastric immunization with *Streptococcus mutans* lasted for a total of approxi-

mately 6 weeks [63]. A secondary immunization gave antibodies of a similar duration though these appeared to give a modified type of secondary response in that the titres were larger (Fig. 15.8), Similar short-lived re-

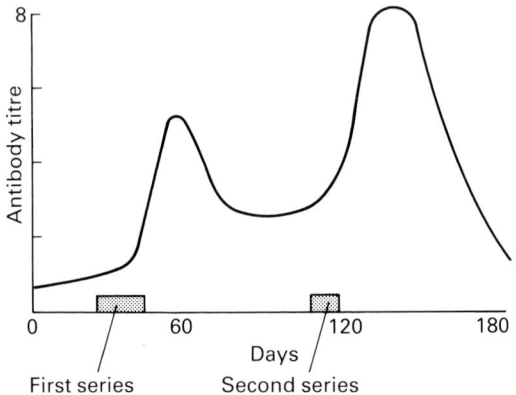

Fig. 15.8 Secretory IgA responses in saliva and lacrimal secretions after intragastric immunization with capsules containing 10^{10} *Streptococcus mutans* in man. Similar responses were found in both secretions. After a second series of immunizations a slightly larger response was seen. Adapted from Mestecky et al [63].

sponses have been found in monkeys [20], and in rabbits secretory responses to the cholera toxin were short-lived after intragastric immunization [50].

These results taken together suggest that, after the migration of antigen-sensitive cells of Peyer's patches to secretory tissues, the cells do not continue to secrete antibodies in the absence of any local or continued antigenic challenge. Amplification of the local antibody response can be induced if antigen is then applied at individual sites [51] (Fig. 15.9).

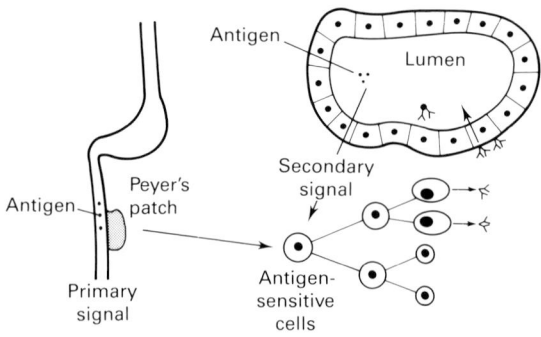

Fig. 15.9 Scheme for optimal induction of secretory responses. Primary signal from antigen in Peyer's patches leads to antigen-sensitive cells in secretory tissues. Secondary signal in the secretory tissue leads to further differentiation and proliferation.

Oral adjuvants

In view of the generally short duration of secretory immune responses after experimental immunization, attention has been focused on methods of prolonging this response. These methods include administering oral adjuvants, and cloning of genes producing protective antigens into gut organisms which are non-pathogenic [27].

The synthetic muramyl dipeptide (*N*-acetylmuramyl-L-alanyl-D-isoglutamine or MDP) has been found to duplicate the adjuvant activity of mycobacteria in Freund's complete adjuvant [33] including administration by the oral route [23]. Taubman et al [96] have shown that MDP given enterically with *Streptococcus mutans* to rats increased the salivary IgA response but had no effect on the serum IgG response. Presumably MDP acts to make the antigen more insoluble and either allows the antigen to be present in the Peyer's patch for longer periods, or is presented in a different way or to different lymphocytes by the Peyer's patch antigen-presenting cells (see Chapter 4).

A recent novel approach has been to clone the gene for streptococcal antigen I/II [85] into *Salmonella typhimurium*. This was based on earlier observations that this organism would invade Peyer's patches in mice [15]. Curtiss et al [27] argued that expression of streptococcal antigen by this particular bacterium would allow longer duration of antigen presentation in Peyer's patches. Although the exact mechanisms have not been confirmed, it seems that this approach has been successful in enhancing the salivary IgA response to streptococcal antigen. This method may allow further elucidation of the mechanisms underlying the induction of secretory antibody responses, and possibly have direct clinical application.

Other adjuvants which have been found useful in enhancing secretory responses are the polycation DEAE-dextran [6] and in the respiratory tract the aerosolization of antigen in a solution of sodium dodecylbenzene sulphate [61]. The use of liposomes containing proteins and administered orally also seems potentially useful [39], especially if combined with MDP (Fig. 15.10).

Mucosal cellular immune responses

It is clear that cell-mediated mechanisms may be activated by antigenic material in the gut. Cells capable of responding to and stimulating mixed lymphocyte reactions have been shown in the lamina propria of the small intestine [42, 87]. Feeding of H2 incompatible cells to mice may lead to the induction of cytotoxic T cells in Peyer's patches and spleen [52]. Local cell-mediated immunity has also been shown in response to various parasites in rats [36], in mice [83] and in chickens [84].

The nature of the intraepithelial lymphocyte (IEL) has been extensively investigated in recent years ([35] and see Chapter 4) and lymphocytes with K cell or NK (natural killer) cell activity have been detected ([68], see Chapter 6). Experimental models of graft-versus-host disease certainly demonstrated the presence of local cell-mediated immunity [58, 59]. The normal bacterial flora in mice has been shown to be an important prerequisite for the capability of mediating a delayed hypersensitivity response to ingested antigen [57]. However, it is not known whether this is a general phenomenon and further work in this area is needed.

Damage by mucosal application of antigen

Various mechanisms by which mucosal application of antigen may lead to unwanted tissue reactions are discussed in Chapter 13. However it is clear that direct application of antigen to the intestinal mucosa may lead to tissue damage and infiltration of polymorphonuclear leukocytes. In pigs it has been demonstrated by Bellamy and Nielsen [8] that exposure of the mucosa to BSA led to the migration of neutrophils into the lumen, but that this was not accompanied by detectable oedema or haemorrhage. This reaction was seen within 4 hours of application of antigen.

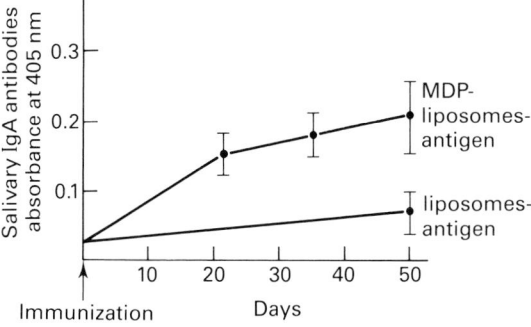

Fig. 15.10 Enhanced salivary IgA response after intragastric immunization with BSA in liposomes containing antigen and muramyl dipeptide (MDP) and antigen, compared with liposomes with antigen alone. Adapted from Genco et al [39].

It was postulated that this was a method by which local immunity might be enhanced by neutrophils, but it is clearly a mechanism by which antigens in the gut may cause damage to the mucosa.

Access of bystander antigens

An interesting phenomenon which may have clinical relevance is the access of bystander antigens during a local immune response to an unrelated antigen. Thus Brandtzaeg and Tolo [12] have shown that in mucosa taken from animals immunized with albumin, the passage of albumin is inhibited. However, the concurrent passage of transferrin was enhanced. The reverse was true in animals immunized with transferrin (Fig. 15.11). This observation may

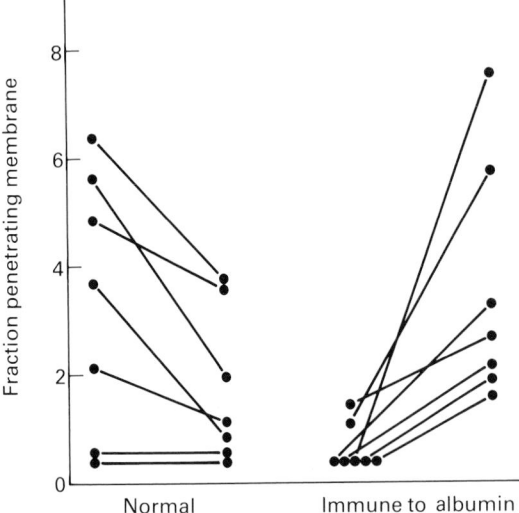

Fig. 15.11 Access of bystander antigens. Passage of albumin across epithelium from animals immunized with albumin was inhibited, but access of transferrin was enhanced. The reverse was seen using epithelium from transferrin-immunized animals. (Redrawn from [12].)

provide an explanation for the observed susceptibility of subjects who are allergic to inhaled antigen to become allergic to foods since allergens/antigens that would normally be excluded, may, at a time of a response to unrelated allergens, cross the mucosa and stimulate reactions.

Implications for the development of vaccines for mucosal infections

It is clear from the previous discussion that there are a great many variables involved in the successful induction of a long-lived secretory response. In fact this has not been achieved convincingly in animal models to date. In the field of oral vaccines, attention has recently turned to immunization with attenuated strains which might colonize the gut such as non-pathogenic strains of *Salmonella typhimurium* which have been used in cows [5]. This approach has been extended to humans and the interesting work with the attenuated strain of *Salmonella typhi* substrain Ty[21a], which lacks an enzyme essential to the utilization of galactose which limits its survival in the host, has been most promising, and it seems also to produce effective protection in man [40, 91].

However, in terms of safety there are obvious advantages in using inactivated oral vaccines and this is the most straightforward and obvious method of oral immunization. In general, the results of feeding inactivated whole organisms on the induction of secretory responses have been much more capricious than using live vaccines. The doses of antigen needed to induce secretory response (see above) have been very large, and with whole bacteria range from 10^{10} organisms in mice [64] to 10^{11} and 10^{12} in pigs and calves [4, 30] and in man [63].

The larger doses needed may reflect the relative inefficiency of sampling in the gastrointestinal tract, or it may indicate that organisms need to adhere to the mucosa to be effective immunogens. It may also reflect that the antigen is greatly diluted in the environment of the gut. The implications of these findings with regard to responses to ingested material are that it would seem that either large doses of antigen or frequent exposure to antigen is needed to have a detectable response in secretions distant from the gut.

The concept of an enteromucosal system in which various mucosal sites are integrated through movement of cells suggests that enteric immunization may provide protection at a number of sites. This may be effective in humans since protection against adenovirus type 4 was found after oral immunization with virus in enteric-coated capsules [88], and oral vaccination with Herpes simplex type 1 has enhanced protection against intravaginal challenge with Herpes type 2 [90].

THE RELATIONSHIP BETWEEN THE SYSTEMIC AND SECRETORY SYSTEMS

General considerations

It has become clear over the last few years that

deposition of antigenic material in the gut may have implications for both the systemic and mucosal immune systems. Several groups of investigators have examined the systemic responses after such immunization and the concept of oral tolerance [98] has arisen to describe the phenomenon of specific systemic hyporesponsiveness to soluble antigens which have previously been given by the oral route [1, 3, 62, 70, 102]. This was first described in the scientific literature by Wells [107] in 1911, expanded in the classical experiments of Chase in 1946 [22] and has received thorough analysis in the last few years [44, 62, 70].

Concurrent activation

The pertinent question of whether both the secretory system and the induction of oral tolerance can be stimulated by the same immunization schedule and whether the conditions are similar for both has been addressed by a few authors. Swarbrick et al [93] showed in rats that feeding of antigen led not only to suppression of the induction of serum antibodies but also to a reduction in the subsequent absorption of antigen in the gut. This was assumed to be a function of local immunity though this was not formally proven. Antigen exclusion after similar immunization schedules has been shown in the elegant experiments of Walker et al [106] and were shown to be due to secretory IgA antibodies in the small bowel.

We [21] examined the induction of salivary antibodies and systemic tolerance after oral immunization, and showed that, in mice, prior feeding of ovalbumin led to a dose-dependent suppression of a proliferative response in draining lymph nodes after a subcutaneous challenge. At the higher doses of antigen, salivary antibodies were detected and thus it seemed that, in these animals, both oral tolerance and salivary IgA antibodies were induced by the same immunization. A single intragastric immunization with 1 mg of ovalbumin led to oral tolerance but did not lead to detectable secretory IgA antibodies whereas 10 mg ovalbumin led to oral tolerance and salivary IgA antibodies. Thus both secretory immunity and systemic tolerance can be induced by the same antigenic challenge (Fig. 15.12).

Possible mechanisms

A possible explanation of how immunity and tolerance can be induced concurrently is that suppressor cells, helper cells and antibody precursor cells are all induced in Peyer's patches by oral immunization. Richman et al [82] using in vitro systems have been able to show that oral immunization led to the induction in Peyer's patches of suppressor cells for IgG and helper cells for IgA responses. An extension of this idea to in vivo would suggest that the suppression of systemic serum IgG responses might be due to suppressor cells whereas helper cells for IgA may explain the secretory IgA responses, particularly if these were to migrate to secretory tissues. However, in other work (discussed in more detail in Chapter 14) it has been reported that serum IgG, IgA and IgM antibody responses may be suppressed at the same time as salivary IgA antibodies are present. This would indicate that suppressor cells are present for systemic IgA responses and that secretory IgA responses escape this suppression, perhaps due to helper cells which are specific for secretory sites. There is some evidence of homing of both T and B cells to secretory tissue as discussed previously.

Possible biological relevance

In man, an inverse relationship between serum IgG and salivary IgA antibodies has also been reported with antibody directed to *Streptococcus mutans* [17]. Sequential studies indicate that as serum IgG antibodies increase in response to the development of dental caries, salivary IgA antibodies decrease. Conversely, when serum IgG antibodies decreased, salivary IgA antibodies were found to increase [17] (Fig. 15.13). These observations indicate some active relationship between the two systems. This inverse relationship and the observation that intragastric immunization may lead

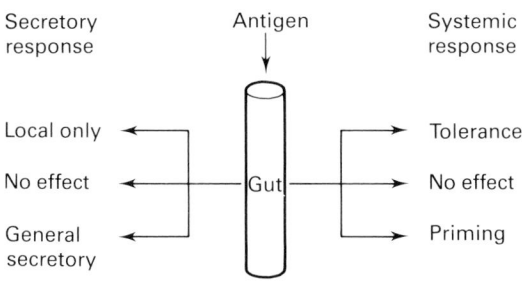

Fig. 15.12 Possible secretory and systemic immune responses after intestinal immunization.

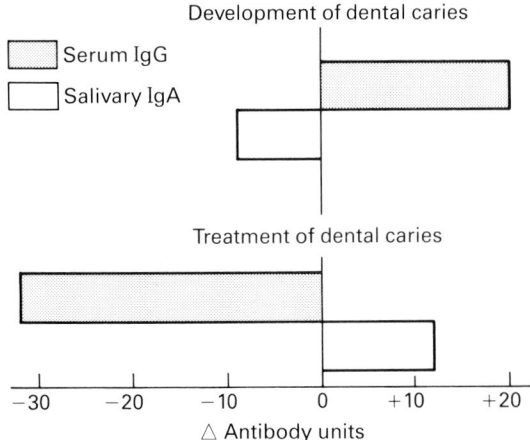

Fig. 15.13 Reciprocal changes in serum IgG and salivary IgA antibodies in humans following development or treatment of dental caries. Antibodies to whole cells of *Streptococcus mutans* assayed by solid-phase radioimmunoassay.

to simultaneous induction of secretory antibodies and systemic suppression raises intriguing speculation as to the relationship between the two systems and the biological relevance of these observations. The occurrence of a secretory immune response after mucosal contact with antigen would appear to be a most useful mechanism with regard to the exclusion of potentially harmful substances from the body [106].

The induction of systemic tolerance could act as a secondary defence to ensure that immunologically damaging reactions to antigens that escape exclusion do not occur. This may be a particularly appropriate response with regard to various allergens [70, 102] which might otherwise have harmful effects on the body. It may also be an appropriate response to antigens that cross-react with self and therefore

might induce autoimmunity, and this is an area which deserves further attention.

CONCLUSIONS

Food antigens, microbiological antigens and chemicals present a normal and enormous daily antigenic challenge throughout the life of the host. The mucosal immune system can be regarded as functioning to counteract and handle this antigenic challenge in a way which results in minimal damage to the host.

There is no doubt that the secretory system can be stimulated independently from the systemic system. It has its own immunoglobulin, secretory IgA, antigen-presenting cells in mucosal-associated lymphoid tissue (MALT) in Peyer's patches and in the lung, and both T and B cells which migrate to or are selectively retained in secretory tissue.

Secretory antibodies may be stimulated either by local application to mucosal surfaces or in the vicinity of secretory tissue, or centrally by GALT or BALT. It is probable that in most cases the induction of effective secretory antibodies requires a primary signal to MALT allowing the release of IgA precursor cells which migrate to secretory tissue, and a secondary signal at the secretory site allowing for further differentiation and proliferation.

Most secretory responses are of short duration. Successful induction of secretory antibodies is dependent on a number of variables including the nature of the antigen, duration of antigenic challenge and prior immune status of the animal. Local or central challenge of secretory tissues may also have an effect on the systemic immune system.

REFERENCES

1 Andre C, Heremans JF, Vaerman JP, Cambiaso CL: A mechanism for the induction of immunological tolerance by antigen feeding: antigen–antibody complexes. *J Exp Med* 1975; 142:1509–19.

2 Andrew E, Hall JG: IgA antibodies in the bile of rats. II. Evidence for immunological memory in secretory immunity. Immunology 1982; 45:177–82.

3 Asherson GL, Zembala M, Perera MACC et al: Production of immunity and unresponsiveness in the mouse by feeding contact sensitizing agents and the role of suppressor cells in the Peyer's patches, mesenteric lymph nodes and other lymphoid tissues. Cell Immunol 1977; 33:145–55.

4 Baljer G: Possibilities and limitations of oral immunisation against *Escherichia coli* in piglets and calves. Fortschr Vet Med 1979; 29:64–72.

5 Baljer G, Hoerstke M, Dirksen G et al: Verglei-

chende Untersuchungen uber die Wirksamkeit einer oralen Immunisierung mit Hitzeinaktivierten und vermehrungsfahigen avirulenten (Gal E)-typhimurium-keimen gegen die Salmonellosi des Kalbes, Zentralbl Vet Med 1981; 28:759–66.

6 Beh KJ: Antibody containing cell response in lymph of sheep after intra intestinal infusion of ovalbumin with and without DEAE-dextran. Immunology 1979; 37:279–86.

7 Beh KJ, Husband AJ, Lascelles AK: Intestinal response of sheep to intraperitoneal immunisation. Immunology 1979; 37:385–8.

8 Bellamy JEC, Nielsen NO: Immune-mediated emigration of neutrophils into the lumen of the small intestine. Infect Immun 1974; 9:615.

9 Besredka A: Local immunisation. Baltimore: Williams and Wilkins, 1927.

10 Bienenstock J, Befus ADM: Musosal immunology. A review. Immunology 1980; 41:249–70.

11 Bienenstock J, McDermott M, Befus AD: A common mucosal immune system. In: Oga PL, Dayton D, eds. Immunology of breast milk. New York: Raven Press, 1979; 135–51.

12 Brandtzaeg P, Tolo K: Mucosal penetrability enhanced by serum derived antibodies. Nature 1977; 266:262–3.

13 Brandtzaeg P, Fjellanger I, Gjeraldsen SJ: Human secretory immunoglobulins. I. Salivary secretions from individuals with normal or low levels of serum immunoglobulins. Scand J Haematol [Suppl] 1970; 12:1–97.

14 Burrows W, Havens I: Studies on immunity to Asiatic cholera. The absorption of immune globulin from the bowel and its excretion in the urine and faeces of experimental animals and human volunteers. J Infect Dis 1948; 82:231–50.

15 Carter PB, Collins FM: Peyer's patch responsiveness to salmonella in mice. J Reticuloendothel Soc 1975; 17:38–46.

16 Cebra JJ, Kamat R, Gearhart PJ et al: The secretory IgA system of the gut. Ciba Found Symp 1977; 46:5–28.

17 Challacombe SJ: Serum and salivary antibodies to *Streptococcus mutans* in relation to the development and treatment of dental caries. Arch Oral Biol 1980; 25:495–502.

18 Challacombe SJ; Salivary antibodies and systemic tolerance in mice after oral immunisation with bacterial antigens. Ann NY Acad Sci 1983; 409:177–92.

19 Challacombe SJ: Systemic tolerance and salivary antibodies after oral immunisation. In: Revillard JP, Voisin C, Wierznicki M, eds. Mucosal immunity: IgA and polymorphonuclear neutrophils. Journées immunologiques. France: Fondation Franco-Allemande, 1985; 73–82.

20 Challacombe SJ, Lehner T: Salivary antibody responses in rhesus monkeys immunised with *Streptococcus mutans* by the oral, submucosal or subcutaneous routes. Arch Oral Biol 1980; 24:917–25.

21 Challacombe SJ, Tomasi B: Systemic tolerance and secretory immunity after oral immunisation. J Exp Med 1980; 152:1459–72.

22 Chase MW: Inhibition of experimental drug allergy by prior feeding of the sensitizing agent. Proc Soc Exp Biol 1946; 61:257–9.

23 Chedid L, Audibert F, Leframcier P et al: Modulation of the immune responses by a synthetic adjuvant and analogs. Proc Nat Acad Sci USA 1976; 73:1472–5.

24 Cooper MD, Lawton AR: The development of the immune system. Sci Am 1974; 2331:59.

25 Crabbe PA, Nash DR, Bazin H: Antibodies of the IgA type in intestinal plasma cells of germ free mice after oral or parenteral immunisation with ferritin. J Exp Med 1969; 130:723–44.

26 Crawford JM, Taubman MA, Smith DJ: Minor salivary glands as a major source of secretory immunoglobulin A in the human oral cavity. Science 1975; 190:1206–9.

27 Curtiss R, Holt RG, Barletta RG: *Escherichia coli* strains producing *Streptococcus mutans* proteins responsible for colonisation and virulence. Ann NY Acad Sci 1983; 409:688–95.

28 Davies A: An investigation into the serological properties of dysentery stools. Lancet 1922; 203:1009–12.

29 Dupont HL, Hornick RB, Synder MJ: Studies of immunity in typhoid fever: protection induced by killed oral vaccines or by primary infection. Bull WHO 1971; 44:667–72.

30 Dziaba KA, Synkiewicz ZM, Binek M, Jakubowski HET: The effect of oral immunisation with *E. coli* vaccine on live weight gain in weaned pigs. Proc Int Vet Soc 1980; 165:121.

31 Ebersole JL, Molinari JA: The induction of salivary antibodies by topical sensitization with particulate and soluble bacterial immunogens. Immunology 1978; 34:969–79.

32 Ebersole JL, Taubman MA, Smith DJ: The effect of neonatal thymectomy on the level of salivary and serum immunoglobulins in rats. Immunology 1979; 36:649.

33 Ellouz F, Adam A, Ciorbaru F, Lederer E: Minimal structural requirements for adjuvant activity of bacterial peptidoglycan derivatives. Biochem Biophys Res Commun 1974; 59:1317–25.

34 Emmings FG, Evans RT, Genco RJ: Antibody response in the parotid fluid and serum of irus monkeys (*Macaca fascicularis*) after local immunisation with *Streptococcus mutans*. Infect Immun 1975; 12:281–92.

35 Ferguson A: Intraepithelial lymphocytes of the small intestine. Gut 1966; 18:921–37.

36 Ferguson A, Jarrett EEE: Hypersensitivity reactions in the small intestine. I. Thymus dependence of experimental 'partial villous atrophy'. Gut 1975;16:114–17.

37 Fubara ES, Freter R: Protection against enteric bacterial infection by secretory IgA antibodies. J Immunol 1973; 111:395–403.

38 Fuhram JA, Cebra JJ: Special features of the priming process for a secretory IgA response. B cell priming with cholera toxin. J Exp Med 1981; 153:534–44.

39 Genco RJ, Linzer R, Evans RT: Effect of adjuvants on orally administered antigens. Ann NY Acad Sci 1983; 409:650–67.

40 Gillman RH, Hornick RB, Woodward WF et al: Evaluation of a UDP-glucose-4-epimeraseless mutant of *Salmonella typhi* as a live oral vaccine. J. Infect Dis 1977; 136:717–23.

41 Goldblum RM Van Bavel J: Immunoglobulin A production by human colostral cells: quantitative aspects. Adv Exp Med Biol 1978; 107:87–94.

42 Goodacre R, Davidson R, Singal D, Bienenstock J: Morphologic and functional characteristics of human intestinal lymphoid cells isolated by a mechanical technique. Gastroenterology 1979; 76:300–8.

43 Hamilton SR, Yardley JH, Brown GD: Suppression of local intestinal immunoglobulin A immune response to cholera toxin by subcutaneous administration of cholera toxoid. Infect Immun 1979; 24:422–6.

44 Hanson DG, Morimoto T: A role of digestion in orally induced tolerance to ovalbumin. J Allergy Clin Immunol 1980; 65:227–36.

45 Hanson LA, Brandtzaeg P: The mucosal defense system. In: Stiehem ER, Fulginiti VA, eds. Immunological disorders in infants and children. Philadelphia: WB Saunders, 1980; 137–62.

46 Hanson LA, Ahlstedt S, Andersson B et al: Mucosal immunity. Ann NY Acad Sci 1983; 409:1–21.

47 Haworth JC, Dilling L: Concentration of γ-globulin in serum, saliva and nasopharyngeal secretions of infants and children. J Lab Clin Med 1966; 67:922–33.

48 Heremans JF, Heremans MT, Schultze HE: Isolation and description of a few properties of the β2A-globulin of human secretion. Clin Chim Acta 1959; 4:96–101.

49 Horsfall DJ, Cooper JM, Rowley D: Changes in the

immunoglobulin levels of the mouse gut and serum during conventionalisation and following administration of *Salmonella typhimurium*. Aust J Exp Biol Med Sci 1978; 56: 727-35.

50 Husband AJ: An immunisation model for the control of infectious enteritis. Res Vet Sci 1978; 25:173-7.

51 Husband AM, Gowans JL: The origin and antigen-dependent distribution of IgA containing cells in the intestine. J. Exp Med 1978; 148:1146-60.

52 Kagnoff MF: Effects of antigen feeding on intestinal and systemic immune responses. I. Priming of precursor cytotoxic T cells by antigen feeding. J Immunol 1978; 120:395-9.

53 Krasse B, Gahnberg L, Bratthall D: Antibodies reacting with *Streptococcus mutans* in secretions from minor salivary glands in humans. Adv Exp Med Biol 1978; 107: 349-54.

54 Linzer R, Evans RT, Emmings FG, Genco RJ: Use of combined immunisation routes in induction of a salivary immunoglobulin A response to *Streptococcus mutans* in *Macaca fascicularis* monkeys. Infect Immun 1981; 31:345-51.

55 Lodinova R, Jouja V, Wagner V: Serum immunoglobulins and copro antibody formation in infants after artificial intestinal colonisation with *Escherichia coli* 083 and oral lysozyme administration. Pediatr Res 1973; 7: 659-69.

56 MacDonald TT: Enhancement and suppression of the Peyer's patch immune response by systemic priming. Clin Exp Immunol 1983; 49:441-8.

57 MacDonald TT, Carter PB: Requirement for a bacterial flora before mice generate cells capable of mediating the delayed hypersensitivity reaction to sheep red blood cells. J Immunol 1979; 122:2624-9.

58 MacDonald TT, Carter PB: Cell-mediated immunity to intestinal infection. Infect Immun 1980; 28:516-32.

59 MacDonald TT, Ferguson A: Hypersensitivity reactions in the small intestine. III. The effects of allograft rejection and of graft-versus-host disease on epithelial cell kinetics. Cell Tissue Kinet 1977; 10:301-12.

60 McGhee JR, Michalek SM, Webb J et al: Effective immunity to dental caries: protection of gnotobiotic rats by local immunisation with *Streptococcus mutans*. J Immunol 1975; 114:300-5.

61 Markham RJF, Wilkie BN: Local adjuvants: the influence of sodium dodecylbenzene sulphonate on immunisation with aerosolized antigen. Experientia 1979; 35:414.

62 Mattingly JA, Waksman BH: Immunologic suppression after oral administration of antigen. I. Specific suppressor cells formed in rat Peyer's patches after oral administration of sheep erythrocytes and their systemic migration. J Immunol 1978; 121:1878-83.

63 Mestecky J, McGhee JR, Arnold RR et al: Selective induction of an immune response in human external secretions by ingestion of bacterial antigen. J Clin Invest 1978; 61:731-7.

64 Michalek SM, McGhee JR Babb JL: Effective immunity to dental caries: dose dependent studies of secretory immunity by oral administration of *Streptococcus mutans* to rats. Infect Immun 1977; 19:217-23.

65 Montgomery PC, Cohen C, Skandera CA, Connelly KM: Evidence for an IgA anamnestic response in rabbit mammary secretions. In: Ogra PC, Dayton D, eds. Immunology of breast milk. New York: Raven Press, 1979;115.

66 Montgomery PC, Connell KM, Cohn J, Skandera

CA: Remote site stimulation of secretory IgA antibodies following bronchial and gastric stimulation. Adv Exp Med Biol 1978; 107:113-22.

67 Montrien B de, Serre A: Etudes des immunoglobulines salivaires après vaccination locale antistreptococcique. Pathol Biol (Paris) 1974; 22:305-12.

68 Mowat A, Tait RC, Mackenzie S et al: Analysis of natural effector and suppressor activity by intraepithelial lymphocytes from mouse small intestine. Clin Exp Immunol 1983; 52:191-6.

69 Newby TJ, Stokes CR, Evans PA, Bourne FJ: The immune response following oral vaccination with *E. coli*. Curr Top Vet Med Anim Sci 1981; 12:377-88.

70 Ngan J, Kind LS: Suppressor T cells for IgE and IgG in Peyer's patches of mice made tolerant by the oral administration of ovalbumin. J Immunol 1978; 120:861-5.

71 Nicklin S, Miller K: Local and systemic immune responses to intestinally presented antigen. Int Arch Allergy Appl Immunol 1983; 72:87-90.

72 Ogra PL, Green HL: Human milk and breast feeding: an update on the state of the art. Pediatr Res 1982; 16:266-71.

73 Ogra PL, Karzon DT: Distribution of poliovirus antibody in serum, nasopharynx and alimentary tract following segmental immunisation of lower alimentary tract with poliovaccine. J Immunol 1969; 102:1423-30.

74 Ogra PL, Ogra SS: Local antibody response to poliovaccine in the human female genital tract. J Immunol 1973; 110:1307-12.

75 Parrott DMV, Ferguson A: Selective migration of lymphocytes within the mouse small intestine. Immunology 1974; 26:571.

76 Parrott DMV, Rose MI: Migration pathways of T lymphocytes in the small intestine. Adv Exp Med Biol 1978; 107:67-74.

77 Peri BA, Theodore CM, Losonsky GA et al: Antibody content of rabbit milk and serum following inhalation or congestion of respiratory syncitial virus and bovine serum albumin. Clin Exp Immunol 1982; 48:91-101.

78 Pierce NF: The role of antigen form and function in the primary and secondary intestinal immune responses to cholera toxin and toxoid in rats. J Exp Med 1978; 148:195-206.

79 Pierce NF, Gowans JL: Cellular kinetics of the intestinal immune response to cholera toxoid in rats. J Exp Med 1975; 142:1550-6.

80 Pierce NF, Koster FT: Parenteral immunisation causes antigen-specific cell-mediated suppression of an intestinal IgA response. J Immunol 1983; 131:115-9.

81 Pierce NF, Cray WC, Sacci JB et al: Oral immunisation against experimental cholera: the role of antigen form and antigen combinations in evoking protection. Ann NY Acad Sci 1983; 409:724-32.

82 Richman LK, Graeff AS, Yarchoan R, Strober W: Simultaneous induction of antigen-specific IgA helper T cells and IgG suppressor T cells in the murine Peyer's patch after protein feeding. J Immunol 1981; 126:2079-83.

83 Roberts-Thomson IC, Mitchell GF: Giardiasis in mice. I. Prolonged infections in certain mouse strains and hypothymic nude mice. Gastroenterology 1978; 75:42-6.

84 Rose ME, Long PL: Immunity to coccidiosis: interaction in vitro between *Eimeria tinnella* and chicken phagocytic cells. In: van de Bossche, ed. Biochem-

istry of parasite and host parasite relationships. 1976; 449-55. Amsterdam: Elsevier/North Holland.

85 Russell MW, Lehner T: Characterisation of antigens extracted from cells and culture fluids of *S. mutans* serotype c. Arch Oral Biol 1978; 23:121-5.

86 Sellwood R: *E. coli* associated porcine neonatal diarrhoea—anti-bacterial activities from colostrum from genetically susceptible and resistant sows. Infect Immun 1981; 35:396-407.

87 Singal DP, O'Neill M, Clancy R, Bienenstock J: Functional T cells in rabbit gut mucosal lymphocytes. Gut 1976; 17:235-43.

88 Smith TJ, Buescher EL, Top FH et al: Experimental respiratory infection with type 4 adenovirus vaccine in volunteers: clinical and immunological responses. J Infect Dis 1970; 122:239-48.

89 Sterzl J, Silverstein AM: Development aspects of immunity. Adv Immunol 1967; 6:337-57.

90 Sturn B, Schneweis KE: Protective effect of an oral infection with herpes simplex virus Type 1 against subsequent genital infection with herpes simplex virus Type 2. Med Microbiol Immunol 1978; 165:119-27.

91 Sutton RGA, Merson MH: Oral typhoid vaccine Ty21a. Lancet 1983; i:523.

92 Svennerholm AM, Holmgren J, Hanson LA et al: Boosting of secretory IgA antibody responses in man by parenteral choleral vaccination. Scand J Immunol 1977; 6:1345-9.

93 Swarbrick ET, Stokes CR, Soothill JF: Absorption of antigens after oral immunisation and the simultaneous induction of specific systemic tolerance. Gut 1979; 20:121-5.

94 Taubman MA, Genco RJ: Induction and properties of secretory IgA antibody directed to group A streptococcal carbohydrates. Immunohistochemistry 1983; 8:1137-55.

95 Taubman MA, Smith DJ: Effects of local immunisation with glucosyltransferase fractions from *Streptococcus mutans* on dental caries in rats and hamsters. J Immunol 1977; 118:710-20.

96 Taubman MA, Ebersole JL, Smith DJ, Stack W: Adjuvants for secretory immune responses. Ann NY Acad Sci 1983; 409:637-48.

97 Tomasi TB: The immune system of secretions. New Jersey: Prentice-Hall; 1976.

98 Tomasi TB: Oral tolerance (an overview). Transplantation 1980; 29:353-6.

99 Tomasi TB, Larson L, Challacombe SJ, McNabb P: Mucosal immunity: the origin and migration patterns of cells in the secretory system. J Allergy Clin Immunol 1980; 65:12-19.

100 Tomasi TB, Tan EM, Soloman A, Predergast RA: Characteristics of an immune system common to certain external secretions. J Exp Med 1965; 121:104-24.

101 Vaerman JP: Comparative immunochemistry of IgA. In: Kwapinski JB, ed. Research in immunochemistry and immunobiology. Baltimore: University Park Press, 1973;234.

102 Vaz NM, Maia LCS, Hanson DG, Lynch JM: Inhibition of homocytotropic antibody responses in adult inbred mice by previous feeding of the specific antigen. J Allergy Clin Immunol 1977; 60:110-15.

103 Waldman RH, Ganguly R: Immunity to infections on secretory surfaces. J Infect Dis 1974; 130:419-25.

104 Waldman RH, Wood JW, Torres EJ, Small PA: Influenza antibody response following aerosol administration of inactivated virus. Am J Epidemiol 1970; 91:575.

105 Walker J: Antibody responses of monkeys to oral and local immunisation with *Streptococcus mutans*. Infect Immun 1981; 31:81.

106 Walker WA, Isselbacher KJ, Bloch KJ: Intestinal uptake of macromolecules: effect of oral immunisation. Science 1972; 177:608-10.

107 Wells HG: Studies on the chemistry of anaphylaxis. III. Experiments with isolated proteins, especially those of the hen egg. J Infect Dis 1911; 9:147-71.

108 Werner GT, Ulm K: Evaluation of oral vaccination against mouse typhoid in a new animal model. Experientia 1981; 37:900-1.

Chapter 16
Animal Models of Food Sensitivity

C. R. Stokes, B. G. Miller and F. J. Bourne

Hypersensitivity reactions in the gastrointestinal tract

The potential for a range of immune hypersensitivity reactions to operate within the gastrointestinal tract is well established, but it is not clear which, if any, of the effector mechanisms may be triggered, either in isolation or in concert, by food antigens. In this chapter we illustrate how in rodents, pigs and calves ingestion of food may lead to immune-mediated gut damage. The mechanisms where characterized are discussed. Since in experimental animals a diagnosis of food allergy is not possible in the absence of either pathological change, weight loss, reduced food intake or diarrhoea, we have restricted our discussion to those studies where gut damage or the consequences of gut damage have been observed. At the outset we must make clear that the investigations in calves and pigs result not from an attempt to develop an animal model for human disease but rather from a desire to understand the pathogenesis of common clinical conditions found in these species.

RODENTS

Evidence of both humoral and cellular mechanisms resulting from reactions to dietary components have been reported.

Humoral-mediated damage

Whilst in a number of rodent systems methods of immunization have been developed to stimulate the production of IgE antibodies [42, 67], few have attempted to demonstrate if such responses lead to intestinal anaphylaxis. Similarly many models have involved parenteral immunization with adjuvants and only rarely has sensitization been achieved by the oral route [5, 28]. Whilst the difficulty in achieving sensitivity via this route is explainable by the induction of oral tolerance (for review see [58] and Chapter 14), the physiological relevance of studies involving 'unnatural' routes of immunization must always be questioned.

Intestinal anaphylaxis

The increase in leakage of plasma proteins into the gut in association with subepithelial oedema [56] has been used as an indicator of intestinal anaphylaxis. Thus Byars and Ferraresi [12] showed that rats sensitized by injection of ovalbumin and *Bordetella pertussis* adjuvant and subsequently injected intravenously with ^{125}I-labelled bovine serum albumin (BSA) immediately before oral challenge with ovalbumin had greatly increased levels of radioactivity in intestinal tissue compared with non-sensitized controls. Since the sera from sensitized rats gave positive 24 hour passive cutaneous anaphylaxis (PCA) tests, reaginic antibody was the likely effector mechanism. Similar studies showed that homologous radiolabelled serum albumin (RSA) could also be used to demonstrate the accumulation of plasma proteins in intestinal secretions and gut segments [40]. Confirmation that IgE antibody could lead to intestinal anaphylaxis was provided by passive transfer studies; serum from rats containing high levels of IgE antiovalbumin being able to promote release of interestinal goblet cell mucus upon intraduodenal challenge [40].

A further indicator of intestinal anaphylaxis is the histamine content of intraluminal contents which rises 15 minutes after antigen challenge and continues to increase for up to 1 hour [38]. Perdue [63] has recently reported a similar study in which a wide variety of parameters were measured following intraluminal perfusion of ovalbumin in parenterally sensitized rats. Absorption of water, sodium, potassium and calcium was reduced within 10 minutes, and markedly so by 40 minutes. There was also a reduction in gut tissue histamine content and in the numbers of granulated mucosal mast cells. Mucosal oedema was observed but there were no changes in villus height or crypt depth, and mucosal permeability was unchanged (Fig. 16.1).

In addition to damage mediated by IgE, other isotypes have also been implicated. Instilling immune complexes (presumably IgG)

in antibody excess into the duodenum of rats has been shown to result in goblet cell mucus discharge [86].

Route of immunization and mucus release

It has been shown [39] that whilst rats orally immunized with 100 mg of BSA on 5 consecutive days and then weekly for 5 weeks showed enhanced release of goblet cell mucus upon intestinal challenge, those immunized by intraperitoneal injection in complete Freund's adjuvant and having high levels of serum antibodies did not. Such studies emphasize not only the importance of the type of adjuvant but also the route of immunization, in determining the clinical outcome.

Cell-mediated hypersensitivity

Evidence that cell-mediated immune reactions may lead to changes in intestinal morphology have come from studies of allograft rejection, graft-versus-host reactions and responses to fed antigens. Whilst it is the intention to concentrate in this chapter on models directly related to food, much of the most compelling evidence has come from studies involving tissue antigens rather than dietary components.

Intestinal graft rejection

It was shown in the early 1970s that rejection of small intestinal grafts in dogs was associated with crypt hypertrophy and villus atrophy [26]. Such studies were extended in the mouse by Ferguson and colleagues who showed that following grafting of allografts of sterile fetal intestine under the kidney capsule of adult mice, rejection occurred within 3 weeks [18, 19]. The earliest morphological signs of rejection were an increase in the number of intraepithelial lymphocytes (IELs) followed by a large increase in the rate of division of cells in the crypt and finally a change in villus architecture [46, 47]. Similar morphological changes have been observed during graft-versus-host reactions, although villus atrophy was not a constant feature [54, 55]. These changes are accompanied by an increased natural killer (NK) cell activity of the IELs and a numerical increase in mucosal mast cells in both epithelium and lamina propria [11, 55]. Since such changes occur in the absence of microorganisms [54] and cannot be elicited by specific cytotoxic cells it has been suggested

---

Leakage of plasma proteins
Subepithelial oedema
Goblet cell mucus release (dependent on regime)
Histamine content: gut lumen ↑
                  gut tissue ↓
Malabsorption: H_2O, K^+, Na^+, Cl^-
Early onset

No change in:

Villus / crypt ratio
Mucosal permeability to [^{14}C] polyethylene glycol

Fig. 16.1 Features of immediate type hypersensitivity reactions described in rodent models of food allergy. (For detailed references see text.)

that lymphokines released by donor T cells responding to host cells in the mucosa are responsible for the changes in mucosal architecture [54]. Cell transfer studies using parental spleen cells depleted of different Lyt subclasses before injection into F_1 mice indicated that the increased IEL count was dependent only on Lyt 1^+2^- T cells whilst enhanced crypt cell mitosis required both Lyt 1^+2^- and Lyt 1^+2^+ T cells [52], thus supporting the concept that the mucosal changes result from a delayed type hypersensitivity (DTH) reaction.

Oral immunization for cell-mediated immunity

Evidence that feeding soluble antigen may lead to a cell-mediated immune reaction capable of causing changes in gut morphology is suggestive but incomplete. One group has shown that feeding a contact sensitizing agent resulted in xylose malabsorption and changes in intestinal morphology in guinea pigs and pigs [10] but others have failed to demonstrate this in mice [22], despite there being clear evidence that such regimes can sensitize for delayed type hypersensitivity reactions at other sites [1, 60].

The question as to whether oral immunization can lead to local cell-mediated immunity and the manifestation of food allergy is not related to any doubt that feeding can stimulate a systemic delayed type hypersensitivity response. This has been shown by feeding a wide range of antigens, including those from infectious agents [20, 21], contact sensitizing agents [1, 60], particulate antigens such as sheep red blood cells [30] and dietary antigens such as ovalbumin [79]. Where doubt remains it relates to whether such responses occur to common dietary components and if so whether

they have local effects within the gastrointestinal tract. The major reason that has been put forward to explain lack of local reactivity is the development of oral tolerance.

Strain differences in delayed type hypersensitivity

Inbred strains of mice differ in their ability to mount DTH skin responses following ovalbumin feeding at a dose rate of 20 mg/day. CBA mice skin tested 2, 3 or 4 days after feeding with ovalbumin gave a positive 24 hour response, whereas similarly treated BALB/c mice did not respond at that time [81] (see Fig. 16.2). It remains to be determined if such differences are reflected locally in response to feeding soluble protein antigens, and the effect that this might have on gut morphology. That this might be so is indicated by the altered ability of mice to respond to a new dietary antigen introduced 2 days after the start of feeding with another unrelated antigen. CBA male mice fed a single tolerizing dose of HSA 2 days after commencing oral immunization with ovalbumin failed to become tolerant to HSA. In contrast, those fed the HSA 4 days after commencing feeding with ovalbumin were made tolerant. No differences were observed in the responses to ovalbumin, both groups developing tolerance [79] (see Fig. 16.3).

The mechanism underlying this change is not clear but since it occurs at a time when DTH reactions can be elicited at distant sites it has been suggested that it may be a consequence of a local CMI reaction to the first oral immunogen (ovalbumin). It is postulated that such reactions cause an 'altered presentation' of antigens [59]. Whatever the mechanism, it does indicate that the manner in which new

Fig. 16.2 Twenty-four hour increase in skin thickness following the injection of 30 μl ovalbumin into the footpad of two strains of mice. Control mice were either unsensitized ($-$ve control) or sensitized by (IP) injection of ovalbumin in complete Freund's adjuvant. The effect of feeding ovalbumin for 2, 3, 4 or 7 days on the ability to mount DTH reactions is compared. Significant responses after feeding were found only in the CBA mice. nd = not determined.

			Change in footpad thickness at 24 h (10^{-3}cm)			
	IP sensitised	$-$ve control	oral ovalbumin			
			2 day	3 day	4 day	7 day
CBA mean	6.4	1.5	3.0	3.0	3.0	1.4
range	5-7	1-3	2-5	2-5	1-4	1-2
Balb/c mean	nd	0.9	nd	1.0	nd	nd
range		0-2		0-3		

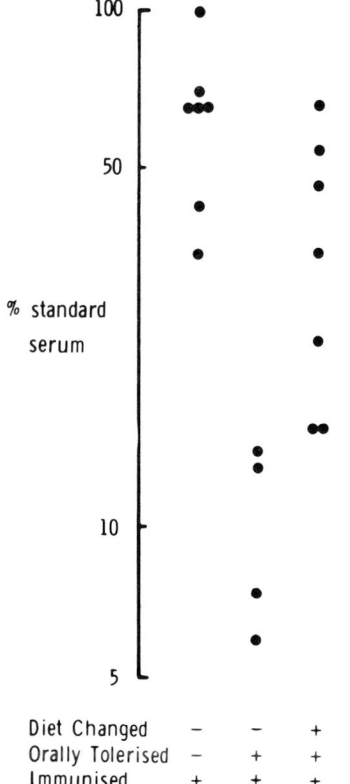

Fig. 16.3 Effect of dietary change on the induction of oral tolerance to an unrelated antigen. Serum IgG antibody response (% standard serum) 14 days after parenteral immunization with human serum albumin (HSA) in complete Freund's adjuvant. The response is compared in three groups of mice: those not tolerized; those tolerized whilst on a stable diet; and those given an orally tolerizing dose of HSA, 2 days after the start of oral immunization with ovalbumin. The data show that the introduction of one novel antigen can prevent the induction of oral tolerance to a second unrelated antigen given within two days of the first antigen. (Reproduced with the kind permission of the editor of *Clinical Experimental Immunology*.)

dietary antigens are introduced can profoundly influence the response and even prevent the induction of oral tolerance, and as such have significant consequences on the development of food allergy.

Oral tolerance (see Chapter 14)

In common with humoral antibody responses [77] it is clear that prior feeding can suppress an animal's specific ability to mount delayed type hypersensitivity reactions to erythrocytes [29], and to viral [72] as well as soluble protein antigens [51, 53]. In order to allow expression of local cell-mediated immunity to fed antigens, recent studies have attempted to abrogate oral tolerance before immunizing for ac-

tive intestinal immunity. In ovalbumin-fed mice, suppressor T cells have been implicated in the resulting tolerance [62, 68, 69] and such cells can be inhibited by cyclophosphamide [2, 71]. In an attempt to prevent tolerance induction, ovalbumin has been fed to cyclophosphamide-treated mice. In these mice both systemic and local delayed type hypersensitivity (DTH) (see Fig. 16.4) was observed.

In the intestine following ovalbumin challenge there was an increase in the rate of crypt-cell division and in the numbers of IELs. Cells isolated from the mesenteric lymph node produced macrophage migration inhibition factor (MIF), indicating that in these mice feeding could result in local cell-mediated immune reactions to dietary antigens and that these led to an altered gut morphology [54]. Further studies have indicated that the cyclophosphamide, whilst having no effect on the intestinal absorption of ovalbumin [83], acts to eliminate the generation of suppressor cells in the local lymph node [24]. In experimental models, a number of factors have been shown to influence the development of oral tolerance. These include genetic differences [80], age [23, 82], liver function [13], bacterial lipopolysaccharide [60, 88] and protein malnutrition [84]. It has been possible by making use of these observations to delay the induction of oral tolerance and allow the expression of local cell-mediated immunity even in the absence of immunosuppressive drugs.

Oral immunization with erythrocytes

In contrast to ovalbumin and other soluble dietary proteins where the period of tolerance induction is relatively short, feeding erythrocytes can lead to a protracted period of DTH sensitivity (of approximately 1 week) [30, 61]

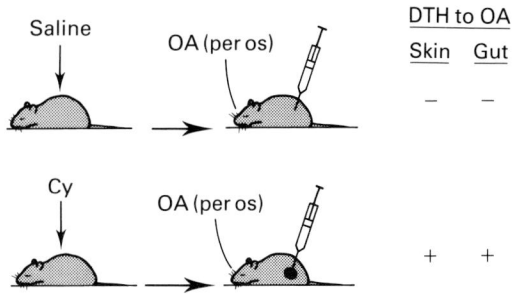

Fig. 16.4 Effect of cyclophosphamide (Cy) on abrogating suppressor cell activity in the induction of oral tolerance. OA = ovalbumin.

prior to the development of the protected state of tolerance. This model therefore provides a method for assessing the effects of local CMI reaction on gut integrity. Groups of eight CBA male mice sensitized by feeding 3×10^9 SRBC (sheep red blood cells) daily for 2 days and then challenged 10 days later on 3 consecutive days with fed SRBC show a significantly impaired capacity to absorb fed xylose compared to unsensitized control animals and those sensitized with the non-cross-reacting horse RBC. Interestingly, in mice that have been fed SRBC for 14 days (and which are tolerant, as judged by their inability to mount DTH skin tests), the ability to absorb xylose was not impaired (Fig. 16.5). This indicates

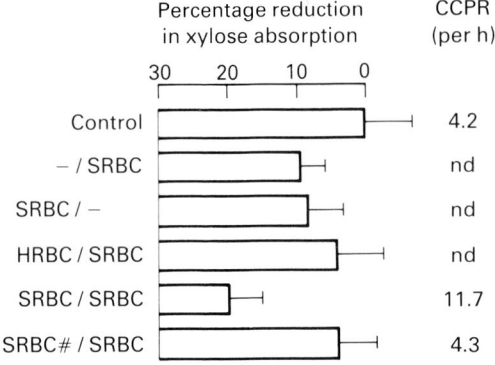

Percentage reduction in xylose absorption   CCPR (per h)

Control	4.2
– / SRBC	nd
SRBC / –	nd
HRBC / SRBC	nd
SRBC / SRBC	11.7
SRBC# / SRBC	4.3

Fig. 16.5 Percentage reduction (± 1 SD) in the ability to absorb xylose and in the rate of production of crypt cells (CCPR/h) in groups of eight male CBA mice. Plasma xylose levels were measured 30 minutes after a single feed of 10 mg of xylose. Mice had been previously sensitized by feeding sheep red blood cells (SRBC) for 2 days (SRBC/−) followed 10 days later by challenge on 3 consecutive days with SRBC (SRBC/SRBC). Xylose tests were performed on the following day and compared with those in unsensitized mice (−/SRBC), mice orally tolerized by feeding SRBC for 14 days (SRBC#/SRBC) and those sensitized with the non-cross-reacting antigen, horse red blood cells (HRBC/). Crypt cell production rates were measured on the same day. nd = not determined.

that a phase of sensitivity during which gut damage can occur precedes the development of the protected state of tolerance.

Histological studies have indicated that the malabsorption was associated with an increase in the rate of production of crypt cells and in the number of intraepithelial lymphocytes. In the SRBC-fed mouse model it is clear that the gut damage is immune mediated. Whilst detailed studies of the mechanism involved remain to be completed, the evidence that damage only occurs during the period when positive skin tests can be elicited would suggest that it is likely to be cell mediated. Preliminary cell transfer studies with mesenteric

lymph node and Peyer's patch cells isolated from the intestine of mice fed SRBC for 2 days would support this view.

PIGS

Humoral-mediated damage

The pig has been used to investigate the immunopathological consequence of antigen-antibody deposition in the intestinal epithelium. Isolated gut loops were prepared in pigs which had been immunized parenterally with BSA and had a high level of circulating antibody. Following challenge with BSA into the intestine, within 4 hours there was an influx of neutrophils into the lumen, epithelium and subepithelial capillaries [8]. Interestingly, however, the neutrophil infiltration into the intestine was not accompanied by haemorrhage, oedema or thrombosis—features typical of an Arthus reaction that could be observed following intracutaneous inoculation of BSA into similarly prepared pigs [7]. No significant effects on fluid and electrolyte movements were caused by the neutrophil response [6]. The ability to mount such responses would appear also to be age related, since attempts to repeat these studies in animals over 8 weeks of age have been unsuccessful [31].

Cell-mediated hypersensitivity

Oral immunization for lymphokine production

There is evidence that local cell-mediated immunity can be detected in the intestine of pigs following oral immunization with both infectious agents [20] and soluble protein antigens [27]. In the latter study, pigs were fed with dinitrophenylated bovine γ-globulin (DNP-BGG) and the immune response assessed using an indirect macrophage migration assay. Two days after the start of oral immunization, cultures of cells from the intestine, but not the mesenteric lymph node or spleen, could be stimulated by antigen to produce MIF. By day 7 all three sites produced MIF, indicating that the ability to mount a cell-mediated immune response had generalized. In this early study the effect of local CMI on mucosal pathology was not examined, but subsequent studies would suggest that it would have been present.

Mucosal damage in unweaned piglets

In unweaned pigs, feeding 100 mg of ovalbumin on 4 consecutive days can sensitize such

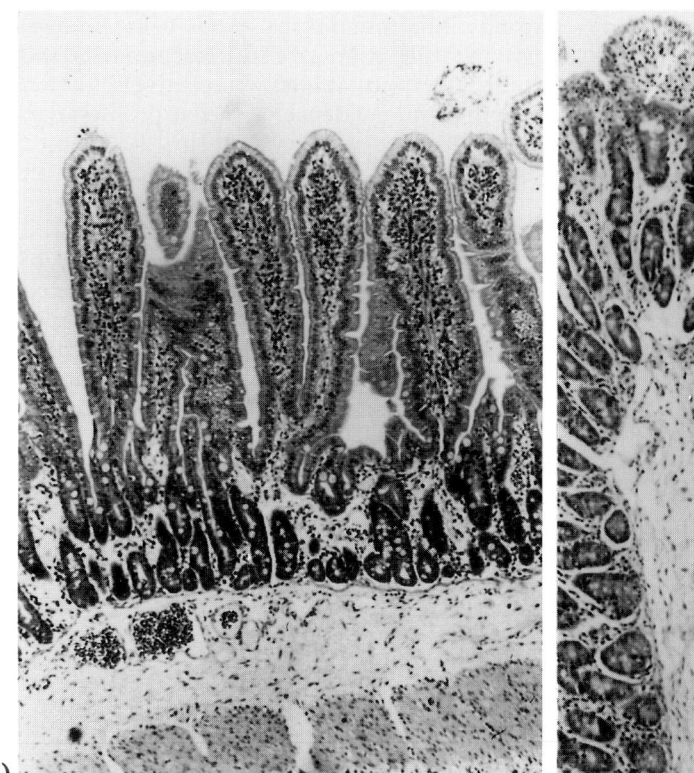
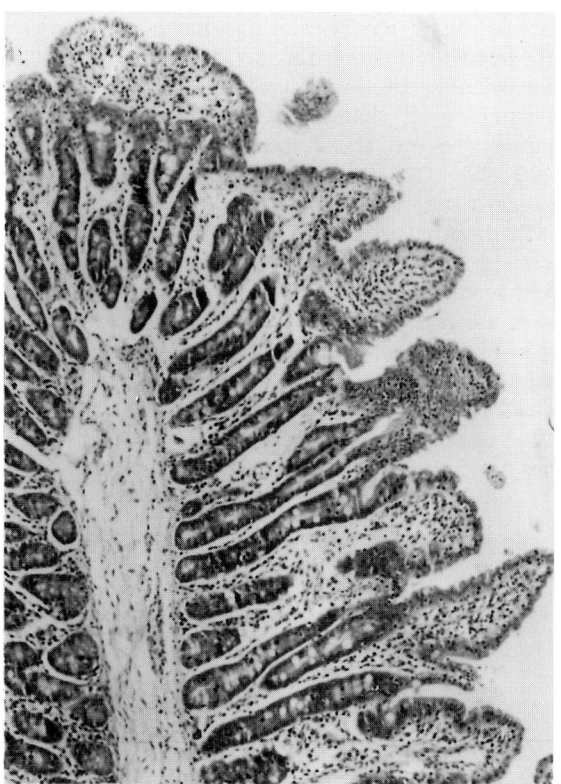

Fig. 16.6 Section of piglet small intestine stained with haematoxylin and eosin. (a) Tissue taken from an unweaned piglet, 26 days old. (b) Tissue taken from a piglet 5 days following weaning at 3 weeks of age on to a soya-containing diet.

that, when challenged 10 days later with ovalbumin 4 g per day for 4 days, they are significantly less able to absorb xylose than either unsensitized controls or those sensitized with an unrelated antigen such as human serum albumin [78]. In these experiments the malabsorption was associated with a change in crypt/villus ratio, the crypt becoming relatively deeper. In subsequent studies in unweaned piglets it has not always been possible to repeat these experiments. This may be related to prior maternal exposure to the fed antigen, and so indicate a protective role for immune milk. A mechanism similar to this has been shown in suckling rabbits where the response to ingested antigens is suppressed [64]. Alternatively the observation that early milk can enhance IgA synthesis by both peripheral blood [66] and cord blood lymphocytes [65] might indicate that in the suckling animal the secretory IgA response to the fed antigen might be promoted so preventing damaging allergic reactions.

Postweaning diarrhoea

At weaning the withdrawal of maternal milk is followed by a period where a vast array of different dietary components are presented, possibly for the first time in large amounts. In the pig, postweaning diarrhoea commonly occurs, but it is not associated with a particular age of pig, rather with the specific event of weaning. It may be controlled by dietary management, such as a reduction in food intake or protein content of the diet [9]. Such practices reduce the severity and incidence of disease.

The initial and characteristic lesion of the disease is a severe villus atrophy (Fig. 16.6) in the small intestine which is associated with a fall in levels of the disaccharidases sucrase and lactase in the enterocyte brush border and with malabsorption. These changes occur within 3–4 days of weaning and a partial recovery occurs after 7–10 days. These enteropathic changes can occur in the complete absence of microbial involvement [32]. The commonly observed proliferation of *Escherichia coli* is subsequent to such change, suggesting therefore that it is acting as an opportunist rather than a primary pathogen [48].

Manipulation of responses to dietary antigens

We have, over the past few years, attempted

to investigate the possibility that a transient hypersensitivity reaction to antigens in the postweaning diet may be the cause of the morphological changes described during this period. To test this hypothesis a number of approaches to manipulating the response to dietary antigens have been employed.

In the first group of experiments pigs were weaned at 3 weeks of age on to a conventional postweaning diet. Prior to weaning, piglets were assigned into three experimental groups so as to receive no supplementary feed, a small amount of feed of the postweaning diet or a large amount of the postweaning diet, such

groups in immunological terms being equivalent to naive animals, sensitized animals and orally tolerized animals respectively. Upon weaning, the incidence of *E. coli* proliferation and diarrhoea was greatest in the primed group, least in the tolerized group, with an intermediate incidence occurring in the naive animals; unweaned animals by comparison showed no change. A reduction in ability to absorb xylose was greatest in the primed group, and in all cases there was a degree of recovery by day 14 postweaning [48]. If such findings have an immunological basis then it should be possible to reduce the incidence of

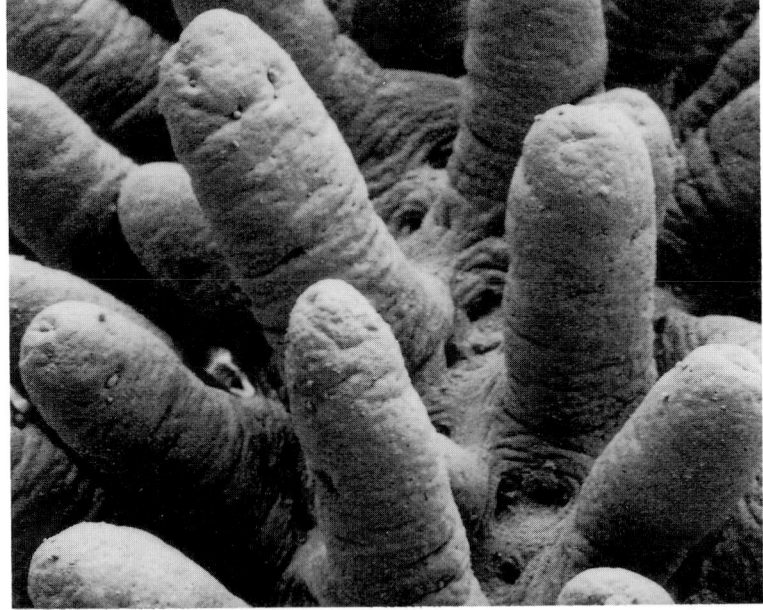

(a)

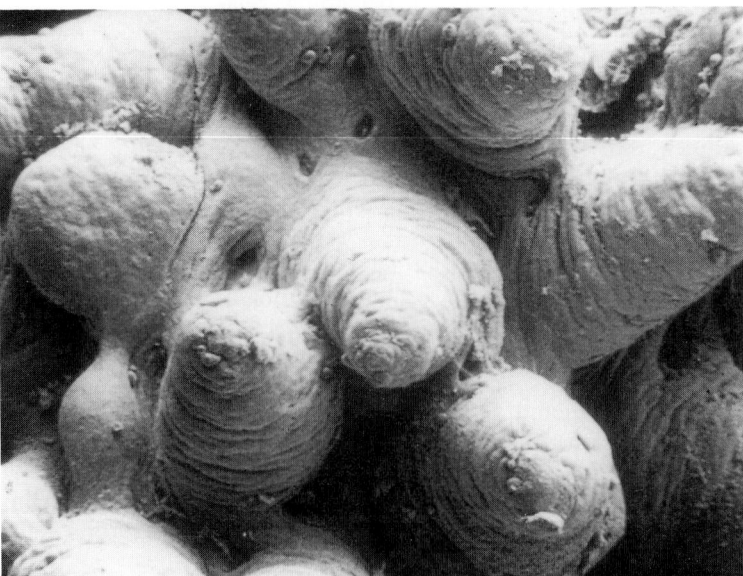

(b)

Fig. 16.7 Scanning electron micrographs of piglet small intestine. (a) Tissue taken from an unweaned piglet 26 days of age. (b) Tissue taken from a piglet 5 days following weaning at 3 weeks of age on to a soya-containing diet.

the disease by lowering the antigenicity of the postweaning diet. To this end animals were weaned on to a diet in which the protein source was either hydrolysed casein or antigenic casein. No increase in faecal water or *E. coli* proliferation was observed in the pigs weaned on to the minimally antigenic diet [48–50]. In these experiments disease was associated with increased crypt depth, villus atrophy and decreased sucrase activities in the brush borders.

Postweaning allergic reactions: effect of different feeds

To further characterize the effect and significance of allergic reactions to antigens in the postweaning diet, a series of experiments have been performed in pigs weaned at 3 weeks of age on to diets containing soya (Fig. 16.7), such pigs having received no prior supplementary feed. Pigs weaned on to a diet in which the sole protein source is a soya protein (which had been treated to remove antinutritional factors) are highly susceptible to an enteritis immediately postweaning. Measurement of absorptive function in vivo by uptake of xylose showed a severe malabsorption by 5 days postweaning which had substantially recovered by 2 weeks postweaning (Fig. 16.8). During this

period a delayed type hypersensitivity response to the soya antigen could be demonstrated by skin test which was at a maximum on day 5 and which had disappeared by day 13 (Fig. 16.9). As in the previous experiments

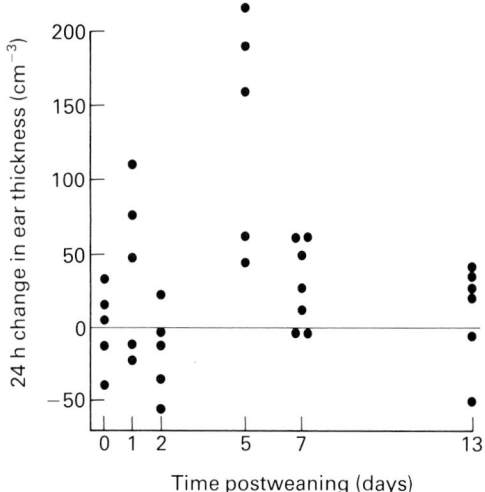

Fig. 16.9 Twenty-four-hour increase in skin thickness following intradermal challenge with an extract of soya in unweaned pigs and those weaned on to a soya-based diet 1, 2, 5, 7 or 13 days earlier.

with casein, adequate feeding of the soya antigen before weaning completely abrogated any malabsorption, or diarrhoea, thus supporting the suggestion that a transient immune response to the dietary antigens may predispose to clinical disease. This indicates that orally induced hyporesponsiveness may protect against changes in gut morphology and therefore disease susceptibility.

Morphological and physiological consequences. The consequences of feeding such diets is profound. There is marked crypt hyperplasia and villus atrophy throughout the small intestine. The crypt hyperplasia can occur prior to the villus atrophy as early as day 2 after weaning. Increased numbers of both goblet cells and intraepithelial lymphocytes were also present from day 5. Thus the morphological picture is similar to both that observed in rodent models of food allergy and in children with cow's milk allergy [87]. In the soya-weaned pig there is a marked malabsorption of carbohydrates which is accompanied by a reduction in the ability of enterocytes to transport amino acids (alanine and lysine) (Fig. 16.10) and to absorb fluid. The weaning procedure also influences brush border disaccharidase development, maltase, isomaltase, sucrase and trehalase activities

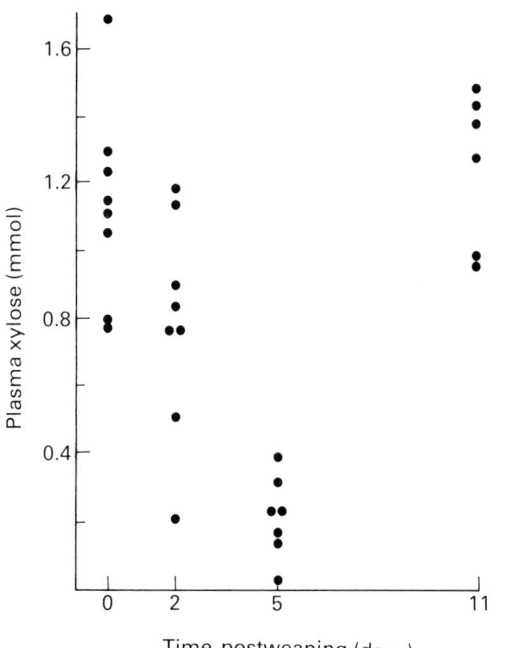

Fig. 16.8 Plasma xylose levels in pigs 60 minutes after a single feed of xylose (100 mg/kg). Pigs were examined sequentially, preweaned, and on days 2, 5 and 11 postweaning on to a soya-based diet.

being lower—a reflection that enzyme development is disturbed.

The changes observed in gut physiology can be explained by a change in the relative maturity of enterocytes present on the villi. Enterocytes arise by division of precursors in the crypts and migrate from the crypt to the tip of the villus. During this migration there is a change from secretory to absorptive function and an increase in the activity of brush border enzymes. Severe changes in the rate of division and migration or length of villi can influence the physiological role of the enterocyte and alter crypt/villus ratios. Water and electrolytes are continuously being secreted into the lumen of the small intestine by crypt enterocytes mainly in the upper and middle small intestine and predominantly by the villi in the posterior ileum (Fig. 16.11). This movement may account for up to 30% of total body water each day [45] and thus any shift in enterocyte maturity could on its own be severe enough to result in diarrhoea.

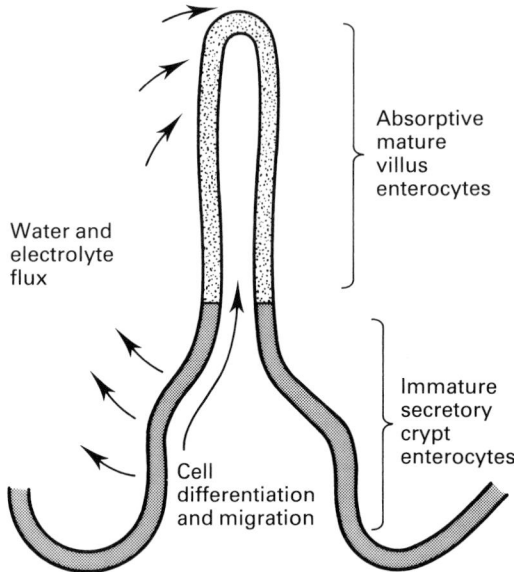

Fig. 16.11 Diagrammatic representation of crypt and villus to show possible function effects of changes in crypt-cell production rate. Enterocytes arise from division of cells in the crypt and then migrate up the villi and are shed at the tips. During this migration they mature and differentiate, changing from immature secretory cells to mature absorptive cells. It has been suggested that an increase in the rate of division of crypt cells will lead to a reduction in the relative maturity of the enterocytes. Such a change would lead to an excess of secretory cells and water imbalance.

Mechanism of cell-mediated hypersensitivity to dietary antigen

The precise mechanism whereby cell-mediated hypersensitivity reactions to dietary antigens within the gut lead to the morphological changes is not clear, but it has been postulated to be lymphokine mediated (for detailed review see [52]). Microbial agents such as rotavirus may also bring about a similar morphological change [41]; however they are unlikely to be significant in the pig model described here since when found, they were exclusive to the upper small intestine and maximum immune-mediated damage was found in the lower small intestine. Furthermore it is difficult to envisage how dietary manipulation preweaning could influence the growth of a virus postweaning.

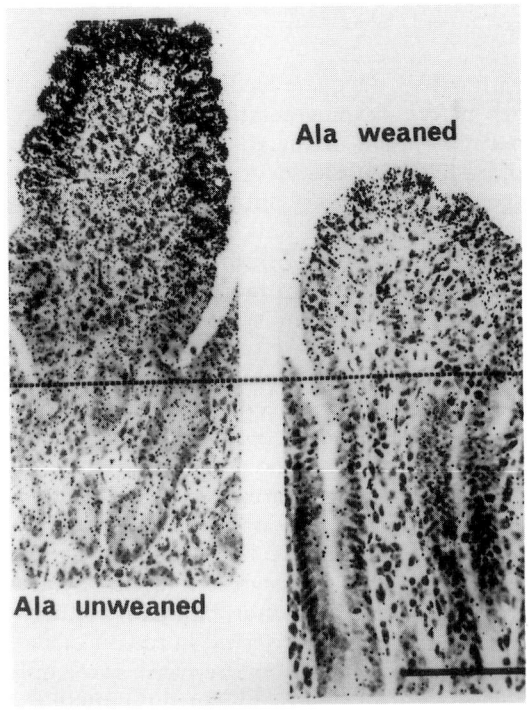

Fig. 16.10 Autoradiographic localization of titrated alanine in small intestinal villi of unweaned and weaned piglets. The horizontal dotted line indicates the crypt-villus junction. The weaned animals show a reduced uptake of alanine, as indicated by the number of grains on the villi. The reduced villus height and increased crypt depth is also clearly shown.

Interaction between diet and bacteria. The interaction between diet and bacteria in the gut should however not be discounted. Following weaning, bacteria can be seen adhering (Fig. 16.12) to the villi on days 5 and 7 postweaning but are absent by day 13. With-

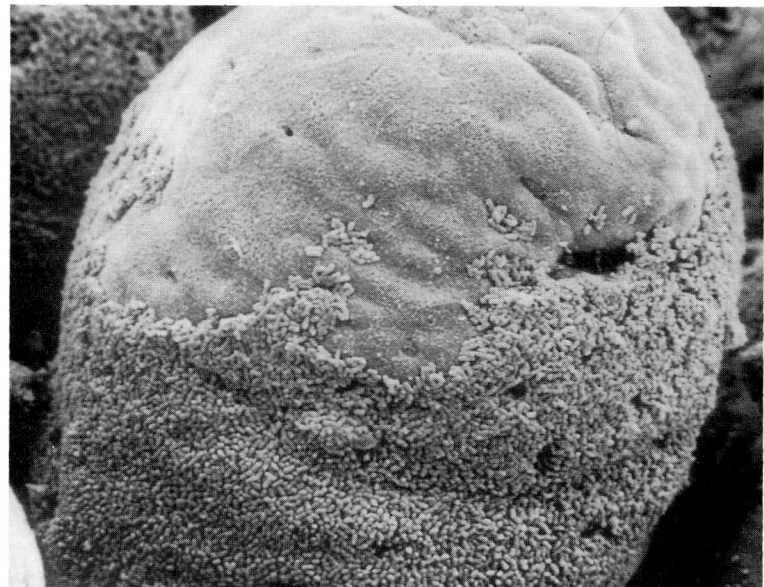

a)

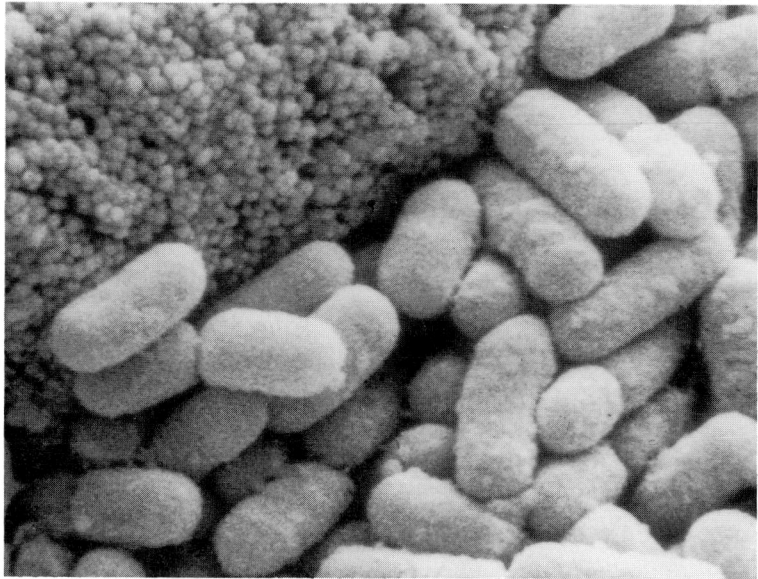

(b)

Fig. 16.12 Scanning electron micrographs of piglet small intestine taken 5 days after weaning. (a) Low power showing *E. coli* covering most of the available surface of a villus. (b) High power showing the bacteria adhering to the brush border, microvillus surface.

drawal of milk antibody is clearly a factor that can influence proliferation, but the delay between weaning and when they appear and the complete lack of appearance in pigs orally tolerized before weaning, suggests that dietary factors are also important. It is possible that a shift in the relative maturity of enterocytes might influence either bacterial adhesion in a manner similar to that shown for the binding of lectins [17] or by altering luminal nutrition for the bacteria as a result of maldigestion. It has also been shown that during the first weeks of life there is a decline in susceptibility of the intestine to the hypersecretory effects of *E. coli* enterotoxin, but immediately after weaning there is a transient, abrupt increase in susceptibility to the levels seen in the neonatal pig [76]. Similarly it has been shown that in parasite-induced villus atrophy the intestine is also more susceptible to enterotoxin [44].

Whilst the mechanism of increased susceptibility has not been determined in either case, the change towards a higher proportion of immature (secretory) cells relative to mature (absorptive) cells would accentuate the effect of enterotoxin by increasing the number of target cells available (enterotoxin acts on secretory cells) and by reducing the capacity of the small intestine to reabsorb. Finally an interaction whereby bacterial lipopolysaccharide can modulate the response to dietary protein [60] will be discussed in detail later.

RUMINANTS

Secretory IgG and tolerance

The ruminant gastrointestinal immune system differs markedly from that of monogastric animals. For example, IgG in cattle is a major secretory immunoglobulin [57]. Furthermore, unlike most other species which are hyporesponsive to skin-test challenge with dietary antigens that they 'tolerate', adult cattle give positive skin test reactions to grass extracts even though they have shown no clinical sensitivity throughout their period of being fed [77].

Since evidence would suggest that gastric secretions have important effects in reducing the antigenicity of fed antigen [36, 37], one might expect that in ruminants with their complex rumen digestive processes this protective effect would be greatest. This is because considerable protein degradation occurs within the rumen itself, and by acting as a reservoir for ingesta it can ensure that the rate of delivery of food into the true stomach is optimal for the digestive process. It is not surprising therefore that problems related to food intolerance are in general restricted to the preruminant period.

Preruminant calves: allergy to soya

Raw soya bean meal contains a variety of antinutritional factors, most of which can be readily inactivated by modern industrial processing [89]. Despite this treatment, feeding preruminant calves with milk replacers containing more than 30% soya can lead to diarrhoea, weight loss and even death [14, 75]. This is associated with the presence of high titres of circulating antibody specific for soya bean antigens [3, 4, 34, 74], and evidence has been put forward to link the changes in gastrointestinal function motility with an allergic response [75]. Morphological changes in gut architecture observed include a broadening and shortening of the villi, a lymphocytic infiltration and an increase in the number of goblet cells [4]. These changes were occasionally associated with small haemorrhages although mucosal thickness generally remained unchanged. Changes in mucosal integrity have also been indicated by functional studies.

Increased intestinal permeability

In soya-sensitized calves, intestinal permeability to β-lactoglobulin increased 1 to 2 hours after ingestion of soya bean proteins and was greatly elevated at 4 to 6 hours, returning to normal by 24 hours [33]. Feeding soya led to increased ileal flow rates [35] which were attributable partly to a decrease in transit time [74] but also to the very large volume of fluid which has been suggested to result from leakage of body fluids into the intestinal lumen [33].

Mechanisms of hypersensitivity

Antibodies found in the sera of soya bean-fed calves include those specific to glycinin and β-conglycinin [35]. Whilst the increased sensitivity of the gut is accompanied by rising IgG, IgA and IgM antibodies in serum, the precise immunological mechanisms responsible for the intestinal changes are uncertain. Both complement-fixing IgG1 [4] and IgE [3, 34] antibodies have been detected, but the appropriate passive transfer studies have not been made to determine the relative importance of each. Similarly the possibility of cell-mediated damage has not been evaluated but the kinetics of change are consistent with a Type I hypersensitivity. Interestingly gut hypersensitivity in preruminant calves is not restricted to those fed on soya, since antibody production and gastrointestinal reactions have also been noted in ovalbumin-fed animals.

OTHER ANIMALS

The rabbit has been used extensively to study the immune response to fed antigens, but little is known of the effect of such responses upon clinical symptoms; therefore they will not be discussed further here. In the guinea-pig pathological changes associated with antigen feeding have been recorded. These effects have been shown at distal sites such as the respiratory tract [16] and within joints [15] following prolonged antigen feeding. Interestingly, in guinea-pigs, the feeding of ovalbumin leads to a persistent serum antibody response and, even after 11 weeks feeding, responsiveness is not fully suppressed, indicating that in this species tolerance is difficult to induce [25].

FUTURE USE OF ANIMAL MODELS

The justification for developing any animal model of human disease must be to bring about an understanding of the pathogenesis of the disease and then to provide indicators for successful treatment, or even better the prevention, of disease. On this basis, how successful have models of food allergy been and what might they provide in the future?

Immune-mediated gut damage following feeding

The evidence that ingestion of food can lead to immune-mediated gut damage is convincing. As to the immune effector mechanisms involved, both Type I and Type IV hypersensitivity reactions have been clearly implicated and the morphological changes detailed above. The role of immune complex (Type III) mediated hypersensitivity is however less convincing; the pathological changes induced in animals are both difficult to reproduce and bear little resemblance to the condition in man.

Non-physiological routes of immunization

In general, animal models of food allergy have required the use of both non-physiological routes of antigen presentation (intraperitoneal) and injection of adjuvants. Whilst such models are of use in the listing of drugs that can prevent or reduce symptoms, they provide little useful information as to how or why an individual becomes hypersensitive to dietary antigens. Similarly they do not indicate how the disease may be prevented. It is perhaps churlish to criticize such models as unphysiological, as it is likely that the same mechanisms that protect in man necessitate the use of parenteral antigen presentation in animal models. The protection afforded by the development of immune exclusion and oral tolerance are discussed in detail elsewhere in this volume (see Chapters 11 and 14).

Maintenance of tolerance

From studies investigating the mechanisms responsible for the maintenance of tolerance it has become clear that prior to the induction of the protected state animals pass through a brief phase of sensitivity. This sequence has been shown following feeding contact sensitizing agents [1, 60] and erythrocytes [29, 79].

With soluble protein dietary antigens, a serum antibody response may also be stimulated [43] which is subsequently suppressed [85], although the local mucosal antibody response persists. In the case of cell-mediated responses following feeding ovalbumin to BALB/c mice, Mowat and Ferguson [53] showed that tolerance resulted and in order to generate DTH responses it was necessary to administer cyclophosphamide. In contrast, in other species such as the pig, feeding DNP-BGG resulted in the appearance of lymphokine-producing lymphocytes in the gut, mesenteric lymph node and spleen [27].

Further, it has subsequently been shown that in other inbred strains of mice, transient sensitivity, as assessed by the ability to mount 24-hour skin test responses, does occur [79]. If a similar pattern of responsiveness occurs in man, one could argue that virtually all individuals pass through a food-allergic phase upon introduction to a new dietary antigen and those which fail to subsequently down-regulate the response develop the clinical manifestations of food allergy.

Mechanisms of tolerance. Feeding contact sensitizing agents stimulates the appearance of effector T cells and suppressor (presumptive B) cells [1]. Similarly, following feeding soluble proteins, effector cells [73] and suppressor cells [62, 68] can be demonstrated in populations of gut lymphocytes. The spleens of mice fed SRBC can be shown, by passive transfer studies, to contain both effectors and suppressors of DTH reactions [61, 77]. Early on in the feeding regime the former predominated, and mice fed SRBC for less than 8 days readily show DTH reactions to SRBC upon challenge. Passive transfer of spleen cells of mice fed for longer periods indicated that subsequently suppressor cells predominated. It is tempting to suggest therefore that agents that enhance the development of suppressor cell population might influence the development of allergy. To this end, results in laboratory animals have shown that adjuvants given either systemically or orally can accelerate the 'tolerization' process [88] and convert what was a sensitizing oral dose of antigen into one that induced tolerance [60].

Development of tolerance. Many factors have been shown to influence the development of oral tolerance (for review see [77] and Chapter 14) including dietary manipulation and bacterial lipopolysaccharide. In the former context it has been shown that in the immediate post-weaning period mice cannot be tolerized [23, 82]. Further, it has been shown that even a minor change, such as the introduction of 20 mg of a new protein into the diet of mice, can prevent the induction of tolerance to a second antigen added to the diet a few days following the first [79]. At weaning, in addition to the introduction of new dietary antigens, milk is withdrawn and the controlling influence of maternal antibody upon gut flora with it. Since bacterial lipopolysaccharides can influence the induction of tolerance [60], this further emphasizes the importance of weaning on subsequent food allergy. The observation that rats reared on 'infant feed formulations' are more readily sensitized with ovalbumin than conventionally reared animals [70] would support this view.

To date, animal models of food allergy have implicated a variety of effector mechanisms and have indicated how damaging allergic reactions can be controlled by oral tolerance and immune exclusion. Their use to provide methods of treatment and prevention should be the future aim.

Acknowledgements

We are indebted to John Walker-Smith, Alan Phillips (Queen Elizabeth Hospital, Hackney) and Mike Smith (Babraham) for providing the photographs used in Figs. 16.7, 16.12 and 16.10, respectively. Financial support was provided by the Agricultural and Food Research Council.

REFERENCES

1 Asherson GL, Zembalan M, Perera MACC, et al: Production of immunity and unresponsiveness in the mouse by feeding contact sensitising agents and the role of suppressor cells in the Peyer's patches, mesenteric lymph nodes and other lymphoid tissues. Cell Immunol 1977; 33:145–55.

2 Attallah AM, Ahmed A, Sell KW: In vivo induction of carrier-specific cyclophosphamide sensitive suppressor cells for cell mediated immunity in mice. Int Arch Allergy Appl Immunol 1979; 60:178–85.

3 Barrett MEJ, Porter P: Immunoglobulin classes implicated in intestinal disturbances of calves associated with soya protein antigens. J Immunol 1979; 123:676–80.

4 Barratt MEJ, Strachan PJ, Porter P: Antibody mechanisms implicated in digestive disturbances following ingestion of soya protein in calves and piglets. Clin Exp Immunol 1978; 31:305–12.

5 Bazin H, Platteau B: Production of circulating reaginic (IgE) antibodies by oral administration of ovalbumin to rats. Immunology 1976; 30:679–84.

6 Bellamy JEC, Hamilton DL: Effects of immune-mediated enteroluminal neutrophil emigration on intestinal function in pigs. Can J Comp Med 1977; 41:36–40.

7 Bellamy, JEC, Nielsen NO: A comparison between the active cutaneous Arthus reaction and immune-mediated enteroluminal neutrophil emigration in pigs. Can J Comp Med 1974; 38:193–202.

8 Bellamy JEC, Nielsen NO: Immune mediated emigration of neutrophils into the lumen of the small intestine. Infect Immun 1974; 9:615–9.

9 Bertshinger HU, Eggenberger E, Jucker H, Pfirter HP: Evaluation of low nutrient, high fibre diets for the prevention of porcine *Escherichia coli* enterotoxaemia. Vet Microbiol 1979; 3:281–90.

10 Bicks RO, Azar MM, Rosenberg EW, et al: Delayed hypersensitivity reactions in the intestinal tract. 1. Studies of 2,4-dinitrochlorobenzene caused guinea pig and swine colon lesions. Gastroenterology 1967; 53:422–36.

11 Borland A, Mowat A McI, Parrott DMV: Augmentation of intestinal and peripheral natural killer cell activity during the graft-versus-host reaction in mice. Transplantation 1983; 36:513–9.

12 Byars NE, Ferraresi RW: Intestinal anaphylaxis in the rat as a model for food allergy. Clin Exp Immunol 1976; 24:352–6.

13 Cantor HM, Dumont AH: Hepatic suppression of sensitisation to antigen absorbed into the portal system. Nature 1967; 215:744–5.

14 Colvin BM, Ramsey HA: Soy flour in milk replacers for young calves. J Dairy Sci 1968; 51:899–904.

15 Coombs RRA, Oldham G: Early rheumatoid like joint lesions in rabbits drinking cows' milk. Int Arch Allergy Appl Immunol 1981; 64:287–92.

16 Coombs RRA, Devey ME, Anderson KJ: Refractoriness to anaphylactic shock after continuous feeding of cow's milk to guinea pigs. Clin Exp Immunol 1978; 32:263–71.

17 Etzler ME: Lectins as probes in studies of intestinal glycoproteins and glycolipids. Am J Clin Nutr 1979; 32:133–8.

18 Ferguson A, Parrott DMV: Growth and development of antigen-free grafts of fetal mouse intestine. J Pathol 1972; 106:95–101.

19 Ferguson A, Parrott DMV: Histopathology and time course of rejection of allografts of mouse small intestine. Transplantation 1973; 15:546–54.

20 Frederick GT, Bohl EH: Local and systemic cell mediated immunity against transmissible gastroenteritis and intestinal viral infection of swine. J Immunol 1976; 116:1000–4.

21 Gadol N, Waldmann RH, Clem WL: Inhibition of macrophage migration by normal guinea pig intestinal secretions. Proc Soc Exp Biol Med 1976; 151:654–8.

22 Glaister JR: Some effects of otal administration of oxazolone. Int Arch Allergy Appl Immunol 1973; 45:828–43.

23 Hanson DG: Ontogeny of orally induced tolerance to soluble proteins in mice. 1. Priming and tolerance in newborns. J Immunol 1981; 127: 1518–24.

24 Hanson DG, Miller, SD: Inhibition of specific immune responses by feeding protein antigens. V. In-

duction of the tolerant state in the absence of specific suppressor T cells. J Immunol 1982; 128:2378–81.

25 Heppell LM, Kilshaw PJ: Immune responses in guinea pigs to dietary protein. 1. Induction of tolerance by feeding ovalbumin. Int Arch Allergy Appl Immunol 1982; 68:54–9.

26 Holmes JT, Klein MS, Winawer SJ, Fortner JG: Morphological studies of rejection in canine jejunal allografts. Gastroenterology 1971; 61:693–706.

27 Huntley JH, Newby TJ, Bourne FJ: The cell-mediated immune response of the pig to orally administered antigen. Immunology 1979; 37:225–30.

28 Jarrett EEE, Haig D, McDougal W, McNulty E: Rat IgE production, II. Primary and booster reaginic antibody responses following intradermal or oral immunisation. Immunology 1976; 30:671–7.

29 Kagnoff ME: Effects of antigen-feeding on intestinal and systemic immune responses. 2. Suppression of delayed type hypersensitivity reactions. J Immunol 1978; 120:1509–13.

30 Kagnoff ME: Effects of antigen feeding on intestinal and systemic immune responses. III. Antigen-specific serum mediated suppression of humoral antibody responses after antigen feeding. Cell Immunol 1978; 40:186–203.

31 Keirby JL: Aspects of the local immune system of the gut and mammary gland. Bristol: University of Bristol, 1983. 176 pp. PhD thesis.

32 Kenworthy R, Allen WD: Influence of diet and bacteria on small intestinal morphology, with special reference to early weaning on *Escherichia coli*. Studies with germ free and gnotobiotic pigs. J Comp Pathol 1966; 76:291–6.

33 Kilshaw PJ: Gastrointestinal hypersensitivity in the preruminant calf. In: Bourne FJ, ed. The mucosal immune system. The Hague: Martinus Nijhoff, 1981;203–19.

34 Kilshaw PJ, Sissons JW: Gastrointestinal allergy to soya bean protein in preruminant calves. Antibody production and digestive disturbances in calves fed heated soya bean flour. Res Vet Sci 1979; 27: 361–5.

35 Kilshaw PJ, Sissons JW: Gastrointestinal allergy to soya bean protein in preruminant calves. Allergenic constituents of soya bean products. Res Vet Sci 1979; 27:366–71.

36 Klipstein FA, Engert RF: Protective effect of active immunisation with purified *Escherichia coli* heat labile enterotoxin in rats. Infect Immun 1979; 23:592–9.

37 Kraft SC, Rothberg RM, Knauer CM et al: Gastric acid output and circulating anti-bovine serum albumin in adults. Clin Exp Immunol 1967; 2:321–30.

38 Lake AM: Experimental models for the study of gastrointestinal food allergy. Ann Allergy 1983; 51:226–8.

39 Lake AH, Block KJ, Neutra MR Walker WA: Intestinal goblet cell mucus release. II. In *vivo* stimulation by antigen in the immunised rat. J Immunol 1979; 122:834–7.

40 Lake AM, Bloch KJ, Sinclair KJ, Walker WA: Anaphylactic release of intestinal goblet cell mucus. Immunology 1980: 39:173–8.

41 Lecce JG, Clare DA, Balsbaugh RK Collier DV: Consequences of maternal exposure to porcine parvovirus at different times during gestation. J Clin Microbiol 1983; 17:689–95.

42 Levine BB, Vaz NM: Effect of combinations of strain, antigen dose on reagin production in the mouse. A mouse model for human atopy. Int Arch Allergy 1969; 39:156–71.

43 Lippard VW, Schloss OM, Johnson PA: Immune re-

actions induced in infants by intestinal absorption of incompletely digested cows milk protein. Am J Dis Child 1936; 51:562–74.

44 Ljungstrom I, Holmgren J, Huldt G et al: Changes in instestinal fluid transport and immune response to enterotoxins due to concomitant parasitic infection. Infect Immun 1980; 30:734–40.

45 Low AG, Partridge IG, Sambrook IE: Studies on digestion and absorption in the intestines of growing pigs. 2. Measurements of the flow of dry matter, ash and water. Br J Nutr 1978; 39:515–26.

46 MacDonald TT, Ferguson A: Hypersensitivity reactions in the small intestine. II. Effects of allograft rejection on mucosal architecture and lymphoid cell infiltrate. Gut 1976; 17:81–91.

47 MacDonald TT, Ferguson A: Hypersensitivity reactions in the small intestine. III. The effects of allograft rejection and of graft-versus-host disease on epithelial cell kinetics. Cell Tissue Kinet 1977; 10:301–12.

48 Miller BG, Newby TJ, Stokes CR, Bourne FJ: Influence of diet on postweaning malabsorption and diarrhoea in the pig. Res Vet Sci 1984; 36:187–93.

49 Miller B, Newby TJ, Stokes CR et al: The role of dietary antigen in the aetiology of post weaning diarrhoea. Ann Rech Vet 1983; 14:487–92.

50 Miller BG, Newby TJ, Stokes CR, et al: The importance of dietary antigen in the cause of postweaning diarrhoea in pigs. Am J Vet Res 1984; 45:1730–3.

51 Miller SR, Hanson DG: Inhibition of specific immune responses by feeding protein antigens. IV. Evidence for tolerance and specific active suppression of cell mediated immune responses to ovalbumin. J Immunol 1979; 123:2344–50.

52 Mowat A Mcl: The immunopathogenesis of food sensitive enteropathies. In: Newby TJ, Stokes CR, eds. Local immune responses of the gut. Roca Baton: CRC Press, 1984;199–225.

53 Mowat AM, Ferguson A: Hypersensitivity in the small intestinal mucosa. V. Induction of cell mediated immunity to a dietary antigen. Clin Exp Immunol 1981; 43:574–82.

54 Mowat A Mcl, Ferguson A: Hypersensitivity reactions in the small intestine.VI. Pathogenesis of the graft-versus-host reaction in the small intestinal mucosae of the mouse. Transplantation 1981; 32:238–43.

55 Mowat A Mcl, Ferguson A: Intraepithelial lymphocyte count and crypt hyperplasia measure the mucosal component of the graft-versus-host reaction in mice small intestine. Gastroenterology 1982, 83:417–23.

56 Murray M, Jarrett EE, Jennings FW: Mast cells and macromolecular leak in intestinal immunological reactions. The influence of sex of rats infected with *Nippostrongylus brasiliensis*. Immunology 1971; 21:17–31.

57 Newby TJ, Bourne FJ: The nature of the local immune system of the bovine small intestine. Immunology 1976; 31:475–80.

58 Newby TJ, Stokes CR, eds. Local immune responses of the gut. Boca Raton: CRC Press, 1984.

59 Newby TJ, Stokes CR, Bourne FJ: Altered polyvinyl-pyrrolidone clearance and immune responsiveness caused by small dietary changes. Clin Exp Immunol 1980; 39:349–54.

60 Newby TJ, Stokes CR, Bourne FJ: Effects of feeding bacterial lipopolysaccharide and dextran sulphate on the development of oral tolerance to contact sensitizing agents. Immunology 1980: 41:617–21.

61 Newby TJ, Stokes CR, Bourne FJ: The effect of orally administered or intraperitoneally injected adjuvant on the generation of oral tolerance in mice. In: Cancellotti

FM, Galassi D, eds. Adjuvants, interferon and non-specific immunity. Luxembourg: CEC, 1984;87–94.

62 Ngan J, Kind LS: Suppressor T cells for IgE and IgG in the Peyer's patches of mice made tolerant by oral administration of ovalbumin. J Immunol 1978; 120:861–5.

63 Perdue MH, Chung M, Gall DG: Effect of intestinal anaphylaxis on gut function in the rat. Gastroenterology 1984; 86:391–7.

64 Peri BA, Rothberg RM: Specific suppression of antibody production in young rabbit Kits after maternal ingestion of bovine serum albumin. J Immunol 1981; 127:2520–5.

65 Pittard WB, Bill K: Differentiation of cord blood lymphocytes into IgA producing cells in response to breast milk stimulatory factor. Clin Immunol Immunopathol 1978: 13:430–4.

66 Pittard WB, Bill K: Immunoregulation by breast milk cells. Cell Immunol 1979; 42:437–41.

67 Revoltella R, Ovary Z: Reaginic antibody production in different mouse strains. Immunology 1969; 17:45–54.

68 Richman LK, Graeff AS, Yarchoan R, Strober W: Simultaneous induction of antigen specific IgA helper T cells and IgG suppressor T cells in murine Peyer's patch after protein feeding. J Immunol 1981; 126:2079–83.

69 Richman LK, Chiller JM, Brown WR, et al: Enterically induced immunologic tolerance. 1. Induction of suppressor T-lymphocytes by intragastric administration of soluble proteins. J Immunol 1978; 121:2429–34.

70 Roberts S, Soothill JF: Provocation of allergic response by supplementary feeds of cows milk. Arch Dis Child 1982; 57:127–30.

71 Rollinghoff M, Starzinski-Powitz A, Pfizenmaier K, Wagner H: Cyclophosphamide-sensitive T-lymphocytes suppress the in vivo generation of antigen-specific cytotoxic T-lymphocytes. J Exp Med 1977; 145:455–9.

72 Rubin D, Weiner HL, Fields BN, Greene MI: Immunologic tolerance after oral administration of reovirus: requirement for two viral gene products for tolerance induction. J Immunol 1981; 127:1697–701.

73 Shields JG, Parrott DMV: Appearance of delayed-type hypersensitivity effector cells in murine gut mucosa. Immunology 1985; 54:771–6.

74 Sissons JW, Smith RH: The effect of different diets including those containing soya bean products, on digesta movement and water and nitrogen absorption in the small intestine of the preruminant calf. Br J Nutr 1976; 36:421–38.

75 Smith RH, Sissons JW: The effect of different feeds, including those containing soya bean products, on the passage of digesta from the abomasum of the pre-ruminant calf. Br J Nutr 1975; 33:329–49.

76 Stevens JB, Gyles CL, Barum DA: Production of diarrhoea in pigs in response to *Escherichia coli* enterotoxin. Am J Vet Res 1972; 33:2511–26.

77 Stokes CR: Induction and control of intestinal immune responses. In: Newby TJ, Stokes CR, eds. Local immune responses of the gut. Boca Raton: CRC Press, 1984; 97–141.

78 Stokes CR, Newby TJ, Bourne FJ: Altered immune function associated with dietary factors. In: Bourne FJ, ed. The mucosal immune system. The Hague: Martinus Nijhoff, 1981; 224–39.

79 Stokes CR, Newby TJ, Bourne FJ: The influence of oral immunisation on local and systemic immune responses to heterologous antigens. Clin Exp Immunol 1983; 52:399–406.

80 Stokes CR, Swarbrick ET, Soothill JF: Genetic differences in immune exclusion and partial tolerance to ingested antigens. Clin Exp Immunol 1983; 52:678–84.

81 Stokes CR, Newby TJ, Miller BG, Bourne FJ: The immunological significance of transient cell-mediated immune reactions to dietary antigens. In: Quinn PJ ed. Cell mediated immunity. Luxembourg: CEC, 1984; 249–59.

82 Strobel S, Ferguson A: Immune responses to fed protein antigens in mice. III. Systemic tolerance or priming is related to the age at which antigen is first encountered. Paediatr Res 1984; 18:588–94.

83 Strobel S, Mowat A, Mcl, Drummond HE, et al: Immunological responses to fed protein antigens in mice. II. Oral tolerance for CMI is due to activation of cyclophosphamide-sensitive cells by gut processed antigen. Immunology 1983; 49:451–6.

84 Swarbrick ET, Stokes CR: The immune effects of ingested antigens in mice. In: Hemmings WA, ed. Protein transmission through living membranes. Amsterdam: Elsevier/North-Holland, 1979; 309–18.

85 Swarbrick ET, Stokes CR, Soothill JF: Absorption of antigens after oral immunisation and the simultaneous induction of specific systemic tolerance. Gut 1979; 20:121–5.

86 Walker WA, Wu M, Bloch KJ: Stimulation by immune complexes of mucus release from goblet cells of the rat small intestine. Science 1977; 197:370–2.

87 Walker-Smith JA: Cow's milk intolerance as a cause of postenteritis diarrhea. J Paediatr Gastroenterol Nutr 1982; 1:163–73.

88 Wannemuehler MJ, Kiyono H, Babb JL, et al: Lipopolysaccharide (LPS) regulation of the immune response: LPS converts germ-free mice to sensitivity to oral tolerance induction. J Immunol 1982; 129:959–65.

89 Wolf WJ, Cowan JC: Soya beans as a food source. Boca Raton: CRC Press, 1971.

PART II

FOOD COMPONENTS AND THEIR REACTIONS

301

Chapter 17
Food Families and Rotation Diets

Jean Monro

THE RATIONALE FOR ROTATION DIETS

Elimination diets followed by challenges remain the most crucial clinical tool for the diagnosis of food sensitivity. Having achieved diagnosis of adverse reactions to food the patient's diet should be constructed positively to minimize reactions from foods, to discourage the production of new sensitivities and to provide optimum nutritional requirements to restore health. The rotation diet assists in this process. It is the chief tool in therapy and could be the health measure beyond any other to minimize the problems of food sensitivities.

Multiple food sensitivities

Most patients who are food sensitive are unlikely to be sensitive to a single food. If the problem is an immunological one, the immune system's dysregulation will not be confined to just milk or wheat. As has been found with allergies producing rhinitis, inhalant sensitivities are unlikely to be single. Prick tests on a patient with hay fever will often show positive reactions not only to grass pollen but also to tree, flower, weed and shrub pollens, as well as animal danders and moulds.

Priming phenomenon

It is well documented that the priming phenomenon occurs in rhinitis. This is the process by which the nasal mucosa when exposed to an allergen, such as pollen, continuously becomes more sensitive to other allergens and indeed to that allergen itself. This is not restricted to pollen sensitivity but also occurs with other allergic nasal conditions throughout the year.

The evidence for this is that symptoms do not start concurrently with a rise in the pollen count. They are delayed and also when they do occur they are maintained long after the

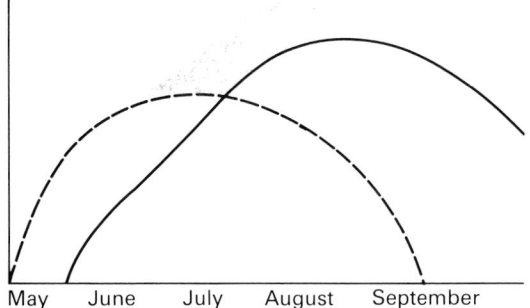

May   June   July   August   September

Fig. 17.1 Diagram of the priming phenomenon. (- - -), pollen season; (——), rhinitis.

pollen count drops once more (Fig. 17.1). It is apparent, therefore, that the symptoms that have been induced are due not only to pollen but also to concomitant sensitivities to other items that are not normally provocants. They are only present at a subclinical level.

Route of concomitant sensitization. At one time it was thought that the concomitant sensitivities would be only to non-food stimuli, such as inhaled allergens, but it has been observed that foods may also be provocants. Thus, some patients who are sensitive to wine or cheese may be able to eat these with impunity in the winter but not during the summer if they are also subject to hay fever when rhinitis will be aggravated by these foods. This concept has been observed by Connell who challenged hay fever patients with ragweed sensitivity out of season with a measured quantity of pollen grains. When challenged on day 1 some nasal blockage occurred. This was more easily provoked over the following 3 days with smaller amounts of pollen. The nasal mucous membrane was thus more sensitive to the pollen having been primed. With a few days without the pollen challenge the original larger dose was required to provoke symptoms. It was also shown that a patient with a positive skin reaction to sorrel pollen showed no symptoms on challenge; however, after 4

days of challenge with ragweed pollen she showed an intense reaction to sorrel pollen on exposure. The nasal mucosa had been primed by ragweed and was much more susceptible to the sorrel pollen.

Reversibility and cross-priming. Both of these reactions show two important features. One is the reversibility of the priming phenomenon and the second is cross-priming. It has been shown that priming also occurs under normal environmental conditions and confirmed by a record of pollen count and symptom score showing that at the beginning of the ragweed season a comparatively high pollen count causes only mild symptoms, whereas later in the season, even though the pollen count has started to fall, the symptom score remains high. This shows that the priming effect causes persistence of symptoms. These principles for rhinitis have been shown also to pertain to food allergy as described by Rinkel in 1934.

MANAGEMENT OF ROTATION DIETS

In the first place the food rotation programme requires a classification of the foods in two ways: (a) by family and (b) by category. There are 23 categories, as shown in Table 17.1. The foods are listed separately in Appendix 17.1. In Appendix 17.2 the categories are the titles of columns in which the foods are then listed. Each food may occur in more than one category; thus scrutiny of the table will show banana listed under both fruit and juice or alcoholic drink. Another example is the cashew family, which appears under fruit (mango), as an alcoholic drink (mango juice) and in the nut column (cashew and pistachio). Approximately 150 food families are listed under the 23 different categories but there is no relationship between the families and category of consumption.

Table 17.1 Categories of foods.

Water	Flour	Starch	Thickener	Raising agent
Oil	Salt	Sweetener	Fruit	Juice/alcoholic drink
Alcohol	Nut/seed	Vegetable	Herb/spice/vinegar	Beverage/tea
Fish	Fowl	Mammal	Other animal	Milk
Fat	Spread	Miscellaneous		

Examples of each category and the variety of ways a single food family can be taken as food are shown in Appendices 17.1–17.3.

Minimum rotation diet: 1 day in 4

The minimum rotation diet is a 1 day in 4 rotation, in which food families eaten on one day may not be consumed for a further 3 days. For people who are more ill it may be necessary to widen the rotation to a 1 in 7, 1 in 14, or even a 1 in 30 day rotation. It is quite possible to extend the variety in this way. Combinations of food used can also be varied so that a single food can be eaten per meal, or two foods per meal, or a wider variety can be combined.

Variations in rotation regimes

Further rotation is possible based on a 3-day-on:4-day-off programme. This enables an individual to select foods in families which can be used over a period of 3 days. They are unlikely to use the same food for the whole 3 days but it means, for example, that chicken eaten on a Sunday evening can also be eaten cold the following day at lunch time; then chicken need not necessarily be eaten again until the following Sunday.

31-Day chart for rotation diets

Appendix 17.3 shows a 31-day chart listing the categories and the families, as well as the days on which the foods can be eaten. In order to ensure variety during the course of the day, a day is taken from 6 p.m. to 6 p.m. In this way the meals in the evening can be different from those taken at lunch time, thus providing a more appetizing choice. The chart provides choice on a 3-day-on:4-day-off rotation but the variety is such that no food need be eaten for more than 1 day of the 3 days and

hence it can also be used for a 7-day rotation diet.

Complexity of rotation diets

The complexity of these rotation diets is frequently unnerving to patients and in the end they tend to stick to a very basic rotation, taking potato as a starch component one day, then wheat, then buckwheat, and then another root vegetable such as parsnips on successive days of the 4-day rotation. This type of rotation, although simple to understand, does not offer the optimum to patients.

THE PURPOSE OF ROTATING FOODS

The purpose of rotating foods is to give the body more variety and to give a rest from each food family; this prevents new or increased sensitivity to foods developing. It also gives freedom from allergic symptoms for a longer period and indeed facilitates the identification of offending foods. It is possible to use a sliding rotation diet for diagnosis; Table 17.2 shows how this can be achieved. However, it is not suggested that this sliding rotation diet is used permanently.

It is crucially important when stressing the value of rotation diets to ensure that the patient does not get bored with a fixed rotation. Rotations can vary with the season and in order to be able to do this it is best to have dietetic guidance.

The World Health Organization states that 'Health is not just the absence of disease, but is the positive presence of emotional, physical and mental well-being.' A rotation diet helps to achieve this in food-sensitive patients.

Table 17.2 Diagnostic sliding rotation diet.

ROTATION DIET

MONDAY		TUESDAY		WEDNESDAY		THURSDAY		FRIDAY		SATURDAY		SUNDAY	
Chicken	(1)	Pork	(2)	Lamb	(3)	Turkey	(4)	Fish	(5)	Rabbit	(6)	Beef	(7)
Sago	(1)	Buckwheat	(2)	Rice	(3)	Parsnip	(4)	Tapioca	(5)	Beans	(6)	Potato	(7)
Pineapple	(1)	Apple	(2)	Banana	(3)	Pear	(4)	Plums	(5)	Grapefruit	(6)	Tomato	(7)
Spinach	(1)	Celery	(2)	Carrots	(3)	Watercress	(4)	Cabbage	(5)	Green beans	(6)	Lettuce	(7)
Pineapple juice	(1)	Apple juice	(2)	Water	(3)	Pear juice	(4)	Plum juice	(5)	Grapefruit juice	(6)	Tomato juice	(7)

SLIDING DIET

MONDAY		TUESDAY		WEDNESDAY		THURSDAY		FRIDAY		SATURDAY		SUNDAY	
Chicken	(1)	Pork	(2)	Lamb	(3)	Turkey	(4)	Fish	(5)	Rabbit	(6)	Beef	(7)
Potato	(7)	Sago	(1)	Buckwheat	(2)	Rice	(3)	Parsnip	(4)	Tapioca	(5)	Beans	(6)
Grapefruit	(6)	Tomato	(7)	Pineapple	(1)	Apple	(2)	Banana	(3)	Pear	(4)	Plum	(5)
Cabbage	(5)	Green beans	(6)	Lettuce	(7)	Spinach	(1)	Celery	(2)	Carrots	(3)	Watercress	(4)
Grapefruit juice	(6)	Tomato juice	(7)	Pineapple juice	(1)	Apple juice	(2)	Water	(3)	Pear juice	(4)	Plum juice	(5)

A rotation diet that can be used in the detection of food allergy

The diet outlined in Table 17.2 has been designed so that each food is eaten 1 day in 7. In this way if a food provokes a reaction this can be confirmed by taking that food on separate days in a 'sliding diet'. A diet eliminating common allergens (e.g. cow's milk, gluten-containing grains, eggs) is used as a basis. Then one food from each category of meat, fruit, vegetable and beverage or juice is included.

Only those foods listed for any day should be eaten. Initially withdrawal symptoms may occur due to the omission of common foods. In the second week there may be immediate reactions on taking a provocative food. If the reactions are to more than one item in a day's diet then on a 'sliding diet' specific reactions may be discerned. If a diet diary and symptom diary are kept at the same time, then the symptoms may be correlated with taking a particular food.

REFERENCES

1 Aiken JR et al: J Allergy Clin Immunol 1981; 67: iii.

2 Connell JT; Quantitative intranasal pollen challenges. Apparatus design and technique. J Allergy 1967; 39: 358–67.

3 Connell JT: Quantitative intranasal pollen challenges. Effect of daily pollen challenge, environmental pollen exposure, and placebo challenge on the nasal membrane. J Allergy 1968; 41: 123–39.

4 Connell JT: The priming effect in allergic rhinitis. J Allergy 1969; 43: 33–4.

5 Van Metre TE, Franklin Atkinson N & Amodio FJ et al: A comparison of immunotherapy schedules for injection treatment of ragweed pollen hay fever. J Allergy Clin Immunol 1982; 69: 181–93.

APPENDICES

Appendix 17.1 Foods.

Food	Biological name	How eaten/remarks
Abalone	*Haliotis* sp. (mollusc)	Shellfish
Acer; maple	*Aceraceae*	Maple sugar
Ackee	*Blighia sapida*	White pulp as fruit/with fish
Acorn	*Quercus robur* (English oak)	After boiling, as nuts
	Quercus ilex (holm oak)	Sweeter—as nuts
	Quercus alba (white oak)	In North America as nuts
		Roasted as chestnuts
		Coffee substitute
		Acorn flour
Adzuki bean	*Phaseolus angularis*	As beans and as flour
Agar-agar; kanten	Number of seaweeds	Vegetable jelly
Ajowan; bishop's weed; omum	*Carum ajowan*	Spice (closely related to caraway)
Alexanders	*Smyrnium olusatrum*	Spring green vegetable; salads
Alfalfa	*Medicago sativa* (legume)	Sprouted seeds as salad and as vegetable
Allspice; Jamaica pepper; myrtle pepper	*Pimenta dioca*	Spice in fruit cakes, mince pies and plum pudding
Almond	*Prunus amygdalus*	Nut; flour
Almond (bitter)	*Prunus amygdalus* var. *amara*	Nut; flour
Amaranthus		Flour
Anchovy	*Engraulis encrasicholus*	Garnish, paste, etc.
Angelica	*Angelica archangelica*	Herb; confectionery; crystallized
Anise; aniseed	*Pimpinella anisum*	Flavouring
Annatto	*Bixa orellana*	Orange-yellow dye for drinks
Apple	*Malus sylvestris*	Fresh fruit; pectin; cider and cider vinegar
Apricot	*Prunus armeniaca*	Fresh fruit; kernels of apricot stones may be poisonous
American aloe; agave	*Agave americana*	Spirit vino mescal; wine
Arrowroot	*Maranta*, mainly *M. arundinacea*	Thickening; starch jelly; arrowroot noodles
	Curcurna angustiflora	
Arum	Aroideae	Flour
Asafoetida	*Ferula asafoetida* (root)	Spice; condiment
Ash	*Fraxinus excelsior*	Nut
Asparagus	*Asparagus officinalis* (Liliaceae)	Young shoots; salad raw
Asparagus bean; yard-long bean	*Vigna sesquipedalis*	A pulse and a green vegetable
Aubergine; eggplant	*Solanum melongena*	Vegetable
Avocado pear; alligator pear	*Persea americana* (laurel family)	Raw
Balm; lemon balm; melissa	*Melissa officinalis*	Flavouring, tea
Bamboo shoots; bambush	Grass (Gramineae)	Vegetable (boil); raw salad
Banana; plantain	*Musa sapientum* (400 varieties)	Raw as fruit—some varieties need cooking; dried for cakes, biscuits etc; flour

Appendix 17.1 Foods continued

Food	Biological name	How eaten/remarks
Barberry	*Berberis vulgaris*	Bright red berries candied, made into jelly or pickled
Barley	*Hordeum vulgare*	Cereal; bread; brewing
Barnacle	*Pollicipes cornucopia* (crustacean)	Boil
Basil; sweet basil	*Ocimum basilicum*	Herb for fish or lamb
Bass; rock fish; striped bass	*Roccus saxatilis*	Fish
Bay; sweet bay; laurel	*Laurus nobilis*	Herb
Beech nut; beechmast	*Fagus sylvatica* (Europe) *Fagus grandifolia* (N. America)	Nut
Beef and veal	*Bos taurus*	Meat
Beefsteak fungus	*Fistulina hepatica*	Cooked or raw
Beet	*Beta vulgaris* (beetroot) *Beta esculenta* (spinach beet) *Beta cicla* (Swiss chard)	Cooked; pickled; leaves cooked when young; beet sugar
Blackberry; bramble	*Rubus fructicosus* (386 species)	Fruit raw; cooked—pies, jams, etc.
Bladderwrack	*Fucus vesiculosus*	Seaweed cooked
Blewits	*Tricholoma saevulum*	Fungus cooked
Boar; wild pig	*Sus scropha*	Meat
Bog myrtle; sweet gale	*Myrica gale*	Aromatic herb
Bombay duck; bummalo	*Harpodon neherius*	Fish eaten fresh or dried
Bonito	*Sarda sarda* (Atlantic bonito) *Katsuwonus pelamis* (skipjack)	Fish (tuna)
Borage	*Borago officinalis*	Boil as vegetable like spinach; flowers can be candied
Brazil nut; papa nut; cream nut	*Bertholettia*	Nut; flour
Breadfruit	*Artocarpu communis*	Fruit; paste or sort of flour
Broad bean; shell bean (US)	*Vicia faba*	Very young pods may be eaten; young beans raw; older beans cooked as vegetable
Broccoli	*Brassica oleracea*	Vegetable
Brooklime	*Veronica beccabunga*	Salad cress
Broom	*Sarothamnus scoparius*	Raw salads
Brussels sprout	*Brassica oleracea*	Vegetable
Buckwheat; beech wheat; brank; Saracen corn	*Fagopyrum esculentum*	Flour; 'grain'
Buffalo		Meat
Bullace (wild plum)	*Prunus domestica*	Fruit
Burdock	*Arctium lappa*	Young leaves and stem may be eaten
Butter bean; Lima bean; Madagascar bean	*Phaseolus limensus*	Bean
Butterfish	*Poronotus striacanthus*	Fish
Butternut; American white walnut	*Juglans cinerea*	Nut
Butter pit; nana nut	*Acanthosicyos horrida*	Nut
Cabbage	*Brassica oleracea*	Vegetable
Cactus	*Echinocactus hamatocanthus*	Fruit

Appendix 17.1 Foods continued

Food	Biological name	How eaten/remarks
Calamus; sweet flag	*Acorus calamus*	Flavouring in liqueurs
Camel	*Camelus* sp.	Meat and milk
Camomile	*Chamaemelum nobile* *Matricaria recutita*	Tea
Campion; bladder campion	*Silene vulgaris*	Herb
Candle nut	*Aleurites moluccana* (spurge) family	When fresh and raw is a violent purgative and poisonous, but when kept the poison dissipates
Caper	*Capparis spinosa* (spiny) *Capparis inermis* (spineless)	Condiment
Capsicum (chilli)	*Capsicum frutescens*	Flavouring
Capsicum (pepper)	*Tetra gonum* *Capsicum annum* (sweet pepper) *Capsicum annum* (cayenne pepper)	Paprika Spices Flavouring; vegetable
Carambola	*Averrhoa carambola*	Fruit
Caraway	*Carum carvi*	Green herb—seeds
Cardamom	*Elettaria cardomomum* (ginger family) *Alpina striata*	Flavouring—whole, like cloves
Cardoon	*Cynara cardunculus*	Leaf stalks—boil
Carob; locust bean	*Ceratonia siliqua*	Pods; have sweet pulp; chocolate substitute
Carp	*Cyprinus carpio*	Fish
Carrageen; Irish moss	*Chondus crispus*	Mucilaginous substance used in ice cream, soups, salad dressing, etc.
Carrot	*Daucus carota* ssp. *sativus*	Vegetable—boil; raw in salad
Cashew	*Anacardium occidentale*	Nut
Cassava; manioc; yuxa	*Manihot ultissima* (spurge family)	Flour; boil as vegetable
Catfish; yellow bullfish	*Ictaturus natalis*	Fish
Catmint; catnip	*Nepeta cataria*	Herb
Cauliflower	*Brassica oleracea*	Vegetable
Celeriac	*Apium rapaceum*	As for celery
Celery	*Apium graveolens*	Herb and vegetable; cooked or raw
Cepe; cep	*Boletus edulis*	Fungus
Chanterelle; girolle	*Cantharellus cibarius*	Fungus
Charlock	*Sinapsis arvensis*	Edible leaves, like spinach
Chayotte; custard marrow; pepinello; choko; vegetable pear	*Sechium edule*	Fruits—young shoot may be boiled; leaves may be eaten as greens; roots similar to yams
Cheese	From milk of various domesticated mammals (e.g. cow, goat, sheep)	Raw or cooked
Cherry	*Prunus avium* *P. ceraasifera* (cherry plum)	Fruit
Chervil	*Anthriscus cerefolium*	Herb
Chestnut, sweet chestnut; Spanish chestnut	*Castanea sativa*	Nut; flour; used in stuffings

Appendix 17.1 Foods continued

Food	Biological name	How eaten/remarks
Chicken	*Gallus gallus*	Fowl
Chick pea; Bengal gram; channa; Egyptian bean; garbanzo; ram's head pea	*Cicer arietinum*	Vegetable
Chickweed	*Stellaria media*	Green vegetable; raw salads
Chicory; endive; sussory	*Chicorium intybus*	Very young shoot used as salad
Chilli; chili; chilly	*Capsicum annuum*	Spice
Chinese artichoke; chorogi	*Stachys sieboldii*	Tubers boiled and eaten
Chinese cabbage	*Brassica pekinensis*	Vegetable; raw salads
Chinese pepper	*Zanthoxylum piperitum*	Dried berry used as spice
Chive	*Allium schoenoprasum*	Flavouring; raw and cooked
Chocolate	*Theobroma cacao*	Paste, with sugar; beverage
Chufa; tiger nut; earthnut; earth almond	*Cyperus esculentus*	Nuts—prepared as a milky drink in Spain; raw nuts
Cinnamon; cassia	*Cinnamomum zeylanicum*	Bark of tree used as spice
Citron	*Citrus medica*	Candied peel and in liqueurs
Citrus fruit	*C. sinensis* (orange) *C. reticulata* (tangerine; mandarin) *C. paradisi* (grapefruit) *C. aurantium* (Seville orange) *C. limon* (lemon) *C. aurantifolia* (lime) *C. medica* (citron) *Fortunella* (kumquat)	Pulp eaten as fruit; peel candied; used in liqueurs; squeezed as beverage
Clam	Bivalve molluscs	Shellfish
Clove	*Eugenia caryophyllata*	Flavouring
Coccus; carmine; cochineal	*Coccus* sp. (insect)	Red colouring
Cockle	*Cardium edule*	Shellfish; pickled
Cocoa; cacao	*Theobroma cacao*	Beans (see chocolate)
Cod/haddock	*Gadus morrhue* (Atlantic cod) *Melanogrammus aeglefinus* (haddock) *Pollachius pollachius* (pollack) *Microgadus tomcod* (tomcod) *Merluccius bilinearis* (silver hake)	Fish
Coffee	*Coffea arabica* *Coffea robusta*	Seeds roasted and ground for beverage
Comfrey	*Symphytum officinale*	Herb
Coriander	*Coriandrum sativum*	Flavouring
Corn	*Sorghum vulgare*	Flour
Cowberry	*Vaccinium vitis-idaea*	Fruit
Cowslip	*Primula veris*	Tea
Crab	*Cancer pagurus* (European edible crab) *C. magister* (Dungeness crab) *Callinectes sapidus* (blue crab)	Shellfish
Cranberry	*Oxycoccus macrocarpus*	Fruit; sauces and pickles
Cucumber	*Cucumis sativus*	Vegetable; salads
Cumin	*Cuminum cyminum*	Flavouring
Custard apple; cherimoya	*Anona cheimolia*	Fresh fruit

Appendix 17.1 Foods continued

Food	Biological name	How eaten/remarks
Dahl lentil	*Cajamis indicus*	Vegetable; flour
Damson	*Prunus damascena*	Fruit
Dandelion	*Taraxacum officinale*	Winter salad; coffee from roots
Dasheen; taro	Aroideae	Flour from root
Date	*Colocasia antiquorum*	Fresh fruit; dried leaves as vegetable
Date palm	*Zizyphus lotus*	Fruit
Deer	*Cervus* sp	Meat (venison)
Dewberry	*Rubus caesium*	Fruit
Dill	*Anethum graveolens*	Herb
Dolphin	*Coryphaena hippurus*	Eaten as fish
Duck	Anatidae	Fowl
Dulse	*Rhodymenia plamata*	Seaweed
Durian; durion	*Durio zibethinus*	Fruit
Eel	*Anguilla anguilla* (common eel) *Conger conger* (conger eel)	Fish
Egg	Various birds, especially domesticated	Cooked (e.g. fried, boiled, poached) or raw
Eggplant	*Solanum melongena*	Vegetable
Elder	*Sambucus nigra* (European) *S. canadensis* (American)	Fruit; flowers used in wine
Endive	*Chicorium endivia*	Salad; roots make coffee flavouring
Epazote; Mexican tea	*Chenopodium ambrosioides*	Strongly flavoured herb
Fennel	*Foeniculum vulgara*	Green herb; seeds used as a spice
Fenugreek	*Trigonella foenumgraecum*	Seeds in flavouring
Fern Patrick fern	*Pteridis aquilina* (bracken) *Matteuccia struthiopteris*	Early shoots as vegetable; may deplete B_1
Feverfew	*Tanacetum Parthenium*	Tea
Fig	*Ficus carica*	Dried or fresh fruit, used in baking
File powder; filet powder	*Sassafras albidum*	Tea
Flatfish	*Scophthalmus rhombus* (brill) *Limanda limanda* (dab) *Platichthys flesus* (flounder) *Hippoglossus hippoglossus* (halibut) *Microstomus kitt* (lemon sole) *Pleuronectes platessa* (plaice) *Solea solea* (sole) *Scophthalmus maximus* (turbot) *Glytocephalus cynoglossus* (witch)	Fish
Flax	*Linum usitatissiumum*	Flaxseed oil
Frog	*Rana esculenta* (edible frog) *R. ridibunda* (marsh frog) *R. lessonae* (pool frog)	Legs (as meat)
Galangal	*Alpinia galanga* (greater galangal) *Alpinia officinarum* (lesser galangal)	Roots used as flavouring
Garlic	*Allium sativum*	Flavouring
Gaur; cluster bean	*Cyamopsis psoraloides*	Vegetable source of gum

Appendix 17.1 Foods continued

Food	Biological name	How eaten/remarks
Geranium	*Pelargonium capitatum* *P. ororatissimum*	Leaves used to perfume jams and jellies
Gherkins	*Cucumis anguria*	Vegetable; pickle
Ginger	*Zingiber officinale*	Vegetable; flavouring
Ginkgo; maidenhair tree	*Ginkgo biloba*	Nut
Globe artichoke	*Cynara scolymus* (thistle) *C. cardunculus* (cardoon)	Vegetable
Goa bean	*Psophocarpus tetragonolobus*	Vegetable
Goat	*Capra* sp.	Meat; milk
Goose	*Anatidae*	Eggs; poultry
Gooseberry	*Ribes uvacrispa*	Fruit
Grape	*Vitis vinifera* (European grape) *V. acetosa* (Australian grape)	Fruit; wine
Grapefruit	*Citrus paradisi*	Fruit; juice
Ground elder; bishopweed; goutweed	*Aegopodium podagraria*	Young leaves—boil; greens in Spring
Ground nut	*Arachis hypogaea*	Nut
Grouse	*Lagopus mutus* (ptarmigan) *Tetrao urogallus* (capercaillie) *Centrocercus urophasianus* (sage grouse) *Lagopus lagopus scoticus* (Scottish grouse)	Fowl
Grunt	*Haemulon macostomum*	Fish
Guava	*Psidium guajava* (myrtle family)	Fruit
Guinea fowl	*Numida*	Fowl
Gum arabic; gum tragacanth; sterculia gum	*Acacia* *Sterculia*	Stabilizer Emulsifier
Hawthorn	*Crataegus monogyna*	Fruit
Hazel nut; cobnut; filbert	*Corylus avellana* *C. maxima* (Barcelona nut) *C colurna* (Turkish hazel)	Nut; Flour
Heather	*Calluna vulgaris*	Tea
Herring	*Clupea harengus* (group including sprat, sardine and pilchard)	Fish
Hibiscus	*H. sabdariffa*	Flour; beverage
Hickory; pecan	*Carya ovata* (shagbark hickory) *C. glabra* (pignut; switchbred hickory) *C. tomentosa* (mocketnut; common hickory)	Nut
Hop	*Humulus lupulus*	Flavouring and preserving beer; young shoots—vegetable
Horse gram; Madras gram; kulthi	*Dolichos biflorus*	Green vegetable and pulse
Horseradish	*Amoractia rusticana*	Flavouring (tap root)
Jack bean; horse bean	*Canavalia ensiformis* *C. gladiata* (sword bean; sabre bean)	Green vegetables; sword bean used ripe as pulse
Jack fruit; jak fruit	*Artocarpus integrifolia* (mulberry family)	Fruit

Appendix 17.1 Foods continued

Food	Biological name	How eaten/remarks
Jamaica flower; roselle; red sorrel	*Hibiscus sabdariffa*	Mexican drink
Jasmine	*Jasminium paniculatum*	Scented tea
Jerusalem artichoke	*Helianthus tiberosus* (sunflower flowers, *not* globe artichoke)	Vegetable
Jujube	*Zizyphus*	Fruits candied or preserved
Juniper	*Juniperus commionis*	Flavouring
Kale; kail; collards; borecole	*Brassica oleracea* var. *acephala* *B. napus* (rape kale)	Vegetable—boil
Kelp	*Laminaria digitata*	Seaweed—boil
Kewra; screwpine	*Pandanus tectorius*	Flavouring—male flowers; soft sweet fruit
Khas-khas; vetiver	*Vetiveria zizamoides*	Flavouring
Kidney bean; French bean; haricot bean; common bean	*Phaseolus vulgaris*	Vegetable
Kiwi fruit; Chinese gooseberry	*Actinidia sinensis*	Raw fruit; juiced
Kohlrabi; knol-kohl	*Brassica oleracea* var. *gongylodes*	Vegetable—boil
Kokum	*Garcinia indica*	Fruit
Korean pine	*Pinus koraiensis*	Nut
Kumquat	*Fortunella margarita* (oval) *F. japonica* (round)	Fruit (small citrus) (eaten whole)
Lablab bean; hyacinth bean; bonavist bean; Egyptian bean	*Dolichos lablab*	Dried or green
Lady's smock; cuckoo flower	*Cardamine pratensis*	Spring salad
Langouste; spiny lobster; southern lobster	*Palinerus elephas* and other species	Shellfish
Laver; laver weed; red laver; tangle	*Porphyra umbilicalis* *P.lacinata* (pink laver)	Seaweed
Leek	*Allium porrum*	Vegetable
Lemon	*Citrus limon*	Fruit
Lentil	*Lens culinaris*	Flour; vegetable
Lettuce	*Lactuca sativa*	Vegetable
Lima bean	*Phaseolus lunatus*	Vegetable
Lime	*Citrus aurantifolia*	Fruit
Lime; linden; basswood	*Tilia europaea* *T. cordata* *T. platyphyllos*	Yellow flowers—tisane or tea
Limpet	*Patella* sp.	Shellfish—boil
Lobster	*Homarus gammarus*	Shellfish
Loquat; Japanese medlar	*Eriobotrya japonica*	Fruit
Lotus; white water-lily	*Nymphaea alba*	Underwater rhizomes
Lovage	*Levisticum officinale*	Herb
Love apple	*Solanum authiopicum*	Fruit
Lychee; litchi	*Litchi chinensis*	Fruit
Macadamia nut; Queensland nut	*Macadamia ternifolia*	Nut
Mace	*Myristica fragrans*	Aril-seed of the nutmeg
Mackerel	*Scomber scombrus* (Atlantic) *S. maculatus* (Spanish)	Fish

Appendix 17.1 Foods *continued*

Food	Biological name	How eaten/remarks
Maidenhair fern	*Adiantum capillus-veneris*	Jelly—boil
Maize; corn (US)	*Zea mays*	Grain
Mallow	*Hibiscus abelmoschus*	Musk flavoured seed
	H. sabdariffa (red sorrel)	Tarts and jams; green leaves
Mango	*Mangifera indica*	Fruit
Mangosteen	*Garcinia mangostana*	Fruit
Marigold	*Calendula officinalis*	Petals—edible yellow colouring
Marjoram	*Origanum* sp.	Herb
Marrow, squash, pumpkin, gourd, etc.	*Cucurbita pepo* (pumpkin, marrow, summer squash, courgette; custard marrow, cymling, etc.)	Vegetable; salads
	Cucurbita maxima (winter squash, hubbard, turban, butternut; and mammoth squash)	
	Cucurbita moshata (cushaw, winter crookneck, Canada crookneck)	
	Citrullus vulgaris var. *fistulosus*	Tiny variety of watermelon
	Tricosanthes cucumerina (snake gourd—native of India)	
	T. dioica (parwal)	Vegetables in the Orient
	Momordica charantia	
	Benincasa hispide (ash gourd)	
	Luffa acutangula (South Indian)	
	Cucumeropsis edulis (West African)	Oily seeds
Marshmallow	*Althaea officinalis*	Cook to extract liquid
Maté; Paraguay tea; yerba maté; yerba	*Ilex paraguayensis*	Beverage
Medlar	*Mespilus germanica*	Winter fruit—raw or cooked
Melilot	*M. officinalis*	Leguminous plant with sweet flavour
Melon	*Cucimis meda*	
	C. vulgaris (watermelon)	
	Cantaloupe melon	
	Casaba melon	
	Musk melon, netted melon, nutmeg, melon or sweet melon	
	Honeydew melon	
	Snap melon	
	Watermelon	
	Cucurbitaceae	
Milk	Various domesticated mammals	Drink
Millet and sorghum	*Echinochloa crusgali* (barnyard millet; bharti)	Porridge
	Pennisetum typhoideum (bulrush millet; bajra; cattail; reedmace)	Flour, bread
	Panicum miliaceum (common millet; broomcorn; proso; Indian millet; hog-millet (US)	Unleavened bread
	Eleusine coracana (finger millet; ragi)	Breads and beer
	Setaria italica (foxtail millet; German millet; Hungarian millet; Italian millet; Siberian millet)	Beer
	Digitalis exilis (Hungary rice)	
	Coix lachrymajobi (Job's tears—not really millet as seeds are large)	
	Panicum miliare (little millet)	
	Sorghum vulgare (sorghum) var. *saccharatum* (white grained sorghum) var. *caffrorum* (kaffir corn) var. *subglabrescens* (milo)	Stem used for juice to make sorghum syrup Bread
	Eragrostis abyssinica (teff)	Bread

Appendix 17.1 Foods continued

Food	Biological name	How eaten/remarks
Mint	*Mentha* sp. *M. piperita* (peppermint) *M. aquatica* (water mint) *M. spicata* (spearmint)	Herb; tea
Monstera, ceriman	*Monstera deliciosa*	Fruit
Moray eel	*Muraena helena*	Fish
Morel	*Morchella esculenta*	Fungus
Moth bean	*Phaseolus aconitifolius*	Vegetable
Mulberry	*Morus nigra*	Fruit
Mullet	*Mullus surmuletus* (red mullet) *M. barbatus* (red mullet) family Mygilidae (grey mullet)	Fish
Mung bean; green gram	*Phaseolus aureus*	Tiny bean
Mushroom	*Agaricus campestris*	Fungus
Mussel	*Mytilis edulis* (edible mussel) *M. galloprovincialis* (Mediterranean mussel) *M. edulis* and *M. californianus* (edible mussel from West Coast of US)	Fresh; cooked; pickled
Mustard	*Brassica nigra* (black mustard) *Sinapis alba* (white mustard) *Brassica juncea* (brown mustard)	Condiment mustard American mustard also used in English mustard Condiment mustard Mustard oil
Mutton and lamb	*Ovis* sp.	Meat
Myrtle	*Murtus communis*	Leaves—for wrapping pork or stuffing small birds; black berries—edible; also for oil
Nasturtium; Indian cress	*Tropaeolum majus*	Leaves for salad; flowers—good to eat and for nasturtium vinegar
Nettle	*Urtica dioica*	Young tops used as vegetable
Nigella	*Nigella sativa*	Black seed used as spice
Nutmeg	*Myristica fragrans*	Flavouring (the aril around the nutmeg is mace)
Oat; oatmeal	*Avena sativa*	Grain
Octopus	Cephalopods (molluscs)	Seafood
Okra; okro; ladies' fingers; gumbo	*Hibiscus esculentus* (mallow family)	Vegetable
Olive	*Olea europaea*	Olive oil
Onion	*Allium cepa*	Flavouring in salads or savouries; vegetable
Orange	*Citrus sinensis* (tight-skinned sweet oranges) *Citrus reticulata* (loose-skinned oranges) *C. aurantium* (bitter oranges; Seville oranges) *C. bergamia* (bergamot) *C. mitis* (calamondin)	Pulp eaten as fruit; peel candied; jam; juices Flavouring
Oregano; wild marjoram	*Origanum vulgare*	Herb
Ostrich	*Struthio camelus*	Fowl

Appendix 17.1 Foods continued

Food	Biological name	How eaten/remarks
Oyster	*Lopha cristagalli* (cock's comb oyster—Pacific) *Ostrea edulis* (flat oyster—British) *Crassostrea angulata* (Portuguese) *Crassostrea virginica* (American)	Shellfish
Palm	Palmae *Borassus flabellifer* *Sabal palmetto* (cabbage palm) *Caryola urens* (jaggery palm)	Dates, coconuts, betel nuts, palm olive, sago, palm sugar Hearts, i.e. terminal buds Palm sugar
Pawpaw	*Asimina triloba*	Fruit
Papaya; pawpaw	*Carica papaya*	Fruit
Paradise nut; sapucaya nut	*Lecythis subasajo*	Nut; flour
Parsley	*Petroselinum crispum*	Herb
Parsnip	*Pastinaca sativa*	Vegetable
Partridge	*Perdix* sp.	Fowl
Passion fruit; purple granadilla	*Passiflora edulis*	Fruit
Pea	*Pisum sativum* var. *saccharatum* (sugar pea; snow pea; mangetout)	Seeds eaten Pods eaten whole
Peach	*Prunus persica*	Fruit
Peacock	*Pavo cristatus*	Fowl
Peanut, groundnut; monkey nut	*Arachis hypogaea*	Flour; nut; oil
Pear	*Pyrus communis*	Fruit
Pecan	*Carya illinoensis*	Nut
Pennyroyal	*Mentha pulegium*	Flavouring
Pepper	*Piper nigrum* *P. cubeb* (cubeb pepper) *Pimenta dioica* (myrtle pepper; Jamaica pepper) *Piper methysticum* (kava pepper) *Lepidium sativum* (pepper grass; garden cress) *L. virginicum* (wild pepper-grass– North America) *L. ruderale* (roadside pepper-grass)	Spice
Persimmon; kaki	*Diospyrus kaki* *D. virginiana*	Fruit
Pheasant	*Phasianus colchicus*	Fowl
Physalis fruit	*Physalis* *P. alkengii* (Chinese lantern plant; bladder cherry) *P. peruviana* (Cape gooseberry) *P. pruinosa* (ground cherry; ground strawberry; ground tomato or dwarf Cape gooseberry)	Fruit
Pigeon pea; red gram	*Cajanus cajan*	Pulse
Pike	*Esox lucius* (northern pike) *E. masquinongy* (muskellunge)	Fish

Appendix 17.1 Foods *continued*

Food	Biological name	How eaten/remarks
Pineapple	*Ananas comosus*	Fruit
Pine nut	*Pinus lambertiana*	Nut
Pistachio nut; green almond	*Pistachio vera*	Nut
Plantain	*Plantago major*	Tea
Plover	Charadriidae family	Fowl
Plum	*Prunus domestica* *P. cerasifera* (cherry plum) *P. insitis* (damson)	Fruit; also dried as prunes
Pomegranate	*Punica granatum*	Fruit
Pompano	*Trachinotus carolinus*	Fish
Poppy	*Papaver somniferum*	Seeds used for flavouring
Pork	*Sus scrofa*	Meat
Porgy	*Pagrus pagrus*	Fish
Potato	*Solanum tuberosum* *Sagittaria sagittifolia* (swamp pot)	Vegetable
Prickly pear; cactus pear; Indian fig; Indian pear; Barbary pear; tuna fig	*Opuntia* sp.	Fruit
Purslane; pussley; pigweed	*Portulaca oleracea*	Raw, as salad
Primrose	*Primula officinalis*	Leaves eaten
Quail	*Coturnix coturnix*	Fowl
Quince	*Cydonia vulgaris*	Fruit
Rabbit and hare	Leporidae	Meat
Radish	*Taphanus sativus*	Roots and tops
Rape	*Brassica napus* var. *napobrassica* (swede) var. *rutabaga*	Spring green vegetable
Raspberry and loganberry	*Rubus* *Rubus R. idaeus* (British) *R. occidentalis* (American)	Fruit
Razor shells	Bivalve molluscs	Shellfish
Redcurrant	*Rheum rubrum*	Fruit
Rhubarb	*Rheum raponticum*	Vegetable
Rice	*Oryza sativa* *Zizinia aquatica* (Indian rice)	Grain
Rice bean	*Phaseolus calceratus*	Pulse
Rice paper	*Tetrapana papyriferum* *Edgeworthia tomentosa* (nakai) *Wickstroemia canescens* (maisin)	Wrapping
Rocket	*Eruca sativa*	Salad
Rose	*Rosa* sp.	Rose water; rose-hip syrup
Rosefish	*Sebastes marinus*	Fish
Rosemary	*Rosmarinus officinalis*	Herb
Rowan and sorb	*Sorbus acuparia*	Jelly
Runner bean	*Phaseolus coccineus*	Vegetable
Rye	*Secale cereale*	Grain

Appendix 17.1 Foods continued

Food	Biological name	How eaten/remarks
Safflower; saffron thistle	*Carthamus tinctosius*	Flowers—food colouring; seeds—safflower oil
Saffron	*Crocus sativus*	Stigmas used as flavouring
Sage; garden sage	*Salvis officinalis*	Herb
Sago	*Metroxylon sagu*	Flour
Salmon	*Salmo salar* (European, Pacific and North American) *Oncorhyncus gorbuscha* (pink salmon) *O. kisutch* (coho salmon) *O. keta* (dog salmon) *O. tschawytscha* (king salmon)	Fish
Salsify; oyster plant	*Tragopogon porrifolium*	Vegetable
Samphire; rock samphire	*Crithmum maritimum*	Vegetable
Sand-eel; sand-lance	*Ammodytes*	Fish
Sapodilla; sapodilla plum; tree potato; sapota; zapote; naseberry; chiku	*Achras sapota*	Fruit
Sassafras	*Sassafras albidum*	Beer; tea
Savory	*Satureja hortensis* (summer savory) *S. montana* (winter savory)	Herb
Scallop; scollop	*Pecten maximus* (great scallop) *P. jacobaeus* (Pilgrim scallop–Mediterranean) *Placopecten magellanicus* (Atlantic deep sea scallop) *Chlamys islandica* (Iceland scallop) *C. opercularis* (queen scallop; quin) *C. varia* (variegated scallop) *C. irradians* (bay scallop)	Shellfish
Scampi; Norway lobster; Dublin Bay prawn	*Nephrops norvegicus*	Shellfish
Sea anemone	*Actinia equina* (beadlet anemone) *Anemonia sulcata* (oplet; snakelocks anemone)	Seafood
Sea cucumber; trepang; bêche-de-mer	*Holothuria*	Seafood
Sea date; date mussel	*Lithophaga lithophaga*	Shellfish
Sea-kale	*Crambe maritima*	Vegetable
Sea urchin	*Echinus esculentus* (edible sea urchin) *Srongylocentrus droebachiensis* (green sea urchin) *Paracentrotus lividus*	Seafood
Seaweed	*Rhodymenia palmata* (dulse) *Laurencia pinnatifida* (pepper dulse) *Porphyra lacinata* (pink laver)	Raw in salads; cooked as vegetable
Sesame	*Sesamum indicum*	Seeds used as flavouring
Shad	*Alosa* sp.	Fish
Shaddock; pomelo; pummelo	*Citrus grandis*	Fruit
Shallot	*Allium ascalonium* (variety of onion)	Flavouring in salads or savouries
Shark, dogfish, ray and skate	Cartilaginous fish	Fish

Appendix 17.1 Foods continued

Food	Biological name	How eaten/remarks
Shrimp and prawn	Small crustaceans *Crangon crangon* (brown shrimp) *Pandalus montagui* (pink shrimp or Aesop prawn) *Palaemon serratus* (common prawn) *Pandalus borealis* (deep water shrimp)	Shellfish
Sloe	*Prunus spinosa* (blackthorn) *P. americana* (wild plum (US))	Sloe gin Jelly for meats
Smelt	*Osmerus mordax*	Fish
Snail	Gastropod (mollusc)	
Snake and gorpad lizard	Reptiles	Meat
Snapper	*Lutjanus aya*	Fish
Snoek; Australian barracuda	*Thyrsites atum* (relative of tunny and mackerel)	Fish
Snook; robalo	*Centropomus undecimales*	Fish
Sorrel	*Oxalis acetosella*	Herb
Soya bean; soybean; soja bean	*Glycine* sp.	Flour; vegetable; 'milk'
Spinach	*Spinacea oleracea* (common spinach) *Chenopodium bonus-henricus* (Good King Henry) *Tetragonia expansa* (New Zealand spinach) *Atriplex hortensis* (orache; mountain spinach) Spinach beet or Swiss chard *Lamium album* (white dead nettle)	Vegetable
Spelt	*Triticum bicorne*	Grain
Spruce	*Picea*	Beer
Squash; pumpkin	*Cucurbita pepo*	Vegetable
Squid	*Loligo pealei* (North American squid)	Seafood
Strawberry	*Fragaria ananassa* (garden strawberry)	Fruit
Sturgeon	*Acipenser sturio* (common sturgeon) *A. guldenstadtii* (Russian sturgeon) *Huso huso* (beluga)	Fish; eggs as caviar
Sugar cane	*Saccharum officinarum*	Sweetener; chewed as fruit
Sumac	*Rhus coriaria* (Mediterranean)	Berries
Sunflower	*Helianthus annuus*	Seeds; oil
Swede; rutabaga	*Brassica napus* (rape) var. *napobrassica* (swede) var. *rutabaga* (rutabaga)	Vegetable
Sweet cicely	*Myrrhis odorata*	Herb
Sweet marjoram; knotted marjoram	*Origanum majorana*	Herb
Sweet pepper; bell pepper; pimento	*Capsicum annuum*	Condiment
Sweet potato	*Ipomoea batatas*	Vegetable
Sweet woodruff	*Galium odoratum*	Herb
Swordfish	*Xiphias gladius*	Fish

Appendix 17.1 Foods continued

Food	Biological name	How eaten/remarks
Tamarind; Indian date	*Tamarinda indica*	Fruity sour taste
Tansy	*Chrysanthemum vulgare*	Herb
Tapioca	*Cassava* sp.	Flour; vegetable
Tarpon	*Tarpon atlanticus*	Fish
Tarragon	*Artemisia dracunculus* (French tarragon) *A. dracunculoides* (Russian tarragon)	Herb
Tea	*Camellia sinensis*	Beverage
Thyme	*Thymus vulgaris*	Herb
Tomato	*Lycopersicon esculentum*	Fruit
Triticale	Cross between wheat and rye	Grain
Trout and char	*Salvelinus fontinalis* (brook trout) *S. gairdneri* (rainbow trout)	Fish
Truffles	*Tuber melanosporum* (black truffle; Perigord truffle) *T. magnatum* (white truffle; Italian truffle)	Fungus
Tuna	*T. thynus* (blue fin tuna) *T. albacares* (yellow fin tuna) *T. alalunga* (long fin tuna; albacore)	Fish
Turkey	*Meleagris gallopavo*	Fowl
Turmeric	*Curcuma longa*	Spice
Turnip	*Brassica rapa*	Vegetable
Turtle and terrapin	*Chelonia mydas* (green turtle)	Meat (reptile)
Valerian	*Centranthus ruber*	Edible young leaves
Vanilla	*Vanilla planifolia* (climbing orchid)	Flavouring
Venison	*Cervus* sp.	Meat
Verbena; lemon-scented verbena	*Verbena tryphilla*	Herb; tea
Vetch	*Vicia sativa*	Animal foodstuff
Vine leaves	*Vitis* sp.	Vegetable
Violet	*Microcosmus sulcatus-tunicate* *Viola odorata*	Crystallized as sweets Flavouring
Viper's bugloss	*Echium vulgare*	Cucumber flavour
Walnut	*Juglans regia*	Nut
Watercress	*Nasturtium amphibium*	Vegetable; salad
Water chestnut	*Trapa natans* *Eleocharis tuberosa*	Vegetable Vegetable
Whale	*Cetacea*	Oil
Whitefish	*Coregonous clupeiformis*	Fish
Whiting	*Cynoscion regalis* (weakfish) *Micropogon undulatus* (Atlantic croaker) *Menticirrhus americanus* (king whiting) *Aplodinotus grunniens* (freshwater drumfish)	Fish

Appendix 17.1 Foods *continued*

Food	Biological name	How eaten/remarks
Wild rice; Indian rice; Tuscarora rice	*Zizania aquatica*	Grain
Winkle; periwinkle	*Littorina littorea*	Shellfish
Woodcock; snipe	*Scolopax rusticola*	Fowl
Wormwood	*Artemisia absinthium*	Flavouring
Yam	*Dioscorea* (250 species) *D. alata* (greater yam; asiatic yam) *Amorphopphallus campanulatus* (Elephant's foot; suram) *Colocasia* (dasheen; taro; eddo; old coco-yam; elephant's ear; avi) *Xanthosoma sagittifolium* (yautia; tannia; new cocoyam) *Pachyrhizus tuberosus* (yam bean) *Oxalis acetosella* *Oxalis tuberosa* (oka; occa; oca) *Tropaeolum tuberosum* (ysano; anu)	Climbing vines Acid leaves
Yarrow; ulluco	*Ullucus tuberosus*	Vegetable
Yeast	*Achillea millefolium*	Herb used as green vegetable or in salads; tea
Zedoary	*Curcuma zedoaria*	Spice

Appendix 17.2 Food families.

Water	Flour	Starch	Thickener	Raising Agent	Oil	Salt	Sweetener	Fruit	Juice/ Alcoholic Drink	Alcohol	Nut/Seed
									Amaryllis Pulque Tequila		
		Arrowroot Maranta	**Arrowroot**								
		Arum Poi	**Arum** Dasheen Taro								
			Banana Musa					**Banana** Banana Plantain	**Banana**		
											Beech Chestnut
								Berries Blackberry Boysenberry Dewberry Loganberry Longberry Raspberry Strawberry Wineberry	**Berries** Blackberry Boysenberry Dewberry Loganberry Longberry (black, purple, red) Strawberry Wineberry		
											Birch Filbert Hazelnut
Brecon Brita											
	Buckwheat										
Buxton											
								Cactus Prickly pear	**Cactus** Prickly pear		

Appendix 17.2 continued

Vegetable	Herb/Spice/Vinegar	Beverage/Tea	Fish	Fowl	Mammal	Other Animal	Milk	Fat	Spread	Misc.
	Acetic acid									
Algae Carrageen Dulse Kelp		**Algae** Dulse								**Algae** Agar-agar
										Amaryllis Agave Mescal
			Anchovy							
Arum Malanga										**Arum** Ceriman Poi Yautia
Banana Banana										
			Bass White perch Yellow bass							
					Bear					
										Beech Chinquapin
	Berry Raspberry	**Berry** Raspberry Strawberry								
										Birch Methyl-salicylate Wintergreen
										Bixa Annatto
			Bluefish							
	Borage Comfrey	**Borage** Comfrey								
					Bovine Beef Bison Buffalo C/cheese C/yoghurt Goat Goat cheese Sheep S/cheese Veal		**Bovine** Cow Ewe Goat	**Bovine** Suet	**Bovine** Butter Oleomarg.	**Bovine** Gelatine Lactose Rennet Rennin Sausage Caseine
	Buckwheat Garden sorrel	**Buckwheat**								
		Buttercup Golden seal								

Appendix 17.2 continued

Water	Flour	Starch	Thickener	Raising Agent	Oil	Salt	Sweetener	Fruit	Juice/ Alcoholic Drink	Alcohol	Nut/Seed
			Canna Queensland								
									Carrot Anise Carrot Kola Parsnip		**Carrot** Cola nut
								Cashew Mango	**Cashew** Mango		**Cashew** Pistachio
	Composite Jerusalem artichoke Sunflower				**Composite** Safflower Sunflower				**Composite** Burdock Dandelion		**Composite** Sunflower
									Conifer Juniper Gin		
Culligan											
								Custard Apple Annona	**Custard Apple** Annona		

Vegetable	Herb/Spice/Vinegar	Beverage/Tea	Fish	Fowl	Mammal	Other Animal	Milk	Fat	Spread	Misc.
Caper										
Carpetweed NZ spinach										
Carrot Carrot Celeriac Celery Fennel Parsnip	**Carrot** Angelica Anise Carroway Celeriac Chervil Coriander Cumin Dill Fennel Parsley Sweet cecily	**Carrot** Celery Fennel Gotu Cola Lovage Parsley								
										Cashew Poison ivy Poison oak Poison sumac
			Catfish Catfish f/w							
						Cephalopod Octopus Squid				
			Cod Cod Cusk Haddock Hake Pollack Scrod							
			Coley							
	Composite Santolina Scorzonesa Tancy Tarragon	**Composite** Bonset Burdock Camomile Chichory Dandelion Golden rod Yarrow							**Composite** Safflower Sunflower	**Composite** Coltsfoot Costmary Escarole Lodnum Pyrethrum Romaine Southern- wood Wormwood
			F/Croaker f/w drum							
			S/Croaker s/w drum s/w trout Silver perch Spot spott. S/trout Weakfish							
Conifer Pine nut Pinon Pinyon		**Conifer** Juniper								**Conifer** Juniper oil
						Crustaceans Crab Crayfish Langustine Lobster Prawn Shrimp Scampi				

Appendix 17.2 continued

Water	Flour	Starch	Thickener	Raising Agent	Oil	Salt	Sweetener	Fruit	Juice/ Alcoholic Drink	Alcohol	Nut/Seed
								Ebony Kaki Persimmon	**Ebony** Kaki Persimmon		
				Fungi Baker's yeast Brewer's yeast							
			Ginger East Indian						**Ginger**		
							Goosefoot Beet sugar				
								Gourd Muskmelon Cantaloupe Caraba Cranshaw Honeydew Persian Watermelon Chinese melon	**Gourd** Muskmelon Cantaloupe Caraba Cranshaw Honeydew Persian Watermelon Chinese melon		**Gourd** Melon Pumpkin

Vegetable	Herb/Spice/ Vinegar	Beverage/ Tea	Fish	Fowl	Mammal	Other Animal	Milk	Fat	Spread	Misc.
					Deer Caribou Deer Elk Moose Reindeer Venison					
			Dolphin							
				Dove Pigeon Squab						
				Duck Duck eggs Goose Goose eggs				**Duck** Goosefat		
			Eel Rock eel							
		Flax Flax seed								
			Flounder Dab Halibut Plaice Sole Turbot							
Fungi Morel Mushroom Puff ball Truffle										**Fungi** Mould
						Frog				
						Gastropod Abalone Snail Whelk Winkle				
	Ginger Cardamon Tumeric									
		Ginseng								**Ginseng**
Goosefoot Beetroot Chard Spinach										**Goosefoot** Lamb's quarters Tampala

Gourd
Acorn
  squash
Buttercup ,,
Butternut ,,
Bostemarrow
Caserta
Cocozelle
Courgette
Crooknock
Cucumber
Cushaw
Gherkin
Golden
  nugget
Hubbard
Marrow
Patypain
Pumpkin
Straightneck
Turban
Veg.
  spaghetti
Zucchini
										Gourd
										Chayote
										  loofah

Appendix 17.2 continued

Water	Flour	Starch	Thickener	Raising Agent	Oil	Salt	Sweetener	Fruit	Juice/ Alcoholic Drink	Alcohol	Nut/Seed
							Grape Raisin	**Grape** Grape Raisin Currant Muscadine Sultana	**Grape** Brandy Champagne Raisin Muscadine Wine		
	Grass Barley Bran Bulgar Corn Hominy grits Millet Oat Rice Rye Wheat Wholewheat	**Grass** Corn Wheat			**Grass** Corn Rice		**Grass** Cane sugar Cane syrup Corn sugar Corn syrup Molasses Raw cane Sorghum		**Grass** Malt Rice Rum		**Grass** Oat Popcorn Rice Rye Wheat
								Heath Bearberry Blueberry Cranberry Huckleberry	**Heath** Bearberry Blueberry Cranberry Huckleberry		
Highland Spring											
								Honey- suckle Elderberry	**Honey- suckle** Elderberry ,, flower		
							Insect Honey				
					Laurel Avocado						
	Legume Soya				**Legume** Peanut Soya		**Legume** Carob syrup	**Legume** Tamarind			**Legume** Soya Peanut

Appendix 17.2 continued

Vegetable	Herb/Spice/ Vinegar	Beverage/ Tea	Fish	Fowl	Mammal	Other Animal	Milk	Fat	Spread	Misc.
	Grape Cream of tartar Wine vinegar									
Grass Bamboo shoots Barley Brown rice Millet Rice Sweetcorn	**Grass** Lemon grass Malt Maltose									**Grass** Citronella Graham Gluten Patent Triticale Wheatgerm
				Grouse Partridge						
				Guinea Fowl G/f eggs						
					Hare Rabbit					
			Harvest Fish Butterfish Harvest fish							
		Heath Bearberry Blueberry Huckleberry								
			Herring f/w Shad							
			Herring s/w Menhaden Pilchard Sea herring Sardine							
		Holly Matte								
					Horse Donkey					
		Horsetail Shavegrass								
						Insect Locust				
	Iris Saffron									
			Jack Amberjack Pompano Yellowjack							
Laurel Avocado	**Laurel** Bayleaf Cassia bark Cinnamon	**Laurel** Sassafras								
Legume Adzuki bean Blackeyed bean	**Legume** Fenugreek	**Legume** Alfalfa Carob Fenugreek Liquorice					**Legume** Soya	**Legume** Peanut Soya	**Legume** Carob Coumarin Gum acacia

Appendix 17.2 continued

Water	Flour	Starch	Thickener	Raising Agent	Oil	Salt	Sweetener	Fruit	Juice/ Alcoholic Drink	Alcohol	Nut/Seed
					Mallow Cotton seed						
								Malpighia Acerola	**Malpighia**		
Malvern											
							Maple Maple sugar Maple syrup				
	Mulberry Breadfruit						**Mulberry** Breadfruit Fig Hop Mulberry	**Mulberry** Hop Mulberry			

Vegetable	Herb/Spice/ Vinegar	Beverage/ Tea	Fish	Fowl	Mammal	Other Animal	Milk	Fat	Spread	Misc.
Legume Butter bean Broad bean Fenugreek Fava bean Field bean Flageolet bean French bean Chickpea bean Kidney bean Lentil Lima bean Mung bean Mung sprout Navy bean Pea Pinto bean Runner bean Soya bean Tonka bean		**Legume** Senna								**Legume** Gum tragacanth Jicama Kudzu Lecithin Liquorice
Lily Asparagus Leek Shallot Yucca	**Lily** Chives Onions	**Lily** Basswood Sarsaparilla								**Lily** Celsevera Sarsaparilla
			Mackerel Albacone Bonito Skipjack Tuna							
		Madder Coffee								**Madder** Woodruff
Mallow Okra		**Mallow** Althea root Hibiscus Roselle								
			Marlin Sailfish							
			Minnow Carp Chubb							
	Mint Applemint Basil Bergamot Marjoram Oregano Peppermint Rosemary Sage Spearmint Summer savory	**Mint** Catnip Chia seed Dittany Horsehound Crissop Lemon balm Pennyroyal Peppermint Spearmint								**Mint** Clary Lavender
					Monkey Opossum					
Morning Glory Sweet potato										
		Mulberry Savory hop								
			Mullett							

Appendix 17.2 continued

Water	Flour	Starch	Thickener	Raising Agent	Oil	Salt	Sweetener	Fruit	Juice/ Alcoholic Drink	Alcohol	Nut/Seed
								Myrtle Guava	**Myrtle** Guava		
					Olive Palm Coconut						
	Palm Coconut	**Palm** Sago starch					**Palm** Date sugar	**Palm** Date	**Palm** Coconut milk		**Palm** Coconut
								Papaya Pawpaw			
								Passion Flower Passion fruit	**Passion Flower** Passion fruit		
Pedalium Sesame					**Pedalium** Sesame						**Pedalium** Sesame
Perrier											

Vegetable	Herb/Spice/ Vinegar	Beverage/ Tea	Fish	Fowl	Mammal	Other Animal	Milk	Fat	Spread	Misc.
Mustard Cardoon cabbage Chinese cabbage Collards/ Broccoli Colza shoots Caivetron-chuob Curlycress Kale/Sprout Kohl-rabi Mustard greens Radish Rape Swede	**Mustard** Horseradish Mustard seed									
	Myrtle Allspice Clove	**Myrtle** Eucalyptus								
Nasturtium English caper										
	Nutmeg Mace									
		Oak Acorn								
Olive Palm Palm cabbage										
	Orchid Vanilla									
									Oxalis Caransoda Oxalis	
									Pedalium Thini	
					Peleopods Clams Cockle Mussel Oyster/ Scallion					
			Perch Sauger Walleye Yell. Perch							
	Pepper Peppercorn Black/White Pepper									
			Pheasant Chicken Chicken eggs Peafowl Pheasant eggs Quail eggs					**Pheasant** Chicken fat		

Appendix 17.2 continued

Water	Flour	Starch	Thickener	Raising Agent	Oil	Salt	Sweetener	Fruit	Juice/ Alcoholic Drink	Alcohol	Nut/Seed
								Pineapple	**Pineapple**		
							Pomegranate Grenadine	**Pomegranate**	**Pomegranate**		
							Pommes Rose-hip syrup	**Pommes** Apple Crab apple Loquat Pear Quince	**Pommes** Apple Cider Crab apple wine Pear Quince		
						Potassium Refined					
	Potato Potato	**Potato** Potato						**Potato** Ground cherry Melon pear	**Potato** Potato wine Tomato		
											Protea Macadamia
						Rocksalt					
								Rue Citron Grapefruit Kumquat Lemon Lime Murcot Orange Pumello Tangello Satsuma	**Rue** Citron Grapefruit Kumquat Lemon Lime Murcot Orange Pumello Tangello Satsuma		
							Saccharine				
							Sapodilla				
											Sapucaya Brazil nut Paradise nut Sapucaya nut
								Saxifrage Currant Gooseberry	**Saxifrage** Currant Gooseberry		

Appendix 17.2 continued

Vegetable	Herb/Spice/ Vinegar	Beverage/ Tea	Fish	Fowl	Mammal	Other Animal	Milk	Fat	Spread	Misc.
			Pike Muskellunge Pickerel							
	Pommes Cider vinegar	**Pommes** Rose hip								**Pommes** Pectin
	Poppy Poppy seed									
			Porgy Northern Carp							
Potato Eggplant Capsicum Potato Tomatillo Tomato Tree tomato	**Potato** Cayenne pepper Chilli Paprika Pimento									**Potato** Tobacco
					Pronghorn Antelope					
	Purslane									**Purslane** Pigweed
	Roseherb Burnet									
						Reptile Python				
			Salmon Trout							
										Sapodilla Chicle
			Scorpian Rose fish Ocean perch							

Appendix 17.2 continued

Water	Flour	Starch	Thickener	Raising Agent	Oil	Salt	Sweetener	Fruit	Juice/ Alcoholic Drink	Alcohol	Nut/Seed
					Seasalt						
											Sedge Chuffa Groundnut
								Soapberry Lychee	**Soapberry** Lychee		
Soda											
	Spurge Tapioca	**Spurge** Tapioca	**Spurge** Tapioca								
											Sterculia Cola
					Stonefruit Almond			**Stonefruit** Apricot Cherry Peach Nectarine Sloe Plum Prune	**Stonefruit** Apricot Cherry brandy Peach Nectarine Sloe gin Plum Prune		
St. Torre											
Swiss											
			Tacca Figi arrowroot								
Tap water											

Vegetable	Herb/Spice/ Vinegar	Beverage/ Tea	Fish	Fowl	Mammal	Other Animal	Milk	Fat	Spread	Misc.
			Sea Bass Grouper							
			Sea Catfish Ocean catfish							
					Seal					
Sedge Chinese water chestnut										
			Shark							
			Silverside Whitebait							
			Skate							
			Smelt							
Spurge Casara Yucca Castor bean										**Spurge** Castor oil
					Squirrel					
		Sterculia Chocolate Cocoa Cola							**Sterculia** Cocoa butter	**Sterculia** Chocolate
			Sturgeon Caviar							
			Sucker Buffalo fish							
			Sunfish Black bass Pumpkin seed Crappi							
					Swine Hog Bacon Ham Pork Pig Wild boar			**Swine** Lard		**Swine** Pork gelatine
			Swordfish							
		Tea								

Appendix 17.2 continued

Water	Flour	Starch	Thickener	Raising Agent	Oil	Salt	Sweetener	Fruit	Juice/ Alcoholic Drink	Alcohol	Nut/Seed
Vichy											
Volvic											

											Walnut
											Black
											  walnut
											Butternut
											English
											  walnut
											Hartnut
											Hickory nut
											Pecan

											Yam Chinese potato Name Yampi

Vegetable	Herb/Spice/ Vinegar	Beverage/ Tea	Fish	Fowl	Mammal	Other Animal	Milk	Fat	Spread	Misc.
			Tilefish							
				Turkey Turkey				**Turkey**		**Turkey** Eggs
						Turtle Terrapin				
										Valerian Fetticus Corn salad
	Verbena Lemon verbena	**Verbena** Lemon verbena								
					Whale					
			Whitefish							
					Yak Yak cheese		**Yak**			

Appendix 17.3 31-day rotation diet.

Evening Morning Afternoon	Animal	Fowl	Fish	Crustacean	Mollusc	Starch Veg.	Non-starch Veg.	Fruit	Seeds/ Nuts	Flours
	Swine Goat		Mullet		Mussel	Potato	Potato	Apple	Cola Nut	Potato
1/2		Grouse	Plaice		Clam	Corn	Caper	Malpighi	Pedalium	Corn Pedalium
2/3	Frog	Turkey	Salmon		Squid	Banana	Algea	Banana	Beech	Wheat
3/4		Pheasant	Sole	Shrimp		Legume	Legume	Date	Legume	Legume
4/5	Rabbit		Sturgeon		Winkle	Morning Glory	Sedge	Stone	Sedge Stone	Spurge
5/6		Partridge	Rock-Eel	Crayfish		Parsley	Carrot	Mulberry	Sapucaya	Barley Mulberry
6/7	Venison	Chicken	Herring		Oyster	Laurel	Olive	Custard Apple	Protea	Millet
7/8		Guinea Fowl	Whitebait	Crab		Rice	Gourd	Gourd	Gourd	Rice
8/9	Beef		Bass		Cockle	Yam	Carpet Weed	Ebony	Birch	Oat
9/10		Moorhen	Cod		Snail	Millet	Fungi	Paw Paw	Walnut	Rye
10/11	Turtle	Wood Pigeon	Trout		Scallop	Potato	Potato	Saxifrage	Conifer	Potato
11/12		Goose	Haddock	Scampi		Corn	Goosefoot	Soapberry	Coconut	Corn Coconut
12/13	Sheep		Flounder		Whelk	Banana	Bamboo	Banana	Cola Nut	Buckwheat
13/14		Woodcock	Skate	Lobster		Legume	Legume	Rue	Legume	Legume
14/15	Hare	Duck	Mackerel		Abalone	Morning Glory	Composite	Cactus	Composite	Composite
15/16		Quail	Tuna	Prawn		Barley	Mallow	Dilenia	Pedalium	Barley Pedalium
16/17	Swine Goat		Mullet		Mussel	Laurel	Lily	Cashew	Cashew	Wheat
17/18		Grouse	Plaice		Clam	Rice	Spurge	Pineapple	Beech	Rice Spurge
18/19	Frog	Turkey	Salmon		Squid	Yam	Mustard	Passion Fruit	Sapucaya	Millet
19/20		Pheasant	Sole	Shrimp		Millet	Caper	Buckwheat	Composite	Buckwheat
20/21	Rabbit		Sturgeon		Winkle	Potato	Potato	Heath	Protea	Potato
21/22		Partridge	Rock-Eel	Crayfish		Corn	Algae	Grape	Birch	Corn

Appendix 17.3 continued

Starch	Fats	Spreads	Oils	Milks	Sweeteners	Herbs/Spices	Waters	Drinks	Beverages
Potato	Swine	Composite	Composite	Goat	Apple	Potato Apple Composite	Brita	Potato Apple Cola Nut	Apple Composite
Corn	Beef	Beef	Corn Pedalium	Beef	Corn	Biva Borage Buckwheat	Saint Lambert	Rue Buckwheat	Beef Borage
Banana Algae Wheat	Turkey	Margarine	Walnut		Cane	Conifer Ginger Pepper	Highland Spring	Amaryllis Conifer	Algae Ginger
Arrowroot	Duck	Legume	Legume	Legume	Legume Date	Iris Lemon Grass Lily	Vichy	Lily	Legume
Spurge	Vitaquel	Vitaquel	Stone		Sorghum	Mustard Myrtle Nutmeg	Buxton	Stone Myrtle	Madder Myrtle
Barley	Sheep	Tomar	Sterculia	Creamer	Maple	Barley Carrot Orchid	Spa	Barley Mulberry	Barley Sterculia Carrot
Arum	Chicken		Olive		Saccharine	Laurel Grape Poppy	Brecon	Grape	Laurel
Canna	Swine		Rice		Fruit	Mint Rose Herb Verbena	Perrier	Rice Mint	Mint Verbena
Cycad	Beef	Beef	Mallow	Beef	Honey	Apple Bixa Borage	Malvern	Dilenia Apple	Beef Mallow Borage
Fungi	Turkey		Walnut	Goat	Cane	Pepper	Quan	Cashew	Ginseng
Potato		Margarine	Conifer		Date	Potato Conifer Iris	Ashbourne	Potato Saxifrage Conifer	Buttercup
Corn	Goose		Corn Coconut		Corn Goosefoot	Lemon Grass Mustard Myrtle	Brita	Coconut Myrtle	Linden Myrtle
Banana	Sheep	Tomar	Stone	Creamer	Sorghum	Buckwheat Borage Carrot	Saint Lambert	Cola Nut Buckwheat Stone	Borage Carrot
Ginger	Chicken	Legume	Legume	Legume	Legume	Ginger Nutmeg Orchid	Highland Spring	Rue Ginger	Legume
Grape	Duck	Composite	Composite		Maple	Composite Grape Mint	Vichy	Grape Mint	Composite Mint
Barley	Vitaquel	Vitaquel	Mallow Pedalium		Saccharine	Barley Poppy Rose Herb	Buxton	Barley Dilenia	Barley Mallow
Wheat	Swine		Olive	Goat	Fruit	Laurel Lily Verbena	Spa	Lily Cashew	Laurel Verbena
Spurge	Beef	Beef	Rice	Beef	Honey	Apple Bixa Conifer	Brecon	Rice Pineapple Apple	Beef Apple Conifer
Sago	Turkey	Margarine	Coconut		Goosefoot	Mustard Lemon Grass	Perrier	Passion Fruit Plum Coconut	Tea
Talla	Goose	Tomar	Sterculia		Apple	Buckwheat Pepper	Malvern	Buckwheat	Sterculia
Potato	Sheep		Stone	Creamer	Cane	Potato Ginger Orchid	Ivan	Potato Heath Stone	Horsetail Ginger
Corn Algae Grape		Composite	Corn Composite		Corn	Grape Composite Mint	Ashbourne	Grape Mint	Algae Composite Mint

Appendix 17.3 continued

Evening Morning Afternoon	Animal	Fowl	Fish	Crustacean	Mollusc	Starch Veg.	Non-starch Veg.	Fruit	Seeds/ Nuts	Flours
22/23	Venison	Chicken	Herring		Oyster	Banana	Sedge	Banana	Sedge	Oat
23/24		Guinea Fowl	Whitebait	Crab		Legume	Legume	Myrtle	Legume	Legume
24/25	Beef		Bass		Cockle	Morning Glory	Carrot	Berry	Walnut	Mulberry
25/26		Moorhen	Cod		Snail	Barley	Olive	Pomegranate	Conifer	Barley
26/27	Turtle	Wood Pigeon	Trout		Scallop	Laurel	Gourd	Gourd	Gourd	Rye
27/28		Goose	Haddock	Scampi		Rice	Carpet Weed	Stone	Stone	Rice
28/29	Sheep		Flounder		Whelk	Yam	Fungi	Apple	Coconut	Coconut
29/30		Woodcock	Skate	Lobster		Millet	Goosefoot	Malpighi	Cola Nut	Wheat
30/31	Hare	Duck	Mackerel		Abalone	Potato	Potato	Date	Pedalium	Potato Pedalium
31/1		Quail	Tuna	Prawn		Corn	Bamboo	Mulberry	Beech	Corn Mulberry

Starch	Fats	Spreads	Oils	Milks	Sweeteners	Herbs/Spices	Waters	Drinks	Beverages
Banana	Chicken		Pedalium		Sorghum	Barley Nutmeg Poppy	Brita	Honeysuckle Barley	Holly Barley
Arrowroot	Duck	Legume	Legume	Legume	Legume	Myrtle Rose Herb Lily	Saint Lambert	Myrtle Lily	Legume Myrtle
Arum	Beef	Beef	Walnut	Beef	Maple	Carrot Bixa Borage	Highland Spring	Berry Mulberry	Beef Carrot Borage
Barley	Vitaquel	Vitaquel	Olive Conifer	Goat	Saccharine	Conifer Verbena Iris	Vichy	Pomegranate Conifer	Verbena
Canna	Turkey	Margarine	Sterculia		Fruit	Laurel Mustard Pepper	Buxton	Amaryllis	Laurel Sterculia
Cycad	Goose	Tomar	Rice Stone		Honey	Buckwheat Lemon Grass Orchid	Spa	Rice Stone Buckwheat	Madder
Fungi	Sheep		Coconut	Creamer	Apple	Apple Grape	Brecon	Apple Coconut Cola Nut	Apple Grape
Ginger	Chicken				Goosefoot	Ginger Mint Barley	Perrier	Ginger Mint Barley	Mint Barley
Potato	Duck	Vitaquel	Pedalium		Date	Potato Lily Myrtle	Malvern	Potato Lily Myrtle	Ginseng Myrtle
Corn	Beef	Beef	Corn	Beef	Corn	Carrot Nutmeg Poppy	Elvan	Mulberry	Beef Carrot

Chapter 18
Cow's Milk and Breast Milk

John W. Gerrard

Introduction

Adverse reactions to cow's milk were first reported more than 2000 years ago when Hippocrates [1] (460–370 BC) noted that cow's milk could cause gastric upset and urticaria. The subject, however, began to attract greater attention after the Second World War when, for the first time, most babies were being brought up on formula feeds. The switch from breast to formula feeding had been associated with an increase in the prevalence of infantile eczema [29] and in mortality rates due to gastroenteritis and pneumonia [30, 66]. With the better understanding of the management of electrolyte disturbances, and appropriate use of antibiotics, mortality rates fell. It then became apparent that not all the gastrointestinal and respiratory problems were infectious in origin; some were due to adverse reactions to cow's milk itself. It was at this juncture that Goldman and his colleagues [27] carried out their now classical studies on cow's milk allergy (CMA). These indicated that cow's milk could cause many problems and that the only sure way of determining in any one case whether cow's milk was or was not responsible was the avoidance and reintroduction of cow's milk; to what extent reactions were due to allergy and to what extent they were due to other factors was not and still is not certain.

There are several reasons which make it difficult for physicians to recognize or realize that some adverse reactions are being precipitated by cow's milk. The first is that many of the symptoms caused by cow's milk resemble those caused by infections; recurrent rhinorrhoea, a persistent nasal stuffiness and repeated spells of wheezy bronchitis resemble infectious colds and bronchiolitis rather than hay fever and asthma. The second is that prick skin tests and RAST (radioallergosorbent test) are usually negative and this suggests that the child is not allergic to cow's milk when in point of fact he may be. The third is that with classical food allergy the patient usually comes to the doctor with the diagnosis already made, knowing that traces of egg cause vomiting or that strawberries cause urticaria. This rarely

344

applies to CMA for the mother does not suspect that the cow's milk which she is giving her child daily may be making him ill.

Although the nature of the reactions, allergy or intolerance, has not yet been entirely resolved, the presence of adverse reactions to cow's milk is not difficult to confirm, for cow's milk can be excluded from and reintroduced into the diet relatively easily. The prevalence of adverse reactions in any given infant population is also easy to determine [8, 26, 31, 35, 38], always provided the manifestations of CMA are recognized for what they are. Almost all children are given cow's milk, usually on a daily basis, and those whose symptoms clear when cow's milk is avoided and return when it is reintroduced can be readily determined.

SYMPTOMS PRODUCED BY CMA IN INFANCY

The symptoms most commonly produced by CMA in infancy are indicated in Table 18.1. The data are derived from three very different sources. Clein [8] was a general paediatrician with a special interest in CMA, Goldman [27] an immunologist whose cases were culled from the practices of many different paediatricians, the diagnosis being confirmed in all instances by three separate challenges, while Gerrard [26] followed an unselected series of normal newborns in order to determine the incidence of CMA in the infant population. Their findings suggest that the manifestations of CMA are relatively uniform.

Eczema

The commonest manifestation of CMA is eczema and though eczema can be precipitated by contact with soaps, wool, diapers etc, foods are important in infancy and cow's milk is probably the commonest precipitating factor. Typically the eczema first starts on the cheeks, chin and forehead, spreading at times to the trunk and limbs, particularly to the flexures, often becoming more severe with the introduction of cereals and fruits.

Gastrointestinal problems

Vomiting, diarrhoea and colic can all be precipitated by cow's milk although they can also

Table 18.1 Manifestations of CMA in percentages as seen in a general paediatric practice (Clein), in a group of children with CMA proven by three repeated challenges (Goldman) and in a series of newborns (Gerrard).

Symptom	Clein	Goldman	Gerrard
Eczema	43%	42%	45%
Vomiting	38	27	22
Colic	31	31	20
Diarrhoea	23	40	40
Irritability	19	13	
Bronchitis	17		20
Asthma	15	31	12
Constipation	3		
Refusing milk	3		
Apathy, cyanosis and collapse	2	4	
Urticaria and angioedema	2	8	
	(n = 209)	(n = 89)	(n = 787)

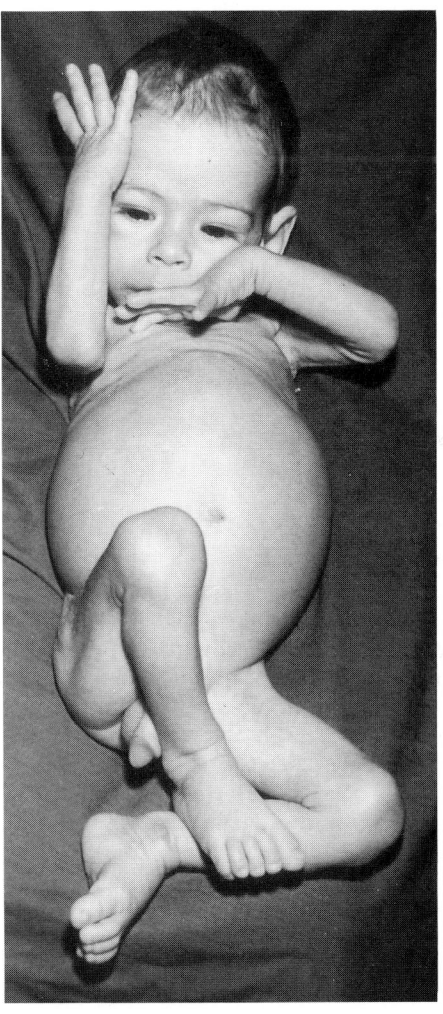

Fig. 18.1 An infant with abdominal distension and muscular wasting due to CMA.

be precipitated by other factors such as pyloric stenosis and infections. Care should be taken to exclude these before incriminating cow's milk. Infants with diarrhoea due to cow's milk may fail to thrive, have wasted limbs and buttocks and abdominal distension (Fig. 18.1). They may also have scalded buttocks (Fig. 18.2) which clear as soon as cow's milk is

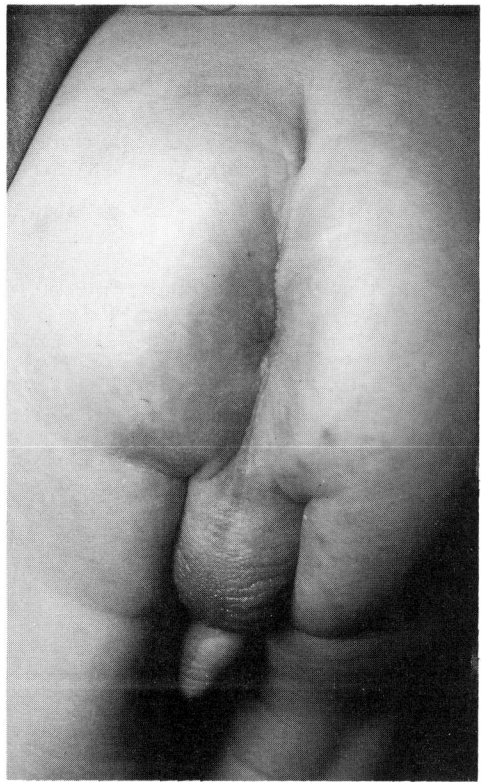

Fig. 18.2 Redness of perianal skin associated with diarrhoea due to CMA.

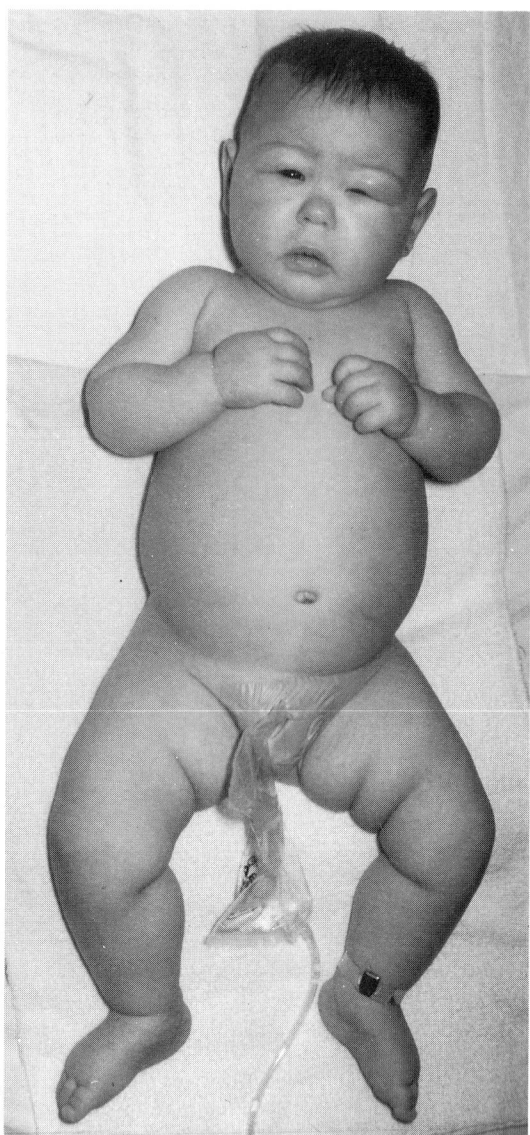

Fig. 18.3 Generalized oedema due to protein-losing gastroenteropathy.

avoided and the diarrhoea has subsided. CMA can also cause hypoalbuminaemia and generalized oedema (Fig. 18.3) due to a protein-losing gastroenteropathy [61] as well as an iron-deficiency anaemia (Fig. 18.4) due to occult or overt blood loss in the stools [65].

The awareness that cow's milk could cause diarrhoea first surfaced at a time when attention was being focused on inborn errors of metabolism and enzyme deficiencies. Infants with diarrhoea due to cow's milk were nearly always placed on formulae containing neither cow's milk protein nor lactose. Their stools often contained reducing substances [19] and lactose tolerance tests were abnormal; it was therefore assumed by many that lactase deficiency was primarily responsible for the diarrhoea [14]. We ourselves felt that this was un-

likely because many of the children continued to have diarrhoea on lactose-free soya formulae. In addition, when babies were found to be intolerant of most or all prepared formulae they frequently tolerated breast milk, a food rich in lactose. The usefulness of breast milk in the management of babies with diarrhoea due to cow's milk and other food intolerances has recently been emphasized by MacFarlane and Miller [45]. This finding confirms what Liu [43] demonstrated; namely, that babies with cow's milk protein intolerance often tolerate lactose as soon as cow's milk proteins have been excluded from the diet. Lactase activities in the jejunal mucosa of babies with

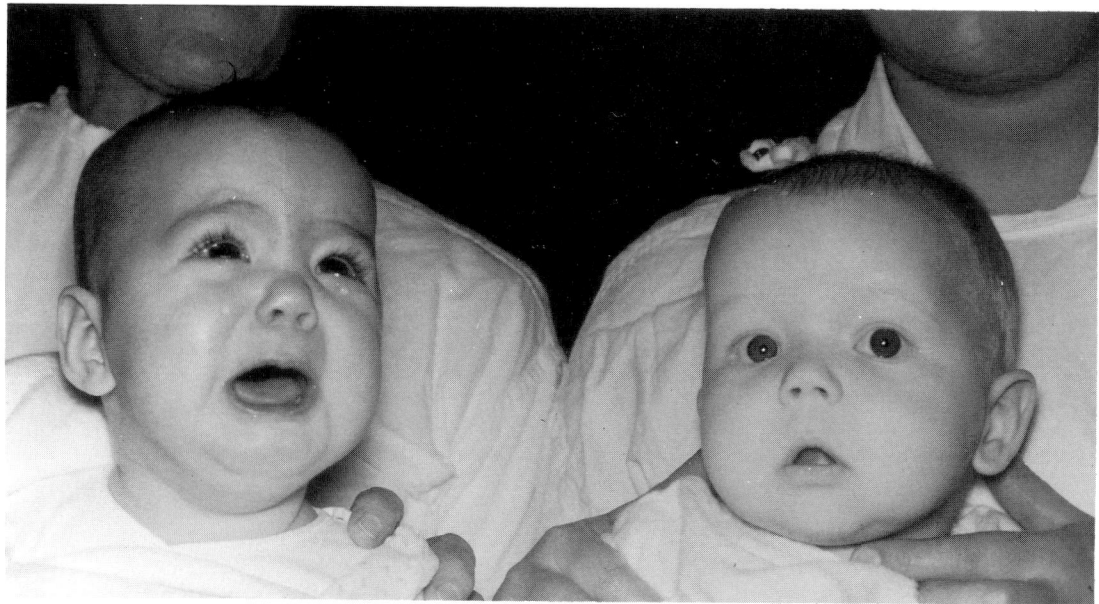

Fig. 18.4 Iron-deficiency anaemia due to CMA.

CMA, though often diminished [62], are not always absent [44]. Such deficiencies seen in these babies may therefore be secondary to CMA [32] and in this respect differ from the lactase deficiencies seen in ethnic groups that do not ordinarily drink milk after weaning.

Respiratory allergies

A recurrent or persistent rhinorrhoea or nasal stuffiness [36], recurrent croup and recurrent bronchitis with or without wheezing are all common manifestations of CMA. Symptoms are sometimes persistent, at other times they are recurrent or episodic, the child appearing to recover from one attack of pneumonia or bronchiolitis only to develop another in spite of the fact that he has remained on his cow's milk formula all along. The most severe manifestation of respiratory CMA is Heiner's syndrome [34]—the child having repeated attacks of pneumonia associated with pulmonary infiltrates, haemosiderosis, anaemia and failure to thrive. Multiple precipitin bands to cow's milk proteins are present in the serum. The disease is not IgE mediated and skin prick and RAST tests to milk are negative [41]. There are more than 25 different proteins in cow's milk and the proteins which most commonly cause allergic reactions are β-lactoglobulin, casein, α-lactalbumin and bovine serum albumin [27].

Neurological manifestations

Irritability and restlessness in babies are not usually thought of as being due to an adverse reaction to a food but they certainly can be, and in infancy cow's milk is the commonest offender [8, 27]. Irritability would appear to be the counterpart in infancy of the tension fatigue syndrome in the child and depression in the adult.

Babies with CMA commonly have more than one symptom, the majority having several, e.g. eczema and rhinorrhoea or recurrent diarrhoea and recurrent bronchitis. Many are also often sensitive to more than one food for they tend to become sensitive to foods which they are given repeatedly. It is probably for this reason that babies sensitive to cow's milk when placed on soya formulae often become sensitive to the latter. Concomitant sensitivities to egg, citrus fruits and tomato are also common [26].

Age at onset of symptoms

One might expect symptoms to start soon after the introduction of cow's milk, sometimes even after the first feed, but this is not always the case. In one series [25] symptoms started in just over a quarter (28%) within three days of the baby starting to take cow's milk or a cow's milk formula, in 41% within seven days and in 68% within a month. Why it is that in some infants symptoms start almost immediately and in others later we do not know, but the later development of allergy seems often to be triggered by infections. This has been shown to be the case by Harrison et al [33]. We, too, have noticed that measles and even ordinary inoculations may trigger the development of an allergy to cow's milk. Viral infections in infancy are often associated with a rise in IgE levels [20]. We would speculate that such infections may act as adjuvants in initiating the development of new allergies. If the patient is seen when he is older and the history indicates that symptoms first started soon after he was placed on a formula and have persisted, milk should be considered a potential cause of his problems.

SYMPTOMS DUE TO CMA IN THE OLDER CHILD AND ADULT

There are no hard and fast data regarding the incidence of CMA in the older child and adult but the following disorders can be milk related, though cow's milk is not necessarily the commonest precipitating factor in any one patient.

Respiratory

Allergic rhinitis

Cow's milk in our experience is as common a precipitating factor of perennial allergic rhinitis in childhood as it is in the infant. It is also common in the adult [21] and should be suspected if symptoms date from infancy, if they are not seasonal and if prick skin tests are negative. Although symptoms usually are perennial they are often more severe in winter than in summer, possibly because of a concomitant house dust allergy which increases the allergic load during the winter months. Another possible reason is because children often prefer juices and carbonated beverages to milk in the summer. Whatever the reason, there appear to be some children who are sensitive to cow's milk in the winter months but not in the summer.

Recurrent bronchitis

This, like a recurrent nasal stuffiness, may be milk related both in children and in adults [21] and should be suspected in the adult if there is a child in the family with a respiratory milk sensitivity, if symptoms are perennial and if the patient is fond of and drinks much milk.

Asthma

Asthma, if seasonal, or by history or prick test is obviously due to inhalants, will probably not have a dietary component. Milk allergy should be considered as a cause when symptoms are perennial, if prick skin tests are negative, if the patient is fond of and drinks much milk together with ice cream and cheese, and if a close relative is known to be allergic to milk (Table 18.2). Under these circumstances the patient should be asked to avoid milk and dairy products for at least two weeks or longer. If his symptoms clear he should be given milk in abundance to see if they return. If they do, milk and dairy products should thereafter be avoided.

Table 18.2 Symptoms indicating milk may be a cause of asthma.

Symptoms are perennial
Skin prick tests negative
A family history of milk allergy is present
Likes and drinks much milk

Wraith [67] studying 119 food-allergic patients of whom 100 had asthma (34 with eczema), 7 had allergic rhinitis and 12 had urticaria, found that symptoms were precipitated by milk in 16 instances (wheat with 24 cases was the commonest food to precipitate a reaction). In no instance did milk cause an immediate reaction, clearly differing in this respect from classical IgE-mediated allergy. In only four was the RAST positive indicating that RAST and prick tests do not usually help to identify the asthmatic whose asthma is triggered by milk. A high index of suspicion combined with positive results in the avoidance and challenge test are the only sure ways of identifying such subjects. Milk may also play a permissive role in facilitating exercise-induced asthma (see Chapter 27).

Gastrointestinal

Milk-induced gastrointestinal problems are relatively easy to identify and treat in infancy. Although it is generally thought that symptoms clear when the child is one or two years old, this is not always the case. The childhood equivalent of the irritable bowel syndrome (IBS)—recurrent spells of abdominal pain, looseness of stools and/or constipation sometimes leading to incontinence and encopresis—

may be milk or lactose induced. Milk should certainly be considered if the child was milk intolerant in infancy and is now drinking large quantities of it, or if he dislikes milk but is encouraged to drink it by well-meaning parents. There are, however, many other important causes of disturbed bowel function in children including coeliac disease, Crohn's disease and ulcerative colitis. Although coeliac disease, Crohn's disease and ulcerative colitis may have dietary components it is important to exclude these disorders before entertaining a diagnosis of CMA (see Chapter 32).

Irritable bowel syndrome

In the adult the IBS comprises a group of symptoms; spells of abdominal pain, flatulence, intermittent diarrhoea and sometimes constipation, with no identifiable pathology. It has been looked on as a functional disorder with a strong psychogenic component [53]. Weser and his colleagues [64] however found that 14 of 27 patients studied had an associated lactase deficiency and eight of these improved remarkably on milk-free and dairy-product-free diets. Bayless et al [2] went on to demonstrate that lactase deficiencies were much more common in North American Blacks (occurring in 19 of 20 patients studied) than in American Whites (present in only two of 20 patients studied). When present it was nearly always associated with symptoms of the IBS with an onset at or around puberty when lactase activity tends to diminish (see Chapter 32).

The racial incidence of lactase deficiency has been mapped out by Kretchmer [40]. It is present in many African groups as well as in the Chinese and Japanese and in most races living in the Orient. If cow's milk ever becomes a staple of the Oriental diet it will almost certainly initiate an outbreak of the IBS.

Jones [39] noting that a patient with the IBS was made worse by bran decided to look into the possibility that foods other than milk and lactose caused this syndrome. She found that 14 of 21 patients with this disorder lost their symptoms on oligoantigenic diets and that when foods were reintroduced wheat caused a relapse in nine, corn in five, milk and dairy products in four and coffee, tea and citrus fruits in nine others. Milk, quite apart from its lactose content, can also cause the IBS. Even Bentley [3] who considers that psychological factors are of primary importance in the aetiology of the IBS found that of 19 patients studied the syndrome was precipitated by foods in three and that in two of these milk, not lactose, was the culprit. Twelve of the 14 patients studied including the three with proven food allergy, were found to have psychiatric problems, depression being the commonest. Although he thought that the psychiatric problem was primary it is possible that it accompanied rather than caused the IBS, for psychiatric problems seem to be a common accompaniment of food intolerances [46].

Vascular: urticaria, purpura and headaches

Milk can, but does not frequently, cause urticaria [8, 27] and purpura [7]. It is however a much more frequent cause of vascular headaches. The latter are not only common but they are commonly triggered by milk. Robert Burton [6] in 'The anatomy of melancholy' published in 1620 stated that: 'Milk and all that comes from milk are not good for those that are subject to headache.'

Headaches, whether manifestations of common or classical migraine, can be triggered by many factors, including inhalants such as perfumes and cigarette smoke, physical factors such as bright lights, noises and weather changes, but also by foods. Speer [58] in a study of 143 cases of headache found that in approximately two-thirds foods were implicated and in half of these foods alone were to blame. The foods implicated most frequently were cow's milk and dairy products which precipitated headaches in 45 of the 143 cases. Monro [49] in her extensive review of the literature on food allergy and migraine found that cow's milk was one of the commonest foods to be implicated. Grant [28] in a series of 60 migraineurs was able to implicate cow's milk in 37% of the cases; Eggar [15] in a more recent study found that 78 of 88 children with migraine were relieved of their headaches by dietary means alone. Cow's milk was the commonest single food to cause a headache (in 27 cases) and cheese caused headaches in 13 (see Chapters 37 and 38).

The urinary bladder: enuresis

There is still no consensus as to the cause of nocturnal enuresis but it is associated with a small bladder capacity [16, 59]. Some enuretics have normal bladder control during the day time but not during the night time (nocturnal enuresis). Others are also caught short during the day time and wet their pants before they can reach the toilet (diurnal enuresis). A few children surprisingly are wet only during the day time, being dry at night. It is probable that all enuretic children with the exception of those presenting with polyuria due to either diabetes mellitus or insipidus have small capacity bladders.

Bray [4] was the first to suggest that enuresis might be allergic in origin and in the four cases he reported foods alone were incriminated in two, foods and inhalants in one and inhalants alone in the fourth. Milk was not one of the foods mentioned by him. Breneman [5] who considers enuresis to be allergic in origin found that milk was the commonest food to be incriminated. McKendry [47] compared the effectiveness of dietary management with imipramine and conditioning with a wet alarm, and found that dietary management was ineffective. Only one child in 64 became dry on dieting whereas 23 of 43 treated with conditioning became dry. It is interesting to note that although just over half the children who were treated with dietary exclusion became dryer, a few actually became wetter. Milk was one of the foods excluded. We have found that the exclusion of milk and dairy products together with a so-called salicylate-free diet frequently leads to an increase in bladder capacity, and in approximately a third of the children to dryness.

The urinary bladder of the enuretic is partially contracted, being in spasm, and in this respect resembles the spasm of the bronchus seen in the asthmatic. The partially contracted bladder is sometimes referred to as the uninhibited bladder for the enuretic cannot, in contrast to the normal child, relax his bladder to accommodate more urine. Spasm is relieved in some instances by dietary exclusion and in others by imipramine [17]. Because the bladder is in spasm the child suffers frequency and urgency and cannot go through the night without emptying his bladder and wetting the bed. Urgency and frequency are often seen in the adult but in the adult they are more frequently due to beverages such as coffee and tea than to milk (see Chapters 23 and 43a).

Neurological and behavioural disorders

Many authors have noted that allergic individuals have disturbances of behaviour, commonly irritability and/or fatigue, which subside with good allergy control. These individuals have been said by some to have 'allergic toxaemia' and by others [57] to have 'the tension fatigue syndrome'. Crook [11] has given details of 50 children with the syndrome suggesting that it is relatively common. Feingold [18], who emphasized the hyperkinetic aspects of the syndrome, has suggested that it is due to salicylates and so-called salicylate-containing foods. The children with this disorder usually have a short attention span, and the syndrome has therefore been renamed 'the attention deficit disorder'. The subject would not have been included in this chapter had not cow's milk been incriminated as a relatively common cause of the problem.

Speer [57], who coined the term 'the tension fatigue syndrome', mentioned in his initial report the foods which precipitated symptoms in the six cases which he reported. In four milk was an important offender precipitating irritability and restlessness; when milk and dairy products together with the other foods to which they were sensitive were avoided, all the children became bright, cheerful and contented. Crook also found milk to be a common offender, the behavioural disturbances being milk-induced in 28 of the 50 patients reported by him. Rapp [54] in a smaller series of eight patients found that milk together with other foods was incriminated in six. In these six, milk caused headache in one, hyperactivity in three, spells of depression and crying in two and respiratory, not neurological, problems in one.

Interestingly, Egger [15] studying the relationship between diet and migraine noted that of 88 patients studied, 41 had associated behavioural disorders. In 36 behaviour improved or normalized on an oligoantigenic diet. No mention was made of the foods responsible for the behavioural changes but cow's milk was the food which most commonly caused migraine, and it is possible that it contributed to the behavioural changes seen in many of the children he studied (see Chapter 38b).

Hyperactivity: attention deficit disorder

There has been much controversy over the aetiology of hyperactivity or the attention deficit disorder [50]. Feingold, while emphasizing the relationship between hyperactivity and food colours and additives unfortunately overlooked the many other foods that have been reported to cause it. The result was that double-blind studies aimed at confirming or disproving his hypothesis found little supportive evidence. Allergies are very individual, some children being sensitive to one food and others to another. Each child must be his own control and diets must be individualized as in Egger's study [15] if they are to be informative.

Food-related disturbances of behaviour also occur in infancy and in the adult. In infancy, irritability and sleeplessness [8, 27] as already mentioned are probably the commonest manifestations, milk being the commonest precipitating factor. In the adult, a sense of profound exhaustion and lassitude is the characteristic component of the 'tension fatigue syndrome'. Weitkamp et al [63] have recently shown that depression in the adult may have an immunological basis—the gene which carries it lies on chromosome 6, closely linked to the HLA locus. Depression, like classical allergic diseases such as asthma and hay fever, also runs in families. The concept that it too may be triggered by environmental antigens, such as milk, may therefore not be too far fetched. Schizophrenia is another relatively common psychiatric disorder which may have a dietary component for it is commoner in coeliacs than would be expected by chance and is sometimes helped by a diet free from milk and cereals [12, 13].

Arthritis

It is well known that polyarthritis and fever can be a manifestation of serum sickness and penicillin allergy. When this is the case, the relationship between the polyarthritis and the injection of either horse serum or penicillin is self-evident. There are only a few reports of foods triggering polyarthritis [10]. This may be because when foods are taken daily and the onset of the arthritis is so gradual, the relationship to diet is not suspected. It is only when there is an unusually brisk response to a food that the relationship between the food and arthritis is obvious (see Chapter 41).

Zeller [68] reported four cases of polyarthritis due to foods, two being triggered by cow's milk and a third by beef. Marshall et al [48], in a study of rheumatoid arthritis, first fasted patients in environmental units and then gave them different foods one by one. Foods were incriminated in all instances. The commonest foods to trigger a relapse of arthritis were red meats and cereals, the best tolerated were vegetables and fruits, and milk and dairy products assumed an intermediate position. Cow's milk given orally has also been shown experimentally to be capable of inducing rheumatoid arthritis-like lesions in rabbits [9] and has also been reported as a cause of rheumatoid arthritis in man [52]. In patients with food-induced rheumatoid arthritis, challenges have been shown to lead to a fall in serotonin and to a rise in serum 5-hydroxyindole acetic acid [42].

ALLERGIES IN THE BREAST-FED BABY

Breast milk in addition to containing the natural ingredients of breast milk contains traces of foods ingested by the mother. This was first shown more than 50 years ago by

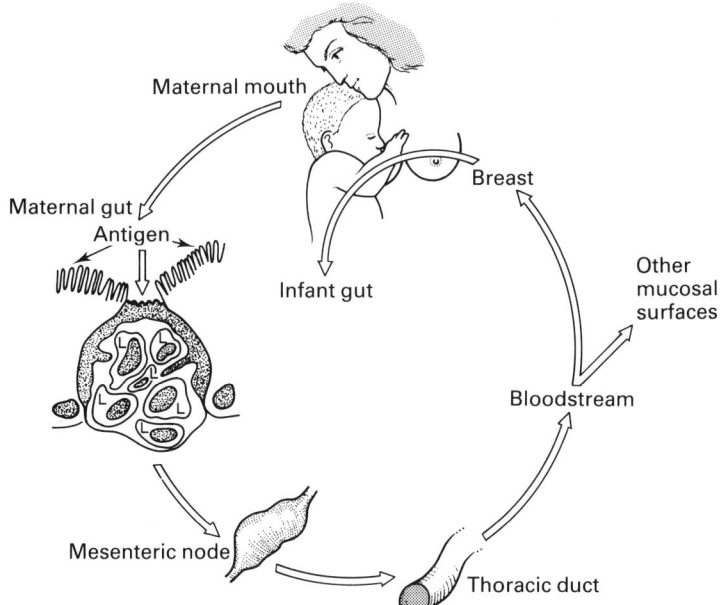

Fig. 18.5 Circulation of possible food antigens. From the mother's gut via M cells, food reaches the mesenteric nodes, thoracic duct and then the bloodstream. From there it is secreted by the breast and thus reaches the infant gut.

Shannon [56]. The traces of food antigen just like the traces of food that are absorbed by all of us do not usually cause problems but may do so in hypersensitive babies. Paediatricians and allergists [51, 60] 60 years ago were very much aware of the development of allergies in breast-fed babies to foods ingested by the mother. The problem became less apparent when formula feeding became fashionable but has become more frequent with the popularization of breast feeding (Fig. 18.5).

Symptoms

The main manifestation of allergy that concerned physicians 60 years ago was eczema and though this was relatively uncommon it became more common by a factor of seven when formula feeding became fashionable [29]. We are now aware that recurrent rhinorrhoea, wheezy bronchitis, vomiting and diarrhoea, and even colic [37] can be manifestations of allergy and in the evaluation of possible allergies in breast-fed babies these are the symptoms that should be looked for.

During the past 25 years 81 breast-fed babies have been seen who developed adverse reactions to foods being ingested by the mother [22]; 35 of the cases were seen during the past four years. The recent increase in cases seen may be due in part to the increase in the prevalence of breast feeding—90% of the babies leaving our hospital at the present time are on the breast—but it is also due to a greater awareness of the problem by nursing mothers and family physicians. The diagnosis was established in each case by first demonstrating relief of the baby's symptoms when the mother avoided the food or foods to which her baby was sensitive and their return when she again took the food.

Table 18.3 Presenting symptoms in 81 breast-fed babies sensitive to foods being taken by the mother.

Symptom	Percentage
Colic	40
Rhinorrhoea	23
Vomiting	21
Diarrhoea	21
Bronchitis	20
Eczema	16
Diaper dermatitis	4
Urticaria	2

The symptoms produced are listed in Table 18.3 and are similar to those seen in formula-fed babies who are allergic to cow's milk. The foods found commonly to precipitate symptoms are listed in Table 18.4. Cow's milk was by far the commonest food to be incriminated (81%), probably because mothers are encouraged to drink large quantities of milk when pregnant or when breast feeding. Egg, wheat and citrus fruits were the next most common foods to cause problems but many foods can precipitate symptoms in the baby.

Table 18.4 Foods taken by the mother which precipitated symptoms in her baby ($n=81$).

Food	Percentage
Cow's milk	81
Egg	15
Wheat	11
Citrus fruits	10
Chocolate	2

Time of onset

Symptoms first develop in some 10% of the affected babies during the first week of life, suggesting that the baby may have already been sensitized in utero. Symptoms develop in another one-third during the next three weeks, in 40% during the second, third or fourth months, and in the remainder at a later date. It is possible that in some babies sensitization is triggered by the inadvertent administration of cow's milk in the nursery but a careful enquiry in our patients suggested that this was rarely if ever the case. Once sensitization has occurred the introduction of formula at a later date always triggers a brisk, immediate, IgE-mediated reaction. Following such an exposure it was not unusual for the baby's symptoms to persist while still on the breast. The mother has then had to avoid cow's milk and dairy products for the baby to be symptom free once more.

Treatment: avoidance

As cow's milk taken by the mother is the commonest food to precipitate symptoms in the baby it is obviously the first food which the mother of a sensitized baby should avoid. It is also, fortunately, an easy food to avoid. In children with eczema, asthma, urticaria or severe vomiting, a prick test and RAST may provide additional confirmation that cow's milk and/or other foods taken by the mother are precipitating symptoms in the baby. It is much better to identify these foods than to take the baby off the breast and to substitute a formula. If the baby is placed on a cow's milk formula he will probably react adversely to it and may also react adversely to other formulae, with his final management being even more troublesome than it was when he was on the breast alone.

Babies who are sensitive via breast milk to foods taken by the mother are ipso facto highly allergic individuals. There is no easy way of distinguishing these babies from others who though apparently equally allergic tolerate foods taken by their mothers. When histories are taken it is often found that the mothers of these allergic babies have consumed, while pregnant, large quantities of the food or foods to which their babies have been sensitized and this may have facilitated their sensitization [55]. However, sensitivities to foods such as peanut and egg can develop in babies whose mothers, because they disliked or were sensitive to these foods, avoided them. The complete exclusion of any one food for at least the last two trimesters of pregnancy is not easy and cross-reactions between foods may nullify the attempt to prevent the sensitization of the baby. It is difficult to be sure that it is no more than coincidence if a mother who having had one baby sensitized to foods that she had eaten and who then avoided these same foods when next pregnant finds that the second baby was free from the allergies. Nevertheless, a programme of food avoidance should be recommended in such cases.

If food avoidance by the mother does not bring relief to the baby a trial of oral cromolyn can be entertained. The starting dose for the baby is 20 mg increasing rapidly if necessary by 20 mg increments to 100 mg dissolved in 5–10 ml hot water 20 minutes before each feed. Cromolyn while not usually helpful has occasionally relieved symptoms dramatically. In two instances, cromolyn given to the mother brought relief to the child, possibly through reducing the mother's absorption of the offending antigen.

Two forms of CMA reaction

Although symptoms produced by cow's milk in the breast- and formula-fed baby are very similar the immunological mechanisms involved are very different [24]. The breast-fed baby is reacting to foods being taken by his mother and to trace amounts of those antigens. If he is given cow's milk as such, he will have a severe IgE-mediated reaction. He is obviously highly atopic and prick skin tests and RAST are usually strongly positive with elevated IgE levels (Table 18.5). The symptoms

Table 18.5 Characteristics of cow's milk allergic responses: route of administration.

	Via breast milk	Directly orally
Quantity of allergen	Trace amounts	Large quantity
Skin prick test	Positive	Negative
RAST	Positive	Negative
IgE	Elevated	Normal
Immediate clinical reaction	+ +	−
Delayed clinical reaction	−	+ +
'Reactivity'	Atopic	Non-atopic

in the formula-fed baby, on the other hand, though essentially the same are triggered by large amounts of antigen and are not associated with severe immediate reactions, or with positive prick and RASTs, or high levels of IgE. These two types of CMA are very clearly delineated and as our understanding of food allergy increases it will no doubt be found that most allergies to foods will fall into one or other of these two categories. The brisk reaction in the breast-fed baby suggests that the hallmark of the atopic individual is his brisk response to low-dose stimulation and though this is a handicap in modern society, for it facilitates the development of atopic disease, it may have given him an advantage in primitive society when his survival was often dependent on the speed of his immunological response to infections [23].

REFERENCES

1 Bahna SL, Heiner DC: Allergies to milk. New York: Grune and Stratton, 1980.

2 Bayless TM, Rosensweig NS: A racial difference in incidence of lactase deficiency. JAMA 1966; 197: 968-72.

3 Bentley SJ, Pearson DJ, Rix KJB: Food hypersensitivity in irritable bowel syndrome. Lancet 1983; ii: 295-7.

4 Bray GW: Enuresis of allergic origin. Arch Dis Child 1931; 6: 251-3.

5 Breneman JC: Nocturnal enuresis, a treatment regimen for general use. Ann Allergy 1965; 23: 185-91.

6 Burton R: The anatomy of melancholy. 1621. In: Dell F, Jordan-Smith, eds. New York: Tudor Publishing Company, 1955; 191. (Quoted by Speer F: The many facets of migraine. Ann Allergy 1975; 34: 273-85.)

7 Caffrey EA, Sladen GE, Isaacs PET, Clark KGA: Thrombocytopenia caused by cow's milk. Lancet 1981; ii: 316.

8 Clein NW: Cow's milk allergy in infants. Pediatr Clin North Am 1954; 1: 949-62.

9 Coombs RRA, Oldham G: Early rheumatoid-like joint lesions in rabbits drinking cow's milk. Int Arch Allergy Appl Immunol 1981; 64: 287-92.

10 Criep LH: Allergy of joints. J Bone Joint Surg [Am] 1946; 28: 276-9.

11 Crook WG, Harrison WW, Crawford SE, Emerson BS: Systemic manifestations due to allergy. Pediatrics 1961; 27: 790-9.

12 Dohan FC: Coeliac disease and schizophrenia. Lancet 1970; i: 897-8.

13 Dohan FC, Grasberger JC: Relapsed schizophrenia: earlier discharge from hospital after cereal-free, milk-free diet. Am J Psychiatry 1973; 130: 685-8.

14 Durand P, ed.: Disorders due to intestinal defective carbohydrate digestion and absorption. Rome: Il Pensiero Scientifico 1964.

15 Egger J, Carter CM, Wilson J et al: Is migraine food allergy? Lancet 1983; ii: 865-9.

16 Esperanca M, Gerrard JW: Nocturnal enuresis. Can Med Assoc J 1969; 101: 324-7.

17 Esperanca M, Gerrard JW: Nocturnal enuresis. Comparison of the effect of imipramine and dietary restriction on bladder capacity. Can Med Assoc J 1969; 101: 721-4.

18 Feingold BF: Why your child is hyperactive. New York: Random House, 1975.

19 Ford JD, Haworth JC: The fecal excretion of sugars in children. J Pediatr 1963; 63: 988-90.

20 Frick OL, German DF, Mills J: Development of allergy in children. I. Association with virus infections. J Allergy Clin Immunol 1979; 63: 228-41.

21 Gerrard JW: Familial recurrent rhinorrhea and bronchitis due to cow's milk. JAMA 1966; 198: 605-7.

22 Gerrard JW: Allergies in breast-fed babies to foods ingested by the mother. Clin Rev Allergy 1984; 2: 143-9.

23 Gerrard JW: Risk factors in developing allergic disease. Immunology and Allergy Practice 1984; 60: 17-24.

24 Gerrard JW, Shenassa M: Food allergy: two common types as seen in breast and formula-fed babies. Ann Allergy 1983; 50: 375-9.

25 Gerrard JW, Lubos MC, Hardy LW et al: Milk allergy: clinical picture and familial incidence. Can Med Assoc J. 1967; 97: 780-5.

26 Gerrard JW, MacKenzie JWA, Goluboff N et al: Cow's milk allergy: prevalence in an unselected series of newborns. Acta Paediatr Scand 1973: (suppl) 234: 3-21.

27 Goldman AS, Anderson DW, Sellars WA et al: Milk allergy. I. Oral challenge with milk and isolated proteins in allergic children. Pediatrics 1963; 32: 425-43.

28 Grant ECG: Food allergies and migraine. Lancet 1979; i: 966-9.

29 Grulee CG, Sanford HN: The influence of breast and artifical feeding on infantile eczema. J Pediatr 1936; 8: 223-5.

30 Grulee CG, Sanford HN, Heron PH: Breast and artificial feeding. JAMA 1934; 103: 735.

31 Halpern SR, Sellars WA, Johnson RB et al: Development of childhood allergy in infants fed breast, soy, or cow milk. J Allergy Clin Immunol 1973; 51: 139-51.

32 Harrison M: Sugar malabsorption in cow's milk protein intolerance. Lancet 1974; i: 360-1.

33 Harrison M, Kilby A, Walker-Smith J et al: Cow's-milk-protein intolerance: a possible association with gastroenteritis, lactose intolerance and IgA deficiency. Br Med J 1976; 1: 1501-4.

34 Heiner DC, Sears JW, Kniker WT: Multiple precipitins to cow's milk in chronic respiratory disease. A syndrome including poor growth, gastrointestinal symptoms, evidence of allergy, iron deficiency anemia and pulmonary hemosiderosis. Am J Dis Child 1962; 103: 634-54.

35 Hide W, Guyer BM: Cow's milk intolerance in Isle of Wight infants. Br J Clin Pract 1983; 37: 285-7.

36 Ingall M, Glaser J, Meltzer RS, Dreyfuss EM: Allergic rhinitis in early infancy. Review of the literature and report of a case in a newborn. Pediatrics 1965; 35: 105-12.

37 Jakobsson I, Lindberg T: Cow's milk as a cause of infantile colic in breast fed infants. Lancet 1978; ii: 437-9.

38 Jakobsson I, Lindberg T: A prospective study of cow's milk protein intolerance in Swedish infants. Acta Paediatr Scand 1979; 68: 853-9.

39 Jones VA, McLaughlan P, Shorthouse M et al: Food intolerance: a major factor in the pathogenesis of the irritable bowel syndrome. Lancet 1982; ii: 1115-17.

40 Kretchmer N: Memorial lecture: lactose and lactase—a historical perspective. Gastroenterology 1971; 61: 805-13.

41 Lee SK, Kniker WT, Cook CD, Heiner DC: Cow's-milk-induced pulmonary disease in children. Adv Pediatr 1978; 25: 39-57.

42 Little CH, Stewart AG, Fennessy MR: Platelet serotonin release in rheumatoid arthritis: a study in food-intolerant patients. Lancet 1983; ii: 297-9.

43 Liu H-Y, Tsao MU, Moore B, Giday Z: Bovine milk-protein induced intestinal malabsorption of lactose and fat in infants. Gastroenterology 1967; 54: 27-34.

44 Lubos MC, Gerrard JW, Buchan DJ: Disaccharidase activities in milk sensitive and celiac patients. J Pediatr 1967; 70: 325-31.

45 MacFarlane PI, Miller V: Human milk in the management of protracted diarrhoea of infancy. Arch Dis Child 1984; 59: 260-5.

46 Mackarness R: Not all in the mind. London: Pan, 1976.

47 McKendry JB, Stewart DA, Khanna F, Netley C: Primary enuresis; relative success of three methods of treatment. Can Med Assoc J 1975; 113: 953-5.

48 Marshall RT, Stroud RM, Kroker GF et al: Food challenge effects on fasted rheumatoid arthritis patients: a multicenter study. Clin Ecol 1984; 2: 181-90.

49 Monro J: Food allergy and migraine. Clin Immunol Allergy 1982; 2: 137–63.

50 National Institutes of Health Consensus Development Panel: Defined diets in childhood hyperactivity. Bethesda, Maryland Office for Medical Applications of Research. NIH Building, No. 1, 1982.

51 O'Keefe ES: The relation of food to infantile eczema. Boston Med Surg J 1920; 183: 569.

52 Parke AL, Hughes GRV: Rheumatoid arthritis and food: a case study. Br Med J 1981; 282: 2027–9.

53 Pearson DJ, Rix KJB, Bentley SJ: Food allergy: how much is in the mind? Lancet 1983; i: 1259–1961.

54 Rapp DJ: Food allergy treatment for hyperkinesis. J Learning Disabilities 1979; 12: 608–16.

55 Rattner B: A possible causal factor of food allergy in certain infants. Am J Dis Child 1936; 36: 277–88.

56 Shannon WR: Demonstration of food proteins in human breast milk by anaphylactic experiments in guinea pigs. Am J Dis Child 1921; 22: 223.

57 Speer F: The allergic tension fatigue in children. Ann Allergy 1954; 12: 168–71.

58 Speer F: Allergy and migraine: a clinical study. Headache 1971; 11: 63–7.

59 Starfield B: Functional bladder capacity in enuretic and non-enuretic children. Pediatrics 1967; 70: 777–81.

60 Talbot FB: Eczema in childhood. Med Clin North Am 1918; 1: 985–96.

61 Waldmann T, Wochner RD, Laster L, Gordon RS: Allergic gastroenteropathy. N. Engl J Med 1967; 276: 761–9.

62 Walker-Smith J, Harrison M, Kilby A et al: Cow's milk-sensitive enteropathy. Arch Dis Child 1978; 53: 375–80.

63 Weitkamp LR, Stancer HC, Persod E et al: Depressive disorders and HLA: a gene on chromosome 6 that can affect behavior. N Engl J Med 1981; 305: 1301–13.

64 Weser E, Rubin W, Ross L, Sleisenger MH: Lactase deficiency in patients with the 'irritable colon syndrome'. N Engl J Med 1965; 273: 1070–5.

65 Wilson JF, Heiner DC, Lahey ME: Milk-induced gastrointestinal bleeding in infants with hypochromic microcytic anemia. JAMA 1964; 189: 122–6.

66 Woodbury RM: The relation between artificial feeding and infant mortality. M J Hyg 1922; 2: 668.

67 Wraith DG, Merrett J, Roth A et al: Recognition of food-allergic patients and their allergens by the RAST technique and clinical investigation. Clin Allergy 1979; 9: 25–36.

68 Zeller M: Rheumatoid arthritis—food allergy as a factor. Ann Allergy 1949; 7: 200–5.

Chapter 19
Fish Allergy and the Codfish Allergen Model

Kjell Aas

Introduction

Allergy to fish plays a classical role in the history of the field of allergology. The passive transfer experiments performed by Prausnitz and Küstner introduced immunological thinking and methods into the field of atopic allergy [35]. Küstner was allergic to fish. His fish allergy was of a rather peculiar type since he reacted only to cooked fish. This kind of fish allergy has never been seen by this author whose approximately 300 fish-allergic patients react to both raw and cooked fish.

Aliquots of Küstner's serum were injected into the skin of Prausnitz. 24 hours later the same sites were injected with fish extract. This produced a flare and wheal reaction. This so-called Prausnitz-Küstner test was the forerunner to the discovery of immunoglobulin E (IgE) and the development of methods for the demonstration and quantitation of IgE antibodies. On the antigen side, the major allergen, allergen M, in codfish represents one of the most advanced allergen models investigated. This purified allergen has been extensively characterized with respect to chemical and immunological properties, as reviewed elsewhere [1, 6, 7, 9, 10–13, 16, 25, 26, 28], and it has served as a model for development and evaluation of immunological methods used in allergy diagnosis and research [8, 15, 17–21]. Furthermore, allergen M is the only natural allergen in which a major allergenic (IgE-binding antigenic) determinant has been characterized and synthesized [7, 26].

CLINICAL ASPECTS OF FISH ALLERGY

Prevalence of fish allergy

Allergy to fish is not a common problem on a worldwide basis but is not infrequent in fish-eating and fish-processing communities. Fish allergens are among the most potent and they may act as both an inhalant and a food allergen. It is possible that it is the inhalation of active allergens which has the greatest sensitizing potency.

In fish-exposed communities, active fish allergens may be demonstrated even in individual house dust samples and in some house dust extracts. In Scandinavian countries fish allergy is among the most predominant allergies in patients allergic to food. Dannaeus and Inganaes found 32 cases of fish allergy among 82 children with food sensitivities (55 were also allergic to egg).

In Norway it is estimated that fish allergy occurs in about one individual per 1000. The incidence is greater in children and young adults. Aas [2] found and investigated 89 cases of fish allergy in 825 children referred for rather severe asthma and/or urticaria (85% of whom were shown to be allergic). Fish was found to provoke asthma in 50 of the children investigated for asthma (6.9%) (Table 19.1). In 76 children exposure to fish resulted in urticaria. Fish hypersensitivity was the only cause of urticaria in 35% of these.

Clinical presentation

The fish-allergic patients investigated suffered as a group from more severe asthma and more multivalent allergies than the average allergic patient in the clinic in question. As this clinic is generally consulted for the more severe allergic diseases, this may have resulted in a higher percentage of patients with fish hypersensitivity than is representative for the total number of asthma and urticaria patients in Norway. Hypersensitivity to fish as the only cause of asthma was demonstrated only in five patients. In three more children fish was the only cause of asthma that could be demonstrated, but in these patients the fish allergy did not provide a satisfactory explanation for all the asthmatic attacks experienced. Additional allergens causing asthma were demonstrated in 85% of the patients. Fish allergy as the only cause of urticaria was found in 32 of the 76 children with urticaria due to fish allergy. Other causes of urticaria were hen's eggs (41 children), peas, nuts, animal dander, cow's milk, wheat, raw potatoes, carrots, beans, strawberries, hips and, in one patient, a special colour pencil. Non-allergic factors contributed to asthma in the majority of patients (Table 19.1).

In 34 children fish acted as an inhalant allergen provoking asthma when odours or vapours from fish were inhaled in sufficient amounts. In an additional eight children such emanations resulted in cough paroxysms without directly provoking asthma. Symptoms related to fish allergy in the patients were as follows: urticaria (76 patients), asthma (50), nasal reactions (25), nausea (24), eczema (23), conjunctival reactions (23), general malaise (20), vomiting (19), cough (19), itching without observed skin eruptions (19), general irritability and nervousness always associated with objective symptoms (12), laryngeal reactions (11), headache (6), abdominal pains (5), diarrhoea (4), bloody stools (1).

Table 19.1 Allergies in patients with asthma and urticaria.

	Number	Percentage of total
Number studied	825	
Allergy to fish	89	10.8
Allergies demonstrated	701	85.0
Asthma with fish provocation	57	6.9
Urticaria with fish provocation	76	9.2
Fish as only cause of asthma	5	0.6
Fish as only cause of urticaria	32	3.9
Urticaria with egg provocation	41	5.0

Natural history

The age of the child at which the hypersensitivity to fish was first observed varied considerably (Fig. 19.1). In most instances fish had been introduced into the diet when the child was 6–12 months old. Twenty-eight children were reported to show hypersensitivity reactions on the very first occasion they were given fish. In two cases the mother reported that the infant had reacted to her breast milk after she herself had eaten fish. During the study period a third infant was seen in whom this phenomenon was observed by the author (see below and Chapter 18). No correlation was found between the use of cod liver oil (whether unwanted reaction had occurred or not) and the early appearance of hypersensitivity reactions to fish.

Kajosaari [32] found no differences in fish allergy between those who had avoided fish during the first year of life and those who had fish introduced earlier. However, the numbers were too small for any conclusions to be made by statistical analysis. In her material, fish allergy subsided during the first six years in the majority of her patients in contrast to the cases reported by Aas [2]. In his material the clinical symptoms of fish allergy disappeared

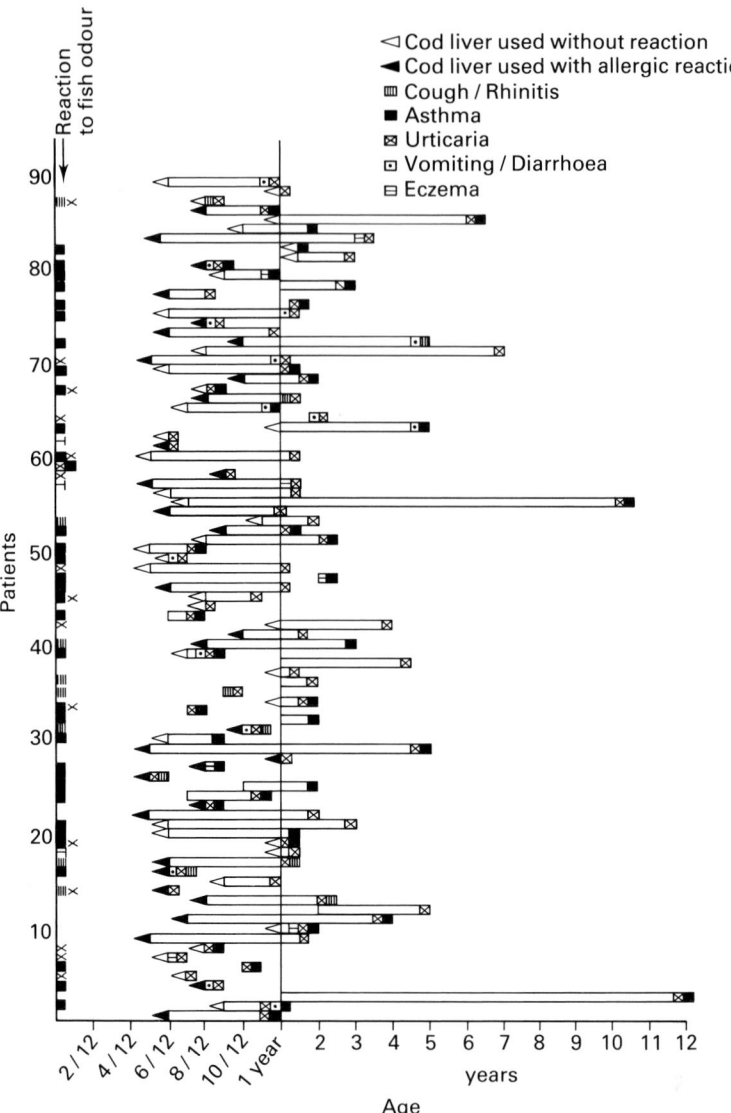

Fig. 19.1 Overview of the author's fish-hypersensitive patients [2]: time when fish was introduced into the diet (left vertical line of each horizontal rod) to first observation of clinical allergy to fish (left vertical border of the symptom symbol in question). Symbols indicate the most prominent symptoms observed for each patient. Symbols along the ordinate indicate reactions to the inhalation of fish emanations. See legend in figure.

spontaneously within a four-year period in only five patients and in a further three it was found that the degree of clinical hypersensitivity had been markedly reduced. The skin test reactions remained unaltered in these eight patients. In two patients the degree of hypersensitivity seemed to be increased during the four-year period. In the majority of patients it was not possible to obtain reliable information about the degree of change of reactivity during the period in question.

In a follow-up study by Dannaeus and Inganaes [23] it was found that most food sensitivities decreased in most patients over a 2–5 year period except allergy to fish (and nuts) which seemed more often to persist or even become more severe with age.

A number of patients (parents) reported that

symptoms of fish allergy appeared on the very first introduction of the item. This has been interpreted by others as a possible result of intrauterine sensitization with the allergens from the mother's diet. Fish allergens are, however, able to pass to the child through the mother's breast milk. They are also found in the indoor air when fish is cooked or fried, and fish allergens may be demonstrated in house dust samples in most homes where fish is often eaten. This is a more likely source for early sensitization than intrauterine sensitization.

Diagnosis

Skin tests. Skin testing was performed with a number of different extracts of fish. With a commercial fish extract, 29% of the skin reactions equal or larger than two plus (+ +) and 21% of those three plus (+ + +) or more were without any clinical significance. This is in accordance with the result of Lessof et al [34] who used the same kind of commercial fish extract. In their patients a clinical diagnosis of fish allergy was made following a skin test reaction of 5 mm or more in 15 out of 19 patients. However, seven patients with no history of intolerance to fish gave a 4 mm reaction to the same extract. When we analysed this extract we found a total protein content of approximately 5 mg/ml. After dilution of the fish allergen extracts to approximately 0.2 mg/ml total protein, three plus (+ + +) scratch test reactions were obtained in 88 of the 89 fish-hypersensitive patients and a positive skin test reaction (+ + + +) was obtained in only one of the control individuals. With a purified codfish allergen material used later on, 100% correct discrimination between fish-allergic and fish-non-allergic individuals was obtained by prick testing [15].

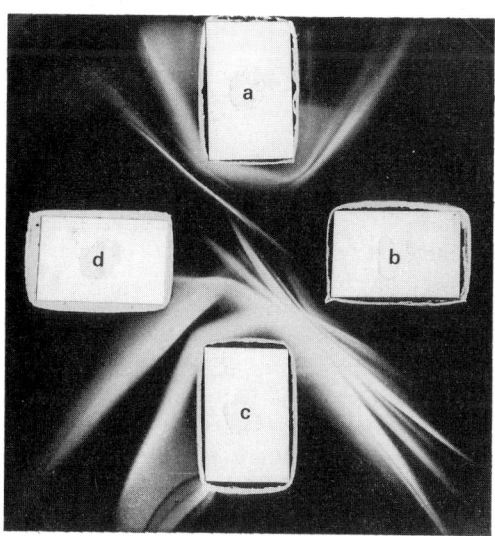

Fig. 19.2 Gel double-diffusion experiment with reference extract from codfish tissue (a) and cod blood serum (c) reacting with rabbit antiserum to the extract (d) and to the cod blood serum (b).

RAST. A similar high degree of diagnostic reliability was obtained with the radio-allergo-sorbent test (RAST) performed with the purified allergen from cod coupled to CNBr-activated cellulose discs [15]. Analysis of serum samples taken at different intervals from codfish-allergic patients revealed that a few patients showed great variations in the content of IgE antibodies to codfish with negative results in some instances.

Approximately 20% of the fish-allergic patients also gave positive skin tests when fish serum was used as the allergen. Immuno-diffusion experiments demonstrated that the fish tissues and blood serum had a number of separate antigens and also some in common (Fig. 19.2).

Treatment of hypersensitivity to fish

Hyposensitization

Avoidance of fish in all forms is advocated as soon as clinical hypersensitivity to fish is suspected or proven. Also emanations from fish should be avoided. When some species are found to be tolerated they should be allowed. In four children who gave severe reactions when exposed to fish and fish emanations, an attempt at hyposensitization was considered worthwhile since they lived in fish-producing areas and could not avoid contact with fish emanations and dust containing fish allergen. No adverse reactions were observed in three of the four children, and with a year's hyposensitization all three tolerated steam from cooking fish which they could not previously; also minute amounts of fish mixed with, for example, mashed potato, could be eaten without discomfort. In a fourth patient, however, a piece of cooked cod put into the mouth immediately resulted in oedema and itching of the mucous membrane and lips. The skin reactions of fish extracts remained unaltered within the limits of reproducibility of the method [2]. Dannaeus and Inganaes [23] reported hyposensitization in one case of fish allergy with a 'satisfactory result'. Hyposensitization is, however, not to be recommended in general but might be considered in extreme cases of fish hypersensitivity where exposure is difficult to avoid.

ANTIGENIC DIFFERENCES BETWEEN FISH SPECIES

Species specificity: clinical responsiveness

Allergy to fish is characterized by a wide range of species specificity with varying patterns of cross-reactivity. Individuals allergic to fish may react to all species of fish and may also react on skin testing with extracts from fish species not usually eaten. From such observations and after closer studies of six fish-hypersensitive patients, Tuft and Blumstein [36] claimed the existence of a fish allergen common to several species. Other authors, however, report important differences in the reactions of some patients to various species of fish [24, 37] and in some instances extreme degrees of species specificity in fish allergy have been reported [24].

Comparative chemical, electrophoretic and immunological studies of fish species have demonstrated distinct differences in the distribution of proteins and in the antigenic composition of extracts from both muscle tissues

and blood serum of various fish species [3]. Specific antisera from rabbits used by the present author for the immunological characterization of allergen extracts from fish have been shown to possess distinct species discrimination capacities (Fig. 19.3). Discrimination between fish species was also prominent in clinical hypersensitivity reactions of several fish-allergic children [3].

In 61 children, two or more different species of fish had been tried in the diet. 34 of these children were reported to react with allergic symptoms to all species tried, whilst 27 tolerated one or more types of fish. Cod was the most common offender with hypersensitivity reactions reported in 78 of 82 children who had tried fish. Fresh-water trout had been tried by 46 children and was tolerated by 21, while 25 experienced hypersensitivity reactions to this species as well. Salmon was tried by 24 patients who were hypersensitive to cod and was tolerated by 11 of them.

Species-specific antigens

Studies of species differentiation were undertaken using direct skin testing, passive transfer experiments and in vivo passive transfer neutralization experiments with simultaneous species differentiation immunodiffusion experiments. The studies indicated the presence of different species-specific antigens in fish that may act as species-specific allergens in a number of fish-hypersensitive individuals. Other patients apparently reacted to common or closely related allergens present in extracts from different species. Complete correlation between clinical reactivity and skin test reactivity was not present. Varying amounts of fish antigens may be found in extracts produced in different ways [4] rendering comparison of skin test results obtained by different investigators difficult.

In 14 cod-allergic patients who had never eaten carp, an extract of this species elicited skin test reactions similar to those obtained by the reference codfish extract. Passive transfer neutralization experiments with two codfish-allergic sera indicated complete cross-reactivity between the two species (for the two serum donors in question). This is particularly interesting since a protein from carp which is very similar to the major allergen M from codfish (see later) has been characterized by X-ray crystallography.

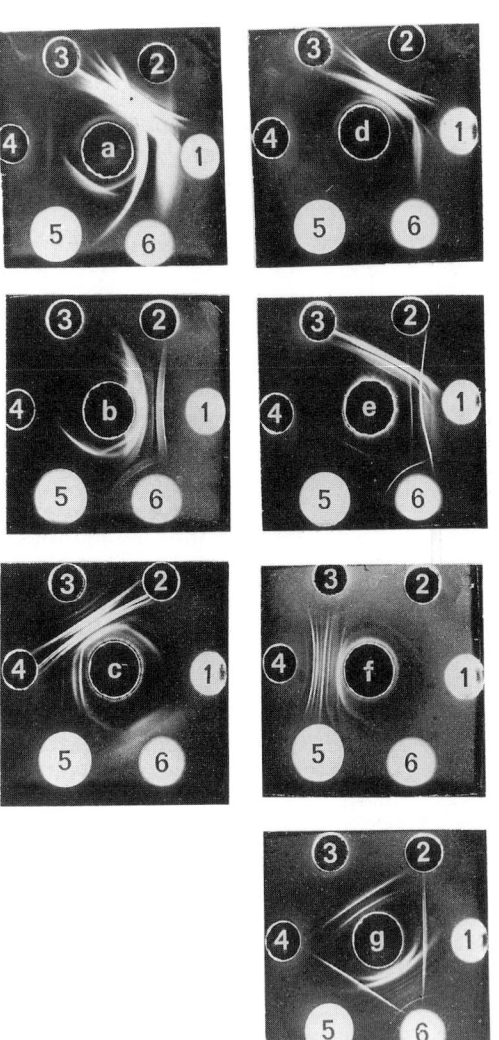

Fig. 19.3 Gel double-diffusion experiments illustrating differentiation between species of fish with the use of antisera from different rabbits immunized with (a) cod blood serum, (b) tissue extract from codfish, (c) salmon blood serum, (d) cod blood serum, (e) tissue extract from cod, (f) mackerel blood serum and (g) salmon tissue extract. The peripheral wells contain (1) tissue extract from cod, (2) cod blood serum, (3) salmon blood serum, (4) mackerel blood serum, (5) tissue extract from mackerel and (6) tissue extract from salmon.

Other immune responses to fish antigens

Fish extracts contain many different antigenic proteins and each of the proteins may present distinct antigenic determinants for different immune reactions. The allergenic determinant binding IgE antibodies may be distinct from IgG antigenic determinants on some of the molecules. Hence a variety of different immune responses would be expected. Dannaeus and Inganaes [23] reported that codfish-allergic patients had both IgE and IgG antibodies to the same (DS 22) purified allergen in codfish. IgG and IgE antibodies to DS 22 were found exclusively in the fish-allergic patients, with parallel concentrations. A patient who underwent immunotherapy showed a marked increase in the IgG antibody level to DS 22. The relief of symptoms continued after the cessation of immunotherapy despite falling IgG antibody levels.

In my own study, haemagglutinating antibodies to a codfish extract were found in two-thirds of 59 cod-hypersensitive children. Positive reactions were also found in 27% of 55 allergic control children tolerating fish and in a third of 65 non-allergic control children. The haemagglutination reactions did not, however, measure the specific IgE antibody in question and also did not engage any of the major allergenic antigens of the fish extract [5] (Fig. 19.4).

In exceptional cases a phenomenon of complement fixation at high dilution may occur in fish allergy cases [22]. The implication of this is not understood.

PURIFICATION AND CHARACTERIZATION OF FISH ALLERGENS AND ANTIGENIC DETERMINANTS

In my laboratory, codfish studies were undertaken not because of their clinical important in Norway but, hopefully, as a model for the characterization of an allergen and allergenic determinants. Purification and characterization of this allergen were not objectives in themselves but a step to providing a much-needed instrument for scientific work in the field of allergy. For this ambitious goal, particularly resistant allergenic molecules were necessary since the way we treat protein molecules in the laboratory during purification procedures is rather rough. The denaturing effects of manipulation may become more pronounced the purer the protein.

Codfish

Codfish was selected for this purpose following clinical observations suggesting that the allergens in question might be particularly resistant to denaturation. A breast-fed infant developed acute atopic exacerbations each time the mother ate fish prior to nursing. The aller-

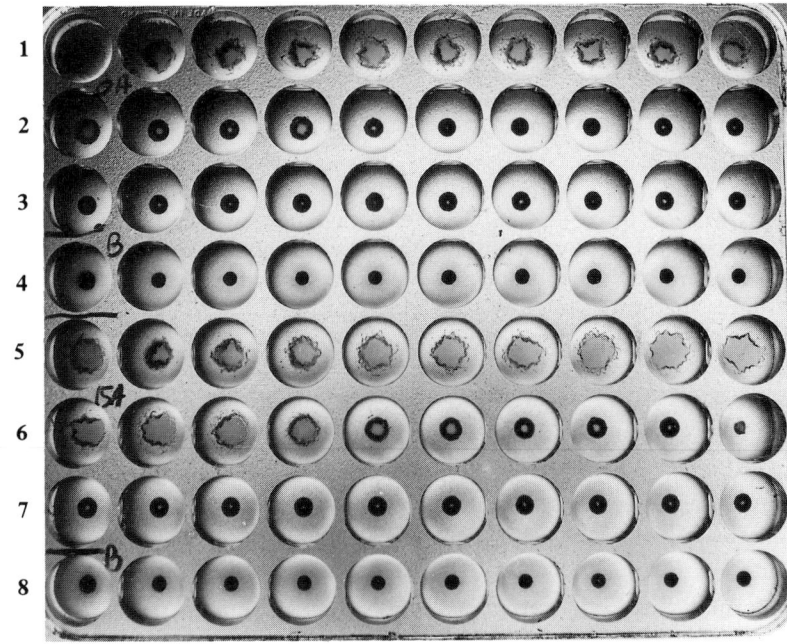

Fig. 19.4 Example of BDB-haemagglutination experiment with a crude codfish extract. Positive reactions in rows 1, 5 and 6; negative reactions in the other rows.

gens in question had resisted prolonged cooking, and the digestive acids and enzymes of the mother. They had passed several biologically active membranes into the mother's milk and then resisted the influence of the infant's digestive juices and had maintained the activity when circulated to sensitized mast cells in the infant's skin and mucosa. Hypothetically, this allergenic activity had to be associated with components which maintained or reorganized the active allergenic determinants in spite of denaturation, or be due to small peptides carrying active allergenic determinants. Results obtained so far have confirmed both hypotheses.

Proteins and antigenic determinants

A protein is made up of a number of amino acids bound together with or without additional carbohydrate residues in the primary structure. Each amino acid has a side chain which is characteristic for it. The side chains together represent chemically active sites in and on the protein molecule. The chain is twisted and is given its final shape through conformational changes of the polypeptide chain due to the chemical forces between the side chains which fold it into its tertiary structure.

Antigenic determinants are defined as the discrete areas of the protein surface structure that combine specifically with the complementary discrete areas of the particular antibody.

Antigenic determinants may be either sequential or conformational. A sequential determinant is organized from a number of amino acids as found directly in a linear sequence in a randomly folded or unfolded form of the molecule. It can thus be picked out directly from the amino acid sequence of the protein. This type of antigenic determinant remains intact following denaturation of the protein. A conformational determinant results from the steric configuration or folding and is made up of amino acid residues that are remote in the unfolded polypeptide chain but are found in juxtapositions in the native structures. Denaturation of the protein will usually break up this type of determinant.

Most protein determinants that interact with humoral IgG antibodies are thought to be conformational but sequential antigenic determinants have been demonstrated for many such protein and polypeptide antigens in the past. The nature of allergenic determinants binding to IgE antibodies has not been eluci-

dated except for some determinants in the major allergen of codfish, as will be described.

THE MAJOR ALLERGEN IN CODFISH

Using various techniques of protein separation and purification, a material (DS 22) was obtained from codfish that could be crystallized (Fig. 19.5) and shown to be extremely potent [14].

Immunodiffusion experiments with antisera from rabbits immunized with the crude extract showed only one precipitation line with the final purification product. This antiserum was shown to be able to absorb out all of the allergenic activity of the extract as shown by direct skin testing and passive transfer tests in eight out of ten codfish-allergic patients. In two of the patients tested, the absorbed extract still had some activity. This suggested the presence of at least one minor allergen in addition to the major one in the semipurified codfish muscle extract. This was later demonstrated directly by means of crossed radioimmunoelectrophoresis (CRIE) and by the use of immunosorbent columns with the particular antiserum [20].

Allergen M

Codfish contains one major allergen (allergen M) and all codfish-allergic patients I have seen react to this allergen. This major allergen is heat stable and quite resistant to proteolytic digestion and several denaturation procedures [27]. This supported the idea that the allergenic activity is found in a linear sequence of certain amino acids and is not dependent on conformational determinants.

The biological relevance of allergen M was established by means of skin testing, double-blind passive transfer testing, release of histamine from chopped human lung sensitized with the appropriate allergic sera, RAST inhibition, CRIE and double-blind controlled food challenges [1, 11, 15, 20]. Extremely small quantities (never exceeding 1 mg) were given concealed in 50 g meat balls or hamburgers. The purified fish material was completely tasteless and without any smell and could not be identified. Allergen M-containing meat elicited rather fierce clinical reactions in the first patients so tested and further provocative feeding was abandoned. With the purified material a close correlation was demonstrated between all the tests mentioned and the presence of allergy to codfish [14].

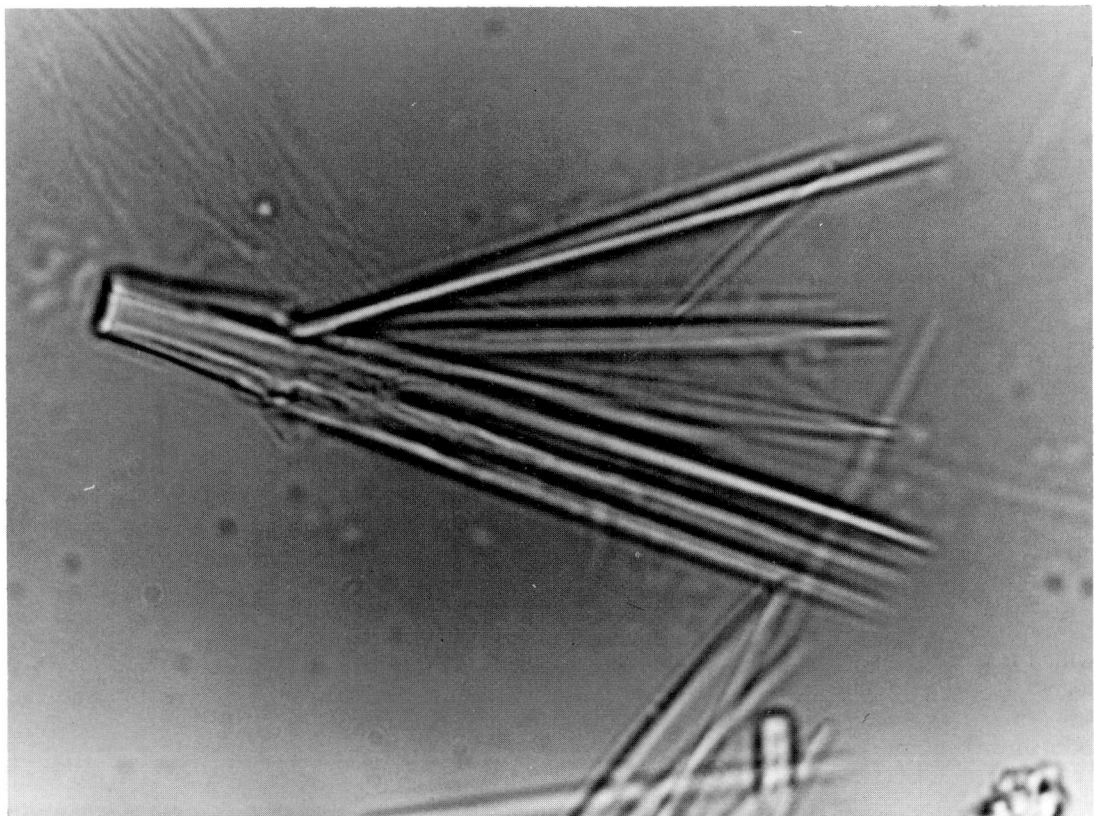

Fig. 19.5 Protein crystals obtained from the purified DS 22 fraction of codfish white muscle tissue extract [14].

In the most sensitive patient system the purified allergenic protein was extremely potent. It could provoke marked whealing reactions in passive transfer or so-called Prausnitz–Küstner experiments in concentrations corresponding to less than 10 000 molecules injected into the sensitized skin [14]. Food challenges with microgram quantities of the purified material given to the recipient of cod-allergic serum into the skin also provoked rather large local swelling.

Potency of allergen M

The extreme potency of this purified material should be noted by all those who now consider production or use of semipurified fish protein for protein enrichment of different mixed foods. It is now possible to produce fish proteins without a fishy taste or smell. The appropriate procedures for this may, however, lead to an enrichment of the major allergenic fraction which represents a risk for sensitization of individuals otherwise not exposed. If produced it is mandatory that such products are labelled in an absolutely clear way to avoid disastrous reactions in fish-allergic individuals. It may also be necessary to organize production, transport, packing and storage under circumstances that protect those who work with it against occupational allergies to fish dust.

Biochemical properties of allergen M

The major allergen is an acidic protein (isoelectric point 4.75) composed of 113 amino acid residues and with a molecular weight of 12 328. In addition, allergen M has a single residue of glucose bound to Cys-18. Neither the glucosidic binding nor Cys-18 makes any contribution to the immunological reactivity of the molecule [7, 13]. Several other members of the parvalbumin group have similarly known amino acid sequences. A detailed tertiary structure analysis of one parvalbumin, namely carp pI 4.25, has been provided by X-ray crystallography [33]. The amino acid sequence of allergen M is known [30].

Allergenic and antigenic determinants of allergen M

A hypothetical model for an allergenic determinant was proposed during the 1975 Nobel Symposium in Stockholm [7] and this model has been substantiated by subsequent experiments [16, 25, 31].

The model was based on the assumptions that a few critical amino acid side chains constitute the determinant but that they may be kept at a critical distance from each other by other amino acids which act only as an inert framework or spacer. Assuming this, the molecule could have six or more similar allergenic determinants made up of two closely connected carboxylic side chains (Asp+Glu or Asp+Asp) kept at a critical distance from the basic residue Lys by one or more residues, the nature of which may be less specific. The sequence Asp-Glu-Leu-Lys and similar configurations pointed themselves out as particularly interesting in this respect (Fig. 19.6).

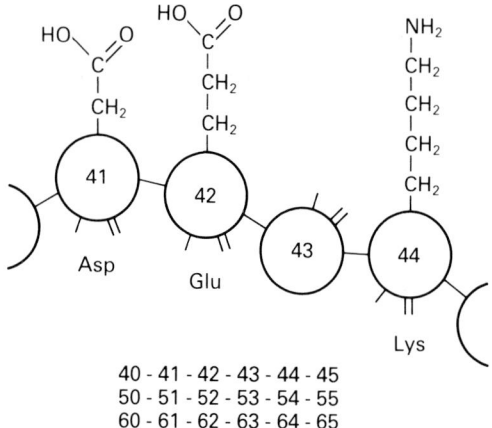

40 - 41 - 42 - 43 - 44 - 45
50 - 51 - 52 - 53 - 54 - 55
60 - 61 - 62 - 63 - 64 - 65

Fig. 19.6 Schematic representation of the essential amino acid (sequential) composition of the major allergenic determinant of the major allergen (allergen M) in codfish.

Synthesis of codfish peptide

A solid phase synthesis (SPPS) hexadecapeptide corresponding to residues 49–64 of allergen M from cod was found to bind IgE antibodies from the sera of cod-allergic individuals. The SPPS peptide was similarly reactive in IgG-mediated reactions; it could interfere with the allergen M precipitate line in rocket-line immunoelectrophoresis, giving a distinct deflection. It is the only reported synthetic polypeptide showing allergenic and antigenic reactivity [26, 31].

The two homologous tetrapeptides (Asp-Glu-Leu-Lys and Asp-Glu-Asp-Lys) and their systematic locations may be mutually critical for the specificity of antibody binding. Furthermore, the region 41–64 of allergen M

encompassed three of these tetrapeptides, interspersed by two segments of six variable amino acid residues [26].

The composition and sequence of the six spacer amino acids between these tetrapeptides were of no importance for the activity. The highest percentage inhibition was obtained by the peptides derived from the primary structure of allergen M. No activity was found in control peptides synthesized under identical conditions. Similar results were shown by Prausnitz-Küstner tests, using two cod-allergic sera and two recipients. In the IgG test system all the four peptides containing the two terminal tetrapeptides showed antigenic reactivity by deflecting the allergen M line in rocket line immunoelectrophoresis. No deflection was given by the control peptides or proteins.

These data indicated that the immunological reactivity of region 41–64 of allergen M is determined by three tetrapeptides. These are repeated in an elegant systematic order in three sites interspaced by six residues in a segment of 24 residues. At least two of these tetrapeptides, one at each of the chain terminals, are necessary for successful interaction with the antibody molecule. The reactivity was independent of both composition and sequence of the six residues of the spacer. However, it remains to be ascertained whether the six spacer residues are a prerequisite for the stereochemical fit of the interaction.

The importance of codfish allergen M

There are few allergen sources that are so suitable as fish for this kind of research. Conformational allergenic determinants are probably much more common in other allergens and are very much more difficult to demonstrate and characterize. Although the methods and results from the codfish model may be useful in principle, there is no room for generalization. The codfish allergen model functions only for certain aspects of our problems. Most other food allergens may behave in a quite different way. Some allergens found in other common allergen sources seem to be as resistant to denaturation as allergen M. Such allergens may prove useful for a similar characterization with respect to allergenic (antigenic) determinants.

The availability of synthetic peptides that represent small molecular fragments taking part in IgE-dependent immune reactions may open the way for studies comprising variable fragments, amino acid substitution, conjugation to inert or active carriers of different kinds and so on. This may open up new fields of research on the nature, immunogenicity and antigenicity of allergenic determinants as combined with various molecules and molecular fragments. More basic knowledge about this may aid the development of better diagnostic and therapeutic material and techniques, hopefully also applicable to occupational allergies and allergies to drugs.

REFERENCES

1 Aas K: Studies of hypersensitivity to fish. Oslo: University of Oslo. Universitetsforlaget, Oslo, 1965. 220 pp. Dissertation.

2 Aas K: Studies of hypersensitivity to fish. A clinical study. Int Arch Allergy 1966; 29:346–66.

3 Aas K: Studies of hypersensitivity to fish. Allergological and serological differentiation between various species of fish. Int Arch Allergy 1966; 30:257–67.

4 Aas K: Studies of hypersensitivity to fish. Characterization of different allergen extracts from fish with respect to content to protein antigens and allergenic activity. Int Arch Allergy 1966; 30:1–14.

5 Aas K: Studies of hypersensitivity to fish. Immunodiffusion and haemaglutination experiments. Int Arch Allergy 1966; 30:190–208.

6 Aas K: Antigens and allergens of fish. Int Arch Allergy 1969; 36:152–5.

7 Aas K: Common characteristics of major allergens. In: Johansson SGO, Strandberg K, Uvnäs B, eds. Molecular and biological aspects of the acute allergic reaction. Nobel Symposium 1976. New York: Plenum 1976; 3–19.

8 Aas K: The diagnosis of hypersensitivity to ingested foods. Reliability of skin prick testing and radio-allergosorbent test with different material. Clin Allergy 1978; 8:39–50.

9 Aas K: What makes an allergen an allergen. Allergy 1978; 33:3–14 (Review).

10 Aas K: Die Natur der Allergene. Die gelben Hefte 1980; 20:77–85.

11 Aas K: The codfish allergen model. In: Oehling A, ed. Advances in allergology and immunology. Oxford: Pergamon Press, 1980; 339–44.

12 Aas K: Antigens in food. Nutr Rev 1984; 42(3):85–91.

13 Aas K, Elsayed SM: Physico-chemical properties and specific activity of a purified allergen (codfish). International WHO-IABS symposium on standardization and control of allergens, administered to man. Geneva 1974. Dev Biol Stand 1975; 29:90–8.

14 Aas K, Jebsen JW: Studies of hypersensitivity to fish. Partial purification and crystallization of a major allergenic component from cod. Int Arch Allergy 1967; 32:1–20.

15 Aas K, Lundkvist U: The radioallergosorbent test with a purified allergen from codfish. Clin Allergy 1973; 3:255.

16 Apold J: The allergenic structure of Allergen M from cod. University of Bergen. Universitetsforlaget, Bergen, 1980. Dissertation.

17 Aukrust L: Immunological techniques in allergen characterization and purification. A methodological study using codfish and *Cladosporium herbarum* as models. University of Oslo. Studentsamskipnaden, Oslo, 1979. Dissertation.

18 Aukrust L, Aas K: A new reference system in crossed radioimmunoelectrophoresis. Scand J Immunol 1977; 6:1093–9.

19 Aukrust L, Almeland TL, Aas K: The specificity of radiostaining in crossed radioimmunoelectrophoresis. Scand J Immunol 1978; 8:421–7.

20 Aukrust L, Grimmer Ø, Aas K: Demonstration of distinct allergens by means of immunological methods. Comparison of crossed radioimmunoelectrophoresis (CRIE), radioallergosorbent test (RAST) and in vivo passive transfer test (PK-test). Int Arch Allergy Appl Immunol 1978; 57:183–92.

21 Aukrust L, Apold J, Elsayed SM, Aas K: Crossed immunoelectrophoretic and crossed radioimmunoelectrophoretic studies employing a model allergen from codfish. Int Arch Allergy Appl Immunol 1978; 57:253–62.

22 Berrens L, Van Dijk AG, Weemaes CMR: Complement consumption in eggwhite and fish sensitivity. Clin Allergy 1981; 11:101–9.

23 Dannaeus A, Inganaes M: A follow-up study of children with food allergy. Clinical course in relation to serum IgE- and IgG-antibody to milk, egg and fish. Clin Allergy 1981; 11:533–9.

24 De Besche A: On asthma bronchiale in man provoked by cat, dog and different other animals. Acta Med Scand 1937; 92:237–55.

25 Elsayed SM: The complete primary structure of Allergen M (cod). University of Oslo. Universitetsforlaget, Oslo, 1975. Dissertation.

26 Elsayed SM: Native and synthetic peptides of cod fish Allergen M. A short review. In: Bostrøm H, Epne H, Ljungstedt N, eds. Theoretical and clinical aspects of allergic diseases. Skandia International Symposium. Stockholm: Almqvist & Wiksell, 1983; 237–53.

27 Elsayed SM, Aas K: Characterization of a major allergen (cod). Observations on effect of denaturation on the allergenic activity. J Allergy 1971; 47:283–91.

28 Elsayed SM, Apold J: The immunochemical analysis of cod fish Allergen M: locations of the immunoglobulin binding sites as demonstrated on the native and synthetic peptides. Allergy 1983; 38:449–59.

29 Elsayed SM, Bahr-Lindstrøm HV, Bennich H: The primary structure of fragment TM_2 of Allergen M from cod. Scand J Immunol 1974; 3:3313–20.

30 Elsayed SM, Sletten K, Aas K: The primary structure of a major allergen (cod). I. N-terminal amino acid sequence of fragment TM_2. Immunochemistry 1973; 10:701–5.

31 Elsayed SM, Titlestad K, Apold J, Aas K: A synthetic hexadecapeptide derived from Allergen M imposing allergenic and antigenic reactivity. Scand J Immunol 1980; 12:171–5.

32 Kajosaari M.: Food allergy in Finnish children 1–6 years of age. Acta Paediatr Scand 1982, 71:815–19.

33 Kretsinger RH, Nockolds CE: Carp muscle calcium binding protein. II. Structure determination and general description. J Biol Chem 1973; 248:3313.

34 Lessof MH, Buisseret PD, Merret J et al: Assessing

the value of skin prick test. Clin Allergy 1980; 10:115–20.

35 Prausnitz C, Küstner H: Studien über die Überempfindlichkeit. Zentralbl Bakteriol Parasitkde 1921; 86:160–9.

36 Tuft L, Blumstein GI: Studies in food allergy. V. Antigenic relationship among members of fish family. J Allergy 1946; 17:329–39.

37 Wenderoth H, Bennecke MM: Zur Frage der Gruppenallergie gegen Fischeiweiss. Dtsch Med Wochenschr 1956; 81:1274–5.

Chapter 20
Allergy to Hen's Egg White: Clinical and Immunological Aspects

Tor Langeland and Kjell Aas

Introduction

Egg is an important source of protein in the human diet, and appears to be among the most common of food allergen sources. It may also produce allergic reactions when found as a contaminant of some virus vaccines. Furthermore, egg proteins may contaminate the house dust in homes where egg is a staple item of the diet. Hen's egg belongs also to the items most thoroughly studied with respect to composition and content of allergenic proteins. In fact the allergenic properties of egg were discussed as early as 1913 by Schloss [42]. Egg proteins and, in particular, ovalbumin have been extensively used as model antigens (and allergens) in experimental animals. Egg proteins have also been used in studies of the permeability of the intestines [43]. Furthermore, the major proteins of egg can be purchased commercially. They are not pure, but represent suitable material for further refined purification. All this makes egg allergy and egg allergens suitable fields of study.

PREVALENCE AND CLINICAL PRESENTATION

Hen's egg white appears to be among the foods that most frequently cause hypersensitivity in children [2, 8, 33]. The incidence varies considerably in different populations. Egg allergy is more frequent in young children than in older children and adults, and tends to subside with age [11, 17].

An attempt to assess the incidence of egg allergy was made by Ratner and Untracht [40]. Among 322 randomly selected children they found only one egg-sensitive child (0.3%), judged on the history and on skin tests. In a group of 500 children with asthma and/or 'eczema' they found about 5% with clinical reactions to egg white.

The incidence reported for different patient populations varies. Major reasons for discrepancies are the type of patient studied and the criteria for inclusion as 'egg-sensitive'. The use of skin testing in patients with atopic eczema will, for example, tend to give an overestimate of the incidence in the population. The incidence seems to be higher in individuals with atopic manifestations in both the skin and the respiratory tract than in individuals with atopic symptoms in just one organ [18, 44, 45, 50]. Among 82 children with food sensitivity, Dannaeus and Inganaes found 55 children with egg allergy [11]. Kajosaari [25] evaluated the prevalence of allergy to egg (as well as to fish, see Chapter 19) in a given community in Finland with a child population of 802. At one and two years of age, the prevalence was 6% and 7%, respectively, based on history. However egg allergy could only be confirmed in half of them by means of oral challenge. At six years of age only 1% of the children were shown to have allergy to egg.

Symptoms of egg allergy

Egg ingestion in hypersensitive individuals has been reported to cause a wide spectrum of symptoms, such as exacerbation of atopic dermatitis, urticaria, angioedema, asthma, vomiting, diarrhoea and anaphylaxis [19, 22, 23]. Egg white proteins have also been reported to cause these reactions following inhalation, for instance in the kitchen when food containing eggs was being prepared [26]. Serious and even fatal reactions have been reported in egg-sensitive patients injected with vaccines containing traces of egg proteins [38, 47].

It is common to find clinically that egg white may cause flare, pruritus and urticarial lesions in the perioral area and in oral mucosa within a few minutes following ingestion, suggesting that these reactions are a manifestation of contact urticaria rather than a symptom of food allergy resulting from intestinal absorption of allergens. Allergic urticaria due to direct skin contact with proteins in food is well documented. Therefore, in clinical studies of egg allergy, generalized reactions should be distinguished from reactions occurring only at the site of contact [49].

Particular interest has been centred on the significance of egg allergy in the pathogenesis of atopic dermatitis [3]. An association between egg allergy and atopic dermatitis is particularly pronounced in infants and young children [39]. It has been suggested that the presence of egg allergy in children with atopic dermatitis leads to a higher risk of developing bronchial asthma [10]. The association between egg allergy and atopic dermatitis may be due to a common disposition to produce high levels of total IgE in the serum [24, 30] (see Chapter 34).

Natural history

IgE antibodies which bind to egg white have been detected in cord blood, supporting theories of the transplacental passage of some allergens and the possibility of occasional in-trauterine sensitization. Egg allergy commonly arises early in life, in many cases during the first one or two years [26].

In a clinical study, 36 out of 63 patients with egg allergy were found to have reacted on the very first occasion they were known to have eaten egg or egg products. This indicates that previous, unnoticed exposure to egg white proteins must have occurred [26]. Such exposure has been assumed to be due to transmittance through the breast milk of egg white proteins ingested by the mother (see Chapter 18) and/or to the ability of such proteins to pass through the placenta and cause sensitization in utero [34]. It is also possible that inhalation of egg white proteins, for instance in house dust, could cause early sensitization.

Hypersensitivity to egg white proteins tends to decrease with age [11, 17, 25]. In 45 of 55 egg-allergic children seen by Dannaeus and Inganaes [11], egg allergy was greatly reduced or had completely disappeared after two to five years. The apparent difference between the decay of, for example, egg and fish allergy, calls for comparative studies to be undertaken of the basic mechanisms involved in the development of tolerance.

DIAGNOSIS

In many instances, the case history gives a good indication of the existence of an allergy to hen's egg. Great care should be taken, however, in sorting out those with true allergy to egg. The tendency to grow out of egg allergy often leaves the question open as to whether or not the individual may still have egg allergy a few years after the last positive observation. According to Ford and Taylor [17], subjects with only one organ system involved are more likely to become tolerant quite quickly compared with those who have multiple organ system involvement. In many, but not all, of the former cases, the skin test may become negative at the time egg is tolerated.

Skin tests

Generally, the reliability of skin tests in the diagnosis of food allergy is disputed. As regards egg allergy, some authors have found a good correlation between clinical hypersensitivity to egg and positive reactions to egg white in skin prick tests (SPT) [2, 8, 19]. This has not been confirmed by others [32, 45].

Lack of characterization of the allergen preparations and lack of standardization of the tests make comparisons of such studies difficult. Skin testing may be particularly unreliable in patients with atopic dermatitis, and especially so when the intradermal technique is employed.

Ratner and Untracht [40] obtained positive skin test reactions to egg in about 20% of 500 children with asthma and/or eczema, but concluded that only one-quarter of those had clinical reactions to egg. Aas [2] found a good correlation between skin testing, the radio-allergosorbent test (RAST) and positive challenge tests in children with proven clinical allergy to egg, as did Dannaeus and Inganaes [11]. The latter found a positive RAST to egg in 96% of egg-allergic individuals, but also in 25% of patients with no clinical symptoms following the ingestion of egg. Clinically insignificant positive RAST results occur most often in patients with a high total IgE serum concentration.

In these series, the skin test reaction subsides more slowly than the serum IgE antibody concentration when the child has outgrown clinical allergy to egg.

There is often a clinical problem with the child who previously had an egg allergy and who now has a positive skin test to egg but a negative RAST. In these circumstances an oral challenge under safe circumstances is often given to exclude current clinical hypersensitivity.

Most commercial test preparations of egg are useful provided they are stored and applied appropriately. Test material can, however, as well be freshly prepared directly from raw eggs [2].

An elimination diet followed by food challenge is the most relevant of the diagnostic procedures. Because the interpretations of reactions observed in the above procedure may be difficult, the necessity for double-blind procedures in food challenge has been emphasized by many [4, 35].

TREATMENT OF EGG ALLERGY

The principal treatment of egg allergy is elimination of egg white proteins from the diet. Cooking the egg may reduce, but not eliminate, the allergenic activity in the egg white since one of the major allergens, i.e. ovomucoid, is resistant to heating [6]. It is advisable to eliminate egg yolk as well because of the possibility of proteins in the yolk cross-reacting with allergens in egg white [29]. Also, it will be difficult to avoid contamination of egg yolk by some egg white proteins when preparing food. Chickens and hens contain proteins demonstrating immunological identity reactions with allergens in hen's egg white. The clinical significance of this will depend upon a number of other factors, such as the ability of the proteins to maintain allergenic activity during heating and digestion.

Peroral hyposensitization has been tried by some clinicians, but the efficacy is hard to evaluate due to the natural history of egg allergy.

Avian-grown vaccines and egg allergy

The safety of using avian-grown vaccines on egg-allergic patients deserves special mention. Miller and co-workers [38] evaluated this in 42 patients with a history of egg sensitivity. Each patient was skin tested with egg antigens and six egg-propagated vaccines. Scratch and intradermal tests to the egg products were positive in 10 patients and 20 patients, respectively. Thirty-two patients underwent oral egg challenge. Twelve of them had no symptoms and no reaction or very weak reactions. Oral egg challenge was omitted in two patients due to a history of severe systemic reaction with any egg exposure. Eight additional patients with negative skin test to egg products were not challenged. Seventeen patients had mild symptoms after egg exposure and three patients had moderate to severe reactions following egg ingestion. Vaccines were withheld from three patients with acute sensitivity to egg proteins. The other patients were immunized with little or no reaction.

A positive reaction to intradermal testing with vaccine prior to immunization was found to be reliable in predicting the patients who should not receive the vaccine [38, 47].

Egg antigens as clinical probes

Egg white and, in particular, ovalbumin, have been used as tracer substances in investigations of the permeability of the intestines to ingested proteins. After ingestion, the serum concentration of ovalbumin can be determined by immunological techniques. As early as 1916 Schloss and Worthen [43] showed that egg proteins pass the intestinal barriers in healthy infants and this has been confirmed many times [21] by investigators using egg proteins as tracers.

Dannaeus and co-workers [13] found that most children with malabsorption disorders showed peak serum concentrations of ovalbumin two hours after the administration, but the concentration varied considerably.

The intestines of healthy adults are also permeable to egg allergenic proteins or peptides. This can be shown by passive transfer to the skin of healthy volunteers using serum from egg allergic individuals followed by the ingestion of egg when a skin reaction can be detected. Due to this absorption, the production of serum IgG antibodies to egg proteins must be considered a normal immune response. They are also found in newborns and reflect the corresponding maternal concentrations [12].

IgE-MEDIATED EGG ALLERGY

IgE-mediated reactions appear to predominate among the immunological events leading to the clinical manifestations of egg allergy. This is indicated by the demonstration of positive immediate skin test reactions to egg white which can also be passively transferred to egg-tolerant individuals, and the presence of specific IgE antibodies in serum from egg-allergic individuals. Such antibodies will usually not be detected in serum from egg-tolerant individuals [2, 8, 23]. In recent years, evidence has been presented suggesting that ingestion of a food allergen may cause formation of immune complexes containing specific IgE antibodies against the allergen in question [9]. Such immune complexes are able to bind complement and have therefore been proposed to be contributing factors to the clinical symptoms of food allergy. Further studies will be required to define the clinical significance of such immune complexes.

In a study of children with allergy to egg Dannaeus and Inganaes [11] found that those with a high IgG/IgE-anti ovomucoid antibody ratio were most likely to develop tolerance during the follow-up period of two to five years. Berrens and co-workers [5] have reported an exceptional case of complement fixation by thermostable IgG antibody to egg white at extremely high antigen dilutions. The clinical significance of this observation remains to be shown.

Occurrence of cross-reacting proteins

Proteins demonstrating complete immunological cross-reactivity with the major aller-gens in hen's egg white have been found in egg yolk and in serum and flesh from hens and chickens. By means of various quantitative immunoelectrophoretic techniques, the amounts of such proteins have been estimated. These proteins were found to bind specific IgE antibodies in serum from egg-allergic patients [29].

Proteins cross-reacting with most allergens in hen's egg white have been demonstrated in egg whites from turkey, duck, goose and seagull, using quantitative immunoelectrophoretic techniques [29]. By means of RAST inhibition, the specific allergenic activity of these egg whites was determined, using hen's egg white as a reference [3]. Considerable variations were found in the specific allergenic activities. Relative to hen's egg white the order of specific allergenic activity in the egg whites studied was found to be: turkey egg white 10^{-1} to 10^{-2}; duck and goose egg whites 10^{-2} to 10^{-3}; and seagull egg white 10^{-3} to 10^{-4} [29].

ANTIGENS AND ALLERGENS IN HEN'S EGG WHITE

The total protein content of egg white is approximately 10% (w/v), and consists of about 40 different proteins [46]. A few of these constitute the majority of the protein content. These are ovalbumin (54%), ovotransferrin (13%), ovomucoid (11%), lysozyme (3–5%) and ovomucin (1.5%). The remaining proteins are minor components.

The antigens in hen's egg white have been subject to a number of studies [7, 14, 27, 37, 41, 42]. More than 20 distinct antigens have been demonstrated in the egg white by means of various immunoelectrophoretic methods [27].

Schloss was probably the first to study individual allergens in hen's egg white, performing skin tests with various fractions of the egg white. He concluded that ovomucoid was the most important skin reactive component in the egg white. Other studies of the allergens in the egg white, chiefly based upon skin testing with various fractions of the egg white, confirmed the importance of ovomucoid as an allergen, but the results were contradictory with respect to the significance of other proteins [7, 36]. Virtue and Wittig [48] working with mast cell degranulation also concluded that ovomucoid was the most important allergen in the egg white.

The development of crossed immunoelec-

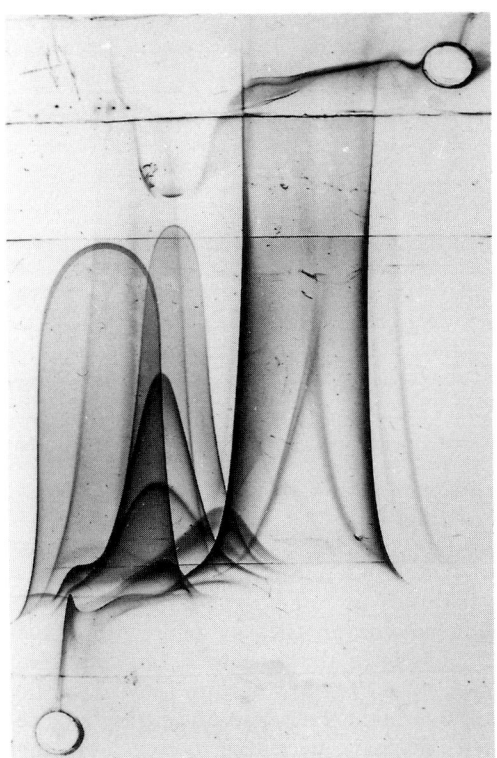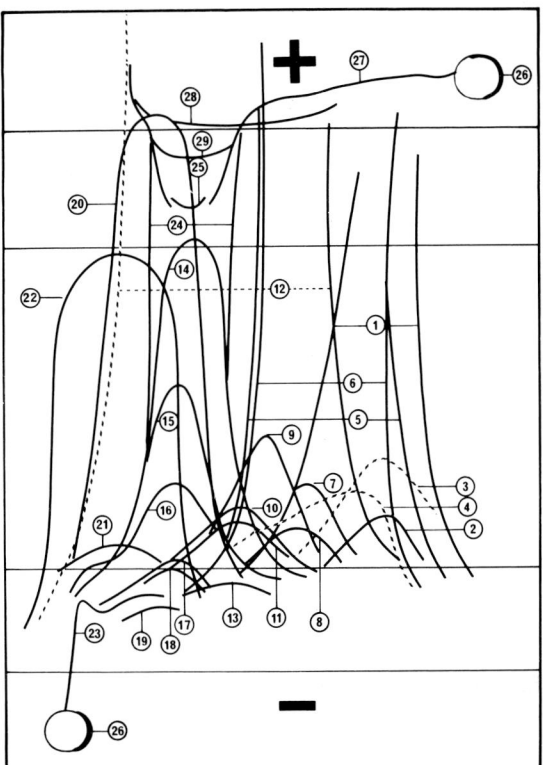

Fig. 20.1 CIE precipitation pattern for hen's egg white. (a) Stained with Coomassie Brilliant Blue. (b) Drawing of (a) (dotted lines: precipitates visible in CRIE only). Gels at top and bottom: primary gels. Antibody-containing gel in the middle of the plate. The antigen (diluted raw egg white) was applied in the wells of the primary gels. The anode was on the right in first-dimensional electrophoresis and at the top in second-dimensional electrophoresis. From [27], with kind permission of the editors of *Allergy* and the publishers, Munksgaard, Copenhagen.

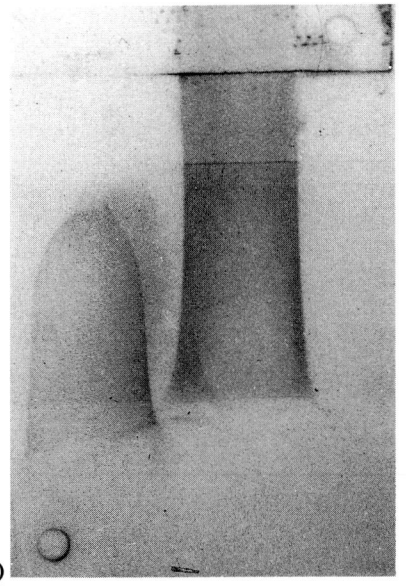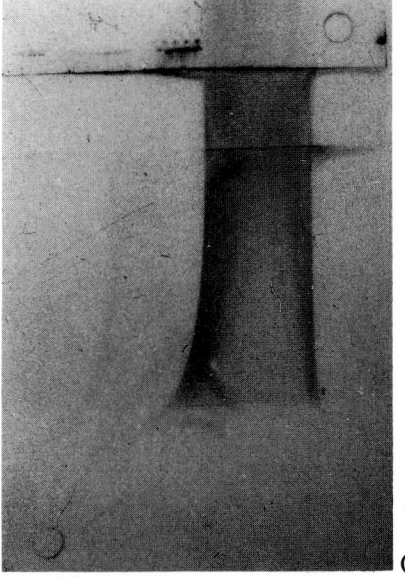

(a)
(b)

Fig. 20.2 CRIE results with sera from two egg-allergic patients, showing photographic films after autoradiography. The radiostaining corresponds to IgE-binding precipitates in the CIE precipitation pattern. From [28], with kind permission of the editors of *Allergy*, and the publishers, Munksgaard, Copenhagen.

trophoresis (CIE) and crossed radioimmuno-electrophoresis (CRIE) represented a breakthrough in studies of distinct allergens in mixed protein solutions. The allergens in hen's egg white have been studied using these methods [22, 27, 28]. By means of CIE, a high resolution of the various antigens in egg white can be obtained (Fig. 20.1a,b). Eighty-four single sera from egg-allergic children were analysed with respect to their contents of specific IgE antibodies to individual allergens in egg white in CRIE (Fig. 20.2).

Thirteen proteins were shown to bind specific IgE antibodies in sera from egg-allergic patients. There were considerable variations among the patients. The percentage of sera reacting to the various proteins and the strength of reaction were used as criteria for classifying the allergens as major, intermediate and minor allergens (Table 20.1).

Table 20.1 Allergens in hen's white determined in CRIE.

Major allergens	Ovalbumin, ovomucoid, ovotransferrin
Intermediate allergens	5, 10, 13, 15, 16
Minor allergens	1, 3, 4, 14, 20

Numbers correspond to precipitates in the CIE reference precipitation pattern for hen's egg white (Fig. 20.1b).

The major allergens were identified as ovalbumin, ovomucoid and ovotransferrin [28, 31] (Table 20.2). This has been confirmed by Hoffman, using radioimmunoelectrophoretic methods [22].

The most striking common characteristic of the major allergens in hen's egg white is the fact that they make up a substantial proportion of the total protein content of the egg white (Table 20.3). For these proteins there seems to be a degree of parallelism between the amount of protein and their allergenicity [28, 31]. Ovalbumin, constituting more than half of the total protein in the egg white, was found to be the most important allergen in the egg white.

Table 20.2 Amounts of proteins[*] in various food items demonstrating complete immunochemical identity reactions with major allergens in egg white.

	Ovalbumin (%)	Ovomucoid	Ovotransferrin (%)
Hen's egg yolk	0.03	Trace	15
Hen serum	0.2	—	50
Hen flesh	Trace	—	0.3
Chicken serum	—	—	15
Chicken flesh	Trace	—	0.1

[*] Relative to amounts in hen's egg white (100%). (Data from [29].)

Lysozyme appears to be of little significance as an allergen [22, 28], in spite of the fact that it constitutes as much as 3–5% of the total protein amount in the egg white [46]. Ovomucin has been reported to be an important allergen based on skin testing [36]. It cannot be excluded that the positive skin reactions reported may have been due to traces of other allergenic proteins contaminating the preparation used.

Allergenic and antigenic determinants

Some of the major allergens in egg white appear to be very resistant to denaturation, as has been shown for the major allergen in cod fish [1]. This suggests that further investigations of molecular characteristics of antigens and allergens present in egg white should be undertaken. It is likely that some essential allergenic determinant is sequential or is repeated in quite short peptides. If so, characterization and synthesis of an antibody-binding peptide could be feasible. This would provide a very valuable tool for further studies of many aspects of the immune reactions in allergy.

Table 20.3 Major allergens in hen's egg white.

	Percentage of total protein in egg white	Molecular weight	Isoelectric point	Antigenicity in rabbits
Ovalbumin	54	45 000	4.5–4.9	Good
Ovomucoid	11	28 000	4.1–4.4	Poor
Ovotransferrin	13	78 000	6.0–6.8	Good

REFERENCES

1 Aas K: Common characteristics of major allergens. In: Johansson SGO, Strandberg K, Uvnaes B, eds. Molecular and biological aspects of the acute allergic reaction. New York: Plenum Press, 1976; 3–22.

2 Aas K: The diagnosis of hypersensitivity to ingested foods. Clin Allergy 1978; 8: 39–50.

3 Atherton DJ: Dietary antigen avoidance in the treatment of atopic dermatitis. Acta Derm Venereol (Suppl) (Stockh) 1980; suppl 92: 99–102.

4 Atherton DJ: Atopic eczema. In: Brostoff J, Challacombe SJ, eds. Food allergy. London: WB Saunders, 1982; 77.

5 Berrens L, Van Dijk AG, Weemaes MR: Complement consumption in egg white and fish sensitivity. Clin Allergy 1981; 11: 101–9.

6 Bleumink E, Young E: Studies on the atopic allergen in hen's egg. I. Identification of the skin reactive fraction in egg-white. Int Arch Allergy 1969; 35: 1–19.

7 Bleumink E, Young E: Studies on the atopic allergens in hen's egg white. II. Further characterization of the skin reactive fraction in egg white: immunoelectrophoretic studies. Int Arch Allergy 1971; 40: 72–88.

8 Bock SA, Lee WY, Remigio LK, May CD: Studies of hypersensitivity reactions to foods in infants and children. J Allergy Clin Immunol 1978; 62: 327–34.

9 Brostoff J, Carini C, Wraith DG, Paganelli R et al: Immune-complexes in atopy. In: Pepys J, Edwards AM, eds. The mast cell, its role in health and disease. Tunbridge Wells, England: Pitman Medical Publishing, 1979; 380–93.

10 Buffum WP, Settipane GA: Prognosis of asthma in childhood. Am J Dis Child 1966; 112: 214–17.

11 Dannaeus A, Inganaes M: A follow-up study of children with food allergy. Clinical course in relation to serum IgE- and IgG-antibody levels to milk, egg and fish. Clin Allergy 1981; 11: 533–9.

12 Dannaeus A, Johansson SGO, Foucard T: Clinical and immunological aspects of food allergy in childhood. II. Development of allergic symptoms and humoral immune response to foods in infants of atopic mothers during the first 24 months of life. Acta Paediatr Scand 1978; 67: 495–504.

13 Dannaeus A, Inganaes M, Johansson SGO, Foucard T: Intestinal uptake of ovalbumin in malabsorption and food allergy in relation to serum IgE-antibody and orally administered sodium cromoglycate. Clin Allergy 1979; 9: 263–70.

14 Deutsch HF: Immunochemical analyses of egg white. Fed Proc 1952; 12: 729–33.

15 Donally HH: The question of the elimination of foreign protein (egg white) in woman's milk. J Immunol 1930; 19: 15–40.

16 Feeney RE: Egg proteins. In: Schultz HW, Anglemiers AF, eds. Proteins and their reactions. Connecticut: The Avi Publishing Company, 1964; 209–24.

17 Ford RPK, Taylor B: Natural history of egg hypersensitivity. Arch Dis Child 1982; 57: 649–52.

18 Freedman SS, Sellars W: Food sensitivity. A study of 150 'allergic' children. J Allergy 1959; 30: 42–9.

19 Gavani UD, Hyde JS, Moore BS: Hypersensitivity to milk and egg white. Skin tests, RAST results and clinical intolerance. Ann Allergy 1978; 40: 314–8.

20 Gerrard JW: Allergy in breast fed babies to ingredients in milk. Ann Allergy 1979; 42: 69–72.

21 Gruskay FL, Cooke RE: The gastrointestinal absorption of unaltered protein in normal infants and in infants recovering from diarrhoea. Pediatrics 1955; 16: 763.

22 Hoffman DR: Immunochemical identification of the allergens in egg white. J Allergy Clin Immunol 1983; 71: 481–6.

23 Hoffman DR, Haddad ZH: Diagnosis of IgE-mediated reactions to food antigens by radioimmunoassay. J Allergy Clin Immunol 1974; 54: 165–73.

24 Juhlin L, Johansson SGO, Bennich H et al: Immunoglobulin E in dermatosis. Arch Dermatol 1969; 100: 12–23.

25 Kajosaari M: Food allergy in Finnish children aged 1 to 6 years. Acta Paediatr Scand 1982; 71: 815–19.

26 Langeland T: A clinical and immunological study of allergy to hen's egg white. I. A clinical study of egg allergy. Clin Allergy 1983; 13: 371–82.

27 Langeland T: A clinical and immunological study of allergy to hen's egg white. II. Antigens in hen's egg white studied by crossed immunoelectrophoresis (CIE). Allergy 1982; 37: 323–33.

28 Langeland T: A clinical and immunological study of allergy to hen's egg white. III. Allergens in hen's egg white studied by crossed radio-immunoelectrophoresis (CRIE). Allergy 1982; 37: 521–30.

29 Langeland T: A clinical and immunological study of allergy to hen's egg white. VI. Occurrence of proteins crossreacting with allergens in hen's egg white as studied in egg white from turkey, duck, goose, seagull and hen's egg yolk, and hen's and chicken's sera and flesh. Allergy 1983; 38: 399–412.

30 Langeland T: Egg allergy and atopic dermatitis. Acta Derm Venereol 1985; suppl 114: 109–12.

31 Langeland T, Harbitz O: A clinical and immunological study of allergy to hen's egg white. V. Purification and identification of a major allergen (antigen 22) in hen's egg white. Allergy 1983; 38: 131–9.

32 Lessof MH, Buisseret PD, Merret J et al: Assessing the value of skin prick tests. Clin Allergy 1980; 10: 115–20.

33 Lessof MH, Wraith DG, Merrett TG et al: Food allergy and intolerance in 100 patients—local and systemic effects. Q J Med New Series XLIX; 195: 259–71.

34 Matsumura T, Kuroume T, Oguri M et al: Egg sensitivity and eczematous manifestations in breast-fed new-borns with particular reference to intrauterine sensitization. Ann Allergy 1975; 35: 221–9.

35 May CD, Bock SA: A modern clinical approach to food hypersensitivity. Allergy 1978; 33: 166–88.

36 Miller H, Campbell DH: Skin test reactions to various chemical fractions of egg white and their possible clinical significance. J Allergy 1959; 21: 522–4.

37 Miller H, Feeney R: Immunochemical relationships of protein of avian egg white. Arch Biochem Biophys 1964; 108: 117–24.

38 Miller JR, Orgel HA, Meltzer EO: The safety of egg-containing vaccines for egg-allergic patients. J Allergy Clin Immunol 1983; 71: 568–73.

39 Rajka G: Atopic dermatitis. London: WB Saunders, 1975: 65–9.

40 Ratner B, Untracht S: Egg allergy in children. Am J Dis Child 1952; 83: 309–16.

41 Rodroquez-Burgos A, Oteiza J: Antigenic composition of hen's (*Gallus domesticus*) egg white. Comp Biochem Physiol 1969; 30: 649–56.

42 Schloss OM: A case of allergy to common foods. Am J Dis Child 1912; 3: 341–62.

43 Schloss OM, Worthen TW: The permeability of the gastro-enterologic tracts of infants to undigested protein. Am J Dis Child 1969; II: 342–60.

44 Shur S, Hyde JS, Wypych JI: Egg-sensitivity and atopic eczema. J Allergy 1974; 54: 174-9.

45 Turner MW, Brostoff J, Mowbray JF, Skelton A: The atopic syndrome: in vitro immunological characteristics of clinically defined subgroups of atopic subjects. Clin Allergy 1980; 10: 575-89.

46 Vadehra DV, Nath KR: Eggs as a source of protein. CRC Critical Reviews in Food Technology, Nov. 1973; 193-309.

47 Van Asperen PP, McEniery J, Kemp AS: Immediate reactions following live attenuated measles vaccine. Med J Aust 1981; ii: 330-1.

48 Virtue CM, Wittig HJ: Allergenicity of egg white fractions as determined by histamine released from human lung tissue. Fed Proc 1970; 29: 576.

49 Von Krogh G, Maibach HI: The contact urticaria syndrome—updated review. Arch Dermatol 1981; 5: 328-42.

50 Wraith DG, Merrett J, Roth A et al: Recognition of food-allergic patients and their allergens by RAST technique and clinical investigation. Clin Allergy 1979; 9: 25-36.

SECTION B
NON-ALLERGIC EFFECTS OF FOOD

Chapter 21
Dietary Lectins and Disease

D. L. J. Freed

HISTORY

That many plants (and some animals) are poisonous when eaten has been known since prehistoric times. Especially notorious in this respect are the seeds of the castor oil plant (*Ricinus communis*, sometimes erroneously termed castor beans), which being large and attractively marked are popular dress orna-ments in some parts of the world, and occasionally cause fatalities when ingested by children.

In 1888 Stillmark was investigating this toxicity by mixing extracts of *R. communis* seeds with blood. He made the curious observation that the red cells were strongly agglutinated, and the serum solidified [191], but appears to have lost interest after that. In 1908 Landsteiner and Raubitschek [108] noted that

375

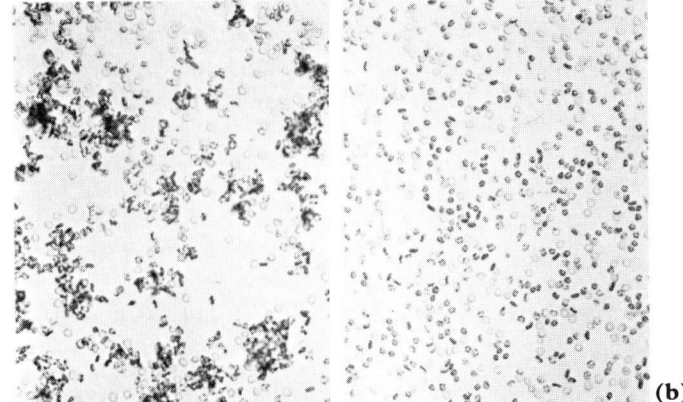

Fig. 21.1 (a) Agglutination of red blood cells by concanavalin A. (b) Control cells. From Tsivion and Sharon [196], with permission.

(a)   **(b)**

the intensity of agglutination caused by a single plant extract can vary with the species of animal, and in the 1940s Boyd [17] and Renkonen [165] independently observed that some plant agglutinins are blood group specific. Boyd and Shapleigh [18] proposed the term 'lectin' for these blood group-specific agglutinins (Latin: *lego, legere, lexi, lectum* = to choose), and this euphonious term has since been generally applied both to group-specific and non-specific plant agglutinins. Synonyms include 'phytoagglutinins' and 'phytohaemagglutinins', although this last term is ambiguous as it also describes one particular group of lectins, i.e. those derived from the common kidney bean *Phaseolus vulgaris*. Many lectins have since been described, and they are used extensively in blood group serology as an alternative to polyclonal antibodies (for review see [87]) (Fig. 21.1).

Plant lectins and 'sugar specificity'

The first lectin obtained in pure form was concanavalin A (con A), from the common jackbean *Canavalia ensiformis*. Sumner and Howell [193] made the key observation in 1936 that purified con A precipitates glycogen and starch from solution, and that its haemagglu-

tinating activity is inhibited by cane sugar. This opened the door to the recognition that, with very few exceptions, the cell surface receptors to which lectins bind are made of carbohydrate, at least in part. The paradigms for such receptors are the blood group antigens, and the techniques and terminology of the blood transfusion laboratory have been adopted wholesale by lectinologists. Thus, although lectin receptors actually contain several monosaccharides and sometimes amino acids as well, we speak of the 'immunodominant sugar', or simply of the 'sugar specificity' of a lectin, when what is really meant is the monosaccharide which inhibits haemagglutination with highest efficiency. The specificities of several common lectins are shown in Table 21.1 though the actual cell surface receptors are far more complex, and there is a degree of cross-reactivity between related sugars. The fact that two lectins share the same 'specificity' does not prove that they will necessarily exert the same effects on intact cells.

Animal lectins

It should also not be forgotten that lectins are not confined to the plant kingdom. Animal lec-

Table 21.1 Specificities of several common lectins.

Name of lectin and abbreviation	Source	'Specificity'
Wheat germ agglutinin (WGA)	Wheat	*N*-Acetylglucosamine
Concanavalin A (con A)	Jackbeans	α-Mannose, α-glucose
Lens culinaris agglutinin (LCA)	Lentils	α-Mannose, α-glucose
Pisum sativum agglutinin (PSA)	Green pea	α-Mannose, α-glucose
Soya bean agglutinin (SBA)	*Glycine max*	*N*-Acetylgalactosamine
Peanut agglutinin (PNA)	*Archis hypogaea*	Galactose
Ulex europaeus agglutinin (UEA1)	Gorse	L-Fucose
Phytohaemagglutinin (PHA)	Kidney beans	No simple sugar inhibitor
Helix pomatia agglutinin (HPA)	Edible snail	*N*-Acetylgalactosamine

tins include the galactose-specific hepatocyte lectins that determine the circulatory half-life of many plasma glycoproteins [183], and the 'electrolectin' of the electric eel (and also of many chordate muscle tissues, including human [112]). Animal lectins have been comparatively poorly studied as they are present in rather low concentrations, whereas up to 10% of some beans is composed of lectin. There is controversy over whether non-agglutinating (i.e. monovalent) molecules having high affinity for carbohydrates should be dignified by the epithet 'lectin', but in this review such substances are included under the same general heading.

Cell surface carbohydrates

Because of the ubiquity of cell surface carbohydrates, virtually all mammalian cells, as well as the majority of enzymes and plasma proteins [100], are susceptible to binding by at least some lectins. Although blood cells had been known in this respect since the turn of the century, Green and Freed in 1975 still found it deplorable [46] that lectin interactions with other cell types had been largely ignored in the literature (with a very few honourable exceptions) [7, 37, 38, 83, 99, 117, 136].

Food and lectins

Since many lectins are highly poisonous—such as the deadly ricin [99]—and since (as shown in Table 21.1) much of the food that we eat is laden with lectins, this omission was a surprising oversight. Perhaps it was then generally assumed (if considered at all) that any food-borne lectins would be destroyed by cooking and digestion—an assumption we now know to be insecure. In the last decade, however, there has been an intense burst of interest in lectin–tissue interactions, so that as doctors we now find ourselves uneasily contemplating the existence of a large field of study, undoubtedly of great pathogenic importance, that we had hitherto been happily unaware of.

In this review the effects on lectins of cooking and digestion are followed by an assessment of lectin–tissue interactions. It will be necessary to enter the caveat that not all lectins exert the same effects on all tissues; lectins are as diverse as prostaglandins. Also, although this review is of dietary lectins, many airborne particles also contain lectins. Jackbeans are not a human food and so con A is not a human

dietary item, but it is so well studied that it is useful to allude to con A as a paradigm for lectins in general.

RESISTANCE TO COOKING AND DIGESTION

Cooking

Many lectin-containing foods evade cooking because they are normally eaten raw, such as the tomato (*Lycopersicon esculentum*), which is now the primary vegetable source of vitamins and minerals in the USA. After mastication of one tomato, its lectin is bound to all oral mucous membranes. This *N*-acetylglucosamine-specific lectin is resistant to pepsin and trypsin and tolerates a pH range of 1.5–9.0 [136]. It inhibits the mitogenic effect (see below) of other lectins on animal lymphocytes, and in their absence suppresses lymphocyte metabolism.

Consumption of raw foods

Raw and relatively unprocessed foods are becoming more fashionable among health-conscious individuals in the Western world. Given the abundance of food in prosperous countries, such persons are therefore exposed to greater doses of dietary lectins than at any time, probably, in human evolution. The current fashion for sprouting beans and grains is therefore to be encouraged in this context, since sprouting in most cases causes a sharp diminution of lectin content within a few days [119]. Nevertheless, occasional outbreaks of food poisoning due to the lectins of uncooked or part-cooked beans are reported [139, 154]. The average American consumes around 200 mg of lectin per year from tomatoes alone [136], and many other salad ingredients are rich in lectins (see below).

Heat-sensitive lectins

Although many lectins are destroyed by normal cooking (which is why grains and beans are edible), many are not. Relative resistance to heat was part of the classic description of wheat germ agglutinin (WGA) made by Aub and colleagues in 1963 [6], and enabled them to distinguish it from the wheat germ lipase from which they got it. WGA in fact is one of the more heat-*sensitive* wheat lectins, being destroyed after 15 minutes at 75°C, whereas the lectins recently reported by Concon et al

[25] in wheat glutenin and gliadin resist auto-claving at 110°C for 30 minutes, and Freed has observed agglutinins in extracts of fresh baked bread (unpublished observations). Purists might object that not all that agglutinates is a lectin because certain plant and other lipids can cause a clumping phenomenon, indistinguishable from true haemagglutination, by partly dissolving portions of the phospholipid bilayer of the red cell membrane [196] (Fig. 21.2). However, although Concon et al [25] did not ascertain a sugar specificity for their autoclave-resistant agglutinins, they had previously removed lipids from the flour by extraction in butanol.

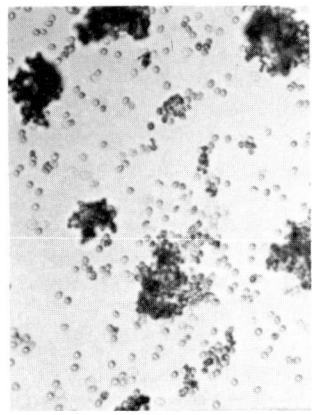

Fig. 21.2 'Agglutination' of rat erythrocytes by calf thymocyte lipids. From Tsivion and Sharon [196], with permission.

Heat-resistant lectins

Three groups of workers [60, 135, 172] have made exhaustive searches of food plants for lectins, identifying over 100 at the last count. Of these, Gibbons and Dankers [60] noted that seven of them were autoclave-resistant (wheat bran, carrot, apple, canned maize, wheat flour, pumpkin seeds and banana). The banana agglutinin was actually enhanced by heating, and was inhibitable by *N*-acetylglucosamine (GNAc) and *N*-acetylgalactosamine (GalNAc). Nachbar and Oppenheim [135] also noted haemagglutinins in dry roasted peanuts, as well as in Corn Flakes, Rice Krispies and Kellogg's Special K (which are all heated during manufacture). Avocado (*Persea americana*) lectin also resists the autoclave [189].

Phytohaemagglutinin.   Phytohaemagglutinin (PHA) in kidney beans (haricot or navy beans) resists mild cooking in the whole beans, surviving up to 4 hours at 70°C with no loss of activity and retaining some activity even at 90°C after 3 hours. Beans that had been pre-soaked overnight before cooking lost all lectin activity after 10 minutes at 100°C, but if they were boiled without this pre-soaking some activity remained after 45 minutes [65] (Fig. 21.3). Young rats reared on a diet that contained part-cooked beans (80°C, 3 hours) went into negative nitrogen balance and lost weight instead of growing. 'Slow cookers', which can cook beans to perfect culinary standards, operate at 60-85°C, which is well within the danger range for PHA. There is however no detectable lectin in textured soya protein (Freed, unpublished observations) or in commercial soya-based infant formula feeds [71], because of the very high temperatures used in the processing.

Several of the above workers have noted year-to-year and batch-to-batch variation in lectin content of various foods, so the occasional lectin accident is likely to occur even with foods normally considered to be safe.

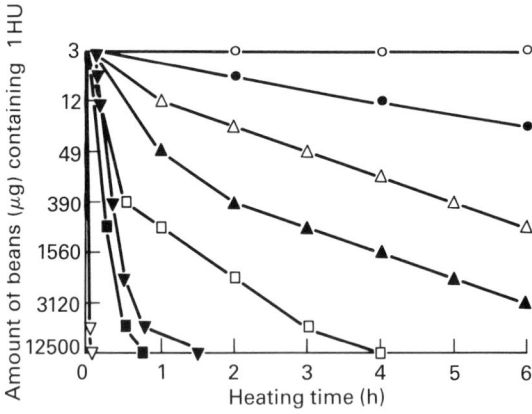

Fig. 21.3 The effect of heat treatment on the haem-agglutination activity of the white kidney bean (*Phaseolus vulgaris* var. Processor). The presoaked samples were heated at various temperatures: ○, 50°C, 65°C or 70°C; △, 80°C; ▲, 85°C; □, 90°C; ■, 95°C; ▽, 100°C; ▼, unhydrated sample heated at 100°C. From Grant et al [65], with permission.

Digestion

Effect of oral administration

Freed ingested a 10 mg dose of con A in tap water [44]. Later that day and on the next day he experienced moderate but quite intrusive small bowel colic, with passage of foul-smelling flatus of unfamiliar odour, and on day 3 passed a stool that was normal in size and texture but unusually thickly coated with mucus. Con A in tap water was administered to 10 rats by intragastric tube, and on killing them 4 days later, pronounced distension of their large bowels with gas and fluid was observed, and a 'mucotractive' effect was evident in their small intestines. Evidently sufficient con A had survived digestion to exert these effects (Fig. 21.4).

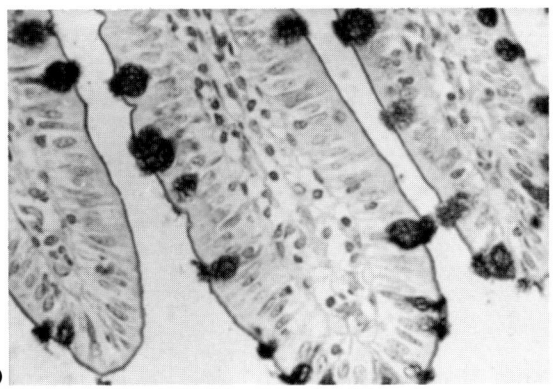

(a)

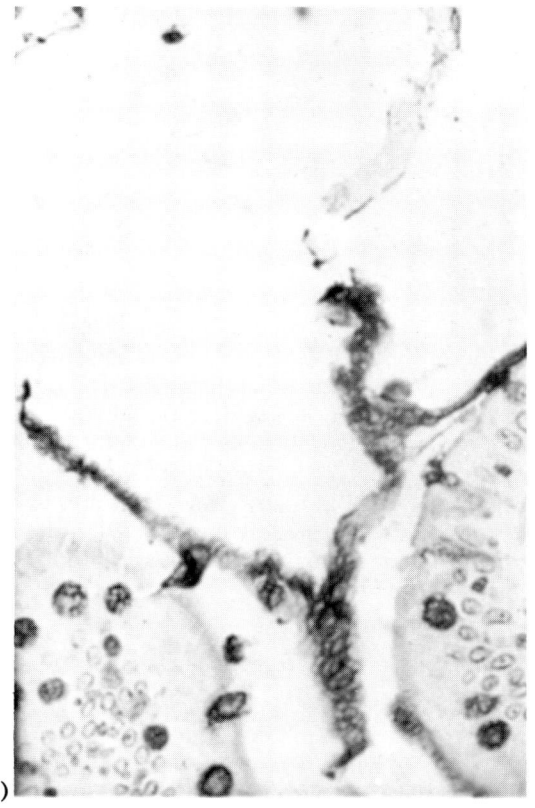

(b)

Fig. 21.4 Mucotractive effect of concanavalin A: (a) normal rat jejunum; (b) con A-fed rat. From [44], with permission.

Recovery of lectin from faeces. Pusztai et al [158] recovered 90% of an ingested dose of PHA from the faeces of experimental rats after oral administration, and also observed [159] circulating antibodies against the lectin in animals that were not producing antibody to other dietary components. Brady et al [19] gave purified WGA to human volunteers and recovered about 0.2% of the dose from the faeces. Recoverability of *added* WGA from faeces was only about 10%, which implies that at least 2.0% of the ingested dose was actually there, mostly irreversibly bound to mucins and other faecal material. A trace of ingested WGA was recovered from faeces (0.013%) even when the wheat germ had been toasted before ingestion. These workers theorized that the lectin escapes digestion by being bound to dietary fibre, and noted (as Freed and Buckley also did [44]) that a high-fibre diet is also, by and large, a high-lectin diet. Haemagglutinins in wheat bran have been noted above [60]. WGA is unusually rich in disulphide bonds and thereby resistant to proteolytic enzymes, as well as detergents, urea, alkalis and acids [119].

Gastrointestinal absorption of lectin. Many other experiments on orally administered lectins (see below) attest to their survival in the gut for long enough to exert several profound effects on the body, and the finding of circulating antibodies noted above [159] is evidence that at least some ingested lectins reach the systemic circulation in undigested form. Plasmacytes and plasmablasts, which are exceedingly rarely found in peripheral blood, were observed to be common in the blood smears of children who accidentally ingested pokeweed [9], so the pokeweed lectin not only reaches the circulation but also stimulates lymphocytes once it arrives.

LECTINS AND THE IMMUNE SYSTEM

Lectins are such an integral tool of immunologists [143] that it is a surprise to remember that it was only in 1960 that Nowell [141], following Li and Osgood [113], added PHA to his blood cultures in order to encourage the removal of erythrocytes (by agglutination) and discovered to his annoyance that the lymphocytes were being stimulated ('transformed') to enter mitosis. Knowledge of mitogenic lectins is now impressive [119, 143]. Most are selective for T cells, though pokeweed mitogen (PWM) also stimulates B cells—even after oral ingestion, as noted above.

Lymphocyte mitogenic response

Various lectins have been noted both to enhance [169] and to suppress ongoing immune responses (both cellular and humoral) to exogenous [72, 138, 188] and endogenous [35, 36, 151] antigens, depending on the time and dosage and other experimental variables. A cluster of Hodgkin's disease cases was observed in a small American town whose main industry was a large navy bean (haricot bean) elevator [151]. Most of the patients lived near to this elevator, and during the harvest season the dust from it covered their homes. Town residents had an elevated mitogenic response (as expected) to the lectin (presumably PHA or a near relative) extracted from the beans, as did mice injected with it. However the mice had a *depressed* mitogenic response to con A.

It may be noted, parenthetically, that immunosuppressive lectins are not necessarily food derived; staphylococcal slime substance inhibits mitogenesis as well [66]. Indeed, immunosuppressive lectins are not necessarily exogenous; human amyloid P component, a normal tissue constituent [90], is itself a galactan-recognizing lectin that inhibits the response of human venous lymphocytes to PPD as well as PHA and PWM [114].

The gut immune system

Anything which encourages the uptake of undegraded protein molecules from the gut, be it alcohol [199], trauma [89] or antiprotease drug, is likely to abrogate the normal gut tolerization mechanism [12] and encourage systemic immunization. Hanson (personal communication) has demonstrated just this phenomenon in mice by the use of the anti-protease aprotinin. Since some ingested lectins are profoundly damaging to the intestinal wall (see below), it is not surprising that a systemic immune response to them is seen [159]. It may be noted that aprotinin, which was used by Hanson in the experiment noted above, is not just an antiprotease; it is also a sialyl- (and uronyl-) specific lectin [81], albeit a non-agglutinating one.

Induction of T suppressor cells

Not all lectins are toxic at all doses, and at subtoxic doses lectins could also have the opposite effect. Con A at such doses induces suppressor T cells more than other T cells, suppressing the production of IgM and IgG by murine lymph node, spleen and Peyer's patch cells [33]. In this in vitro study con A was also found to suppress IgA production by spleen cells, had no effect on IgA production by lymph node cells and *enhanced* IgA production by Peyer's patch B cells [33] by a factor of 2–10 (Fig. 21.5). Peyer's patch T cells enhanced IgA—but not IgM or IgG—production when added to lipopolysaccharide (LPS)-driven spleen cells.

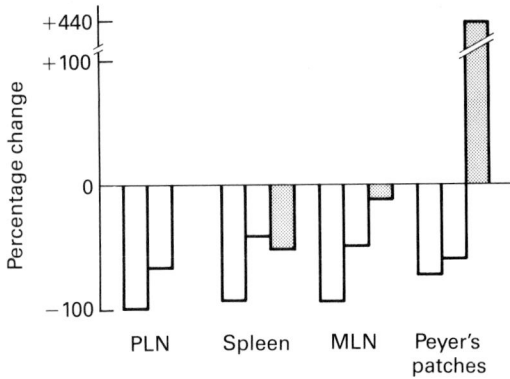

Fig. 21.5 Con A stimulates IgA production from Peyer's patch cells while suppressing other isotypes and cells from other tissues. Unshaded blocks: IgG and IgM; stippled blocks: IgA. From Elson et al [33].

The IgE system

Of particular pertinence to allergic diseases is the finding that PWM, a B cell mitogen, can directly drive human B cells in vitro to produce IgE as well as IgG, especially if the donor of the lymphocytes is atopic [211]. Pokeweed is not normally a food, but it is an indigenous weed in many American states and is occasionally ingested by children [9]; indeed it is used medicinally in some parts of the world.

Effects of lectins on IgE production in vivo

Other mitogenic lectins also modulate IgE production, presumably indirectly via an effect on T cells. When given 2 days before antigen, PHA enhanced reaginic antibody formation to that antigen while not affecting the titre of non-reaginic antibody to it. Curiously, when PHA was given 1 day before antigen, it exerted the opposite effect [5]. Injection of con

A before or together with ovalbumin into mice enhanced the reaginic antibody response to ovalbumin, though this effect was not seen with other antigens, nor with a different mitogen (endotoxin) [176]. Con A is also an allergen in its own right, provided that the recipient animal is genetically equipped to produce good reaginic responses [132]. Haptens coupled to con A induce, in such mice, an antihapten reaginic response. It may be noted in passing that *Bordetella pertussis*, itself a haemagglutinin [177], is one of the classic IgE adjuvants [73, 146]. It would not be surprising if influenza virus, another haemagglutinating organism, showed the same effect in some cases—influenza A virus is a lymphocyte mitogen [21]. Some patients with food intolerance relate the onset of their illness to an attack of influenza.

Histamine release from mast cells and basophils

Several lectins are capable of triggering degranulation and histamine release by mast cells and basophils, either by cross-linking cell-bound IgE molecules [185], by cross-linking the membrane IgE receptors [70], by themselves acting as allergens [109, 132] or by all these mechanisms. IgE-sensitized cells release more histamine than non-sensitized cells [109, 185]. WGA is particularly active in this regard [109]. Under different dosage conditions, the same lectins can *desensitize* mast cells and basophils, preventing their response to antigen, anti-IgE and compound 48/80 [7, 185]. Other lectins can only desensitize. The triggering role of infections may be important; bacteria commonly isolated from the respiratory tract during acute flare-ups of 'intrinsic' asthma were shown to cause direct histamine release from the basophils of asthmatic children (and to a lesser extent from those of normal children), being inhibited by a cocktail of simple monosaccharides [140].

Platelet aggregation

WGA aggregates human platelets (in autologous plasma but not when washed) and stimulates serotonin release [51]. This phenomenon is different from agglutination, though cross-linking of receptors is required [52-54]. A number of lectins can also block the aggregation of platelets by thrombin or other agents, given different experimental conditions [52, 68] (Fig. 21.6). Once activated, platelets develop the ability to agglutinate with other pla-

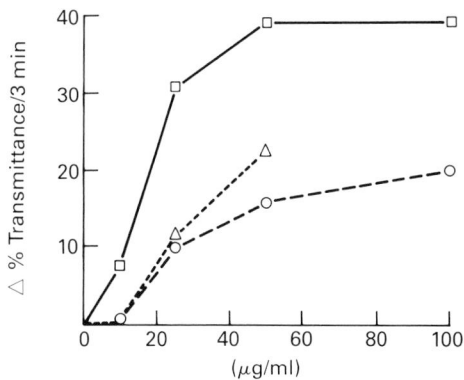

Fig. 21.6 Effect of lectin concentration on aggregation of platelets. □, wheat germ agglutinin; △, *Ricinus communis*; ○, *Phaseolus coccineus*. From Greenberg and Jamieson [68], with permission.

telets and with erythrocytes; this is due to an endogenous platelet lectin, thrombospondin [56, 82]. In addition to these direct effects, WGA also enhances the effect of thrombin on platelets by increasing the number of high-affinity receptors, whereas LCA and PHA reduced thrombin binding [88].

Tissue histiocytes. Peanut agglutinin (PNA) is a highly specific marker for human tissue histiocytes [76], though this has not (yet) been reported to have a biological consequence.

Inflammation and phagocytosis

Inhalation of con A

Con A, when injected [184] or inhaled [205], is powerfully inflammatory. In addition to causing interstitial pneumonitis when inhaled alone (Fig. 21.7), it caused a severe pneumonia with granulomatous vasculitis and areas of parenchymal necrosis in the lungs of rabbits when given in conjunction with a previously inhaled antigen, bovine serum albumin (BSA) (Figs. 21.8, 21.9). If this experiment was repeated, in the same animals, much worse damage occurred, with acute necrotic areas developing followed by interstitial fibrosis as well as deposition of antigen, antibody and complement. The authors of this experiment [205] likened the less severe picture to human extrinsic allergic alveolitis, and the more severe picture (seen after repetition of the inhalation) to Wegener's granulomatosis. Mann and Freed, while investigating the mucotractive effect of con A, inhaled 2 mg and 20 mg of con A, respectively, using a commercial powder-inhalation device. Mann, who took the smaller dose, felt rather ill later that day.

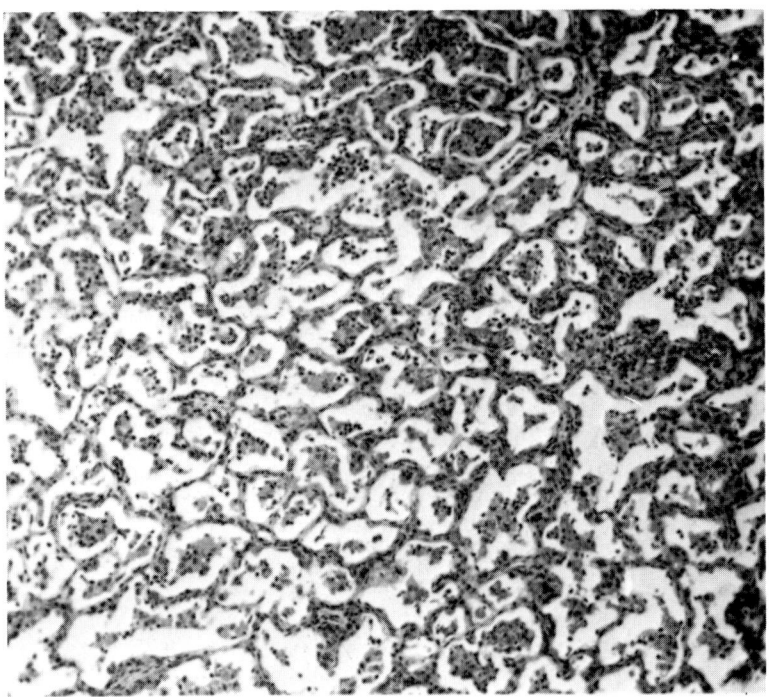

Fig. 21.7 Interstitial inflammation in a non-immunized rabbit given con A aerosol. Haematoxylin and eosin, × 110. From Willoughby et al [205], with permission. © 1979 US-Canadian Division of the IAP.

Freed developed a high fever and an illness clinically indistinguishable from acute bronchopneumonia, except that it came on within 4 hours of the inhalation, was maximal at 8–10 hours and had virtually disappeared next morning (unpublished observations). The experiment has not been repeated.

Effects in vitro

At the cellular level, con A induces microtubule assembly in, and granule discharge from, human polymorphs [74, 109] and release of arachidonic acid from human mononuclear cells and lymphocytes [145]. Like the respiratory bacteria noted above [79, 140], con A can activate the alternative pathway of complement. This is sometimes the reason why supraoptimal concentrations of mitogen inhibit lymphocyte transformation, since the effect can be blocked by the use of heated serum or zymosan in the medium [41]. The same is also presumably true of some other mitogenic lectins that show the phenomenon of inhibition at supraoptimal concentrations.

Lectin-induced cellular cytotoxicity (LICC)

Human lymphocytes and polymorphs can be stimulated by PHA to kill target cells non-specifically. This process (lectin-induced cellular cytotoxicity, LICC) [208] is therefore analo-

gous to antibody-dependent cellular cytotoxicity (ADCC) except that in the case of LICC it is thought to be the cytotoxic cell, rather than its target, that is the prime recipient of the lectin (this assumption has not been closely examined and may turn out to be erroneous). PHA-stimulated porcine alveolar macrophages are also cytotoxic, though they are able to discriminate self from non-self [170]. Indeed, 'spontaneous' cellular cytotoxicity (natural killer cell activity) was shown in one report to be inhibitable by simple sugars (ribose, lactose, GalNAc), which implies that this 'spontaneous' cytotoxic activity is in fact being driven by lectins, either exogenous or endogenous [124]. ADCC was not inhibited by the same or other sugars.

Variable susceptibility to lectin effects

All of the above-mentioned effects are determined to some extent by genetic and environmental influences acting on the individual recipients. Gauthier-Rahman et al [57] noted 20-fold variations in PHA mitogenesis between different strains of mice. These differences were reflected in mixed-lymphocyte and graft-versus-host reactivity. Paradoxically, the high responders required 10-fold *greater* doses of antigen to induce delayed hypersensitivity than did low responders.

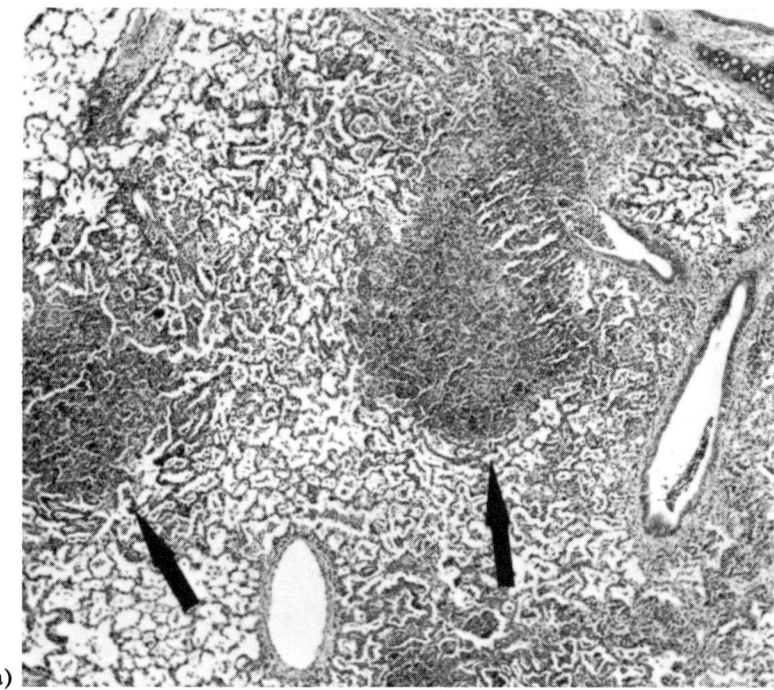

(a)

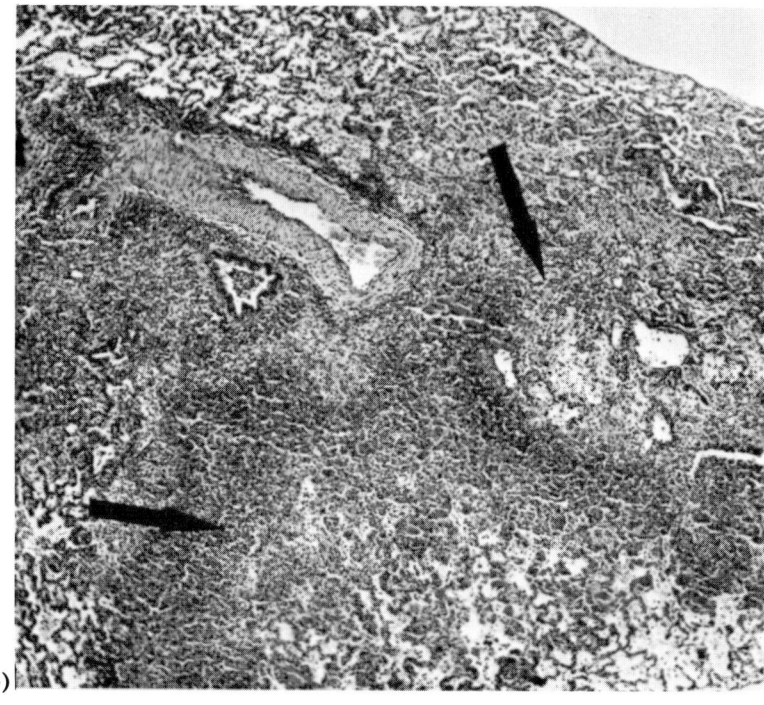

(b)

Fig. 21.8 (a) Areas of parenchymal necroses (arrows) in the lung of a BSA-immunized rabbit challenged with BSA–con A aerosol mixture. Note also the presence of interstitial inflammation affecting necrotic areas. Haematoxylin and eosin, × 45. (b) Bland infarcts (arrows) occurring in the lung of a BSA-immunized rabbit challenged with BSA–con A aerosol. Haematoxylin and eosin, × 45. From Willoughby et al [205], with permission. © 1979 US-Canadian Division of the IAP.

(a)

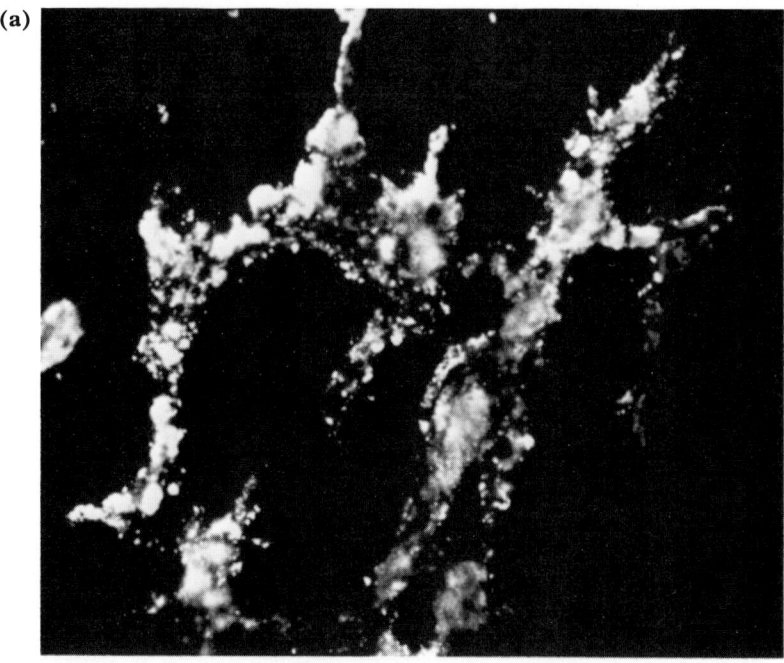

(b)

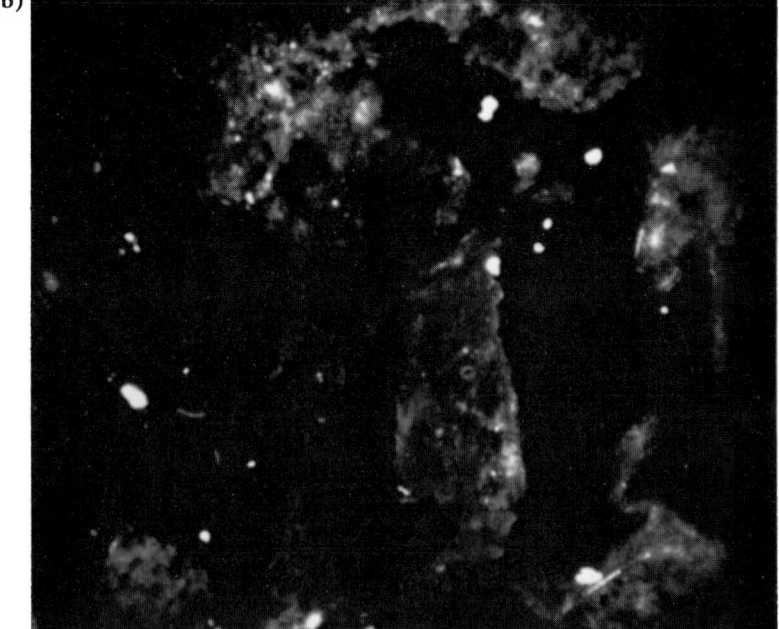

Fig. 21.9 (a) Immunofluorescent demonstration of rabbit IgG in a BSA-immunized rabbit challenged with BSA–con A aerosol. Note the granular pattern of localization within the thickened septa. (b) Complete inhibition of staining by prior absorption of the FITC–goat antirabbit IgG with purified rabbit IgG, × 300. From Willoughby et al [205], with permission. ©1979 US-Canadian Division of the IAP.

Intradermal PHA and immune response

The response of humans to an intradermal injection of PHA (a general test of immune responsiveness popular in Continental Europe though not in English-speaking countries) varies widely between patients. In one French intensive care unit 81% of PHA-anergic patients died while on the unit, whereas only 10% of PHA-responsive patients died [104]. Such differences are related to nutritional status [104], and to the levels of zinc [42, 64] and (at least in pigs) of vitamin E and selenium [110], as well as to intake of corticosteroids [105].

Mitogenesis in diabetes: effect of insulin

The lymphocytes of diabetics respond to PHA, con A and PWM subnormally; this defect can be partly normalized in vitro by insulin, and by tight clinical control in vivo [62, 142]. Insulin also enhances con A stimulation of normal mouse lymphocytes [187]. A single report in Russian notes a subnormal lymphocyte response to PHA and con A in schizophrenics [150]; the English abstract of this paper does not speculate as to whether this is cause or effect, or the effect of an institutional diet.

LECTINS AND THE ALIMENTARY CANAL

Mouth

As noted above, all buccal mucous membranes are coated with lectin after the mastication of one tomato [136] (see Table 21.2). After eating 2–7 g of raw wheat germ, or 25 g of raw peanuts, WGA and PNA respectively were found adherent to buccal and lingual epithelial cells; binding was inhibitable by the appropriate monosaccharides [61]. In mouse oral mucosae, PNA, WGA and SBA all had a histological affinity for basement membrane [167]. Basement membranes are in general rich in sugars such as glucose, galactose, fucose and galactosamines (a point which is also pertinent to the kidney, as will be noted below).

Precipitation of saliva

WGA and PNA [61], as well as crude extracts of various foods (tomato, lettuce, cucumber, wheat bran and whole wheat, sesame and sunflower seeds, vanilla yoghurt, coconut, banana and babyfood banana, carrot, onion, apple, alfalfa and soya protein) [60], also bound to and in some cases precipitated with components of human saliva, including cellular debris and

bacteria. This is in agreement with the ability of saliva to inhibit the binding of various lectins to experimental tooth pellicles in vitro [61]. This is important because in vivo, pellicle (a glycoprotein coating on teeth adsorbed from saliva) is the first component of dental plaque. The next step is when caries-associated bacteria such as *Streptococcus mutans* and *S. sanguis* bind to the pellicle, a process that is enhanced by sucrose. The bacteria then synthesize the extracellular slime which is mainly polyglucan and a main component of the plaque.

Lectins and caries

Binding of *S. mutans* and *S. sanguis* to experimental hydroxyapatite–saliva pellicles was inhibited by the various foods, noted above [60], that precipitated human saliva. Avocado lectin [189] also inhibited the sucrose-dependent adherence of *S. mutans* to experimental pellicle, so it seems possible that dietary lectins could protect against caries. Purists will argue that avocado lectin is not a true lectin as it binds to basic proteins and not apparently to carbohydrates. Lectins that bind directly to pellicle, such as con A, PNA, SBA and WGA, might also inhibit bacterial adhesion by masking pellicle receptor sites. However, this protective effect is not seen with all lectins [60], and indeed con A has been reported to *enhance* bacterial adhesion [189], though this is controversial.

Stomach

As with the small intestine (see below), various lectins tend to bind patchily to gastric mucosal cells of various types, varying from one cell to

Table 21.2 Binding of various dietary lectins to human alimentary-tract cells and cell products.

Site	Lectins	Bind to:	Reference
Mouth	WGA PNA	Buccal and lingual epithelial cells and salivary sediment	61
Stomach	PNA	Some but not all epithelial, neck, parietal, chief, antral gland, Brunner's gland, goblet and columnar cells	106, 147, 207
Stomach	PHA	Gastrin-secreting cells	77
Small bowel	WGA	Mucin in goblet cells and in process of extrusion, especially at tips of villi	80
Small bowel	PHA	Brush-border enzymes (sucrase–isomaltase, maltose glucoamylase, lactase, neutral and acid aminopeptidases, oligopeptidyl peptidases)	195
Large bowel	PNA	Epithelial cells	34
Pancreas, liver, duodenum	WGA	γ-Glutamyltransferase	179

its neighbouring cell even when these are of the same type, and from one patient to another unrelated to blood group [147]. This heterogeneity is evidence of variable maturity of surface glycoproteins. Parietal cells in general do not bind PNA, though a number of nondietary lectins do bind [147]. PNA did bind, however, to mucus-producing cells at the surface epithelium and in the glands [106].

One finding of note was an 'extraordinary affinity' for PHA of gastrin-secreting cells as opposed to other stomach cells (Fig. 21.10) and other endocrine cells of pancreas, thyroid and parathyroid [77]. As at other histological

sites [166], the binding of lectins is crucially determined by the method of fixation and processing of the section.

Small and large intestine

WGA and various non-dietary lectins bind to rat intestinal epithelia in different patterns. WGA binds to microvilli in the crypts and along the villi except in the distal reaches of the ileum where binding is weak and confined to the bases of the villi [37]. Binding to goblet cells increases from proximal to distal small intestine in the rat [37]. Binding capacity of rat intestine for various lectins exhibits considerable changes over the first weeks of life, in line with 'gut closure' [126]. Rat mucus and goblet cells also bind SBA, PNA, con A and LCA [47].

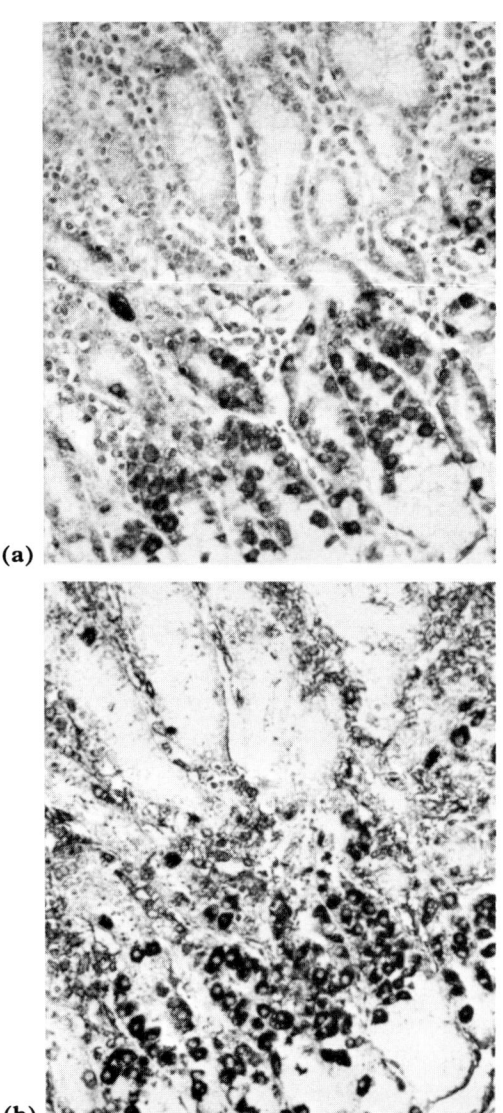

(a)

(b)

Fig. 21.10 Lectins and the stomach: human antropyloric mucosa (a) stained for gastrin, (b) stained by *Phaseolus vulgaris* agglutinin. From Hsu and Raine [77], with permission.

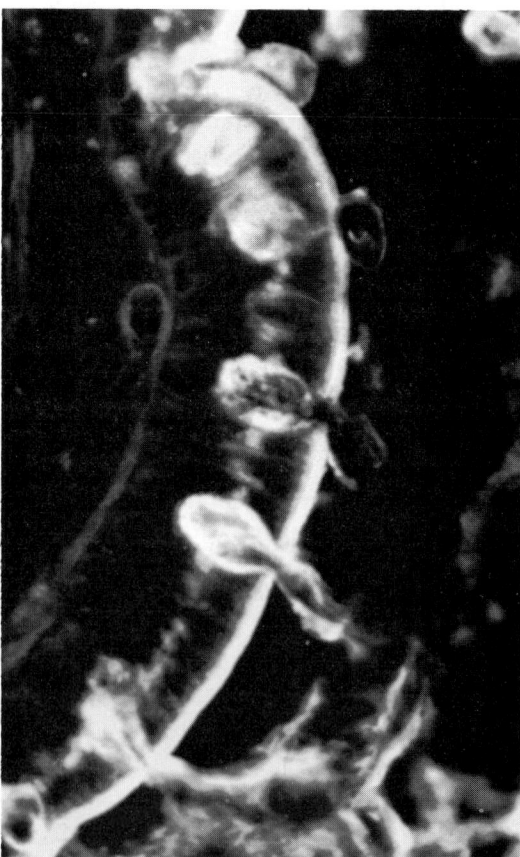

Fig. 21.11 Lectins and the intestine: base of jejunal villus from a cystic fibrosis small bowel biopsy, labelled with fluorescein isothiocyanate–*Triticum vulgare* agglutinin. Release of mucin from goblet cells into the intervillous space is seen. Intracellular staining of epithelial cells in the supranuclear region appears to be localized to the Golgi apparatus. × 400. From Jacobs et al [80], with permission.

Binding of WGA to goblet cells

The predilection of WGA for goblet cells is also seen in human intestine (Fig. 21.11), but in the human this is not shared by PNA or SBA [80]. PNA binds variably in the human duodenum (Fig. 21.12) [207], and rather more generally in the human large bowel, probably as a result of bacterial action on the mucus (see below [27].

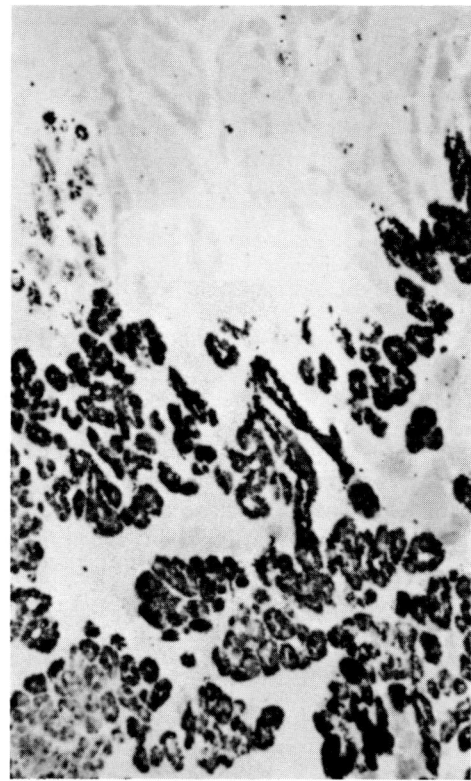

Fig. 21.12 Lectins and the intestine: *Arachis hypogaea* agglutinin positivity of Brunner's glands. No staining in goblet cells and striated columnar cells. × 63. From Wurster et al [207], with permission.

Lectin binding to intestinal enzymes and secretory immunoglobulins

Various rat [34] and human [179, 195] intestinal enzymes can be bound and in some cases precipitated by con A, WGA, PHA and *Helix pomatia* lectin. Sandholm and Scott [175] observed that con A, PWM and raw soya beans interfered with the adsorption of chicken pancreatic enzymes to chicken intestinal mucosa, and released enzymes that had already been adsorbed. This is important because digestion of foods at the brush border is nutritionally far more important than is digestion in the gut lumen. This inhibitory effect was not universal; PHA actually increased adsorption of amylase. These authors speculated that gut mucosal turnover is the biological price paid by animals in order to rid the intestine of unwanted lectins. Binding of gut secretory immunoglobulins by lectins (IgA and IgM are precipitated by LCA, PSA and several other lectins in preference to IgG) [171] might also interfere with any digestive function of gut antibodies [48, 67]. However it should be noted that the mere binding of a lectin to an enzyme does not necessarily obstruct the enzyme's catalytic properties [121].

Damage to gut structure and function

Antinutritive effects of ingested lectins

That uncooked legumes are of poor nutritive value, and sometimes cause scours in farm animals and humans [139, 154], has been known to livestock farmers since antiquity. Legumes contain many potentially antinutritive factors such as antiproteases, antiamylases and saponins [26, 116, 163], and the first suggestion that lectins might be responsible is attributable to Jaffe in 1960 [83]. He suggested that dietary lectins might interfere with the absorption of nutrients by coating the intestinal epithelium and passively obstructing uptake—a suggestion that is still current although we now know other mechanisms that also operate. The adsorption of vitamin B_{12}–intrinsic factor complex to the distal ileal mucosa of guinea pigs was inhibited by PHA—although WGA and con A enhanced adsorption [15]. In the rabbit jejunum, the attachment of glycinin (the main protein of soya beans) was enhanced by the simultaneous presence of SBA and soya saponin [1]. It seems therefore that lectins can sometimes act in favour of nutrition.

PHA effect on gut mucosa

But these two papers [1, 15] stand isolated in the literature, in stark contrast to the many papers that indict lectins as being antinutritive. In a careful series of studies in which uncooked kidney beans or PHA were fed to rats, Pusztai and colleagues showed that the rats entered negative nitrogen balance, with increased faecal and urinary nitrogen and sometimes death, and also showed that this was caused not by the antiproteases or other factors but by the lectin [94–96, 157, 158, 160, 162, 206]. The lectin binds to the microvilli

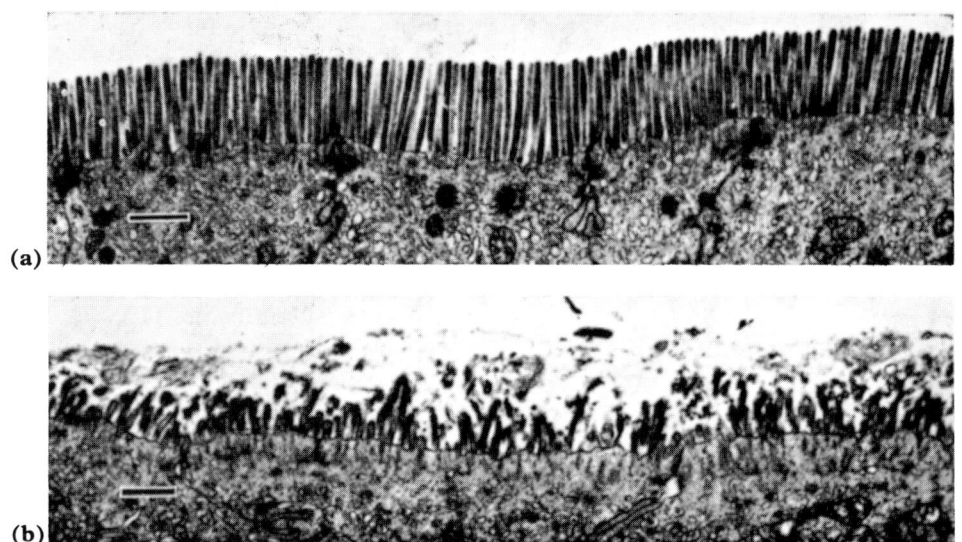

Fig. 21.13 (a) Jejunum of a rat fed for 10 days on a diet containing 10% cooked *Phaseolus vulgaris* var. Processor bean protein, showing the normal appearance of the microvilli. Bar = 1.0 μm. (b) Jejunum of a rat fed for 3 days on a diet containing 10% raw Processor bean protein, showing stunted microvilli. Bar = 1.0 μm. From King et al [96], with permission.

on the enterocytes and there causes severe disruption of tissue architecture both at light- and electron-microscopic level (Fig. 21.13). This does not happen in the ileum but reappears in the caecum and slightly in the colon. These results were confirmed by Banwell et al [8], using lower doses of lectin, and these workers observed reduced mucosal enzyme levels, with malabsorption of lipids and vitamin B_{12} even at dose levels too low to produce overt intestinal damage. Other workers showed that oral WGA and con A are equally antinutritive for the rat, and observed another possible antinutritive mechanism, namely an increase of exfoliation of the mucosal surface such that at high doses there was shortening of the villi with a net reduction of absorptive surface area [122]. Freed and Buckley [44] observed yet another possibly antinutritive mechanism of intragastric con A in rats, namely a 'mucotractive' effect on small-intestinal goblet cells associated with intestinal hurry.

SBA and coeliac disease: effect of sugars

In man, a number of workers have noted that soya bean intolerance can produce a syndrome that is indistinguishable from coeliac disease [2, 131]. Textured soya protein is just as cytotoxic in vitro to Hela cells as is a bread extract [45], although the soya protein did not have detectable haemagglutinin (unpublished observations); on the other hand, Donovan

and Torres-Pinedo [31] described a patient with soya intolerance whose severe diarrhoea was ameliorated by ingestion of the sugar inhibitors of SBA (galactose or lactose) whereas glucose and sucrose made it worse. It therefore seems that heated soya protein, even if no longer haemagglutinating, can still interact with sugars and cause intestinal disease.

Lectins and bacterial overgrowth: experiments in germ-free animals

Several workers have observed that in quail [84] and rats [8, 162, 206] the antinutritive effect of PHA and con A is largely abrogated when the experiment is performed with germ-free animals, or when conventional animals are treated with antibiotics. The PHA-damaged areas of jejunum noted above [8, 206] were heavily infected by coliform bacteria, and when gnotobiotic quail were monocolonized with quail coliforms, the antinutritive effect of con A returned. Lectins in the small intestine therefore appear to encourage bacterial overgrowth, in marked contrast to the effect in the mouth (see above). It is worth noting that most human intestinal microbial parasites—viruses, bacteria and bacterial toxins—are able to overcome normal gut motility by their own lectin-like properties [59]. Forsdyke [40] has put forward the plausible hypothesis that those ingested lectins which are cytotoxic (e.g. by alternative pathway complement activation or directly) are likely to damage first the lymphocytes in the mesenteric lymph nodes, thus making more likely both bacterial overgrowth and eventual food allergy.

Similar effects of other agents. Of course, none of the pathological effects noted in this section are unique to lectins. A mucotractive effect, for example, can also be stimulated immunologically by administration of antigen to a pre-immunized animal, or by preformed immune complexes [107], and several other food-borne toxins (alkaloids, saponins, antienzymes, hormone mimics and so on) [26, 116, 163] are also directly damaging to tissues.

Coeliac disease

The lectin hypothesis

It was shown over 20 years ago that a component of wheat gliadin binds preferentially to the crypt epithelial cells in human coeliac disease, and this binding is only rarely seen in healthy volunteers [173]. This lectin hypothesis of coeliac disease really owes its popularization to Weiser and Douglas [202], who in 1976 put forward the suggestion that a gluten lectin binds preferentially to coeliac enterocytes because their surface carbohydrates are of an immature pattern. They based this idea on the agglutinability of human fetal—but not adult—intestinal cells by con A [201], and on the demonstration of a glycoprotein isolated from gluten (and shown to be toxic by feeding to a coeliac volunteer, although it was not gliadin) that was able to bind better to coeliac jejunal mucosa than to normal mucosa [32]. Con A, in contrast, binds less well to coeliac mucosa than it does to normal [198].

This work has since been confirmed by other workers [25, 102, 103], strongly supporting the lectin hypothesis. All workers are agreed that WGA, the classic wheat lectin, is *not* the coeliac lectin [25, 32, 102, 103]. Final proof of the lectin hypothesis waits upon a therapeutic trial of the appropriate sugar inhibitor (once this has been identified) in otherwise untreated coeliac disease patients. At present a mannosyl oligosaccharide (possibly an enteric-coated preparation) seems to be the most promising candidate [102, 103], although this is not universally agreed [32]. Far from contradicting the other theories of coeliac disease causation—the 'defective enzyme' hypothesis and the 'allergy' hypothesis—the lectin theory marries them harmoniously together, since lectins can inhibit enzyme activity [8,

175, 179, 195], and being themselves antigenic are prime targets for antibody deposition and immune complex inflammation.

LECTINS AND OTHER ORGANS

Kidney

Both human [39, 75] and animal [75, 134, 148] kidneys contain essential structural glycoproteins that offer binding sites for various lectins (Fig. 21.14). WGA binds to the glomerular capillary wall in all 14 animal species studied [75] including man, and in man also to the inner surfaces of collecting ducts, Henlé's loops and proximal and distal convoluted tubules. SBA and PNA also bind to various sites in human kidney, but not as much as WGA. Any disturbance of function at these sites would have important consequences; glomerular permeability and tubular transport are to a large extent determined by their glycoproteins [134] (Table 21.3).

Heymann nephritis

Heymann nephritis in rats is an immune complex nephritis that has a striking histological and immunochemical similarity to human idiopathic membranous glomerulonephritis [91, 92, 127, 130]. It can be actively induced by immunization with syngeneic kidney cortex in complete Freund's adjuvant, and passively transferred using the autoantibodies eluted from kidney at pH 3.2. The antibodies bind in characteristic granular pattern to the lamina rara externa of the glomerular basement membrane, even though the exciting antigen is typically found in the proximal convoluted tubule.

Heymann 'antigen'. However, the use of monoclonal antibodies demonstrates that the antigen is also to be found in the glomerular epithelial cells, under and in the foot processes, in and between their points of application to the basement membrane [92]. The antigen splits into several bands on sodium dodecyl sulphate-polyacrylamide gel electrophoresis [91], but only one of these is bound by Heymann antibody. This antigen is a glycoprotein of molecular weight 330 000 that binds strongly to WGA and con A [127, 130] but has an 'extraordinarily high affinity' for LCA [91]—being eluted from it only by a combination of 500 mM α-methyl mannoside, 10 mM EDTA and 6.0 M urea. A very few

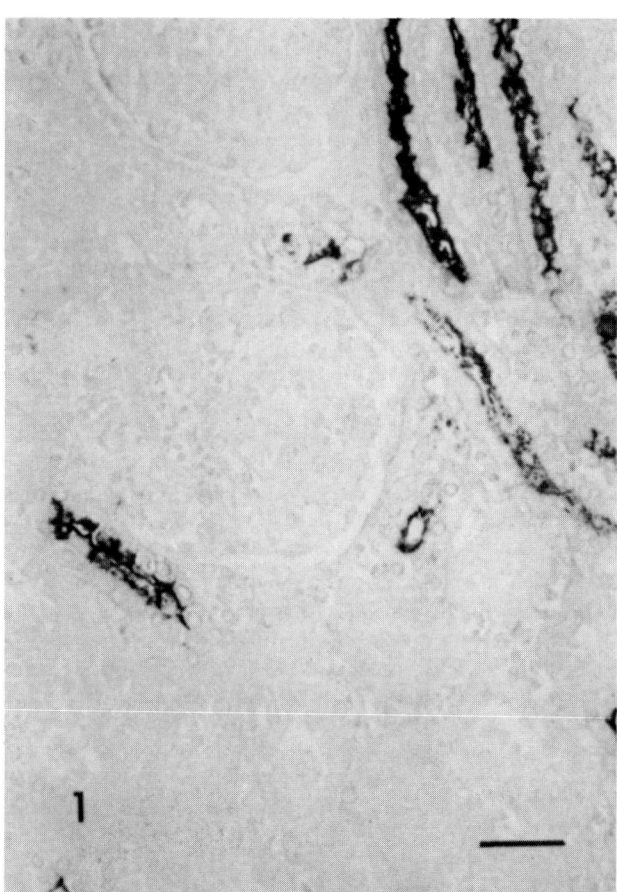

Fig. 21.14 Lectins and the kidney: normal human kidney following formalin fixation, paraffin embedding, peanut lectin–peroxidase incubation, and diaminobenzidine–H_2O_2 reaction. There is strong binding of the lectin to the collecting ducts and loops of Henlé and a lack of staining in the glomeruli and proximal convoluted tubules. Bar = 100 μm. From Faraggiana et al [39], with permission. Copyright 1982 by The Histochemical Society, Inc.

Table 21.3 Binding of various dietary lectins to non-alimentary human tissues.

Site	Lectins	Cells bound	Reference
Kidney	WGA SBA PNA	Proximal tubule, distal tubule Distal tubule	75
Kidney	WGA	Inner surfaces of collecting ducts, Henlé's loops, vascular endothelium, proximal convoluted tubules (lysosomes and brush borders), glomerular capillary walls, collagen fibres, basement membranes	39
Kidney	PNA	Lumen of collecting ducts, distal convoluted tubules	39
Kidney	WGA	Embryonic kidney epithelial cells adhere to and grow well on WGA-coated plastic, though soluble WGA is toxic	148
Brain	LCA PHA WGA	Membranes and myelin of white matter	78
Brain	PNA	Choroid plexus after neuraminidase treatment	133
Skin	PNA WGA	Keratinocytes (more so in psoriatic plaques)	63
Breast	WGA PNA SBA	Mammary epithelial cells, duct lumina	43
Syncytial trophoblast	WGA	Surface membrane and coated pits	203

molecules of this or similar lectin, if presented to the kidney in vivo, would bind virtually irreversibly into the filtration apparatus of the glomerulus, disrupting its function and attracting immunological attack.

Lectin-induced cellular cytotoxicity (LICC). Although Heymann nephritis is a rat model, of unproven relevance to human nephritis, there is a clue in the study of lectin-induced cellular cytotoxicity (LICC), which as discussed above is rather similar to 'spontaneous' natural killer (NK) cell activity and may in fact be being driven by lectins. PHA-induced LICC activity was 17% higher in patients awaiting kidney transplants than in normals, in spite of the fact that the cytotoxic cells themselves were no different (ADCC levels were normal) [200].

Triggering role of infections

The Thomson–Friedenreich antigen (T anti-

gen) is not generally found on human cells but can be exposed on many cell types after terminal sialic acid molecules have been stripped off by the action of neuraminidase (Fig. 21.15). This apparently improbable occurrence is actually very common, since pneumococci, *Vibrio cholerae* and *Clostridium perfringens*—not to mention the ubiquitous influenza virus—all contain active neuraminidase.

Action of neuraminidase and the T antigen. Antibodies against T antigen are universal in humans after the first few months of life and T antigen itself is usually to be found on human colonic mucosa [27], presumably as a result of bacterial action. The carbohydrate structure of the T antigen is well worked out—and PNA is specific for it. After neuraminidase exposure, PNA-binding sites are exposed on human erythrocytes, lymphocytes, thrombocytes, breast epithelium and milk fat-globule membranes, glomeruli (on the ep-

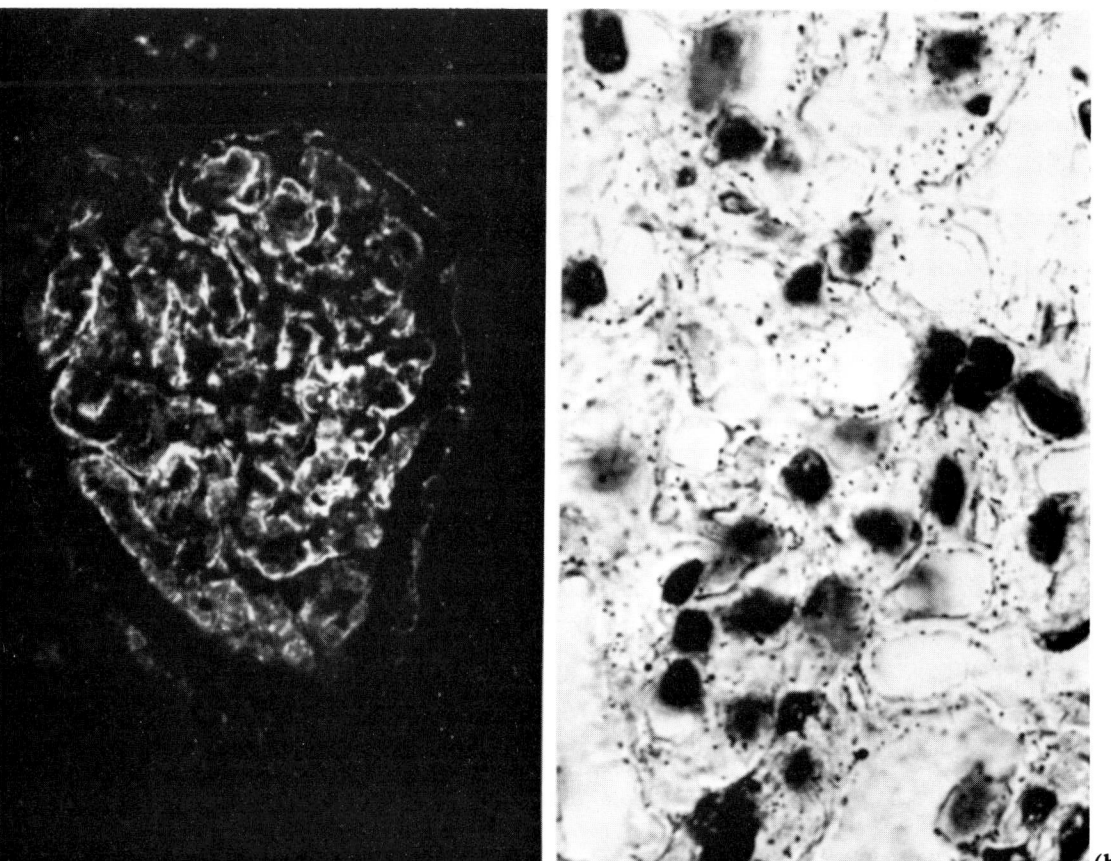

(a)   (b)

Fig. 21.15 Demonstration of Thomsen–Friedenreich antigen on kidney glomeruli after treatment with neuraminidase as shown by (a) fluorescein-labelled peanut agglutinin and (b) autoradiography using ³H-labelled peanut agglutinin (part of a glomerulus). The receptors are arranged along the basement membrane of capillary loops, as clearly shown by the autoradiographic technique. From Klein et al [98], with permission.

ithelial cell foot processes along the external surface of the basement membrane) and on many serum glycoproteins [98]. Klein et al [97] reported two children in whom pneumococcal sepsis was followed by severe haemolytic–uraemic syndrome, in whom T antigen had been uncovered on both erythrocytes and glomeruli. This was associated with renal cortical necrosis, presumably due to attack by anti-T antibodies and perhaps also by T specific food lectins, such as PNA.

Nervous system

Axonal transport of lectin

Although mature neurons do not divide, it would be wrong to think of them as metabolically inactive. Neurons face the problem of keeping axon terminals, that may be over a metre away, supplied with nutrients and metabolites, and are in fact the most actively synthesizing of cells [24].

There is a vigorous axonal transport mechanism, in both directions, and if the cut end of a living nerve is dipped into a solution of WGA or SBA, the lectin is transported to the other end of the axon within 1–2 days [16, 58, 111]. The same phenomenon occurs after injection of lectin into nerves or brain. These procedures are of course highly improbable in normal life, and the suggestion has been made that uptake of lectins does not occur in undamaged nerves [20].

Lectin binding to myelin.   Both rat and human myelins have a strong affinity for con A, WGA, PHA and LCA [78, 125, 161], as do nicotinic acetylcholine receptors of rat brain [174], and after injection of lectins into the rat lateral ventricle they were found within periventricular neurons within 48 hours [149]. In this context it is noteworthy that whereas normal human choroid plexus does not take up PNA, neuraminidase treatment (such as occurs in various infections) uncovers multiple PNA-binding sites [133]. Whether lectin uptake by neurons causes the cell any harm is unknown, although 'suicide transport' by neurons, after persuading them to imbibe toxic lectins like ricin and abrin, is popular among some neuroanatomists as a tool for tracing nerve connections [204].

Skin and mammary tissue

Normal human keratinocytes bind con A, WGA, PNA and HPA strongly; psoriatic ker-

atinocytes bind the first three even more [63]. Normal human breast tissue binds WGA, PNA, SBA and con A, especially at the apices of the mammary epithelial cells [43], from which the milk fat globules form by budding.

The binding of PNA is greatly increased on both mammary epithelial cells and on milk fat-globule membranes after neuraminidase treatment [98]. It is possible that after infections such as influenza, the breast, its milk and all other tissues that express the T antigen may become more susceptible to binding by PNA and similar lectins (not to mention the universal anti-T antibody). Perhaps in this context the naturopaths' practice of starving patients during acute infectious illnesses makes some sense.

Miscellaneous tissues

Con A and WGA bind to both mouse embryos [101] and human syncytial trophoblast [203]. Con A and WGA interfere with the binding of nerve growth factor to human fibroblasts [23] and rabbit sympathetic ganglia [28], and con A also binds to follicle-stimulating hormone [13]. Multiple interactions with normal plasma enzymes [121] and glycoproteins [197], including immunoglobulins [171, 210], have already been noted. α_2-Macroglobulin (α_2M) is a major plasma component comprising 8.5% of total plasma carbohydrate, and binds con A and WGA.

Cystic fibrosis

The α_2M of cystic fibrosis (CF) patients binds more con A and WGA molecule for molecule, than the α_2M of normals, with heterozygotes falling between. The same is true of IgM and IgG molecules. Curiously, CF α_2M also binds more limulin (a non-dietary sialic acid-binding lectin), although it actually possesses less sialic acid than the normal molecule [11, 144, 178]. Lectin studies in CF are long overdue in view of the affinity of many lectins for mucins [129], and the suggestion made by Freed and Buckley [44] that con A therapy might be worth investigating in CF because of its mucotractive effect. However, the evidence so far appears to weigh against this suggestion, since CF serum already has at least one mucotractive factor of its own [14], which could well be the pathognomonic fructose-inhibitable haemagglutinin for murine cells noted by Lieberman et al [115] in the serum of CF patients, associated with (but not the same as) IgM.

This is an exciting development, but it has yet to be determined whether this endogenous CF lectin is pathogenic, or whether it represents the body's attempt to compensate for abnormally adherent mucus. Only a therapeutic trial of the sugar inhibitor—ethically very difficult—would decide the matter.

LECTINS AND THE DIET OF DIABETICS

Many workers have noted that carbohydrates differ in their glycaemic effects, in both normals and diabetics, depending on the physical form of the food. Thus, high-fibre diets, including the use of pectins and guar gum are frequently recommended [3, 85, 168]. Cooked dried beans are especially recommended [86, 128], which will not by now surprise the reader in view of the multiple antinutritive effects of lectins noted above.

Lectin binding to insulin receptors

In addition to these effects, many lectins including WGA, LCA, PSA and con A, bind to both rat and human insulin receptors and mimic insulin. WGA is as effective in molar terms as is insulin at enhancing glucose oxidation and transport in isolated adipocytes (Fig. 21.16), and enhances the affinity of in-

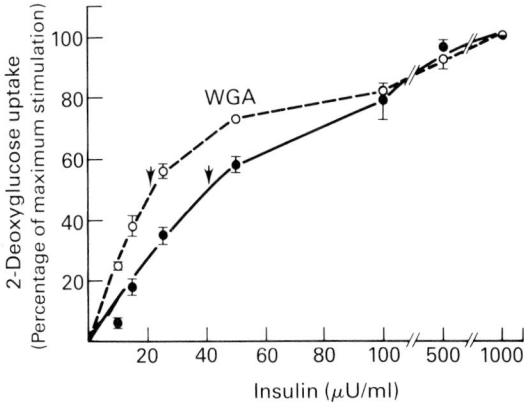

Fig. 21.16 Effect of a low wheat germ agglutinin (WGA) concentration on insulin dose–response curve for stimulation of 2-deoxyglucose uptake. Fat cells were incubated for 60 minutes in the presence (○) or absence (●) of 1 µg/ml WGA with indicated concentration of insulin. Rate of 2-deoxyglucose uptake was determined and expressed as a percentage of maximum insulin stimulation. Arrows represent concentrations of insulin needed to stimulate half-maximal activation of 2-deoxyglucose uptake. Results are mean ± SE of four separate experiments. From Livingston and Purvis [120], with permission.

sulin itself for its receptors [30, 69, 120]. This low-dose insulin-facilitating effect is also seen with LCA. WGA also increases the rate of synthesis of new insulin receptors [29]. These effects remain after the cell surfaces have been washed [180, 186], unlike the effect of insulin itself. The waxbean lectin is also insulinomimetic, although in this case a different receptor is involved [181]. Once bound by its target cells, insulin is internalized and proceeds to bind to the nuclear membrane, where by regulating phosphorylation it increases the efflux of mRNA from nucleus to cytoplasm. PHA and con A also do this, albeit in doses rather too high (10 µg/ml) to be entirely biologically credible [156]. The interaction between insulin and lectins works both ways, as noted above; insulin enhances con A mitogenesis of mouse T lymphocytes, and once they are activated by con A, insulin can replace the lectin for continuing stimulation [187].

POSSIBLE BENEFICIAL EFFECTS OF DIETARY LECTINS IN NORMAL HUMAN PHYSIOLOGY

Although this review has been largely concerned with potentially damaging effects of dietary lectins, there are also possible beneficial effects. Some have already been mentioned, such as an anticariogenic effect in the mouth, the occasional promotion of specific immune responses, promotion of immune surveillance by driving 'spontaneous' NK cell activity, regulation of the intestinal immune response by promoting IgA and suppressing IgG and IgM, and the insulin-sparing effect. Five other possible benefits deserve a mention.

Maintaining cell architecture

Con A, WGA, SBA, PNA and PHA all exhibit the curious phenomenon of 'positive cooperativity' when incubated with lymphocytes. This becomes apparent when trying to work out the affinity of lectins by using the Scatchard equation [190] in the hump-back plots that result [153]. These graphs are a flagrant violation of the Law of Mass Action, and can only mean that the Law's basic assumptions do not apply. In molecular terms it means that as the first few molecules of lectin begin to bind to a cell, they rearrange that cell's surface in such a way as to facilitate the binding of subsequent lectin molecules.

Decreased cell fluidity. Monomeric (non-mitogenic) derivatives of these lectins do not exhibit this outrageous behaviour, which at the level of the whole cell makes itself apparent, usually, by an increased rigidity and reduced lateral fluidity of the cell surface [50, 198]. The effect is all-or-nothing; having switched in at critical lectin concentration it cannot be raised by using higher lectin concentrations. Thus, human erythrocytes are prevented from assuming 'echinocyte' morphology under conditions of physicochemical distress [123], isolated adipocytes are protected against 'nutritional stepdown' when serum is removed from the culture medium [186] and Hela cell monolayers are protected against the toxic effect of bread extract [45]. Positive cooperativity has been elegantly demonstrated in artificial liposomes containing transmembrane glycophorin, when incubated with WGA in the presence of albumin. The lectin appears to rearrange the receptors into a polydentate form that encourages further lectin adhesion [93].

Increased cell fluidity. However, in other experimental conditions it should be noted that lectins can exert the opposite effect on cells, increasing fluidity [10, 194]. Thus, WGA and con A induce redistribution of filopodia on the growth cones of chick neurons [22], and induce the expression of DR transplantation antigens on cultured human follicular thyroid cells [155].

Increasing gut mucosal turnover

Although it is possible almost to abolish defecation by the use of the low-fibre diets used by astronauts (and many teenagers), the fibre hypothesis makes it clear that there are risks entailed in this. Some turnover of gut mucosa is evidently desirable, although in excess it is likely to lead to malabsorption and malnutrition. In the light of the effects on the gut noted above, at least some of the effects of a high-fibre diet can be attributed to the concomitant lectins. In the affluent and obese north-west quadrant of the world, a judicious intake of antinutritive lectins is probably no bad thing, as witnessed by the 'starch blocker' episode [4, 55].

Anticancer effect

Apart from the possible effect on NK activity noted above, many lectins exert noteworthy direct antitumour effects both in vitro and in vivo (reviewed in [118]). This effect is additive with that of specific antitumour immunity [152]. It has been suggested that a high intake of dietary lectins would probably protect against colonic cancer [46], a suggestion that still seems plausible, though hard to test.

Prevention of autoimmunity

Experimental autoimmune thyroiditis in mice can be prevented by the administration of PHA if the dose and timing are right (though existing disease is not cured) [35, 36]. On the other hand, if the dose and timing are not just right, the disease is potentiated, so the value of this observation is doubtful.

Prevention and treatment of virus infections

WGA prevents herpes simplex virus from adhering to rat sensory neurons, by binding to the cell surface and presumably obstructing the virus's 'landing pad' receptor. Con A also prevents herpesvirus attachment, though in this case by attaching to the virion rather than the cell [209]. Con A also inhibits influenza virus release from infected human cells in tissue culture, presumably by increasing cell surface rigidity (as noted above) and preventing the virus from budding off [192].

POSSIBLE THERAPEUTIC ROLES FOR LECTINS

The possible uses for lectins in diabetes mellitus, cystic fibrosis, virus infections and obesity have already been noted. These are all very speculative ideas, but in one area of therapy—transplantation—lectins have been tested in animals and are already in use for humans.

Transplantation

Lentil lectin induces striking allotransplantation tolerance in mice [72], as do several other lectins albeit to a lesser extent. This was not due to general immunosuppression, and indeed 'third party' grafts were rejected normally. Human bone-marrow transplantation is bedevilled by the problem of graft-versus-host disease (GVHD). T cells can be removed from the graft by soy bean agglutinin (SBA), followed by rosetting with sheep red cells [164], and the remaining stem cells have now been successfully used to reconstitute immunodeficient patients without GVHD [49]. PNA has been used to isolate suppressor T cells, these having been first induced by con A [137].

CONCLUSIONS

Dietary lectins are causes in search of diseases. They are second only to bacteria and viruses in their pathogenic potential. Like microorganisms, many or most are excluded from the body by digestion and cooking, but some survive or evade these defences and gain access. Having done so, they can affect virtually every cell in the body. Again like microorganisms, some may play a part in maintaining body health, or may act as opportunist pathogens when the way is opened by a predisposing infection, e.g. the T antigen effect. The role of lectins has not yet been proven in any disease with the exception of one case of soya intolerance, but it seems probable that coeliac disease, perhaps some cases of idiopathic glomerulonephritis, and other chronic inflammatory conditions will in due course be shown to be lectin-induced.

Of the various lectins, WGA stands out as binding particularly strongly to human tissues. This may be relevant to the popularity of wheat as a foodstuff.

The treatment of a lectin-induced disease is in principle easy, since virtually all lectin effects can be abolished by the administration of the appropriate sugar inhibitors.

REFERENCES

1 Alvarez JR, Torres-Pinedo R: Interactions of soybean lectin, soya-saponins and glycinin with rabbit jejunal mucosa in vitro. Pediatr Res 1982; 16:728–31.

2 Ament ME, Rubin CE: Soy protein—another cause of the flat intestinal lesion. Gastroenterology 1972; 62:227–34.

3 Anonymous editorial: High fibre diets and diabetes. Lancet 1981; i:423–4.

4 Anonymous: Much interest in new 'starch-blockers'. Pharmaceut J 1982; 229:124

5 Astorquiza MI, Sayago S: Modulation of IgE response by phytohemagglutinin. Int Arch Allergy Appl Immunol 1984; 73:367–9.

6 Aub JC, Tieslau C, Lankester A: Reactions of normal and tumor cell surfaces to enzymes. I. Wheat-germ lipase and associated mucopolysaccharides. Proc Natl Acad Sci USA 1963; 50:613–19.

7 Bach MK, Brashler JR: Inhibition of IgE and compound 48/80-induced histamine release by lectins. Immunology 1975; 29:371–86.

8 Banwell JG, Boldt DH, Meyers J et al: Phytohemagglutinin derived from red kidney bean (*Phaseolus vulgaris*): a cause for intestinal malabsorption associated with bacterial overgrowth in the rat. Gastroenterology 1983; 84:506–15.

9 Barker BE, Farnes P, LaMarche PH: Peripheral blood plasmacytosis following systemic exposure to *Phytolacca americana* (pokeweed). Pediatrics 1966; 38:490–3.

10 Barnett RE, Scott RE, Furcht LT, Kersey JH: Evidence that mitogenic lectins induce changes in lymphocyte membrane fluidity. Nature 1974; 249:465–6.

11 Ben-Yoseph Y, Defranco CL, Nadler HL: Decreased sialic acid and altered binding to lectins of purified α2 macroglobulin from patients with cystic fibrosis. Clin Chim Acta 1979; 99:31–5.

12 Bienenstock J: Cellular and secretory aspects of the gastrointestinal tract. In: Brostoff J, Challacombe SJ, eds. Clinics in immunology and allergy. Vol. 2, No. 1. Food allergy. Eastbourne: WB Saunders, 1982; 5–14.

13 Bleustein BI, Sickel MA, Schmid K, Vaitukaitis JL: Heterogeneity of FSH receptor complexes and their interactions with selected lectins. Biol Reprod 1981; 24:671–81.

14 Boat TF, Polony I, Cheng PW: Mucin release from rabbit tracheal epithelium in response to sera from normal and cystic fibrosis. Pediatr Res 1982; 16:792–7.

15 Boedecker EC, Boldt DH: Effect of plant lectins on the binding of human intrinsic factor-vitamin B_{12} complex (IF-B_{12}) to isolated guinea pig brush border membranes. Gastroenterology 1975; 68:A-9/866.

16 Borges LF, Sidman RL: Axonal transport of lectins in the peripheral nervous system. J Neurosci 1982; 2:647–53.

17 Boyd WC: Lectins. Ann NY Acad Sci 1970; 169:168–90.

18 Boyd WC, Shapleigh E: Diagnosis of subgroups of blood groups A and AB by use of plant agglutinins (lectins). J Lab Clin Med 1954; 44:235–7.

19 Brady PG, Vannier AM, Banwell JG: Identification of the dietary lectin wheat germ agglutinin in human intestinal contents. Gastroenterology 1978; 75:236–9.

20 Brodal P, Dietrichs E, Bjaalie JG et al: Is lectin-coupled horseradish peroxidase taken up and transported by undamaged as well as by damaged fibers in the CNS? Brain Res 1983; 278:1–9.

21 Butchko GM, Armstrong RB, Martin WJ, Ennis FA: Influenza A viruses of the H2N2 subtype are lymphocyte mitogens. Nature 1978; 271:66–7.

22 Carbonetto S, Argon Y: Lectins induce redistribution of receptors on the surface of cultured neurons. Dev Biol 1980; 80:364–78.

23 Carpenter G, Cohen S: Influence of lectins on the binding of ^{125}I-labelled EGF to human fibroblasts. Biochem Biophys Res Commun 1977; 79:545–52.

24 Cavanagh JB: The problems of neurons with long axons. Lancet 1984; i:1284–7.

25 Concon JM, Newberg DS, Eades SN: Lectins in wheat gluten proteins. J Agric Food Chem 1983; 31:939–41.

26 Conning DM, Lansdown ABG, eds: Toxic hazards in food. London: Croom Helm, 1983.

27 Cooper HS: Peanut lectin binding sites in large bowel carcinoma. Lab Invest 1982; 47:383–90.

28 Costrini NV, Kogan M: Lectin induced inhibition of nerve growth factor binding by receptors of sympathetic ganglia. J Neurochem 1981; 36:1175–80.

29 Cuatrecasas P: Interaction of concanavalin A and wheat germ agglutinin with the insulin receptor of fat cells and liver. J Biol Chem 1973; 248:3528–34.

30 Cuatrecases P, Tell GPE: Insulin-like activity of concanavalin A and wheat germ agglutinin—direct interactions with insulin receptors. Proc Natl Acad Sci USA 1973; 70:485–9.

31 Donovan K, Torres-Pinedo R: Effect of D-galactose on the fluid loss in soybean protein intolerance (abstract). Pediatr Res 1978; 12:433.

32 Douglas AP: The binding of a glycopeptide component of wheat gluten to intestinal mucosa of normal and coeliac human subjects. Clin Chim Acta 1976; 73:357–61.

33 Elson CO, Heck JA, Strober W: T cell regulation of murine IgA synthesis. J Exp Med 1979; 149:632–43.

34 Erickson RH, Kim YS: Interaction of purified brush-border membrane aminopeptidase N and dipeptidase IV with lectin-Sepharose derivatives. Biochim Biophys Acta 1983; 743: 37–42.

35 Esquivel P, Mena M, Folch H: Autoimmune thyroiditis in mice: effect of phytohemagglutinin. Immunology 1982; 47:233–8.

36 Esquivel P, Mena M, Folch H: Suppression of auto-immune thyroiditis by phytohaemagglutinin. Cell Immunol 1982; 67:410–13.

37 Etzler ME, Branstator ML: Differential localization of cell surface and secretory components in rat intestinal epithelium by use of lectins. J Cell Biol 1974; 64:329–43.

38 Evans RJ, Pusztai A, Watt WB, Bauer DH: Isolation and properties of protein fractions fron navy bean (*Phaseolus vulgaris*) which inhibit growth of rats. Biochim Biophys Acta 1973; 303:175–84.

39 Faraggiana T, Malchiodi F, Prado A, Churg J: Lectin-peroxidase conjugate reactivity in normal human kidney. J Histochem Cytochem 1982; 30:451–8.

40 Forsdyke DR: Role of complement in the toxicity of dietary legumes. Med Hypotheses 1978; 4:97–100.

41 Forsdyke DR, David CM: Comparison of enhancement of heated serum and 2-mercaptoethanol of lymphocyte transformation induced by high concentrations of concanavalin A. Cell Immunol 1978; 36:86–96.

42 Fraker PJ: Zinc deficiency: a common immunodeficiency state. Surv Immunol Res 1983; 2:155–63.

43 Franklin WA: Tissue binding of lectins in disorders of the breast. Cancer 1983; 51:295–300.

44 Freed DLJ, Buckley CH: Mucotractive effect of lectin. Lancet 1978; i: 585–6.

45 Freed DLJ, Cooper RJ: Cytotoxicity of bread and soya protein in tissue culture. Lancet 1977; i:371.

46 Freed DLJ, Green FHY: Do dietary lectins protect against bowel cancer? Lancet 1975; ii: 1261.

47 Freeman HJ, Lotan R, Kim YS: Application of lectins for detection of goblet cell glycoconjugate differences in proximal and distal colon of the rat. Lab Invest 1980; 42:405–12.

48 Freier S, Lebenthal E, Freier M et al: IgE and IgD antibodies to cow milk and soy protein in duodenal fluid: effect of pancreozymin and secretin. Immunology 1983; 49:69–75.

49 Friedrich W, Goldmann SF, Vetter H et al: Immunoreconstitution in severe combined immunodeficiency after transplantation of HLA-haploidentical, T-cell-depleted bone marrow. Lancet 1984; i:761–4.

50 Gall WE, Edelman GM: Lateral diffusion of surface molecules in animal cells and tissues. Science 1981; 213:903–5.

51 Ganguly P, Fossett NG: Evidence for multiple mechanisms of interaction between wheat germ agglutinin and human platelets. Biochim Biophys Acta 1980; 627:256–61.

52 Ganguly P, Fossett NG: Inhibition of epinephrine-induced platelet aggregation by a derivative of wheat germ agglutinin. Biochim Biophys Res Commun 1981; 98:297–302.

53 Ganguly P, Fossett NG: Induction of serotonin secretion by cross-linking of surface receptors of a derivative of wheat germ agglutinin on human platelets. Biochim Biophys Res Commun 1981; 99:176–82.

54 Ganguly P, Fossett NG: Inhibition of thrombin-induced platelet aggregation by a derivative of wheat germ agglutinin. Evidence for a physiologic receptor of thrombin in human platelets. Blood 1981; 57:343–52.

55 Garrow JS, Scott PF, Heels S et al: 'Starch blockers' are ineffective in man. Lancet 1983; i:60–1.

56 Gartner TK: The endogenous lectin of human platelets is an α-granule component. Blood 1981; 58:153–7.

57 Gauthier-Rahman S, El Rouby S, Liacopoulos-Briot M et al: Delayed hypersensitivity and migration inhibition in two lines of mice genetically selected for high or low responsiveness to phytohemagglutinin. Cell Immunol 1983; 77:249–65.

58 Gerfen CR, O'Leary DDM, Cowan WM: A note on the transneuronal transport of wheat germ agglutinin-conjugated horseradish peroxidase in the avian and rodent visual systems. Exp Brain Res 1982; 48:443–8.

59 Giannella RA: Pathogenesis of acute bacterial diarrheal disorders. Annu Rev Med 1981; 32:341–57.

60 Gibbons RJ, Dankers I: Lectin-like constituents in foods which react with components of serum, saliva and *Strep. mutans*. Appl Environ Microbiol 1981; 41:880–8.

61 Gibbons RJ, Dankers I: Association of food lectins with human oral epithelial cells in vivo. Arch Oral Biol 1983; 28:561–6.

62 Glassman AB, Lindsay JH, Bennett CE, Hodges ER: Effects of insulin on PHA-P, Con A and PWM in diabetic and nondiabetic lymphocytes. Ann Clin Lab Sci 1981; 11:9–14.

63 Gommans JM, Van den Hurk JJMA, Bergers M et al: Studies on the plasma membrane of normal and psoriatic keratinocytes. V. Lectin binding. Br J Dermatol 1982; 106:317–22.

64 Good RA: Nutrition and immunity. J Clin Immunol 1981; 1:3–11.

65 Grant G, More LJ, McKenzie NH, Pusztai A: The effect of heating on the haemagglutinating activity and nutritional properties of bean (*Phaseolus vulgaris*) seeds. J Sci Food Agric 1982; 33:1324–6.

66 Gray ED, Peters G, Verstegen M, Regelmann WE: Effect of extracellular slime substance from *Staph. epidermidis* on the human cellular immune response. Lancet 1984; i:365–7.

67 Green FHY, Freed DLJ: Antibody-facilitated digestion and the consequences of its failure. In: Hemmings WA, ed. Antigen absorption by the gut. Lancaster: MTP Press, 1978; 189–97.

68 Greenberg JH, Jamieson GA: The effects of various lectins on platelet aggregation and release. Biochim Biophys Acta 1974; 345:231–42.

69 Hedo JA, Harrison LC, Roth J: Binding of insulin receptors to lectins: evidence for common carbo-

hydrate determinants on several membrane receptors. Biochemistry 1981; 20: 3385–93.

70 Helin RM, Froese A: Binding of the receptors for IgE by various lectins. Int Arch Allergy Appl Immunol 1981; 65:81–4.

71 Hervada AR: Soybean formulas. In: Freed DLJ, ed. Health hazards of milk. Eastbourne: Baillière Tindall, 1984; 158–69.

72 Hilgert I, Hořejší VA, Angelisová P, Krištofová H: Lentil lectin effectively induces allotransplantation tolerance in mice. Nature 1980; 284:273–5.

73 Hoffman DR, Yamamoto FY, Geller B, Haddad ZH: Specific IgE antibodies in atopic eczema. J Allergy Clin Immunol 1975; 55:256–67.

74 Hoffstein S, Soberman R, Goldstein I: Concanavalin A induces microtubule assembly and specific granule discharge in human polymorphonuclear leukocytes. J Cell Biol 1976; 68:781.

75 Holthöfer H: Lectin binding sites in kidney. A comparative study of 14 animal species. J Histochem Cytochem 1983; 31:531–7.

76 Howard DR, Batsakis JA: Peanut agglutinin: a new marker for tissue histiocytes. Am J Clin Pathol 1982; 77:401–8.

77 Hsu SM, Raine L: Discovery of a high affinity of *Phaseolus vulgaris* agglutinin (PHA) with gastrin-secreting cells. Am J Clin Pathol 1982; 77:396–400.

78 Hukkanen V: Lectin-reactive components in white matter membranes from normal and multiple sclerosis brains. J Neurochem 1982; 38:1537–41.

79 Ingham E, Gowland G: Complement, histamine release and treatment of upper respiratory tract infection. Lancet 1983; ii:1027.

80 Jacobs LR, DeFontes D, Cox KL: Cytochemical localization of small intestinal glycoconjugates by lectin histochemistry in controls and subjects with cystic fibrosis. Dig Dis Sci 1983; 28:422–8.

81 Jacobson W, Stoddart RW, Collins RD: Lectin staining of carbohydrates of haemic cells. II. The cells of normal lymphoid origin, of lymphatic leukaemias and related diseases. Histopathology 1980; 4:491–506.

82 Jaffe EA, Laing LLK, Nachman RL et al: Thrombospondin is the endogenous lectin of human platelets. Nature 1982; 295/5846: 246–8.

83 Jaffe WG: Über Phytotoxine aus Bohnen (*Phaseolus vulgaris*). Arzneimittelforsch 1960; 10:1012–6.

84 Jayne-Williams DJ: Influence of dietary jack beans and of con A on the growth of conventional and gnotobiotic Japanese quail (*Coturnix coturnix japonica*). Nature 1973; 243: 150–1.

85 Jenkins DJA, Wolever T, Leeds AR et al: Dietary fibres, fibre analogues, and glucose tolerance: importance of viscosity. Br Med J 1978; 1:1392.

86 Jenkins DA, Wolever TMS, Taylor RH et al: Exceptionally low blood glucose response to dried beans: comparison with other carbohydrate food. Br Med J 1980; 281:578–80.

87 Judd WJ: The role of lectins in blood group serology. CRC Crit Rev Clin Lab Sci 1980; 12:171–214.

88 Jung SM, Ordinas A, Jamieson GA: Synergistic effects of lectins in the interaction of thrombin with human platelets. Biochim Biophys Acta 1981; 673:312–22.

89 Kessel D, Cuthbert AW: Sidedness of the reaction to β-lactoglobulin in sensitised colonic epithelia. Int Arch Allergy Appl Immunol 1984; 74:113–9.

90 Kendall CH, Walker F: Amyloid P component in human thyroid. Virchows Arch [Cell Pathol] 1984; 45:75–8.

91 Kerjaschki D, Farquhar MG: The pathogenic anti-

gen of Heymann nephritis is a membrane glycoprotein of the renal proximal tubule brush border. Proc Natl Acad Sci USA 1982; 79:5557–61.

92 Kerjaschki D, Farquhar MG: Immunocytochemical localization of the Heymann nephritis antigen (GP 330) in glomerular epithelial cells of normal Lewis rats. J Exp Med 1983; 157:667–86.

93 Ketis NV, Girdlestone J, Grant CWM: Positive cooperativity in a (dissected) lectin–membrane glycoprotein binding event. Proc Natl Acad Sci USA 1980; 77:3788–90.

94 King TP, Pusztai A, Clarke EMW: Immunocytochemical localization of ingested kidney bean (*Phaseolus vulgaris*) lectins in rat gut. Histochem J 1980; 12:201–8.

95 King TP, Pusztai A, Clarke EMW: Kidney bean (*Phaseolus vulgaris*) lectin-induced lesions in rat small intestine. I. Light microscope studies. J Comp Pathol 1980; 90:585–95.

96 King TP, Pusztai A, Clarke EMW: Kidney bean lectin induced lesions in rat small intestine. III. Ultrastructural studies. J Comp Pathol 1982; 92:357–73.

97 Klein PJ, Bulla M, Newman RA et al: The significance of the Thomsen–Friedenreich antigen in haemolytic-uraemic syndrome. Lancet 1977; ii: 1204–5.

98 Klein PJ, Newman RA, Muller P et al: Histochemical methods for the demonstration of Thomsen–Friedenreich antigen in cell suspension and tissue sections. Klin Wochenschr 1978; 56:761–5

99 Knight B: Ricin—a potent homicidal poison. Br Med J 1979; i:350–1.

100 Kohn J, Whicher J, Warren C, O'Kelly T: The use of lectins to measure acute phase proteins in the serum or plasma of man and animals during inflammation and tissue breakdown. FEBS Lett 1980; 109:257–60.

101 Konwinski M, Vorbrodt A, Solter D, Koprowski H: Ultrastructure study of concanavalin-A binding to the surface of preimplantation mouse embryos. J Exp Zool 1977; 200:311–23.

102 Köttgen E, Kluge F, Volk B, Gerok W: The lectin properties of gluten as the basis of the pathomechanism of gluten sensitive enteropathy. Klin Wochenschr 1983; 61:111–2.

103 Köttgen E, Volk B, Kluge F, Gerok W: Gluten, a lectin with oligomannosyl specificity and the causative agent of gluten sensitive enteropathy. Biochem Biophys Res Commun 1982; 109:168–73.

104 Krojevitch A, Nal JN: Intérêt prognostique de l'intradermo réaction a la phyto-hémagglutinine chez des malades d'un service de réanimation polyvalente. Ann Anesthesiol Fr 1981; 22:245–9.

105 Kruszewski J, Plusa T, Szezylik C, Wiktor-Jedrzejczak W: Reaction to intradermally applied phytohaemagglutinin in asthma patients in relation to corticosteroid therapy. Allergy 1983; 38:201–5.

106 Kuhlmann WD, Peschke P, Wurster K: Lectin peroxidase conjugates in histopathology of gastrointestinal mucosa. Virchows Arch [Pathol Anat] 1983; 398:319–28.

107 Lake AM, Bloch KJ, Neutra MR, Walker WA: Intestinal goblet cell mucus release. II. In vivo stimulation by antigen in the immunized rat. J Immunol 1974; 112:834–7.

108 Landsteiner K, Raubitschek H: Beobachtungen uber Hämolyse und Hämagglutination. Zentralbl Bakteriol 1907; 45:660–1.

109 Lansman JB, Cochrane DE: Wheat germ agglutinin stimulates exocytotic histamine secretion from rat

mast cells in the absence of extracellular calcium. Biochem Pharmacol 1980; 29:445–58.

110 Larsen HJ, Tollersrud S: Effect of dietary vitamin E and selenium on the PHA response of pig lymphocytes. Res Vet Sci 1981; 31:301–5.

111 Lechar RM, Nestler JL, Jacobson S: Immunohistochemical localization of retrogradely and anterogradely transported wheat germ agglutinin (WGA) within the CNS of the rat. J Histochem Cytochem 1981; 29:1255–62.

112 Levi A, Tarrab-Hazdai, Teichberg VI: Electrolectin therapy of myasthenia gravis in rabbits. Eur J Immunol 1983; 13:500–7.

113 Li JG, Osgood EE: A method for the rapid separation of leucocytes and nucleated erythrocytes from blood or marrow with a phytohemagglutinin from red beans (*Phaseolus vulgaris*) Blood 1949; 4: 670–5.

114 Li JJ, Pereira MEA, DeLellis KA, McAdam KPWJ: Human amyloid P component; a circulating lectin that modulates immunological response. Scand J Immunol 1984; 19:227–36.

115 Lieberman J, Costea NV, Jakulis VJ, Kaneshiro W: Detection of a lectin in the blood of cystic fibrosis homozygotes and heterozygotes. Trans Assoc Am Physicians 1979; 92:121–9.

116 Liener IE, ed: Toxic constituents of plant foodstuffs. New York: Academic Press, 1969.

117 Liener IE: Phytohemagglutinins: their nutritional significance. J Agric Food Chem 1974; 22:17–22.

118 Lis H, Sharon N: The biochemistry of plant lectins (phytohemagglutinins). Annu Rev Biochem 1973; 42:541–74.

119 Lis H, Sharon N: Lectins in higher plants. In: Marcus A, ed. Proteins and Nucleic Acids. (The Biochemistry of Plants, Vol. VI). New York: Academic Press, 1981.

120 Livingston JN, Purvis BJ: Effects of wheat germ agglutinin on insulin binding and insulin sensitivity of fat cells. Am J Physiol 1980; 238: E267–75.

121 Lorenz K, Flatter B, Kolle FW: Lectine als Reagentien zür Differenzierung von Enzymen im Serum. J Clin Chem Clin Biochem 1979; 17:757–65.

122 Lorenzsonn V, Olsen WA: In vivo response of rat intestinal epithelium to intraluminal dietary lectins. Gastroenterology 1982; 82:838–48.

123 Lovrien RE, Anderson RA: Stoichiometry of wheat germ agglutinin as a morphology controlling agent and as a morphology protective agent for the human erythrocyte. J Cell Biol 1980; 85:534–48.

124 MacDermott RP, Kienker LJ, Bertovich MJ, Muchmore AV: Inhibition of spontaneous but not antibody dependent cell-mediated cytotoxicity by simple sugars. Immunology 1981; 44:143–52.

125 McIntyre LJ, Quarles RH, Brady RO: Lectin-binding proteins in central-nervous system myelin. Biochem J 1979; 183:205–12.

126 Mahmood A, Torres-Pinedo R: Postnatal changes in lectin binding to microvillus membranes from rat intestine. Biochem Biophys Res Commun 1983; 113:400–6.

127 Makker SP: Evidence that the antigen of autologous immune complex glomerulonephritis of rats is a mannose- or glucose-containing glycoprotein. Proc Soc Exp Biol Med 1980; 163:95–9.

128 Mann JI: What carbohydrate foods should diabetics eat? Br Med J 1984; 288:1025–6.

129 Mazzuca M, Lhermitte M, Lafitte JJ, Roussel P: Use of lectins for detection of glycoconjugates in the glandular cells of the human bronchial mucosa. J Histochem Cytochem 1982; 30:956–66.

130 Miettinen A, Tornroth T, Tikkanen I: Heymann nephritis induced by kidney brush border glycoproteins. Lab Invest 1980; 43:547–55.

131 Mike N, Haeney MR, Goodwin BJF et al: Soya protein antibodies in man: their occurrence and possible relevance in coeliac disease. In: The second Fisons food allergy workshop. Oxford: Medicine Publishing Foundation, 1983; 35–8.

132 Mitchell GF, Charles AE: Allergenicity of concanavalin A in mice. Int Arch Allergy Appl Immunol 1979; 58:391–401.

133 Muller W, Klein PJ, Vierbuchen MJ, Uhlenbruck G: Lectin binding sites in the choroid plexus and choroid plexus papillomas. Neurosurg Rev 1980; 3:57–65.

134 Murata F, Tsuyama S, Suzuki S et al: Distribution of glycoconjugates in the kidney studied by use of labelled lectins. J Histochem Cytochem [1A Suppl] 1983; 31:139–44.

135 Nachbar MS, Oppenheim JD: Lectins in the US diet: a survey of lectins in commonly consumed foods and a review of the literature. Am J Clin Nutr 1980; 33:2338–45.

136 Nachbar MS, Oppenheim JD, Thomas JO: Lectins in the US diet. Isolation and characterization of a lectin from the tomato (*Lycopersicon esculentum*). J Biol Chem 1980; 255:1056–61.

137 Nakamura T, Tanimoto K, Nakano K, Horinchi Y: Isolation of human suppressor T cells by peanut agglutinin. Int Arch Allergy Appl Immunol 1982; 68:338–41.

138 Nirmul G, Severin C, Taub RN: In vivo effects of con A. I. Immunosuppressive effects. Transplantation 1972; 14:91–5.

139 Noah ND, Bender AE, Reaidi GB, Gilbert RJ: Food poisoning from raw red kidney beans. Br Med J 1980; ii:236–7.

140 Norn S, Stahlskor P, Jensen C et al: Intrinsic asthma and bacterial histamine release via lectin effect. Agents Actions 1983; 13:210–12.

141 Nowell PC: Phytohemagglutinin: an initiator of mitosis in cultures of normal human leukocytes. Cancer Res 1960; 20: 462–6.

142 Omar MAK, Pudifin DJ, Coovadia HM, et al: The PHA response of young blacks and Indians with insulin dependent diabetes mellitus. S Afr Med J 1983; 63:776–8.

143 Oppenheim JJ, Rosenstreich DL, eds: Mitogens in immunobiology. New York: Academic Press, 1976.

144 Owens-Williams L, Shapira E: Increased binding of limulin to α2-macroglobulin and immunoglobulin M from cystic fibrosis patients. J Pediatr Gastroenterol Nutr 1982; 1: 567–70.

145 Parker CW: Pharmacologic modulation of release of arachidonic acid from human mononuclear cells and lymphocytes by mitogenic lectins. J Immunol 1982, 128:393–7.

146 Pauwels R, Van der Straeten M, Platteau B, Bazin H: The non-specific enhancement of allergy. I. In vivo effects of *B. pertussis* vaccine on IgE synthesis. Allergy 1983; 38: 239.

147 Peschke P, Kuhlmann WD, Wurster K: Histological detection of lectin binding sites in human gastrointestinal mucosa. Experientia 1983; 39: 286–7.

148 Phillips SG, Lui SL, Phillips DM: Binding of epithelial cells to lectin-coated surfaces. In Vitro 1982; 18:727–38.

149 Phillipson OT, Griffiths AC: Antegrade and retrograde labelling of CNS pathways. Brain Res 1983; 265:199–207.

150 Pivovarova AI, Kolyaskina GI: [Effect of various doses of phytomitogens on blood lymphocyte proliferation in schizophrenia.] Biull Eksp Biol Med 1980; 90:552-4.

151 Plouffe J, Lofgren R, Silva J et al: Suppression of immune response in mice by navy bean lectin. J Clin Lab Immunol 1979; 3:189-90.

152 Poduval TB, Seshadri M, Sundaram K: Lectin potentiation of BCG-contact mediated antitumor action. J Natl Cancer Inst 1980; 65:909-12.

153 Prujansky A, Ravid A, Sharon N: Cooperativity of lectin binding to lymphocytes and its relevance to mitogenic stimulation. Biochim Biophys Acta 1978; 508:137-46.

154 Public Health Laboratory Service: Unusual outbreak of food poisoning. Br Med J 1976, ii:1268.

155 Pujol-Borrell R, Hanafusa T, Chiovato L, Bottazzo GF: Lectin-induced expression of DR antigen on human cultured follicular thyroid cells. Nature 1983; 304:71-3.

156 Purrello F, Burnham DB, Goldfine ID: Insulin receptor antiserum and plant lectins mimic the direct effects of insulin on nuclear envelope phosphorylation. Science 1983; 221:462-4.

157 Pusztai A, Palmer R: Nutritional evaluation of kidney beans (*Phaseolus vulgaris*): the toxic principle. J Sci Food Agric 1977; 28:620.

158 Pusztai A, King TP, Clarke EMW: Recent advances in the study of the kidney bean (*Phaseolus vulgaris*) lectins in rats. Toxicon 1982; 20: 195-7.

159 Pusztai A, Clarke EMW, Grant G, King TP: The toxicity of *Phaseolus vulgaris* lectins. Nitrogen balance and immunochemical studies. J Sci Food Agric 1981; 32:1037-46.

160 Pusztai A, Clarke EMW, King TP, Stewart JC: Nutritional evaluation of kidney beans (*Phaseolus vulgaris*): chemical composition, lectin content and nutritional value of selected cultivars. J Sci Food Agric 1979; 30: 843-8.

161 Quarles RH, McIntyre LJ, Pasnak CF: Lectin-binding proteins in CNS myelin. Binding of glycoproteins in purified myelin to immobilized lectins. Biochem J 1979; 183:213-21.

162 Rattray EAS, Palmer R, Pusztai A: Toxicity of kidney beans (*Phaseolus vulgaris* L) to conventional and gnotobiotic rats. J Sci Food Agric 1974; 25:1036-40.

163 Rechcigl M, ed: Handbook of naturally-occurring food toxicants. Boca Raton, Florida: CRC Press, 1983.

164 Reisner Y, Pahwa S, Chiao JW et al: Separation of antibody helper and antibody suppressor human T cells by using soybean agglutinin. Proc Natl Acad Sci USA 1980; 77:6778-82.

165 Renkonen KO: Studies on hemagglutinins present in seeds of some representatives of family of leguminoseae. Ann Med Exp Biol Fenniae 1948; 26:66-72.

166 Rittman BR, Mackenzie IC: Effects of histological processing on lectin binding patterns in oral mucosa and skin. Histochem J 1983; 15:467-74.

167 Rittman BR, Mackenzie IC, Rittman GA: Lectin binding to murine oral mucosa and skin. Arch Oral Biol 1982; 27:1013-9.

168 Rivellese A, Giacco A, Genovese S et al: Effect of dietary fibre on glucose control and serum lipoproteins in diabetic patients. Lancet 1980; ii:447-9.

169 Romball CG, Weigle WO: the enhancing effect of mitogens in the in vivo immune response in rabbits. J Immunol 1975; 115:556-60.

170 Rothlein R, Yoon Berm Kim: Porcine alveolar macrophages discriminate between self and nonself

171 Rougé P, Chatelain C, Père D: Interactions entre les hémagglutinines des graines de diverses espèces de légumineuses et les immunoglobulines (IgG, IgA et IgM) du sérum humain normal. Ann Pharm Fr 1978; 36:143-7.

172 Roy S, Bhalla V: Haemagglutinins and lysins in plants and their application in characterising human and animal red cells. Aust J Exp Biol Med Sci 1981; 59:195-201.

173 Rubin W, Fauci AS, Sleisenger MH et al: Immunofluorescent studies in adult coeliac disease. J Clin Invest 1965; 44: 475-85.

174 Salvaterra PM, Gurd JM, Mahler HR: Interaction of the nicotinic acetylcholine receptor from rat brain with lectins. J Neurochem 1977; 29:345-8.

175 Sandholm M, Scott ML: Binding of lipase, amylase and protease to intestinal epithelium as affected by carbohydrate and lectins in vitro. Act Vet Scand 1979; 20:329-42.

176 Sastry-Gollapudi VS, Kind LS: Enhanced reaginic antibody formation to ovalbumin in mice given repeated injections of con A. Int Arch Allergy Appl Immunol 1977; 53:569-73.

177 Sato Y, Kimura M, Fukumi H: Development of a pertussis component vaccine in Japan. Lancet 1984; i:122-6.

178 Shapira E, Menedez R: Increased binding of concanavalin A to α2-macroglobulin, IgM and IgG from cystic fibrosis plasma. Biochem Biophys Res Commun 1980; 93: 50-6.

179 Shaw LM, Petersen-Archer L: Interaction of gamma-glutamyltransferase from human tissues with insolubilized lectins. Clin Biochem 1979; 12:256-60.

180 Schechter Y: Bound lectins that mimic insulin and produce persistent insulin-like activities. Endocrinology 1983; 113:1921-6.

181 Schechter Y, Sela BA: Insulin-like effects of wax bean agglutinin in rat adipocytes. Biochem Biophys Res Commun 1981; 98:367-73.

182 Schlessinger J,. Elson EL, Webb WW et al: Receptor diffusion on cell surfaces modulated by locally bound concanavalin A. Proc Natl Acad Sci USA 1977; 74:1110-14.

183 Sharon N: Carbohydrates. Sci Am 1980; 243:90-116.

184 Shier WT: Concanavalin A as in inflammogen. In: Bittiger H, Schnebli HP, eds. Concanavalin A as a tool. London: John Wiley and Sons, 1976; 573-9.

185 Siraganian RP, Siraganian PA: Mechanism of action of concanavalin A on human basophils. J Immunol 1975; 114:886-93.

186 Smith JD, Liu AYC: Lectins mimic insulin in the induction of tyrosine aminotransferase. Science 1981; 214:799-800.

187 Snow EC, Feldbush TL, Oaks JA: The role of insulin in the response of murine T lymphocytes to mitogenic stimulation in vitro. J Immunol 1980; 124:739-44.

188 Spreafico F, Lerner EM: Suppression of the primary and secondary immune response of the mouse by phytohemagglutinin. J Immunol 1967; 407-16.

189 Staat RH, Doyle RJ, Langley SD, Suddick KP: Modification in in vitro adherence of *Streptococcus mutans* by plant lectins. Adv Exp Med Biol 1978; 107:639-47.

190 Stavard MW, Steensgaard J: The experimental determination of antibody affinity. In: Antibody affinity: thermodynamic aspects and biological significance. Boco Raton, Florida: CRC Press, 1983; 59-97.

in lectin-mediated cellular cytotoxicity. Cell Immunol 1982; 68:368-76.

191 Stillmark H: Über Rizin, ein giftiges Ferment aus Samen von *Ricinis communis* L., und einigen anderen Euphorbiaceen. Dorpat (Tartu), 1888. Inaugural dissertation.

192 Stitz L, Reinacher M, Becht H: Studies on inhibitory effect of lectins on myxovirus release. J Gen Virol 1977; 34:523–30.

193 Sumner JB, Howell SF: Identification of hemagglutinin of jack bean with concanavalin A. J Bacteriol 1936; 32:227–37.

194 Toyoshima S, Osawa T: Lectins from *Wistaria floribunda* seeds and their effect on membrane fluidity of human peripheral lymphocytes. J Biol Chem 1975; 250:1655–60.

195 Triadou N, Audran E: Interaction of brush border hydrolases of the human small intestine with lectins. Digestion 1983; 27:1–7.

196 Tsivion Y, Sharon N: Lipid-mediated hemagglutination and its relevance to lectin-mediated agglutination. Biochim Biophys Acta 1981; 642:336–44.

197 Uhlenbruck G, Newman R, Steinharsen G, Schwick HG: Further studies on the interaction of lectins with human serum glycoproteins. Z Immun-Forsch 1977; 153:183–7.

198 Vasmant D, Feldmann G, Fontaine JL: Ultrastructural localization of concanavalin A surface receptors on brush-border enterocytes in normal children and during celiac disease. Pediatr Res 1982; 16:441–5.

199 Walzer M: Allergy of the abdominal organs. J Lab Clin Med 1941; 26: 1867.

200 Wasik M, Gradswska L, Rowinska D et al: Diagnostic and prognostic value of antibody-dependent cellular cytotoxicity and lectin-induced cellular cytotoxicity tests for renal graft rejection. Transplantation 1981; 32:217–21.

201 Weiser MM: Concanavalin A agglutination of intestinal cells from the human fetus. Science 1972; 177:525–6.

202 Weiser MM, Douglas AP: An alternative mechanism for gluten toxicity in coeliac disease. Lancet 1976; i:567.

203 Whyte A: Lectin binding by microvillus membranes and coated-pit regions of human syncytial trophoblast. Histochem J 1980; 12:599–607.

204 Wiley RG, Blessing WW, Reis DJ: Suicide transport: destruction of neurons by retrograde transport of ricin abrin and modeccin. Science 1982; 216:889–90.

205 Willoughby WF, Willoughby JB, Cantrell BB, Wheelis R: In vivo responses to inhaled proteins. II. Induction of interstitial pneumonitis and enhancement of immune complex mediated alveolitis by inhaled concanavalin A. Lab Invest 1979; 40: 399.

206 Wilson AB, King TP, Clarke EMW, Pusztai A: Kidney bean (*Phaseolus vulgaris*) lectin-induced lesions in rat small intestine. II. Microbiological studies. J Comp Pathol 1980, 90:597–603.

207 Wurster K, Peschke P, Kuhlmann WD: Cellular localization of lectin-affinity in tissue sections of normal human duodenum. Virchows Arch [Pathol anat] 1983; 402:1–9.

208 Yue CL, Tanimoto K, Horinchi Y: Characterization and possible mechanisms of mitogen-induced cell-mediated cytotoxicity. Scand J Immunol 1981; 14:397–408.

209 Ziegler RJ, Pozos RTS: Effects of lectins on peripheral infections by HSV of rat sensory neurons in culture. Infect Immun 1981; 34:588–95.

210 Ziska P, Franz H: The lectin from garden cress (*Lepidum sativum*). Isolation and characterization. In: Bog-Hansen TC, ed. Lectins: biology, biochemistry and clinical biochemistry, Vol. II. Berlin; Walter de Gruyter, 1982; 511–9.

211 Zuraw BL, Nouaka M, O'Hair C, Katz DH: Human IgE ab synthesis in vitro: stimulation of IgE responses by pokeweed mitogen and selective inhibition of such responses by human suppressor factor of allergy (SFA) J Immunol 1981; 127:116–77.

Chapter 22a
Uptake, Measurement and Elimination of Synthetic Chemicals by Man

D.B. Seba, M.J. Milam and J.L. Laseter

Introduction

On a daily basis the human population comes into contact with thousands of chemicals that are the products of human endeavour. This influx of xenobiotic ('foreign to life') [88] chemicals and their biological and abiological breakdown products into modern society has long concerned both health professionals and citizens. In most instances there is a lack of scientific information which might allow the effect of acute exposures on health to be accurately assessed. The effects of chronic exposures are even less well understood. Almost no information exists on the consequences of exposure to mixtures of environmental toxins. As a result, it is not surprising that there exist today frustrated regulatory agencies, irritated industrialists, concerned health professionals and a worried public sector. A list of food additives and their known or suggested effects are shown in Appendix 22a.1.

This chapter will discuss aspects of the sources, uptake, detoxification and measurement of anthropogenic xenobiotic organic chemical agents which may be found in food. Because of the enormous scope of the subject, inorganic toxic compounds such as cadmium [101], lead [91] or mercury [5] which are sometimes found in food have been excluded from discussion.

Categories of organic chemicals

This chapter will discuss two broad categories of organic chemical agents: those that are deliberately added to food, i.e. additives; and those that are inadvertently added, i.e. pesticide and toxic man-made contaminants. Both are medically important. The increasing contamination of our food and drinking water by man-made organic compounds, some of whose adverse health effects may only be measured after decades of exposure, represents an epidemiological experiment of grand proportions and a profound medical challenge to diagnose and treat what can truly be said to be the man-made illness of the 20th century—chemically induced environmental disease.

Quantity ingested

It has been suggested that the average consumer in the United States ingests more than 8.8 kg per year of preservatives, stabilizers, colourings, flavourings and other intentional additives. These estimates are independent of the numerous contaminants and man-made chemical agents also found in foods. More than 700 such agents have been identified in the finished drinking waters of the United States [47, 64].

Sources of chemicals

Ott [70] emphasizes that an assessment of the public health risk from environmental pollutants requires a knowledge of the sources, transport, exposure levels, doses received and health effects of those substances. In addition, an understanding of the means by which pollutants are absorbed, metabolized and dispersed within the human body is important in treatment of disease states related to chemical exposure. The opportunity for exposure occurs not only under extraordinary environmental conditions, such as chemical spills and accidents, but through our everyday experiences. Contacts with substances and situations long taken for granted as 'safe' can, because of widespread mishandling of chemicals, no longer be overlooked as insignificant sources of contamination.

FOOD ADDITIVES

Sources of exposure and degree of contamination

To some degree all commercial food is contaminated with synthetic chemicals in the form of additives. Fresh foods are grown with chemical fertilizers and treated with pesticides, and many have been sprayed with chemicals in the store to maintain freshness. Other foods may be processed, which generally refers to the addition of chemicals and artificial components [83].

Definition of food additive

The US Food and Drug Administration (FDA) defines a food additive as any substance that becomes part of a food product when

Table 22a.1 Functional classes of additives to foods.

Class	Number of compounds in each class
Preservatives	30
Antioxidants	28
Sequestrants	44
Surfactants	85
Stabilizers	31
Bleaching and maturing agents	24
Buffers	66
Colours	35
Special sweeteners	9
Nutrient supplements	116
Flavouring compounds	720
Natural flavouring materials	357
Miscellaneous	158

Source [56, 63].

added directly or indirectly. These substances are present in processed foods in much larger quantities than pesticides and therefore may cause many more general toxicity problems. A listing by functional class reveals many different categories as shown in Table 22a.1.

Reasons for adding chemicals to food

Chemicals are added to foods for many reasons, the major ones being (a) to maintain or improve nutritional value, (b) to prevent spoilage and maintain freshness, (c) to aid in processing or preparation and (d) to make food more appealing [63]. Many foods are often enriched and fortified with nutrients such as vitamins and minerals that are lost in processing or deficient in the average diet. The addition of iodine, iron, thiamine and other nutritional supplements usually represents an important and appropriate use of food additives. Substances used to preserve foods (ascorbic acid, potassium propionate, etc.), retard bacterial fungal and mould growth which, left untreated, would spoil food quickly. Colour, flavour and nutrients are maintained and shelf life extended as a result. Antioxidants prevent undesirable changes produced by oxidation such as rancidity of fats and enzymatic browning of fruits and vegetables. Some commonly used antioxidants include butylated hydroxyanisole (BHA), citric acid, ethylene diamine tetraacetic acid (EDTA) and propyl gallate.

Aids to processing

Examples of chemicals that aid in the preparation or processing of foods include cellulose, calcium alginate, carrageenan, sodium stearyl fumarate, phosphoric acid, calcium silicate and propylene glycol. These substances may control pH, stabilize, thicken, emulsify, leaven, bleach or condition.

Flavour enhancers

To make food more appealing or palatable, manufacturers add sweeteners, flavour enhancers, flavourings and colours. Some are synthetic while others are natural. Many flavour enhancers supplement, magnify or modify the original taste of food while others work by temporarily deadening certain nerves—those responsible for perception of bitterness, for example, thereby increasing the perception of other tastes. Substances falling into this fourth group are the FD&C (Federal Drug & Cosmetic) dyes, sorbitol, sugar and monosodium glutamate (MSG).

Acceptable levels?

All food additives in the United States are regulated by governmental agencies and any chemical that is shown to be harmful in small amounts is judged unacceptable as a food additive. These controls may not be sufficient for a variety of reasons. Only a single chemical is tested at a time; in real life we eat combinations of hundreds of chemicals which may interact. Testing chemicals on laboratory animals does not necessarily predict the human response nor individual differences. In the daily consumption of prepared foods, a toxic substance may be obtained from several different sources and intake over a 24-hour period may be much larger than would be acceptable by FDA standards.

DRINKING WATER

Drinking water contains many of the same chemicals seen in food and air. Study results for tap water in two US cities combined are shown in Table 22a.2 [73]. Another study of selected organic contaminants in drinking water in three cities along the Mississippi River is shown in Appendix 22a.2. A third study shows similar results for measurements in 13 US cities [45].

Source of contamination

Contaminants may enter water supplies from contact with polluted air and soil, from improperly disposed of industrial and commercial waste, and from home disposal of chemicals. Many of these compounds persist through raw water treatment procedures. Some may be formed by reactions with chlorine during treatment and still others are picked up from materials used in distribution systems [53].

The man-made compounds most commonly found in ground water are principally traceable to industrial wastes, municipal land fills, agricultural chemicals, defective septic tanks, animals' wastes, leaks from petroleum pipelines, underground storage tanks etc. [17,18]. Table 22a.3 shows the extent to which the water can be contaminated through soil leaching [48].

Contaminants have also been measured in rain water [38], in commercially bottled water and in filtered tap water [49]. While the filtered source showed reduced concentrations of compounds such as chloroform and benzenes, others were increased (tetrachloroethylene)

Table 22a.2 Weighted summary statistics for water (ng/ml) with Bayonne and Elizabeth combined.

Compound	Arithmetic mean	SE	Median	Range
Vinylidene chloride	0.25	0.03	0.03	0.03– 2.36
Chloroform	69.90	1.49	66.80	0.03–168.00
1,1,1-Trichloroethane	0.59	0.08	0.03	0.03– 5.34
Trichloroethylene	0.56	0.08	0.06	0.03– 4.18
Bromodichloromethane	13.60	0.16	13.40	0.06– 23.40
Dibromochloromethane	2.45	0.06	2.38	0.06– 8.39
Toluene	0.42	0.04	0.31	0.31– 2.73
Tetrachloroethylene	0.42	0.06	0.06	0.03– 3.22

Estimate population size: 128 603.
Minimum sample size: 265.
Maximum sample size: 354.
Note: ng/ml is equivalent to ppb; samples were collected from potable water in Bayonne and Elizabeth, New Jersey (USA)

Table 22a.3 Organic chemicals observed in ground water adjacent to an abandoned chemical waste site.

	Concentration ppb (μg/l)
Dichloroethylene	138
Chloroform	86
Trichloroethylene	194
Benzene	95
Tetrachloroethylene	62
Toluene	5
Chlorobenzene	18
Ethylbenzene	4

and still others, methylmethacrylate and styrene, had not been present in the unfiltered source.

PESTICIDES

The predominant route of exposure to pesticides is probably food. This has been found to be true on a regional basis for the Great Lakes basin of North America [65]. Episodes of gross food contamination by pesticides do occur, such as the poisoning of 1,000 persons who ate watermelons tainted with Temik [57]. Another regional effect is the strongly positive correlation (0.967) between Parkinson's disease and the use of the herbicide paraquat in the nine hydrographic regions of Quebec Province [54].

Acceptable daily intake (ADI)

Contaminants in foods are measured yearly in 20 different areas in US cities by the FDA

Table 22a.4 Number of pesticides and other man-made agents observed in total diet samples in the United States during 1980–1982 sample period.

Class of food products tested	Chemicals	
	Number of chemicals detected	Total chemical residues detected
Dairy products	8	71
Meat, fish and poultry	17	157
Grain and cereal products	15	91
Potatoes	19	80
Leafy vegetables	16	89
Legume vegetables	9	13
Root vegetables	19	81
Garden fruits	26	91
Fruits	22	82
Oil/fats	20	218
Sugar and adjuncts	16	72
Beverages	0	0
All groups	60	1045

[34, 35]. A typical grocery basket of a wide range of foods is collected and analysed for pesticides and industrial chemicals. Table 22a.4 summarizes the number of man-made organic chemicals and the total residues detected in various food groups characterized during the 1980–1982 sample period [34, 35].

Polychlorinated biphenyls (PCBs)

PCB levels in Canadian beef are much higher in the Great Lakes basin than in the Atlantic or Western provinces [82] and can also be detected in dairy products, eggs, potatoes, oysters, crabmeat, candy, meat, poultry and cereals [74]. The average concentration of PCB in whole milk from southern Ontario in 1983 was 0.889 parts per billion (ppb), which, for an intake of 1 litre/day, would result in an annual intake of 327 ng [32]. It has also been shown that maternal serum PCB levels can be positively associated with infectious illnesses in newborn infants [94].

Infant feeding

Studies of pesticides and/or industrial chemicals in the diets of infants and toddlers have shown that 37 different pesticides and industrial chemicals (including degradation products) can be identified in the infant diet [29, 34, 35, 84, 95]. The greatest variety of such man-made organic compounds was found in oils and fats and potato groups of foods. On a daily intake per unit body weight of each organic chemical observed during 1978–79 survey, none approached the acceptable daily intakes (ADIs) proposed by the United Nations Food and Agriculture Organization and the World Health Organization [30]. However, the chlorinated pesticide dieldrin was between 36% and 48% of the ADI in toddler and infant diets.

LD_{50} values in the newborn

Because LD_{50} values in newborn animals are often higher than for adults [39], it remains an open question as to whether children are at greater risk [3]. Studies on PCB uptake by infants in Canada from mother's milk showed average levels of 17 ppb [58], and 45 ppb for fish-eating women in Sheboygan, Wisconsin [94]. This would result in the children's annual intake being 2190 ng and 9855 ng, respectively, which would exceed the maximum daily PCB dose rate for adults [65].

Routes of exposure of chemicals

Chemicals enter the body by three routes: inhalation of airborne molecules and contaminated particulates, absorption through skin contact with chemical substances, and ingestion from contaminated and/or chemically treated foodstuffs and water. It would appear that for both animals and man, ingestion is the major source of exposure for the general population, particularly so for highly lipophilic hydrocarbons which have long half-lives and accumulate in fat tissue [69].

Ingestion

Chemicals regularly enter the body via the ingestion of contaminated or treated foods, beverages, by licking the lips or placing contaminated non-food objects in the mouth [23]. These compounds may be absorbed throughout the gastrointestinal tract. Absorption depends upon the availability of the ionized form of the chemical [9].

Modification of absorption. Several factors work to modify gastrointestinal uptake of chemical compounds. The amount of chemical that is already dissolved and its degree of solubility may affect the current ingested dose. A high protein or high fat meal may delay absorption, but absorption may be increased by increasing gastric emptying time.

Metabolism of organic pollutants

Although each organic compound may be treated individually by the body, most compounds in general show broad similarities in the ways they are metabolized. This process involves two basic steps: firstly, conversion of lipophilic compounds by various enzyme systems into simpler products which are then conjugated to form readily excretable, water-soluble derivatives [26] (Fig. 22a.1) (see also Chapter 24).

The resulting products are usually highly water soluble, biologically inactive, non-toxic and readily excreted. Excretion through sweat, bile, respiration, lactation or urine may occur at any time following intake [102].

Metabolic response to contaminants

The metabolic response to chemical contaminants may vary under certain conditions. The cytochrome P-450 enzyme systems may be dependent, to a great extent, upon sufficient ascorbic acid levels in the organism [13]. These systems also have a tendency to shift to accommodate toxins. Saturation of a particular system may also result in higher levels of unmetabolized chemicals in the blood stream, and the excretion rate may plateau.

MEASUREMENT IN BODY TISSUES AND FLUIDS

Techniques

The combined use of gas chromatography and mass spectrometry in the measurement of organic compounds in human tissues and fluids has made such analyses rapid, comprehensive, sensitive and inexpensive. Information about chemicals in parts per billion can now be obtained [25]. Hundreds of substances have been measured to date from a variety of sources such as urine, breath, milk, blood and other body fluids [76, 102]. These contaminants are the same chemicals that are found in food, water, air, industry, agriculture and private use. The predominant storage compartment within the body is fat tissue.

Fat solubility

Most toxic chemicals in adipose tissue are usually biologically persistent or frequently used materials such as dichlorodiphenyltrichloroethane (DDT), PCBs and dioxin [27]. The goal in detoxification is often fat mobili-

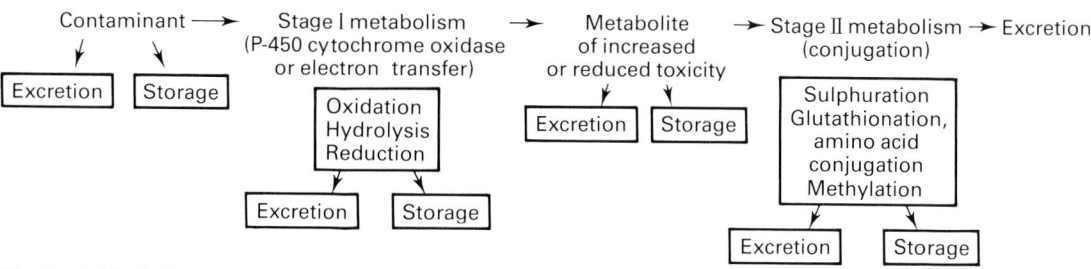

Fig. 22a.1 Typical metabolic pathway of organic contaminants.

zation of these stored contaminants. In one study, 16 organohalides were identified in the adipose tissue of the participants. These included PCBs, polybrominated biphenyls (PPBs) and DDE, heptachlor epoxide and dieldrin. Concentrations range from none detected to high levels of 2.72 ppm [86].

Blood

Blood analysis, although an invasive technique requiring careful collection methods, provides an accurate reflection of xenobiotic compounds present in the body. The path of organic contaminants from food, water, air, etc. into the human body is easily traced through the use of blood analysis. Blood levels analysed in 21 subjects living in New Orleans area, showed measurable amounts of the same pollutants found in their water supply [49]. Cord blood samples taken from newborns illustrate the potential for toxic compounds to cross the placental barrier [25].

Urine

Urine analysis generally, although not always, involves a metabolite. Since many factors affect rate and quality of metabolism, there may be great difficulty in relating the results of urinary analysis to exposure levels. A comprehensive view of those factors has been published [20].

Breast milk

The lactating mother appears to be an excellent source of contaminants for young infants [102] who are a high-risk population representing a higher trophic level than adults and who are exposed to contaminants at sensitive stages of development. Breast-milk sampling offers an easy way of measuring contaminants in the human body, although the subjects are of course limited to women of child-bearing age and so are poorly representative of the general population [72].

Nonetheless, a number of studies have shown widespread contamination of mother's milk, a supposed perfect human food, sometimes at levels that exceed maximum governmental permissible levels for toxic compounds [32, 58, 65, 94, 103].

Other body fluids

Other body fluids have been examined for chemical components as well. These include cerebrospinal fluid, human gastric juice, stool water, amniotic fluid, saliva and sweat [76, 102]. Each of these body fluids offers its own benefits for examination, although blood, urine and mother's milk tend to be more appropriate for a wide range of reasons.

EXPOSURE MECHANISMS

The health effects of chemical contamination have been well documented [20, 26, 41]. Generally, the research has focused on acute rather than chronic exposure, so that the symptoms usually relate to high dosages with direct effect. Chronic toxicity may occur under different circumstances from those that produce acute reactions and may be of great importance because of continued exposure to low levels of a host of chemical substances in the environment including food [26].

Synergistic effects

There may be a synergistic enhancement of chemical toxicity which may be *additive*, where the subtoxic doses of several chemicals combine to produce toxic effects, or *potentiative*, where the effect is greater than that expected from the sum of the individual components. Alternatively, the interaction may be *antagonistic* in that the effects of the combination are less than those expected from the sum of the individual substances [44].

Competition for storage

Some substances may compete mechanically for storage in tissues. This interaction is seen with the combined administration of two organochlorine pesticides, DDT and dieldrin. The storage of DDT is increased while that of dieldrin is decreased, compared with that expected for each administered separately [96]. Other substances may compete for enzyme sites and metabolic function. Typically an enzyme with multisubstrate capability will preferentially metabolize one substrate over another. For example, in cases where exposure to ethanol and methanol occurs concurrently, ethanol will be monopolized initially so that methanol circulates largely unmetabolized in the blood stream [52].

Bioaccumulation

Perhaps the most important problem of repeated low-level exposures is the process of bioaccumulation. The accumulation of a single agent in the body is dependent upon three factors—the dose, the dose interval and the half-life of the agent [26]. A chemical with a short half-life can be rapidly eliminated prior to the next exposure. This is assuming that the dose is at a level manageable by the body's metabolic system. Blood and tissue concentrations can return to zero or near zero in such a case. However, should the chemical have a long half-life (such as polybrominated biphenyls) the body burden never returns to zero. Therefore each successive dose builds the body burden to a higher level [71] (Figure 22a.2).

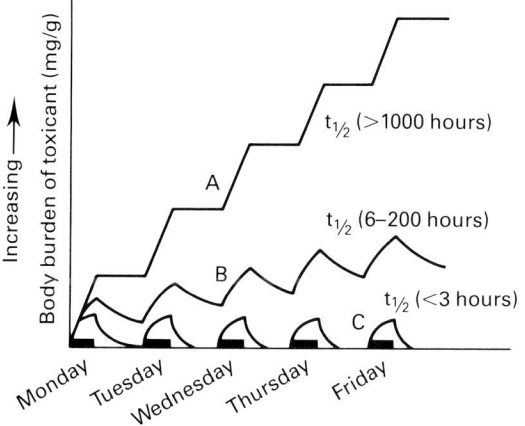

Fig. 22a.2 Body or tissue burden as a function of a chemical's uptake and elimination rate (i.e. biological half-life). From Paustenbach [71].

Bioaccumulation usually reaches a plateau level in cases where fairly constant dosage of the compound is being administered and absorption rate is equal to elimination rate [36]. That plateau level may or may not be above the level of toxicity. The half-lives and sources of some common organic substances are shown in Appendix 22a.3.

Biological half-life. Biological half-life estimates may not accurately reflect the decomposition in the body of toxic materials. Metabolism is rapid for high doses of the toxic material but as the concentration drops, the rate of removal is slower [26, 37]. Thus, residuals may remain in the blood and tissues for extended periods not predicted by half-life.

With continuous or repeated exposure (from the same or several different sources) a substance may accumulate to many times the level seen following a single exposure. This slow build-up of toxic concentrations may result in

symptoms which may be 'similar to or distinctly different from the symptoms expected for an acutely toxic dose' [26]. Several factors may influence chemical accumulation: low solubility quotient, storage in poorly perfused tissues such as fat, poor glomerular filtration, intensive tubular reabsorption and slow biotransformation. Highly lipid-soluble compounds are stored easily in adipose tissue and therefore may show an increased tendency to accumulate [71].

Susceptibility

Subtoxic doses of chemicals, particularly those that tend to bioaccumulate, while sometimes not affecting normal individuals, may produce symptoms in the susceptible or sensitive individual [46]. Several factors can affect metabolism and excretion of toxic materials.

Genetic and individual variation. Genetic and individual variations in enzymes and protein synthesis may lead to individuals missing an enzyme or showing abnormal enzyme activity, who could thus, if exposed to a chemical demanding performance of that enzyme for metabolism and excretion, manifest symptoms of toxic accumulation [51, 102].

Diet and nutritional state. A high protein or high fat diet appears to result in enhanced metabolism and storage of some chemicals in humans [2], while a low protein diet may inhibit metabolism in rats [66]. Brussels sprouts, cabbage, cauliflower [55] and diets high in corn oil and low in starch and sugar have, in rats [104], been reported to result in increased liver enzyme activity. It is likely that a diet deficient in any individual nutritional component could affect chemical metabolism [102].

Fat/muscle ratio. For both water- and fat-soluble chemicals, an increase of 50–100% in body half-life has been reported in obese individuals. In such persons, more fat is available for distribution and storage of fat-soluble materials. The increased volume of distribution also reduces the elimination rate of water-soluble chemicals [1].

Age. A 50–100% increase in body half-life for medicinal chemicals was seen in disease-free elderly subjects compared with young subjects [99]. This may be due to a reported 35% decrease in glomerular filtration rate [81] and/or a reported 40–45% decrease in hepatic blood flow with age [67]. Newborns may be more susceptible to toxicity since the hepatic excretory system is not fully functional [9].

Disease state. Any disease such as cirrhosis or abnormal renal function is likely to affect metabolism and/or excretion of chemicals [79, 102]. Likewise, many genetically transmitted diseases, such as sickle-cell anaemia, may affect the toxic response [62].

Sex. Many of the organophosphate pesticides are three to four times more lethal to one sex than to the other. Which sex is the more sensitive tends to vary with the chemical [22] (Table 22a.5).

Hormonal status. Several conditions may alter the hormonal balance with resulting untoward responses to many toxic agents [6, 19, 24, 42, 89, 90].

Environmental stress. Environmental stress conditions [75], such as cold [33, 75], heat [4], dehydration [4] (response similar to that of temperature elevation), hypoxia and noise [22] seem to affect toxicity and to produce typical stress responses.

FACTORS ENHANCING ELIMINATION

Removal from source

While seemingly a commonsense approach, this method may be fairly complex due to the ubiquitous nature of organic chemicals in our society. However, if there is a single major

Table 22a.5 Differential toxic and carcinogenic responsiveness toward xenobiotics between females (F) and males (M).

Compound and species	Type of adverse response	Susceptibility record	Origin of the susceptibility difference and comments
Benzene (various species)	Haematopoietic disturbance, myeolotoxic action	F > M	F show higher rate of conversion of benzene into toxic phenols (catechol) and lesser ability of conjugation of metabolites
Chloroform (mouse)	Renal damage	M > F	Hormone-dependent effect, enhanced by androgens
Trichloroethylene (humans)		Undertermined	Differential rate of excretion of trichloroethanol (TCE) and trichloroacetic acid (TCA); TCE: M > F, TCA: F > M
Aliphatic nitriles (rat)	Acute toxicity	M > F	F more efficient in detoxication by thiocyanate elimination
Fluoroacetate (rat)	Acute toxicity (convulsive action)	F > M?	Sex-dependent difference in fluorocitrate accumulation
Pesticides Aldrin, heptachlor, isodrin (rat)	Chronic toxicity, accumulative tendency	M > F	Related to greater conversion by M into toxic epoxides, as compared to F; sex-linked differential partition of the pesticides amongst erythrocytes and plasma in humans
Endrin		F > M	Higher retention of endrin in F
Warfarin (rat)	Clotting impairment	F > M	Higher degree of metabolic hydroxylation in M
Parathion (rat)	Anti-ChE action	F > M	Relatively, enhanced conversion of parathion into paraoxon in F; paraoxon degradation is not influenced
Schradan (OMPA) (rat)	Anti-ChE action	M > F	More rapid detoxication of the toxic intermediate Schradan N-oxide in F
Dimethylnitrosamine (mouse)	Hepatoma induction	M > F	Related to sex-linked difference in microsomal dealkylation, also modulated by age
Aflatoxin B$_1$ (rat)	Neoplasm, response	M > F	Higher detoxication of aflatoxin B$_1$ into aflatoxin metabolites in F, as compared to M
Acetylaminofluorene	Mammary cancer, liver tumorigenesis	M > F	Probably related to higher extent and rate of N-hydroxylation in M
Polycyclic hydrocarbons (e.g. benzopyrene)	Epidermal cancer	M > F or F > M	Variable sensibility related to the phenomenon that the epidermis of females passes through cycles of different thickness
4'-Amino-2,3'-dimethyl azobenzene	Hepatoma induction	F > M	Probably mediated by differential biotransformation

Source: [22].
ChE = cholisterase.

source which is well defined, then elimination of that single source may allow the body time to metabolize and excrete much of the offending substance, a process technically known as depuration. In more difficult cases where the patient is exposed to offending contaminants from many sources or is suffering serious medical and/or psychological symptoms as a result, hospitalization in a relatively chemical-free environment such as an environmental control unit (ECU) has been effective [50] (See Chapter 55).

Dietary/nutritional treatments

Starvation (fasting) can mobilize fat-stored chemical contaminants. Obviously, mobilizing such chemicals could have deleterious consequences if other measures are not utilized to aid in the rapid excretion of these harmful toxins. Oils may also assist in chemical reduction. The introduction of polyunsaturated oils into the diet has been observed to mobilize lipids by replacing existing adipose tissue [93].

Exercise

Exercise may help in toxic chemical reduction by directly hastening toxic excretion in sweat, urine and stool and by indirectly speeding up metabolic excretory functions by stimulating the adrenal glands in production of adrenaline (epinephrine) and noradrenaline (norepinephrine) [98]. Also, like starvation, exercise mobilizes fat in which toxic chemicals are stored, thus allowing them to be metabolized and excreted [28].

Elevated body temperature

The sauna has been used in some chemical reduction regimens in order to force sweating so that excretion through perspiration would be enhanced [43, 87].

Drugs and vitamins

Several substances have been observed to bind toxins in the blood stream and assist in their elimination from the body. These substances include various vitamins, including ascorbic acid [10, 12, 14, 61, 92], vitamin E [92], niacin [8, 11, 85, 86], selenium [60, 78, 92] and/or drugs, including cholestyramine [7, 15, 16] and phenobarbital [21, 41, 68].

Chemical reduction programmes

Controlled hospital facilities provide an optimal environment for the recovery of the contaminated patient under medical supervision. Fig. 22a.3 shows the levels of DDT/DDE for

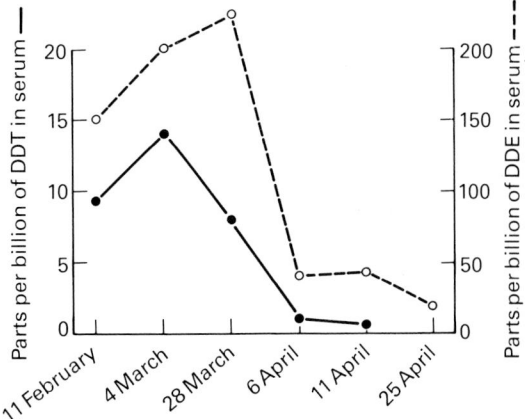

Fig. 22a.3 Levels of DDT and DDE in a female patient treated in a comprehensive chemical reduction programme in an environmental control unit.

a female patient treated in a comprehensive chemical reduction programme in an environmental control unit. This illustrates the initial spontaneous increase in pesticide blood level due to fat mobilization following fasting when there was no opportunity for the patient to receive any outside source of pesticide while in this protected environment. Significant reductions in the blood levels of the pesticides heptachlor, endosulfan I, γ-chlordane and DDT have been found in a series of 40 patients treated in the ECU [77].

Conclusion

Food additives

For some time food additives have been an issue for concern [31, 40, 97], especially since the discovery that the addition of anthropogenic compounds to food can cause serious health problems. This was recognized as early as 1965 by the National Research Council [63] and continues to stimulate regulatory action and research today on a worldwide basis [59, 100]. By 1972, a number of dye salts had already been banned. However, several hundred compounds are still recognized as safe by the FDA's GRAS (generally regarded as safe) list, many of which have not been adequately tested for harmful effects [80, 83].

These ingredients are still widely used in the preparation of foods for the general public. Health effects have proved so significant that many physicians are using chemical reduction methods to clear symptoms in toxic patients, although another effective therapeutic approach is simple avoidance. Certainly, in cases where a patient is reacting to additives, those chemicals that are intentionally added can be intentionally avoided by using foods that have not been processed.

Chemicals. The connection between the availability of low-dose chemical contaminants in our society, body load of chemical and health effects should not be ignored. The peoples of the modern world can be regarded as being engaged in a mass epidemiological experiment, which would never be approved by any governmental agency or human subjects committee. It may be many years before the implications of the combined and sustained intake of low-level toxic chemicals are known. Certainly, vast numbers of these chemicals are available and too little is understood about the interactions involved.

However, there are avenues by which to control and measure chemical exposure in patients who are suffering the physical and behavioural consequences of that exposure. Extremely sensitive measurements can be made and treatment techniques and/or treatment facilities are available for the toxic patient. Various treatments have been successful in bringing about changes in body load of contaminants. Physicians may benefit from being alert to specific chemical sources in their own areas and by utilizing the specific treatment modes effective with chemicals common to their area.

APPENDICES

Appendix 22a.1 Food additives and health effects

Artificial colourings. Blue Nos 1 and 2, Citrus Red No 2, Orange B—cause cancer in laboratory animals. Green No. 3 is poorly tested and may be carcinogenic. Red No. 3 induces hyperactivity in children and may cause cancer. Red No. 40 may cause cancer in mice. Yellow No. 5 is a potent allergen and possible carcinogen. Yellow No. 6 is related to allergic reactions.
Artificial flavours. May cause hyperactivity in children.

Benzoic acid. A mild irritant to skin, eyes and mucous membranes; toxicity increases when combined with other additives.
Brominated vegetable oil (BVO). Toxic residues of BVO stored in body fat; possible organ damage.
Butylated hydroxyanisole (BHA). Claimed to protect human liver from toxic chemicals; known to cause allergy, affect liver and kidney function, increased incidence of stomach cancer.
Butylated hydroxytoluene (BHT). Credited for declining incidence of stomach cancer; same negative effects as BHA but more toxic to liver, some studies show that BHT promotes lung tumours in mice; accumulates in human fat.
Caffeine. Stimulant (see Chapter 23).
Calcium (or sodium) propionate. Provokes reactions in allergic persons; inhibits assimilation of calcium.
Carrageenan (seaweed). Causes ulcers, liver lesions and birth defects in animals.
Cellulose gum (sodium carboxymethylcellulose). Causes cancer in mice.
Calcium disodium edetate (EDTA). In large amounts, causes kidney damage and gastrointestinal problems.

Heptyl paraben. Has not been tested in the presence of alcohol to which it is commonly added.
Hydrogenated or partially hydrogenated fat. As a saturated (hard) fat, it elevates cholesterol and is strongly linked to heart disease.

Mannitol, sorbitol, xylitol. Have laxative effect in large doses.
Modified starches. High levels cause abnormalities in rats.
Monosodium glutamate (MSG). Contains wheat, corn and beet sugar by-products which are common allergens; may be contaminated with *Aspergillus* mould; destroys brain cells in every species of laboratory animal, especially newborn; can cause headache, chest tightness, burning sensation in neck and arms and possible seizures (Chinese restaurant syndrome).

Phosphoric acid, phosphates. Contribute to dietary imbalance that may lead to osteoporosis.
Propyl gallate. Poorly tested; increases risk of cancer in mice.

Quinine. Can cause vomiting, disturbances in vision, dizziness, ringing in ears; related to birth defects.

Saccharin. Promotes bladder cancer in rats.
Sodium chloride. Associated with hypertension, heart disease, cerebrovascular accidents.
Silicates. Some are a form of asbestos with carcinogenic potential.
Sodium bisulphite. Destroys vitamin B_1 (thiamine); produces gastric distress and diarrhoea; is a potent allergen capable of causing anaphylactic shock.
Sodium nitrate. Readily converts to sodium nitrite in the body.
Sodium nitrite. Combines with other substances in the digestive tract to form nitrosamines, strong carcinogens; can also trigger diabetic attacks.
Sugar. Contributes to poor nutrition, obesity, tooth decay.
Sulphur dioxide. Causes gastric distress, headaches and diarrhoea; destoys vitamins A and B_1.

Source: [83].

Appendix 22a.2 Volatile and base-neutral extractable organics found in potable water from three US cities.§.

	New Orleans (ppt)¶	East St. Louis (ppt)	Minneapolis (ppt)
1 Chloroform*‡	45	37	4.7
2 Bromodichloromethane*	96	57	9.7
3 Dibromochloromethane*	15	4.1	0.12
4 1,2-Dichloropropane*	1.3	ND	ND
5 Trichlorofluoromethane*	ND	ND	ND
6 Bis(2-chloreothyl) ether*‡	1.3×10^2	ND	ND
7 Dichlorobenzene* (isomer)‡	22	ND	ND
8 Dichlorobenzene* (isomer)‡	0.72	ND	ND
9 1,1-Oxybis(3-chloro)-propane	9.2×10^2	ND	ND
10 Naphthalene*	58	ND	ND
11 1-Chloro-3-nitrobenzene	51	ND	ND
12 1-Bromo-2,3-dichloropropane	66	ND	ND
13 Methylnaphthalene	ND	ND	15
14 1,3,5-Triazine-2,4,6-trion-1,3,5-trimethyl	30	ND	15
15 (Butylhexyl)benzene	ND	26	ND
16 4-Chlorophenyl phenyl ether*	ND	ND	4.5×10^2
17 Fluorene*	32	ND	ND
18 Diethylphthalate*	2.1×10^3	2.1×10^3	3.0×10^3
19 1,2-Dimethyl-4-(phenylmethyl)benzene	2.0×10^2	ND	2.7×10^2
20 Tributyl phosphate	3.5×10^2	3.3×10^2	0.48×10^2
21 (1-Methyldecyl)benzene	78	77	84
22 (4-Bromophenyl) phenyl ether*	ND	ND	0.24
23 Hexachlorobenzene*‡	ND	ND	0.28
24 1,1,3-Trimethyl-3-phenylindan	11	40	ND
25 (1-Penthylheptyl)benzene and (1-butyloctyl)benzene	73	1.3×10^2	1.1×10^2
26 (1-Propylnonyl)benzene	22	22	ND
27 (1-Ethyldecyl)benzene	43	25	25
28 Dibutylphthalate*	ND	2.0×10^3	1.7×10^3
29 2-Hydroxy-4-methoxybenzophenone	ND	2.0×10^3	1.2×10^3
30 Fluoranthene*	32	ND	ND
31 1,2,3-Propanetricarboxylic acid, (2-acetyloxy) tributylester	15	19	61
32 1-Phenanthrenecarboxylic acid-1,2,3,4,4a,9,10,10a-octahydro-1, 4a-dimethyl	ND	ND	6.1
33 Bis(2-ethylhexyl)phthalate*	24	7.8	ND
34 Di-n-octylphthalate*	ND	ND	50

* EPA priority pollutant.
† Carcinogenic.
‡ Potentially carcinogenic.
ND = None detected.
¶ ppt is equivalent to pg/ml or ng/l.
§ Data developed at the Center for Bio-organic Studies at the University of New Orleans.

Appendix 22a.3 Organic compounds, blood concentrations, half-life estimates and sources.

Compound	Arithmetic mean	Frequency of occurrence per 100	Body half-life (single exposures) estimates*	Common environmental sources†
Chlorinated pesticides				
Aldrin	0.02	1.6		Agricultural insecticide
Dieldrin	0.17	66.8	50–266 days (human)	Metabolite of aldrin
α-BHC	0.02	3.3		Agriculture—lindane, termite control
β-BHC	1.20	71.5		Termite control
γ-BHC	0.02	2.8		Termite control
δ-BHC	0.01	0.2		Termite control
DDT	0.28	54.3	2+ years (humans)	Illegal use and contaminated imported products
DDE	5.64	97.3	2+ years (humans)	Metabolite of DDT
DDD	0.02	2.8	2+ years (humans)	Metabolite of DDT
α-chlordane	0.01	1.4	21–88 days (humans)	Agriculture, termite control
γ-chlordane	0.01	1.6	21–88 days (humans)	Agriculture, termite control
Heptachlor	0.01	0.5	21–88 days (humans)	Agriculture, termite control
Heptachlor epoxide	0.43	78.5	21–88 days (humans)	Metabolite of heptachlor
trans-Nonachlor	0.21	80.7	21–88 days (humans)	Termite control
Endosulfan I	0.01	2.8	235 hours (rabbits)	Agriculture
Endosulfan II	0.01	1.1	597 hours (rabbits)	
HCB	0.54	95.3	Up to 3 years (Rhesus monkeys)	Fungicide, by-product of chlorinated solvent manufacture
Mirex	0.01	1.1	3–4 months (rats)	Fire ant insecticide
Endrin	0.01	3.7	3–4 days (rats)	Agricultural crops
Chlorinated phenols				
Penta	13.5	92.9	Approx. 8 days (humans)	Fungicide, bacteriocide, herbicide, packaging, shoe leather, etc.
2,3,5,6-Tetra	0.1	0.6		Fungicide, insecticide, contaminants of pentachlorophenol
2,3,4,5-Tetra	0.1	2.4		Fungacide, insecticide, contaminants of pentachlorophenol
2,4,6-Tri	0.10	0.50		Biocidal, herbicide, germicides
2,3,6-Tri	0.10	0.50		Biocidal, herbicide, germicides
2,3,5-Tri	0.10	0.50		Biocidal, herbicide, germicides
2,4,5-Tri	0.10	0.50		Biocidal, herbicide, germicides
2,3,4-Tri	0.10	0.50		Biocidal, herbicide, germicides
3,4,5-Tri	0.10	1.20		Biocidal, herbicide, germicides
Total dichloro	0.10	0.50		Herbicide 2,4-Di
Polychlorinated biphenyls (PCBs)				
PCBs	2.01	100.00	? years (humans)	Insulating coolants in electrical transformers, paints, coatings, lubricants

* These are, in most cases, only gross estimates of the half-life of the parent chemical. There is increased evidence that the parent and/or metabolites may persist for considerably long periods of time in the tissues of the exposed animal or human. Recurrent symptoms (of subclinical symptoms) may occur for much longer than expected based on simple half-life calculations.

† Major source is residence of USA.

REFERENCES

1 Abernethy D, Greenblatt D, Divoll M et al: Alterations in drug distribution and clearance due to obesity. J Pharmacol Exp Ther 1981; 217:681-5.

2 Alveres A, Anderson K, Conney A, Kappas A: Interactions between nutritional factors and drug biotransformations in man. Proc Natl Acad Sci USA 1976; 73:2501-4.

3 Babich H, Davis DL: Food tolerances and action levels: do they adequately protect children? Bioscience 1981; 31:429-38.

4 Baetjer AM, Joardar SND, McQuary WA: Effect of environmental temperature and humidity on lead poisoning in animals. Arch Environ Health 1960; 1:463-77.

5 Barber RT, Whaling PJ, Cohen DM: Mercury in recent and century-old deep sea fish. Environ Sci Techno 1984; 18:552-5.

6 Booth J, Gillette JR: The effect of anabolic steroids on drug metabolism by microsomal enzymes in rat liver. J Pharmacol Exp Ther 1962; 137:374-9.

7 Boylan J, Egle J, Guzelian P: Cholestyramine: use as a new therapeutic approach for chlordecone (Kepone) poisoning. Science 1978; 199:893-5.

8 Brown O, Heitkamp M, Song C: Niacin reduces paraquat toxicity in rats. Science 1981; 212: 510-1.

9 Bus J, Gibson J: Body defense mechanisms to toxicant exposure. In: Cralley LJ, Cralley LV, eds. Patty's industrial hygiene and toxicology. 2nd ed. New York: John Wiley and Sons, 1985.

10 Cameron E, Pauling L, Leibowitz B: Ascorbic acid and cancer: a review. Cancer Res 1979; 39:663.

11 Carlson L: Nicotine acid and inhibition of fat mobilizing lipolysis. Adv Exp Med Biol 1978; 109:225-38.

12 Chadwick RW, Peoples AJ, Cranmer MF: The effect of ascorbic acid deficiency and protein quality on stimulation of hepatic microsomal enzymes in guinea pigs. Toxicol Appl Pharmacol 1982; 20:308.

13 Chakrabortz O, Bhattacharyya A, Majumdar K et al: Studies on L-ascorbic acid metabolism in rats under chronic toxicity due to organophosphorus insecticides: effects of supplementation of L-ascorbic acid in high doses. J Nutr 1978; 108:973-80.

14 Chow CK: Nutritional influence on cellular antioxidant defense systems. Am J Clin Nutr 1979; 32:1066-81.

15 Cohn W, Blanke R, Griffith F, Guzelian P: Distribution and excretion of Kepone in humans. Gastroenterology 1976; 71: A-8/901.

16 Cohn W, Boylan J, Blanke R et al: Treatment of chlordecone (Kepone) toxicity with cholestyramine. N Engl J Med 1978; 298: 243-8.

17 Committee on Government Operations: Ground water contamination. Hearing before a Subcommittee of the Committee on Government Operations, House of Representatives, First Session. Washington DC: GPO, 1984

18 Committee on Government Operations: Review of ground water contamination and depletion problems in the Northwest. Hearing before a Subcommittee of the Committee on Government Operations, House of Representatives, First Session. Washington DC: GPO, 1985.

19 Conney AH, Garren L: Contrasting effects of thyroxin on zoxazolamine and hexobarbital metabolism. Biochem Pharmacol 1961; 6:257-62.

20 Cralley LJ, Cralley L: Patty's industrial hygiene and toxicology. New York: John Wiley and Sons, 1985.

21 Davies JE, Edmundson WF, Maceo A et al: Reduction of pesticide residues in human adipose tissue with diphenylhydantoin. Food Cosmet Toxicol 1971; 9:413-23.

22 DeBruin A: Biochemical toxicology of environmental agents. Amsterdam: Elsevier/North-Holland, 1976.

23 Derman B: The mode of entry and action of toxic materials. In: Clayton G, Clayton F, eds. Patty's industrial hygiene and toxicology. 3rd ed. New York: John Wiley and Sons, 1978; 135-64.

24 D'Iorio A, Mavrides G: Actions of the thyroid hormones and analogues in vitro on catechol-o-methyltransferase. Biochem Pharmacol 1963; 12:1307-13.

25 Dowty BJ, Storer J, Laseter JL: The transplacental migration and accumulation in blood of volatile organic constituents. J Pediatr Res 1976; 10:696.

26 Ecobichon D, Joy R: Pesticides and neurological diseases. Boca Raton: CRC Press, 1982.

27 Environmental Protection Agency: Chemicals identified in human biological media, a database. US EPA. Washington DC: EPA 560/13-80-036B, PB 81-161-176, 1980.

28 Essen B: Intramuscular substrate utilization during prolonged exercise. Ann NY Acad Sci 1977; 301:30-44.

29 Food and Agriculture Organization (FAO) Working Party on Pesticide Residues: Evaluation of some pesticide residues in food. Rome: Food and Agriculture Organization of the United Nations, 1967.

30 Food and Agriculture Organization/World Health Organization (FAO/WHO) Code Alimentarium Commission: Summary of acceptances of recommended worldwide and regional codex standards and recommended code maximum limits for pesticide residues (as to 30 October 1978). Rome: Food and Agriculture Organization of the United Nations, 1979; 28.

31 Federation of American Societies for Experimental Biology. Select Committee of GRAS Substances: Evaluation of health aspects of GRAS food ingredient: lessons learned and questions unanswered. Fed Proc 1977; 37: 2519-62.

32 Frank R, Rasper J, Braun HE, Smout MS: Organochlorine residues in human adipose tissues, blood and milk from Ontario residents, 1976-1982. Ontario Ministry of Agriculture and Food, unpublished data, 1985.

33 Fuhrman GJ, Fuhrman FA: Effects of temperature on the action of drugs. Ann Rev Pharmacol 1961; 1:65-78.

34 Gartrell M, Craun J, Podrebarac D, Gunderson E: Pesticides, selected elements and other chemicals in adult total diet samples. J Assoc Off Anal Chem 1986 (in press).

35 Gartrell M, Craun J, Podrebarac D, Gunderson E: Pesticides, selected elements and other chemicals in infant and toddler total diet samples. J Assoc Off Anal Chem 1986 (in press).

36 Gibaldi M, Perrier D: Pharmacokinetics. New York: Marcel Dekker, 1975.

37 Gibaldi M, Weintraub H: Some considerations as to the determination and significance of biologic half-life. J Pharm Sci 1971; 60:624-6.

38 Giger W, Reinhard M, Schaffner C, Zarcher F: Analysis of organic constituents in water by high resolution gas chromatography in combination with specific detection and computer-assisted mass spectrometry. In: Keith L, ed. Identification and analysis

of organic pollutants in water. Ann Arbor: Ann Arbor Service, 1977.

39 Goldenthal ES: A compilation of LD50 values in newborn adult animals. Toxicol Appl Pharmacol 1971; 18:185–207.

40 Harkins RW: Food additive safety evaluation. Food Drug Cosm Law J 1977: 32:182–93.

41 Hayes W: Pesticides studied in man. Baltimore: Williams and Williams, 1982.

42 Hsia DYY, Riabov S, Dowben RM: Inhibition of glucoconosyl transferase by steroid hormones. Arch Biochem Biophys 1973; 103:181–5.

43 Johnson J, Maibach H: Drug excretion in human eccrine sweat. J Invest Dermatol 1971; 56:182–8.

44 Kato R, Gillette JR: Effects of starvation on NADPH-dependent enzymes in liver microsomes of male and female rats. J Pharmacol Exp Ther 1985; 150:279–84.

45 Keith L, Garrison A, Allen F et al: Identification of organic compounds in drinking water from thirteen US cities. In: Keith L, ed. Identification and analysis of organic pollutants in water. Ann Arbor: Ann Arbor Science, 1976.

46 Kelly W, Harris E: Protection of the sensitive individual. Ann Am Conf Govern Indust Hyg 1982; 3.

47 King J: Troubled water. Emmaus, Pennsylvania: Rodale Press, 1982; ix–xiii.

48 Lao R, Thomas R, Baston R et al: Analysis of organic priority and non-priority pollutants in environmental samples by GC/MS computer systems. In: Albargie J, ed. Anal Tech Environ Chem 2. Proc Second Int Congr. Barcelona, Spain: Pergamon Press, 1981

49 Laseter J, Dowty B: Association of biorefractions in drinking water and body burden in people. Ann NY Acad Sci 1977; 298:547–56.

50 Laseter J, DeLeon I, Rea W, Butler J: Chlorinated hydrocarbon pesticides in environmentally sensitive patients. Clin Ecol 1983; 2:3–12.

51 Lathe GH, Walker M: The synthesis of bilirubin glucuronide in animal and human liver. Biochem J 1958; 70:705–12.

52 Leaf G, Zarman LJ: A study of the conditions under which methanol may exert a toxic hazard in industry. Br J Ind Med 1952; 9:19–31.

53 Leahy JS: The determination of organics in drinking water. In: Albargie J, ed. Anal tech environ chem 2. Proc Second Int Congr Barcelona, Spain. Oxford: Pergamon Press, 1981.

54 Lewin R: Parkinson's disease: an environmental cause. Science 1985; 229:257–8.

55 Loub W, Wattenburg L, Davis D: Aryl hydrocarbon hydroxylase induction in rat tissues by naturally occurring indoles of cruciferous plants. J Natl Cancer Inst 1975; 54:985–8.

56 Marmion DM: Handbook of US colorants for foods, drugs and cosmetics. 2nd edn. New York: Wiley-Interscience, 1984; 466.

57 Marshall E: The rise and decline of Temik. Science 1985; 229:1369–71.

58 Mes J, Davies DJ: Presence of polychlorinated biphenyl and organochlorine pesticide residues and the absence of polychlorinated terphenyls in Canadian human milk samples. Bull Environ Contam Toxicol 1979; 21:381–7.

59 Millstone E: Food additive regulation in the UK. Food Policy 1985; 10:237–52.

60 Milner JA: The effect of selenium on carcinogenesis. In: Xenobiotic metabolism: nutritional effects. Washington DC: American Chemical Society, 1985.

61 Mirvish SS, Wallcave L, Eagen M, Shubik P: Ascor-

bate–nitrate reaction: possible means of blocking the formation of carcinogenic N-nitroso compounds. Science 1972; 177:65–8.

62 Mullick FG, Delage C, Nelson SI: Arch Environ Health 1973; 26:221.

63 National Research Council, Food Protection Committee, Food and Nutrition Board: Chemicals used in food processing, Publication 1274. Washington DC: National Academy of Sciences, 1965; V–XV.

64 National Research Council. Safe Drinking Water Committee: Drinking water and health. Washington DC: National Academy of Sciences, 1977; 2.

65 National Research Council of the United States and the Royal Society of Canada: The Great Lakes water quality agreement—an evolving instrument for ecosystem management. Washington DC: National Academy Press, 1985; 55–63.

66 Newberne P: Dietary factors affecting biological responses to esophageal and colon chemical carcinogenesis. In: Finley J, Schwess D, eds. Xenobiotic metabolism: nutritional effects. Washington DC: American Chemical Society, 1985.

67 Nomiyama K, Nomiyama H: Sex differences in benzene uptake of man. Chem Abstr 1970; 72: 82685a.

68 Ohtsuji H, Ikeda M: The metabolism of styrene in the rat and the stimulatory effect of phenobarbital. Toxicol Appl Pharmacol 1971; 18:321–8.

69 Oliver BG, Niiomi AJ: Bioconcentration factors of some halogenated organics for rainbow trout: limitations in their use for prediction of environmental residues. Environ Sci Technol 1985; 19:842–9.

70 Ott WR: Total human exposure. Environ Sci Technol 1985; 19:880–6.

71 Paustenbach D: Occupational exposure limits, pharmacokinetics, and unusual work schedules. In: Cralley LJ, Cralley LV, eds. Patty's industrial hygiene and toxicology. New York: John Wiley and Sons, 1985; 111–277.

72 Pellizzari E, Hartwell T, Harris B et al: Purgeable organic compounds in mother's milk. Bull Environ Contam Toxicol 1982; 28:322–8.

73 Pellizzari E, Hartwell T, Sparacinio CM et al: Interim report on the total exposure assessment methodology (TEAM) study: first season, northern Jersey. Research Triangle Institute, Report No. RTI/2392/03-035, 1985.

74 Pinn LR: The invisible additives. Toronto, Canada: Doubleday, 1981.

75 Platonow N, Coldwell BB, Dugal LP: Rate of metabolism of radioactive ethanol in cold environment. Q J Stud Alcohol 1963; 24:385–96.

76 Politzer I, Dowty B, Laseter J: Use of gas chromatography and mass spectrometry to analyze underivatized volatile human or animal constituents of clinical interest. Clin Chem 1976; 22: 1775.

77 Rea W, Butler J, Laseter J, DeLeon I: Pesticides and brain-function changes in a controlled environment. Clin Ecol 1984; 2: 145–9.

78 Reddy CC, Thomas CE, Scholz RW: Effects of inadequate vitamin E and/or selenium nutrition on enzymes associated with hydroperoxide metabolism. In: Xenobiotic metabolism: nutritional effects. Washington DC: American Chemical Society, 1985.

79 Reidenbur MM: Effects of disease states on plasma protein binding of drugs. Med Clin North Am 1974; 58: 1103–9.

80 Ribicott A: Chemicals and the future of man. Washington DC: Hearings on the Committee on Government Operations, US Senate, 1972.

81 Rowe J, Andres R, Tobin J et al: Age adjusted stan-

dards for creatinine clearance. Am Int Med 1976; 84:567.

82 Saschenbrecker PW: Levels of terminal pesticide residues in Canadian meat. Can Vet J 1976; 17:158-63.

83 Saifer P, Zellerbach M: Detox. Los Angeles: Jeremy P Tarcher, 1984.

84 Savage EP et al: National study of chlorinated hydrocarbon insecticide residues in human milk, USA. Am J Epidemiol 1981; 113:413-22.

85 Schlief G, Dorow E: Diurnal patterns of triglycerides, free fatty acids, blood sugar, and insulin during carbohydrate induction in man and their modification by nocturnal suppression of lipolysis. J Clin Invest 1973; 52: 732-40.

86 Schnare D, Denk M, Shields M: Reduction of human organohalide body burdens. Final research report. Los Angeles: Foundations for Advancements in Science and Education, 1983.

87 Schnare D, Denk M, Shields M, Brunton S: Evaluation of a detoxification regimen for fat stored xenobiotics. Med Hypotheses 1982; 9:265-82.

88 Schwass DE, Finley JW: Overview: the influence of nutrition on xenobiotic metabolism: nutritional effects. In: Finley JM, Schwass DE, eds. Xenobiotic metabolism: nutritional effects. Washington, DC: American Society Society Symposium Series 277, 1985.

89 Selyé H: Catatoxic steroids. Can Med Assoc J 1969; 101:51-2.

90 Selyé H: Resistance to various pesticides induced to catatoxic steroids. Arch Environ Health 1970; 21: 706-10.

91 Settle M, Patterson CC: Lead in albacore: guide to lead pollution in Americans. Science 1980; 207:1167-76.

92 Shamberger RJ: Relationship of selenium to cancer. I. Inhibitory effect of selenium on carcinogenesis. J Natl Cancer Inst 1970; 44:931-6.

93 Shepherd J, Stewart J, Clark J, Carr K: Sequential changes in plasma lipoproteins and body fat composition during polyunsaturated fat feeding in man. Br J Nutr 1980; 44:265-71.

94 Smith BJ: PCB levels in human fluids: Sheboygan case study. Report funded by University of Wisconsin Sea Grant Institute. WIS-SG-83-240, 1984.

95 Smith R: Hawaiian milk contamination creates alarm: a sour response by state regulators. Science 1982; 217: 137-40.

96 Street JC: Metabolism of animal responses to toxicants. In: Hodgson J, ed. Enzymatic oxidations of toxicants. North Carolina University, Raleigh, North Carolina: 1968; 197.

97 Stumpf SE: Culture, values, and food safety. Bioscience 1978:186-90.

98 Swartz R, Sidel F: Effects of heat and exercise on the elimination of pralidoxime in man. Clin Pharmacol Ther 1972; 14:83-9.

99 Triggs E, Nation R, Long A, Ashley J: Pharmacokinetics in the elderly. Eur J Clin Pharmacol 1975; 8:55-62.

100 US Department of Defense, Defense Technical Information Center Defense Logistics Agency: Technical Report Summaries. Search Control NO. DJK/51L, 1985.

101 Varma M, Katz HM: Environmental impact of cadmium. J Environ Health 1978; 40:308-14.

102 Waritz RS: Biological indicators of chemical dosage and burden. In: Cralley LJ, Cralley LV, eds. Patty's industrial hygiene and toxicology. 2nd edn. New York: John Wiley and sons, 1985.

103 Wickiyer TM, Brilliant LB, Copeland R, Filden R: Polychlorinated biphenyl contamination of nursing mothers' milk in Michigan. Am J Public Health 1981; 71:132-7.

104 Yaffe S, Sonawane B, Lau H et al: Influence of dietary carbohydrates on liver microsomal drug metabolism. Fed Prog Fed Am Soc Exp Biol 1980; 39:751.

Chapter 22b
Clinical Detection of Sensitivity to Preservatives and Chemicals

Phyllis L. Saifer and Mark Saifer

Introduction

Chemical contamination of food is to this century what microbial contamination was to the last. The intent of this chapter is to apprise the medical practitioner of intentional and unintentional chemical food additives (hidden ingredients) so that the task of explaining some erratic responses to foods may be less puzzling. Awareness of the practice of dipping apples into paraffin for cosmetic purposes, for example, may help to explain a patient's ability to eat his own home-grown apples with impunity but suffer reactions from ingestion of supermarket apples.

Discussion of mechanisms is the purview of other contributors. We will simply review the food-processing chain to demonstrate chemical contaminants of foods and water as sources of hidden ingredients in foods and similarly consider unlisted 'inert' ingredients in drugs. Some food additives are well known as causes of adverse reactions: monosodium glutamate, nitrates, BHA (butylated hydroxyanisole) and BHT (butylated hydroxytoluene), tartrazine and metabisulphites, for example. Others are

suspected but not yet as well documented. We will attempt to review more of them as a guide to potential troublemakers.

Environmentally directed history

It is essential for the clinician to identify through environmentally directed history-taking the patient who is most likely to react adversely to chemical food additives and contaminants. We will list some of the most essential clues. We will also present a workable system to enable the clinician to separate reactions to

Table 22b.1 Unintentional food and water contaminants.

Herbicides
Fungicides
Insecticides
Natural gas residues
Antimicrobials
Antibiotics
Hormones
Artificial flavourings
Artificial colourings
Texture modifiers
Packaging plasticizers

foods from responses to contaminants by means of elimination and challenge.

Chemicals, intentionally and unintentionally, can enter water and food chains at multiple levels: growing, processing, packaging and cooking, so that the final product may contain quite a large variety (Table 22b.1).

For naturally occurring toxins and carcinogens the reader is referred to an excellent review article by Ames.

Degree of contamination

It helps in presenting this material to classify foods into categories based on degree of contamination:

1 Organic foods ('biodynamic' in Australia).
2 Natural foods.
3 Junk foods.

Organic or biodynamic foods

By these, we refer to fruits, vegetables and grains grown without pesticides or fertilizers other than untreated manure. Cattle and sheep are grass-grazed and given no hormones, antibiotics or pesticided grains. Poultry are fed 'organic' grains, free of hormones, antibiotics, colourants or pesticides. Ocean fish might qualify as 'organic' whereas pond-fed trout, catfish, tilapia and cultured shrimp would not. The degree of chemical contamination of wild game depends on where they have fed. There are no chemicals added between picking or slaughtering and when the consumer purchases the groceries. We would include here chlorine-free and chemical-contaminant-free water, i.e. spring or distilled water bottled in glass as opposed to plastic containers.

Natural foods

By these are meant fruits, vegetables, grains, cattle, sheep, poultry, pigs and fish that are grown with the usual pesticides, hormones and antibiotics but suffer no further chemical processing or contamination before reaching the consumer.

Junk foods

These are grown with pesticides, hormones and antibiotics and then heavily processed (by smoking with nitrates, for example). The list of intentional additives is long (Table 22b.2).

They may have been packed in plastics that leach plasticizers into the foods, or in packages

Table 22b.2 Intentional food and water contaminants.

Preservatives	Humectants
Colourants	Leavening agents
Flavourings	Lubricating agents
Extenders	Neutralizers
Acidulants	Sweeteners
Aerators	Nutrient supplements
Bleaching agents	Oleoresins
Thickeners	Preservatives
Buffers	Propellants
Carriers	Sequestrants
Clarifiers	Solvents
Anticrystallization agents	Stabilizers
Curing agents	Vegetable gums
Conditioners	Washing agents
Emulsifiers	Waxes
Enzymes	Yeast foods

that contain leachable preservatives or pesticides. Banana crates, for example, are treated with thiobendazole which can contaminate the contents. Lead solder in cans has been shown to dissolve in foods; plastic or phenolic linings in cans may also present leaching problems.

To identify the particular offending agent for any one patient, given the enormous list of contaminants, could make even Sherlock Holmes quake.

Labelling

Inadequate labelling is a major problem for the hypersensitive patient and the physician. At the time of this writing, American drug companies are not required to list excipients, the so-called inert fillers in most drug preparations. The US Federal 'Standard of Identity' is a rule stating what is required and what may optionally be present in many prepared foods such as catsup, mayonnaise, ice cream, etc. Foods which meet the 'Standard of Identity' are not required to specify their ingredients on the label. The patient or physician must resort to the Federal Register to learn what might be in a prepared food, but to be certain about any particular product he would have to write to the manufacturer and even then there could be an uncertainty factor. If soya oil was cheap in a particular week, the mayonnaise might contain soya. Then again, if cottonseed oil was a bargain, it might be cottonseed. Labelling now often says 'vegetable oil (cottonseed or soya)' but one can never be certain which one is in any one jar.

Incomplete labelling

This presents another problem. The manufacturer of potato crisps (US: chips) puts 'potatoes, vegetable oil (soya or palm) and salt' on the label. The vegetable oil may have come in a container bearing the label 'soya oil and BHA (an antirancidity preservative)'. This preservative is carried into the potato crisps but the potato crisp producer calls his crisps 'all natural' because he did not add any preservatives intentionally.

Metabisulphite. The labelling problem goes further. The preservative and antibrowning (antioxidant) agent, metabisulphite, used on shrimp, fresh produce, wine and so on, is well established as a cause of life-threatening bronchospasm in sensitive individuals. There are as yet no laws requiring that restaurants using foods already containing this material or restaurants adding this material notify the consumer of its presence. Produce stores may spray it on their fruits and vegetables without announcing it to the shopper. (The US Food and Drug Administration is considering a ban on the use of sulphiting agents in foods.)

Pesticides, antibiotics and hormones

Information regarding the presence of specific pesticide residues derived from growing and preserving fruits, vegetables and grains and in animal feeds does not reach the consumer directly. Antibiotics and hormones in feed of cattle, poultry and cultivated fish are not announced to the purchaser of these products. The penicillin content of milk, which may be adequate to trigger allergic reactions in sensitive individuals, is not revealed on labels. In Puerto Rico excessive amounts of diethylstilboestrol (DES) introduced into chicken feed caused disastrous premature telarche and pubarche in infants and young children.

Preservatives in packaging materials are not labelled and can leach into the foods, so that recycled paper containing polychlorinated biphenyls is not permitted for use in food packaging (Federal Register) for example.

IDENTIFICATION OF THE ADDITIVE-SENSITIVE PATIENT

There are aspects of the patient's history that should alert the physician to the possibility of an additive/contaminant-sensitive patient.

Clinical history

On specific questioning patients will often re-

Table 22b.3 Chemical fumes.

Cigarette smoke
Perfumes
Car exhaust
Gasoline
Pesticides
Fresh newsprint
Household cleaning agents
Scented toilet tissue
Soap aisle of grocery stores
Tar
Fresh paint
Formaldehyde in clothing and fabric shops
Chlorine in indoor pools
'New building odour'
'New car odour'
Synthetic clothing and fabric finishes
Wood smoke
Toiletries
Natural gas

port multiple drug sensitivities or tolerance of only very small doses of analgesics, for example. They are likely to complain about dislike for or actual reactions to certain chemical fumes (see Table 22b.3). These people exhibit a preference for open windows and out-of-door activities. They would prefer an ocean vacation rather than a trip to Paris. They may report feeling ill more often after eating in restaurants. Specific questioning is sometimes required to elicit this information.

Early clinical signs

One of the first signs of onset of this disorder is the development of intolerance for alcohol. Tolerance for red wine and beer is lost first, and then white wine and distillates become a problem. Chemical sensitivity tends to include inhalants as well as ingestants and so specific questioning regarding the patient's adverse reactions to certain odours should lead the clinician to suspicion of sensitivity to chemicals in foods as well.

Symptoms alone do not provide many clues since there is not a unique symptom complex which is characteristic of food additive sensitivity. The presence of multisystem responses and a preponderance of central nervous system symptoms on review might tilt suspicions towards chemical sensitivity. Headache, fatigue, poor concentration and muscle weakness in addition to skin and respiratory symptoms may be present.

Chemical exposure

The chemically sensitive patient may report

onset of symptoms after an especially heavy chemical exposure such as being caught in a pesticide spraying, home fumigation, moving into a new mobile home with high formaldehyde levels, moving to work in a new airtight energy-efficient 'sick building' and so on. The highly susceptible patient may be sensitized to specific chemicals by such exposures to the degree that he remains ill and susceptible even after elimination of the initiating exposure. We further observe that one excessive exposure may trigger sensitivity to other even unrelated chemicals as if perhaps there had been a toxic effect on the immune system and/or overload of the enzyme detoxifying systems (see Chapter 42).

We are now cognizant of a number of predisposing factors in individual susceptibility to chemical sensitivity but a discussion of these is beyond the scope of this chapter.

DETECTING REACTIONS TO CHEMICALS IN FOODS

Whether a reaction is caused by toxic, allergic or other mechanisms, when the physician suspects a chemical contaminant in the diet as the offending agent the only practical approach is to begin with dietary manipulation.

Finding and preparing chemically less contaminated foods is the most desirable alternative to challenging the patient with an enormous number of individual additives for two reasons. Firstly, from a practical point of view, labelling in grocery stores and restaurants is inadequate, and, secondly, most patients have multiple sensitivities.

It is most logical to begin with a diet of less allergenic foods in less chemically contaminated forms. Ideally one would construct a diet of organically grown foods and exclude those most suspected as allergenic offenders. (See Appendices 22b.1–7 for diet and patient instructions.)

Handling

If the foods are wrapped in plastic, they should be permitted to stand for 24 hours following removal from the plastic and then be stored in glass containers. Cooking should be done in glass, stainless steel or porcelain-coated pots.

Cooking and drinking water should be charcoal-filtered, spring water stored in glass, or water that has been boiled and cooled to room temperature before using. Triple distilled water may also be used.

Dietary elimination and challenge

The patient should maintain the elimination diet for 6 days. At that juncture one new organic food may be added each day at lunch and the same food repeated at dinner. If no reaction has occurred by noon the next day, the food introduced the previous day may be presumed 'safe'. If a reaction occurs, no new foods should be introduced until symptoms subside. When the patient has enough variety of 'safe' organic foods, he may then try fresh fruits, vegetables, meat, poultry and fish and unmixed grains that are grown with pesticides and chemical fertilizers. It may take a 4-day accumulated exposure before the most subtle reactions occur to the traces of organophosphates and halogenated hydrocarbon pesticides, hormones and antibiotics.

Junk foods. If there are no untoward effects from natural foods, the patient may then want to try junk foods like lunch meats, canned soups, sodas, baked goods, breakfast cereals, powdered drinks, salad dressing mixes, airplane food, flavoured and coloured medications and so on. Many of these items have multiple additives. By noting which foods cause reactions and what the additives are, one may eventually be able to isolate a particular offender. Quite often, the chemically sensitive patients will react to multiple additives so the isolation of particular offenders becomes futile and the patients do best with organic or natural foods.

The patient must also test his tap water as a separate item and he may also want to test food stored for 24 hours or more in plastic containers.

Abstinence from exposure to these items for approximately a 2-year period will usually allow the patient some latitude to break the diet for travel and special occasions.

One might speculate that participation in a medically supervised 'detoxification' programme like the one devised for the victims of the kepone spill accident in the 1970s would decrease the level of fat-soluble accumulated chemicals thus allowing occasional exposures which would not precipitate reactions be they toxic or allergic.

CONCLUSION

The importance of adverse effects of additives to the public health cannot be accurately deduced from available evidence. The incidence of such adverse effects would be grossly underestimated if calculated from reports in the medical literature, since few practitioners are aware of the value of making such a diagnosis to the wellbeing of their patients. The authors hope that this exposition will increase awareness of the nature and occurrence of contaminants, thereby facilitating diagnosis.

It is unfortunate that quantitative information regarding doses of additives consumed by a patient is usually totally lacking. A particular additive may occur at unknown concentration in each of several commonly eaten foods, resulting in a higher total dose than would be predicted from the average intake of any one food.

It is extraordinarily difficult to assess the magnitude of sensitivity to additives and residues because so often both physician and patient are unaware of the presence of miniscule amounts of contaminants to which they might attribute symptoms. The same contaminant, for example a common halogenated hydrocarbon pesticide like heptachlor, might be found in pineapples, in the milk of cattle fed on pineapple leaves and in the aquifers filled by run-off water from the heptachlor-treated pineapple fields. The patient who reacts to pineapple, milk and water could certainly present a confusing picture. To add to the difficulty of assessing the extent of these sensitivities is the cumulative nature of some of these reactions. This effect may be compounded further when several different, chemically related additives are being consumed.

A diversity of potential mechanisms of reaction may operate in any given patient. They include allergic, enzymatic, pharmacological, toxic and psychological responses. The relative importance of biochemical and immunological mechanisms in adverse reactions to food additives is worthy of investigation. If an important role could be demonstrated for impaired detoxification capacity due to enzymatic defects (whether genetic or nutritional in origin), diagnosis and therapy would be facilitated (see Chapter 24).

RECOMMENDED READINGS AND RESOURCES FOR PATIENTS

Ames B: Dietary carcinogens and anticarcinogens. Science 1983; 24: 1256–64.

Considine D, Considine GD: Foods and food production encyclopedia. New York and London: Van Nostrand Reinhold, 1982.

Golos N: Coping with your allergies. New York: Simon and Schuster, 1979.

Hunter BT: The great nutrition robbery. New York: Charles Scribner's Sons, 1978.

Hunter BT: Additives book. New Canaan, CT: Keats Publishing, 1980.

Lipske M: Chemical additives in booze. Washington, DC: Center for Science in the Public Interest, 1982.

Ministry of Agriculture, Fisheries and Food: Look at the label. England: Colibri Press, 1982.

Mott L: Pesticides in food: what the public needs to know. San Francisco, CA: Natural Resources Defense Council, 1984.

Office of the Federal Register, Code of Federal Regulations: Food and Drugs, 21, Parts 1–499. Washington, DC: National Archives and Records, 1984.

Randolph T, Moss R: An alternative approach to allergies. New York: Lippincott and Crowell, 1986.

US Department of Health and Human Services: FDA consumer. Rockville, Maryland: Public Health Service, Food and Drug Administration, ongoing publications.

Weir D, Schapiro M: Circle of poison. San Francisco, CA: Institute for Food and Development Policy, 1978.

APPENDICES

Appendix 22b.1 Some processing contaminants.

1 *Natural gas residues* from roasting and baking
Coffee and chocolate beans
Baked goods
Roasted and broiled meats

2 *Solvents* (chlorinated hydrocarbons)
Decaffeination of coffee
Extracting agents for oils, fats, waxes—from seeds, grains

3 *Fumigants*
Tea, spices, herbs, grains, fruits, chocolate, coffee beans, imported nuts

4 *Lubricants*
Releasing agents for hard candies, baked goods

5 *Additives in alcoholic beverages*
Asbestos, clay, seaweed, polyvinylpyrrolidine, citric, tannic, fumaric acids, potassium sorbate, sulphurs-bisulphite, captan, and arsenic for filtering wine
EDTA, glycerin, peptones, alginate, vitamin C, sulphites, flavours, colours, preservatives, monosodium glutamate for beer and liquors

Appendix 22b.2 Processing chemicals that remain in foods (a partial list).

1 *Cosmetic oils or petroleum-derived waxes*
Cucumbers, peppers, apples (not water-soluble and do not wash off)

2 *Ethylene gas*
Bananas and Florida oranges for ripening and colour development (breakdown products remain in fruit)

3 *Dyes*
Oranges, pistachios

4 *Spoilage retardants*
Eggs and chickens dipped in phenol or penicillin to retard spoilage

5 *Bleaches*
Sulphur dioxide, chlorine in sugar, flour, fats, oils, cheeses

Appendix 22b.3 Chemical contaminants from cooking.

1 *Teflon*
Breakdown products include fluorides

2 *Metals*
Iron—cast iron pots
Lead—glazes on pottery
Aluminium—pots, foils

3 *Plasticizers*
Plastic storage containers and plastic cookware for microwave ovens

4 *Residues of natural gas*

5 *Oven cleaner residues*

6 *Acrolein*
And other products of toasting, burning, broiling and frying at high temperatures (nitrosamines, for example)

Appendix 22b.4 Water contaminants.

1 *Chlorine*
Combines with methane from decomposition of organic matter to form chloroform, carcinogen

2 *Pesticides*
From agricultural run-off

3 *Industrial pollutants*
Sulphites from paper industry, organic mercurial compounds in the Great Lakes, trichloroethylene in Silicon Valley wells

4 *Plasticizers*
Polyvinylchlorides from plastic pipes in homes
NB Spring water may be delivered to bottling plants in plastic-lined trucks or in plastic bottles to the consumer
Distilled water may be contaminated by volatile chemicals

Appendix 22b.5 Hidden ingredients in drugs.

1 *Colours*
Coal-tar derivatives like tartrazine

2 *Glazes*
Plastics, petroleum-derived waxes

3 *Humectants*
In soft gelatin capsules

4 *Flavouring, sweeteners, solvents* (alcohol, propylene-glycol)
In syrups

5 *Inks*
Identifying marks on tablets and capsules

6 *Preservatives*
Benzyl alcohol, phenol, thimerosal, benzalkonium chloride, metabisulphite for injectables
NB Epinephrine (adrenaline) is preserved with the antioxidant metabisulphite

7 *Plasticizers*
In flexible intravenous bags and tubing

8 *Ethylene oxide*
In plasma from sterilization of disposable bags

NB Multidose vials are required by law to contain a bacteriostatic agent. Single dose vials may be free of these agents
There are paraben-free dental analgesics available

Appendix 22b.6   The basic organic menu.

All of the sources mentioned below should be organic (free of pesticides).

Protein
    Lamb, turkey

Grains
    Barley, rice, rye

Fruits
    Apricots, peaches, pears, cranberries

Vegetables
    Artichokes, avocados, beets (beetroot), carrots, chard, okra, sweet potatoes, yams, broccoli, lettuce

Oils
    Olive oil, safflower oil

Condiments
    Sea salt

Dessert
    Pudding—made from tapioca beads or agar agar flakes

Beverages
    Safe water (see Appendices 22b.4 and 22b.7) Organic juice from any of the above-mentioned fruits

---

Basic organic elimination diet instructions

1 Begin your investigation by eating only the foods listed on your menu for 5 days. Keep a diary of your entire experience, listing the date, time, food eaten and how you feel. You will need to plan to shop ahead, having plenty of appropriate foods on hand. You may get bored, but you won't go hungry. There is no restriction on calorie intake unless you intentionally wish to lose weight.

2 You'll notice that the menu is quite simple, without spices, butter or condiments. So don't start at Christmas or during the holiday season or around birthday parties.

3 By eliminating questionable variables, your observation will be much more accurate. Use as many organic food sources as possible; unsprayed is the next best choice. You will be provided with a list of places to shop.

4 Drink, cook and wash your food with only a safe source of water, which is obviously not tap water. See Appendix 22b.7 for advice on what is 'safe water'.

5 Use pots and pans that do not contain aluminium, Teflon or silverstone interiors. These are 'little toxic additions' that can confuse a possible food reaction with a chemical reaction.

6 Avoid sources of chemicals in the following:

chewing gum	over-the-counter medications (unless you really need them)
breath mints	coffee
mouth wash	tea
cigarettes	diet drinks

7 Remember that most food allergies are 'masked' or 'hidden' and only become obvious when you take out the commonly eaten food allergens for a period and reintroduce them. If this is the case for you, then you may notice a period of withdrawal on the first through third days of beginning your menu. Lots of rest, vitamin C, alkali salts and water will help to minimize this experience. You may also notice that some of your symptoms start to clear and you should be free of food reactions by the fifth or sixth day. Keep track of these experiences in your diet diary.

8 Follow the instructions on the allergic foods sheet as to which foods are added in the first week. Eat a large serving of the food at lunch with other foods on your menu, and again at dinner, if you don't react at lunch.

9 Wait until the next morning to see if there's a delayed reaction upon waking. If nothing has happened, then consider the food now part of your menu and continue to eat it as desired.

10 If you do clearly react to the food at lunch, then do not eat it again at dinner; try to clear the reaction right away by using the alkali salts. If you are clear by noon the next day, you may go on to add another food.

11 If you have a severe reaction, then taking unflavoured milk of magnesia (2–4 tablespoons) or the alkali salts (1–2 teaspoons) will help you to eliminate the food as soon as possible. (You could react for up to 4 days if you don't do this.) Use your antiallergy or antiasthma medications if necessary.

12 Weigh yourself every morning after emptying your bladder and before eating. Failure to drop a pound or two overnight indicates that the food you introduced yesterday may be an allergen and cause fluid retention.

13 The symptoms that you may experience can be any one of the items you checked on your symptom check list when you first came to see the doctor.

14 Focus on adding back the major food groups—proteins, grains, legumes, milk products, vegetables and fruits—as opposed to chocolate, sugar and alcohol in the beginning. Use only single ingredient foods (wheat as opposed to bread) and wait to add spices until you are done with this entire investigation. Once you eat a meal that you know you don't react to, you can always season it with a spice and observe whether or not you react.

15 Vitamins from sources that are hypoallergenic, not containing milk products, yeast, corn, wheat or soya may be taken through the entire investigational period.

16 When you have completed your investigation you will be asked to challenge your 'safe' foods from the regular grocery store. This will determine whether or not your diet needs to remain organic.

17 To handle social eating situations: eat your own meal before joining others; bring your own food; invite them to your home for a meal.

Allergenic foods★

1: Often cause allergies	2: Sometimes cause allergies	3: Seldom cause allergies
Alcoholic beverages	Apples	Apricots
Beans	Avocados	Artichokes
Berries	Bananas	Asparagus
Buckwheat	Beef (beef gelatin)	Barley
Chocolate	Beets (beetroot)	Broccoli
Cola products	Cabbage	Carrots
Coconut	Cauliflower	Chard
Corn	Celery	Cranberries
Egg	Cherries	Grapes
Fish—all types including crab, lobster,	Chicken	Honey
shrimp and soft fish	Coffee	Lamb
Milk products	Cottonseed	Lettuce
Mustard	Cucumber	Oats
Nuts—oil and extract	Garlic	Peaches
Oranges and other citrus fruits	Green and red peppers	Pears
Peanut and peanut butter	Mangos	Poi (taro root from Hawaii)
Peas	Melons	Raisins
Pineapple	Mint	Rice
Pork (pork gelatin)	Mushrooms	Rye
Soya bean products	Onion	Sugar (maple, sorghum, beet)
Sugars (cane, corn, molasses)	Plums	Sweet potatoes
Tomato products	Prunes	Tapioca
Vinegar	Safflower	Tea
Wheat	Sesame	
Wine	Spinach	
Yeasts	Squash	
	String beans	
	Turkey	
	Yams	

Begin by adding back one food a day on the sixth day of your programme. Focus on the foods that were common in your diet or the ones that fall in column 1. For the seriously allergic, some caution may need to be used in how to add back foods. This will be discussed before you begin.

There are several lists of allergenic foods available. One person's body will react differently from another's; there are always exceptions in the field of allergy.

★ Modified from Rapp D: Allergies and your family. New York: Sterling Publishing, 1982.

Appendix 22b.7 Water information.

The offending elements in water are most often:
Chlorine
Pesticides and other organic chemicals
Minerals (fluoride, sulphur, copper, aluminium, lead etc.)
Particulate (asbestos, etc.)
Organisms (bacteria, parasites, viruses).
To minimize these elements the following alternatives to 'tap water' are available:

Spring or bottled water
You can reasonably expect glass- or ceramic-bottled spring waters to be free of chlorine only. The source of origin will determine whether they are pesticide-free and which minerals are present. Trace minerals are essential to normal metabolism; however, excesses may be harmful. Some people demonstrate sensitivity to certain minerals even in small amounts. You will have to experiment to determine your sensitivities. The company should be able to provide you with a quantitative analysis of organic and inorganic residues.

Bottled water should come in glass or ceramic containers, not plastic or resin. Plastic containers leach out components of plastic into the water, therefore you are simply trading one poison for another. Ensure that the water was not shipped to your area in a plastic-lined tank truck or that chlorine residues from sterilization of containers are not present. Be aware that popular bottled brands can contain offending substances (Perrier has many natural phenols; Calistoga and Calso are mineral laden).

Well water
Well water may be contaminated by agricultural or other run-off and cannot be assumed safe. Test for yourself as you would test for food and other exposures. A professional analysis for organic and inorganic contamination is strongly advised.

Distilled water
Professionally triple-distilled water should be free of chlorine, pesticides and *all* minerals. It will not provide essential trace elements which cannot be totally replaced by mineral supplementation. Again, it should be purchased in glass or ceramic containers. The problems with distilled water are inadequate distillation:

1 It must be triple distilled.
2 The first batch must be discarded.
3 The still must be thoroughly cleansed between uses because of the non-volatile residues left behind.

Boiled water

Bringing the water to a boil, boiling uncovered for 10 minutes and allowing it to cool until no more steam comes off removes some of the chlorine and volatile pesticides only. It is satisfactory to start water testing or for use in emergencies when better water is not available. (It is better than tap water.)

Filtered water

Before purchasing a water filter the following questions should be considered:

1 *What type of filter do I need?*

Basically, there are three means of purifying water by filtration: mechanical, activated charcoal and reverse osmosis.

(a) Mechanical filtering will remove only particulate matter, the minimum size depending on the filter medium. Along with this method is the danger of introducing a contaminant from the filter medium.

(b) Activated charcoal will remove chlorine and pesticides adequately for most people. It will not remove all of the minerals or fluoride. Charcoal filtration depends on the following variables: surface area of charcoal granule, time of contact with charcoal (flow rate, geometry of bed, etc.) and type of charcoal (mainly due to possible residues introduced into the water). There are two methods of charcoal packing. The water can be passed through a loose bed of charcoal gravel, or through a porous core of solid charcoal. The core method is more expensive to manufacture but has a smaller volume for the same surface area. This type of filtration is also subject to the growth of bacteria and mould in the bed. This problem is reduced by several methods: back flushing with hot water, silver impregnation of charcoal (not recommended due to possibly leaving a silver residue in water), replacement of bed more often and thorough regular cleaning of the unit.

(c) Reverse osmosis filtration works by way of diffusion across a membrane. The membrane allows water molecules to migrate through the membrane but prevents passage of contamination. For this process to work the 'dirty' side of the membrane must be constantly flushed with new water. Reverse osmosis is only for very sensitive people. It removes essentially all organics and fluoride. The inherent drawbacks to this system are in the limited quantity of water it will produce (up to 5 gallons/day), the wasted water used (up to 10 gallons for every gallon produced) and the need to store the water continuously. Possible contamination can occur from the membrane itself or in some units from the polychloroprene bladder used in conjunction with the storage system and reverse osmosis units do not work well on chlorine; therefore, we recommend the use of a charcoal filter at the outlet of the reverse osmosis.

2 *How much of my water supply do I need to filter?*

Several systems are available. You may choose to filter all of your water supply. This will require a large filter at the inlet to your house (before the hot water heater as charcoal filtration does not handle hot water efficiently). Or you may choose to filter only your cooking and drinking water with a filter installed in your kitchen. There is also an option for filtering your shower water alone. We advise patients to at least filter cooking and drinking water. For the person who is extremely sensitive to chlorine fumes, filtration of the entire house may be necessary.

3 *What installation best meets my needs?*

If you are renting or planning to move in the near future, you may wish to purchase a self-contained unit. These units require much less installation and usually consist of a device that sits on your counter top. An under-the-counter permanent installation can be much more practical for people who own their home. These filters usually have a third tap (faucet) mounted on the sink board. For people who travel a lot there are small portable units available that can be packed in your luggage.

4 *What materials should the water filter be made from?*

Water filters are constructed of many materials but predominantly from plastic, fibreglass or metal. We recommend you purchase one with a stainless housing and outlet hardware. A plastic inlet line is adequate in that the water passes through the filter element afterwards. All parts and lines should be well cleaned before use with approved cleaning solutions. Make sure the final drinking water is not in contact with plastic containers or tubing.

5 *Do I want to buy or rent my filter?*

Several companies will rent their filters. This option reduces the initial outlay of money and provides for maintenance, but it may cost considerably more in the long run.

Testing

Samples of different waters should be tested just like foods in a rotary diet until a safe one is found. Safe water should be used for drinking, cooking and brushing teeth. For the more sensitive person, safe water should be used for washing food. For the extremely sensitive person, safe water should be used for bathing. Prior to testing you need to be off 'tap water' for 3 weeks. The challenge process then consists of 3 hours of abstinence from drinking and eating, followed by drinking two full glasses of the water you wish to challenge, followed by a 3 hour wait to see if any symptoms develop.

Chapter 23
Pharmacological Actions of Foods

Ronald Finn

Introduction

Pharmacological reactions to foods can cause symptoms of food intolerance similar to those produced by true food allergy. Moreover, the resolution of symptoms on an exclusion diet does not distinguish between food allergy and a pharmacological reaction. True food allergy can only be diagnosed when associated with typical allergic phenomena or with laboratory evidence of an immunological reaction. In contrast to allergic reactions, pharmacological reactions are more likely to be dose dependent, and usually occur when large quantities of the affected food are taken.

COMPOUNDS THAT CAN CAUSE ADVERSE REACTIONS

Caffeine

The most important cause of pharmacological symptoms is excessive caffeine consumption. Caffeine is the most widely used cerebral stimulant drug in the world, and is widely distributed in 63 species of plant. For many centuries, man searched for stimulant drugs and originally found caffeine in the coffee bean in Arabia (Fig. 23.1), the tea leaf in China, the kola nut in West Africa, the cocoa bean in Mexico and the christmas berry tree in North America. Caffeine is a methyl xanthine and is mainly taken as tea (50–80 mg per cup), coffee (40–150 mg per cup) and to a lesser extent in coca cola. It is addictive and has widespread

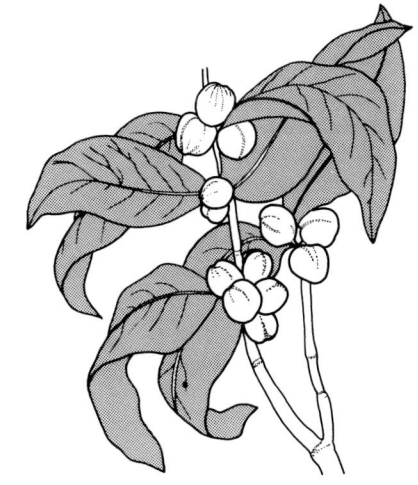

Fig. 23.1 Beans growing on a coffee plant.

pharmacological actions including stimulation of the central nervous system, cardiac muscle and gastric secretion. Because of these varied actions, a wide range of clinical symptoms can be produced. It should, however, be pointed out that coffee contains about 300 organic substances, and hence any clinical symptoms due to drinking large quantities of coffee are not necessarily always due to caffeine.

When originally introduced to the Western world as coffee or tea, it was considered an intoxicating drink that was dangerous to health. Many attempts were made to suppress it but it has become over the years a socially acceptable beverage. Caffeine has similar pharmacological effects to amphetamines which are banned in competitive sport. Caffeine itself was banned for use in athletic competition in Italy in the 1960s, but it was removed from the list of restricted drugs by the International Olympic Committee before the 1972 Olympic Games. It should be emphasized that, taken in moderate quantities, caffeine is an innocuous stimulant, but problems arise when it is taken in excessive amounts. There is also a clinical suspicion that certain individuals are particularly sensitive to the effects of large quantities of caffeine.

Chronic anxiety state. Large quantities of coffee and tea can produce a clinical picture indistinguishable from a chronic anxiety state [13], with anxiety, mood changes, weight loss, palpitations, tremor and sweating. Insomnia and changes of sleep pattern are frequently concomitant and may occur on their own. The anxiety state may be accompanied by a chronic hyperventilation syndrome with difficulty in breathing, muscle and chest pains, tingling in the extremities which can be unilateral, dizziness and syncopal attacks. In patients with any of these manifestations, the daily intake of coffee, tea and coca cola should be ascertained, and if in excess of eight cups, a gradual withdrawal should be advised, and this will often produce a major clinical improvement.

It is possible that the so-called 'total allergy syndrome' (Table 23.1) is due to the simultaneous occurrence in the same subject of the symptoms of allergy and of hyperventilation.

Table 23.1 Total allergy syndrome.

Allergy	Hyperventilation
Eczema	Breathlessness
Joint pains	Chest pains
Rhinitis	Dizziness
Urticaria	Headache
Wheezing	Fatigue
	Palpitations
	Paraesthesiae
	Syncope

Caffeine probably binds to receptor sites in the brain normally reserved for adenosine, thus blocking the action of adenosine [11, 12, 21]. Adenosine given to rats has a quietening effect which is reversed by giving caffeine. In rats given caffeine over a period of time, the number of adenosine receptors increases to compensate. If caffeine is then suddenly withdrawn, the excessive number of free adenosine receptors makes the animal very sensitive to adenosine. This may produce severe headache due to cerebral vasodilation as adenosine is a potent vasodilator. Withdrawal of caffeine should therefore be gradual.

Insomnia. As little as two cups of coffee can disturb the EEG sleep pattern, and hence caffeine is a potent cause of insomnia, and caffeine consumption, particularly in the evening, should always be assessed in patients presenting with this complaint.

Palpitations. Palpitations can be part of an anxiety state or can occur independently as a primary complaint. Extrasystoles and even paroxysmal tachycardia can occur, and can be mistaken for primary cardiac disease [10]. Sudden alteration of rhythm can produce unsteadiness and faintness. Patients with coronary artery disease, particularly following a myocardial infarction, should be advised to avoid excessive caffeine consumption, because the induction of extrasystoles could precipitate a fatal arrhythmia in an ischaemic and hence irritable myocardium.

Headache. Excessive coffee and tea consumption is a common cause of headache and will precipitate classical migraine in predisposed subjects. Headache due to caffeine often occurs at weekends, and is due to a sharp reduction of caffeine consumption at the weekend, compared with that taken during the week [13]. Such caffeine withdrawal headaches are responsible for so-called 'weekend migraine'. Physical dependency or addiction is common with caffeine and sudden withdrawal leads to a group of symptoms including headache, which can be very severe, and irritability, lassitude and occasional nausea. It is therefore important to advise patients who take large quantities of coffee and tea to slowly reduce the quantity over a few weeks.

Gastrointestinal tract. Caffeine stimulates gastric acid secretion but coffee, including decaffeinated coffee, is a stronger simulant of acid secretion than caffeine [4]. The non-caffeine acid stimulants in coffee have not been identified. Excess coffee consumption should therefore be discouraged in patients with peptic ulcers, but there is no evidence that excessive caffeine consumption can cause ulcers in man, although prolonged stimulation by caffeine, administered in beeswax, provoked the development of gastric ulcers in cats and guinea-pigs [20]. Excessive tea consumption can produce recurrent vomiting, which is often projectile, and may be due to an underlying gastritis. Excess caffeine consumption should always be looked for in patients with unexplained vomiting, as caffeine withdrawal is often beneficial [10].

Caffeine may reduce lower oesophageal sphincter pressure and so exacerbate oesophagitis [6], but the evidence is conflicting, and there is a suggestion that coffee and caffeine have different effects. Thus coffee may exacerbate the symptoms of oesophageal reflux and oesophagitis.

Caffeine stimulates small intestinal water secretion [22] but the effects of caffeine may again be dissimilar to caffeine-containing compounds such as coffee, since coffee does not influence salt and water transport when infused into the jejunum.

Thus it will be seen that the effects of caffeine and caffeine-containing compounds on the gastrointestinal tract are not clear-cut, but a clinical trial of caffeine withdrawal is always worth considering in patients with abdominal symptoms which have not responded to standard treatments. Unexplained projectile vomiting will often respond to tea withdrawal, but other symptoms such as heartburn, abdominal pain and diarrhoea may also improve.

Restless legs. This syndrome was originally described by Thomas Willis in 1685 [23]. Willis is, of course, better known for his identification of the circle of Willis at the base of the brain. He wrote that 'wherefore to some, when being in bed, they betake themselves to sleep, presently in the arms and legs, leapings and contraction of the tendons, and so great a restlessness and tossings of their members ensue, that the diseased are no more able to sleep, than if they were in a place of the greatest torture.'

This syndrome was studied in detail by Ekbom [8], and is often known as Ekbom's syndrome. It is of interest that coffee first entered Europe via Venice in 1615, and by 1685, when Willis first described the syndrome of restless legs, coffee had spread widely throughout Europe.

The main symptom is an unpleasant creeping sensation in the lower legs between knee and ankle. It can also occur in the shoulder girdles and the arms. The discomfort occurs at rest and produces an irresistible need to move the limbs. It mainly occurs in the evening and at night, and the patient has to get up and walk about to relieve his discomfort; this may cause severe insomnia.

Treatment. On the basis of therapeutic experience with 62 patients over an 11-year period, Lutz [16] concluded that caffeine is a major factor in this syndrome. Many patients had symptoms of anxiety and depression which may also be due to excess caffeine consumption. Lutz suggests that caffeine is responsible for the increased nervous system arousal responsible for the toxic sensory experience of restless legs. Treatment consisted of the withdrawal of caffeine and other xanthines such as coffee, tea, cola, cocoa and chocolate, as well as analgesic preparations containing caffeine which are often taken by these patients, but which only exacerbate the symptoms. Diazepam can be used on a temporary basis. All patients are advised to withdraw the offending substance slowly to minimize withdrawal reactions. Providing patient compliance is obtained, Lutz claims a high success rate in the treatment of this otherwise intractable condition.

Tannic acid and anaemia

Tannic acid in tea forms a complex with iron rendering it unavailable for absorption [1]. The effect of tea as an inhibitor of iron absorption is specific for non-haem iron. The inhibition in one study varied from 41% to 95%. It has been suggested that tea could be used to decrease iron absorption from the gut in thalassaemia, as chronic iron overload is a major complication in this condition. Large quantities of tea can likewise inhibit iron absorption in normal subjects, and particularly when combined with a poor diet is a major cause of anaemia and general ill-health. This situation is not uncommon in middle-aged females who consume large quantities of tea. Withdrawal of tea in these subjects usually leads to an improvement in the anaemia.

Vasoactive amines

Vasoactive amines are contained in a variety of foods including cheese (tyramine and histamine), chocolate (phenylethylamine) and citrus fruits (octopamine and phenylephrine (synephrine)). They act directly on blood vessels or indirectly by liberating adrenaline and noradrenaline from nerve endings. They can precipitate headache in predisposed subjects and a trial [14] indicated that 125 mg of tyramine produced headache in 80 of 100 predisposed subjects, whereas placebo lactose tablets only produced headache in 6 of 66 similar subjects. The trial was double-blind in that neither subject nor observer knew whether the tablet was tyramine or the lactose placebo. Many patients are aware that these foods, particularly chocolate and cheese, precipitate migraine attacks, and are much improved when they are avoided.

NON-IMMUNOLOGICAL RELEASE OF VASOACTIVE AMINES (FALSE FOOD ALLERGY)

In this condition [17] symptoms are clinically indistinguishable from those found in true food allergy, but the histamine and other vaso-active amines are released by mechanisms other than antibodies. It is probably far more common than true food allergy.

Symptoms can also be caused by excessive consumption of foods which contain large quantities of histamine or other vasoactive amines (Table 23.2), or by foods which act as

Table 23.2 Foods rich in histamine (μg/g).

Fermented cheeses	up to 1330
Fermented drinks (wine)	20
Fermented foods	
Sauerkraut	160 mg/kg
	(a portion of 250 g = 40 mg)
Dry pork and beef sausage	225
Pig's liver	25
Tinned tuna	20
Tinned anchovy fillets	33
Tinned smoked herring's eggs	350
Tinned foods	from 10 to 350
Meats	10
Vegetables	traces
Tomato	22
Spinach	37.5
Deep-frozen fish	1
Fish, fresh shellfish	0.2
Fish	
Tuna	5.4
Sardine	15.8
Salmon	7.35
Anchovy fillets	44

Data taken from Quevauviller et al [18].

histamine releasers (Table 23.3). Increased intestinal permeability, and an abnormal tendency to release histamine or react to histamine, are contributory factors. It is therefore common in atopic subjects. Thus, eczema, where there are large numbers of mast cells in the skin, is often exacerbated by such foods, but it should be stressed that this is not a true allergic phenomenon.

Symptoms can include chronic urticaria, recurrent vasomotor headaches, facial flushing

Table 23.3 Histamine releasing foods.

Egg white
Shell fish
Strawberries
Tomatoes
Chocolate
Fish
Pineapple
Alcohol

and intestinal problems such as abdominal pain and recurrent diarrhoea. In contrast to true food allergy, in which symptoms are precipitated by even minute quantities of the allergenic food, large quantities of the offending food have to be taken, and immunological tests such as RASTS (radioallergosorbent tests) are uniformly negative.

Management comprises taking a dietary history to identify amine-releasing or -containing foods (see Tables 23.2 and 23.3) and advising a major reduction in their intake. Total avoidance is not necessary.

Starch-containing foods. These foods taken in excess increase the intestinal flora leading to excessive fermentation. The bacteria produce histamine which is irritant to the gut mucosa, and can be absorbed leading to symptoms. This is probably the explanation of what used to be called carbohydrate dyspepsia.

Alcohol. Reaction to excessive amounts of alcohol is common. Consumption of ethanol can result in release of histamine, and there is also a high concentration of histamine in certain wines. Aldehyde dehydrogenase is deficient in 50% of Japanese who are therefore intolerant to alcohol [15].

Scombroid fish poisoning. Histidine is converted to histamine in certain stored foods. This occurs particularly in scombroid fish such as mackerel in which histamine levels can reach 100 mg per 100 g, if the fish are not stored properly at 0°C. Symptoms of scombroid fish poisoning include headache, flushing, urticaria, thirst, abdominal pain and vomiting, and are due to histamine toxicity.

Tyramine reaction. Tyramine is produced by decarboxylation from tyrosine and is found in high concentrations in fermented cheeses. Tyramine releases noradrenaline from tissue stores and causes a rise in blood pressure. Tyramine is normally destroyed by monoamine oxidases but this does not occur in patients with depression when treated with monoamine oxidase inhibitors. If such patients take large quantities of cheese, the blood pressure may rise to dangerous levels leading to headache, nausea, dizziness and even cerebral haemorrhage. Tyramine is also found in chocolate, yeast extract, liver, sausages, broad beans and pickled herrings, and these foods should be avoided by patients treated with monoamine oxidase inhibitors for depression.

Monosodium glutamate

Monosodium glutamate is often used in Chinese cooking as a flavour-enhancing agent, and may produce the Chinese restaurant (Kwok's) syndrome. The symptoms include tightness, pain and tingling in the front of the chest, radiating to the arms, often associated with palpitations and faintness. The mechanism is uncertain and the condition has to be distinguished from myocardial infarction.

Additives

Food additives are used as preservatives, colouring agents and to provide odour, taste and texture. They include colouring agents such as tartrazine and erythrosin, preservatives such as benzoates and sulphur dioxide, and antioxidants such as butylated hydroxytoluene. Sodium nitrite is an antioxidant which reacts with myoglobin to form the pink colour of cooked pork meats and is responsible for many so-called allergic reactions to pork.

It has been estimated that 0.1% of the population react to additives [5], the clinical reactions including urticaria, asthma, rhinitis, angioedema, headache and irritable bowel syndrome. Nasal polyps and asthma can be associated with sensitivity to acetylsalicylic acid. Feingold [9] has suggested that hyperactive children are often sensitive to colouring agents and salicylates but this view is not entirely accepted, although it does seem to be of clinical importance in some cases. Rapp [19] has reported similar results, and a trial of the Feingold diet (Table 23.4) is worth trying in hyperactive children. Recent data (see Chapter

38) have shown that hyperactivity can be associated with sensitivity to colours, preservatives and many foods.

The untoward action of additives is not understood, although it is considered that most reactions are pharmacological rather than immunological. Thus although tartrazine can act as a hapten, this is not thought to be clinically relevant. Asthma due to acetylsalicylic acid or tartrazine may be due to inhibition of prostaglandin E_2 which usually acts as a bronchodilator. Patients with aspirin-sensitive asthma can also be sensitive to non-steroid anti-inflammatory drugs which also inhibit prostaglandin synthesis. Colouring agents such as erythrosin alter the membrane permeability of neurones, and animal experiments indicate that it facilitates the release of neurotransmitters at the neuromuscular junction [3]. This action could possibly be related to behaviour disorders in man. Butylated hydroxytoluene also provokes behaviour disorders in animals.

Additives, and particularly colouring agents, are a common cause of urticaria, and patients with this condition often respond to an additive-free diet. Such a diet is always worth trying in patients with other intractable problems such as asthma, rhinitis, behaviour disturbances and irritable bowel syndrome.

Exorphins

Peptides derived from gluten can be detected in brain tissue and could act as exorphins [24]. Claims have been made that wheat and rye may predispose to schizophrenia [7], but these suggestions have not been confirmed. High-carbohydrate, low-protein meals elevate brain tryptophan, which accelerates the synthesis of the neurotransmitter serotonin, which is associated with an increase in fatigue [2].

The possibility therefore exists that certain small food molecules may cross the blood-brain barrier and, by influencing cerebral neurotransmitters, cause a change in brain function, but at the present time there is no firm scientific evidence to confirm that diet is a major cause of psychiatric disease.

Table 23.4 Modified Feingold diet.

Avoid:
Fruits: Almonds, apples, apricots, blackberries, gooseberries, raspberries, strawberries, cherries, currants, grapes and products such as wine, nectarines, oranges, peaches, plums, prunes
Vegetables: Tomatoes and tomato products, cucumbers, green peppers
Artificial colours: Avoid all artificially coloured foods
Keep to natural foods

REFERENCES

1 Alarcon PA, Donovan ME, Forbes GB et al: Iron absorption in the thalassemia syndrome and its inhibition by tea. N Engl J Med 1979; 300:5-8.

2 Anderson GM: Diet neurotransmitters and brain function. Br Med Bull 1981; 37:95-100.

3 Augustine JR, Levitan H: Neurotransmitter release from a vertebrate neuromuscular synapse affected by a food dye. Science 1980; 207:1489-90.

4 Cohen S, Booth GH: Gastric acid secretion and lower oesophageal pressure in response to coffee and caffeine. N Eng J Med 1975; 293:897-9.

5 Commission of the European Communities: Report of a working group on adverse reactions to ingested additives, 111, 556-81-EN. Brussels: Commission of the European Communities, 1981.

6 Dennish GW, Castell DO: Caffeine and the lower oesophageal spincter. Am J Dig Dis 1972; 17:993-6.

7 Dohan FC: Cereals and schizophrenia: data and hypothesis. Acta Psychiatr Scand 1966: 42:125-52.

8 Ekbom KA: Restless legs. Acta Med Scand [Suppl] 1945; 158:1-123.

9 Feingold B: Why your child is hyperactive. New York: Random House, 1975.

10 Finn R, Cohen HN: Food allergy—fact or fiction. Lancet 1978; i:426-8.

11 Fredholm BB: Are the actions of methyl xanthines due to antagonism of adenosine? Trends Pharmacol Sci 1980; 1:129-32.

12 Gattin A, Rall TW: The effect of adenosine and adenine nucleotides on the cyclic adenosine 3-5 phosphate content of guinea pig cerebral cortex slices. Mol Pharmacol 1970; 6:13-23.

13 Greden JF: Anxiety or caffeinism—a diagnostic dilema. Am J Psychiatry 1974; 131:1089-92.

14 Hanington E: Migraine. Trans Med Soc Lond 1970; 87:32-9.

15 Harada S, Agarwal DP, Goedde HW: Aldehyde dehydrogenase deficiency as cause of facial flushing reaction to alcohol in Japanese. Lancet 1981; ii:982.

16 Lutz EG: Restless legs. Anxiety and caffeinism. J Clin Psychiatry 1978; 39:693-8.

17 Moneret-Vautrin DA: False food allergies: nonspecific reaction to foodstuffs. In: Lessof MA, ed. Clinical reactions to food, New York: John Wiley, 1983; 135-54.

18 Quevauviller A, N'Guyen Van Hoa: L'histamine dans quelques produits alimentaires d'origine occidentale ou extreme-orientale. Bull Soc Sci Hyg Alim 1965; 53:284-94.

19 Rapp DJ: Allergies and the hyperactive child. New York: Sovereign Books, 1979.

20 Roth JA, Ivy AC: Comment. Caffeine and peptic ulcer. Gastroenterology 1946; 7:576-82.

21 Snyder SH, Katims JJ, Annau Z et al: Adenosine receptors and behavioural reactinthines. Proc Nat Acad Sci USA 1981; 78:3260-4.

22 Wagner SM, Mekhjian HS, Caldwell JH, Thomas FB: Effects of caffeine and coffee on fluid transport in the small intestine. Gastroenterology 1978; 75:379-81.

23 Willis T: The London practice of physick, 1st edn. London: Thomas Bassett and William Cooke, 1685; 404.

24 Zioudrou C, Streaty RA, Klee WA: Opioid peptides derived from food proteins. The exorphins. J Biol Chem 1979; 254:2446-9.

PART III
END-ORGAN EFFECTS

SECTION A
MECHANISMS

Chapter 24
Mechanisms: An Introduction

Jonathan Brostoff

Introduction

In some respects there has not been a quantum leap in our clinical understanding of food-allergic responses over the last 50 years, perhaps since the first edition of Rowe's classic textbook on food allergy [72], or indeed since that of Rinkel et al in 1951 [70]. Of course, our understanding of immediate Type I hypersensitivity reactions has immeasurably increased since the definition of the reaginic activity in serum as a new class of immunoglobulins—IgE [41]. However, from the doctor's point of view, it is the patient who makes the diagnosis of food allergy when the mechanism is IgE mediated because the time interval between ingestion and allergic reaction is short. This reaction also represents a rather fixed allergic response. When the symptoms are chronic and the reaction to food is delayed, the patient is normally unaware of the time relationship between ingestion of the food and the appearance of symptoms.

This chapter is not designed to be a complete account of all the possible mechanisms of food intolerance but is rather a general outline of some known mechanisms of producing symptoms of food allergy with descriptions of possible mechanisms of food intolerance looking for their disease. Three topics will be discussed in this chapter:

1 Immunological mechanisms with special reference to Type III hypersensitivity.
2 Enzyme defects: a known classic defect leading to a definite clinical syndrome—alactasia—and two enzyme deficiencies looking for clinical syndromes.
3 Brain and opioid effects and the immune system with special reference to hypersensitivity mechanisms.

433

The cornerstone of diagnosis

The cornerstone of diagnosis of food sensitivity is the removal of that food from the patient's diet with concomitant improvement in the patients symptoms which then reappear when that food is added back—preferably in a double-blind manner. At the clinical level, pragmatism is all important to the patient, the mechanism of the allergic reaction being less so. However, the more that is understood about mechanisms, the closer one can come to truly diagnostic tests.

Definition. The classification of food allergy and intolerance is difficult but the scheme outlined in Table 24.1 is roughly in accord with that suggested by others [55, 73] and is by no means perfect.

Table 24.1 Classification of food allergy and intolerance.

1 *Food intolerance*
   Pharmacological action, e.g. caffeine, tyramine
   Foods releasing mediators
   Toxic substances
   Irritants to the mucosa
   Fat—bile salt deficiency

2 *Food idiosyncrasy*
   Enzyme defects
      e.g. lactase deficiency
         lipase deficiency

3 *Food fads*
   'Popular' diets
   Anorexia nervosa
   Bulimia

4 *True food allergy*
   Immunologically mediated reactions
      Antibody mediated
      Immune complex mediated
      Cell mediated

IMMUNOLOGICAL MECHANISMS

Hypersensitivity may be classified according to the scheme of Gell and Coombs into reactions of Types I to IV (see also Chapter 14). These divisions are useful for discussion but may not necessarily occur as single entities in vivo. There is good evidence that Types I and III hypersensitivity can cause food-allergic symptoms and some evidence that Type II mechanisms can be associated with gut disease. In contrast to the considerable body of literature on antibody-mediated reactions to foods there is less direct evidence of cell-mediated reactions to food antigens in man.

There are, of course, data on lymphocyte transformation and migration inhibition in food allergy but this is not necessarily direct evidence of lymphocyte involvement in the disease. Experimental cell-mediated immunity to an antigen introduced into the gut lumen can produce chronic colitis but this is not produced as a result of natural exposure [69]. Coeliac disease and other villus atrophies and their relationship to Type IV hypersensitivity are discussed in the relevant chapters (Chapters 30, 33 and 36).

Type I hypersensitivity

In Type I reactions, mast cells sensitized with IgE antibody degranulate and release mediators when the antibodies are cross-linked by the relevant antigen (Fig. 24.1). The occurrence of Type I reactions to foods is undisputed and symptoms may include anaphylaxis, urticaria, rhinorrhoea, asthma, diarrhoea and vomiting [52].

These occur shortly after food ingestion and are usually associated with positive skin prick tests and positive radioallergosorbent tests (RAST) to the relevant food. These reactions are more common in children and it is suggested that 7–12% of all infants are allergic to cow's milk [7]. There is a tendency for these immediate reactions to disappear with age.

Fc_ε receptor-mediated mast-cell triggering

Mast cells are triggered when the Fc receptors for IgE ($Fc_\varepsilon R$) are cross-linked. This may occur with both specific, e.g. antigen, or non-specific agents such as lectins. It is the perturbation of the mast-cell membrane caused by cross-linking of the Fc_ε receptors that is the first stage of mast-cell activation (see also Chapter 5).

Mast-cell activation. In addition to the immunological stimuli which cross-link Fc_ε receptors, mast cells can be activated by other stimuli such as anaphylatoxins (C3a, C5a) and by non-physiological secretagogues such as compound 48/80, mellitin and calcium ionophore A23187 [67]. As can be seen in Fig. 24.2 drugs such as codeine, morphine and synthetic adrenocorticotropic hormone (ACTH) can also activate mast cells directly [25]. More recently, opioids, somatostatin and substance P have been shown to have mast-cell activating capacity thus providing a link between the central and peripheral nervous systems and the allergic response [65].

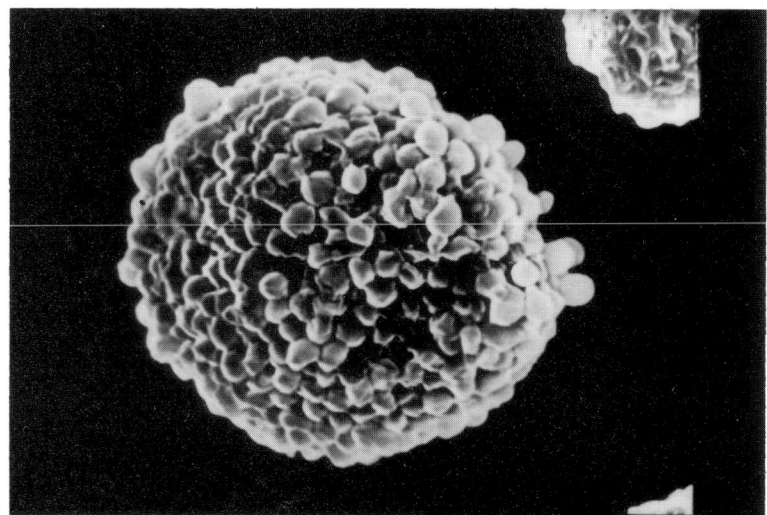

(a)

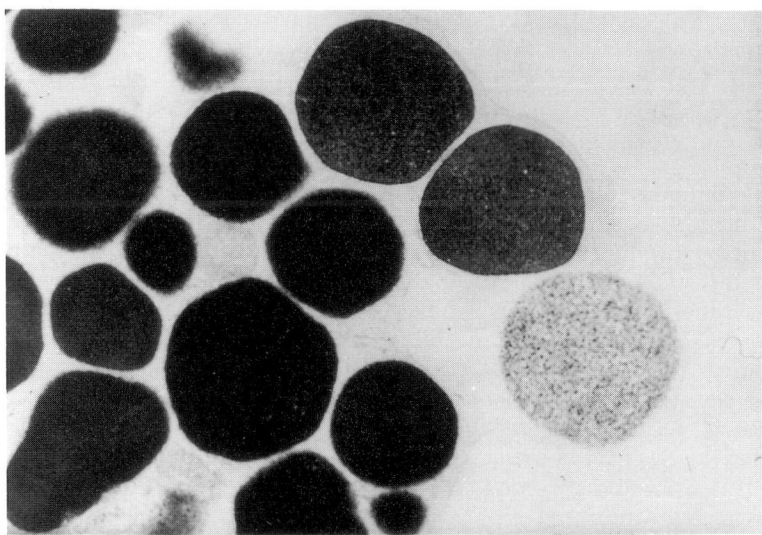

(b)

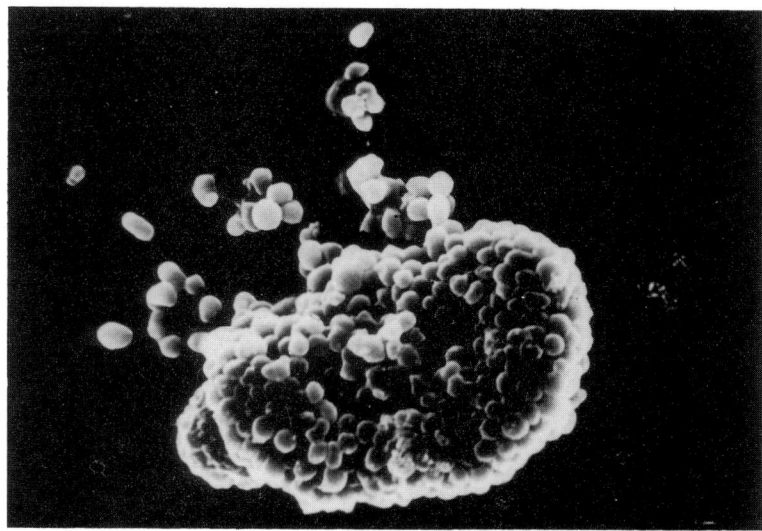

(c)

Fig 24.1 Electron micrographs (EM) of peritoneal mast cells (rat) showing an undegranulated cell (a, scanning EM × 1500); granule in the process of exocytosis (b, transmission EM × 15 000) and (c) exocytosis of granules following incubation with anti-IgE at 37°C for 30 seconds (EM × 1500). (Photographs by courtesy of Dr T.S.C. Orr and reproduced with the permission of Gower Medical Publishing Ltd., publishers of *Immunology* (edited by Roitt, Brostoff and Male).)

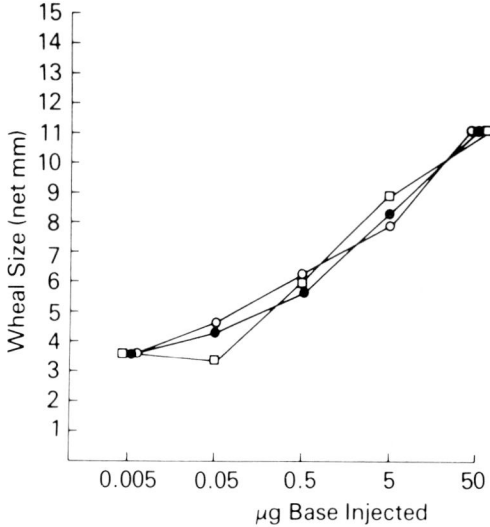

Fig. 24.2 Opiate skin tests in humans. Six human volunteers were skin tested with morphine (●), codeine (○) or meperidine (□); maximal diameter of whealing was measured after 15 minutes. Results are the mean of six skin tests on each subject, corrected for whealing indued by diluent alone. Data from [25].

actions can be obtained from cyclooxygenase inhibitors such as aspirin [24] as well as sodium cromoglycate (SCG) [22].

Populations of mast cells

It has long been suggested that mast-cell morphology not only varies from species to species but between different sites in the same animal [1]. In addition to morphological differences there are also functional differences between different populations of mast cells. The major differences between the two populations are summarized in Table 24.2.

Of major interest from a clinical point of view is the fact that SCG does not block histamine release from mucosal mast cells (MMC) whereas it does inhibit the release from connective tissue mast cells (CTMC) [67]. It may also be significant that MMC are T cell dependent and are recruited following antigen challenge, especially by parasitic antigens (see Chapter 5).

Central role of the mast cell in the gut. Whether gut mast cells are triggered by IgE-mediated, or other, mechanisms, they play a central role for focusing a variety of inflammatory events in the gut wall (Fig. 24.4). Mediators will provoke smooth muscle contractions, small vessel permeability, chemotaxis and cell activation. The release of mediators may also lead to an increase in gut permeability that has been seen in food-allergic subjects [3] and to the increased entry of antigen and immune complexes [22].

Mast-cell mediators. Following antigen-IgE-mast-cell interaction, degranulation occurs and a variety of mediators can be produced (Fig. 24.3). Some are preformed in the mast-cell granules and some newly synthesized following activation of arachidonic acid metabolism in the mast-cell membrane.

These latter mediators consist of cyclooxygenase and lipoxygenase products, i.e. prostaglandins and leukotrienes. There is clear evidence of histamine release [9] as well as prostaglandin production following activation, and protection from some food-allergic re-

Fig. 24.3 Following triggering, preformed and newly synthesized mediators are released. Histamine and various chemotactic factors are preformed. Following activation, phospholipase A₂ releases arachidonic acid (AA) which can then be metabolized by lipoxygenase (Lipox) or cyclooxygenase (Cyclox) pathways depending on the mast-cell type.

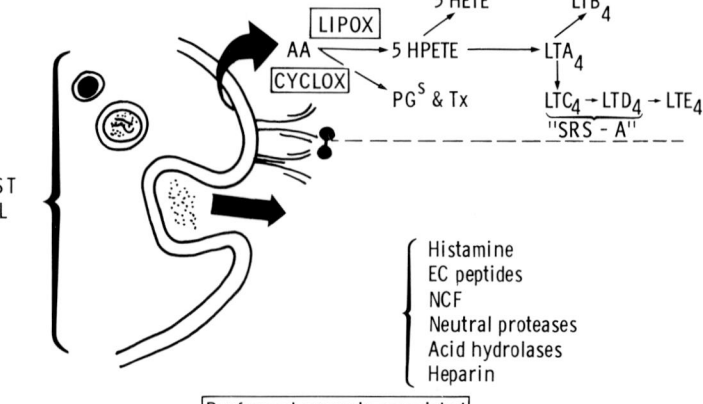

Table 24.2 Differences between mast-cell populations.

	Mucosal mast cell (MMC)	Connective tissue mast cell (CTMC)
Location in vivo	Gut and lung	Ubiquitous
Life span	40 days (?)	40 days (?)
T cell dependent	+	−
Number of Fcε receptors	2×10^5	3×10^4
Histamine content	+	+ +
Cytoplasmic IgE	+	−
Major arachidonic acid metabolite LTC$_4$/PGD$_2$ ratio	25:1	1:40
SCG/theophylline inhibits histamine release	−	+
Major proteoglycan	Chondroitin sulphate	Heparin

Type II hypersensitivity

In cytotoxic hypersensitivity, antibody is directed against a cell-surface tissue antigen or a hapten associated with a tissue (e.g. a drug). Complement activation leads to the generation of inflammatory mediators with resulting tissue damage and chemotactic activity bringing cells out of the circulation to the site of inflammation (Fig. 24.5).

Circulating antibodies have been described in inflammatory bowel disease [19]. These are autoantibodies to colonic epithelium which can cause cytotoxic reactions in vitro [80]. It is thought that these autoantibodies were primarily directed against gut bacteria but cross-react with colonic epithelial symptoms and lead to damage [46].

Antibodies against food proteins are seen in inflammatory bowel disease but also in other gut diseases and in normal controls [32]. This suggests that they are of minimal significance at least in the intestinal lesions of inflammatory bowel disease. However, this increased level of antibodies against food might be relevant in Type III immune complex-mediated reactions.

Type III hypersensitivity

The removal of antigen from the circulation is achieved by the formation of immune com-

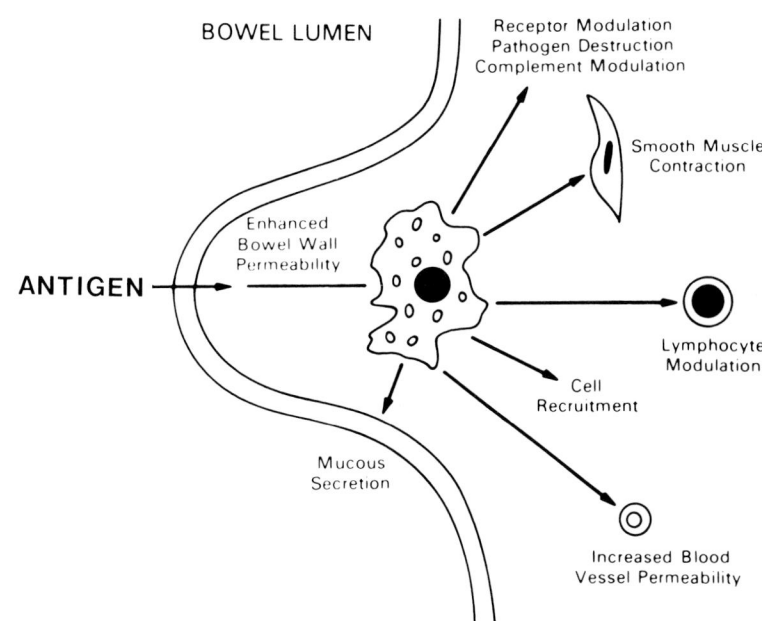

Fig. 24.4 Degranulation of the intestinal mast cell can lead to a variety of responses leading to local inflammation and increased gut permeability.

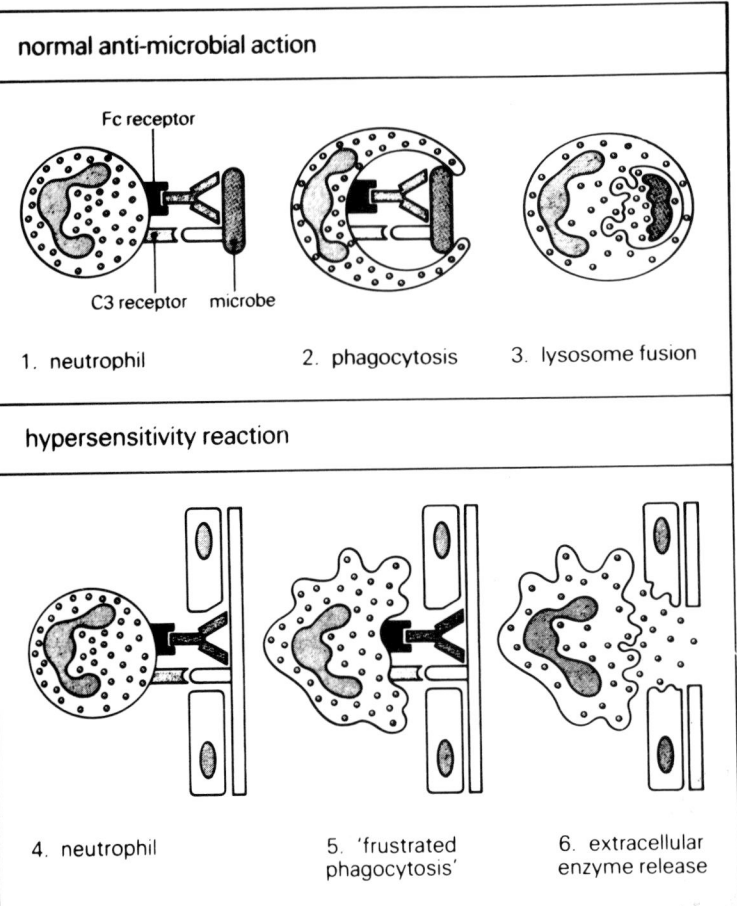

Fig. 24.5 Damage mechanisms: neutrophil-mediated damage is a reflection of normal antibacterial action. If the target is large, e.g. a solid tissue, the neutrophils suffer from 'frustrated' phagocytosis and release their enzymes causing local damage. From Roitt, Brostoff and Male (eds) *Immunology*, with the permission of Gower Medical Publishing Ltd.

plexes which can then be cleared by the reticuloendothelial system. Thus, immune complex formation is a normal physiological event after eating, for removing antigen from the circulation.

If the formation of immune complexes is excessive or if the quality of the complex is abnormal or if reticuloendothelial function is impaired, then these complexes can cause disease. Immune complex disease can occur with persistent infection, in autoimmune disease or as a result of allergen challenge at body surfaces, e.g. the lung, or following food ingestion.

The Arthus reaction

The skin reaction typical of Type III hypersensitivity is the Arthus reaction seen clinically in patients with precipitating antibodies, e.g. to *Aspergillus fumigatus*. The Arthus reaction takes place at a local site, e.g. in the skin following antigen injection, where immune complexes activate complement and cause an inflammatory cascade involving poly-

morphs, platelets and mast cells (Fig. 24.6). This form of immune complex disease is rarely seen in the allergic patient although the possibility of it being present must exist in patients with IgA deficiency who have precipitating antibodies to milk (see Chapter 12).

Why do complexes persist? Normally, complexes are removed by the phagocytic system in the liver, spleen and lungs. Large complexes are removed quickly whereas smaller ones circulate for longer periods of time. There is evidence that the phagocytic system becomes overloaded in chronic immune complex disease and this favours prolonged circulation. Further, if the antibody affinity is low, smaller complexes will be produced which will be cleared less readily.

Why do complexes deposit in tissue? The circulation of immune complexes is not in itself harmful. Damage only occurs when they are deposited in tissues.

This may occur because of increased vascular permeability whether induced by com-

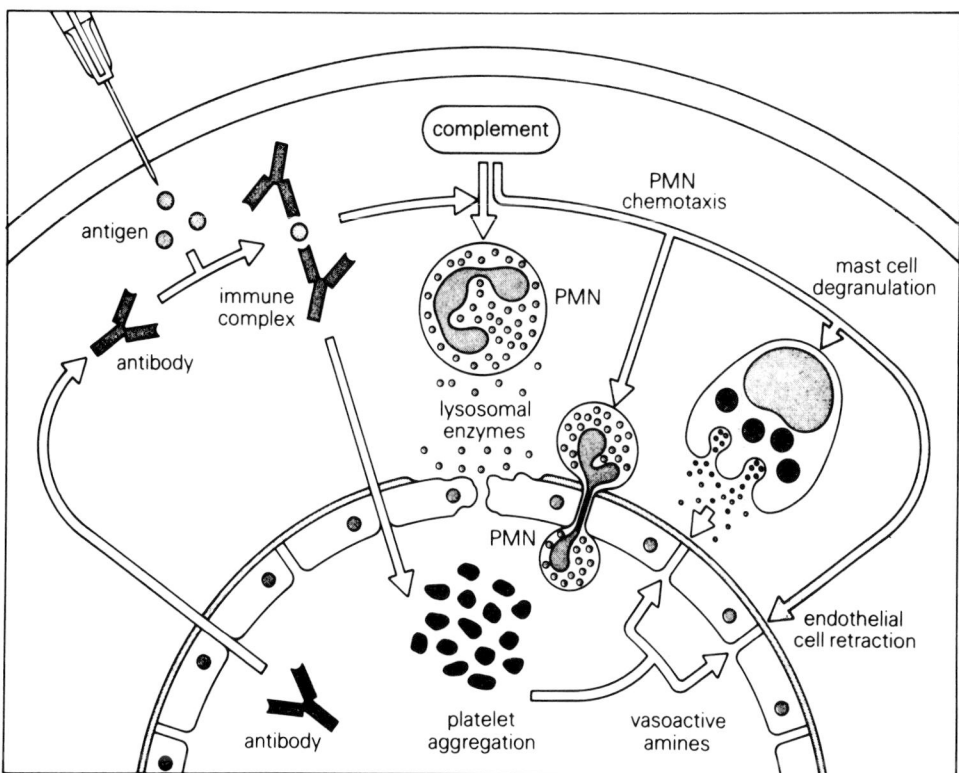

Fig. 24.6 The Arthus reaction. Antigen injected intradermally forms complexes in the skin which then activate complement with the production of inflammatory mediators. The reaction is potentiated by enzyme release from the polymorphs. From Roitt, Brostoff and Male (eds) *Immunology*, with the permission of Gower Medical Publishing Ltd.

plement activation, platelet aggregation or mast-cell degranulation. Increased turbulence of blood flow in small vessels will also favour deposition as in the glomerular capillaries. Lastly, the antigen in the complex may bind to specific tissues directly as can DNA to collagen in the glomerular basement membrane in patients with systemic lupus erythematosus (SLE).

Immune complexes containing IgE

Of particular interest to the understanding of disease mechanisms in the allergic patient is the possibility that they make abnormal immune complexes, in this instance, containing IgE.

There have been suggestions that high molecular weight reaginic activity does occur in atopic patients [38] and a rheumatoid factor IgM anti-IgE was shown by Williams et al using agglutination techniques [84]. The first direct demonstration of immune complexes containing IgE was made using ultracentrifugation techniques [21] in sera from classical

atopic patients (Fig. 24.7). Of particular interest is the observation that a considerable proportion of the total IgE in such patients could be complexed (Fig. 24.8).

The relevance of IgE-containing immune complexes in food allergy. Normal individuals form immune complexes between food allergens and IgG and IgA and these are harmless, playing their part in antigen elimination. In contrast, we [62] and others [4] have shown that food-allergic individuals form immune complexes containing allergens and specific IgG and IgA in concentrations exceeding those detectable in normal subjects. We have also shown that these immune complexes are both quantitatively and qualitatively different from those formed in normal individuals, in particular with respect to their content of IgE [23].

The role of the gut in IgE complex formation

A patient given an oral egg challenge can become asthmatic within 2 hours. If sodium cromoglycate (SCG) is given orally before the

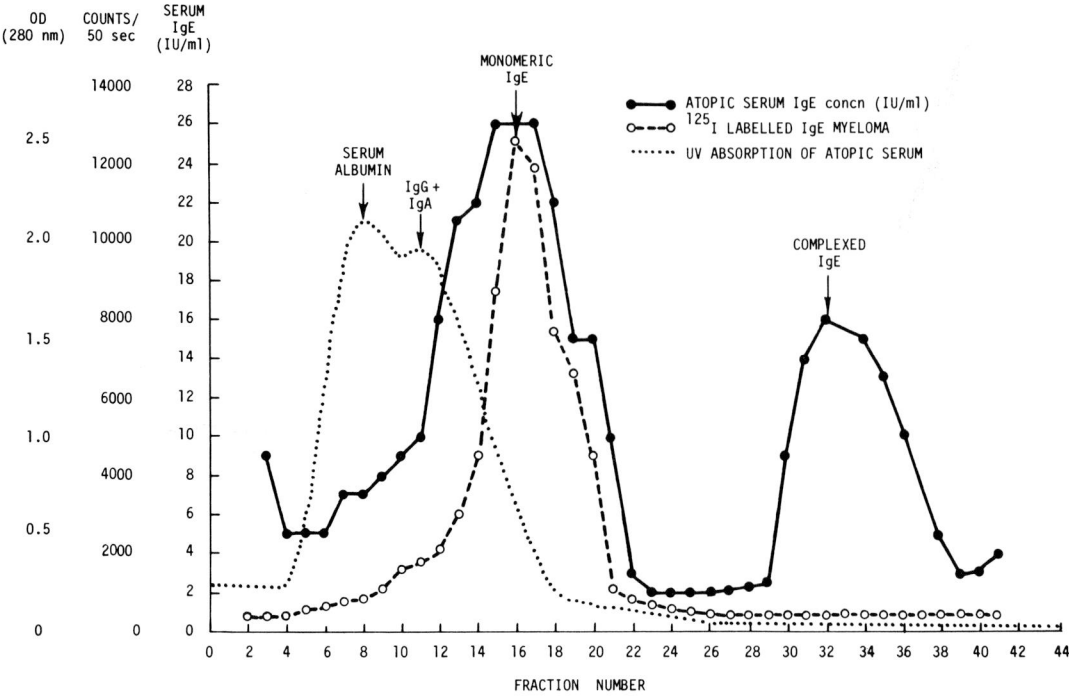

Fig. 24.7 A typical density gradient ultracentrifugation profile of serum from a patient with atopic eczema and asthma, showing distribution of IgE expressed as radioactive ^{125}I counts per fraction. Normal sedimentation distribution of a radiolabelled IgE myeloma protein, ultracentrifuged under identical conditions, has been superimposed for comparison.

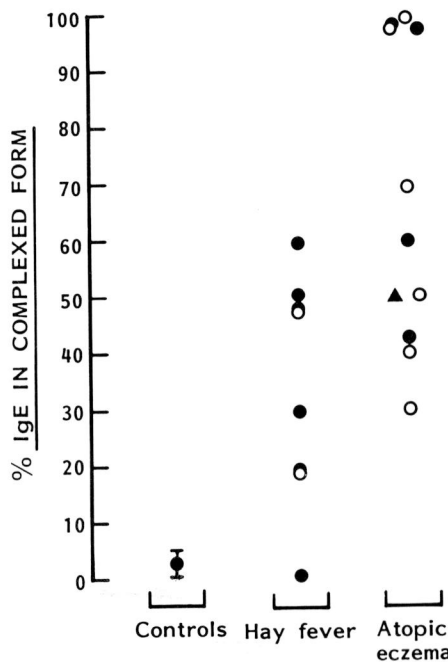

Fig. 24.8 The percentage of complexed IgE in non-atopic controls is less than 5%. In atopics, greater than 50% of the total IgE can be complexed, occasionally very much more in subjects with eczema. ○ Asthma; ▲ Hayfever.

challenge, no asthma results (Fig. 24.9). This protection by SCG shows the role of hypersensitivity reactions at the level of the intestinal mucosa as being the trigger for the systemic allergic response. In this patient the shock organ was the lung [22] but it could also be the nose [79], joints [63], skin [5] or cerebral vasculature [57].

IgE complexes following food challenge. In the patient described in Fig. 24.9, complexes were detectable with a time course similar to that for the production of her asthma (Fig. 24.10). Of note is the considerably reduced level of circulating immune complexes when the patient is pretreated with SCG. This reduction in immune complexes is paralleled by a decreased level of circulating antigen when SCG pretreatment is given (Fig. 24.11).

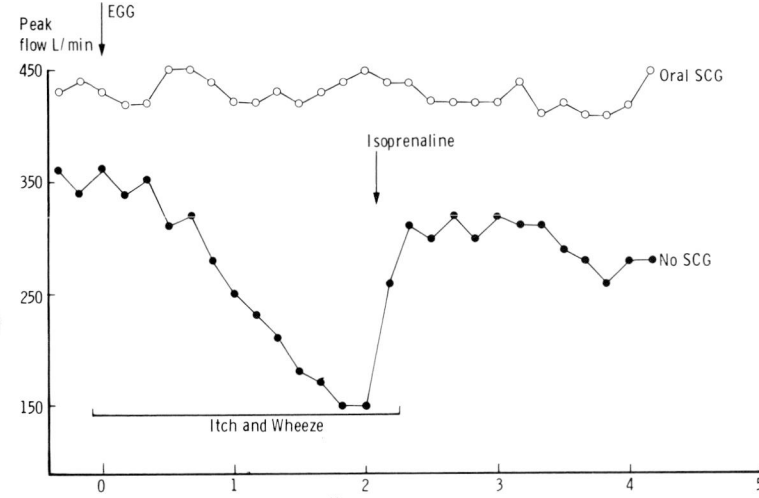

Fig. 24.9 A patient orally challenged with egg developed asthma within hours. This was prevented by oral SCG. This emphasizes the importance of the mucosal hypersensitivity response in the gut opening the 'gate' to systemic effects.

Bystander effect. There is evidence from animal models that absorption of antigens from the gastrointestinal tract is increased if an IgE-mediated hypersensitivity is present locally [13]. This can be shown by increased absorption of the specific antigen and also bystander molecules into the circulation [45]. This mechanism may help to explain the so-called 'spreading phenomenon' in food-allergic patients where the patient becomes intolerant of an increasing range of foods over a short period of time having been previously sensitive to only one or two.

Withdrawal symptoms on elimination diets: the precipitin curve. If the patient with delayed onset food allergy (the majority) has a form of chronic serum sickness with few or many organ systems involved, then this would provide an explanation for the polysymptomatology of the condition, the lack of abnormal

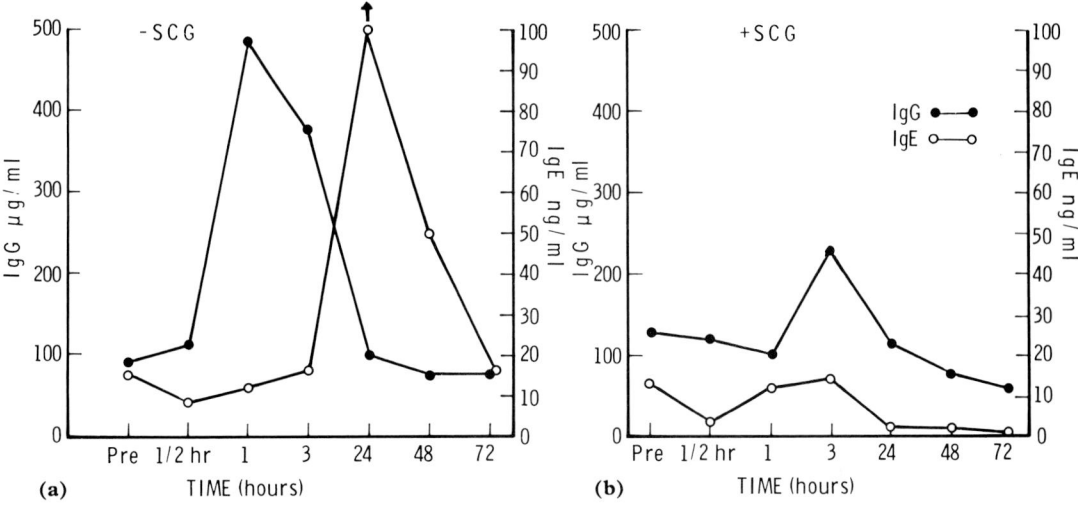

Fig. 24.10 IgG and IgE (total) following food challenge. Polyethylene glycol (PEG) precipitable IgE and IgG. The serial serum samples were precipitated with PEG and the pellets assayed for total IgE and IgG. (a) Considerable peaks of complexed IgG and IgE are seen. (b) In the presence of SCG, only small amounts of IgG complexes were seen, slightly later in time at 3 hours, but no precipitated IgE was detectable.

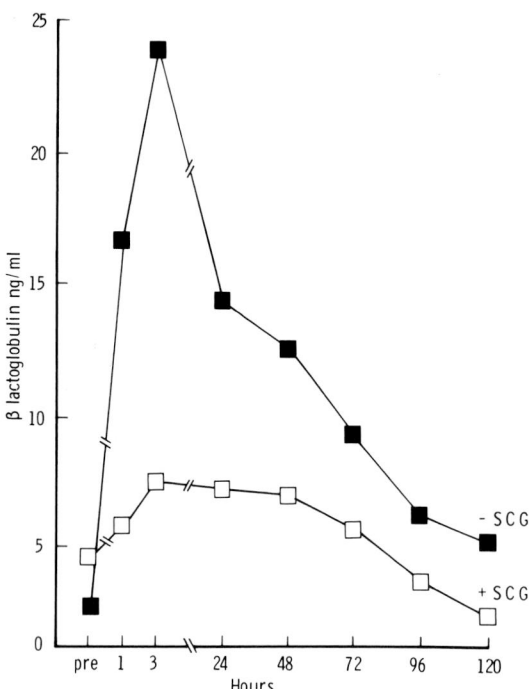

Fig. 24.11 There is an increase in serum antigen (β lacto-globulin) level following milk challenge, peaking at 3 hours (with a level of 24 ng/ml) and then returning to normal levels over the next 3 days. Pretreatment with SCG leads only to a modest increase (~ 8 ng/ml), with a similar gradual fall.

laboratory tests and the exacerbation of symptoms on dietary exclusion.

As long as the patient is eating the food, often in large amounts, immune complexes are formed in antigen excess and are therefore soluble (see Fig. 24.12). These would cause relatively mild but chronic symptoms. On dietary exclusion, antigen concentration falls, optimally precipitable immune complexes are formed and acute 'serum sickness' results, i.e. withdrawal symptoms. When the antigen is finally cleared, any complexes formed will be in antibody excess and soluble again, and symptoms will also clear.

This hypothesis would also suggest a logical approach to the management of the condition and the possibility of devising model systems in the human to understand further the mechanisms producing the symptoms. What governs the selection of the target organ by the complexes is still a mystery.

A concept of food allergy as chronic serum sickness

In allergic patients we [22] and many others (e.g. [26, 27]) have shown the presence of immune complexes following food challenge and the protective effect of oral SCG on both symptoms and the appearance of immune complexes. These data suggest that an IgE-mediated mechanism acts as a trigger by altering the permeability of the gut mucosa.

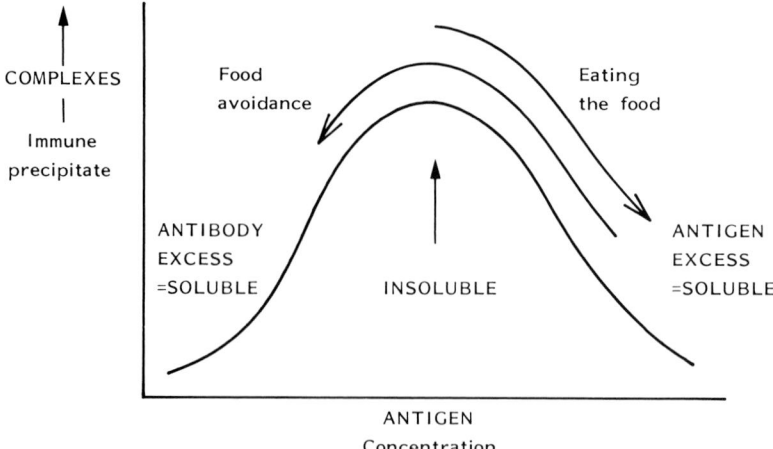

Fig. 24.12 A hypothetical 'clinical' precipitin curve: when a patient eats large quantities of an allergenic food, complexes are found in antigen excess and are soluble. When they avoid that food, antigen concentration falls and they 'climb-up' their precipitin curve and develop serum sickness shown as withdrawal symptoms which clear on antigen elimination.

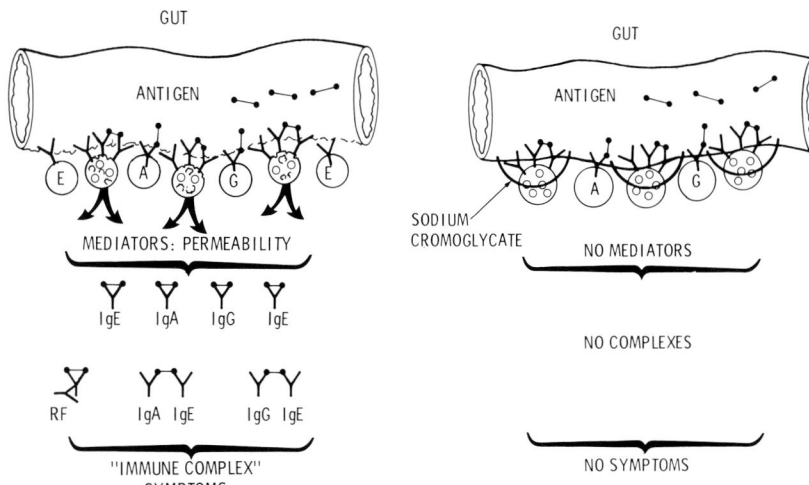

Fig. 24.13 A model of food allergy and the action of sodium cromoglycate. (a) Release of mediators from sensitized mast cells by ingested food leads to increased gut permeability and absorption of antigen with the formation of immune complexes and symptoms. (b) Prior treatment with sodium cromoglycate inhibits degranulation and mediator release, reduces antigen absorption and immune complex formation and thus symptoms are prevented.

This increase in permeability may not necessarily be reflected in histological or ultrastructural abnormality in the gut mucosa[68] but is clearly adequate to allow increased entry of antigen and complexes and to cause symptoms. A scheme for this concept[20] is shown in Fig. 24.13.

ENZYMES

Inborn errors of metabolism may affect many organ systems and as regards the gut may affect the digestion and absorption of carbohydrate, fat and protein. There are also enzyme systems involved in general detoxification and metabolism that may be abnormal. An enzyme may be present but only slowly metabolically active, thus at least potentially allowing the build-up of toxic products.

In this section three enzymes will be mentioned. Firstly, a classical enzyme—lactase—because its deficiency, either primary or secondary, leads to classical gastrointestinal symptoms. Secondly, an enzyme associated with oxidative biotransformation of drugs. The debrisoquine hydroxylation locus can regulate or influence the metabolism of many drugs and possibly foods. Thirdly, the enzyme phenol sulphotransferase which sulphates phenolic compounds. This may have particular application to food sensitivity as many foods contain considerable quantities of phenolic compounds, which have been said to cause sensitivity reactions.

There will surely be more enzyme deficiencies discovered in the coming years which may provide an explanation for many of the food intolerances that are seen today.

Lactase deficiency

Congenital alactasia

Congenital lactase deficiency persists in the neonatal period with collapse when milk feeds containing lactase are given. This is often associated with watery diarrhoea[48] (see also Chapter 2).

Acquired alactasia

The acquired form presents later and although there seems to be an inverse correlation between the quantity of milk drunk and the incidence of alactasia in the population it is generally accepted that the deficiency is genetically based and not due to environmental factors[36]. There are extreme variations in lactase activity[35] with some adult populations showing an almost complete absence of enzyme activity (Fig. 24.14). Transient lactase deficiency may occur after an episode of diarrhoea but will recover on a dairy-free diet. Man is probably the only animal (apart from the domestic cat) that drinks milk after weaning and thus adult alactasia could be considered the normal state.

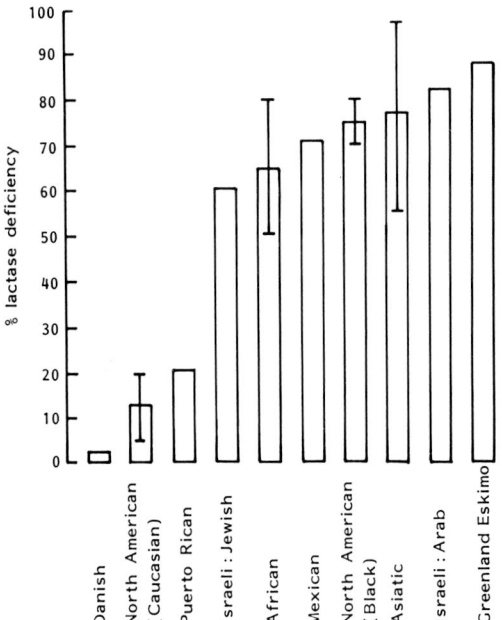

Fig. 24.14 The geographical and ethnic variation in lactase deficiency. Adapted from Gray [35].

Cytochrome P-450 oxidative reactions

The metabolism of drugs and other chemicals displays marked interindividual variation. Many contributing factors have been identified and it appears that interindividual differ-

ences in drug metabolism have their origins in variations of the functional expression of the cytochrome P-450 isozymes as regulated and influenced by a variety of genetic, environmental, physiological and pathological factors. Where the P-450 enzyme system fits in to the detoxification metabolic pathways is shown in Fig. 24.15.

Genetic polymorphism

The oxidative metabolism of a number of drugs has been shown to be under single gene control, variable oxidation patterns arising from the occurrence of allelomorphic variant forms of the gene in the population.

It has been suggested that there is a relationship between enzyme function and polymorphism [43] and that the polymorphism is more prevalent with enzymes that metabolize environmental substrates than with those that are concerned with endogenous metabolic processes [44]. If environmental factors changed, in that the external chemical load increased, it would make sense for the enzymes that relate to the chemical to maintain a high degree of polymorphism and therefore flexibility. Such polymorphism does seem to be a feature of drug-metabolizing enzymes.

Significance of the debrisoquine oxidation locus

The debrisoquine hydroxylation locus has been shown to regulate the metabolism of many other drugs such as phenformin [61], nortriptiline [54] and phenacetin [81]. Of special interest is that this particular locus also influences events related to oxidative metabolism which in turn affect the likelihood of developing exaggerated or adverse responses to drugs and chemicals. Genetically determined oxidation status may be an important susceptibility factor in certain diseases related to exposure to toxic environmental chemicals as well as cancer [40] and Balkan nephropathy [71].

Metabolic phenotype. Population studies have shown that the metabolic reaction of debrisoquine hydroxylation is under single gene control and exhibits polymorphism both within families [31] and in the population [51]. Two alleles (DH and DL) govern extensive and poor oxidation [53] and reflect the two phenotypes in the population, i.e. extensive metabolizers (EM) and poor metabolizers (PM) respectively.

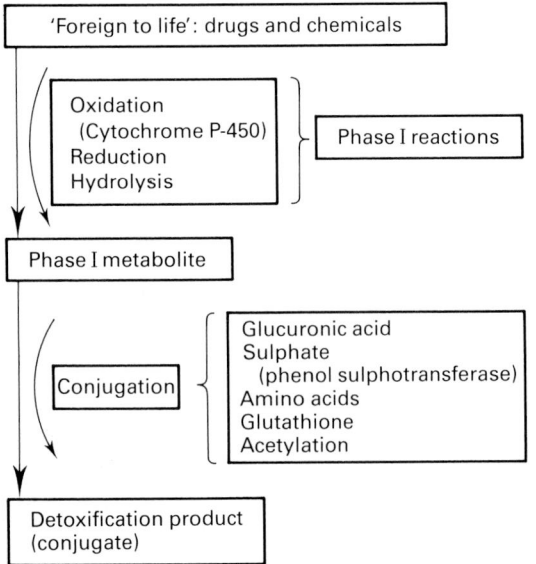

Fig. 24.15 The relationship of the cytochrome P-450 oxidation system to the other major metabolic enzyme systems involved in detoxification.

Population differences in poor-metabolizer phenotype. Poor metabolizers have been seen in all populations studied but there is considerable heterogeneity with respect to metabolic status. As can be seen in Fig. 24.16 there is an increase in the frequency of poor metabolizers as one moves from Eastern to Western population groups—one might speculate that this is perhaps related to increased chemical and drug exposure.

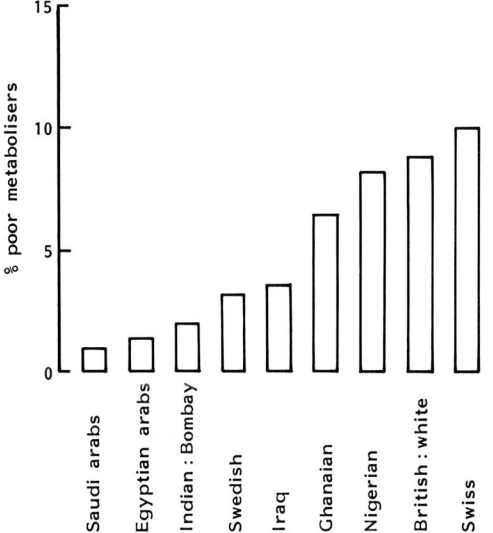

Fig. 24.16 Ethnic differences in the frequency of poor metabolizers of debrisoquine. The frequency increases from East to West.

Sulphoxidation reactions. Genetic polymorphism for the sulphoxidation of *S*-carboxymethylcysteine has also been described [83]. The sulphoxidation indices (ratio of total sulphide to total sulphoxide in urine following 750 mg of *S*-carboxymethyl-L-cysteine, a mucolytic drug, taken orally) show that in a White European population, less than 20% are slow metabolizers. A bimodal model is most probable and family studies suggest a genetic effect with overlying environmental influences (see below).

Occurrence of poor metabolizers in patients with food allergy

Genetic variation in the ability to metabolize various drugs is likely to be reflected in the handling of foods and associated chemicals and could explain, in fact, susceptibility of

certain individuals to environmental agents and foods. This possibility is at present being investigated by us in a group of food-sensitive patients. The preliminary results are shown in Fig. 24.17, where the increased incidence of poor metabolizers compared to the normal volunteer population is notable. Since vitamin C may have an effect on cytochrome P-450 [76], six patients have been retested after a week on a small dose, 200 mg/day and, interestingly, two patients showed a reduction in sulphoxidation index, i.e. increased metabolic activity, but in only one of these did it return to within the normal range of 0.7 to 5.9.

It is possible that an increased dosage of vitamin C may have a greater effect on the enzyme activity. This would provide a rationale for the large doses of vitamin C given to some allergic patients.

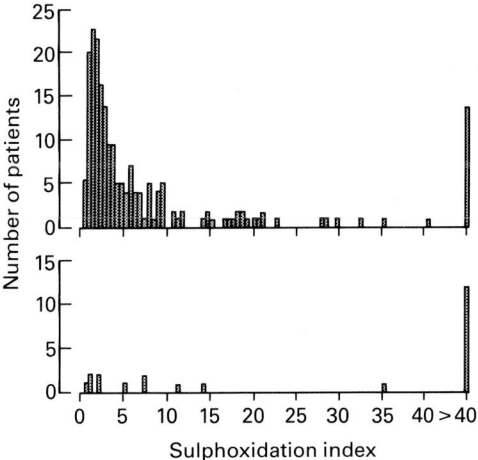

Fig. 24.17 The sulphoxidation index in a normal population (top panel) and in a group of patients with food allergy (bottom panel). The efficient metabolizers (to the left) are in the majority in the normal population whereas poor metabolizers form the majority of the food-allergic group.

Environmental causes for disease

Food allergy. There is preliminary evidence that poor metabolizer status is associated with food allergy (Fig. 24.17). This would suggest that the enzyme phenotype of the patients makes them more or less susceptible to foods, chemical constituents of the foods or chemicals added to the foods. It is this last aspect that also causes particular concern to environmentalists.

Parkinson's disease. Recent reports have suggested that there might also be environmental causes for Parkinson's disease [49]. Barbeau [8] in a study of more than 5000 cases has collected data showing a surprising correlation of 0.967 between the level of pesticide use and disease incidence. The incidence of Parkinson's disease in areas of high pesticide use was 0.89 per 1000 compared with 0.13 per 1000 where use was low. His group has further shown an increase in the frequency of poor metabolizers in the patient group (more than half) compared with controls [9].

As Parkinson's disease is not a homogeneous entity, it does suggest that a subgroup of patients, due to their enzyme phenotype, may be at risk from environmental chemicals.

Phenol sulphotransferase

Migraine, headache and monoamine oxidase inhibitors

The particular association of tyramine-containing foods and migraine was suggested because of the similarity of foods prohibited to patients taking monoamine oxidase inhibitors and those that have been said to cause migraine [39]. However, although cheese may be rich in tyramine, other foods known to provoke migraine such as chocolate and citrus fruit have very low levels although they do contain other pressor amines. In addition, tyramine challenge has in general not been successful in provoking headaches [56, 75] although Hanington was successful [39]. Thus, tyramine is unlikely to be the main cause of migraine.

Food phenolic compounds

Naturally occurring phenolic compounds in food have been suspected of playing a role in allergic reactions in both animals [10] and man. Chlorogenic acid (a phenol) which is found in green coffee, castor bean and oranges can produce an immediate wheal and flare reaction in sensitized subjects [33]. This would suggest that not only this compound but other related plant phenolics may be the allergic constituent of other foods, pollens, dusts or moulds. As can be seen from Table 24.3, phenolic compounds are widespread in many of the foods that we eat.

If simple chemical 'allergens' could be isolated from foods and pollens then we might have easily standardized materials for the diagnosis of common allergic disorders.

Phenol sulphotransferase

Sulphate conjugation of an oral tryamine load is abnormal in some patients with migraine. Phenol sulphotransferase (PST) occurs in two forms in man: PST-M inactivates monoamines such as tyramine whereas PST-P adds sulphate to a wide variety of endogenous and dietary phenols (Fig. 24.18).

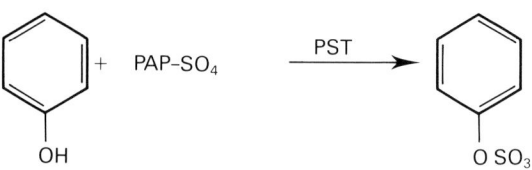

Fig. 24.18 The action of phenol sulphotransferase (PST).

PST-P deficiency in migraine. If tyramine were the main cause of migraine one might hope to find an especial susceptibility to it in affected patients, perhaps by reduced PST-M enzyme activity. If on the other hand, poor metabolic handling of phenolic compounds was the major factor, low levels of PST-P might be found. In a study by Littlewood et al [47], 46 patients with migraine were studied and divided into those who thought dietary factors might be important and those who had discovered no provoking factor. As can be seen in Fig. 24.19, there was no difference in PST-M levels between either of the groups but the so-called 'dietary' migraine patients had significantly lower levels of PST-P ($P < 0.01$), suggesting decreased ability to metabolize phenolic compounds.

It is interesting that wine almost totally inhibits PST-P thus potentially compounding the insult of having low levels of the enzyme to begin with.

Clinical significance of PST-P deficiency

The results of enzyme assays in migraine are of profound interest as they suggest a possible mechanism by which patients may be sensitive to particular foodstuffs. It may well be that a primary or acquired enzyme deficiency may also alter antigen handling so that the antigen becomes more immunogenic. A double defect, i.e. an enzyme defect as well as an immune response gene may make the patient very susceptible to environmental allergens and chemical haptens.

Table 24.3 Phenolic compounds in foods.

	Capsaicin	Cinnamic acid	Coumarin/Scopoletin	Eugenol	Gallic acid	Malvin (anthocyanidins)	Menadione (naphthoquinones)	Nicotine	Phenyl(benzyl) isothiocyanate	Phlorizin or phloridzin	Piperine	Piperonal	Rutin—quercetin (Flavonol)	Vanillylamine	Apiol
Almond				•	•							•		•	•
Apple		•	•		•	•	•			•			•	•	
Banana		•	•												
Beef			•	•				•	•	•	•	•	•	•	•
Beet sugar		•			•					•	•	•	•		
Cabbage					•	•			•			•			
Cane sugar			•		•								•		
Carrot			•	•	•	•							•		•
Celery		•	•	•	•	•	•						•		•
Cheese		•	•	•	•					•	•		•	•	•
Chicken			•			•			•			•	•		
Egg			•		•	•	•		•	•			•		
Grape		•			•	•	•			•	•		•	•	
Lamb			•			•			•	•	•	•	•	•	
Lettuce		•	•		•	•	•			•		•	•	•	
Milk (cow)	•	•		•	•	•		•	•	•	•	•	•	•	•
Onion	•	•			•	•	•		•			•	•	•	
Orange		•	•	•	•					•			•	•	•
Pea		•	•	•	•		•		•		•		•		•
Potato	•		•		•			•			•		•	•	
Rice			•										•		
Soya bean			•	•		•			•	•	•		•	•	•
Tomato	•	•	•	•	•	•		•	•		•	•	•	•	•
Wheat			•		•								•		
Yeast			•					•	•		•	•	•	•	

Adapted from Robert Gardner, Brigham Young University.

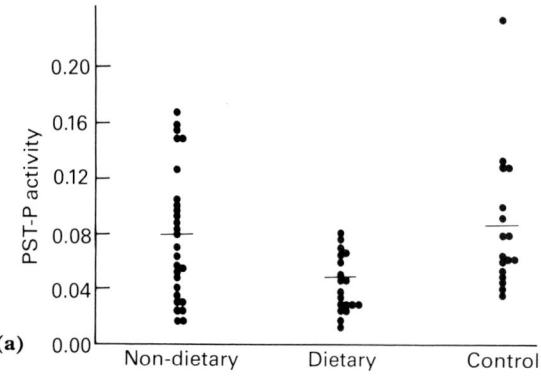

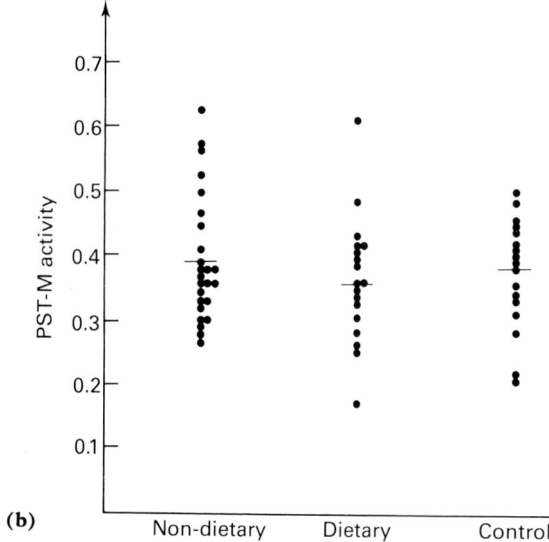

Fig. 24.19 A comparison of PST-P (a) and PST-M (b) activity in control subjects and patients with dietary and non-dietary migraine. Patients with dietary migraine have significantly less PST-P activity ($P < 0.01$). Data from [47].

RAST cross-reactivity and phenolic compounds. As can be seen in Fig. 24.20, many foods and pollens which are not members of the same botanical family seem to cluster in the RAST assay and this is also reflected in RAST cross-inhibition [14]. Other possibilities for cross-reaction may be through cross-reacting carbohydrate determinants [1] or other chemical compounds such as phenolics. It is interesting to compare the RAST cross-reactivity with the phenolic content of these foods. There is a remarkable similarity in phenolic content paralleling the RAST cross-reactivity. The comparison is incomplete as data for the phenolic content of foods are qualitative and those for pollen are not available. This must be a fruitful area to explore both in vivo and in vitro.

Possible protective effect of plant phenols. Among the potentially damaging components of foods are their lectin (see Chapter 21) and phenolic content. There are, of course, many other possible candidates. If lectins were continually to degranulate inestinal mast cells our homeostatic mechanisms would be severely strained.

Interestingly, data from Pearce et al [66] suggest that some food phenolics may act similarly to sodium cromoglycate (SCG) and protect mast cells. In Fig. 24.21 can be seen the effect of quercitin on mast cells, it being equally effective against both mucosal and connective mast cells where SCG is only effective against the later.

Clearly, these compounds may have a protective effect on the intestinal mast cell as well as potential for causing adverse clinical reactions.

Summary

These data reflect the possibility that cross-reactivity among foods and other allergens may be through their phenolic content and that the clinical reaction may be immunologically or biochemically mediated or need both mechanisms.

What is badly needed are secure clinical data examining the clinical and in vitro response to these phenolic compounds.

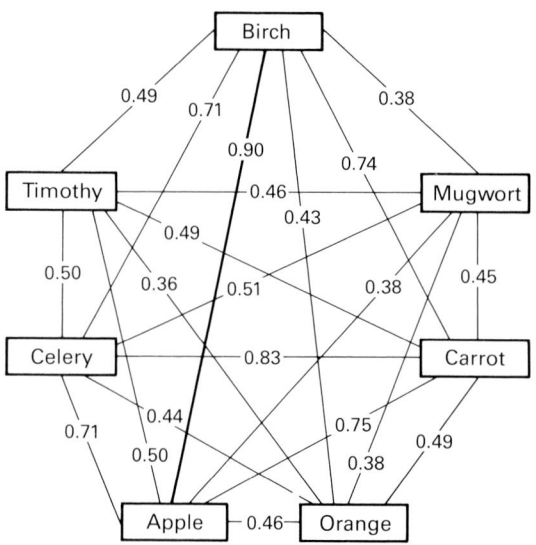

Fig. 24.20 Clustering of positive RAST results in 90 sera. Each pair of source materials is joined by a line and an associated number which indicates the probability that the second source material yields a positive result when the first one has given a positive result. Data from [14].

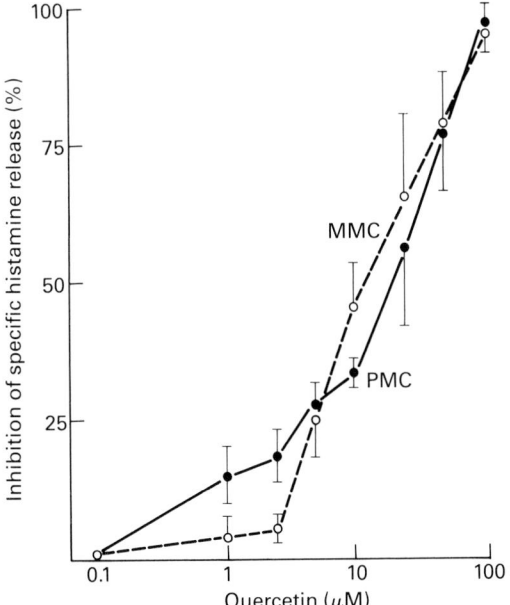

Fig. 24.21 The phenolic compound quercitin is able to inhibit histamine release from both peritoneal mast cells (PMC) and mucosal mast cells (MMC). Data from [66].

OPIOID PEPTIDES

Endorphins

Endorphins consist of a family of endogenous peptides which occur naturally in the brain and bind to morphine receptors. There are now at least five groups of naturally occurring opioid peptides [59] and three distinct opioid receptors [64] which are closely related to the opioid peptides.

In addition to the well-known physiological roles, opioids have prominent effects on mood and behaviour. Of particular interest to the allergist are three areas of positive action of opioid peptides, namely mood and behavioural changes, their effect on immune function and their interaction with allergic responses. The literature in these areas is now substantial and the following is intended as an hors d'oeuvre rather than a main course.

Immunity, stress and emotions

Lymphocyte function. The classic paper by Bartrop et al in 1977 was the first essay into psychoneuroimmunology and showed that lymphocyte transformation was depressed in bereaved spouses although no change was noted in the absolute number of T and B cells [12]. Further studies confirmed these findings in hospitalized patients with major depressive illnesses. Interestingly, ambulatory depressed patients, schizophrenics and surgical in-patients had normal T cell function (Fig. 24.22) suggesting that these changes were a feature of a severe depression and not related to a stay in hospital [82]. From the purely in vitro point of view β-endorphin and other opioids significantly inhibit rosette formation between human T lymphocytes and sheep red blood cells [28]. This effect is blocked by naloxone whereas naloxone itself does not influence rosette formation. This reflects a further factor linking the immune and neuroendocrine system.

Antibody secretion. Stress can also be seen to affect antibody production in particular secretory IgA [42]. Dental students were tested for personality type and followed through stressful examination periods, measuring the amount of salivary IgA produced. The IgA

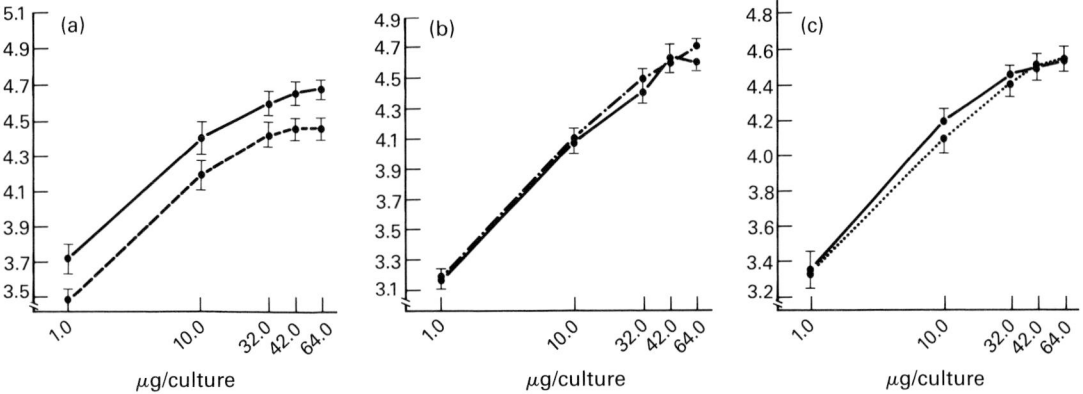

Fig. 24.22 Lymphocyte transformation by concanavalin A (Con A) in patients with severe depression is reduced (a), but when the depression is milder (b) or in patients with schizophrenia (c), lymphocyte function is normal. (Redrawn from original artwork published in the *Archives of General Psychiatry* (Scheifer et al, 1985; 42:131). © 1985 American Medical Association.)

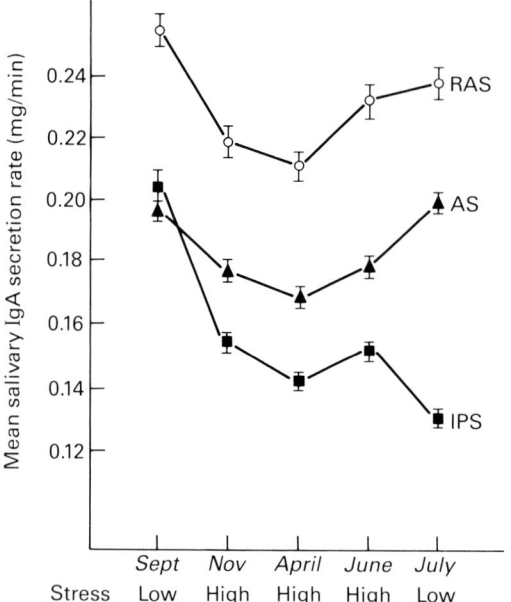

Fig. 24.23 Mean salivary immunoglobulin A secretion rate in high and low stress periods for all subjects (AS), those with the relaxed affiliative motive syndrome (RAS) and those with the inhibited power motive syndrome (IPS). Vertical bars = standard error of the mean. IgA secretion is significantly reduced during periods of high stress. Data from [42].

secretion rate was significantly lower in high stress periods, coinciding with exams, than in low stress periods (Fig. 24.23) and as can be seen, there was also an effect of personality characteristics.

Emotions versus immunity. These data and many others raise the question as to the clinical importance of the relationships between emotions and immunity [30]. Maybe the answer is that psychological counselling in the acute phase of disease may be as important to the outcome of that disease as many of the therapeutic measures we now undertake.

Opioids and the allergic response

Mast-cell histamine release. It is well known that opiate drugs such as morphine and codeine are able to release histamine from mast cells both in vivo [25] and in vitro [78] (Fig. 24.2) and it was reasonable to assume that endorphins could act similarly. This is indeed the case as can be seen in Fig. 24.24. Interestingly, the histamine release induced by the opioids could be blocked by SCG at a rather high concentration (10^{-4} M), and by naloxone, which was also able to block antigen-induced secretion. The opioid effects were only seen

on connective tissue and not on mucosal mast cells.

This lack of response of intestinal mucosal mast cells to endorphins may be useful teleologically since these cells may be exposed to high levels of biologically active peptides derived from foods—exorphins which may otherwise lead to degranulation and histamine release by direct action on the cell membrane. Protection of other potentially responsive mast cells may be by the action of other food chemicals such as quercitin [66] which can block histamine secretion (Fig. 24.21).

Exorphins

The original stimulus in this area came from the observations of Dohan [29] where he suggested that gluten or possibly peptides derived from gluten could be implicated in the pathogenesis of schizophrenia.

Two groups, those of Zioudrou et al [86], and Brantl and Teschemacher [18], have investigated proteinase-resistant peptides that have endorphin-like activity. These exogenous peptides have been called exorphins to be compared with their endogenous counterparts, the endorphins. Active peptides can arise during the digestion of several dietary proteins including wheat, milk and maize [18, 86]. The activity of gluten exorphin in binding to brain receptors was similar to that of morphine and inhibitable by naloxone [85].

Clinical relevance

There is no doubt that potent pharmacological

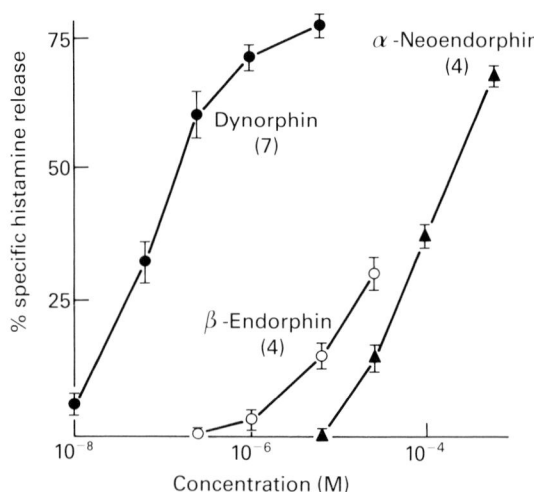

Fig. 24.24 Opioids (dynorphin, β-endorphin and α-neoendorphin) can release histamine from mast cells although with greatly differing efficiencies. Data from [78].

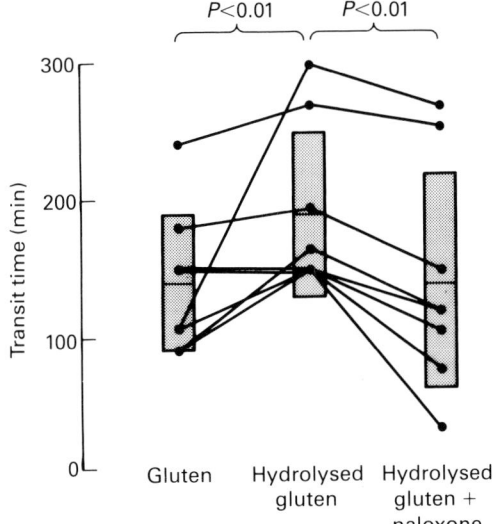

Fig. 24.25 The effect of gluten on intestinal transit time. Intestinal transit was measured by the appearance of breath hydrogen after ingestion of a non-absorbable sugar (lactulose). The transit time was increased significantly when hydrolysed gluten was fed and this effect was substantially blocked by naloxone. Data from [60].

peptides can be produced using enzyme digestion of common dietary proteins in vitro. There is a strong supposition that this also occurs in vivo.

Gastrointestinal function: irritable bowel syndrome. Administration of hydrolysed gluten in humans [60] consistently increased intestinal transit times (Fig. 24.25). There was also an increase in somatostatin-like immunoreactivity, both of which actions were inhibited by naloxone. It is interesting to speculate that exorphins could be causative factors in irritable bowel syndrome, especially as somatostatin is

able to release histamine from mast cells [65], thus producing an allergic picture perhaps similar to 'asthma of the gut', superimposed on the exorphin effect.

Perhaps in future, gastrointestinal diseases may be managed not by food elimination but by exorphin elimination as has been suggested by Morley [58].

Water retention. A feature of many food-sensitive patients is the complaint of water retention or bloating. Water load studies have suggested that food-sensitive subjects on their presenting diet excrete a standard water load poorly, whilst on a successful dietary elimination regime water handling capacity improves (Brostoff and Scadding, unpublished observatons).

An explanation for this may be the action of opiates on vasopressin release [6]. Small doses of morphine (in rats) not only led to an increase in plasma vasopressin (Fig. 24.26) but also to a marked antidiuresis (Fig. 24.27). It has been suggested that radiolabelled peptides of gliadin can reach the brain after oral administration, bind to opiate receptors and trigger their function [70]. Thus, the ingestion of foods which on digestion produce active peptides may lead to a variety of clinical effects such as changes in gut motility, increased somatostatin-like reactivity and possibly an effect on mucosal permeability (not related directly to exorphin activity) as well as a direct effect on the brain.

The complexity of the brain–allergy axis

Aspects of the complex interrelationship between the brain and the psyche with the im-

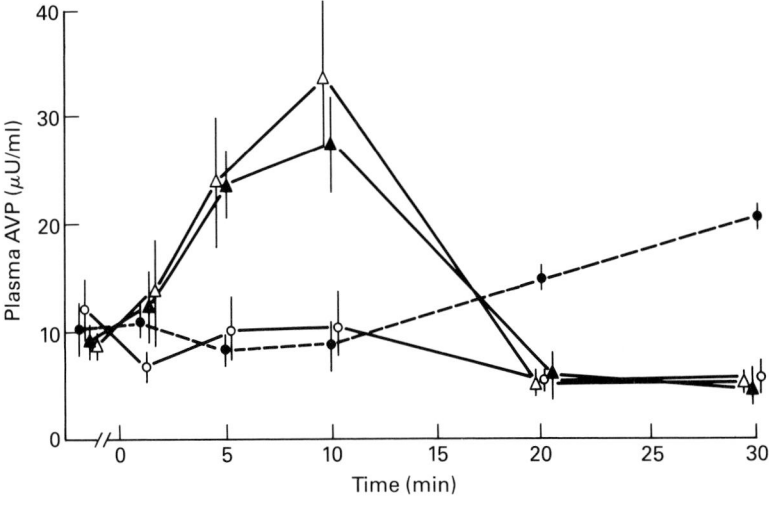

Fig. 24.26 The effect on plasma vasopressin concentrations of doses of 10 μg ($\bigcirc$), 50 μg ($\blacktriangle$) and 150 μg ($\triangle$) of morphine given intracerebroventricularly ($\bullet$ control). The saline controls are represented by the closed circles and dashed line. Each value represents the mean of six observations, vertical bars indicate SE. With optimal dosage, a threefold increase in plasma AVP was seen at 10 minutes. Data from [6].

Fig. 24.27 The effect of intracerebroverticular morphine and intravenous infusion of vasopressin on urine flow in the anaesthetized, water-loaded rat. The effect of morphine and AVP on antidiuresis was similar. Data from [6].

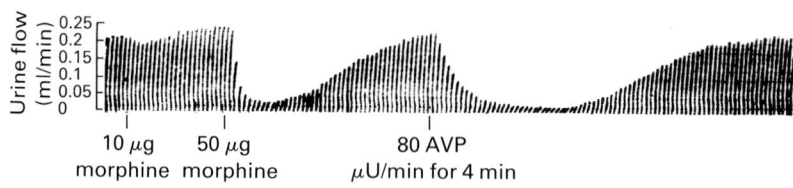

Urine flow (ml/min) — 0.25, 0.2, 0.15, 0.1, 0.05, 0

10 µg morphine   50 µg morphine   80 AVP µU/min for 4 min

mune system and the allergic response have been discussed. Hypnosis and Pavlovian conditioning can alter both antibody- and cell-mediated immunity (see [2]). However, experimental data have not been readily available to show that conditioning can actually produce allergic responses.

Conditioned responses

The report from Russell et al [74] shows that guinea pigs immunized with a foreign protein—bovine serum albumin—and conditioned with an odour at the same time, subsequently released histamine when presented with the odour alone in the absence of the antigen. This is further evidence that immune responses can be enhanced through activity of the central nervous system.

Sex hormones

Grossman [37] has reviewed the regulation of the immune system by gonadal steroids such as oestrogen, progesterone and androgen. Circulating levels of these hormones can also be affected by the immune system itself. For example, in animals, castration can lead to a doubling of the thymus weight and, conversely, thymectomy can lead to oophoritis.

Sinistrality

The left-handed, sinister, subject has been viewed with suspicion over the centuries. Broca demonstrated that although the two symmetrical hemispheres looked similar from the anatomical point of view, they were functionally distinct. Aphasia follows left but not right hemisphere lesions in the majority of individuals. From this followed the concept of further functional asymmetry, i.e. handedness.

Complicating further the brain–allergy axis are the observations by Geschwind [34] who has shown that left-handers have an increased frequency of immune disorders, e.g. migraine, Hashimoto's thyroiditis, coeliac disease and ulcerative colitis. Handedness should be another question added to the history taking.

Lymphokines

Blalock [16] has shown in a series of elegant studies that a lymphokine (interferon) can act as a hormone with ACTH-, melanocyte-stimulating hormone (MSH)- and thyroid-stimulating hormone (TSH)-like activates. Further, interferon has endorphin-like activity in its ability to bind to opiate receptors. The ability of neuropeptide hormones to function as lymphokines and of lymphokines to cause hormonal changes raises the possibility that the neuroendocrine and immune systems may share signals that have common structures [17]. This seems to be the case since lymphocytes have been shown to produce ACTH- and endorphin-like peptides concomitantly with interferon. TSH- and human chorionic gonadotropin (HCG)-like molecules can also be shown to be produced by lymphocytes.

These studies suggest that the immune and neuroendocrine systems represent a totally integrated circuit by sharing a common set of signals and their receptors.

Summary

It could be said that the relationship between the nervous system and peripheral immune function began almost 60 years ago with the description of the triple response in the skin by Sir Thomas Lewis [50]. This was followed by the work of Selye on the many interactions between stress and the immune response [77]. Apart from one well-controlled study by Humphrey showing that the tuberculin reaction could be inhibited by posthypnotic suggestion [15] there was a general lack of interest in these interactions for a number of years until the recent surge of publications.

CONCLUSION

In this chapter I have outlined three areas which reflect the interaction of patients with the food they eat. Immune reactions are clearly important in protecting the patient from antigen and clearing it from the circulation. When these mechanisms go 'wrong' or are exaggerated, hypersensitivity can result. Apart from Type I reactions, there are too few immunological tests to help the clinician make a diagnosis of food allergy which suggests that either the tests will be developed in the future or that many of the reactions that we think of as food allergy are in fact mediated by other mechanisms.

Enzyme deficiencies would also provide a mechanism for food intolerance. Alactasia is well understood and leads to clear-cut clinical symptoms. Of the many potential enzyme defects, I have discussed two others which are centrally involved in detoxification of external chemicals and drugs (xenobiotics). Defects in both these are now described in 'food-allergic' patients. These findings raise the interesting question as to which compound in food is the substrate for these deficient enzymes. For phenol sulphotransferase P the answer is clear: phenolic compounds. For the cytochrome P-450 enzyme system the answer is not so clear. What is sorely needed now are quantitative data on the phenolic content of foods.

Lastly, everyone can appreciate the effect of stress and the psyche on immune function. The profound interaction of the nervous system with the immune system is now becoming clearer. Both systems share messengers and receptors and provide a truly integrated circuit. 'It's not all in the mind'—but some of it might be!

We now have to realize that there is enormous complexity even in the simplest allergic response and the understanding of these complexities will lead to exciting developments in the diagnosis and treatment of our patients.

REFERENCES

1 Aalberse RC, Koshte V, Clements JGJ: IgE antibodies that cross react with vegetables foods, pollens and hymenoptera venom. J Allergy Clin Immunol 1981; 68: 356.

2 Ader R, ed: Psychoneuroimmunology. New York: Academic Press 1981.

3 Andre C, Colin L, Descos L, Daniere J: Non invasive evaluation of intestinal permeability in food allergy. Coeliac disease and inflammatory bowel disease. Gut 1984; 25: A1189.

4 Andre C, Heremans JF, Vaermann JP, Cambiasco CL: A mechanism for the induction of immunological tolerance by antigen feeding: antigen–antibody complexes. J Exp Med 1975; 142: 1059.

5 Atherton DJ, Sewell M, Soothill JF, et al: A double blind controlled crossover trial of an antigen avoidance diet in atopic eczema. Lancet 1978; i: 401.

6 Aziz LA, Forsling ML, Woolf CJL: The effect of intracerebroventricular injections of morphine on vasopressin release in the rat. J Physiol 1981; 311: 401.

7 Bahna SL, Heiner DC: Cows milk allergy. Adv Pediatr. 1978; 25: 1.

8 Barbeau A: The eighth international symposium on Parkinson's disease. New York: 9–12 June, 1985.

9 Barbeau A, Cloutier T, Roy M, et al: Ecogenetics of Parkinson's disease: 4 hydroxylation of debrisoquine. Lancet 1985; ii: 1213.

10 Barratt MEJ, Strachan PJ, Porter P: Antibody mechanisms implicated in digestive disturbances following ingestion of soy-protein in calves and piglets. Clin Exp Immunol 1978; 31: 305.

11 Barrett KM, & Metcalfe DD: (1984) Mast cell heterogeneity: evidence and implications. J Clin Immunol 1984; 235–61.

12 Bartrop RW, Lazarus L, Luckhurst E, Kiloh LH: Depressed lymphocyte function after bereavement. Lancet 1977; i: 834.

13 Belut D, Moneret-Vautrin DA, Nicolas JP, Grilliat JP: IgE levels in intestinal juice. Dig Dis Sci 1980; 25: 323.

14 Bjorksten B: Food sensitivity. Nut Rev 1984; 42: 131.

15 Black S, Humphrey JH, Niven JS: Inhibition of Mantoux reaction by direct suggestion under hypnosis. Br Med J 1963; 534: 1649.

16 Blalock JE: The immune system as a sensory organ. J Immunol 1984; 132: 1067.

17 Blalock JE, Harbour-McMenamin D, Smith EM: Peptide hormones shared by the neuroendocrine and immunologic systems. J Immunol 1985; 135: 858S.

18 Brantl V, Teschemacher H: A material with opioid activity in bovine milk and milk products. Naunyn-Schmeideberg's Arch Pharmacol 1979; 306: 301–4.

19 Broberger O, Perlmann P: Autoantibodies in human ulcerative colitis. J Exp Med 1959; 110: 657.

20 Brostoff J, Carini C, Wraith DG: Food allergy: an IgE complex disorder. Theoretical and clinical aspects of allergic disease. Stockholm: Almquist and Wiksell International, 1983.

21 Brostoff J, Johns P, Stanworth DR: Complexed IgE in atopy. Lancet 1977; ii: 741.

22 Brostoff J, Carini C, Wraith DG, Johns P: Production of IgE complexes by allergen challenge in atopic patients and the effect of sodium cromoglycate. Lancet 1979; ii: 1268.

23 Brostoff J, Carini C, Wraith DG, et al: Immune complexes in atopy. In: Pepys J, Edwards AM, eds. Mast cell. London: Pitman. 1979; 380.

24 Buisseret PD, Youlten LJF, Heinzelmann DL, Lessof M: Prostaglandin synthesis inhibitors in prophylaxis of food intolerance. Lancet 1978; i: 906.

25 Casale TB, Bowman S, Kaliner M: Induction of human cutaneous mast cell degranulation by opiates and endogenous opioid peptides: evidence for opiate and non-opiate receptor participation. J Allergy Clin Immunol 1984; 73: 775.

26 Dahl R, Zetterstrom O: The effect of orally administered sodium cromoglycate on allergic reactions caused by food allergens. Clin Allergy 1978; 8: 419.

27 Dannaeus A, Inganas M, Johansson SGO, Foucard T: Intestinal uptake of ovalbumin in malabsorption and

food allergy in relation to serum IgG antibody and orally administered sodium cromoglycate. Clin Allergy 1979; 9: 263.

28 De Carolis C, De Sanctis G, Perricone R et al: Evidence for an inhibitory role of beta-endorphin and other opioids on human total T rosette formation. Experientia 1984; 40: 738.

29 Dohan FC: Is celiac disease a clue to the pathogenesis of schizophrenia? Ment Hygiene 1969; 53: 525-9.

30 Editorial: Emotion and immunity. Lancet 1985; ii: 133.

31 Evans DAP, Mahgoub A, Sloan TP et al: A population and family study of the genetic polymorphism of debrisoquine oxidation in a British white population. J Med Genet 1980; 17: 102-5.

32 Falchuk KR, Isselbacher KJ: Circulating antibodies to bovine albumin in ulcerative colitis and Crohns disease. Gastroenterology 1976; 70: 5-8.

33 Freedman SO, Siddiavi JH, Krupey JH, Sehon AH: Identification of a simple chemical compound (chlorogenic acid) as an allergen in plant material causing human atopic disease. Am J Med Sci 1962; 244: 548.

34 Geschwind N, Behan P: Left handedness: association with immune disease, migraine and developmental learning disorder. Proc Nat Acad Sci USA 1982; 79: 5097.

35 Gray GM: Absorption and malabsorption of dietary carbohydrates. In: Nutrition and gastroenterology. New York: Wiley, 1980. Winick M, ed.

36 Gray GM: Intestinal disaccharidase deficiencies and glucose-galactose malabsorption. In: Stanbury JB, Wyngaarden JB, Fredrickson DS et al, eds. The metabolic basis of inherited disease, 5th edn New York: McGraw Hill, 1983; 1729-42.

37 Grossman CJ: Interactions between the gonadal steroids and the immune system. Science 1985; 227: 257.

38 Gyenes L, Gordon J, Sehon AH: Ultracentrifugation characterisation of antibodies in sera of ragweed sensitive individuals. Immunology 1961; 4: 177.

39 Hanington E, Harper AM: The role of tyramine in the aetiology of migraine and related studies on the cerebral and extracerebral circulations. Headache 1968; 8: 84-97.

40 Idle JR, Mahgoub A, Sloan TP et al: Some observations on the oxidative phenotype status of Nigerian patients presenting with cancer. Cancer Lett 1981; 11: 331-8.

41 Ishizaka K, Ishizaka T, Hornbrook MM: Physiochemical properties of human reaginic antibody. IV. Presence of a unique immunoglobulin as a carrier of reaginic activity. J Immunol 1966; 97: 75.

42 Jemmott JB, Borysenko JZ, Borysenko M et al: Academic stress, power motivation and decrease in secretion rate of salivary secretory immunoglobulin A. Lancet 1983; i: 1400.

43 Johnson GB: Importance of substrate variability to enzyme polymorphism. Nature 1973; 243: 151-3.

44 Johnson GB: Enzyme polymorphism and metabolism. Science 1974; 184: 28-37.

45 Kilshaw PJ, Hester-Slade H: Passage of ingested protein into the blood during gastrointestinal hypersensitivity reactions experiments in the preruminant calf. Clin Exp Immunol 1980; 6: 45.

46 Lagerkrantz R, Hammarstrom S, Perlmann P, Gustafsson: Immunological studies of ulcerative colitis. IV. Origin of autoantibodies. J Exp Med 1968; 128: 1339.

47 Littlewood J, Glover V, Sandler M et al: Platelet phenolsulphotransferase deficiency in dietary migraine. Lancet 1982; i: 983.

48 Levin B, Abraham JM, Burgess EA, Wallis PG: Congenital lactose malabsorption. Arch Dis Child 1970; 45: 173-7.

49 Lewin R: Parkinson's disease: an environmental cause. Science 1985; 229: 257.

50 Lewis T: The blood vessels of the human skin and their responses. London: Shaw and Sons, 1927.

51 Mahgoub A, Idle JR, Dring LG et al: Polymorphic hydroxylation of debrisoquine in man. Lancet 1977; ii: 584-6.

52 May CD: Objective clinical and laboratory studies of immediate hypersensitivity reactions to foods in asthmatic children. J Allergy Clin Immunol 1976; 58: 500.

53 Mbanefo C, Bababunmi EA, Mahgoub A et al: A study of debrisoquine hydroxylation polymorphism in a Nigerian population. Xenobiotica 1980; 19: 819-25.

54 Mellstrom B, Bertillson L, Sawe J et al: E- and Z-10-hydroxylation of nortriptyline: relationship to polymorphic debrisoquine hydroxylation. Clin Pharmacol Ther 1981; 30: 189-93.

55 Metcalfe DD: Food hypersensitivity. J Allergy Clin Immunol. 1984; 73: 749.

56 Moffett A, Swash M, Scott DF: Effect of tyramine in migraine: a double blind study. J Neurol Neurosurg Psychiatry 1972; 35: 496-9.

57 Monro J, Carini C, Brostoff J, Zilka K: Food allergy in migraine. Lancet 1980; ii: 1.

58 Morley JE: Food peptides. A new class of hormones? J Am Med Assoc 1982; 247: 2379.

59 Morley JS Chemistry of opioid peptides. Br Med Bull 1983; 39: 5.

60 Morley JS, Levine AS, Yamada T et al: Effect of exorphins on gastrointestinal function, hormonal release, and appetite. Gastroenterology 1983; 84: 1517-23.

61 Oates NS, Shah RR, Idle JR, Smith RL: Genetic polymorphism of phenformin 4-hydroxylation. Clin Pharmacol Ther 1982; 32: 81-9.

62 Pagnelli R, Levinsky RJ, Brostoff J, Wraith DG: Immune complexes containing food proteins in normal and atopic subjects after oral challenge and the effect of sodium cromoglycate on antigen absorption. Lancet 1979; i: 321.

63 Parke AL, Hughes GRV: Rheumatoid arthritis and food: a case study. Br Med J 1981; 282: 2027.

64 Paterson SJ, Robson LE, Kosterlitz HW: Classification of opioid receptors. Br Med Bull 1983; 39: 31.

65 Payan DG, Levine JD, Goetzl EJ: Modulation of immunity and hypersensitivity by sensory neuropeptides. J Immunol 1984; 132: 1601.

66 Pearce FL, Befus AD, Bienenstock J: Mucosal mast cells. Effect of quercitin and other flavonoids on antigen induced histamine secretion from rat intestinal mast cells. J Allergy Clin Immunol 1984; 73: 819.

67 Pearce FL, Ali H, Barrett KE et al: Mast cell heterogeneity: frontiers in histamine research. Oxford: Pergamon Press, 1984.

68 Perkkio M: Immunohistochemical study of intestinal biopsies from children with atopic eczema due to food allergy. Allergy 1980; 35: 573.

69 Rabin BS, Rogers SJ: A cell mediated immune model of inflammatory bowel disease in the rabbit. Gastroenterology 1978; 75: 29.

70 Rinkel HJ, Randolph TG, Zeller M: Food allergy. Springfield, Ill: Charles C Thomas, 1951.

71 Ritchie JC, Crothers MJ, Idle JR et al: Evidence for an inherited metabolic susceptibility to endemic (Balkan) nephropathy. In: Strahinjic S, Stefanovic V, eds. Proceedings of the 5th Symposium on endemic (Balkan) nephropathy.

72 Rowe AH: Food allergy. Springfield, Ill: Charles C Thomas, 1931.

73 Royal College of Physicians and the British Nutrition Foundation: a joint report: Food intolerance and food aversion. J R Coll Physicians 1984; 18: 3.

74 Russell M, Dark KA, Cummins RW et al: Learned histamine release. Science 1984; 225: 733.

75 Ryan RE Jr: A clinical study of tyramine as an aetiological factor in migraine. Headache 1974; 14: 43–8.

76 Sattaur O: New roles for 'vitamin C'. New Scientist 1985; 11 July: 23.

77 Selye H: The story of the adaptation syndrome. Montreal: Acta Inc Medical Publishers, 1952.

78 Shanahan F, Lee TDG, Binenstock J, Befus AD: The influence of endorphins on peritoneal and mucosal cell secretion. J Allergy Clin Immunol 1984; 74: 499.

79 Shiada H, Mishima T, Yamada S et al: Nasal smears in the diagnosis of food allergy. In: Pepys J, Edwards AM, eds. Mast cell. London: Pitman. 1979; 422.

80 Shorter PC, Cardogan M, Spencer RJ et al: Further studies of in vitro cytotoxicity of lymphocytes from patients with ulcerative and granulomatous colitis for allogeneic colonic epithelial cells, including the effects of colectomy. Gastroenterology 1969; 56: 304–9.

81 Sloan TP, Mahgoub A, Lancaster R et al: Polymorphism of carbon oxidation of drugs and clinical implications. Br Med J 1978; 655–7.

82 Stein M, Keller SE, Schleifer SJ: Stress and immunomodulation. The role of depression and neuroendocrine function. J Immunol 1984; 135: 8275.

83 Waring RH, Mitchell SC, Shah RR et al: Polymorphic sulphoxidation of S-carboxymethyl-L-cysteine in man. Biochem Pharmacol 1982; 31: 3151–4.

84 Williams RC, Griffiths RW, Emmons JD, Field RC: Naturally occurring human antiglobulins with specificity for gamma E. J Clin Invest 1972; 51: 455.

85 Zioudrou C, Klee WA: Possible roles of peptides from food proteins in brain function. In: Wurtman RJ, Wurtman JJ, Eds. Nutrition and the brain. New York: Raven Press, 1979; 125–58.

86 Zioudrou C, Streaty RA, Klee WA: Opioid peptides derived from food proteins. The exorphins. J Biol Chem 1979; 254: 2446–9.

Chapter 25
Anaphylaxis in Relation to Food Allergy

A. W. Frankland

Definition

Anaphylaxis is the most urgent of clinical immunological events but, as will be discussed, it is often incorrectly treated. It results from an explosive generation and release of a variety of potent, biologically active mediators and their concerted effects on various tissue organs. It has been defined to denote an IgE-mediated antigen-induced reaction in animals and humans but this definition is too narrow, so that it is better to think of anaphylaxis as a clinical descriptive term for symptoms producing a severe, abrupt, untoward event often with unknown immunological significance. Essentially, therefore, anaphylaxis is a clinical syndrome with a multiplicity of inciting aetiological agents and a variety of pathological mechanisms.

It is of some interest that the first research in immunology was carried out by a food (fish)-sensitive individual. Küstner had been highly sensitive to fish since the age of six years. What is strange about Küstner's fish allergy was that he was sensitive to cooked fish but not to raw fish. Usually cooking destroys, or partially destroys, the allergenicity of foods for many of those patients allergic to foods. Küstner's serum, when injected into the non-fish-sensitive Prausnitz's skin, sensitized the skin locally by passive transfer of fish antibodies. Strangely, they were unable to do the reverse, i.e. passively sensitize Küstner's skin with Prausnitz's pollen allergy [25].

Anaphylaxis has both a clinical meaning and an immunological meaning. The clinical usage of the term tends to be restricted to generalized shock and possibly collapse occurring when a patient reacts to a food (or drug) to which he is anaphylactically sensitive. Anaphylaxis as an immunological term designates those allergic reactions which are initiated by antigen (allergen) reacting with anaphylactically sensitized mast or basophil cells in the tissue. This is often referred to as an immediate Type I reaction because the signs and symptoms appear within minutes of reaction with the antigen. However, many food reactions that will be discussed are not immediate and are not IgE mediated. It is unfortunate that there is no experimental model that compares exactly to anaphylaxis in man. Some of the problems in investigating and treating anaphylaxis in man have been recently reviewed [12].

ANAPHYLACTOID REACTIONS

IgG reaginic antibody

The classical anaphylactic antibody in man is the IgE reagin and man may also form an IgG anaphylactic antibody. However, in many clinical conditions which appear to be mediated by anaphylactic changes especially in skin and lung, no antigen or indeed specific antibody can be demonstrated. The patient may or may not be atopic and although the same pharmacological substances may be released to cause the symptoms, the stimulus for their release differs. Therefore, clinically we must distinguish between anaphylactic reactions and anaphylactoid (anaphylaxis-like) reactions. It must be admitted that when someone reacts quickly and quite severely to a food, yet the reaction is not IgE mediated, there is a tendency to refer to all such non-immunologically mediated reactions as anaphylactoid. Some anaphylactoid reactions result from aggregation and mediator release from platelets when induced by antigen–antibody complexes. It seems likely that this may be a possible mechanism of some food allergic reactions (see Table 25.1).

Table 25.1 Some causes of anaphylactoid reactions.

IgG reaginic antibody
Aspirin sensitivity
Food-induced anaphylaxis (non-IgE mediated)
Urticaria and hereditary angioedema
Food additives and preservatives

Aspirin sensitivity

In the aspirin-sensitive asthmatic, although we can measure many of the very active substances that are released in an anaphalactoid reaction, the changes are measured indirectly by mediator release. There may be an immunological mechanism which can be measured because specific anti-salicylol IgE and IgG levels can often be measured. It could be argued that immunological reactions are related clinically to the mediator release of many very active substances. It would be the hope of immunologists, however, to know by what mechanisms the reactions are initiated and to

be able to demonstrate that the food (or drug) is acting as an antigen.

Food-induced anaphylaxis

When an immediate reaction due to a food is IgE mediated, the measurement of specific IgE and the demonstration of specific skin tests is not difficult. The difficulty arises when there may be a severe anaphylactic or anaphylactic-like reaction to a food and there are no positive tests for IgE antibody.

Food antigens in breast milk

It is interesting that over 60 years ago, Shannon [30] demonstrated the presence of food antigens in breast milk by inducing anaphylactic reactions in guinea pigs sensitized to egg protein by challenging them with breast milk from a woman taking eggs in her diet. We know that cow's milk and other food proteins may be detectable in breast milk, and this may explain not only why breast feeding may not protect the infant from allergic disease, but also why an infant may have an anaphylactic response the first time it receives such foods as milk or eggs. There may be other reasons that explain why a child reacts to a food the first time it ever attempts to eat it. A few million molecules of peanut butter which become airborne when a parent eats it may be enough to sensitize a young child to the food, so that the first time it eats a peanut (groundnut), it will experience an allergic reaction (Fig. 25.1). This could manifest itself as gross facial oedema followed by diarrhoea, vomiting and shock. We must use the word anaphylaxis when we can demonstrate that the reaction is mediated by IgE antibodies but may use the word anaphylactoid when antigen–antibody reactions cannot be demonstrated.

Urticaria and hereditary angioedema

Urticaria may occur in a patient who also has an unrelated hereditary angioedema associated with C1 esterase inhibitor deficiency. The latter condition, occurring independently, might be thought to be a manifestation of food-induced anaphylaxis when severe abdominal symptoms occur. It must, therefore, be remembered that allergic urticaria and hereditary angioedema can occur independently in the same patient, so that food elimination and anabolic steroids are required for successful treatment in such a patient [21].

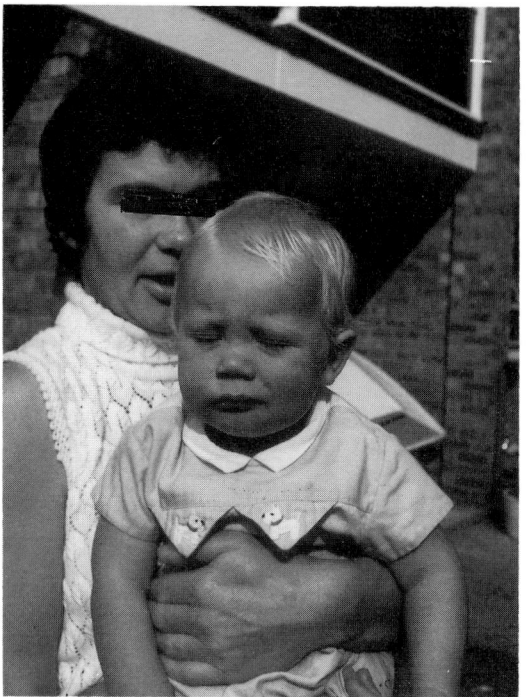

Fig. 25.1 Acute allergic reaction to peanut. Photograph taken 5 minutes after eating and before onset of generalized urticaria and shock.

Food additives and preservatives

When someone has a severe, and often unexpected, anaphylactic reaction during or just after a meal, particularly a restaurant meal, it is easy to say that the reaction was 'allergic'. However, this may often be impossible to prove and it is better to limit the use of the term 'allergic' to those reactions that are immunologically mediated or can be presumed to be. Very often anecdotal accounts with no documented proof have blamed serious reactions on various food additives. Food additives and preservatives are examples of substances that have been used for years but have recently been recognized as being hazardous to some people. Metabisulphate may cause anaphylaxis [26]. It may be that sulphur dioxide, rather than the bisulphate, is what causes the acute symptoms. This is known to be the case in some asthmatics who use aerosols that contain bisulphate. The asthma may become worse or anaphylaxis may occur [34].

Normally the ubiquitous tissue enzyme, sulphite oxidase, converts sulphite (HSO_3) into the inactive sulphate (SO_4). It seems that 5 mg of sulphite orally may induce asthma in those patients who are very sensitive to sulphate or sulphur dioxide. It would seem that the sulphite oxidase enzyme is substantially reduced in the sulphite-sensitive asthmatic [15]. It may be, but it has yet to be proved, that it is this group that is particularly liable to have an anaphylactic response after eating in restaurants. It will be the large amount of preservatives in the food rather than an individual food that causes the reaction. It has been found that the patients shown to be most sensitive to oral challenge were not the same patients most sensitive to inhalation challenge. It has been shown [24] that all asthmatic subjects have bronchoconstriction after inhalation exposure of 1 to 5 ppm of sulphur dioxide. The mechanism for this reaction has been demonstrated to be a direct stimulation of different receptors in the bronchi by inhaled sulphur dioxide. A lot more work remains to be done to find out whether sulphite preservatives in food may not cause both asthma and food anaphylaxis.

CLINICAL ASPECTS OF FOOD-INDUCED ANAPHYLAXIS

Age of onset

Anaphylaxis due to foods is commoner in infancy and early childhood but it can occur in adults when, for unknown reasons, an acute IgE reaction may develop to a food which previously has been enjoyed for years. Such a patient, seen recently, became acutely allergic to sesame seed at the age of 50. In the past, she had often had bread with sesame seed on it and had used sesame in soups and biscuits. She noticed that a biscuit she was eating seemed to cause tingling of the buccal mucous membrane and irritation of the throat. In a few minutes she had developed a mild urticaria which disappeared in an hour. Two weeks later, she had another sesame biscuit. In five minutes, she realized her lips and eyelids were becoming swollen; she then developed a gross generalized urticaria, felt very ill and phoned for her husband to come immediately. He found her unconscious on the floor. She gave a positive wheal and flare response to a sesame skin prick test. It would seem that some people after many years can become anaphylactically allergic to a food in the same way that it may be years before the bee keeper, after many stings, becomes anaphylactically allergic to the venom. This contrasts to most food anaphylactic responses which may begin in infancy and generally, but not always, disappear. Death in infancy from food anaphylaxis is rare but was described by Finkelstein [11].

Development

Quite often the acute reaction occurs the first time the child eats some food containing egg or drinks some milk. Maternal dietary antigens can cross the placenta to enter the fetal circulation so that IgE food antigens have been detected in newborn infants [17, 20]. But we know that food antigens such as egg and cow's milk are also found in human milk and this may be the more likely way that babies are sensitized. The smell of food can provoke rhinitis and asthma in someone sensitized to the food and inhalation may be one of the ways a patient becomes sensitized. Parents or other children eating peanut butter could sensitize the baby if it repeatedly inhales a few million molecules of peanut from peanut butter.

Parish et al [23] suggested that some sudden cot deaths might be due to an anaphylactic reaction to cow's milk. This might happen with a regurgitation of cow's milk during an upper respiratory tract infection. Using the same model, it was shown that the sensitizing capacities of infant milk formulae varied [4]. If the results of these experiments were extrapolated to human infants, the observations could be very important.

Severity of response

There are varying grades of severity of anaphylaxis. These have been described in patients who are venom allergic [13], and similar grades occur in food anaphylactic reactions. Although the reactions can be very severe, death from a food anaphylactic reaction is very rare. In its mildest form, the responses are entirely cutaneous with erythema, pruritis, urticaria and angioedema. The latter may be amazingly unilateral on the face. Only half of the upper or lower lip may be involved or only one eyelid. But both eyelids may be so swollen that the patient cannot see. Beside lip swelling which is easily seen, there is often gross oedema of the buccal mucosa. The tongue may become so swollen that the patient has to keep the mouth open and the tongue protrudes through the teeth. The soft palate and particularly the uvula may become very swollen, speaking becomes difficult and it is about this time that there is difficulty in breathing, not only from the oedematous throat but because asthma has supervened. The respiratory difficulty can be made worse by acute abdominal pain and vomiting which may be followed by diarrhoea. When there is an associated generalized urticaria, hypotension with loss of consciousness may occur.

Case history 1: Fish allergy. I have no knowledge that anyone has required a tracheotomy because of food anaphylaxis; arrangements were made for such an operation—but not used—on a small boy aged six years who was made to eat fish in hospital. He had always been very fish allergic, but his mother forgot to impart this fact to the Ward when her son was admitted for a minor operation. It is as well to remember that a deeply unconscious patient can still have severe food anaphylaxis. This happened in an intensive care unit where a girl aged 14, (who was unconscious from a fractured base of skull as a result of a riding accident), was tube fed with egg. She had had eczema and asthma since infancy and had always been very acutely allergic to eggs.

Natural history

Most, but not all, children seem to grow out of their reaction after a few years [27]. Unfortunately, some patients retain their acute food allergy throughout life. One such patient, aged 76, who has had lifelong eczema and severe asthma, still retains her acute fish sensitivity.

However, the natural history of anyone with an IgE-mediated food allergy is unknown. Although most IgE reactions to foods disappear with increasing age [27], those that do not, remain a social rather than a medical problem. Many adult patients who have food anaphylaxis react to the food that has always caused an immediate reaction. These patients nearly always retain the atopic stigmata of eczema and asthma that have been present since early childhood. Adults, not children, develop shellfish anaphylaxis. This is perhaps because children have not eaten shellfish and it may take two or three decades before shellfish reactions suddenly appear. It must be remembered that patients may not necessarily be atopic for them suddenly to develop, at any age, an acute food allergy.

Common food allergens

The basic treatment for all IgE-proven reactions is, without doubt, to identify the allergen that produces the reaction and avoid it. This is often possible with inhalant allergens, but can be very difficult on occasions when a common food allergen is involved. A patient aged 18 knew that a minute amount of mustard, when ingested, would cause immediate anaphylactic shock. As a result of bitter experience, with many hospital admissions, she had decided never to eat away from home. To celebrate her birthday, she had dinner at a restaurant and ate some salmon with mayonnaise which, she was assured, contained no mustard. Unfortunately, the waiter who served her and who had said he double checked with the chef, was not speaking the truth. The mustard in a very small amount of mayonnaise caused immediate anaphylactic symptoms requiring emergency hospital treatment.

An infant under the age of one year will instinctively spit out egg that is causing an immediate reaction in the mouth. But egg, fish, nuts (including peanut which is a pulse) and, occasionally, milk can all cause immediate and severe anaphylactic shock with gross oedema of the face, abdominal pain, vomiting and diarrhoea, wheezing and urticaria. Skin prick tests with the appropriate food allergen that causes anaphylaxis are quite safe and confirm the diagnosis, even in an infant aged three months. If a child has more than one acute food allergy, it might be prudent to prick test only one food at a session. The individual response may be very specific so that patients sensitive to one nut are not necessarily allergic to all nuts or, if to fish, to all fish. Peanut, which is a not uncommon allergen in very young children, may be the only food allergen causing acute anaphylaxis. Measles vaccine appears safe in the egg-sensitive child [16], but vaccines produced in ova, like influenza, have caused anaphylactic reactions in people with egg allergy [7]. Virtually any food can cause anaphylaxis (Table 25.2).

Table 25.2 Foods causing anaphylaxis.

Egg	Fish
Shellfish	Nuts
Peanut	Milk
Milk products	Chocolate
Bananas	Citrus fruits
Sesame	Mango
Vegetables	Grains
Meats	Seeds
Chinese	Others

Case history 2: Cow's milk allergy. A female, followed up for 25 years, remains anaphylactically sensitive to cow's milk. She is an interesting case because the first time cow's milk was spilt on her leg when she was four months old, the mother thought she had scalded her infant. She then realized that the local response was only urticarial, as it disappeared quickly. When still breast feeding her 14-month-old child, she put a drop of milk with a pipette into a glass of water and gave a teaspoonful of this very diluted milk to her daughter to drink. The child had an immediate anaphylactic response. This patient, at the age of 16, was successfully hyposensitized but, on discontinuing the injections, she relapsed and still cannot eat any dairy product. Socially, she finds her acute allergy to a common ingredient of the diet very embarrassing.

Uncommon causes

Case history 3: Hazel and silver birch. A patient aged 46 had had seasonal allergic rhinitis due to grass pollen but also an increasing amount of Spring hay fever with an associated asthma usually beginning about the third week in April and lasting two or three weeks. Grass pollen in June and July caused only mild hay fever and no associated asthma. Skin tests confirmed that she reacted to all the catkin-bearing tree pollens, including hazel (*Corylus*) and silver birch (*Betula*) pollens. After eating a hazel nut, she immediately developed swollen lips, itchy palate and urticaria which became so alarming that she required treatment at a hospital emergency department. About 50% of patients who are hazel-pollen-allergic will also react to the hazel nut.

Fresh fruit sensitivity

Some patients have mild reactions of irritation of the buccal mucous membrane and of the lips and itchy throat when they eat raw celery, apples or carrots. These sensitivities could be confirmed by vast wheal and flare responses using the prick method, the needle having previously just been plunged into a fresh apple, carrot or celery.

Fresh fruit sensitivity, which occurs in association with various specific pollen allergies, is probably more common than is realized (Table 25.3). The immunological and clinical reactions have recently been reviewed [1]. In spite of the very large prick skin responses that can be obtained with fresh extracts, such sen-

Table 25.3 Fresh fruits, vegetables and nuts causing immediate reactions in patients allergic to silver birch pollen.

Almond	Celery	Melon	Raisins
Apple	Currants	Orange	Raspberry
Apricot	Gooseberry	Peach	
Blackberry	Grapes	Plum	
Carrot	Hazelnut	Potato	

sitivities normally cause only local discomfort in the mouth, rarely mild generalized urticaria and, only very occasionally, anaphylaxis.

Case history 4: Fructose intolerance. Allergists are often asked to see patients with possible food intolerances causing many different kinds of symptoms, but it must be very unusual to be asked to see a patient with 'food anaphylaxis' who was not anaphylactic and whose symptoms had nothing to do with allergy. The lady, when first seen aged 33, knew that she had not been able to eat puddings, fruit or sweets since early infancy without severe abdominal pain followed by vomiting and diarrhoea. On a few occasions she had become unconscious at the end of the attacks—from hypoglycaemia. She was suffering from hereditary fructose intolerance which, strangely, had never been diagnosed [8].

Chinese food

Although the same clinical conditions can be induced by immunological mechanisms, the pathways which also lead to the non-immunological causal event often remain to be established. Chinese food has been reported to cause many allergic reactions and monosodium glutamate seems in some established asthmatic individuals to produce asthmatic attacks [3]. An important component in Chinese food is tangeh, a sprouted small green bean which makes up a typical Chinese egg-roll. A patient is described [33] who had reactions to various inhalant and food allergens as well as exercise-induced urticaria and angioedema, and who developed generalized urticaria and angioedema within 15 minutes of eating tangeh in a Chinese restaurant. She gave a specific positive skin prick test to tangeh as well as showing a specific histamine release and RAST (radioallergoabsorbent test). Some patients with IgE to peanut also have IgE antibodies against tangeh. As peanut is one of the commonest foods causing some IgE-related

symptoms, it may be that this group of patients is especially liable to have an allergic reaction after eating Chinese food. However, it must be admitted that many of the often late rather than immediate reactions that occur after eating Chinese food are not immunologically produced and should be called pseudo-allergic and not anaphylactic.

Anaphylaxis to antibiotics in food

Beef cattle are often treated with antibiotics before being sold for the market. Moreover, antibiotics, particularly penicillin and streptomycin, are readily available in feed stores or obtainable from veterinary surgeons for various reasons. Different countries have various laws to deal with the potential hazard of antibiotics in food. It is recommended that there is a withdrawal of all antibiotics for a stated interval prior to slaughter for market. Milk must not be sold from a cow receiving penicillin for mastitis.

Case history 5: Antibiotic allergy. A case had been described of a 14-year-old girl who had had four anaphylactic reactions from beef over a period of a year. It was puzzling because she often could eat beef without difficulty. It was found from prick and Prausnitz–Küstner tests that she was allergic to streptomycin. She had had an injection of streptomycin at the age of three years. The authors make the point that 'idiopathic' anaphylaxis is not always idiopathic [32].

Penicillin has been estimated to be responsible for 75% of anaphylactic deaths [9]. Anaphylaxis has been reported [35] from penicillin added to a soft drink and from hidden sources of penicillin in foods. Anaphylaxis has been described in a patient known to be allergic to penicillin who had a severe anaphylactic reaction after eating a frozen steak dinner which was shown to contain penicillin or penicilloyl groups [29].

Penicillin in milk

Legal requirements are that milk should not be sold which might contain more than 0.02 i.u./ml penicillin. A farmer may treat one infected udder of a cow with penicillin and he may not want to stop selling the milk from this cow for a week or longer. So quite large amounts of penicillin would be in the milk from the treated cow. The large milk distributors in a city such as London, will carry out daily penicillin estimations on their bulk supplies. This is not to protect the potential penicillin-allergic individual but because, if penicillin is present, any unsold milk cannot be made into cheese or yoghurt. The whole subject of the supposed reactions—usually urticaria, and not anaphylaxis—has recently been reviewed [10]. It was pointed out that cases of so-called penicillin allergy due to milk as reported in the literature are very poorly documented and do not seem to pose a significant public health problem, although anaphylaxis due to penicillin in milk occurred in the patient who also reacted to penicillin in soft drinks [36].

TREATMENT OF FOOD-INDUCED ANAPHYLAXIS

Hyposensitization

Rush desensitization

Incremental hyposensitization therapy (high dose) can be considered experimental and potentially hazardous. Clinically, the results of immunotherapy can be successful, and were in the milk-allergic patient described above as long as the patient continued the injections. In another patient, with an acute egg allergy, treatment was partially successful, in that it allowed him to eat foods containing egg but not eggs themselves. He persisted with his injections once a month until, after a gap of no injections for two months, a repeat dose caused a worrying anaphylactic response.

Food allergens used for skin tests are largely unstandardized and the label of a commercially made extract may be very uninformative as to its content. Although a purified allergen is available from codfish [2] (see Chapter 19), we do not know whether a patient may have reactions to other antigenic determinants which do not cross-react with the pure allergen. Clinically, patients may note that some, but not all, fish cause an immediate reaction.

Case history 6. This was well established by the patient who, in 1971, was the first to be successfully immunized against his acute egg allergy. This was done by rush desensitization in hospital over a period of 12 days. At the end of the course of injections, he could, for the first time in his life, eat eggs. One or two of the very low doses caused mild generalized urticaria as did the first dose out of the strongest bottle (0.1 ml of whole egg 1/10 w/v) (Table

25.4). He did not attend for follow-up but two years later reported that he wanted to be desensitized now to fish which, all his life, had caused anaphylactic reactions. Kissing his new girl friend, half an hour after she had eaten fish, caused him acute mouth and lip swelling. He was again successfully hyposensitized to cod using the rush method. After 14 days in

Table 25.4 Rush desensitization schedule.

Day	Dose (ml)	Dilution (w/v)
1 every 4 hours (5/day)	0.01	10^{-10}
	0.10	↓
↓		10^{-7}
3	0.01	10^{-6}
	0.10	↓
↓	0.50	10^{-2}
6	0.01	10^{-1}
	0.10	
↓	0.20	
12	0.30	
	↓	
	1.0	

hospital, he had a meal of cod which he had never before tasted, without any reaction. Three days later, he had one mouthful of herring and had to have emergency treatment in hospital for anaphylactic shock. This patient shows both the success and failure of treatment with immunotherapy in the anaphylactically food-allergic patient.

Fungal spore sensitivity

There are many substances taken as drinks which can cause an allergic reaction but only rarely anaphylaxis. Some patients who have allergic symptoms to inhalant fungal spores may be allergic to various yeasts. It is such patients who may find that even a small amount of champagne will cause almost immediate severe asthma. One such patient had a drink of 'Marmite' which is basically a brewer's yeast extract. As she finished drinking she had an immediate severe anaphylactic attack and became unconscious with asthma as the presenting symptom, followed by generalized urticaria.

Symptomatic treatment

The diagnosis of acute anaphylaxis should not be difficult even if the immediate cause of the reaction is not known. The physician is dealing with an urgent medical emergency and the

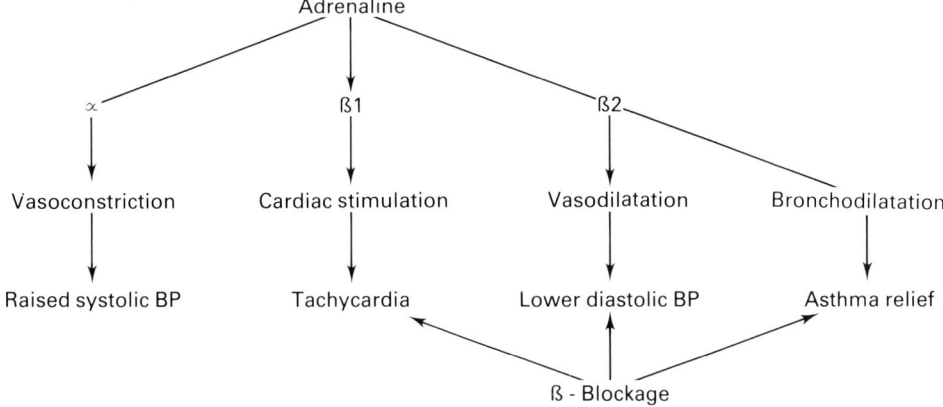

Fig. 25.2 Adrenaline helps anaphylaxis unless patient is on β-blocking drugs.

immediate treatment is an injection of adrenaline 1:1000 (Table 25.5, Fig. 25.2). This is usually given in a dose of 0.5 ml, deep subcutaneously. This dose can safely be repeated in 15 minutes and again after another 30 minutes if necessary. The blood pressure should be continuously recorded until it is normal. When there is gross urticaria, with or without facial oedema, it may be decided to give an injectable antihistamine, such as diphenhydramine. The dose of this antihistamine is 10 mg given either i.m. or i.v. This may be followed by 100 mg hydrocortisone i.m. or i.v. It must

Table 25.5 Drugs for the treatment of acute anaphylaxis.

Adrenaline 1:1000
0.5 ml s.c. and repeat in 15 minutes and again after 30 minutes if necessary

Antihistamine e.g. diphenhydramine 10 mg i.v. or i.m.
Hydrocortisone 100 mg i.v. or i.m.

Isoprenaline or adrenaline aerosol
5–10 puffs every 5 minutes

Isoprenaline tablet 10 mg under the tongue

---

be stressed that antihistamines and corticosteroids are not acutely anti-anaphylactic but may be given to suppress any non-immediate symptoms that might occur [6] (Fig. 25.3).

It is unfortunate that so often after an acute anaphylactic response due to a food, the treatment given is a steroid injection, presumably

Erythema ⇨ Pruritus ⇨ Urticaria ⇨ Angio-oedema

⇨ Laryngeal oedema ⇨ Difficulty in breathing

⇨ Asthma ⇨ Vomiting ⇨ Diarrhoea

⇨ Hypotension ⇨ Unconsciousness

TREAT with ADRENALINE

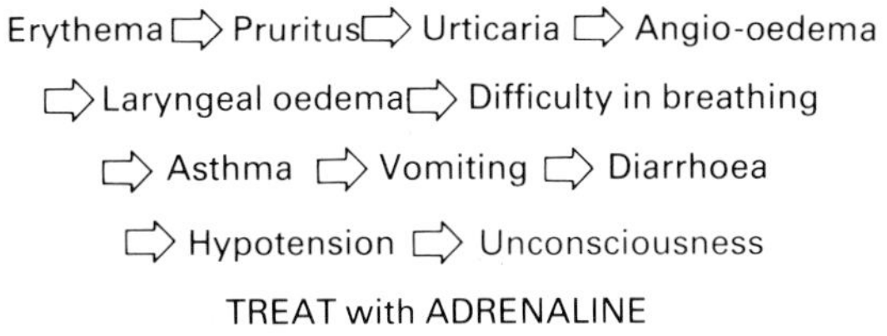

Fig. 25.3 Anaphylactic reaction.

on the basis that the reaction is an immunological one. Sometimes the patient remains in a state of shock with the blood pressure almost unrecordable so that volume replacement and α-adrenergic agonists will be necessary. Isoprenaline tablets, chewed into fragments and dissolved under the tongue, provide an easily available treatment that the patient can carry around at all times. Another practical first aid measure is to use a pressurized atomizer, such as asthmatics use, of isoprenaline or adrenaline. Five to ten puffs can be used every five minutes, if such an atomiser is available (Table 25.5).

β-Blockers and anaphylaxis

Some patients may be on continued β-blockers—these may include propranolol, stenolol, oxprenolol, nadolol, pindolol, timolol and solatol. β-Adrenergic drugs may be used in hypertension, angina pectoris, cardiac arrhythmias, phaeochromocytoma, thyrotoxicosis and migraine. Patients taking these drugs may have very severe anaphylaxis which does not respond to conventional treatment with adrenaline [14]. This effect has now been well documented in patients with venom anaphylaxis [13]. Adrenaline, when given alone, has an α-adrenergic effect (causing vasoconstriction), and causes β_1 stimulation (causing cardiac stimulation) and β_2 stimulation (causing vasodilation and bronchodilatation). The increase in heart rate with a rise of systolic and fall in diastolic blood pressure, can be measured after an adrenaline injection. But when the patient is receiving a non-selective β-adrenergic blocker, both the β_1 and β_2 stimulating effects would be inhibited and only the α (vasoconstrictor) effects of adrenaline would predominate. The pharmaceutical companies are working on more selective β-blocker preparations, such as metoprolol (Lopresor), and such β-selective drugs should be used in patients who are at risk from analphylaxis, whatever the cause. For hypertension, there are now available effective drugs which are not β-blockers.

FOOD-DEPENDENT EXERCISE-INDUCED ANAPHYLAXIS

This syndrome has also been called post-prandial exercise-induced anaphylaxis [22]. In the original description of 16 patients [31], it was realized that, because anaphylaxis did not always follow exercise, it was likely that there was some other factor in addition to the exercise required for the reaction to occur. In the original account of the 16 patients with exercise-induced anaphylaxis, only three patients thought the symptoms occurred after eating food. In subsequent accounts, it has been realized that a specific food or foods must first be ingested for anaphylaxis to occur.

Serum IgE concentrations were not elevated in four of the five atopic patients assessed. Five of the patients who had ingested aspirin before the exercise, and two who had taken caffeine, had symptoms induced out of proportion to the modest exercise, whereas normally, without exercise, these substances did not produce symptoms. It seems important that anyone with this syndrome must be warned against taking aspirin at any time because, in some patients, the exercise that produced the attack was not at all strenuous—for example, a mild tennis warm-up or while jogging, particularly when it was warm. The hallmark of the syndrome is exercise-induced urticaria which generally progresses to angioedema involving face, palms and soles. Twelve of the 16 patients collapsed. Choking developed in 10 patients but wheezing was mild. Nausea, colic and diarrhoea may occur. Late sequelae are headaches persisting for 24 to 72 hours.

Role of skin tests

It may be that when an offending food is recognized, a positive skin test will be obtained to this food which perhaps would not normally be tested. In an account of food-dependent exercise-induced anaphylaxis [18], three of the four cases produced anaphylaxis only if celery had been eaten prior to the exercise. The patients gave positive skin prick tests to celery.

In the other case, a meal had to be eaten within two hours before exercise—no specific food seemed to be important.

Patients who have this rare form of anaphylaxis are advised not to take any strenuous exercise within two (and preferably four) hours of a meal. Obviously, they would not partake of a food known to be a possible precipitating factor but, quite often, more than one—or no known food—is involved, rather the anaphylaxis seems to be related to a meal. It is for this reason that the syndrome has been called post-prandial exercise-induced anaphylaxis. The different types of exercise producing the symptoms can be very varied.

Case history 7: Exercise-induced anaphylaxis. One patient aged 30 was taken to hospital before half time when playing his first game of football for three years. His next attack occurred when playing strenuous table tennis, his third attack when taking part in old time dancing.

The foods that may give rise to exercise-induced anaphylaxis are very varied. An athlete only had a reaction if he ate shellfish before going on a long distance run [19].

HISTAMINE

Plasma histamine levels

In evaluating subjects thought to be allergic to foods, we can obtain information from skin testing but it must be remembered that only 40–70% of patients with positive skin tests will develop symptoms on challenge. Food challenge in children with atopic eczema [35] and in adults with anaphylaxis [5] causes a rise in blood histamine. This indicates the participation of mast cells (and basophils) in food-induced allergic reactions. However, even with positive skin tests and a positive challenge, not all patients show a rise in the plasma histamine level. Moreover, it was found that elevations in plasma histamine levels did not always correlate with symptoms. Therefore, plasma histamine levels cannot be used as a criterion of a positive or negative response. These studies in no way solve any of the problems of possible non-IgE-mediated food reactions.

Foods, histamine and histamine release

Theoretically, food additives and contaminants, as well as the foods themselves, could interfere with the synthesis of prostaglandins and leukotrienes or might activate bradykinin. Also, reactions due to histamine from those foods that have a histamine-releasing activity are probably quite common. Many foods possess this property, including egg white, shellfish, strawberries, tomatoes, chocolate, fish and pork. These foods may also make an eczematous skin, rich in mast cells, produce histamine and the scratching accentuates the eczematous lesion in children. In an adult, histamine shock may develop. Some foods, however, are rich in histamine, so that eating such foods as cheese or tuna fish can cause an immediate shock-like condition (see Chap. 23).

Alcoholic drinks

Alcohol, especially the preprandial drink, allows rapid passage of foods across the intestinal mucous membrane. Ethanol is also a potent histamine releaser and many red and white wines are themselves rich in histamine. There are, therefore, many reasons why alcoholic drinks in some people may potentiate or cause not only mild, but sometimes severe, pseudo-allergic reactions.

It is clear that many problems remain to be solved in our understanding of the pathogenesis of the anaphylactically food-allergic patient.

REFERENCES

1 Aalberse RC, Kuslete V, Clements JOS: Cross reactions between vegetable foods, pollen and bee venom due to IgE antibodies to an ubiquitous carbohydrate determinant. Int Arch Allergy Appl Immunol. 1981; 66 (Suppl): 259-60.

2 Aas K, Lunkkvist U: The radioallergosorbent test with a purified allergen from codfish. Clin Allergy 1973; 3: 255.

3 Allen DH, Baker GJ: Asthma and MSG. Med J Aust. 1981; 2: 576.

4 Anderson KJ, McLauchlan P, Devey ME, Coombes RRA: Anaphylactic sensitivity of guinea pigs drinking different preparations of cows milk and infant formulae. Clin Exp Immunol 1979; 35: 454.

5 Atkins FM, Steinberg SS, Metcalf PD: Evaluation of immediate adverse reactions to foods in adults. A detailed analysis of reaction patterns during oral food challenge. J Allergy Clin Immunol (in press).

6 Austen KF: The anaphylactic syndrome. In: Samter M, ed. Immunological diseases. Boston: Little Brown, 1978; 2: 885-9.

7 Bierman CW, Shapiro G, Pierson WE et al: Safety of influenza vaccination in allergic children J Infect Dis 1977; 136: (suppl) 652.

8 Cox TM, O'Donnell MW, Camilleri M: Allergic heterogeneity in adult hereditary fructose intolerance. Mol Biol Med 1983; 1: 393-400.

9 Delage C, Grey ND: Anaphylactic deaths: a clinic study of 43 cases. J Forensic Sci 1972; 17: 525.

10 Dewdney JM, Edwards MG: Penicillin hypersensitivity—is milk a significant hazard? A review. J R Soc Med 1984; 77: 866-77.

11 Finkelstein H: Kuhmilch als Ursach Akuter Ernahrungsstoerungen beir Sauglingen. Monatsssch Kinderheilk 1905; 4: 65-72.

12 Frankland AW: Anaphylaxis—Past and present. In: Molina C, ed. Proceedings of the tenth annual meeting of the European Academy of Allergology and Clinical Immunology. Paris: Technique and Documentation Lavoisier, 1981; 1: 417-23.

13 Frankland AW: Allergy to insects and arachnids. In: Lessof MH, ed. Allergy: immunological and clinical aspects. Chichester: J Wiley, 1984; 425-45.

14 Hannaway PJ, Hopper GDK: Severe anaphylaxis and drug induced beta-blockage. N Engl J Med 1983; 308: 1536.

15 Jacobson DW, Simon RA, Singh M: Sulphite oxidase deficiency and cobalamine projection in sulphite-sensitive asthmatic. J Allergy Clin Immunol 1984; 73: 135.

16 Katz SL: Safety of measles vaccine in egg sensitive individuals. J Pediatr 1978; 92: 859.

17 Kauffman HS, Hobbs JR: Immunoglobulin deficiencies in an atopic population. Lancet 1971; 2: 1061.

18 Kidd JM, Cohen SH, Sosman AJ, Fink JN: Food-dependent exercise-induced anaphylaxis. J Allergy Clin Immunol 1983; 71: 407-11.

19 Maulitz RH, Pratt DS, Schorbet AL: Exercise-induced anaphylactic reaction to shellfish. J Allergy Clin Immunol 1979; 63: 433-4.

20 Michel FB, Bousquet J, Greillier P et al: Comparison of cord blood immunoglobulin E concentrations and maternal allergy for prediction of atopic diseases in infancy. J Allergy Clin Immunol 1980; 65: 422-30.

21 Mowbray JF, Brostoff J: Allergic urticaria and hereditary angiooedema. Clin Allergy 1984; 14: 589-92.

22 Noveg HS, Fairshter R, Salness K et al: Post-prandial exercise-induced anaphylaxis. J Allergy Clin Immunol 1983; 71: 498-504.

23 Parish WE, Richards CB, France AE, Coombs RRA: Further investigations on the hypothesis that some cases of cot deaths are due to a modified anaphylactic reaction to cow's milk. Int Arch Allergy 1964; 24: 215.

24 Peppard D, Wong WS, Uepara CF et al: Lower threshold and greater bronchomotor responsiveness of asthmatic subjects to sulphur dioxide. Am Rev Respir Dis 1980; 122: 873.

25 Prausnitz C, Kustner H: Studien über Uberemfindlichkeit. Centralbl Bakteriol 1921; 1 Abt Orig 86: 160-9. [Translated from the German by Carl Prausnitz In: Gell PGH, Coombs RRA, eds. Clinical aspects of immunology. Oxford: Blackwell Scientific Publications, 1962; 808-16.]

26 Prenner BM, Stevens JJ: Anaphylaxis after ingestion of sodium bisulphate. Ann Allergy 1976; 37: 180.

27 Price JF: Allergy in infancy and childhood. In: Lessof MH, ed. Allergy: immunological and clinical aspects. Chichester: J Wiley, 1984; 161.

28 Sampson HA, Jolie PL: Increased plasma histamine concentrations after food challenge in children with atopic dermatitis. N Engl J Med 1984; 311: 372-6.

29 Schwartz HJ, Sher PH: Anaphylaxis to penicillin in a frozen dinner. Ann Allergy 1984; 53: 342-3.

30 Shannon WR: Demonstration of food proteins in human breast milk by anaphylactic experiments on guinea pigs: Am J Dis Child 1921; 22: 223.

31 Sheffer AL, Austen KF: Exercise-induced anaphylaxis. J Allergy Clin Immunol 1980; 66: 106-11.

32 Tenkelman DG, Bock SA: Anaphylaxis presumed to be caused by beef containing streptomycin. Ann Allergy 1984; 53: 243-4.

33 Toorenberger AW, Dieges PH: IgE-mediated hypersensitivity to tangeh (sprouted small green beans). Ann Allergy 1984; 53: 239-42.

34 Twarog FJ, Leung PK: Anaphylaxis to a component of Isoetharine (sodium bisulphite). JAMA 1982; 248: 2030.

35 Wicher K, Reisman RE: Anaphylactic reaction to penicillin (or a penicillin-like substance) in a soft drink. J Allergy Clin Immunol 1980; 66: 155-7.

36 Wicher K, Reisman RE, Aarbesman CE: Allergic reactions to penicillin in milk. JAMA 1969; 208: 143.

Chapter 26
Rhinitis and Secretory Otitis Media: A Possible Role of Food Allergy

Zdenek Pelikan

Introduction

The role of food allergy and of food in general in subjects with allergic disorders, especially in those suffering from rhinitis, otitis media and sinusitis, is still underestimated by clinicians. This is because (a) these allergic disorders in the past have been attributed to immediate (Type I) hypersensitivity mechanisms only and the allergens suspected have been those acquired by the inhalational route; (b) there may be many mechanisms by which foods can cause clinical disorders in patients of which hypersensitivity mechanisms are only one; (c) the diagnosis of food allergy and its confirmation in the symptomatology of patients is difficult and requires both experience and a clear system of diagnosis, as well as patience from both clinician and patient [13, 47].

Definition

Food allergy or hypersensitivity may be defined as the clinical manifestation of an immunological process in which foods or their ingredients are able to act as antigens or haptens to stimulate the production of antibodies which then interact with cells of the immune system, in this way resulting in an allergic reaction. Foods may be responsible for immunological injury by any of the classical types of hypersensitivity reaction [5, 58] (see Chapter 13).

Differential diagnosis. A distinction must be made between a true food allergy which is due to an immunological process and other disorders which can also be caused by foods, their ingredients or factors related to them which can produce similar symptoms but which are due to completely different mechanisms (Table 26.1) [5, 45, 51, 73] (see Chapter 48).

Table 26.1 Survey of the disorders caused by foods, their ingredients or factors relating to them, which can lead to symptoms similar to those due to the food allergy mechanism.

1 Idiosyncrasy
2 Intolerance (e.g. enzymatic)
3 Non-specific hyperreactivity (e.g. histamine or other mediator liberators, food additives)
4 Toxicity
    (a) by non-controlled chemical compounds (e.g. insecticides, contaminants)
    (b) by microorganisms
    (c) by products of microorganisms
       (i) bacterial toxins
       (ii) mycotoxins
    (d) by controlled chemical compounds exceeding their permitted threshold or individual subjects having increased susceptibility to these compounds (e.g. disinfectants) caused by other metabolic disorders
5 Adverse non-immunological reaction to additives (controlled chemical compounds)
    (a) preservation and conservation compounds
    (b) colouring compounds
    (c) flavouring compounds
    (d) consistency correcting compounds, emulsifiers and stabilizers
    (e) antioxidants
    (f) adjuvants
6 Psychological disorders

Forms of food allergy. There are two basic forms of food allergy [58]:

1 Primary, where the food alone via an immunological process causes the defined clinical symptoms. Here the food is the primary and sole cause of the hypersensitivity mechanism and the resulting symptoms.

2 Secondary, where one or more foods potentiate an already existing hypersensitivity mechanism caused by different antigens (e.g. inhalants, etc.). The foods may act via different pathways in potentiating the response. Here the food allergy is only complementary to another hypersensitivity state which is the primary and basic one. This secondary form of food intolerance occurs more frequently than the primary and is regularly overlooked.

Immunological characteristics of food allergy

1 Foods normally enter into the body via the digestive tract, i.e. by ingestion. Foods can also cause hypersensitivity reactions by contact with the skin, gingiva, lips or tongue, and also by inhalation in the nasal or bronchial mucosa.

2 The antibodies involved in food allergy are classically those of the IgE class. However, antibodies of other classes, for example IgG, IgM as well as IgA and immune complexes [15, 55] may also be involved. There is evidence that T lymphocytes may also be involved in hypersensitivity mechanisms [19, 36, 49].

3 All four basic types of hypersensitivity, i.e. Types I–IV, may be involved in food allergy

and can lead to clinical symptoms. However, the immediate (Type I) and late phase (? Type III) reactions have mostly been documented and investigated [15, 21, 35, 58a, 71].

The terms 'food allergy' or 'hypersensitivity' imply an immunological mechanism but in many instances the exact immunopathological mechanism producing symptoms is unknown. It would therefore be more appropriate to speak of 'adverse reactions to foods', real food hypersensitivity being only one of the suspected mechanisms [5, 47, 58].

Food additives. Chemical additives in foods present a very special problem, not only with respect to their frequent occurrence in manufactured foods and their heterogeneity, but also because of the lack of understanding concerning their mode of production of clinical symptoms. There is clear evidence in various organ systems that additives may cause symptoms, this being demonstrated by clinical oral challenge studies [39, 73, 74, 75, 80]. Although clinical manifestations are associated with the ingestion of additives, antibodies of the IgE or other classes or indeed sensitized lymphocytes have not yet been unequivocally found in the clinically affected patients [5, 40, 51].

Although disodium cromoglycate is effective in preventing symptoms following challenge with foods there is little evidence to date to suggest that this drug can prevent the symptoms following oral challenge with additives (see Chapter 56). This suggests that additives produce their symptoms through non-immunological mechanisms. It may be that the additives produce symptoms through non-specific mechanisms, such as mediator release or direct effects on the effector organs, or indeed through pharmacological action (e.g. subtoxic effects) [9, 45, 87] (see Chapter 23).

Isolated adverse reactions to additives are usually diagnosed in only a small number of patients reporting adverse reactions to foods. In the majority of patients food hypersensitivity only, or a parallel role of food intolerance and adverse reactions to the additives are found. Diagnostic confirmation that additives are the cause of the patient's symptoms is often difficult to obtain. A review of the additives appearing most frequently in foods which may also play a role in adverse reaction to foods in rhinitis patients is shown in Table 26.2.

body interactions which lead to the release of mediators which then act on the various effector organs (e.g. smooth muscle, mucosal glands, goblet cells, etc.). The combined response of the effector organs results in the clinical symptoms of the disease.

The allergic mechanism may be seasonal or non-seasonal depending on the kind of allergens involved. Of the four basic types of hypersensitivity reaction, three (Type I—immediate, Type III—late and Type IV—delayed) can be involved in the production of symptoms in the rhinitis patient. However, immediate hypersensitivity (Type I) is the most commonly involved in these patients leading to the so-called 'immediate nasal response'.

Table 26.2 Review of the additives appearing most frequently in foods.

Colouring agents	Flavouring agents	Preservatives	Stabilizers/emulsifiers
Tartrazine	trans-Anethole	Benzoic acid	Calcium salts
Coccine	Malic acid	EDTA derivatives	Agar-agar
Amaranth	Acetic acid	o-Phenylphenol	Carbonates
Sunset Yellow	Benzaldehyde	Formic acid	Diacetyl tartaric acid
Pyrazole	Benzyl compounds	Nitrate compounds	Phosphate compounds
Hydrozy aromatic acids	Cyclamate	Propionic acid	Glycerol derivatives
Annatto	Ethylmaltol	Sulphites	Lecithin
Anthocyanins	Ethylvanillin	4-Hydroxybenzoic acid	
Azorubine	Fumaric acid	Benzene sulphuric acid	Antioxidants
Brilliant Blue FCF	l-Glutamates	Sodium sulphuric acid	Butylated hydroxyanisole
Brilliant Black PN	Maltol	Sodium benzoate	Acetone peroxide
Brilliant Black	Amylbutyrate		Citric acid
Food Green S	Benzyl acetate	Consistency corrigents	Gallates
Allura Red AC	D-Camphor		
Chlorophyll	Citronellol	Carrageenan	
Citral	Ethyl acetoacetate	Aluminium compounds	Others
Ponceau 4R	Ethyl propionate	Cellulose compounds	Bacitracin
Food Green 3	Alpha ionone		
Food Red 14	Gamma undecanone		
Indigotin	2,4-Undecadienal		
Carminic acid	Delta nonalactone		
Patent Blue	Propyl propionate		
Indigo Carmine	Methyl thiopropionate		
Wool Green B	2-Pentenol		
	n-Heptenal		

RHINITIS

Allergic rhinitis is a non-infectious disorder characterized by nasal obstruction due to swelling of the nasal mucosa, hypersecretion, sneezing and itching [5, 57]. Nasal symptoms may be caused by two different mechanisms— an allergic component and a non-specific hyperreactivity component. These may both participate in the same patient to various degrees.

The allergic component

The allergic component is due to antigen-anti-

This occurs within 120 minutes after allergen exposure. In addition to the immediate nasal response, so-called 'non-immediate nasal responses' also occur. The 'late nasal response' appearing 4–24 hours after allergen exposure could be due to either a late phase response or Type III hypersensitivity. The 'delayed nasal response' occurring 30–56 hours after allergen challenge suggests that delayed type hypersensitivity (Type IV) may be involved. Allergic reactions of all types can be demonstrated by the simple use of nasal provocation tests with allergen [56, 57].

The 'non-specific hyperreactivity' component

The non-specific hyperreactivity component may lead to a similar spectrum of nasal symptoms as that caused by an immunological mechanism. These non-specific agents, mostly small molecular chemical compounds, physical factors such as temperature differences or mechanical factors such as non-organic dusts, either (a) influence the immunocompetent or target cell directly causing non-specific release of mediators; (b) act via the stimulation of mediator precursors leading firstly to stimulation of mediator production which then acts directly on the effector organs and, secondly, to feedback inhibition of these mediators on immunocompetent cells; or (c) act on the effector organs directly, thus causing the clinical effects. Nasal challenge with histamine is an indication for the involvement of non-specific hyperreactivity in the rhinitis patient.

In the majority of patients with rhinitis (70%) both the allergy component as well as an element of non-specific hyperreactivity are usually found. In the remaining patients only one of these components is found. Cases of rhinitis where the non-specific hyperreactivity component is dominant can be called vasomotor rhinitis. The role of foods in producing symptoms in patients with allergic rhinitis is regularly discussed in the literature, sometimes from controversial points of view. More recently the role of food has been recognized and confirmed by clinical challenge [58, 77, 78]. This does not imply that all the clinical responses to food are via immunological hypersensitivity mechanisms, but certainly some of them may be.

Diagnostic procedures in vivo

History and physical examination

In all patients with rhinitis, otitis media and sinusitis a case history should be taken with special emphasis on dietary history. In our clinical experience approximately 18% of patients with rhinitis, 7% with otitis media and 5% with sinusitis have a history suggestive of food allergy. The positive history for food intolerance in rhinitis patients reported by Wilson (16%) [83] and Eriksson (24%) [25] is in accordance with the author's findings. In practice, sufficient attention is not paid to the dietary history in the diagnosis of these patients [58, 64].

In addition, other symptoms and signs may also be suggestive of food allergy in these patients. When there is other organ involvement, such as urticaria, erythema, irritable bowel or gingivitis, foods may be indicated as possible causative agents.

Laboratory and X-ray examination

A basic laboratory screening and also X-ray of the sinuses are important in these patients from the point of view of differential diagnosis. In addition, mildly abnormal blood tests, such as sedimentation rate, leukocytosis and eosinophilia, are frequently present as is oedema of the mucosa of the maxillary sinuses.

Skin tests

Dermal (scratch and prick) and intracutaneous tests have been used. However, there are very definite problems concerning skin tests with food extracts including (a) the standardization of the food extract itself, (b) the technology and purification of the allergen and (c) the method of testing and the correlation with the clinical picture. There is also much debate as to the clinical value of such skin tests with food extracts [5]. The reported correlation between skin testing and clinical symptoms varies widely in the literature. In patients with rhinitis where there is a presumed food allergy, skin testing with food allergens was found to be a useful diagnostic test by some authors [5, 14, 46, 82], while other authors were not able to confirm this [4, 6, 8, 16, 54, 64, 84].

In our own department skin tests with food extracts in patients with allergic rhinitis due to food allergy correlated with other diagnostic parameters in only 60%, which is unsatisfactory [58]. The immediate skin response was positive in only 55% of the immediate nasal responders. The late skin response (LSR) was positive in 48% of those with late nasal response and the delayed skin response was positive in only 42% of those with a clinical delayed nasal response [58] (Table 26.3).

Schedule for skin testing. Our schedule for skin testing is as follows. Cutaneous (scratch or prick) tests are performed and after 20 minutes are measured. If they are negative, as they are in approximately 95% of the patients, then intracutaneous tests are carried out and evaluated after 20 minutes (for immediate response) (Fig. 26.1a), and then every 4 hours up to 12 hours. They are then examined after

Table 26.3 The association of the various types of nasal response to food ingestion challenge with other diagnostic parameters.

	Nasal mucosa response to food ingested			
	Immediate (n = 267)	Late (n = 203)	Delayed (n = 164)	Negative (n = 309)
Positive skin response	146 (55%)			48 (16%)
		98 (48%)		11 (4%)
			69 (42%)	3 (1%)
Increase in total serum IgE (PRIST)	11 (4%)	1 (0.5%)	0 (0%)	3 (1%)
Increase in specific serum IgE (RAST)	38 (14%)	3 (1.5%)	1 (0.6%)	4 (1.3%)
Increase in blood eosinophils	14 (5%)	17 (8%)	2 (1%)	2 (0.3%)
Increase in blood leukocytes	10 (4%)	18 (9%)	11 (7%)	3 (1%)
Aspects of the nasal mucosa:				
hyperaemia	97 (36%)	47 (23%)	1 (0.5%)	5 (1.5%)
lividity	168 (63%)	55 (76%)	163 (99.5%)	0 (0%)
Nasal mucosa haemorrhages	0 (0%)	42 (21%)	2 (1%)	0 (0%)
Nasal secretions Changes in count of:				
eosinophils	201 (75%)	128 (63%)	53 (32%)	21 (7%)
mast cells/basophils	53 (20%)	30 (15%)	6 (4%)	0 (0%)
neutrophils	208 (78%)	182 (90%)	41 (25%)	15 (5%)
goblet cells	113 (42%)	49 (24%)	14 (8.5%)	2 (10.6%)
lymphocytes	9 (3%)	5 (2%)	46 (28%)	0 (0%)

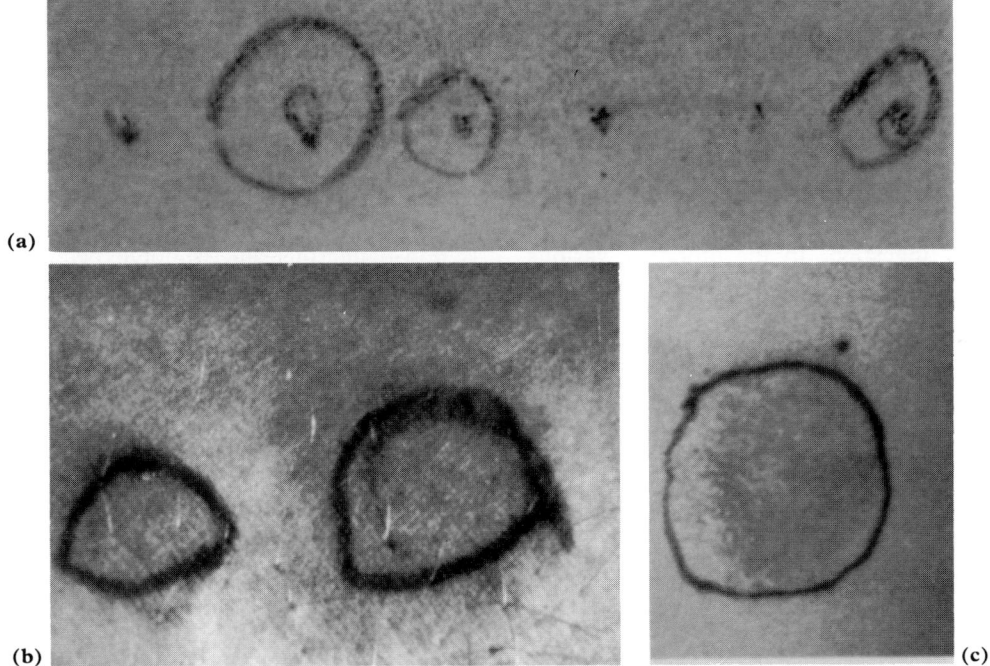

Fig. 26.1 Skin responses after intracutaneous tests with food extracts: (a) immediate skin response (after 20 minutes); (b) late skin response (after 8 hours); (c) delayed skin response (after 56 hours).

24 hours for the late skin response (Fig. 26.1b) and assessed after 36, 48, 60 and 72 hours (for delayed skin response) (Fig. 26.1c). If necessary the skin is examined for longer periods up to the disappearance of the wheal or induration.

It should be emphasized, as has been mentioned above, that skin tests alone are not sufficient for diagnosis of food allergy but should be followed by food ingestion challenge to definitively confirm the role of food in the rhinitis patient [6, 8, 54, 58, 84].

Provocation tests with foods

Challenge with the appropriate foods should be considered the cornerstone of diagnosis for the role of food allergy in the rhinitis patient [1, 34, 87]. Provocation tests should demonstrate the appearance of the patient's substantive symptoms, in this case nasal symptoms after the ingestion of the suspected food [53, 58]. The challenge should be regarded as a model investigation and as a simulated reproduction of the patient's complaints following exposure to their particular allergen (in this case food).

There are two main principles involved in the provocation tests. (a) The qualitative aspect—the test should demonstrate that the particular organ does indeed react to the suspected allergen by the typical response; (b) the quantitative aspect—the test should confirm that the suspected allergen (food) in a particular dose and following single or repeated introduction causes the specific organ response. This is the time- and dose–response principle.

A most important aspect of the provocation test is the comparison of objective measurements before and after challenge with the allergen by ingestion. In the literature various modifications of the provocation tests with foods have been described. Ingestion challenge with foods in their natural form, so-called 'open oral challenge', is frequently used [5].

The challenge can be accompanied by various measurements, such as clinical symptoms [5], pulse rate [64], nasal or lung function and so on [6, 58a, 84, 85]. Other authors prefer a single-blind challenge [5], open challenge with disguised foods [16, 64], double-blind challenge with foods processed in capsules [46] or so-called 'sublingual testing' where the foods in their natural form or their extracts in dilutions are placed under the tongue [28, 31, 64]. Elimination diets and rotation diets [5, 64],

where the food is reintroduced after specific times following elimination, can also be used for diagnostic purposes (see Chapter 46).

There are few published data concerning the role of foods and food allergy in patients with allergic rhinitis or secretory otitis media. Especially uncommon are reports of the investigation of the nose, conjunctiva, sinuses or middle ear response following food ingestion challenge by quantitative objective measurements [84, 85].

Precautions for oral challenge. The following requirements should be met before oral provication tests are carried out.

1 The tests should be safe, reproducible and sufficiently sensitive to show positive results. The patient should not be able to influence the result by some knowledge of the challenging agent.

2 A careful system for the evaluation of indications and contraindications for the specific patient is necessary. This involves a detailed disease history, general physical examination and laboratory screening before oral challenge is carried out.

3 The absolute contraindication for this test is a presumption that the patient may develop an anaphylactic reaction to the specific food [6, 33]. Pregnancy or any state or disorder which can lead to irreversible damage in the patient or to an emergency situation is contraindicated.

4 Any medication which may mask or influence the result of the challenge is contraindicated. Specifically the patient should be tested while he/she is not receiving any medication and has no intercurrent illness or other relevant allergic symptoms [6].

5 Oral challenges where the clinical response is non-dangerous and is not expected to be severe (e.g. mild diarrhoea), can be performed in Out-Patients. Other challenges where lung function or severe gastrointestinal upsets may occur or where a late onset reaction is expected, should be performed as an in-patient in hospital. The challenge should be carried out under direct supervision of the medical staff. Facilities for resuscitation and intensive care must be available if necessary.

6 Allergens (foods or extracts) should be continually checked for standardization and quality.

7 The foods or additives suspected of causing the adverse reactions should be excluded from the diet for a sufficient period before the challenge. Opinions concerning this exclusion period vary. Some authors recommend 1–2 weeks' elimination [45, 47]. However, our clinical experience suggests that if a large number of foods need to be excluded, 3 days' avoidance before the challenge is sufficient.

Techniques for oral provocation with foods

The two basic techniques for oral provocation tests with foods are the double-blind challenge and the open challenge with natural foods. Both of these methods have advantages and disadvantages.

In many cases we prefer open challenge with foods, our results being comparable with those obtained by the double-blind technique. Open challenge is satisfactory where objective measurements of the responses to the ingested food can be made, such as in those cases where there is bronchial, nasal, skin or middle ear involvement [58]. The double-blind or cross-over technique is important where drug effects are being investigated or in such cases of food allergy where objective measurements cannot be recorded, as in migraine, headache, gastro-intestinal complaints, arthralgia or pruritus or where there may be a psychosomatic component to the symptoms.

Double-blind challenge

In cases where the double-blind challenge is performed with lyophilized food in capsules, there are a number of disadvantages, namely:

1 The maximum content of capsules is 500 mg which is considerably less than the quantity of food normally eaten. If the quantity of freeze-dried food in the capsules is to be comparable with a natural meal-size portion (e.g. 100 g of meat), more than 200 capsules would be necessary [6, 20, 34].

2 Ideally, the food should be colourless, odourless and tasteless. The processing of the foods to make them suitable for such administration will inevitably lead to changes in their physical properties, and in some cases to changes in their chemical structure.

3 By administering the food in capsules, contact with buccal mucosa, tongue, oesophagus and also stomach is totally excluded. In a number of patients with food allergy problems these organs play a most important role or are indeed the site of the clinical response, i.e. oedema of the tongue, vesicular eruption of the buccal mucosa, gingivitis, epiglottal oedema and oesophageal dysfunction [64, 83].

4 By administering the food in capsules the digestive process, which begins in the mouth, may be prolonged and the expected response may appear later than that in practice under natural conditions.

5 Providing a suitable placebo that matches the offending food in quantity, consistency, colour and taste is not always possible [6].

6 The long dietary restriction for 1 or 2

Table 26.4 Survey of the food quantities used for ingestion challenge.

Food	Quantity used for ingestion challenge
1 Basic foods of 'solid consistency' consumed in various quantities, usually more than 100 g at one time: cheese, chocolate, peanuts, walnuts, almonds, apple, shrimps, spinach, tomato, strawberries, Dutch sweets, honey, pear, cabbage, mussels, banana, pork, cocoa powder, meat, molluscs, crustacea, grain, flour, fish, jams, marmalades, other vegetables and fruits	up to 100 g of each
2 Basic foods of 'fluid consistency' consumed in various quantities, usually more than 100 g at one time: milk, yoghurt, Coca-cola, 7-Up, coffee, tea, and other non-alcoholic beverages	200 ml of each

3 Foods, parts of foods or foodstuffs, usually with a well-defined flavour or taste, only added to the basic foods in very small quantities:
     Spices (paprika powder, mustard, ginger, nutmeg, vanilla, onion, garlic, etc.)
     Vegetables (garlic, onion, paprika, chilli, horseradish, etc.)
     Varia (casein, lactose, glucose, sucrose, olive oil, butter, margarine, herbs, vinegar, dressing, etc.)
	5 g of each on brown bread with butter

4 Alcoholic beverages:
     Soft: beer, wine sherry, port, shandy, etc.
     Liquor: whisky, gin, cognac, etc.
	100 ml of each
	 5 ml of each

5 Additives are used in quantities corresponding with those occurring in 100 g or 100 ml of the basic foods or in 5 g or 5 ml of the 'flavouring' foods (e.g. vinegar, ketchup, dressings, etc.)	usually 1–10 mg, sometimes more

weeks as suggested by some authors [13, 46] can sometimes cause other problems.

Excluding a large number of foods for 1 or 2 weeks can be stressful for the patient, is sometimes impractical and, lastly, during this time various uncontrolled factors can influence the patient's response. Moreover, the standard elimination diet itself as suggested by some authors [47] contains foods which have regularly been found by us to be responsible for the complaints in our patients (e.g. pineapple, apricots, peaches, pears, lamb, asparagus, honey, spice, white vinegar) [58, 58a].

The following schedule of food ingestion challenge in patients with rhinitis is used by the author. After a 72-hour avoidance of the appropriate food and food family, the ingestion challenge is performed with the food in its natural form. This is accompanied by rhinomanometry (resistance, pressure difference, flow and so on). If necessary, other measurements are also made, such as nasal secretions histology, nasal mucosa biopsy, tympanometry, lung function, sinus X-ray and so on. There is always an interval of 1 hour following food challenge before measurements are made to allow digestion of food. For control challenges (placebo) we used cooked rice, glucose or potatoes, depending on the patient's symptomatology.

The amounts of various foods used for ingestion are shown in Table 26.4. In general we prefer quantities of foods for the oral provocation tests which correspond to the normal consumption of that food by the patient.

Diagnostic procedures in vitro

Serum immunoglobulins

Total IgE (radioimmunosorbent test, RIST). The level of total IgE has not been found to be significantly related to rhinitis, sinusitis or otitis media where food allergy has been the cause [6, 27].

Specific IgE (radioallergosorbent test, RAST). This is the most frequently used technique [17, 37, 70] but also one of the most controversial techniques in patients with food allergy. This is especially so because of (a) its unsatisfactory correlation with the clinical state and other in vivo diagnostic parameters [1], (b) the interpretation of the results [2] and (c) the methodology, which raises several questions as to its value [3, 20, 26, 27].

The author has investigated the correlation of RAST and other diagnostic parameters with the clinical state of patients with rhinitis due to food allergy. A positive RAST in the serum was found in only 14% of the patients who showed an immediate nasal response following oral provocation and who also had a positive disease history relevant to that food (Table 26.3). There was a better correlation between a negative oral provocation test and negative RAST (Fig. 26.2). Total IgE in the serum was found to be unchanged in most patients with an immediate nasal response to food ingestion challenge (Tables 26.3 and 26.5). We conclude that the RAST has little value in the diagnosis of the food-allergic patient with rhinitis. Our conclusion is in accordance with the findings and experience of other investigators [17, 70, 72].

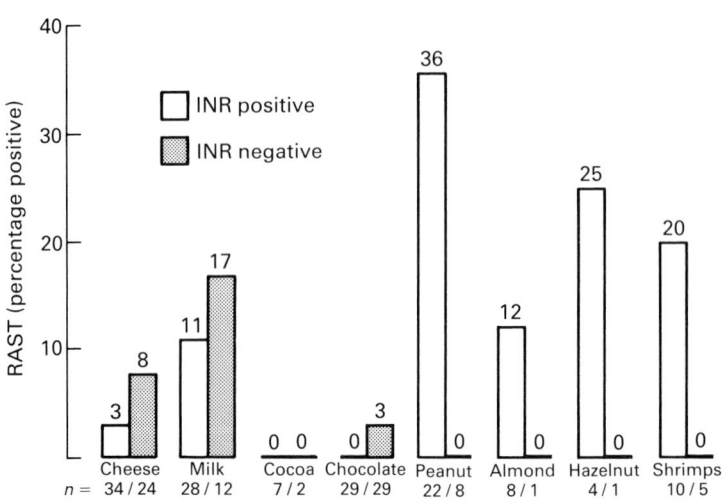

Fig. 26.2 Serum-specific IgE antibodies in patients with immediate nasal response (INR) following food challenge.

Table 26.5 Survey of the total serum IgE antibodies (PRIST) in the patients with positive immediate nasal responses (INR) to the ingestion challenge with foods.

	PRIST				
	0-50 IU/ml	50-100 IU/ml	100-500 IU/ml	500-1000 IU/ml	>1000 IU/ml
Subjects (n = 134)	84 (63%)	39 (29%)	7 (5%)	2 (1.5%)	2 (1.5%)

Interpretation of the PRIST results, modified by the author: ≤ 100 IU/ml = not increased (negative); 100–500 IU/ml = slightly increased (doubtful); > 500 IU/ml = increased (positive).

Other immunoglobulins. There is evidence that at least in part the nasal response to foods involves antibodies of other classes, e.g. IgG and IgM [29, 36]. These immunoglobulins seem specially relevant to the late nasal response following food challenge [36, 57, 84]. There is also evidence for other non-immediate types of hypersensitivity, e.g. Type III or Type IV, in food-induced reactions (see Chapters 13 and 24).

Mucosal production of IgE

The role of specific IgE produced locally in the nasal mucosa must contribute to the particular character of allergic reactions in the nose and possibly also to the unsatisfactory correlation of the serum RAST and the clinical state [61].

Nasal secretions

The study of nasal secretions and the cellular content is a useful supplement to rhinomanometry techniques following oral provocation. The patient blows his nose into a polythene sheet before and after food ingestion and the air-dried specimens are processed using polyethylene glycol and stained by a modified Hansel's technique [60]. Changes in the number of eosinophils, increase in the number of goblet cells and decrease in the number of basophils

suggest involvement of food in the positive nasal response [60, 77] (Fig. 26.3, Table 26.3).

Leukocyte and eosinophil response in blood. There can be increases in leukocytes and eosinophils after a positive food ingestion challenge. However, their relationship to a positive nasal response following oral provocation is not significant [5] (Table 26.3).

Other laboratory tests. Lymphocyte transformation, leukocyte migration inhibition, leukocyte histamine release and cytotoxic tests have been discussed in the literature but their diagnostic value has not been confirmed for patients with rhinitis, secretory otitis media and sinusitis due to food allergy.

Clinical studies

We have investigated the role of food allergy in patients with rhinitis, some of whom had associated symptoms of sinusitis, headache, conjunctivitis and otitis media [59]. Of the patients with rhinitis where an allergic component was suspected, the role of foods was confirmed in two-thirds. In 19% of these cases food was found to be the sole cause of the rhinitis. In half these patients the rhinitis was caused by various inhalant allergens with foods also having an effect ('secondary' food allergy).

Table 26.6 The time course of the individual clinical types of nasal response to the food ingestion challenge.

	Onset	Maximum	Resolving
Immediate	10–20 minutes	30–45 minutes	90–120 minutes
Late	4–6 hours	6–10 hours	12–24 hours
Delayed	24–28 hours	32–36 hours	48–52 hours

The time is expressed in minutes or hours after a 60-minute waiting interval following the ingestion challenge.

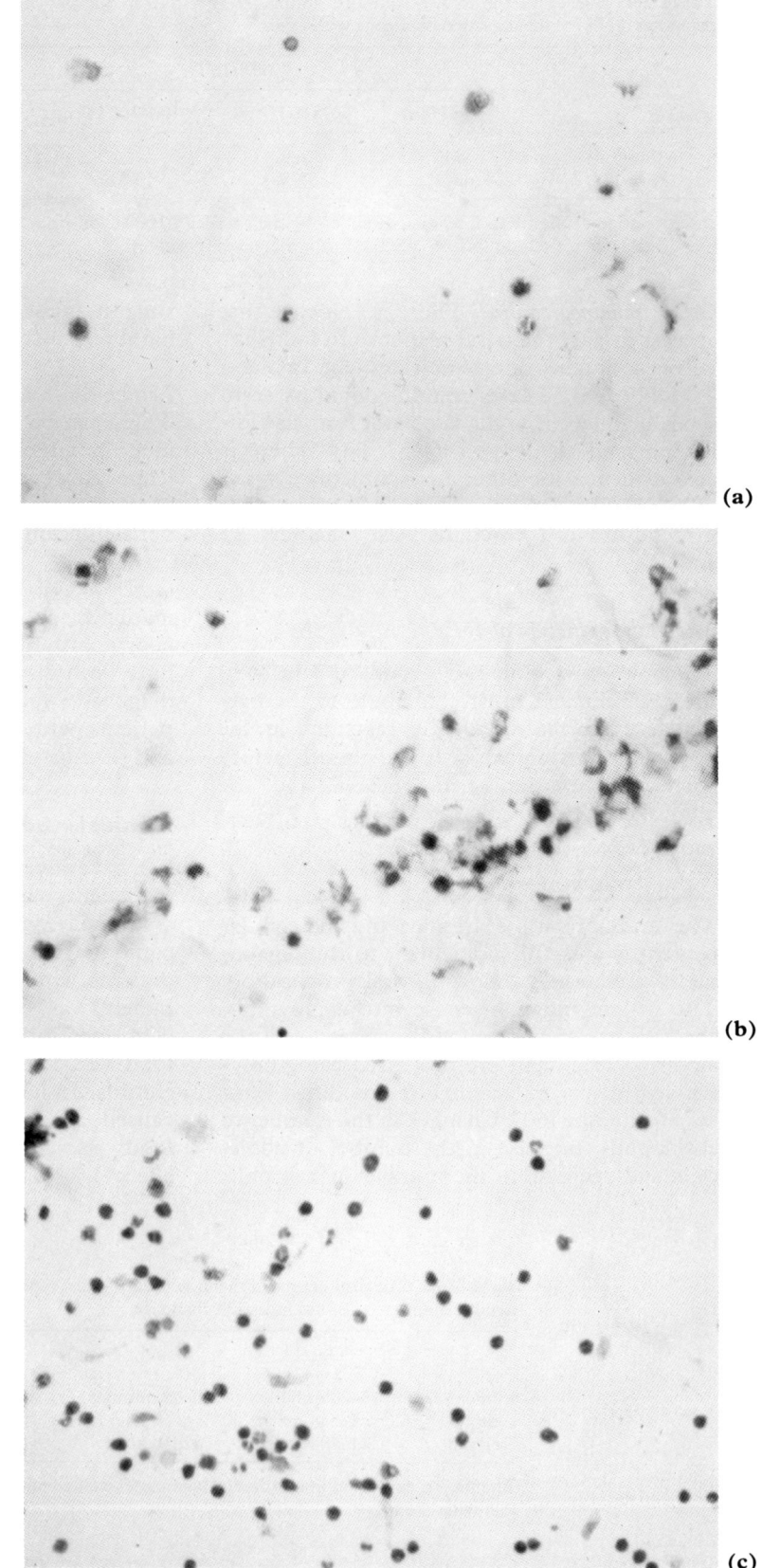

Fig. 26.3 Eosinophils in the nasal secretions (a) before food ingestion challenge, (b) 120 minutes after food ingestion challenge and (c) 180 minutes after food ingestion challenge.

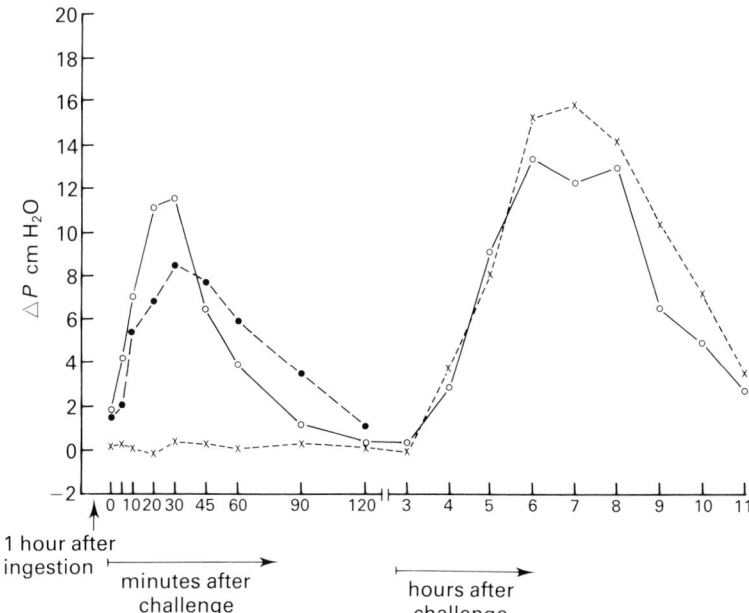

Fig. 26.4 Types of nasal mucosa response recorded in patients after ingestion of selected foods. The mean NPG values after food ingestion with respect to the appropriate 'Coca's solution' NPG values were always calculated from all patients developing the same type of nasal response. ($\bullet - - \bullet$), immediate nasal mucosa response ($n = 67$); ($\circ - - \circ$), dual (immediate + late) nasal response ($n = 21$); ($\times - - - \times$), isolated late nasal response ($n = 14$).

Types of nasal response

Three types of nasal response following food challenge were recorded (Table 26.6).

1 An immediate response occurring within 10 minutes of challenge, peaking at 45 minutes and resolving by 120 minutes (Fig. 26.4).
2 A late response starting 6 hours after challenge, peaking at 10 hours and resolving by 24 hours (Fig. 26.4).
3 The delayed response started at 24 hours, was at its maximum at 36 hours and resolved by 52 hours (Fig. 26.5).

The late and delayed responses could be observed in either an isolated form or in combination with the immediate type—so-called 'dual late' or 'dual delayed' responses (Figs. 26.4 and 26.5). The time course was recorded after an interval of 1 hour following challenge with a particular food. The frequency of the individual nasal responses to food ingestion was as follows: (a) isolated immediate type—30%; (b) isolated late type—20%; (c) dual late type—35%; (d) isolated delayed type—5%; (e) dual late type—10% of all cases. The combined data are shown in Table 26.3.

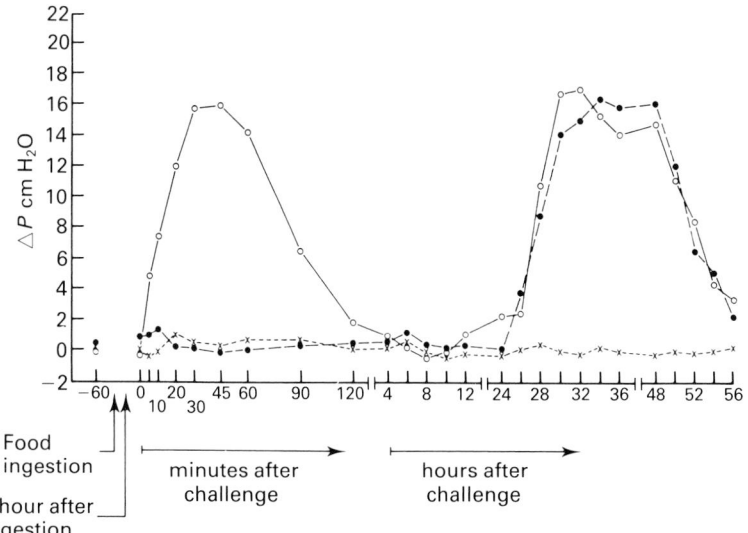

Fig. 26.5 Dual and isolated delayed nasal response due to ingestion challenge with foods. The mean NPG values recorded after the food ingestion challenge with respect to the appropriate control NPG values were calculated from all patients developing the same type of nasal response. ($\bullet - - \bullet$), isolated delayed response ($n = 31$); ($\circ - - \circ$), dual delayed (immediate + delayed) response ($n = 56$); ($\times - - - \times$), control test ($n = 87$).

The frequency with which individual foods cause nasal or middle ear symptoms after ingestion challenge is very varied, but the most common foods implicated are dairy produce, chocolate, peanuts and alcoholic drinks.

Association with other allergic disorders

Food-induced rhinitis may be associated with other clinical disorders and with other organ system as a result of similar allergic mechanisms [12, 16, 81] (Table 26.7). This association may be of two kinds. Firstly, it may be of the 'independent type' where the food itself causes not only the nasal response but also a response in another organ system. Secondly, it may be of the 'dependent' type where the food ingestion leads primarily to the nasal response, which then induces a secondary response in another organ. The 'independent' type response has been observed by us in a number of diseases, such as sinusitis, stomatitis, conjunctivitis, secretory otitis media, asthma, eczema, urticaria, arthralgia, migraine

and in association with a variety of abdominal symptoms. The 'dependent type' of association has been observed by us to induce secondary organ responses such as sinusitis, secretory otitis media, migraine and rarely bronchial asthma (Table 26.7).

Treatment

The management of the patient with allergic rhinitis due to food allergy has two main avenues: (a) the avoidance of the incriminating foods (dietary treatment), and (b) pharmacological treatment.

Elimination diet

This is the most important part of the management of food allergy, especially where only a small number of foods are involved. Two precautions are important: (a) diagnostic procedures must have confirmed the involvement of these foods in the patient's complaints, and (b) it must be possible for the incriminating

Table 26.7 Review of the nasal complaints and other organs' complaints accompanying the various types of nasal response to food ingestion challenge.

	Nasal mucosa response to food ingested			
	Immediate ($n=267$)	Late ($n=203$)	Delayed ($n=164$)	Negative ($n=309$)
Nasal complaints				
obstruction	267 (100%)	203 (100%)	164 (100%)	0 (0%)
sneezing	19 (7%)	1 (0.5%)	0 (0%)	1 (0.3%)
hypersecretion	193 (72%)	166 (82%)	39 (24%)	16 (15%)
itching	181 (68%)	75 (37%)	145 (88%)	13 (4%)
General malaise complaints	22 (8%)	54 (27%)	49 (30%)	1 (0.3%)
Conjunctival irritation	35 (13%)	18 (9%)	6 (4%)	0 (0%)
Middle ear response (otalgia, decrease of hearing, change of middle ear pressure)	31 (12%)	19 (9%)	13 (8%)	10 (3%)
Pressure in the sinuses (maxillary and frontal, acute oedema of sinus mucosa)	45 (17%)	32 (16%)	33 (20%)	7 (2%)
Cephalgia	56 (21%)	91 (45%)	125 (76%)	42 (14%)
Urticaria	4 (1.5%)	7 (3%)	8 (5%)	5 (1.5%)
Angio-oedema (labial, palpebral or elsewhere)	9 (3%)	6 (3%)	3 (2%)	3 (1%)
Increase in body temperature	4 (1.5%)	21 (10%)	1 (0.6%)	0 (0%)
Bronchial complaints	13 (5%)	15 (7%)	12 (7%)	8 (3%)
Other complaints	2 (0.7%)	1 (0.5%)	2 (1%)	0 (0%)

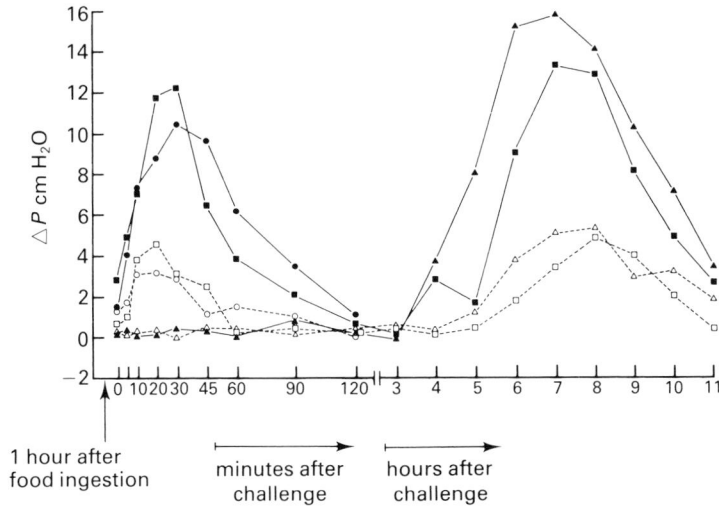

Fig. 26.6 Protective effects of oral disodium cromoglycate (DSCG) on the nasal response due to the ingestion challenge with food. The mean NPG values after non-pretreated and pretreated nasal mucosa responses due to the food ingestion challenge, with respect to the appropriate 'Coca's solution' NPG values, were always calculated from all patients developing the same type of nasal response. Isolated immediate response ($n = 1$): (●) non-pretreated and (○) pretreated with DSCG. Isolated late response ($n = 2$): (▲) non-pretreated and (△) pretreated with DSCG. Dual response (immediate + late) ($n = 22$): (■) non-pretreated and (□) pretreated with DSCG.

food or food group to be fully avoided by the patient.

There are many reported schedules and modifications of the elimination diet (see Chapters 46 and 57).

Pharmacological treatment

Oral disodium cromoglycate (DSCG). Disodium cromoglycate administered orally in a dose of 100–200 mg four hours daily has been found to be effective in patients with rhinitis, sinusitis, otitis media and conjunctivitis where food allergy has been involved [7] (Fig. 26.6). Our data suggest that oral DSCG showed significant protection ($P < 0.001$) against both the immediate (83%) as well as the late (79%) nasal response to food ingestion challenge (Fig. 26.6). We are currently studying the effect of this drug on the delayed nasal response to food ingestion.

Local treatment. Disodium cromoglycate is also useful as a local treatment for the nasal mucosa. Rynacrom (10 mg capsule four times daily intranasally, divided between both nostrils), or its aerosol form, Lomusol (6 × 1 puff in each nostril daily), in addition to topical corticosteroids (e.g. beclomethasone dipropionate, Viarin R, Vancenase R, Beconase R) and topical decongestants (e.g. xylomethazoline hydrochloride) are useful in the treatment of rhinitis. These latter drugs should be added to the armamentarium when oral DSCG is not able to fully prevent the nasal symptoms caused by ingested food or when late or delayed nasal responses are present.

Supplementary treatment. In some patients where a combination of food and inhalant allergy causes the symptoms, supplementary treatment may be needed to achieve optimal control of the nasal complaints. The most frequently used drugs in this group are antihistamines, anticholinergics or alpha-sympathomimetics.

Controversial and unproven procedures

The basic requirements and necessary conditions for every diagnostic as well as therapeutic procedure are a scientific basis, reasonable effectiveness and minimal risk for the patient. It must be added that some tests are performed where the scientific basis is not clear but where the clinical response is consistent. The controversial (unproven) methods related to the diagnosis of food allergy include:

Leukocytotoxic testing (cytotoxicity test). This test, modified by Bryan and Bryan, was found to be ineffective for diagnosis of food allergy and therefore unproven [4, 5, 27, 42, 79].

Peripheral leukocyte count. This was not found to be of significant value for the diagnosis of food allergy [5] or of nasal response to foods (Table 26.3).

The indirect skin test (passive transfer, Prausnitz–Küstner test). This should not be performed because of the inherent risk of transferring serum hepatitis [5, 79].

The skin-test end-point titration. This test, introduced by Rinkel [67] as an indicator for immunotherapy and as a provocative test, and later improved by some authors [64, 82], has been considered by the American Academy of Allergy [4] and others [5, 6, 79] as an unproven method and therefore not recommended for practice.

Immunotherapy with food extracts. This procedure in all its modified forms such as subcutaneous neutralization [48], intracutaneous neutralization [41, 48, 67], sublingual neutralization [41, 52] or oral immunization, has not been found to be effective [5, 30]. It is considered an unproven method and therefore not recommended for the treatment of food allergy [4] (but see Chapters 54 and 56).

Skin-test end-point titration, provocation neutralization and sublingual provocation will be discussed more fully in the relevant chapters. Another technique known as autologous urine immunization has been reviewed by Van Metre [79] and was found not only to be unproven but, moreover, to be potentially dangerous [4, 5].

SECRETORY OTITIS MEDIA

Secretory otitis media (SOM), or otitis media with effusions, is especially common in children and adolescents [24, 65] and can be divided with respect to appearance into (a) acute and (b) chronic forms. It can also be classified according to the middle ear fluid produced— either serous, mucoid (both non-suppurative) or purulent (so-called 'glue ear'). The purulent (suppurative) forms of the acute as well as of the chronic otitis media are generally caused by bacterial agents [e.g. *Streptococcus pneumoniae* (40%), *Haemophilus influenzae* (20%), *Streptococcus pyogenes* (5%), etc.]. In approximately 25% of cases no bacteria can be identified in the middle ear effusions [10, 12]. The most common cause of acute serous secretory otitis media is presumed to be bacterial infection whereas, in contrast, hypersensitivity mechanisms, and in particular allergy, are presumed to be the most important cause of chronic secretory otitis media [12].

Epidemiology of SOM

The estimates reported in the literature concerning the incidence of SOM vary widely from 15% to 64% of children [12, 24, 38, 66, 76]. SOM occurs mainly unilaterally, bilateral secretory otitis media being rare. Epidemiological data concerning SOM in adults are difficult to find. SOM is more frequent during the first 2 years of life and then decreases slowly in incidence towards the teenage years. There is no sex difference but there is a greater frequency during the winter and early spring than in the summer [12].

Pathophysiology and aetiology of SOM

SOM is an accumulation of serous or sometimes mucoid fluid in the middle ear with an associated possible increase in the local pressure and with dysfunction of the middle ear structures [5]. It has multiple aetiologies as discussed above.

The eustachian tube

The pathogenetic mechanism of otitis media and of the secretory component appears to be related to abnormal function of the eustachian tube [10].

The eustachian tube has three basic functions: (a) protection of the middle ear from the nasopharyngeal secretions; (b) ventilation of the middle ear to equilibrate air pressure in the middle ear with atmospheric pressure; and (c) drainage of secretions from the middle ear into the nasopharynx.

The major types of abnormal function of the eustachian tube that can cause SOM are obstruction, abnormal patency or a combination of both.

Obstruction. Obstruction of the eustachian tube can be caused by various factors including:

1 Mechanical obstruction: extrinsic causes, e.g. adenoids; intrinsic causes, e.g. infection or allergy.
2 Functional obstruction: caused by increased compliance, by an abnormally active opening mechanism or by nasal obstruction (so-called Toynbee phenomenon). In this form allergy is usually involved [10, 12].

Bluestone [12] suggested that persistent high negative middle ear pressure was associated with a collapse or retraction of the tympanic membrane called 'atelectasis'. If ventilation of the eustachian tube occurs when there is high negative middle ear pressure, nasopharyngeal secretions could be aspirated into the middle ear and result in an acute otitis media with effusion. In the case where ventilation of the eustachian tube does not occur, the persistent obstruction of the tube could also result in an otitis media with effusion. The occurrence of otitis in this example may be dependent on the degree and duration of the negative pressure as well as on middle ear hypoxia or hypercapnia, which can also lead to the stimulation of secretion and local exudation [63].

Nasal obstruction

Nasal obstruction may also be involved in the pathogenesis of SOM. This can lead to either oedematous obstruction of the eustachian tube or increased negative pressure in the nasopharynx resulting in an increase in the negative pressure of the middle ear with the known consequences, i.e. Toynbee phenomenon.

The corollary is that nasal obstruction can lead to an increase in positive nasopharyngeal pressure causing the aspiration of nasopharyngeal secretions into the middle ear [12].

The relationship of SOM with other allergic diseases, especially of the nose, has long been recognized [12, 44]. Allergy is presumed to be one of the most important aetiological factors in SOM because SOM occurs so frequently in subjects with other allergic disorders [62, 81]. In addition, management of the allergic condition regularly leads to a distinct improvement in the SOM. The majority of patients with secretory otitis media also have a nasal allergy both to inhalant allergens and to food [82]. In these patients treatment and management focused on the food-allergic component is extremely successful [10, 18, 68].

The involvement of allergy in secretory otitis media

In spite of the manifold evidence of the involvement of allergy in SOM, the exact mechanism of this involvement is not yet fully understood and the alternative views are controversial [22]. Reisman and Bernstein [66] and Mogi [50] found the IgE levels in SOM effusions lower than IgE levels in the serum.

From this they concluded that allergy is not a major cause of SOM.

In contrast, Phillips et al [62] and Lim et al [43] found distinctly higher levels of IgE in the middle ear effusions than in the serum and concluded that Type I allergy is the major cause of SOM—a view endorsed by Dockhorn [23]. However, the findings of high concentrations of IgG and IgA antibodies in middle ear effusion suggest that other hypersensitivity mechanisms are involved. Hall et al [32] suggested that allergy was not the primary aetiological factor in chronic SOM but only a contributing factor. Williams [82], Ruokonen [68, 69] and Clemis [18] concluded that foods and food allergy are regularly involved in SOM and, moreover, Clemis [18] believes that foods are more significant factors in allergic diseases of the upper airway and in SOM than inhalant allergens.

Author's clinical studies

In approximately 80% of patients with SOM, allergic rhinitis is also present. The corollary is that 5% of patients with allergic rhinitis also have SOM. In a few of our patients with allergic rhinitis an increase in negative middle ear pressure has been recorded after allergen challenge. Increased negative pressure in the middle ear after intranasal challenge can be found in patients with a clinically negative nasal response.

We have also found that some patients with both positive and negative nasal provocation tests with allergen can report a sharp pain in the middle ear (otalgia) or a sudden decrease in hearing after allergen challenge, while the middle ear pressure as measured by tympanometry remains unchanged.

Thus our observations implicate two possible mechanisms of involvement of food allergy in SOM. The middle ear response can be caused by foods either directly through the bloodstream or, rarely, through the topical contact in the nasopharynx without any involvement of the nasal mucosa, or indirectly through the nasal mucosa being the primary site of the hypersensitivity reaction and thus the primary effector organ. The nasal mucosa response (oedema and hypersecretion) then leads to the swelling of the peritubal tissue and lymphatics of the pharyngeal orifice of the Eustachian tube, resulting in its partial or full obstruction with the known consequences.

Diagnostic procedures

1 (a) A detailed case history, (b) a physical examination, (c) laboratory screening tests, (d) X-ray examination.

2 Ear, nose and throat examination: this should consists of (a) otolaryngologic physical examination including otoscopy, (b) tympanometry and (c) if necessary, pneumatoscopy, audiometry and diagnostic aspiration of middle ear effusions [12].

3 Allergy investigations: (a) skin testing with basic inhalant and food allergens; (b) RAST may sometimes be of diagnostic value in SOM. Total IgE does not seem to be of diagnostic value (Table 26.8); (c) repeated nasal secretions for cytogram especially with respect to eosinophils; and (d) nasal provocation tests with inhalation allergens and/or food ingestion challenges. The combination of nasal challenge with tympanometry before and after challenge is a useful diagnostic procedure in some patients.

Management and treatment

Otitis media due to infection

Acute otitis media. Antibiotics (systemic and local) and analgesics with nasal decongestants if indicated may be used and if fever and pain persist for longer than 24–48 hours then myringotomy may be indicated. In the case of recurrent otitis media, the insertion of ventilation tubes at least temporarily may be helpful [12].

Chronic otitis media. Prophylactic antimicrobial therapy, nasal decongestants and myringotomy with insertion of ventilation tubes may be used in treatment and occasionally inflation of the middle ear (Politzer's manoeuvre) may be helpful and prevent further complications [12].

Secretory otitis media with an allergic component

Acute SOM. The isolated form (where the confirmation of allergy is usually difficult) needs nasal decongestants, antihistamines and the elimination of the presumed allergen. The forms associated with, or induced by, the nasal mucosal response due to hypersensitivity suggest the use of disodium cromoglycate complemented with antihistamines, nasal decongestants, rinsing of the nose with sterile saline and, if necessary, intranasal topical corticosteroids, as described above for rhinitis. If the acute SOM due to the allergy mechanism is accompanied by the production of middle ear effusions, in addition to the antiallergy treatment, myringotomy should also be considered [11, 12, 22, 69].

Chronic SOM. When there is no associated nasal mucosal allergic state (rare), antihistamines and, if necessary, myringotomy may be indicated. With associated nasal allergy (common), treatment consists of long-term disodium cromoglycate intranasally supplemented by antihistamines and possibly hyposensitization. Occasionally additional anticholinergic drugs (e.g. thiazinamium hydrochloride) or a sustained action oral combination of these preparations may be useful. Where a non-immediate nasal response to allergen occurs, topical corticosteroid aerosols intranasally should be used (e.g. beclomethasone dipropionate). Every effort should be made to eliminate the allergens involved. If middle ear effusions occur, myringotomy should be considered, with the possible insertion of ventilation tubes or other surgical procedures.

Table 26.8 Survey of the total serum IgE antibodies (PRIST) of 29 patients with positive immediate middle ear response to the food ingestion challenge.

	PRIST				
	0–50 IU/ml	50–100 IU/ml	100–500 IU/ml	500–1000 IU/ml	>1000 IU/ml
Subjects (*n* = 29)	16 (55%)	9 (31%)	1 (3.5%)	2 (7%)	1 (3.5%)

Interpretation of the PRIST results, modified by the author: $\leqslant 100\,\text{IU/ml}$ = not increased (negative); 100–500 IU/ml = slightly increased (doubtful); >500 IU/ml = increased (positive).

SOM induced by the nasal mucosa response due to food allergy. In this situation topical intranasal disodium cromoglycate with supplementary antihistamines is effective in a large proportion of patients. Where the existence of the late nasal response is predominant, topical intranasal corticosteroids should also be used. If topical intranasal DSCG is not effective then treatment with the oral preparation (100–200 mg four times daily) should be considered.

SOM due directly to the food allergy without involvement of the nasal mucosa. In these cases prophylactic treatment with oral disodium cromoglycate is the treatment of choice.

The involvement of food allergy in SOM

The avoidance of the incriminating foods or their constituents should be the first step in the management of this disorder [68]. Other steps such as the pharmacological control of SOM depend on the involvement of food allergy in the disease process [76, 86].

SOM induced by the nasal mucosal response to foods and inhalants in combination with non-specific nasal hyperreactivity. In these cases intranasal and oral disodium cromoglycate is indicated, sometimes accompanied by antihistamines.

Conclusion

The involvement of food and inhalant allergens in the production of secretory middle ear disease is becoming more widely recognized. A diligent search for extrinsic causes should be pursued in all cases of SOM because removal of such aetiologic agents results in resolution of the disease. Other therapeutic manoeuvres are obviously necessary when the invoking agents are not discovered or when their elimination is not fully possible.

REFERENCES

1 Aas K: The critical approach to food allergy. Ann Allergy 1983; 51: 256-9.

2 Adkinson NF: The radioallergosorbent test: uses and abuses. J Allergy Clin Immunol 1980; 65: 1-4.

3 Adkinson NF: The radioallergosorbent test. J Allergy Clin Immunol 1980; 66: 174-5.

4 American Academy of Allergy: Position statements— controversial techniques. J Allergy Clin Immunol 1981; 67: 333-8.

5 Anderson JA, Sogn DD: Committee on adverse reactions to foods of the American Academy of Allergy and Immunology and National Institute of Allergy and Infectious Disease. In: Adverse Reactions to Foods. Washington: US Department of Health and Human Services, 1984; NIH Publication No. 84-2442.

6 Bahna SL, Ghandi MD: Milk hypersensitivity. II. Practical aspects of diagnosis treatment and prevention. Ann Allergy 1983; 50: 295-301.

7 Berman BA: Cromolyn: past, present and future. Pediatr Clin North Am 1983; 30 (5): 915-30.

8 Bernstein M, Day JM, Welsh A: Double blind food challenge in the diagnosis of food sensitivity in the adult. J Allergy Clin Immunol 1982; 70: 205-10.

9 Bernstein IL, Johnson CL, Gallagher JS et al: Are tartrazine reactions mediated by IgE? J Allergy Clin Immunol 1978; 61: 191.

10 Bluestone ChD: Eustachian tube function and allergy in otitis media. Pediatrics 1978; 61: 753-60.

11 Bluestone ChD: Recent advances in the pathogenesis, diagnosis and management of otitis media. Pediatr Clin North Am 1981; 28: 727-55.

12 Bluestone ChD, Douglas DS, Bernstein JM: Otitis media. In: Middleton E, Reed ChE, Ellis EF, eds. Allergy, principles and practice, St Louis: CV Mosby; 1023-38.

13 Bock S: Clinical aspects of food sensitivity. In: Kerr JW, Ganderton MA, eds. Proceedings of the XIth International Congress of Allergology and Clinical Immunology. London: Macmillan, 1983; 181-5.

14 Bock S, May D, Remigio L: Clinical manifestations and immunological findings in food sensitivity confirmed objectively. In: Pepys J, Edwards AM, eds. The mast cell—Its role in health and disease. Tunbridge Wells: Pitman Medical, 1979; 411-15.

15 Brostoff J, Carini C, Wraith DG et al: Immune-complex in atopy. In: Pepys J, Edwards AM, eds. The mast cell—Its role in health and disease. Tunbridge Wells: Pitman Medical, 1979; 380-93.

16 Buisseret PD: Common manifestations of cow's milk allergy in children. Lancet 1978i: 304-5.

17 Chua YY, Bremner K, Lakdawalla N et al: In vivo and in vitro correlates of food allergy. J Allergy Clin Immunol 1976; 58: 299.

18 Clemis JD: Identification of allergic factors in middle ear effusions. Ann Otol Rhinol Laryngol 1976; 23: 234-7.

19 Coombs RRA: Pathogenesis and mechanisms. In: Coombs RRA, ed. Proceedings of the First Food Allergy Workshop. Oxford: Medical Education Services, 1980; 7-8, 13-27.

20 Dannaeus A: Management of food allergy in infancy. Ann Allergy 1983; 51: 303-6.

21 Delire M: Detection of circulating immune-complexes in infants fed on cow's milk. In: Pepys J, Edwards AM, eds. The mast cell—Its role in health and disease. Tunbridge Wells: Pitman Medical, 1979; 375-9.

22 Derlacki EL: Otologic allergy. Am J Otol 1982; 3: 379-83.

23 Dockhorn RJ: Otolaryngologic allergy in children. Otolaryngol Clin North Am 1977; 10: 103-12.

24 Draper WL: Secretory otitis media. Laryngoscope 1967; 78: 636.

25 Eriksson NS: Food sensitivity reported by patients with asthma and hay fever. Allergy 1978; 33: 189–96.

26 Evans R III: Variability in the measurement of specific immunoglobulin E antibody by the RAST procedure. J Allergy Clin Immunol 1982; 69: 245–52.

27 Freed DLJ: Laboratory diagnosis of food intolerance. In: Brostoff J, Challacombe SJ, eds. Clinics in immunology and allergy—Food allergy. Philadelphia: WB Saunders, 1982; 181–203.

28 Gerrard JW: The diagnosis of the food-allergic patient. In: Pepys J, Edwards AM, eds. The mast cell—Its role in health and disease. Tunbridge Wells: Pitman Medical, 1979; 416–21.

29 Gleich GS, Sachs MI, O'Connel EJ: Hypersensitivity reactions induced by foods. In: Parker Ch W, ed. Clinical immunology. Philadelphia: WB Saunders, 1980; 1261–83.

30 Golbert TM: A review of controversial diagnostic and therapeutic techniques employed in allergy. J Allergy Clin Immunol 1975; 56: 170–90.

31 Green M: Sublingual provocative testing for food and FD and C dyes. Ann Allergy 1974; 33: 274.

32 Hall LJ, Asuncion J, Lukat M: Allergy skin testing under general anesthesia with treatment response in ninety-two patients with chronic serous otitis media. Am J Otol 1980; 2: 150–7.

33 Halpern GM: Alimentary allergy. J Asthma 1983; 20(4): 251–84.

34 Heiner DC: Food allergy and respiratory disease. Ann Allergy 1983; 51: 273–4.

35 Heiner DC, Sears JW: Chronic respiratory disease associated with multiple circulating precipitins to cow's milk. Am J Dis Child 1960; 100: 500–2.

36 Heiner DC, Spears JW, Kuiker WT: Multiple precipities to cow's milk in chronic respiratory disease. Am J Dis Child 1962; 103: 634.

37 Hoffman DR, Haddad ZH: Diagnosis of IgE-mediated reactions to food antigens by radioimmunoassay. J Allergy Clin Immunol 1974; 54: 165–73.

38 Ingvarsson L, Lundgren K, Olofsson B, Wall S: Epidemiology of acute otitis media in children. Acta Oto-Laryngol [Suppl] (Stockh) 388: 1–52.

39 Juhlin L: Incidence of intolerance to food additives. Int J Dermatol 1980; 19: 548–51.

40 Juhlin L, Michaelsson G, Zetterstrom O: Urticaria and asthma induced by food- and drug-additives in patients with aspirin hypersensitivity. J Allergy Clin Immunol 1972; 50: 92–8.

41 Lee CH, Williams RI, Binkley EL: Provocative testing and treatment for foods. Arch Otolaryngol 1969; 90: 87–94.

42 Lehman CN: The leukocytotoxic food allergy test: a study of its reliability and reproducibility. Effect of diet and sublingual food drops on this test. Ann Allergy 1980; 45: 150.

43 Lim DJ, Liu YS, Schram J, Birck HG: Immunoglobulin E in chronic middle ear effusions. Ann Otol Rhinol Laryngol 1976; 85(25): 119.

44 McGovern JP, Haywood TJ, Fernandes A: Allergy and secretory ototis media. J Am Med Assoc 1967; 200: 134.

45 May CD: Immunologic versus toxic adverse reactions to foodstuffs. Ann Allergy 1983; 51: 267–8.

46 May CD, Bock SA: A modern clinical approach to food hypersensitivity. Allergy 1978; 33: 166–88.

47 May CD, Bock SA: Adverse reactions to foods due to hypersensitivity. In: Middleton E Jr, Reed CE, Ellis EF, eds. Allergy, principles and practice. St Louis: CV Mosby, 1978; 1159–71.

48 Miller JB: A double-blind study of food extract injection therapy: a preliminary report. Ann Allergy 1977; 38: 185–91.

49 Minor JD, Tolber SG, Frick OL: Leukocyte inhibition factor in delayed-onset food allergy. J Allergy Clin Immunol 1980; 66: 314–21.

50 Mogi G: Secretory IgA and antibody activities in middle ear effusion. Ann Otol Rhinol Laryngol 1976; 85(25): 97.

51 Moneret-Vautrin DA: Non specific reactions to foodstuffs: false food allergies. In: Kerr JW, Ganderton MA, eds. Proceedings of the XIth International Congress of Allergology and Clinical Immunology. London: Macmillan, 1982; 175–9.

52 Morris DL: Use of sublingual antigen in diagnosis and treatment of food allergy. Ann Allergy 1969; 27: 289–94.

53 Ogle KA, Bullock JD: Children with allergic rhinitis and/or bronchial asthma treated with elimination diet. Ann Allergy 1977; 39: 8–11.

54 Ogle KA, Bullock JD: Children with allergic rhinitis and/or bronchial asthma treated with elimination diet: a five-year follow-up. Ann Allergy 1980; 44: 273–8.

55 Paganelli R, Levinsky RJ, Brostoff J, Wraith DG: Immune complexes containing food proteins in normal and atopic subjects after oral challenge and effect of sodium cromoglycate on antigen absorption. Lancet 1979; i: 1270–2.

56 Pelikan Z: Late and delayed nasal mucosa response to allergen challenge. Ann Allergy 1978; 41: 37–47.

57 Pelikan Z: The role of immediate, late and delayed reactions in allergic nasal disease. In: Pepys J, Edwards AM, eds. The mast cell—Its role in health and disease. Tunbridge Wells: Pitman Medical, 1979; 772–7.

58 Pelikan Z: Occurrence of food allergy and the correlation of skin tests with disease history and with the effect of the elimination diet. In: Nelemans FA, Quarles van Ufford WJ, Schwietert HR, eds. Food allergy. Haarlem: HAL Allergy Service, 1980; 59–70.

58a Pelikan Z: The effects of disodium cromoglycate and beclomethasone dipropionate on the delayed nasal mucosa response to allergen challenge. Ann Allergy 1984; 52: 111–14.

59 Pelikan Z: Allergic conjunctivitis—relationship to allergic rhinitis and the effect of disodium cromoglycate (DSCG). In: Abstracts of the XIth International Congress of Allergology and Clinical Immunology, London, Oct. 17–22, 1982. London: Macmillan, 1982; Abstract No. 392P.

60 Pelikan Z: The changes in the nasal secretions of eosinophils during the immediate nasal response to allergen challenge. J Allergy Clin Immunol 1983; 72: 657–62.

61 Pelikan Z: The diagnostic approach to the immediate hypersensitivity in patients with allergic rhinitis: a comparison of nasal challenges and serum RAST. Ann Allergy 1983; 59: 283–92.

62 Phillips MJ, Knight NJ, Manning E et al: IgE and secretory otitis media. Lancet 1974; ii: 1176.

63 Pulec JL, Horwitz MJ: Diseases of the Eustachian tube. In: Paparella MM, Schumrich DA, eds. Otolaryngology. Philadelphia: WB Saunders, 1973; 75–92.

64 Radcliffe MJ: Clinical methods for diagnosis. In: Brostoff J, Challacombe SJ, eds. Clinics in immunology and allergy—Food allergy. London: WB Saunders, 1982: 205–20.

65 Rapp DJ, Fahey DJ: Allergy and chronic secretory

otitis media. Pediatr Clin North Am 1975; 22: 259-64.

66 Reisman ER, Bernstein J: Allergy and secretory otitis media. Pediatr Clin North Am 1975; 22: 251-7.

67 Rinkel HJ, Lee CH, Brown DW et al: The diagnosis of food allergy. Arch Otolaryngol 1964; 79: 71-9.

68 Ruokonen J, Paganus A, Lehti H: Elimination diets in the treatment of secretory otitis media. Int J Pediatr Otorhinolaryngol 1982; 4: 39-46.

69 Ruokonen J, Holopainen E, Palva T, Backman A: Secretory otitis media and allergy. Allergy 1981; 36: 59-68.

70 Sachs MI: Value of food antigen specific IgE-RAST and immediate reaction skin test. Ann Allergy 1983; 51: 264-6.

71 Sampson HA: Role of immediate food hypersensitivity in the pathogenesis of atopic dermatitis. J Allergy Clin Immunol 1983; 71: 473-80.

72 Sampson HA, Albergo R: Comparison of results of skin tests, RAST and double-blind, placebo controlled food challenges in children with atopic dermatitis. J Allergy Clin Immunol 1984; 74: 26-33.

73 Schlumberger HD: Pseudo-allergic reactions to drugs and chemicals. Ann Allergy 1983; 51: 317-24.

74 Schwartz HJ: Sensitivity to ingested metabisulfite: variation in clinical presentation. J Allergy Clin Immunol 1983; 71: 487-9.

75 Settipane GA, Chafee FH, Postman IM et al: Significance of tartrazine sensitivity in chronic urticaria of unknown etiology. J Allergy Clin Immunol 1976; 57: 541-6.

76 Shanon E, Englender M, Beizer M: A clinical pilot study of disodium cromoglycate in the treatment of secretory otitis media. In: Pepys J, Edwards AM, eds. The mast cell—Its role in health and disease. Tunbridge Wells: Pitman Medical, 1979: 791-4.

77 Shioda H, Mishima T, Yamada S, et al: Nasal smears in the diagnosis of food allergy. In: Pepys J, Edwards AM, eds. The mast cell—Its role in health and disease. Tunbridge Wells: Pitman Medical, 1979: 422-30.

78 Soothill J: Food allergy. In: Pepys J, Edwards AM, eds. The mast cell—Its role in health and disease. Tunbridge Wells; Pitman Medical, 1979; 367-70.

79 Van Metre TE: Critique of controversial and unproven procedures for diagnosis and therapy of allergic disorders. Pediatr Clin North Am 1983; 30: 807-17.

80 Weber RW, Hoffman M, Raine DA, Nelson HS: Incidence of bronchoconstriction due to aspirin, azo-dyes, non-azo dyes and preservatives in a population of perennial asthmatics. J Allergy Clin Immunol 1979; 64: 32-7.

81 Whitcomb NJ: Allergy therapy in serous otitis media associated with allergic rhinitis. Ann Allergy 1965; 23: 232-6.

82 Williams RI: Hypersensitivity problems in otorhinolaryngology. Ann Otol Rhinol Laryngol, 1978; 87: 670-4.

83 Wilson CMW: Food sensitivities, taste changes, aphthous ulcers and atopic symptoms in allergic disease. Ann Allergy 1980; 44: 302-7.

84 Wraith DG: Asthma and rhinitis. In: Brostoff J, Challacombe SJ, eds. Clinics in immunology and allergy—Food allergy. Philadelphia: WB Saunders, 1982; 101-12.

85 Wraith DG, Young GVM, Lee TH: The management of food allergy with diet and Nalcrom. In: Pepys J, Edwards AM, eds. The mast cell—Its role in health and disease. Tunbridge Wells: Pitman Medical, 1979; 443-6.

86 Zanussi C: Food allergy treatment. In: Brostoff J, Challacombe SJ, eds. Clinics in immunology and allergy—Food allergy. Philadelphia; WB Saunders, 1982; 221-40.

87 Zanussi C, Ortolani C, Pastorello E: Dietary and pharmacologic management of food intolerance in adults. Ann Allergy 1983; 51: 307-10.

Chapter 27
Asthma

D. G. Wraith

Introduction

Food allergy is a very important cause of asthma but is often overlooked. It is important because it may cause severe symptoms and asthma still has a high mortality despite improvements in drug treatment. It is overlooked because the usual skin (prick) tests are often negative and the history is often not of help as symptoms appear gradually, hours or days after ingestion of the food (Fig. 27.1). Avoidance of the cause would prevent much disability and also lessen the amount of drugs needed, which is important considering their expense and potential side-effects.

CLINICAL FEATURES SUGGESTING FOOD INTOLERANCE

There are often some clinical features which suggest that food intolerance may be a cause of asthma and suggest that further investigation should be undertaken.

Table 27.1 gives the features which were found in a series of patients which suggest the possibility of food intolerance. The majority of patients had other symptoms besides asthma and it was these multiple symptoms which were characteristic of food intolerance (food intolerance syndrome). This was more likely if there was an allergic background, with

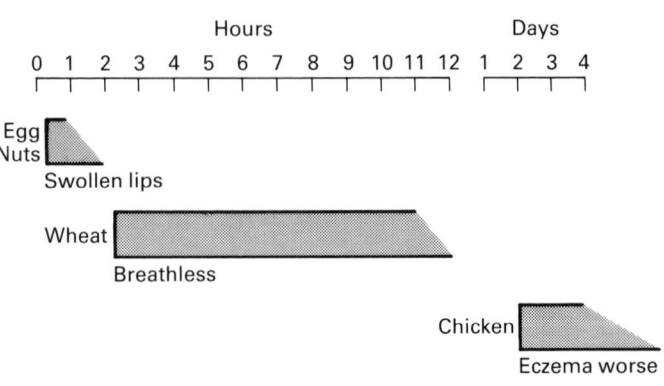

Fig. 27.1 Male, 24 years: the different time delays of symptoms of asthma and eczema following ingestion of certain foods. Immediate symptoms and positive skin tests were obvious but breathlessness and wheeze did not appear until over 2 hours after wheat ingestion and there was no exacerbation of eczema until 3 days after ingestion of chicken. The latter two foods were confirmed by their elimination and reintroduction on several occasions, but skin tests were negative. From Wraith [45], with permission.

486

Table 27.1 Features suggesting food intolerance.

1 Multiple symptoms

2 Family history of allergy or food intolerance

3 Other atopic symptoms

4 If one food is known, others are likely

a family history or other known allergies. If one food was already known to trigger a response there would probably be others, as multiple foods were usually involved in asthma.

Skin tests

In a group of 180 patients with asthma caused by foods, 65% gave a positive skin (prick) test with one or more inhalants. Not all these positive tests were associated with symptoms, some being the result, for example, of previous exposure to the allergen.

Skin tests (538 tests) were positive for only 39% of food extracts causing 'non-immediate' asthma symptoms (more than 1 hour after the food) but also there were 12% positive tests with foods not causing asthma symptoms. These were positive in most of those with 'im-mediate' symptoms. In a previous report [28] skin tests with foods were positive in 32% of 43 patients with non-immediate asthma symptoms. Some patients had symptoms from chemical food additives but tests with these were not practicable.

Case report. A male, aged 12 years, had severe asthma in the summer. This was considered to be due to grass pollen allergy because he had a positive skin test to pollen but his asthma cleared when he stopped drinking orange squash containing artificial colouring, of which he had more than usual in the summer.

Total IgE

Fig. 27.2 shows the total IgE values in 128 patients with non-immediate symptoms from foods. There is much variation in these values depending on whether the asthma is associated with eczema and inhalant allergies, inhalants alone or neither. In those with eczema and inhalant allergies, for example, the majority of the values are above 500 IU/ml, but in those with neither of these, the majority of the values are normal, i.e. below 120 IU/ml.

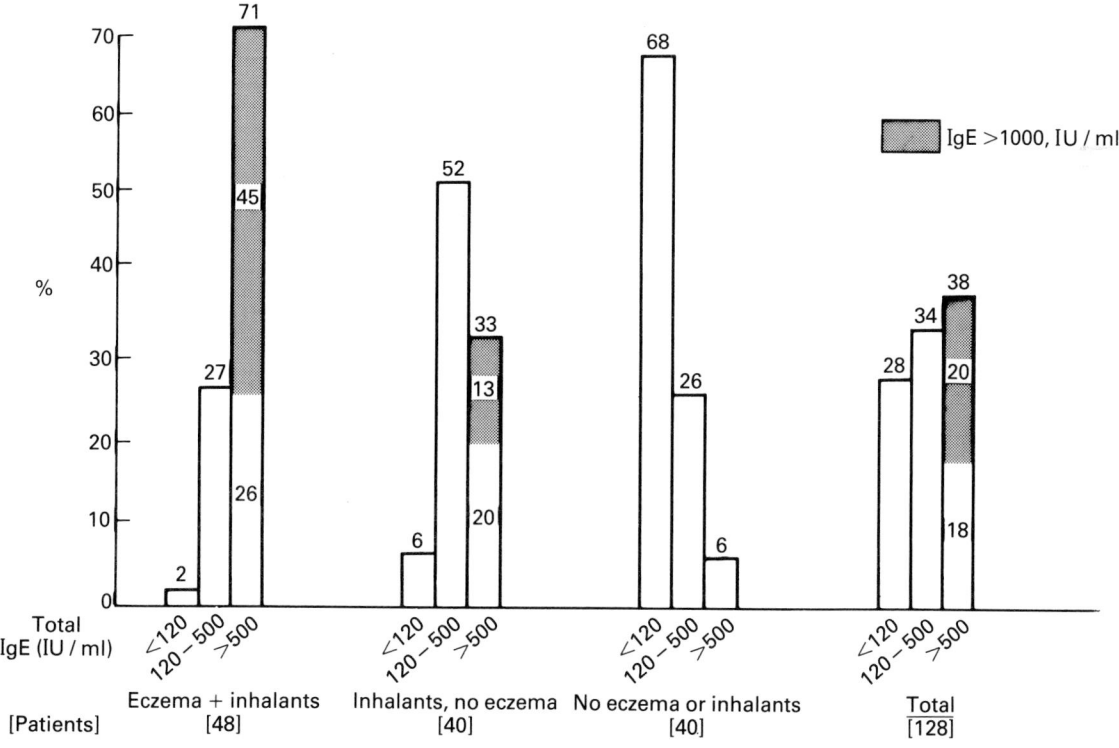

Fig. 27.2 Total IgE values in 128 patients with non-immediate symptoms of asthma from foods, subdivided into those with eczema and inhalation allergies, inhalation allergies alone and neither of these. There is a much higher number of patients with eczema with raised values than without eczema or inhalation allergies.

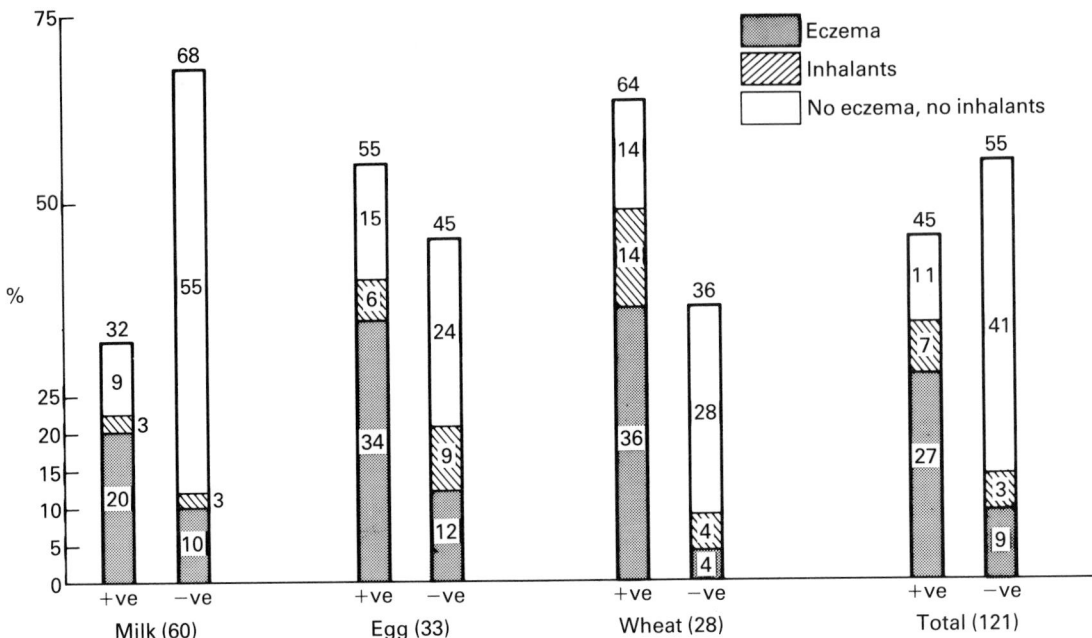

Fig. 27.3 Specific IgE (RAST). The proportions of positive and negative radioallergosorbent test results (RAST) with milk, egg and wheat in patients with symptoms of asthma from these foods. In general there is a higher proportion with eczema associated with the asthma with positive RAST than in those without eczema. There is a higher proportion with negative RAST (<1.2) and symptoms with milk, compared with other foods.

RAST

Figure 27.3 shows the results of radioallergosorbent tests (RAST) performed with milk, egg and wheat extracts in 87 patients with asthma caused by one or more of these foods. The figure gives the proportions with negative RAST (less than 1.2 times the background counts) and positive RAST with each of the foods that caused symptoms. It is seen that (a) there was a higher proportion of positive results in those in whom eczema was associated with the asthma and (b) there was a difference between the foods, and milk produced a higher proportion of symptoms and negative tests. Also (not shown in the figure) there was a small proportion of positive tests with foods which did not cause symptoms (8%).

The results of these tests illustrate the limitation of RAST in the diagnosis of food intolerance. The variations, due to presence or absence of eczema, and the particular foods involved, give rise to difficulties in making comparisons with other reported studies. In a previous report [47] a higher number (64%) or patients with symptoms of asthma had a positive RAST, possibly due to more of the patients having eczema and also differences in foods. In that study, milk was less often im-plicated but cereals and nuts were more frequently implicated.

INVESTIGATION OF FOOD INTOLERANCE

Elimination diets

Investigation of which specific foods and additives were responsible for inducing asthma was carried out in these patients by elimination diets and provocation tests (Table 27.2).

Table 27.2 Investigation of food intolerance.

1 Selected foods stopped for 2 weeks and reintroduced one at a time

2 Hypoantigenic diet

3 Record diary of daily food intake and symptoms with breathing tests (peak expiration flow rate)

4 Confirmation if necessary by repeating tests, in some cases 'blind'

Elimination of foods for about 2 weeks enhances the patient's sensitivity so that their reintroduction, one at a time, will give a more clear-cut reaction for those that are relevant, as recorded by serial breathing (peak flow) tests.

The foods selected for testing were those

considered to be the most likely causes of the asthma. Those taken in relative excess were found to be the most frequent causes, e.g. specific likings (sometimes cravings). Habits and customs, such as racial differences or vegetarianism, need to be analysed. Those foods disliked but still consumed are also possible causes. This way of selecting foods is more practical than a single standardized elimination diet—merely stopping foods and waiting takes longer and the results may be indistinct because several foods are usually involved.

Reintroduction of foods

Each food or group of foods is reintroduced one at a time for about 5 days before proceeding to the next one, but stopped again if symptoms become worse or if there is a fall in the serial peak flow values. A small amount of the food is taken at first and then gradually increased amounts are taken; this is because those patients who are very sensitive will react almost immediately, but those less sensitive may require several days and larger amounts of the food to elicit a reaction which might otherwise be missed.

Restricted diet

A very restricted hypoantigenic diet consisting of, for example, lamb, rabbit, cauliflower, pears and spring water, is taken for 5 days and foods reintroduced as before. This is more comprehensive than the previous method but takes longer and 'withdrawal' symptoms may sometimes be severe (Fig. 27.4).

Daily food diary

A daily record of all foods consumed and a record of symptoms and serial breathing tests may be sufficient to identify specific foods. This takes time and since many foods are often involved some foods causing symptoms can be missed. Stopping and restarting foods may sometimes enable the relevant ones to be found (Fig. 27.5).

Confirmation of food allergy

1 The reaction to a food may be so obvious that the patient does not want to repeat it or a food may be taken by mistake and identified by the reaction.

2 Where there is doubt, the challenge should be repeated with a larger amount of the food for a longer time because foods to which one is not very sensitive may be missed.

3 'Blind' testing is not very practicable with the very large numbers of patients attending clinics, especially as a large amount of food may have to be disguised and taken for several days, and as several foods are usually involved. Blind challenges may be necessary with colouring in capsules or with foods disguised (Fig. 27.6). Pretreatment with either oral sodium cromoglycate or placebo before challenge can be a useful method of defining an allergic response in some cases (Figs. 27.7 and 27.8).

The results with repeated tests may vary as there may be a refractory period after the previous test or sensitivity may change during the menstrual cycle, or as a result of exercise and psychological stresses.

Difficulties and hazards

1 With cases of severe asthma, especially in

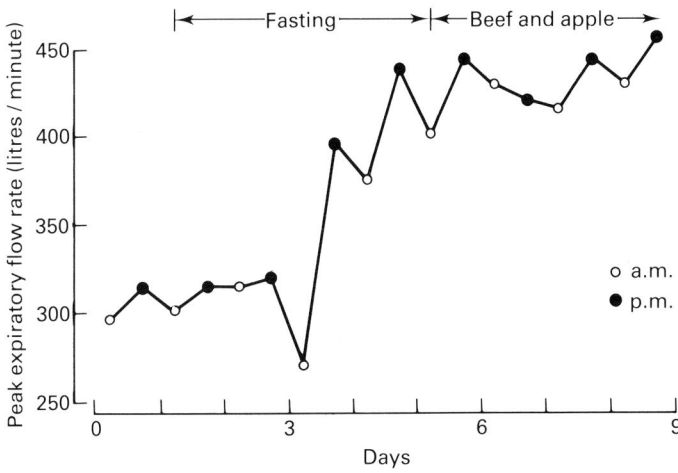

Fig. 27.4 Male, 24 years, with severe asthma and eczema since childhood. The figure shows results of a 5-day fast. There was an initial decrease of peak flow values (withdrawal symptoms) and then a considerable increase. Foods were then gradually added. Milk and wheat were found to be the main foods responsible (skin tests negative). Despite the long history, a great improvement was achieved on an elimination diet. Reproduced from Wraith [44] with permission.

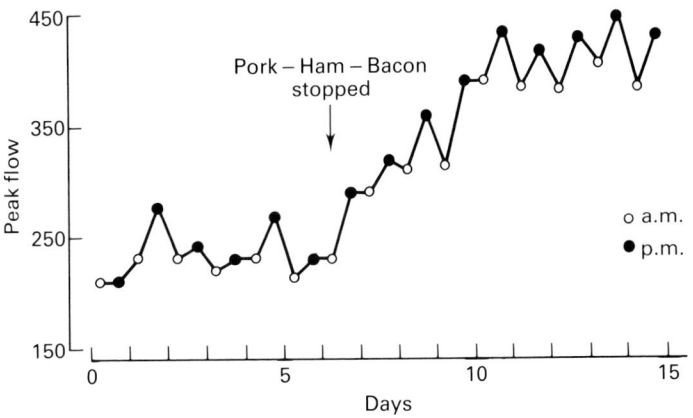

Fig. 27.5 Male, 40 years: morning and evening peak flow breathing tests and a diary of all foods, etc. The patient showed improved values when pork, ham and bacon were stopped. Several other allergenic foods were found later and all were confirmed by a fall in peak flow values on their reintroduction. From Wraith [45], with permission.

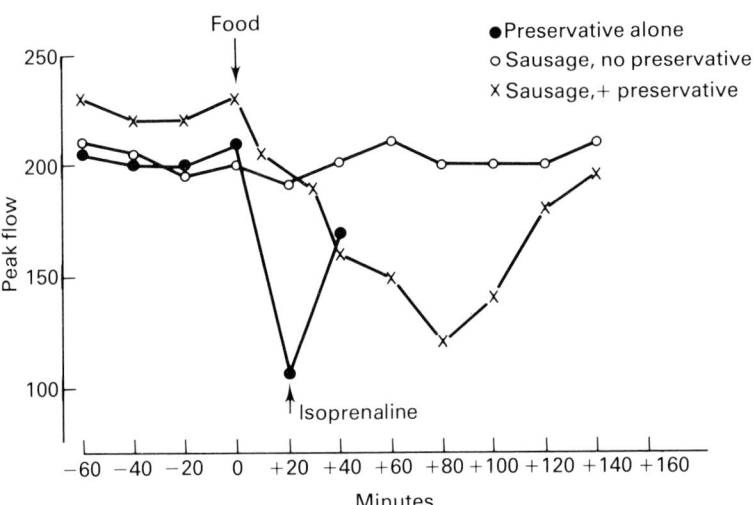

Fig. 27.6 Female, 57 years, with recent onset of severe asthma considered to be 'intrinsic'. Skin tests were negative. Food tests confirmed preservatives as the cause. There was a rapid and big drop in peak flow values and severe breathlessness after lemonade containing preservatives (sodium benzoate and sulphur dioxide). On other days, sausages with identical appearances with and without preservatives caused fall (○) and no fall (×) in peak flow values. From Wraith [45], with permission.

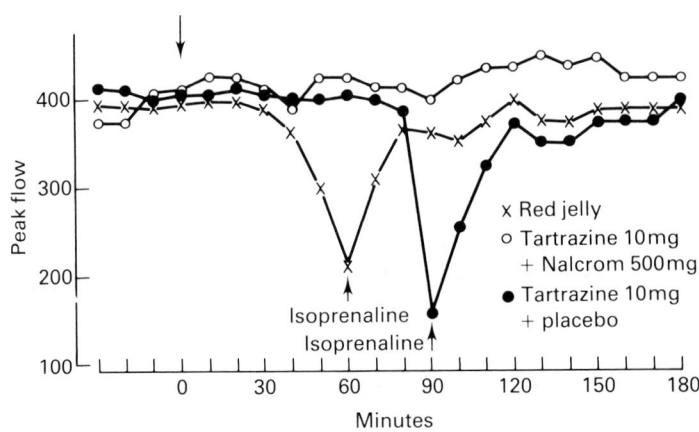

Fig. 27.7 Female, 47 years, with recent onset of asthma considered to be 'intrinsic'. Peak flow values fell after red jelly containing artificial colour and also tartrazine, 10 mg. This was prevented by pretreatment with Nalcrom, 500 mg, 15 minutes and 2 hours before eating, but not by a placebo drug. This shows the ability of Nalcrom to prevent symptoms due to sensitivity to food colourings. There was no fall (not in figure) when placebo was substituted for tartrazine. From Wraith [45], with permission.

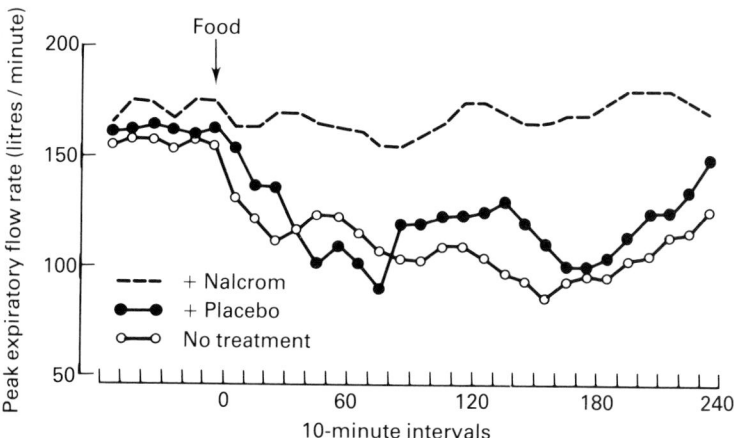

Fig. 27.8 Female, 38 years, with a long history of asthma, but recently found to be sensitive to a number of foods: milk, eggs, wheat and coffee; skin tests were negative. The figure shows a fall in peak flow values after two eggs. This was prevented by pretreatment with Nalcrom, 500 mg, 10 minutes and also 2 hours before eating, but not by a placebo drug. Reproduced from Wraith [44], with permission.

children, tests should be carried out under medical supervision, e.g. in hospital.

2 Withdrawal symptoms: a temporary increase of asthma or other symptoms may occur for a few days after stopping the foods.

3 In children and those on already restricted diets, alternative foods or supplements are necessary.

4 Practical difficulties with stopping foods include cravings, sweets from friends, school meals and so on, so careful explanation is necessary. Tablets and medicines containing colouring may need to be changed.

A STUDY OF PATIENTS WITH ASTHMA

In a series of 265 patients with asthma found to be caused by foods or food additives, just over half, 151, were aged less than 15 years. There was a preponderance of males (65%) in the younger group and of females (75%) in the older patients.

Treatment had included continuous or intermittent oral steroids in about a quarter (26%) and regular bronchodilators in just under half (44%). This reflects the degree of severity of asthma in these patients. The steroid treatment was mainly in the older patients. The reduction of medication in the group after food avoidance, with steroids down from 26% to 3%, and regular bronchodilators from 44% to 20%, illustrates the value of food avoidance. This also resulted in a considerable decrease in the expense of drug treatment.

The majority of these patients also had other symptoms combined with their asthma which will be briefly described. The individual case histories in the accompanying figures illustrate many points, such as duration and severity of the asthma (e.g. Figs. 27.8, 27.11, 27.12–27–14).

Foods causing asthma

Figure 27.9 shows the main foods found to cause asthma in those aged less than 15 years and in those aged 15 years and above. In the younger group, milk, egg and artificial colouring stood out as being the chief culprits; in the older patients there was a much wider range of foods incriminated, with milk and wheat being the main ones. There was considerable individual variation depending very much on habits of eating, and foods taken regularly in relatively larger amounts were found to be the chief offenders. This would explain the frequency of involvement of artificial colouring in the younger patients and the obvious implication that a decreased intake at an earlier age in those with an allergic background would have helped to prevent the symptoms. Colours and preservatives are difficult to avoid as they occur in so many foods, drinks, sweets and also in medicines. In those patients, mainly adults, who were sensitive to wheat, other cereals (rye, oats, corn) were also frequently implicated. In adults especially, a very wide variety of foods were involved in addition to the main ones included in Fig. 27.9. Multiple food sensitivities were usual. Figs 27.7 and 27.14 show that additives were an important cause of asthma and Fig. 27.6 gives an example of intrinsic asthma caused by preservatives.

Intrinsic asthma

Intrinsic asthma describes the condition in patients who have negative skin (prick) tests and no cause apparent from their history; they have also been termed 'cryptogenic'. Asthma

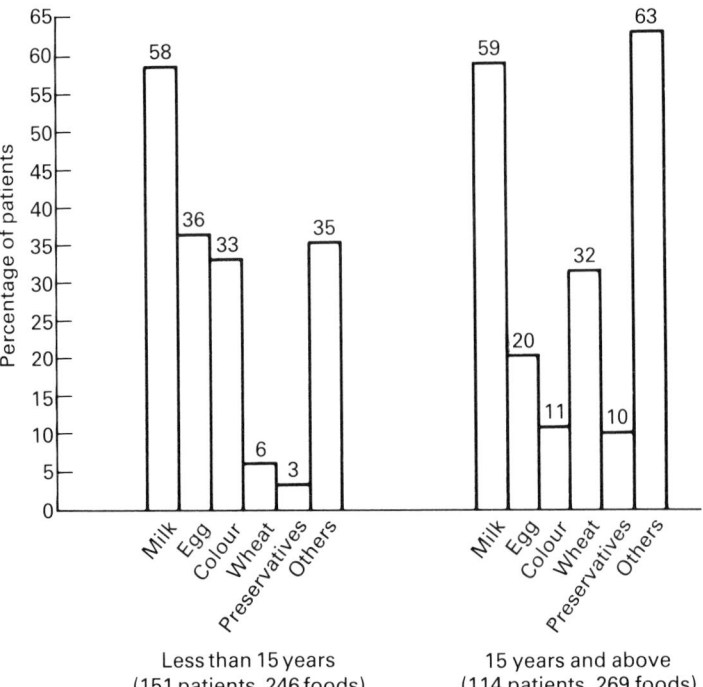

Fig. 27.9 Foods causing asthma. The figure shows the percentages of patients in the two age groups with asthma caused by the main foods. In the younger group, milk, egg and artificial colouring were the main ones. In the older patients, milk is also the main one, and wheat the next most frequent cause. There is a much greater variety of implicated foods in the older group. Other foods included cheese, fish, chocolate, soya, citrus fruit and nuts in the younger group and yeast, other cereals (rye, oats, corn, etc.), pork, cheese, chocolate, coffee and many others in the older patients.

is often severe. In our study there were 30 patients with onset over the age of 40 years, half of whom required continuous or intermittent steroids.

The main foods implicated were milk, wheat, egg, yeast, preservatives, colouring, coffee and cheese. Avoidance of these resulted in a marked improvement and enabled the steroids to be stopped in the majority. Figs 27.6 and 27.7 give typical examples.

About half of these patients had other symptoms, such as rhinitis, including some with nasal polyps, joint and gastrointestinal symptoms.

Other reports showing the importance of food allergy and intolerance as a cause of asthma have included those of Rowe [39], Gerrard [23], Ogle and Bullock [33], Papageorgiou et al [35], Kniker and Rodriguez [27], Dahl and Zetterstrom [13] and Dahl [12]. The latter two reports have also shown the value of oral sodium cromoglycate in the prevention of symptoms. Additives in foods, artificial colouring and preservatives have been shown to be causes of asthma by Stenius and Lemola [42], Freedman [19,20], Baker et al [4], Stevenson and Simon [43] and Ortolani et al [34].

OTHER SYMPTOMS CAUSED BY FOODS IN PATIENTS WITH ASTHMA

The majority of patients in this study, 65%, had other—often several—symptoms caused by foods. Fig. 27.10 shows the proportions of these. They were often caused by different foods than those causing the asthma. These various symptoms which are associated with asthma are emphasized because their combination is a characteristic feature of food intolerance and so is of diagnostic value. The symptoms are also important in their own right, illustrating the wide range that may be caused by food intolerance. These were found in patients attending allergy and chest clinics with asthma so one would expect many similar symptoms to be found in other specialized clinics caused by food intolerance which may be overlooked.

Eczema

Eczema was the most frequent in the younger age group caused mainly by milk, artificial colouring and egg. The importance of foods as a cause has been shown in a controlled trial by Atherton et al [2]. Infants and children with eczema seem more likely to develop asthma later (see Chapter 34).

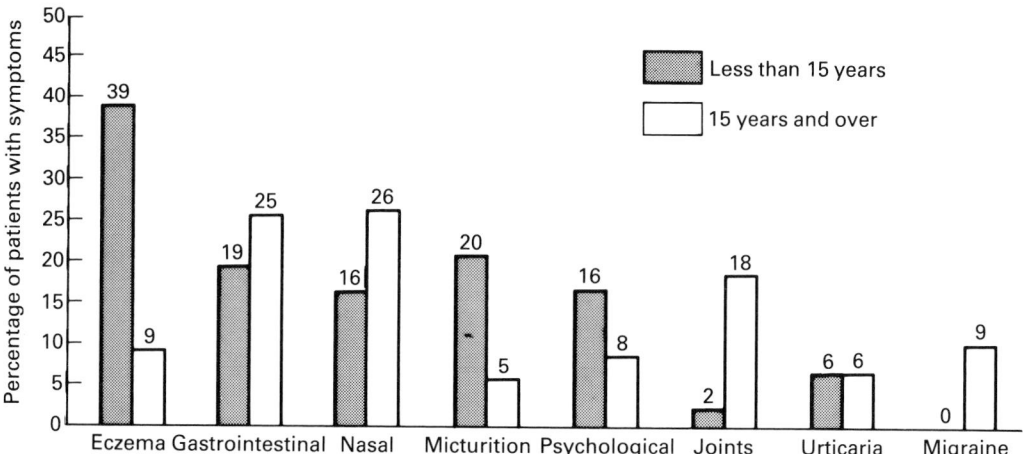

Fig. 27.10 Other symptoms. The figure shows the percentages of the different symptoms in the younger and older age groups. Under 15 years 102 patients (67%) and over 15 years, 114 patients (64%) had one or more symptoms.

Gastrointestinal symptoms

Abdominal pain and discomfort and diarrhoea were caused mainly by milk, colouring and egg in the younger patients. In adults, wheat was the main cause, followed by milk, egg and yeast. Distension and flatulence were prominent features. The importance of food intolerance in causing gastrointestinal symptoms has been shown by Alun Jones et al [1], who found the main foods associated were wheat, dairy produce and corn (see Chapter 32).

Rhinitis and nasal polyps

These were caused mainly by milk, egg and wheat. Fourteen per cent of patients studied had nasal polyps. About half had inhalant allergies associated with the foods [41] (see Chapter 26). In nasal allergy due to inhalants a proportion of patients have negative skin tests as the nasal mucosa may be locally sensitive [26], so the history of environmental exposure is all the more important. Careful questioning is necessary to find out if there is any potential source of allergen, such as animal pets, or old pillows which may contain large numbers of mites [46].

Micturition symptoms

In children, bed-wetting and diurnal frequency were associated mainly with milk and colouring and in adults with wheat. Allergy as a cause of nocturnal enuresis in children has been recorded by Bray [5], Breneman [6,7] and Gerrard [24], and symptoms in adults by McAllen (1980, personal communication).

Arthralgia

In the majority of those affected, several joints were involved, being painful and sometimes swollen (Fig. 27.11) but a few had pain and swelling of multiple symmetrical joints. Approximately a third of these were severely disabled and unable to work, a third moderately disabled and a third had mild symptoms. The main foods associated were wheat, milk,

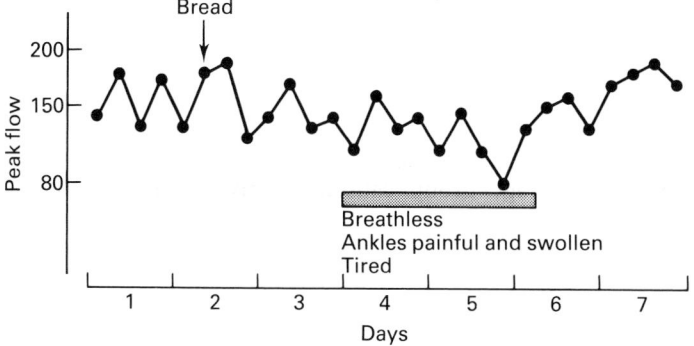

Fig. 27.11 Female, 35 years, with a long history of asthma and recent attacks of severe pain and swelling of ankles. She was found to be sensitive to yeast. The figure shows the gradual fall of peak flow values to a minimum level 3 days after eating bread, with the associated recurrence of pain and swelling of ankles. From Wraith [45], with permission.

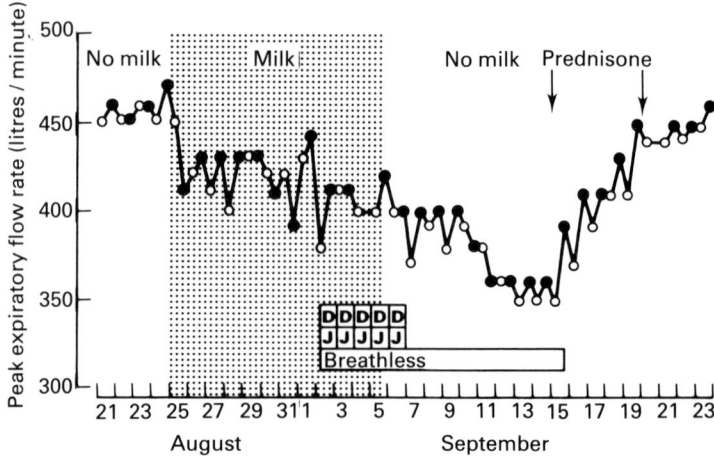

Fig. 27.12 Male, 63 years, with asthma, pains in joints (fingers and knees), diarrhoea and depression for 12 years. Milk was found to be the cause (skin test negative, although positive to house dust) and the patient was symptom-free on stopping milk. On taking milk for 12 days there was a gradual fall in peak flow values, but severe breathlessness, joint pain (and swelling of knees) (J) and diarrhoea (D) appeared only after 8 days. Peak flow values continued to fall despite stopping milk, until prednisone was given. All symptoms were confirmed by repeated blind tests with milk disguised. Reproduced from Wraith [44], with permission.

yeast, preservatives, sugar and also tap water. Avoidance of these resulted in complete clearance or considerable improvement in the symptoms. Most were rechecked by repeated challenge tests. In some, taking foods by mistake caused relapse. In a number of subjects tests were repeated 'blind' or with pretreatment with oral sodium cromoglycate or placebo (Figs. 27.12 and 27.13). Some of these results have been previously reported [9, 44]. There have been many reports in the literature of joint symptoms caused by foods [25, 36, 49, 50] and experimental production of joint lesions [10] (see Chapter 41).

Psychological symptoms

Ill-defined symptoms of fatigue, irritability and depression were a characteristic feature in many patients and improved with avoidance of specific foods. Those patients included in Fig. 27.10 had more severe symptoms (and see Fig.

27.12). In children there were behaviour problems, tantrums and hyperactivity, in many cases interfering with school performance. In adults symptoms found included depression, aggression and panic feelings as well as difficulty with concentration and forgetfulness. The main causes were artificial colouring and milk in children and wheat in adults. Symptoms cleared or were much improved when these and other relevant foods were avoided. The importance of food intolerance as a cause of these symptoms in children has been reported by Buisseret [8], Feingold [17], Rapp [37, 38], Crook [11] and Egger et al [16], and in adults by Finn and Cohen [18] (see Chapters 38 and 39).

Urticaria

This was found in a small proportion of patients and was caused mainly by artificial colouring and preservatives in both age

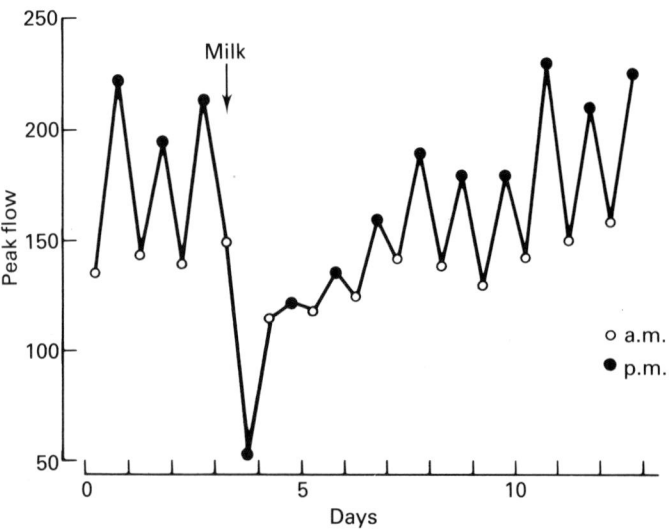

Fig. 27.13 Male, 55 years, with 15 years' persistent and severe asthma causing much disability and necessitating steroid therapy. Skin tests for inhalants and foods were negative. Symptoms improved on stopping milk and deteriorated on restarting it. The figure shows a fall in peak flow values which persisted for a week after taking half a pint of milk only. From Wraith [45], with permission.

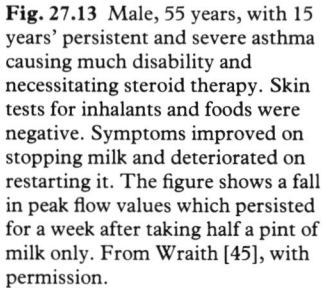

groups. The importance of these additives has been reported by Lockey [29, 30], Michaelsson and Juhlin [32], Doeglas [15] and August [3] (see Chapter 35).

Migraine

This was caused mainly by chocolate, cheese, milk and wheat. A fuller assessment of the association of migraine and ingestion of foods is given in Chapters 37 and 38.

MANAGEMENT

Food avoidance

It was found that foods to which the patient was very sensitive should be very strictly avoided because even very small amounts (such as corn starch in tablets and artificial colouring in medicines) could provoke symptoms. Those to which a patient was not so sensitive could be taken in small amounts every few days in a system of rotation.

Balanced diet

If alternative foods were taken in large amounts there was a likelihood that a relapse would occur due to an intolerance developing to these. Thus a balanced diet without particular emphasis on any one food or food group is important.

Nutrition

This is especially important in children and in those on restricted diets, such as vegetarians. A careful assessment of intake of nutrients is necessary, preferably by a dietitian, with advice about suitable alternatives and supplements.

Use of oral sodium cromoglycate (Nalcrom)

This was very useful in a small group of patients in whom it was difficult to avoid the incriminating foods, especially if many were involved. It was also useful on special occasions when it was difficult to adhere to diets such as when on holiday. In a few patients there was a temporary increase of symptoms if the full dose was started at once so it was started gradually; a dose of 400 mg four times daily was found to be optimal in adults, but there was some individual variation in this. Opening the capsule, dissolving the powder in hot water and rinsing round the mouth before swallowing before meals was found to give better results than swallowing the capsules whole [14, 22, 48].

PREVENTION

A more detailed account of prevention of food allergy is given in Chapter 61 but some brief points with respect to asthma are made here.

Early diagnosis

Investigation and avoidance of the causes (usually multiple, including inhalants and foods) at an early stage can prevent much subsequent disability. Symptomatic treatment with bronchodilators may be of some help but does not (as is shown by the morbidity and mortality) prevent the ultimate disability. Inhalant allergies, e.g. to house dust and animal pets, may be obvious and avoidable but foods and food additives, often a more potent cause, are often neglected due to lack of awareness and because skin tests are usually negative.

Early allergen avoidance

In families with a background of allergic symptoms avoidance of exposure to potential allergens (e.g. animal pets, excessive dust) is obviously necessary. A balanced diet without excess of any particular foods is also important because those foods or additives taken in excess due to habit or restricted diets were frequently found in our study to be causes of asthma. The very high number of children in whom artificial colouring was implicated is an example of this (Fig. 27.14), especially in families with an allergic history and with early symptoms of allergies (e.g. eczema or asthma). Artificial colourings should be avoided in foods, drinks, sweets and medicines as much as possible.

Breast feeding

There is a lower incidence of allergic disease in infants who are breast fed [31, 40] so clearly breast feeding should be encouraged. In addition mothers who are breast feeding (as well as pregnant mothers) should be advised not to have excessive amounts of any food, e.g. cow's milk, as it is possible for the infant to become sensitized to this [21] (see Chapter 18).

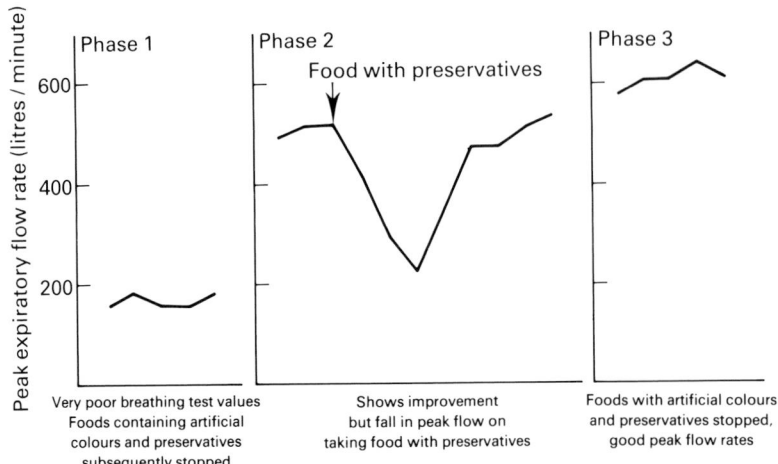

Fig. 27.14 Peak values in a boy aged 9 with severe asthma. Skin (prick) tests positive with house dust but negative with foods so the latter had not been considered as a cause. Avoidance of foods etc. containing artificial colouring and preservatives resulted in considerable improvement. From Wraith, *Mims Magazine*, October 1984, p. 11.

CONCLUSIONS

1 Food intolerance is a very substantial cause of asthma as well as of other symptoms. This fact is very much neglected due to lack of awareness that foods and food additives may be responsible and because skin (prick) tests with foods are often negative or not practicable with food additives. Asthma may be ascribed solely to inhalants or considered to be 'intrinsic'.

2 Certain features have been shown to be of help in suggesting the possibility of food intolerance. Multiple symptoms (food intolerance syndrome) are characteristic of food intolerance, especially if there is an allergic background or a family history of other allergic symptoms.

3 Elimination and challenge tests are useful in the confirmation of the diagnosis.

4 The importance of ensuring adequate nutrition is emphasized. Oral sodium cromoglycate (Nalcrom) is very useful if avoidance of foods is difficult.

REFERENCES

1 Alun Jones V, McLaughlin P, Shorthouse M, et al: Food intolerance, a major factor in the pathogenesis of irritable bowel syndrome. Lancet 1982; ii:115–7.

2 Atherton DL, Sewell M, Soothill JF, et al: A double blind cross over trial of an antigen avoidance diet in atopic eczema. Lancet 1978; i:401–3.

3 August PJ: Successful treatment of urticaria due to food additives with sodium cromoglycate and an exclusion diet. In: Pepys J, Edwards AM, eds. The mast cell. Tunbridge Wells: Pitman, 1979; 584–90.

4 Baker GJ, Collett P, Allern DH: Bronchospasm induced by metabisulphite-containing foods and drugs. Med J Austr 1981; ii:614–6.

5 Bray CW: Enuresis of allergic origin. Arch Dis Child 1931; 6:25.

6 Breneman JC: Nocturnal enuresis; a treatment regimen for general use. Ann Allergy 1965; 23:185.

7 Breneman JC: Primary nocturnal enuresis. In: Basics of food allergy. Springfield: Charles C Thomas, 1978; 54–66.

8 Buisseret PD: Common manifestations of cow's milk allergy in children. Lancet 1978; i:304.

9 Carini C, Brostoff J, Wraith DG: Food allergy as a cause of arthralgia. Immun Clin Sper 1984; iii: 31–40.

10 Coombs RRA, Oldham G: Early rheumatoid-like joint lesions in rabbits drinking cow's milk. Int Arch Allergy Appl Immunol 1981; 64: 287.

11 Crook WG: Can your child read? Is he hyperactive? Jackson, Tenn: Pericenter Press, 1975.

12 Dahl R: Oral and inhaled sodium cromoglycate in challenge tests with food allergens or acetylsalicylic acid. Allergy 1981; 36:161–5.

13 Dahl R, Zetterstrom O: The effect of orally administered sodium cromoglycate on allergic reactions caused by food allergens. Clin Allergy 1978; 8:419–22.

14 Dannaeus A, Foucard T, Johansson SGO: The effect of orally administered sodium cromoglycate on symptoms of food allergy. Clin Allergy 1977; 7:109.

15 Doeglas HMG: Reactions to aspirin and food additives in patients with chronic urticaria. Br J Dermatol 1975; 93:135.

16 Egger J, Graham PJ, Carter CM, et al: Controlled trial of oligoantigenic treatment in the hyperkinetic syndrome. Lancet 1985; i:540–5.

17 Feingold BF: Why your child is hyperactive. New York: Random House, 1975.

18 Finn R, Cohen HN: 'Food allergy': fact or fiction. Lancet 1978; i:426–8.

19 Freedman BJ: Asthma induced by sulphur dioxide,

benzoate and tartrazine contained in orange drinks. Clin Allergy 1977; 7:407-15.

20 Freedman BJ: Sulphur dioxide in foods and beverages. Its use in preservatives and its effect in asthma. Br J Dis Chest 1980; 14:128-34.

21 Gerrard JW: Allergy in breast fed babies to ingredients of breast milk. Ann Allergy 1979; 42:69.

22 Gerrard JW: Oral sodium cromoglycate: its value in the treatment of adverse reactions to foods. Ann Allergy 1979; 42:135.

23 Gerrard JW: Food induced respiratory disease. In: Gerrard JW, ed. Food allergy; new perspectives. Springfield: Charles C Thomas, 1980; 85-98.

24 Gerrard JW: Nocturnal enuresis. In: Gerrard JW, ed. Food allergy: new perspectives. Springfield: Charles C Thomas, 1980; 169-85.

25 Hicklin JA, McEwen LM, Morgan JE: The effect of diet in rheumatoid arthritis. Clin Allergy 1980; 10:463.

26 Huggins KG, Brostoff J: Local production of specific IgE antibodies in allergic rhinitis patients with negative skin tests. Lancet 1975; ii:618.

27 Kniker WT, Rodriguez LM: Non-IgE mediated and delayed adverse reactions to food or additives. In: Breneman JB, ed. Handbook on food allergies. New York: Marcel Dekker, 1985.

28 Lessof MH, Wraith DG, Merrett TG, et al: Food allergy and intolerance in 100 patients. Local and systemic effects. Q J Med NS, 1980; XLIX (no. 195):259-71.

29 Lockey SD: Reactions to hidden agents in foods, beverages and drugs. Ann Allergy 1971; 29:461.

30 Lockey SD: Hypersensitivity to tartrazine and other dyes and additives present in foods and pharmaceutical products. Ann Allergy 1977; 38:206-10.

31 Matthew DJ, Norman AP, Taylor B, et al: Prevention of eczema. Lancet 1977; i:321.

32 Michaelsson G, Juhlin L: Urticaria induced by preservatives and dye additives in food and drugs. Br J Dermatol 1973; 88:525-32.

33 Ogle KA, Bullock JD: Children with allergic rhinitis and/or bronchi asthma treated with eliminated diet, a five year follow-up. Ann Allergy 1980; 44:273-8.

34 Ortolani C, Pastorello E, Laraghi MT, et al: Diagnosis of intolerance to food additives. Ann Allergy 1984; 53: 587-91.

35 Papageorgiou N, Lee TH, Nagakura T, et al: Neutrophil chemotactic activity in milk-induced asthma. J Allergy Clin Immunol 1983; 72:75-82.

36 Parke AL, Hughes GRV: Rheumatoid arthritis and food: a case study. Br Med J 1981; 282:2027-9.

37 Rapp D: Hyperactivity and the tension-fatigue syndrome. In: Gerrard JW, ed. Food allergy: new perspectives. Springfield: Charles C Thomas, 1980; 186-208.

38 Rapp D: Allergies and the hyperactive child. New York: Cornerstone, 1980.

39 Rowe AH: Bronchial asthma because of food and inhalant allergy and less frequent drug and chemical allergy. In: Rowe AH, ed. Food allergy. Springfield: Charles C Thomas, 1972; 169-210.

40 Saarinen UM, Backman A, Kajosaari M, Simes MA: Prolonged breast feeding as prophylaxis for atopic disease. Lancet 1979; ii:163.

41 Shioda H, Mishima T, Yamada S, el al: Nasal smears in the diagnosis of food allergy. In: Pepys J, Edwards AM, eds. The mast cell. Tunbridge Wells: Pitman Medical, 1979; 422-30.

42 Stenius BSM, Lemola M: Hypersensitivity to acetylsalicylic acid and tartrazine in patients with asthma. Clin Allergy 1976; 6:119-29.

43 Stevenson DD, Simon RA: Sensitivity to ingested metabisulphites in asthmatic subjects. J Allergy Clin Immunol 1981; 68:26-32.

44 Wraith DG: Diagnostic methods and criteria: respiratory diseases. In: Coombs RRA (Chairman) Proceedings of the First Food Allergy Workshop. Medical Education Services: Oxford, 1980; 64.

45 Wraith DG: Asthma and rhinitis. Clin Immunol Allergy 1982; 2:101-12.

46 Wraith DG, Cunnington AM: The mite and childhood asthma. Lancet 1975; iii:766.

47 Wraith DG, Merrett J, Roth A, et al: Recognition of food allergic patients and their allergens by the RAST technique and clinical investigation. Clin Allergy 1979; 9:25.

48 Wraith DG, Young GVW, Lee TH: The management of food allergy with diet and Nalcrom. In: Pepys J, Edwards AM eds. The mast cell, 1979; 443.

49 Zeller M: Rheumatoid arthritis. Food allergy as a factor. Ann Allergy 1949; 7:200.

50 Zussman BM: Food hypersensitivity simulating rheumatoid arthritis. South Med J 1966; 59:935.

Chapter 28
Alveolitis

D. J. Hendrick and A. G. Bird

Introduction

An earlier book edited by Brostoff and Challacombe concerning food allergy included contributions from 19 authors, four countries and both sides of the Atlantic [11]. It was published as recently as 1982 and was followed in 1984 by the report on food intolerance and food aversion by the joint committee of the Royal College of Physicians and the British Nutrition Foundation [27]. Both publications provide testimony to the increasing awareness and respect that the subject of food allergy has commanded over the last decade, a decade that began with the very existence of food allergy being described in editorial comment as 'beyond the fringe of credibility' [35]. Neither publication, however, acknowledged even the possibility that food allergy could produce a direct effect in the gas-exchanging tissues of the lung. Our task is therefore a limited one—

to consider whether alveolitis attributable to food allergy lies within the fringe of credibility.

THEORETICAL CONSIDERATIONS

Could food allergy cause alveolitis?

There are excellent theoretical reasons for supposing that food allergy could indeed cause alveolitis (and its end stage, diffuse pulmonary fibrosis), a good deal of which is currently considered to be idiopathic or 'cryptogenic' in origin. The most important aetiological agents in conventional types of extrinsic allergic alveolitis (EAA) are derived from vegetable (and microbial) dusts and from birds. With both, relevant antigens are likely to find their way into food products. Food processing and cooking will, in many instances, destroy or modify much of the antigenic specificity, and that which survives will be further degraded by digestive processes within the alimentary tract. On the other hand, the magnitude of an ingested antigenic challenge may be substantially larger than that which is experienced in the alveoli following airborne exposure. Furthermore, not all antigenic food is fully denatured by cooking or digestion, and it is now well recognized that many macromolecules cross the intestinal mucosa antigenically intact [29, 50]. These can be identified in the milk of nursing mothers whose infants may occasionally suffer allergic symptoms as a consequence [1, 26, 48]. The fact that food allergy may present in any organ beyond the gut is itself supportive evidence that food proteins may be absorbed with preserved antigenicity and distributed systemically. That this distribution can be of clinical significance to the lungs is shown by numerous reports of asthma following the ingestion of foods or food additives.

Food additives

With food additives (such as the colouring agent tartrazine, benzoate preservatives and salicylates) the chances of heat or enzymic denaturation are much less than with antigens in food itself, and these are, perhaps, the more important cause of asthma provoked by foodstuffs. With agents of this type there is little evidence that specific immunological mechanisms are responsible and with salicylates (which occur naturally in certain fruits and vegetables, and are added to flavour a variety of food products) the major mechanism probably involves inhibition of prostaglandin synthesis and the direct release of mast-cell mediators.

Antibiotics

Antibiotics may contaminate food, and with penicillins there is interesting confirmation that once the airways are sensitized by the inhalation route, further asthmatic reactions can be produced when the provoking agent is ingested [15]. The subjects concerned were employed in the manufacture of ampicillin from benzylpenicillin and developed occupational asthma as a result of continual exposure to fine airborne dust containing these antibiotics. Inhalation provocation tests lasting 30 minutes using an airborne dust from a mixture of 250 g lactose containing 1–10 g of antibiotic powder led to typical and reproducible late asthmatic responses which were duplicated when 500 mg of each drug were ingested (see Fig. 28.1). It is interesting that the ingested challenges provoked, in addition, late reactions in the gastro-intestinal tract (diarrhoea) and skin (urticaria). It is difficult to estimate the actual dose deposited in the lungs and absorbed systemically following the airborne challenges, but this must have been substantially less than that responsible for the orally provoked responses.

Relevance to alveolitis

The possible relevance of these observations to food-induced alveolitis is twofold. Firstly, many airborne dusts which induce EAA (and which induce asthma also) are likely to contribute or share relevant antigens with compo-

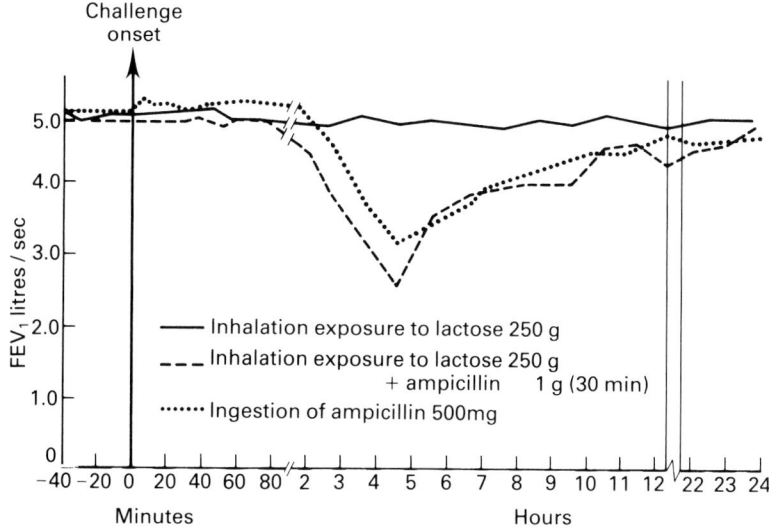

Fig. 28.1 Inhalation and ingestion provocation tests with ampicillin in a 26-year-old production worker. (Reprinted, with permission, from Occupational lung disease. In: Simmons DH, ed. Current pulmonology, Vol. 3. New York: John Wiley, 1981. Data originally published in ref. 15 are reproduced with permission of Blackwell Scientific Publications.)

nents or contaminants of foodstuffs. Flour and grain dust with bread; avian bloom, urine and faeces with egg; yeasts and other fungi with various food 'extracts' and alcoholic beverages, are examples. In each case ingestion of the end product is known to provoke asthma in some individuals, not necessarily those sensitized initially by the inhalation route. Secondly, a number of drugs, including a further antibiotic—nitrofurantoin—may cause alveolitis when ingested [10, 45]. This occurs in the absence of apparent prior sensitization by the respiratory route, a point of potential importance. The drugs and doses involved are not, however, likely to be encountered in everyday foods. Most are cytotoxic agents and some, such as bleomycin, exert their effects largely through toxic mechanisms. With others, such as methotrexate, hypersensitivity mechanisms appear more probable, though the definite participation of immunological processes has not yet been confirmed. Nevertheless the clinical picture of the alveolitic response to many of these agents is identical to that observed in classical types of EAA, and its mechanism may well be that responsible for the late type of asthmatic response.

IMMUNOLOGICAL CONSIDERATIONS

Before considering further the clinical evidence that immunological reactions against food antigens might induce alveolitis, it is important to consider the immunological responses which may be relevant. Earlier chapters which have dealt with immunological mechanisms have stressed the preoccupation of bowel mucosal immunity with local defence. Thus, local antigen challenge, whether with microbial, chemical (haptenic) or environmental antigens such as foods, induces local immunity only. Systemic immunization does not normally occur even if the antigens traverse the bowel mucosa, as occurs frequently in the case of food antigens. This failure of systemic priming applies to both systemic humoral (mainly IgG) and cellular (principally T lymphocyte) limbs of the immune response system and a principal mechanism is active suppression by T lymphocytes [47].

Route of antigen presentation

The route of initial antigenic presentation to the specialized cells of the monocyte/macro-

phage series, now referred to as antigen-presenting cells, appears crucial to the outcome of mucosal compared to systemic antigen challenge. For systemic immunization to follow antigen penetration of the bowel mucosa the antigen must not only evade local mechanisms for generating suppression but must also run the gauntlet of the liver reticuloendothelial system. The latter is also responsible for induction of specific systemic suppression following immunization with certain soluble antigens and haptens by the hepatic portal vein route [12]. Consideration of these observations is of particular relevance to alveolitis. For such distant disease to occur as a result of food absorption, either the mechanisms for systemic suppression must have been bypassed, or prior sensitization of the systemic immune system by another route of presentation must have occurred.

Abrogation of systemic suppression

Possible ways in which the first criterion might be met include failure of local immune mechanisms (e.g. IgA deficiency), inflammatory bowel disease permitting a generalized increase in mucosal permeability, local immunological disorders of the bowel (e.g. coeliac disease) or generalized immunological disorders associated with abnormal immune responses.

Primary sensitization via airways

In the context of parenchymal lung disease, the most likely route for primary systemic sensitization would be via the airway mucosa itself. There is sparse information available about local and systemic immune responses generated as a result of bronchial antigenic challenge. The bronchial tree possesses a secretory mucosal immune system similar to that of the gastrointestinal tract, but from the limited experimental data available it appears unlikely that antigen presentation via this route is geared to the induction of systemic immune suppression to quite the same degree. This probably reflects the nature of the antigenic challenge to which the respiratory mucosa is normally exposed—inhaled pathogenic microorganisms rather than non-pathogenic food. Clinical evidence supports this view. IgG antibodies directed against vegetable and animal antigens associated with EAA are found in serum and alveolar fluid in both asymptomatic and clinically affected individuals exposed to the relevant antigens. The levels are generally greater in those who are clinically affected, however.

It therefore appears that airway exposure to food antigens would provide a more immunogenic form of antigen presentation than would their absorption through healthy bowel. These considerations do not apply if the bowel is diseased and there is increased absorption of food antigens (see Table 28.1)

Table 28.1 Factors increasing gut absorption of food antigens.

Immature gut
IgA deficiency
Inflammatory bowel disease
Local immunological disorders of the bowel, e.g. coeliac disease
Post-diarrhoea states

Neonatal antigen challenge

Antigenic challenge in the neonate is worthy of special consideration. IgA production increases after a variable period following birth, and in the immediate postnatal period a number of immunological responses remain immature. In particular, food antigen penetration of the bowel is liable to occur to a greater degree at this age. This immaturity of mucosal immune exclusion in the neonate is compounded by an inherent increased permeability of the neonatal gut, which may represent the residuum of a primitive absorption mechanism [51]. A third relevant consideration is that in early infancy aspiration of food is frequent, creating the possibility of an alternative route of sensitization prior to the development of specific tolerance. These three factors probably combine to induce the high levels of precipitating (IgG) antibodies directed against food antigens, which are invariably found in normal infants. Such antibodies generally persist in readily detectable quantities for about three years after which their concentration and prevalence drop sharply [19].

IgE-mediated mechanisms

This discussion of gastrointestinal and respiratory immune responses to food antigens and their interrelationships has to this point excluded IgE. This class of antibody is not thought to be of major importance in the initiation or perpetuation of parenchymal lung disease. Nevertheless, IgE antibodies against food antigens will, in some cases, form part of the humoral immune response generated at gastrointestinal mucosal surfaces, particularly in atopic subjects. This antibody, though synthesized locally in the gut mucosa and mesenteric lymph nodes, will disseminate systemically sensitizing mast cells in other mucosal and epithelial surfaces. It could then be responsible for distant immediate reactions following food ingestion. IgE antibody production is under separate class-specific regulatory control, and is very dependent upon the concentration of sensitizing antigen. Therefore, in genetically predisposed subjects exposed to antigen under appropriate conditions, specific IgE responses may occur with resulting distant consequences, even though the other major limbs of the immune response outside the gut mucosa are not primed to the same antigen.

MECHANISMS RESPONSIBLE FOR THE INDUCTION OF EXTRINSIC ALLERGIC ALVEOLITIS (EAA)

Conflicting evidence for Type III hypersensitivity

The possible pathogenic immunological mechanisms responsible for the induction of EAA are of interest and importance. The similar time course of response to exposure to that of the experimental Arthus reaction, and the almost invariable finding of precipitating antibodies to provocation antigens in the serum of affected subjects, initially encouraged the belief that the disease was the result of immune complex formation at sites of antigen deposition. To accommodate the view that IgG-class antibody and complement were largely responsible for the associated parenchymal lung damage, certain conflicting pieces of evidence were overlooked. In particular, evidence of local vasculitis, a cardinal feature of the experimental Arthus reaction, is lacking in most cases of EAA, while evidence of immune complex and complement deposition in affected tissue is unconvincing. The histological findings in EAA of granulomatous lesions associated with mononuclear infiltration of alveoli and interstitial tissue are also atypical of immune complex-induced disease and are more consistent with T-cell-mediated hypersensitivity. Finally, precipitating antibodies cannot always be demonstrated in the serum of affected subjects, although they may be found in similarly exposed individuals, who have no symptoms.

T cell-mediated hypersensitivity

The preoccupation with antibody-mediated mechanisms has undoubtedly resulted from the ease with which these specific immunoglobulins can be detected when contrasted with the difficulty, until recently, of studying specific T lymphocytic responses in humans. Animal models of disease are now increasing our understanding. They have confirmed that whilst acute necrotizing lesions associated with polymorph infiltration can be readily induced experimentally by humoral immunization or serum transfer into immunologically naive, antigenically challenged animals, T lymphocyte responses induced by adjuvant sensitization are essential to produce the clinical and histological features of hypersensitivity alveolitis.

Summary

In summary, asthma and alveolitis may arise in similar circumstances in response to challenge from inhaled common allergens and ingested pharmaceutical agents; although toxic and pharmacological mechanisms may play a role in some circumstances, most cases are probably the result of hypersensitivity mechanisms. In the case of asthma, symptoms may also develop following the ingestion of common food allergens, and in some instances prior respiratory sensitization to airborne pharmaceutical agents leads to asthmatic reactions when the drug is ingested in conventional therapeutic dosage. Whether an alveolar response can also occur when foods or food additives/contaminants are ingested is not established. Logic would argue that this is feasible, but the current lack of confirmatory evidence suggests it must be a rare phenomenon if it exists at all. Such rarity is, however, to be expected in view of the immunological considerations already discussed.

Systemic sensitization to ingested food antigens is unlikely to occur in the presence of mature local and systemic immune systems, and normal gastro-intestinal mucosal permeability. Nevertheless, food allergy could account for a proportion of the alveolitic dis-

orders whose aetiology is currently unknown. To explore this possibility further, we shall turn to three related topics: (a) an alveolar disorder of children resembling pulmonary haemosiderosis which has been attributed to milk allergy; (b) the alleged association between alveolitis and coeliac disease; (c) the speculative suggestion that bird fancier's lung could be exacerbated or even initiated by egg allergy.

PULMONARY HAEMOSIDEROSIS AND MILK ALLERGY

Pulmonary haemosiderosis is a rare disorder characterized by pulmonary haemorrhage at alveolar level. Its major clinical features are haemoptysis and iron-deficient anaemia. These features may also be prominent in systemic lupus erythematosus (SLE) and Goodpasture's syndrome—diseases which are known to be mediated by immune complexes. In SLE, circulating complexes are selectively deposited in pulmonary capillaries by a mechanism which remains unclear. Deposition in other sites leads to the multisystem dysfunction so typical of this disease. In Goodpasture's syndrome the immune complexes are formed in situ by the complexing of a specific circulating IgG with basement membranes of capillaries in both alveoli and renal glomeruli. When pulmonary alveolar haemorrhage occurs in isolation, these immunological abnormalities are less often found (or sought), and the disorder is conventionally labelled idiopathic pulmonary haemosiderosis.

In 1962, Heiner and colleagues reported the curious case of an eight-month-old North American infant who had a severe and persistent cough, recurrent diarrhoea and failure to thrive [20]. Investigation revealed recurrent pulmonary infiltrates on chest radiographs and a persistent iron-deficiency anaemia. No infecting microorganisms were discovered and cystic fibrosis was excluded. Although skin tests for tuberculosis, histoplasmosis, blastomycosis and coccidioidomycosis proved to be negative, the child's serum gave a strong precipitin reaction with a culture filtrate of a virulent strain of *Mycobacterium tuberculosis*. With culture filtrates from five other virulent strains of *M. tuberculosis* no immunological reactions were observed. It transpired that the filtrate giving the positive reaction had been cultured from a medium containing bovine serum, the latter sharing antigens with raw cow's milk. An appropriate exclusion diet was recommended and the child improved dramatically.

As a result of this experience, these investigators studied sera from 65 further children with respiratory diseases of uncertain aetiology and an additional 1980 subjects who were either well or had diseases of established cause. Seven gave precipitin responses to cow's milk that closely resembled those from the index case. That is, strong precipitin lines were seen to at least five components of cow's milk. A further 18 sera gave precipitin reactions to 1–3 components of cow's milk only. One child with a strong precipitin response could not be evaluated fully but the other six, together with the index case, were found to exhibit a remarkable constellation of similar clinical features. Those with less strong responses did not.

Clinical features

The seven affected subjects were infants aged 13 days to six months when they became ill. They were troubled by chronic cough and rhinitis, persistent tachypnoea and recurrent fever. In six, poor weight gain and pallor together with recurrent diarrhoea and otitis media were associated features. In addition, five experienced recurrent vomiting and four recurrent haemoptysis. Investigation confirmed the presence of recurrent pulmonary infiltrates in all the children. Six had hypochromic anaemias and six had weights below the 10th percentile. Eosinophilia was seen in six also. All seven underwent aspiration of gastric or bronchial secretions which on examination revealed an excess of iron-laden macrophages in four. A similar excess was noted following the one needle aspiration of lung. These findings led the authors to suggest the iron-deficient anaemias were due to bleeding from gut and lungs. The pulmonary component of the syndrome therefore resembled pulmonary haemosiderosis.

In six of these infants major changes in diet were introduced. Five received evaporated or boiled milk but no raw cow's milk, and two became symptom-free within two days. The four who remained symptomatic were then given soy bean substitute feeds and cow's milk was withdrawn altogether. All recovered fully. After 3–6 months, cow's milk was reinstituted in the diet of each infant. Two developed a recurrence of all former symptoms but four appeared to have become partially tolerant.

The authors believed the syndrome described was caused by allergy to ingested cow's milk. It is interesting that as many as six of the seven infants were breast fed initially, which did not therefore confer protection.

Precipitins to cow's milk

The authors remarked that precipitins to cow's milk are also commonly observed in children with coeliac disease but the absence of precipitins to wheat made this diagnosis unlikely in their particular cases. They did, however, refer to a further case in which pulmonary haemosiderosis (proved at autopsy) and coeliac disease appeared to have coexisted. Precipitins were detected to both cow's milk and gliadin. They also remarked that precipitins to cow's milk are not always found with pulmonary haemosiderosis, implying that milk allergy is simply one possible cause of this disorder in childhood. Finally, this landmark publication briefly reported the outcome of a further survey of 1284 sera obtained from subjects with some clinical suspicion of this interesting syndrome. Strong precipitin responses to cow's milk were noted in 26. With 10 there was iron-deficiency anaemia but no evidence of pulmonary disease. With 8, both gastrointestinal and pulmonary disorders were evident and these improved with cow's milk avoidance.

The evidence presented by these investigators is very persuasive and their conclusions are broadly accepted today, 20 years later. It is possible, however, that sensitization could have resulted from regurgitation and aspiration of ingested milk into the lungs. Subsequent experience suggests this may indeed occur in infants with this syndrome, but it is not a uniform finding, and it is now generally accepted that milk allergy in childhood can be manifested at alveolar level producing both inflammatory changes and bleeding.

Mechanism of pulmonary damage

The mechanism of pulmonary damage in this syndrome has not been investigated by immunopathological techniques, but the evidence that circulating immune complexes can initiate similar effects in a small proportion of patients with SLE suggests the possibility that circulating food containing immune complexes could be responsible. The low incidence of this complication in milk-allergic infants in general would then illustrate the recognized variability between individuals in sites of immune complex deposition.

In adults with idiopathic pulmonary haemosiderosis (IPH) there is no direct evidence suggesting an association with food hypersensitivity, although occasional case reports have suggested a link with malabsorption [4, 32]. In a recent study designed to investigate this possible association in more detail, jejunal biopsies revealed abnormal morphological appearances in two of six patients with IPH [53]. IPH is an uncommon disease, however, and further studies are needed before its possible association with coeliac disease can be verified and quantified.

ALVEOLITIS AND COELIAC DISEASE

Interest in a possible association between a true diffuse alveolitis and coeliac disease (and hence food allergy) was first kindled in the early 1970s. The report by Hood and Mason described two patients with both disorders but gave no indication of the size of the population from which they had emerged [25]. Whether the association could have been one of chance alone could not consequently be assessed. Lancaster-Smith and colleagues reported alveolitis in three of a selected group of 24 patients with coeliac disease [30], but when the group was increased to 57 no further cases of diffuse lung disease were noted [31]. Following the suggestion of Berrill and colleagues from Southampton that coeliac disease was associated specifically with bird fancier's lung (BFL) [7, 8], case reports have emerged linking coeliac disease with farmer's lung also [43, 44], and there is now much speculation that this intestinal food allergy may be associated with both cryptogenic fibrosing alveolitis and EAA [2, 3, 13].

Clinical significance of precipitins to bird serum

Sera from the initial 24 patients reported by Lancaster-Smith et al were examined for a number of antibodies to both auto and extrinsic antigens. Faux (personal communication, 1976) found a high proportion (7/24) to have precipitins directed against the sera of many species of bird, but these did not cross-react with the appropriate droppings extracts. This response pattern is not characteristic of BFL [18]. Furthermore, none of the patients concerned appeared to be exposed to birds at the

time, and when avian inhalation provocation tests were performed on two of the three with alveolitis no reactions were produced [5]. It was concluded that these precipitins to bird serum were 'non-specific'. Similar observations were reported independently by Morris and colleagues at about the same time [38].

The presence of precipitins to bird serum was an important diagnostic feature in the Southampton study of Berrill et al, although their 'specificity' was unknown. These investigators reported a high prevalence of villous atrophy in small bowel biopsies taken from patients with presumed BFL [7]. Of 16 patients thought to have BFL, nine underwent jejunal biopsy, and villous atrophy was demonstrated in five. No inhalation provocation tests were performed with avian antigens, and only one of the five subsequently achieved an adequate and persisting pulmonary response from bird avoidance alone. The specific diagnosis of BFL could therefore be questioned, as could the strength of the suggested association with coeliac disease. That villous atrophy should have been found so commonly in the patients with diffuse pulmonary disease of whatever cause is, however, surprising and it is possible selection bias may have confounded the matter.

The clinical significance of the 'non-specific' precipitin response to bird sera has now been clarified by Faux and her colleagues in Oxford [18, 23]. Precipitin responses to bird serum, droppings and egg from a number of species were examined in current and former bird fanciers, patients with BFL proved by inhalation provocation tests, control subjects unexposed to birds and patients with biopsy-proved coeliac disease. Two patterns of response were distinguished.

Bird fancier's lung associated precipitins

The response illustrated in Fig. 28.2 shows reactions of identity (or partial identity) between the bird serum and droppings of exposure. Although there is some cross-reactivity with other species, the responses are most marked to the species of exposure. Their strength is also dependent on the degree of current exposure (i.e. number of birds). This pattern proved to be significantly related not only to current bird exposure but to BFL itself. The immunologically identical antigens of the birds' blood and excreta that are responsible were consequently termed 'BFL-associated' and the corresponding antibodies

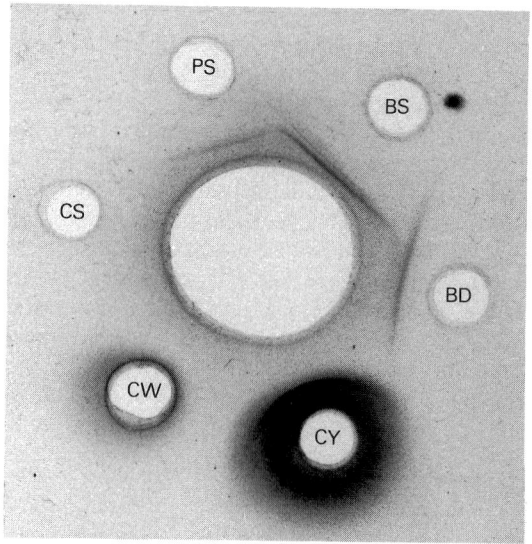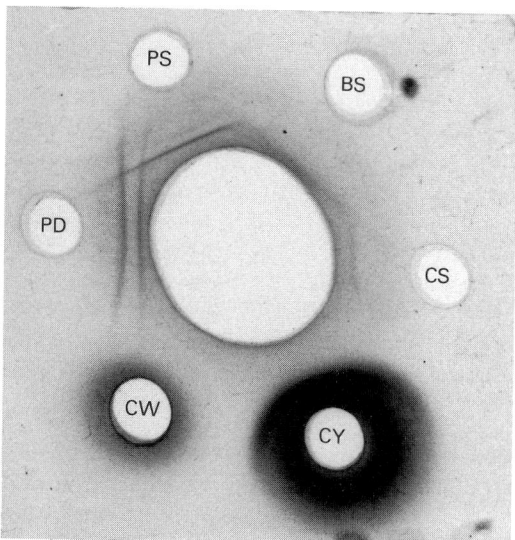

Fig. 28.2 Bird fancier's lung-associated precipitins from a budgerigar fancier (single bird) and pigeon breeder, respectively. BD = budgerigar droppings, BS = budgerigar serum, CS = chicken serum, CW = chicken egg white, CY = chicken egg yolk, G = gluten, PD = pigeon droppings, PS = pigeon serum.

'BFL-associated precipitins'. A number of different antigens may be involved, some of which may be found in egg.

Coeliac disease associated precipitins

Fig. 28.3 shows the second pattern of response which involves a single reaction and presumably a single antigen. The common reaction observed indicates it is present equally in the sera of a number of avian species and in chicken egg yolk, but not in droppings. This pattern was not related to BFL or even bird exposure but it was closely related to coeliac disease. The precipitins were therefore termed 'coeliac disease-associated'.

It was assumed that this antibody response to the coeliac disease-associated antigen was provoked by dietary egg, and a relationship was sought between its presence and the degree of derangement of the small bowel mucosa [23]. Precipitin tests were carried out on the sera of 25 patients with coeliac disease who had undergone initial or follow-up small bowel

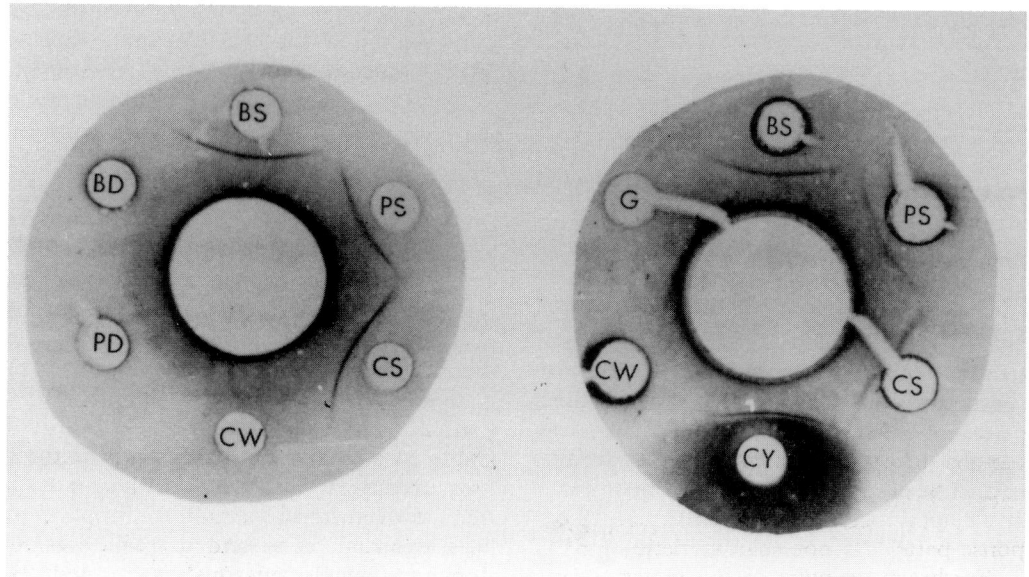

Fig. 28.3 Coeliac disease-associated precipitins. For abbreviations, see legend to Fig. 28.2. From ref. 21.

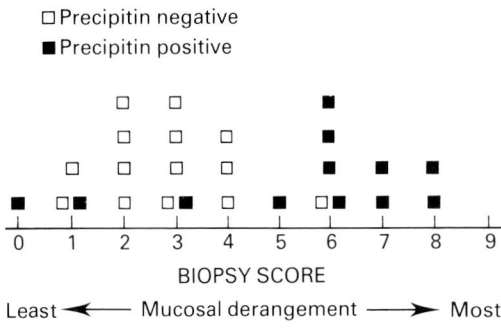

Fig. 28.4 Distribution of small bowel biopsy scores in subjects with and without coeliac disease-associated precipitins. From ref. 21.

biopsies within the preceding three years. Each biopsy was paired with the temporally most closely related precipitin test, and a 0–9 point scoring system was devised to quantify the mucosal abnormalities. The villi, crypts and lamina propria were scored independently 0–3 by a pathologist with special interest in coeliac disease. He had no prior knowlege of the source of each biopsy. The coeliac disease-associated precipitins were indeed found chiefly among the patients with the greater degrees of mucosal derangement (Fig. 28.4), and the mean scores of the precipitin-positive patients proved to be significantly greater than those who were precipitin-negative (Table 28.2).

Table 28.2 Mean small bowel biopsy scores of subjects with and without coeliac disease-associated precipitins.

Coeliac disease-associated precipitins	Precipitin test/biopsy intervals	
	36 months (mean 6.0 months) 26 paired results*	3 months (mean 1.1 months) 11 paired results
Present	5.3	6.2
Absent	2.9	3.0
$P<$	0.05	0.05

Statistical significance from Mann–Whitney test.
* One subject contributed two pairs.

Patients with active coeliac disease are consequently likely to show positive precipitin test results to bird serum irrespective of bird exposure or lung disease, and special care should be taken in interpreting the results when BFL is suspected in such patients.

Effect of smoking

The results of precipitin tests may also be ser-

iously confounded by cigarette smoking. A number of investigators have now shown that precipitin responses to aetiological agents of EAA are diminished in smokers [9, 36, 37, 52]. Some suggest that EAA is itself less common in smokers, but this is not easily confirmed or excluded in the absence of a precipitin response unless inhalation provocation tests are performed. Definitive tests of this type were widely used in the Oxford studies of BFL, irrespective of the results of precipitin tests. Although precipitin responses were indeed less common in the smokers, it was less clear that BFL itself was associated with non-smoking (Table 28.3).

Table 28.3 Relation of smoking to bird fancier's lung (BFL) in 24 current bird fanciers (BF) undergoing diagnostic inhalation provocation tests with avian antigens.

	BF ($n=24$)	BFL confirmed ($n=15$)
Current smokers	7	4 (57%)
Current non-smokers	17	11 (65%)

These proportions are not significantly different.

Bird fancier's lung and coeliac disease

Inhalation provocation tests were also used to re-examine the suggested association between BFL and coeliac disease [23]. Thirteen consecutive patients proved to have BFL by these tests were invited to undergo small bowel biopsy, and 12 obliged. No biopsy was suggestive of coeliac disease. The mean biopsy score was 0.4 (compared with a maximum possible of 9.0), the range being 0–2. In a parallel study of 61 patients with biopsy-established coeliac disease, seven were found to be currently exposed to birds [23]. Three of these reported the onset of undue breathlessness during the period of bird exposure, and all three underwent inhalation provocation tests with appropriate avian antigens. The one with several clinical features of EAA gave reproducible positive results. She was one of four currently exposed to budgerigars, a proportion which may be compared to a prevalence of BFL predicted among current budgerigar fanciers in general of 0.5–7.5% [22].

Little significance can be attached to this single case in a statistical sense, and the Oxford investigators concluded that an association between these interesting disorders must be a weak one if it existed at all. Curiously, they have since reported a second patient with both disorders [39]. Tarlo and colleagues have, however, failed to find any evidence of an excess of diffuse alveolitis (of any cause) in a sample of 18 (of 28) patients with coeliac disease compared with 18 control subjects [49], while the Southampton investigators have reported villous atrophy in three of 26 further patients presumed to have BFL [16].

More recently the British Thoracic Society has published its findings from a multicentre national survey of BFL [42]. Jejunal villous atrophy was demonstrated in five of 143 subjects thought to have BFL, a mild but significant excess over the expected prevalence in a normal population. The diagnostic criteria for BFL were not strict, however, and collaborating physicians were alerted to possible markers of coeliac disease at the time they entered patients into the study. This could have introduced a mild but important selection bias.

The strength (or validity) of the suggested association between coeliac disease and alveolitis therefore remains controversial, and it may be that chance alone accounts for many of the reported cases where these two disorders co-exist.

Possible mechanisms for an association between alveolitis and coeliac disease

Is coeliac disease the primary disorder?

Regardless of this persisting controversy, it is tempting to consider the mechanism by which coeliac disease could be associated with alveolitis. A number of interesting hypotheses have been advanced. Scott and Losowsky suggest that coeliac disease is the primary disorder, and that antigen–antibody complexes originating in damaged intestinal mucosa could give rise to immune complex disease in various distant sites of deposition [46]. A variety of immunological disorders could result including cryptogenic fibrosing alveolitis, and both intrinsic (gut) and extrinsic (food) antigens could be involved. Ingested egg could contribute the appropriate antigens as readily as gluten or milk, and patients with coeliac disease could develop avian allergic alveolitis (egg eater's lung) irrespective of bird exposure. The report of McColl and colleagues lends some support to this possibility [33]. They described acute diffuse interstitial lung disease following inoculation with influenza vaccine raised in chicken embryo. Their patient had coeliac disease and had showed precipitin responses to a variety of food antigens including

chicken serum. They suggested that precipitins to the latter formed immune complexes with common avian antigens of the vaccine.

Is lung disease the primary disorder?

The possibility that the lung disease could precede the intestinal disease was suggested by Purtilo and colleagues [40]. They demonstrated that patients with BFL have antibodies which react with intestinal mucosal cells of the avian species involved. They consequently postulated that the same antibodies might react with the patient's own intestinal mucosa causing villous atrophy. They did not, however, investigate this interesting possibility any further, and it is not known whether these antibodies do in fact react with human intestinal cells. It seems more likely that the reaction they observed was species-specific rather than organ-specific, and that the antibodies involved would react with tissue from other organs of the avian species of exposure. On the other hand, we have seen that once the airways are sensitized to inhaled antibiotics, gastrointestinal responses may occur when the relevant antibiotic is ingested. It is therefore conceivable that once BFL has arisen in a subject exposed to birds, gastrointestinal allergy to ingested egg (and perhaps villous atrophy) could follow.

A common defect?

Finally, a number of authors have suggested that both coeliac disease and alveolitis could develop as a result of a common basic defect or circumstance, and that the one is not a direct effect of the other. A genetic HLA predisposition to autoimmunity/hypersensitivity has been a popular suggestion but BFL, unlike coeliac disease, does not appear to be associated with any specific histocompatibility locus [6, 39]. MacGregor suggested that sarcoidosis may be responsible for both diffuse alveolitis and villous atrophy [34], but the diagnostic specificity of the Kveim test can be questioned in these circumstances [28] and the diagnosis of sarcoidosis may itself have been inaccurate. This leaves the intriguing possibility that food allergy could be the common denominator causing both disorders in some cases.

BIRD FANCIER'S LUNG AND EGG ALLERGY

Route of sensitization

We have mentioned the theoretical possibility that ingested egg could exacerbate or even initiate BFL. BFL-associated antigens can be demonstrated in chicken egg, and ingested chicken egg (and inhaled avian dust) can provoke asthmatic reactions in the lungs of sensitized individuals [24]. In most cases asthmatic sensitization probably results from gastrointestinal challenge, though occupational asthma attributable to allergy to inhaled egg has been described [17]. The affected workers used a spray system to coat meat rolls with egg solution. One also reported intolerance of ingested egg, but this was noted by a similar proportion of the unaffected workers.

Allergy to ingested egg appears to be the chief if not sole cause of adverse reactions to systemically administered vaccines that are raised in egg and contaminated by it [14, 41]. Since they include skin rashes, asthma, angioedema, alveolitis and even fatal anaphylaxis, it seems undeniable that ingested egg, like cow's milk, can occasionally lead to a systemic hypersensitivity state. That BFL could become a consequence of childhood egg allergy in subjects who later become exposed to birds is thus an intriguing idea, but it is an idea that currently lacks any published confirmatory evidence. Similarly, the suggestion of a number of authors that ingested egg could adversely affect lungs that have become sensitized to inhaled avian dust is essentially unsupported by published clinical experience. This has stimulated us to review our data concerning possible egg intolerance among the Oxford patients investigated for possible BFL [21].

Dislike of chicken egg

Like or dislike of chicken egg was compared in three groups of patients: the 15 in whom BFL was confirmed by inhalation provocation tests, the 12 in whom BFL was excluded using these tests and 20 control patients who were selected at random from a respiratory ward. Seven of the BFL group (47%) reported a dislike of eggs compared with one (8%) and two (10%) respectively in the other two groups (Table 28.4). The difference is significant at the 1% level, but the circumstances under which the questions were asked could have

Table 28.4 Egg preference in patients with bird fancier's lung (BFL).

Suspected BFL	Dislike of egg	
Proven	47%	
Disproven	8%	$p = 0.01$
Control respiratory subjects	10%	

introduced a degree of bias. The BFL patients were more likely to have appreciated the significance of the questions and may have admitted to egg aversion more readily as a result. Not all those disliking eggs admitted to definite adverse reactions, whereas two subjects who did describe adverse reactions claimed to enjoy eating eggs. Overall six of the BFL group (40%) claimed adverse reactions compared with three (9%) from the other two groups. Most reported abdominal discomfort or diarrhoea, but some complained of nausea, an unpleasant taste, malaise or even (in two cases) increased breathlessness on exertion. It is interesting that some strongly related the onset of their intolerance to egg to the onset of their respiratory diseases, while others claimed the intolerance to be lifelong.

CONCLUSIONS

The conclusions that can be drawn from studies such as these are very limited because the data are meagre and almost entirely subjective. They are not without interest however, and they may provide a useful stimulus for more definitive egg-ingestion tests. They may also stimulate the development of animal models of avian hypersensitivity. It would be interesting to sensitize animals systemically to avian droppings on the one hand and egg on the other, and then assess the effects of egg ingestion and droppings inhalation respectively.

Studies such as these might provide convincing evidence linking food allergy with alveolitis. Until this is available, we can merely conclude that alveolitis attributable to food allergy does lie within the fringe of credibility—but only just.

Acknowledgements

We are grateful to Dr J. A. Faux for Figs. 28.2 and 28.3 and for her collaboration in much of the work we have quoted.

REFERENCES

1 Anonymous. Antigen absorption by the gut [Editorial]. Lancet 1978; 2: 715.

2 Anonymous. Bird fancier's lung and jejunal villous atrophy [Editorial]. Med J Aust 1976; 1: 813.

3 Anonymous. Coeliac lung disease [Editorial]. Lancet 1978; 1: 917.

4 Bailey P, Groden BM: Idiopathic pulmonary haemosiderosis: report of two cases and review of the literature. Postgrad Med J 1979; 55: 266–72.

5 Benson MK, Lancaster-Smith MJ, Perrin J et al: Serum immunoglobulins, autoantibodies and avian precipitins in adult coeliac disease, and avian antigen inhalation provocation tests in patients with adult coeliac disease and diffuse interstitial lung disease. Arch Fr Mal App Digestif T 1972; 61:398.

6 Berrill WT, van Rood JJ: HLA-DW6 and avian hypersensitivity (corresp). Lancet 1977; 2: 248.

7 Berrill WT, Eade OE, Fitzpatrick PF, et al: Bird-fancier's lung and jejunal villous atrophy. Lancet 1975; 2: 1006.

8 Berrill WT, Eade OE, Macleod WM et al: Proceedings: bird fancier's lung and coeliac disease. Gut 1975; 16: 825–6.

9 Boyd G, Madkour M, Middleton S, Lynch P: Effect of smoking on circulating antibody levels to avian protein in pigeon breeder's disease. Thorax 1977; 32: 651.

10 Brettner A, Heitzman ER, Woodin WG: Pulmonary complications of drug therapy. Radiology 1970; 96: 31.

11 Brostoff J, Challacombe SJ, eds: Food allergy. Clinics in immunology and allergy. London: WB Saunders, 1982.

12 Cantor HM, Dumont AE: Hepatic suppression of sensitization to antigen absorbed into the portal system. Nature 1967; 215: 744–5.

13 Cummiskey J, Keelan P, Weir DG: Coeliac disease and diffuse pulmonary disease (corresp). Br Med J 1976; 1: 1401.

14 Davies RJ, Pepys J: Egg allergy, influenza vaccine and immunoglobulin E antibody. J Allergy Clin Immunol 1976; 57: 373.

15 Davies RJ, Hendrick DJ, Pepys J: Asthma due to inhaled chemical agents: ampicillin, benzyl penicillin, 6 amino penicillanic acid and related substances. Clin Allergy 1974; 4: 227.

16 Eade OE, Hodges JR, Berrill WT et al: Immunofluorescent antibodies in patients with bird fancier's lung. Clin Exp Immunol 1978; 32: 263.

17 Edwards JH, McConnachie K, Trotman DM et al: Allergy to inhaled egg material. Clin Allergy 1983; 13: 427–32.

18 Faux JA, Hendrick DJ, Anand BS: Precipitins to different avian serum antigens in bird fancier's lung and coeliac disease. Clin Allergy 1977; 8: 101.

19 Gunther M, Aschaffenberg R, Matthews RH et al: The level of antibodies to proteins of cow's milk in the serum of normal infants. Immunology 1960; 3: 296–306.

20 Heiner DC, Sears JW, Kniker WT: Multiple precipitins to cow's milk in chronic respiratory disease. Am J Dis Child 1962; 103: 634.

21 Hendrick DJ: Bird fancier's lung—clinical, epidemiological and laboratory features. MD Thesis, University of London, 1979.

22 Hendrick DJ, Faux JA, Marshall R: Budgerigar-fancier's lung: the commonest variety of allergic alveolitis in Britain. Br Med J 1978; 2: 81.

23 Hendrick DJ, Faux JA, Anand B et al: Is bird fancier's lung associated with coeliac disease? Thorax 1978; 33: 425.

24 Hoigne R, Scherrer M: An attack of bronchial asthma produced by egg-white and studied by means of lung function tests. Int Arch Allergy 1960; 17: 152.

25 Hood J, Mason AMS: Diffuse pulmonary disease with transfer defect occurring with coeliac disease. Lancet 1970; 1: 445.

26 Jakobsson I, Linberg T: Cow's milk as a cause of infantile colic in breast-fed infants. Lancet 1978; 2: 437.

27 Joint Report of the Royal College of Physicians and the British Nutrition Foundation. Food intolerance and food aversion. R Coll Physicians Lond J 1984; 18: 83–123.

28 Karlish AJ, Cox EV, Hampson F, Hemsted EH: The Kveim test in Crohn's disease, ulcerative colitis, and coeliac disease (corresp). Lancet 1972; 1: 438.

29 Kuroume T, Oguri M, Matsumura T et al: Milk sensitivity and soybean sensitivity in the production of eczematous manifestations in breast-fed infants with particular reference to intrauterine sensitization. Ann Allergy 1976; 37: 41.

30 Lancaster-Smith MJ, Benson MK, Strickland ID: Coeliac disease and diffuse interstitial lung disease. Lancet 1971; 1: 473.

31 Lancaster-Smith MJ, Swarbrick ET, Perrin J, Wright JT: Coeliac disease and autoimmunity. Postgrad Med 1974; 50: 45.

32 Lane DJ, Hamilton WS: Idiopathic steatorrhoea and idiopathic pulmonary haemosiderosis. Br Med J 1971; 2: 89–90.

33 McColl KEL, Addis GJ, Thomson TJ, Kirkwood EM: Coeliac lung disease and influenza vaccination. Lancet 1978; 2: 434.

34 MacGregor GA: Coeliac disease and diffuse pulmonary disease (corresp). Br Med J 1976; 2: 106–7.

35 May CD: Food allergy—a commentary. Pediatr Clin North Am 1975; 22: 217.

36 Morgan DC, Smyth JT, Lister RW, Pethybridge RJ: Chest symptoms and farmer's lung: a community survey. Br J Ind Med 1973; 30; 259–65.

37 Morgan DC, Smyth JT, Lister RW et al: Chest symptoms in farming communities with special reference to farmer's lung. Br J Ind Med 1975; 32: 228–34.

38 Morris JS, Read AE, Jones B et al: Coeliac disease and lung disease. Lancet 1971; 1: 754.

39 Muers MF, Faux JA, Ting A, Morris PJ: HLA-A,B,C, and HLA-DR antigens in extringic allergic alveolitis (budgerigar fancier's lung disease). Clin Allergy 1982; 12; 47–53.

40 Purtilo DT, Bonica A, Yang JPS: Bird-fancier's lung and coeliac disease (corresp). Lancet 1978; 1: 1357.

41 Ratner B, Untracht S: Allergy to virus and rickettsial vaccines. 1. Allergy to influenza A and B vaccine in children. JAMA 1946; 132: 899.

42 Report to the Research Committee of the British Thoracic Society: A national survey of bird fancier's lung: including its possible association with jejunal villous atrophy. Br J Dis Chest 1984; 78: 75–88.

43 Robinson TJ: Coeliac disease with farmer's lung. Br Med J 1976; 1: 745.

44 Robinson TJ: Coeliac disease with farmer's lung (corresp). Br Med J 1976; 2: 593.

45 Rosenow EC: The spectrum of drug-induced pulmonary disease. Ann Intern Med 1972; 77: 977.

46 Scott BB, Losowsky MS: Coeliac disease: a cause of various associated diseases? Lancet 1975; 2: 956.

47 Strobel S, Mowat AM, Drummond HE et al: Immunological responses to fed protein antigens in mice. 2. Oral tolerance for CM1 is due to activation of cyclophosphamide sensitive cells by gut processed antigen. Immunology 1983; 49: 457–66.

48 Stuart CA, Twiselton R, Nicholas MK, Wilde DW: Passage of cow's milk protein in breast milk. Clin Allergy 1984; 14: 533–5

49 Tarlo SM, Brodes I, Prokipchuk EJ et al: Association between coeliac disease and lung disease. Chest 1981; 80: 715–8.

50 Walker WA: Antigen absorption from the small intestine and gastrointestinal disease. Pediatr Clin North Am 1975; 22: 731.

51 Walker WA: Antigenic uptake in the gut: immunological implications. Immunol Today 1981; 2: 30–4.

52 Warren CPW: Extrinsic allergic alveolitis: a disease commoner in non-smokers. Thorax 1977; 32: 567–9.

53 Wright PH, Menzies IS, Pounder RE, Keeling PWN: Adult idiopathic pulmonary haemosiderosis and coeliac disease. QJ Med 1981; 50: 95–102.

SECTION C
GASTROINTESTINAL TRACT

Chapter 29
Oral Manifestations of Food Allergy and Intolerance

S.J. Challacombe

Introduction

The oral manifestations of food allergy and intolerance have been observed relatively frequently but rarely investigated. One of the most frequent oral mucosal lesions is ulceration of which there are at least 35 distinct types. Food allergy is often cited as a cause of recurrent aphthous stomatitis which affects some 10% of the population. However, there is no evidence that food allergy is the cause of ulceration in the majority of these patients. Oral lesions in food allergy may be local, as in oral pruritus, may be part of a systemic disease thought to be related to food allergy such as coeliac disease, or part of a generalized reaction to food, such as angioedema in anaphylactic reactions to food.

LOCAL ORAL DISEASE

Aphthous ulcers

Characterization

Recurrent aphthous stomatitis (RAS) (or recurrent oral ulceration, ROU) is characterized by oral ulcers, occurring singly or in crops

Table 29.1 Characteristics of different types of recurrent oral ulceration.

	Minor	Major	Herpetiform
Sex ratio F:M	1.5:1	2:1	2:1
Peak age of onset	10–19	0–19	20–29
Number of ulcers	1–5	1–10	10–100
Size	<10mm	>10mm	1–2mm
Duration	4–14 days	10–30 days	7–14 days
Recurrence	1–4 months	<monthly	>monthly
Sites	Non-keratinized mucosa (lips, cheeks, sides of tongue)	Lips, cheeks, palate, dorsum of tongue, pharynx	As MiAU and floor of mouth and gums
Healing by scar	No	Yes	Some

which usually last for 7–21 days before healing spontaneously. These ulcers recur after a variable period of time which may be a few days or several weeks. ROU can be separated clinically into three types: minor aphthous ulcers (MiAU), major aphthous ulcers (MjAU) and herpetiform ulcers (HU) (Table 29.1) [24]. There has been a tendency for clinicians to describe any ulcer occurring in the mouth as aphthous. However, aphthous ulcers have been carefully defined to allow differentiation from the many other types of ulcers occurring in the oral cavity (Table 29.2).

The exact pathogenesis of recurrent aphthous stomatitis has not been defined though many causes have been suggested (Table 29.3 and Fig. 29.1). The prevalence of ROU is in the order of 10% of the population with a wide range reported in the literature [31]. The peak age of onset of MiAU is in the second decade of life, MjAU in the first decade of life and herpetiform ulcers in the third decade of life. Thus some 85% of patients have developed ROU in the first three decades.

Genetic aspects

A family history of ulcers is found in approximately 40% of patients [31] and the highest incidence is found in siblings of parents both of whom have RAS [29]. Identical twins show a 90% concordance, implicating a genetic component [25] and this has been further confirmed by HLA studies showing a relationship with A2 and B12 [7].

Aetiology of aphthous ulceration

There is no evidence that food allergy is causative in the majority of cases of aphthous ulceration though it is likely that food allergy or intolerance can initiate some cases of oral ulceration. It is not clear whether these can be distinguished clinically from the majority of cases of aphthous ulceration. An impressive

Table 29.2 Diagnosis of 295 patients presenting with oral ulceration.

Diagnosis	No.	Percentage of total	Diagnosis	No.	Percentage of total
Recurrent oral ulceration	198	67.1	Viral	15	5.1
Minor aphthous ulceration	103	34.9	Herpes simplex	7	
Major aphthous ulceration	42	14.2	Herpes zoster	1	
Herpetiform ulceration	36	12.1	Hand, foot and mouth disease	2	
Behçet's syndrome	17	5.8	Others	5	
Pseudo-recurrent oral ulceration*	13	4.4	Trauma	14	4.7
Pseudo-minor aphthous ulceration	5	2.0	Carcinoma	3	
Pseudo-major aphthous ulceration	4	1.4			
Pseudo-herpetiform ulceration	4	1.4	Oral Crohn's disease	4	
Erosive lichen planus	16	5.4	Acute necrotizing stomatitis	3	
Erythema multiforme	11	3.7	Agranulocytosis	2	
Pemphigus vulgaris	8	2.7	Sarcoidosis	1	
Mucous membrane pemphigoid	5	1.7	Epidermolysis bullosa	1	
			Wegener's granulomatosis	1	

* Pseudo—secondary to haematological deficiencies.

Table 29.3 Aetiology of recurrent oral ulceration.

Food allergy
Viruses
L forms of bacteria
Mycoplasma
Hormones
Trauma
Immunological
Haematological

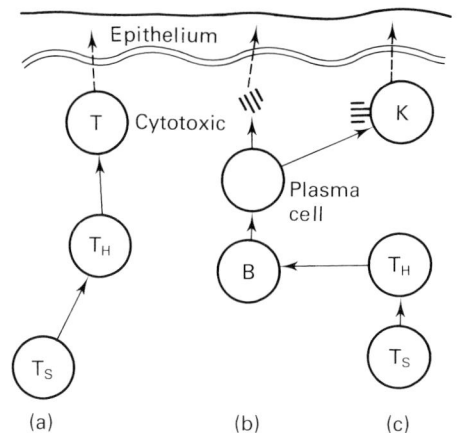

Fig. 29.1 Pathogenesis of recurrent aphthous ulceration. The possible mechanisms include (a) lymphocytes which are cytotoxic for oral mucosa, regulated by T_H and T_S cells, (b) autoantibodies against oral mucosa, and (c) antibody-dependent cellular cytotoxicity (ADCC).

array of factors has been implicated as being potentially causative in RAS although it is likely that many influence the nature of the disease rather than cause it. These include hereditary factors as discussed above, hypersensitivity predisposition, socioeconomic status, psychological factors [29, 30] endocrine factors [5, 15], microbial agents [4] and chemical factors in food stuffs [37, 38] (Table 29.3).

Other factors associated with aphthous ulceration. Haematological deficiencies [6, 41] may not only cause some types of oral ulceration but may also influence susceptibility to other types of ulceration. In addition, lesions consistent with RAS are encountered in association with systemic or multisystem illnesses of an immunopathological nature including Behçet's syndrome, cyclical neutropenia, vitamin B_{12} deficiency and idiopathic inflammatory bowel disease.

Viral aetiology. There is little evidence to support a viral aetiology for RAS. Typical RAS lesions fail to show any significant relationship to herpesvirus on the basis of histopathology, culture or serological investigations

[24]. However, recent deoxyribonucleic acid (DNA) hybridization experiments have indicated some homology between the DNA of herpes type 1 virus and the DNA in mitogen-transformed lymphocytes from some cases of Behçet's syndrome and MiAU [13]. Adenovirus has been identified in some aphthous lesions by immunofluorescence techniques but no causative role has been implicated [28].

Theory of pathogenesis of RAS

Whilst no definitive infective microorganism has been identified, a currently accepted hypothesis of RAS is that patients are exposed to an unidentified infective agent which, in susceptible patients, triggers an autoimmune response against oral mucosa [12, 24]. The agent is thus either in, or cross-reacts with, oral mucosa in these patients. Autoantibodies, cytotoxic lymphocytes and circulating sensitized lymphocytes to oral mucosa can be demonstrated in RAS patients (Fig. 29.1) [24]. There is a significant association with the formation of antiepithelial antibodies which are cytotoxic to oral epithelial cells [10, 24].

Treatment of oral ulceration with cromoglycate. Several authors have examined the use of sodium cromoglycate in the treatment of recurrent aphthous ulceration [11, 19]. In general the results have been disappointing with no consistent benefit in patients. However, it seems that in a subset of patients treatment with sodium cromoglycate did help in aborting ulceration.

Basophil histamine release to food allergen

Wray et al [40] studied the histamine release in response to food antigens in patients with RAS (Table 29.4). Of 60 patients tested, 23 showed significant histamine release to food antigens. Only five of these subjects had given a history of allergy to food antigens whilst three subjects who gave a history did not show

Table 29.4 Correlation of in vitro histamine release to food antigens in atopic and non-atopic patients with RAS and controls.

Groups	Non-atopic			Atopic		
	+	−	n	+	−	n
Aphthous	9	33	42	14	4	18
Controls	6	65	71	71	32	108
Significance	$P = <0.05$			n.s.		

Data from Wray et al [40].

significant histamine release. Overall the ability of patients to correlate clinical food allergy to the histamine assay was less specific than for respiratory allergies.

An interesting finding was that a higher proportion of non-atopic patients showed histamine release from leukocytes in response to food antigens compared with non-atopic controls. Atopic patients and atopic controls both showed a high prevalence of histamine release to foods and were not statistically significantly different. Overall no difference was found between patients and controls.

Effect of elimination of specific foods

This study was extended to the elimination of specific foods in those patients who had shown histamine release to foods, in an attempt to correlate the in vitro histamine release to the development of oral ulcers. Of the patients, 30% had a decreased incidence of ulcers after eliminating foods which had induced in vitro histamine release. On rechallenge in a double-blind manner, 30% of the foods which caused histamine release also correlated with an increased incidence of oral lesions (though 70% did not) and in eight patients, ingestion of specific foods was correlated with oral ulceration by food challenge and then elimination on an open trial basis.

These results suggest that sensitivity to food may play a minor role in the development of some cases of recurrent aphthous stomatitis though it should be noted that dietary manipulation did not eliminate the ulceration in any of the patients.

Food challenge in RAS patients

Some studies have shown a statistical relationship between atopy and RAS [33], though this is not always found [14]. This latter group challenged RAS positive and RAS negative subjects with selected food agents which included tomatoes, strawberries and walnuts, but these foods did not induce an exacerbation of ulceration in the patient group (Table 29.5).

Table 29.5 Prevalence of ulcers in patient and control groups challenged with specific food.

Food	Patients	Controls	Significance
Walnuts	3/58	1/57	n.s
Strawberries	4/40	0/43	?
Tomatoes	2/26	1/30	n.s.

n.s. = not significant.

There was subjective correlation between specific foods and the onset of RAS but this was probably due to pain and discomfort associated with the acidic nature of certain foods rather than stimulating ulcers themselves.

Elimination diet and aphthous ulcers

The involvement of components of food in the causation of RAS was tested in 17 selected patients by Hay and Reade [18]. Seventeen patients with RAS who had been resistant to other forms of treatment were studied with the aid of a strict elimination diet. Five patients abandoned the diet and five patients had a remission of ulcers whilst on the diet. In four of the five patients, a particular food was identified which when eliminated from the subsequent normal diet, lead to either marked improvement or resolution. The elimination diet had been maintained for 8 weeks or so in patients who were not free of ulcers for more than a few days. The results of this study indicate that in a small proportion of cases of recurrent aphthous stomatitis, reactions to food components may participate in the aetiology of the oral ulceration.

Conclusions from elimination of specific foods and dietary challenge. The evidence from the three published trials of food elimination and challenge in RAS patients suggests that allergy or intolerance to foods may play a role in the ulceration in a small number of patients (Table 29.6). They also suggest that such allergy or intolerance to food does not play a role in the aetiology of the majority of cases of RAS.

Table 29.6 Effect of food challenge on incidence of RAS.

	Observations	Number with ulcers
RAS challenge	124	9 (7.3%)
RAS unchallenged	77	5 (6.5%)

It remains to be seen whether oral ulceration secondary to allergy or intolerance can be clinically distinguished from the more classical minor or major aphthous ulceration. Clearly more work is needed to identify the exact proportion of patients presenting with RAS which is secondary to food allergy, and also to determine whether these can be distinguished in some way from the majority of cases of ulcers.

Oral and pharyngeal pruritus

Oral and pharyngeal pruritus is itching of the mouth, palate and throat following food ingestion. Patients with inhalant allergies may spontaneously describe symptoms of oropharyngeal pruritus or hoarseness after ingestion of certain foods. These symptoms may be part of a generalized anaphylactic reaction or they may be isolated local reactions. In one series of ragweed-sensitive patients, 6.2% reported oral pruritus after ingestion of melons or bananas. Although this may have been due to cross-reaction between ragweed and bananas, in vitro assay systems have not been able to confirm this.

The correlation between patients allergic to inhalant antigens and to food antigens is common and oral symptoms have been reported in patients allergic to bee venom who also reacted to carrots, parsnips, apples, potatoes and hazel nuts [21]. Cross-reacting antigens remain a possibility though other mechanisms are discussed elsewhere in this volume and Aalberse et al [1] have described a carbohydrate side chain component of glycoproteins common to a variety of plants.

Taste changes and food

It can be argued that the oral cavity is physiologically designed to provide a precise taste function which determines ingestion or refusal of all foods. Alteration of this function as detected by abnormalities in sensation following consumption of food allergens can provide, according to some authors, a sensitive method for the detection and identification of allergenic foods.

Thus Wilson [38] examined 61 atopic patients with hay fever and found that 65% of foods tested would induce a positive buccal reaction as defined by changes in taste and feeling when food was introduced into the mouth by the patient. Fifty of these 61 patients gave a positive skin test to foods. Fifty-six per cent gave a history of aphthous ulceration and 18% associated their ulcers with specific foods. Introduction of these specific foods into the diet resulted in a burning sensation of the buccal mucosa and ulceration in three of the patients (5%) some 12–48 hours later.

This paper therefore suggested that foods introduced into the oral cavity could give rise to a buccal sensation and in some instances to aphthous-type ulceration. These findings were in atopic patients but in the absence of a control group it is not possible to say whether these findings have any significance with regard to the role of food sensitivity in aphthous ulceration generally.

Non-specific perioral rashes

These are rather ill-defined specific perioral rashes which are usually self-limiting. The perioral reddening is often found after the ingestion of tomatoes, fruits and/or soft drinks. There are no defined studies examining the incidences of this rash in regard to food allergy. Typically, the perioral reddening is noted after ingestion of tomatoes and particularly after citrus fruits. Occasionally the rashes become secondarily infected. The reactions are not proved to be IgE mediated. Often on rechallenge with the incriminated foods at a later date, the signs cannot be reproduced. It is possible that acid content or irritant qualities of food or preservatives coming into contact with the skin may be responsible for the symptoms.

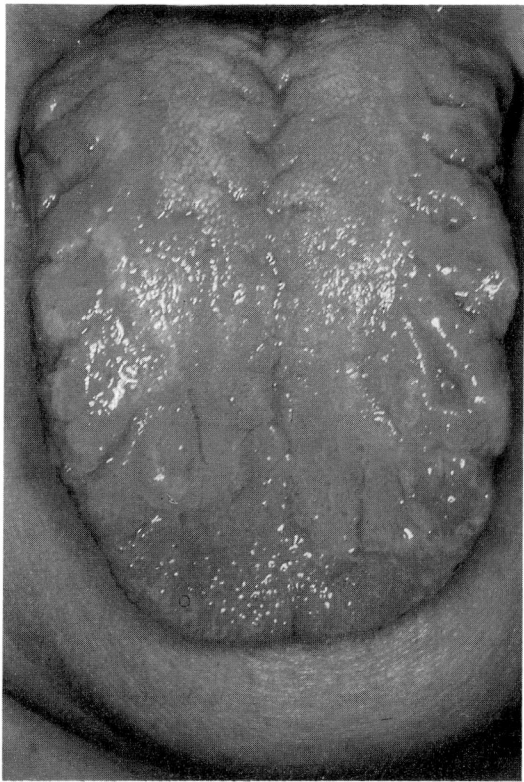

Fig. 29.2 Severe erythema migrans showing lateral fissures. Erythema migrans is common but the aetiology is unknown. Fissured tongues can be exacerbated by, or caused by, allergies including those to food.

Hypersensitivity-fissured mouth

Fissuring of parts of the mouth such as the tongue, mucosa and pharynx and lips in association with food ingestion has been reported. Fissured tongue on its own as an isolated finding has been described as a congenital anomaly and has certainly been found in various syndromes such as the Melkersson-Rosenthal syndrome and in some cases of severe erythema migrans (Fig. 29.2). Quite extensive furrows or fissures appearing over much of the oral mucosa can occur with food ingestion [3]. Evaluation of these patients has shown positive prick skin tests, elevated salivary IgE and marked eosinophils using the Rebuck skin window technique. It is possible that IgE-mediated release of mediators is responsible for the fissures [3].

Mucosal reaction to spices

It is possible for spices to induce mucosal reactions. In a large series of over 1000 atopic and 380 non-atopic patients tested with common spices, positive skin test reactions were seen almost exclusively in atopics. These spices included curry and paprika although coriander, cayenne and mustard were responsible for the majority of skin reactions. Of the 35 unselected patients with positive skin tests, 14 showed a local reaction in the oral mucosa when small amounts of spices were spread on the mucosa. In agreement with the study of Amlot [2], oral challenges with spices in gelatin capsules were negative in 20 non-selected patients [26].

Mucosal contact dermatitis

Delayed hypersensitivity reactions can occur in the oral mucosa. Thus classical contact dermatitis reactions have been described in association with heavy metals involved in dentures. The situation with regard to food components is less clear. One study has examined the mucosal contact dermatitis due to the application of instant coffee [32] and this is an area which clearly requires further evaluation.

ORAL MANIFESTATIONS OF DISTANT FOOD-ALLERGIC REACTIONS

Gastrointestinal diseases. Food allergy and coeliac disease, ulcerative colitis and Crohn's disease are discussed in Chapters 30–32. Each of these gastroenteropathies has been associated with oral ulceration.

Coeliac disease

It is reported that some 25% of patients with coeliac disease may give a history of oral ulceration. However the converse is not true and in recent studies of the incidence of coeliac disease in patients presenting with recurrent aphthous stomatitis a figure of 2–4% was found on the basis of jejunal biopsy [8, 16]. The oral ulcers of those patients with coeliac disease often respond extremely well to correction of underlying haematological deficiencies, particularly folate and iron. It seems that the oral ulceration is often due to the associated deficiencies rather than a direct response of the oral mucosa to the allergen.

Gluten sensitivity without coeliac disease

Cooper et al [9] have described adult female patients suffering from abdominal pain and chronic diarrhoea who responded immediately to a gluten-free diet and in whom symptoms returned on gluten challenge. Recurrent oral ulceration was described in three of the eight patients and macroglossia was found in five patients. Jejunal biopsies were normal in these patients as were enzyme levels of lactase and maltase. When these patients were put on a gluten-free diet, the diarrhoea, abdominal symptoms and the ulceration or macroglossia improved. Reversion to a gluten-containing diet resulted in a return in symptoms including a sore mouth in two of the eight patients. The results of this paper suggest that oral signs and symptoms can be associated with gluten in the absence of coeliac disease, and that such oral symptoms are accompanied by varying abdominal problems.

Crohn's disease

Many cases of oral Crohn's disease have been reported over recent years with or without accompanying gastrointestinal Crohn's. Crohn's disease in the mouth may present either as thickened rubbery lips and cheeks with deep fissures and with enlarged gingiva, or as ulcers and epithelial tags in the buccal sulcus (Fig. 29.3). In both these clinical manifestations, biopsy of the affected areas will show granulomata. A number of cases of swol-

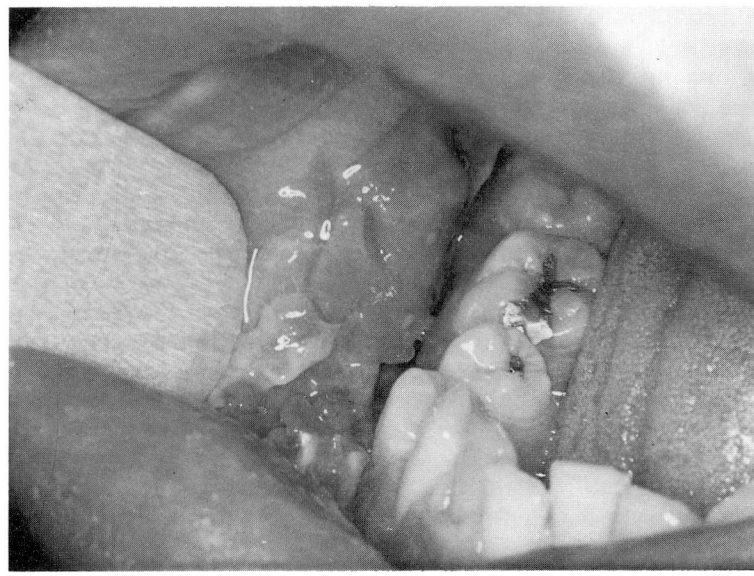

Fig. 29.3 Oral Crohn's disease showing swollen gingiva, cobblestone mucosa and enlarged rubbery lips. Biopsy of any of these sites will usually show granulomata containing multinucleate giant cells. These can be found in the absence of any detectable bowel disease.

len lips without any intraoral signs have been reported and these also have been classified as oral Crohn's by some workers though the term cheilitis granulomatosa would be more appropriate. The role of food allergy in these subjects has not been fully investigated (Fig. 29.4).

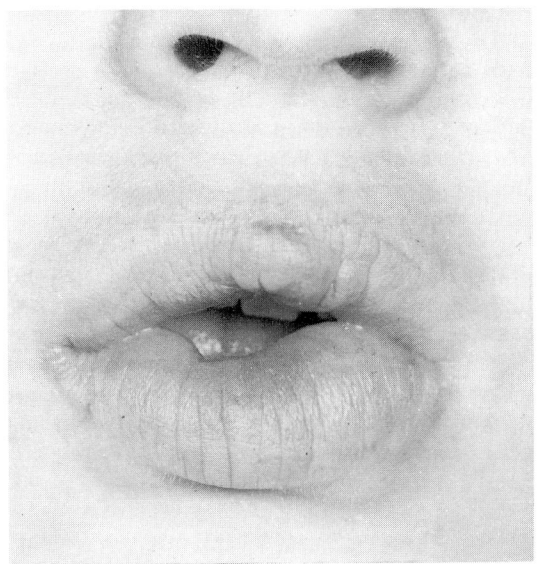

Fig. 29.4 Cheilitis granulomatosa (orofacial granulomatosis). Swollen lips containing granulomata can be found as a reaction to antigens or as part of Crohn's disease. In the majority the cause is unknown.

Ulcerative colitis

Oral ulceration is frequently associated with ulcerative colitis and may be one of at least four types: (a) aphthous, (b) pyostomatitis

necrotica, (c) pyostomatitis vegetans or (d) haemorrhagic. The incidence of oral lesions in patients with ulcerative colitis is approximately 20%. The oral ulcers of groups (b), (c) and (d) are readily distinguishable from the more common types of aphthous ulceration. Unlike Crohn's these lesions do not appear to occur in the oral cavity in the absence of any bowel symptoms. The role of allergy or intolerance to foods in these subjects remains to be elucidated.

Anaphylaxis

Oral signs and symptoms as part of food-allergic reactions elsewhere have been described frequently in individual patients. Thus swollen lips or itching of the palate after eating hazel nuts or other foods is a recognized phenomenon. These symptoms may occur as part of a generalized anaphylactic reaction (see Chapter 25) or urticarial syndrome [20]. However, there are few if any studies which have looked systematically at swelling of the lips in relation to food allergy.

IN VITRO INVESTIGATION OF FOOD ALLERGY

Food lectins and oral epithelial cells

There have been no studies directly associating food lectins with oral disease. However, this remains a possibility which is discussed in some detail in Chapter 21. Gibbons and Dankers [17] examined the association of food lectins with human oral epithelial cells in vivo. They asked patients to chew either wheat germ or peanuts and then used an enzyme assay to detect wheat germ agglutinin or peanut agglutinin on epithelial cells. Interestingly, the lectin could be found for some hours after ingestion and both lectins were also detected in preparations of salivary bacteria where they persisted for up to 6 hours.

The binding appeared to be specific since it could be reduced by prior incubation with *N*-acetylglucosamine or galactose. Sufficient quantities of wheat germ agglutinin became associated with oral epithelial cells to influence bacterial attachment. It is not clear at this stage whether these findings have any relevance to oral disease but clearly more work is needed.

Fluoresceinated lectins were used to examine the carbohydrates on epithelial cell surfaces of oral mucosa and skin from mice by Rittman et al [27]. The study showed that lectin binding to oral epithelial cells was present in other species also and might be used as a convenient method of detecting functional changes in normal cells.

Antibodies to foods in oral diseases

The prevalence of serum antibodies to foods in patients with oral aphthous ulceration was first examined by Taylor et al [34], who found a raised prevalence. In a more recent paper by Thomas et al [36], this basic finding was confirmed. However, the latter paper not only

Table 29.7 Food antibodies in ulcerative oral diseases.

	Aphthous ulcers	Other oral ulcers	Controls
Number tested	25	22	50
Antibodies to:			
food antigens	13 (52%)	12 (54%)	2 (4%)
avian antigens	4 (16%)	4 (18%)	0

compared the prevalence of food antibodies in aphthous patients with controls but also with another group of patients with other oral ulcerative diseases which include pemphigus, pemphigoid, erosive lichen planus and acute ulcerative gingivitis. Interestingly, the prevalence of food antibodies was also significantly raised in this group in comparison with controls to a level similar to that found in the RAS patients (Table 29.7).

Primary or secondary sensitization

It is certainly possible that patients may become sensitized to a single food antigen and as a result of the damage to the mucosa caused by this hypersensitivity reaction, increased amounts of other food antigens may be absorbed and these may stimulate additional antibodies. However, since patients with a variety of other types of oral ulcerative disease showed a similar pattern of antibodies to food antigens, it seems unlikely that they are all caused by primary hypersensitivity to food antigens. It thus seems much more likely that the presence of antibody to food antigens in patients with aphthous ulceration is merely an indication of increased mucosal permeability secondary to other factors.

Salivary IgA

In view of the possibility that increased access of antigens is found in IgA deficiency (see Chapter 12), serum IgA levels though not salivary IgA were examined in the subjects and all were found to be normal. Salivary IgA levels have been examined in patients with minor aphthous ulceration and have been found to be normal [24].

An increased prevalence of antibodies to food antigens is found in patients with coeliac disease and ulcerative colitis (see Chapters 30, 31), but in these diseases a large surface area may be damaged. With oral disease a much smaller area of mucosa is damaged but there still appears to be sufficient absorption of antigen to cause immunization in subjects with oral ulceration. This may be partly due to the high concentration of antigen in the mouth but also to the fact that antigens absorbed from the mouth enter the systemic circulation, whereas those entering via the gut pass through the liver where the more immunogenic components of foods may be removed.

IN VIVO INVESTIGATION OF FOOD ALLERGY

Comparison of buccal challenge with skin, nasal and gastric challenge

The oral cavity can be used as a site for testing type 1 allergy. Amlot et al [2] compared skin prick tests with buccal challenge and also nasal and gastric provocation. As well as the observation that the skin test could be positive in the absence of symptoms, they found overall that the high responders (that is those who responded to very low amounts of allergen on titration) showed a good correlation with symptoms. In terms of sensitivity, the skin and nose were much more sensitive than the buccal cavity and the buccal cavity was much more sensitive than the stomach.

Method of testing. The method of testing was to take 2 ml of food solution and hold it in the lower buccal sulcus between the lower teeth and lip for 5 minutes. At the end of this time, the 2 ml was spat out and the patient observed for 30 minutes. A positive reaction was taken as blanching and swelling in the lip which were described as granular by the patient. These appeared clinically as raised white spots which lasted for an hour or so. A positive reaction was also accompanied by a complaint of irritation or tingling by the patient.

Lip swelling was not a reliable parameter and was not clinically observed in any of the positive patients. Of patients showing positive skin test, 90% also showed positive nasal test at about the same antigen dose. Only 45% of patients showing a skin positive test could be induced to show a buccal reaction and this was usually at a dose 10–1000 times greater than that inducing a skin reaction. Interestingly, in only 15% of patients who were positive in the skin tests, could a reaction be induced by a gastric challenge. The antigens used were egg and milk and in a few patients, fish.

This careful study shows clearly that buccal reactions can be induced in allergic patients and could prove useful in assaying oral reactions to a number of other allergens.

CONCLUSIONS

Allergies to foods may certainly be manifest in the oral cavity. They may present with a variety of oral signs and symptoms including a perioral rash, swelling of the lips, oral pruritus, fissuring of the tongue or oral ulceration. Aphthous ulceration affects approximately 10% of the population and there are many other types of oral ulceration. It is unlikely that food allergy or intolerance is responsible for more than a very small proportion of these cases, perhaps less than 1%.

Overall, oral symptoms are most likely to be found in the atopic patient and in these subjects allergy to foods should be entertained as a possible diagnosis in the absence of other definitive diagnoses and in the absence of disease elsewhere.

REFERENCES

1 Aalberse RC, Koshte V, Clements JGJ; IgE antibodies that cross react with vegetable foods, pollen and hymenoptera venom. J Allergy Clin Immunol 1981; 68:356–64.

2 Amlot PL, Urbanek R, Youlten LJ, et al: Type 1 allergy to egg and milk proteins: comparison of skin prick tests with nasal buccal and gastric provocation tests. Int Arch Allergy Appl Immunol 1985; 77: 171–3.

3 Anderson LB Jr, Dreyfuss EM, Logan J et al: Melon and banana sensitivity coincident with ragweed pollinosis. J Allergy 1970; 45:310–19.

4 Barile MF, Graykowski EA, Driscoll EJ, Riggs DB: L forms of bacteria isolated from recurrent aphthous stomatitis lesions. Oral Surg 1963; 16:1395–402.

5 Bishop PMF, Harris PWR, Trafford JAP: Oestrogen treatment of recurrent aphthous mouth ulcers. Lancet 1967; i:1345–7.

6 Challacombe SJ, Barkhan P, Lehner T: Haematological features and differentiation of recurrent oral ulceration. Br J Oral Surg 1977; 15:37–48.

7 Challacombe SJ, Batchelor JR, Kennedy LA, Lehner T: HLA antigens in recurrent oral ulceration. Arch Dermatol 1977; 113:1717–9.

8 Cooke BED, Challacombe SJ, Rose M et al: Recurrent oral ulceration. Proc R Soc Med 1977; 70:354–7.

9 Cooper BT, Holmes GKT, Ferguson R et al: Gluten-sensitive diarrhoea without evidence of coeliac disease. Gastroenterology 1980; 79:801–6.

10 Dolby AE: Mickulicz's recurrent oral aphthae: the effect of antilymphocyte serum upon the in vitro cytotoxicity of lymphocytes from patients for oral epithelial cells. Clin Exp Immunol 1970; 7:681–6.

11 Dolby AE, Walker DMA: A trial of cromoglycic acid in recurrent aphthous ulceration. Br J Oral Surg 1975; 12:292–5.

12 Donatsky O: Comparison of cellular and humoral immunity against streptococcal and adult oral mucosa antigens in relation to exacerbation of recurrent aphthous stomatitis. Acta Pathol Microbiol Immunol Scand 1976; 84:270–82.

13 Eglin RP, Lehner T, Subak-Sharpe JH: Detection of RNA complementary to Herpes simplex virus in mononuclear cells from patients with Behçet's syndrome and ROU. Lancet 1982; ii:1356.

14 Eversole LR, Shopper TP, Chambers DW: Effects of suspected foodstuff challenging agents in the aetiology of recurrent aphthous stomatitis. Oral Surg 1982; 54:33–8.

15 Ferguson MM, Hart DMcK, Lindsay R, Stephen KW: Progesterone therapy for menstrually related aphthae. Int J Oral Surg 1978; 7:463–70.

16 Ferguson MM, Wray D, Carmichael HA et al: Coeliac disease associated with recurrent aphthae. Gut 1980; 21:223–36.

17 Gibbons RJ, Dankers J: Association of food lectins with human oral epithelial cells in vivo. Arch Oral Biol 1983; 28:561–6.

18 Hay KD, Reade PC: The use of an elimination diet in the treatment of recurrent aphthous ulceration of the oral cavity. Oral Surg 1985; 57:504-7.

19 Kowolik MJ, Muir KF, MacPhee IT: Di-sodium cromoglycate in the treatment of recurrent aphthous ulceration. Br Dent J 1974; 136:452-4.

20 Kresmer K, Lindemayr W: The frequency of the apple contact urticaria syndrome in patients with birch pollinosis. Z Hautkr 1983; 58:543-52.

21 Lahti A, Bjorksten F, Hannuksela M: Allergy to birch pollen and apple, and cross-reactivity of the allergens studied with the RAST. Allergy 1980; 35:297-300.

22 Lehner T: Pathology of recurrent oral ulceration in Behçet's syndrome. Light, electron and fluorescence microscopy. J Pathol 1969; 97:481-94.

23 Lehner T: Immunoglobulin estimation of blood and saliva in human recurrent oral ulceration. Arch Oral Biol 1969; 14:351-64.

24 Lehner T: Immunological aspects of recurrent oral ulceration and Behçet's syndrome. J Oral Pathol 1978; 7: 424-30.

25 Miller MF, Garfunkel AA, Ram CC, Ship II: Inheritance patterns in recurrent aphthous ulcers: twin and pedigree data. Oral Surg 1977; 43:836-91.

26 Niinimaki A, Hannuksela M: Immediate skin test reactions to spices. Allergy 1981; 36:487-93.

27 Rittman BR, MacKenzie IC, Rittman GA: Lectin binding to murine oral mucosa and skin. Arch Oral Biol 1982; 27:1013-9.

28 Sallay K, Kulcsar G, Nasz I et al: Adenovirus isolation from recurrent oral ulcers. J Periodontol 1973; 44: 712-4.

29 Ship II: Inheritance of aphthous ulcers in the mouth. J Dent Res 1965; 44:837-44.

30 Ship II: Epidemiologic aspects of recurrent aphthous ulcerations. Oral Surg 1972; 33:400-6.

31 Sircus W, Church R, Kelleher J: Recurrent aphthous ulceration of the mouth: a study of the natural history aetiology and treatment. Q J Med 1957; 26:235-49.

32 Sonnex TS, Dawber RP, Ryan TJ: Mucosal contact dermatitis due to instant coffee. Contact Dermatitis 1981; 7:298-300.

33 Spouge JD, Diamond HF: Hypersensitivity reactions in mucous membranes. Oral Surg 1963; 16:412-21.

34 Taylor KB, Truelove SC, Wright R: Serological reaction to gluten and cow's milk proteins in gastrointestinal disease. Gastroenterology 1964; 46:99-109.

35 Taylor KB, Thomson DL, Truelove SC, Wright R: An immunological study of coeliac disease and idiopathic steatorrhoea. Br Med J 1961; ii:1727-31.

36 Thomas HC, Ferguson A, McLennan JG, Mason DK: Food antibodies in oral disease: a study of serum antibodies to food proteins in aphthous ulceration and other oral diseases. J Clin Pathol 1973; 26:371-4.

37 Tuft L, Ettleson LN: Canker sores from allergy to weak organic acids (citric and acetic). J Allergy 1956; 27:536-43.

38 Wilson CW: Food sensitivities, taste changes, aphthous ulcers and atopic symptoms in allergic disease. Ann Allergy 1980; 44:302-7.

39 Wray D: Gluten-sensitive recurrent aphthous stomatitis. Dig Dis Sci 1981; 26:737-40.

40 Wray D, Vlasopoulos TP, Sirasanian RP: Food allergens and basophil histamine release in recurrent aphthous stomatitis. Oral Surg 1982; 54:388-95.

41 Wray D, Ferguson MM, Mason DK, et al: Recurrent aphthae. Treatment with vitamin B_{12}, folic acid and iron. Br Med J 1975; ii:490-3.

Chapter 30
Gluten Toxicity in Coeliac Disease and its Role in Other Gastrointestinal Disorders

Nigel Mike and Peter Asquith

Introduction

There can be little doubt that the momentous observation made by Dicke that gluten played a central role in the causation of coeliac disease provided an enormous stimulus to further studies of the gastrointestinal tract pathophysiology [43]. This chapter explores the mechanism of gluten toxicity in coeliac disease in considerable detail but also examines non-responsive coeliac disease and soya sensitivity, transient gluten intolerance, gluten and atopic diseases and finally the effect of wheat protein in non-coeliac gluten sensitivity and in healthy controls.

GLUTEN AND FLOUR PROTEIN

Coeliac disease was accurately described by Samuel Gee in 1888 though its cause, namely sensitivity to gluten, was not demonstrated until 1950 when Dicke showed that removal of wheat from the diet resulted in clinical remission [43]. Since then there has been great interest in the toxic fraction of wheat which mediates the intestinal damage but to date it has eluded exact definition.

Chemistry of wheat proteins and gliadin
(Fig. 30.1)

The endosperm of the wheat kernel is milled to wheat flour which consists of 70–75%

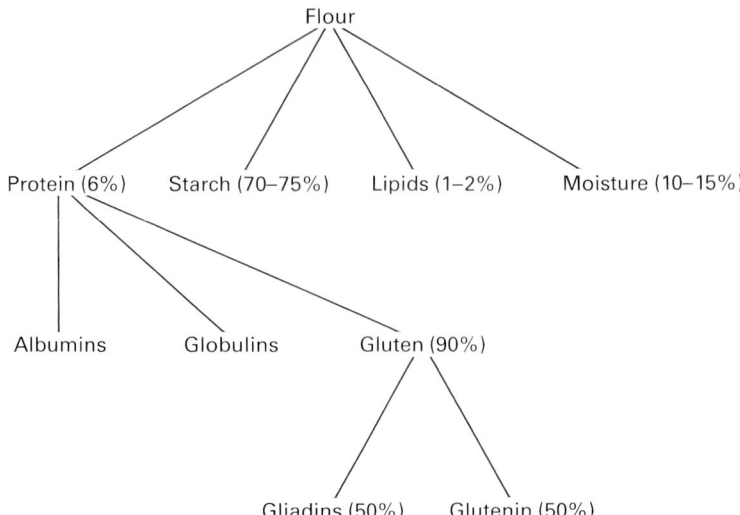

Fig. 30.1 The composition of wheat flour.

starch, 10–15% moisture, 6–8% protein and 1–2% lipids [133]. The flour protein consists of gluten (90%), albumins and globulins whilst gluten itself is made up of glutenin (soluble in alkali) and gliadin (soluble in aqueous alcohol) in approximately equal amounts.

The gliadins have been extensively investigated; there are four separate groups (α-, β-, γ- and ω-gliadins) separated on the basis of their mobility on starch-gel electrophoresis at pH 3.2 [91] with the α-, β- and γ-gliadins each contributing 30% of the total gliadin, and ω-gliadin 10%. The molecular weights of α-, β- and γ-gliadin range from 31 000 to 44 000 [55] and ω-gliadins around 70 000. The α-, β- and γ-gliadins have single polypeptide chains, with disulphide bonding. Their amino acid composition is unusual with approximately 40% glutamine and 15% proline. Furthermore, N-terminal sequence studies have been difficult because of the problems in isolating pure protein fractions. However, these studies show that large regions of the polypeptide chain are similar in different proteins, suggesting that gliadin proteins have evolved from a common parent [90].

Gluten—the toxic fragment

The chemical nature of the damaging fraction of gluten remains unknown. Frazer [70] considered that a toxic intermediate breakdown product of gluten, possibly because of lack of a specific peptidase, injured the intestinal mucosa. In the last 30 years, a number of fragments and digests have been investigated.

Glutamine. Glutamine, the major amino acid in gliadin, was the original suspect [165]. Its toxicity was thought to be due to its binding to some other substance, or alternatively becaue of its ability to become cyclized to pyrrolidone carboxylic acid. Conversion of glutamine into glutamic acid by hydrochloric acid renders it non-toxic. Frazer and his co-workers [71] made a peptic-tryptic digest of gluten, and were thus able to prepare six separate fractions. Of these, the soluble fraction III has been most extensively studied. Fraction III possesses all the amino acids present in gluten, and is as harmful to coeliacs as the parent material. The toxicity even persists after autoclaving and an ultrafiltrate of fraction III, containing 6–8 amino acids including glutamine and proline, remains damaging [99].

Effect of enzymes. Proteolytic enzymes do not make gluten harmless. This may be because the toxicity resides in a small peptide resistant to proteolytic cleavage. Alternatively the destructiveness could exist in non-peptide material. In this respect Phelan et al [136] separated the carbohydrate moiety of gliadin from the protein–glycoprotein using carbohydrases. The removal of bound carbohydrate destroyed the toxicity of the gliadin to coeliac jejunal mucosa, suggesting that the carbohydrate material bound to gliadin was vital for its action. These authors subsequently showed that gliadin toxicity could also be abolished using enzymes from *Aspergillus oryzae* and *Bacillus subtilis* [137]. This work still remains to be confirmed, and it is of interest that Bernardin and colleagues [17] were unable to detect carbohydrate in the toxic fragment of gliadin.

Components of gliadin. Of the components of gliadin, α, β and γ are toxic, α being the most toxic, while ω-gliadin is non-toxic. Using enzymatic degradation, followed by ion exchange chromatography, Cornell [39] has demonstrated at least 10 subfractions of α-gliadin. Of these, subfraction 9 was the most damaging to coeliac jejunal mucosa, and this fraction also elicited the most extreme antibody response from untreated coeliac patients [161]. Fraction 9 is particularly rich in glutamic acid, glutamine and proline [40].

Gluten fraction III. Ultrafiltration of Frazer's original gluten fraction III has produced three subfractions; fraction A with small molecular weight peptides (less than 1,000), fraction B with peptides of molecular weight 8,000 and fraction C with larger peptides. Fractions B and C proved to be toxic to coeliac jejunal mucosa [44] whilst a subfraction of B also gave positive intradermal skin tests in coeliac patients [2].

Studies using cultured jejunal mucosa

Organ culture techniques have provided an alternative method for understanding gluten toxicity, intestinal mucosa being viable for 24–28 hours in this system [162]. The morphology of the mucosa, and the activity of brush border enzymes can both be studied (Fig. 30.2). In healthy human intestine cultured in vitro, alkaline phosphatase activity increases due to maturation of the relatively immature crypt cells (Table 30.1). This is true also if jejunal tissue from an untreated coeliac is placed in a gluten-free medium [60]. The epithelial cells show normal morphology and enzyme activity. In contrast, when intestine from a patient with untreated coeliac disease is culture with gluten, the jejunal epithelial cells remain abnormal, and the increase in alkaline phosphatase activity is considerably reduced. Falchuk suggested that this represents perpetuation of the disease state in vitro [59].

Co-culture experiments. When intestinal tissue from coeliac patients in remission is cultured with gluten, the mucosa is unaffected and behaves normally [89] suggesting that gluten is not directly cytotoxic to coeliac jejunal mucosa but requires an effector mechanism. In subsequent co-culture experiments, Strober et al [158] demonstrated that jejunal tissue from a coeliac in remission, when cultured in the same chamber as jejunal tissue from a coeliac in relapse, became susceptible to the toxic effects of gluten. This implies that the mucosa of coeliacs in relapse produces either an antibody, lymphokine or activated cells which can traverse the medium and sensitize the remission coeliac mucosa. This is taken as strong evidence for the role of immune mechanisms in the pathogenesis of coeliac disease [60].

The lesions seen are specific to gluten and are not seen when other dietary antigens, such as casein, are added to the medium. The specific effects of gluten on coeliac intestine in vitro, could, however, be abolished by adding cortisol to the organ culture medium [93]. This further suggests that the reaction is indeed an immune one, because of the known effects of cortisol on immunoglobulin secretion and T cell function. The organ culture technique is supposedly so specific for coeliac disease, that Katz and Falchuk [92] have used it as a diagnostic test; when used prospectively

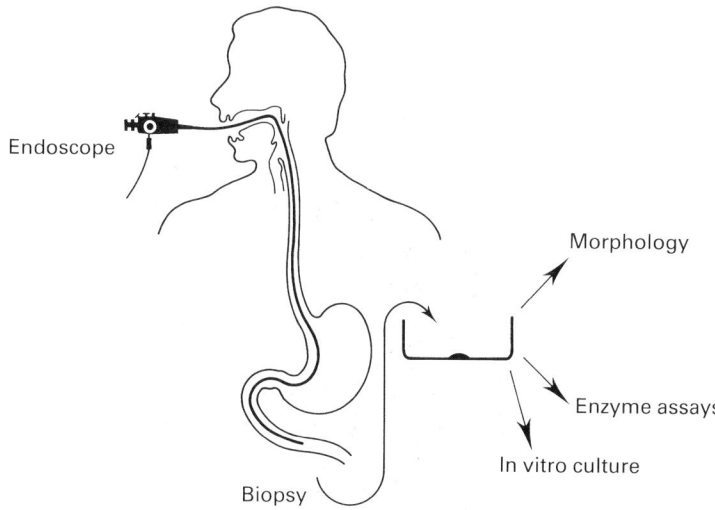

Endoscope

Morphology

Enzyme assays

In vitro culture

Biopsy

Fig. 30.2 Investigation of jejunal mucosa. The patient is endoscoped and a biopsy of jejunum taken with a Crosby capsule. Modern in vitro techniques allow culture of the jejunal mucosa as well as immunocytochemistry and enzyme assays.

Table 30.1 Culture of jejunal mucosa.

Assay	Healthy	Coeliac		Treated or in remission
		Untreated		
		Medium alone	Medium + gluten	Medium
Alkaline phosphatase	↑	↑	↓	↑
Maturation of crypt cells	+	+	−	+
Epithelial cells				
Morphology	Normal	Normal	Abnormal	Normal
Enzyme activity	Normal	Normal	Abnormal	Normal

in 75 patients with diarrhoea or malabsorption, the technique correctly established the diagnosis in all, but with a false-positive rate of 7% and false-negative rate of 15%. Similar findings have been described by others [84]. However, it is noteworthy that Hauri et al [78] were unable to demonstrate toxicity with the in vitro system using four fractions of gluten which had been shown to be toxic in vivo. Furthermore, in children, a number of gluten digests produced non-specific direct damaging effects [89].

Gluten: dose and type

Wheat, rye, barley and possibly oats are harmful in coeliac disease. Different patients show unequal susceptibility to the toxic effects of gluten; as little as 100 mg of gliadin has been shown to cause jejunal mucosal damage in vivo in a patient with coeliac disease [33], although 10 mg was non-toxic. Normal bread contains about 1.25 g gliadin per 30 g slice [32]. Even gluten-free products contain a small quantity of gluten (0.2–0.4 g/slice). Fortunately, this dose is not toxic to coeliacs.

In addition to the quantity of gluten, its source may also be important. The peptide mixtures in the gliadin fraction from hexaploid wheat such as used in bread differ significantly from those of tetraploid gliadins such as in durum wheat. Auricchio et al [10] confirmed the toxic effect of peptic–tryptic–Cotazym digests of bread wheat gliadin on in vitro cultured small intestinal mucosa from patients with active coeliac disease. However, the peptides from durum wheat gliadins are significantly less toxic in the in vitro organ culture system than those from bread, a fivefold higher concentration of durum being required to induce damage. Durum wheat gliadins are mainly found in spaghetti and pasta products, and are possibly better tolerated by coeliacs, though the results of formal trials are still awaited.

One of the unfulfilled hopes in coeliac disease is that if the toxic fragment in gluten could be identified it might be possible to breed plants which did not possess this fragment and thus eliminate coeliac disease.

COELIAC DISEASE

Clinical features

The main clinical features of coeliac disease are summarized in Table 30.2. Coeliac disease may be diagnosed at any age including in childhood; however, there is a peak of newly diagnosed adults in the third decade. The disease varies in severity, from the totally asymptomatic patient diagnosed as part of a family study to the severely affected patient presenting with complications; for example, with pathological fractures from osteomalacia. Diarrhoea, or frank steatorrhoea, is the com-

Table 30.2 Clinical features of coeliac disease.

Gastrointestinal
  Diarrhoea (occasionally constipation)
  Abdominal distension and gas
  Recurrent oral ulcers
  Glossitis
  Angular stomatitis
  Nausea and vomiting
General
  Malaise and weakness
  Weight loss
  Finger clubbing
  Short stature
Skin
  Dermatitis herpetiformis
  Vasculitis
Vitamins
  Vitamin K deficiency
  Calcium and vitamin D malabsorption
Typical facies
  Prominent forehead
  Narrow jaw
  Blue eyes
  Fair hair
  Premature greying

monest mode of presentation, though rarely patients may be constipated. Malaise and weakness, often expressed as 'not being 100%', along with abdominal distension and flatulence are also commonplace [36].

Oral ulceration. Patients with untreated coeliac disease may have recurrent mouth ulcers. However, 5–10% of the general population also suffer this affliction. Ferguson et al [67] found that 8 of 33 patients with severe recurrent aphthous stomatitis had coeliac disease. This high figure has, however, not been substantiated in other studies. Thus, in a series of 100 unselected patients with oral ulceration of varying degrees of severity, Bateman et al [15] found only four with coeliac disease, and Lehner [103] an incidence of 2%. This lower figure seems a more likely incidence. Glossitis, with a smooth, red, denuded tongue, and additionally angular stomatitis and cheilosis, are further oral manifestations of untreated coeliac disease.

Abdominal symptoms. Nausea and vomiting are also found surprisingly often. Weight loss is almost invariable in symptomatic patients, though the occasional obese coeliac is seen. Up to one-quarter of coeliac patients complain of abdominal pain. In some this is due to volvulus or intussusception, or other abdominal conditions unrelated to coeliac disease. It is striking that in a percentage of coeliacs stabilized on a gluten-free diet, accidental or deliberate ingestion of gluten can rapidly lead to severe symptoms with mouth ulcers, colicky abdominal pain, nausea, vomiting and diar-

rhoea. This lasts from 3 to 7 days and is incapacitating. In the most severely affected individuals, a state of 'gluten shock' occurs, with hypotension and bronchospasm.

There are a number of extraintestinal manifestations of coeliac disease, mostly related to the malabsorption. These include vitamin K deficiency with petechiae and ecchymoses, and calcium and vitamin D malabsorption with rickets or osteomalacia (Table 30.2)

Characteristic facial appearance. It is common for coeliac patients to have blue eyes and fair hair and premature greying is often found. A characteristic facies has also been described, with a triangular appearance due to a prominent forehead and narrow jaw [36].

Other features. Up to 20% of adult coeliacs are below their expected height. Finger clubbing also occurs [16] though it is not usually marked, whilst oedema is found in more ill patients. The abdomen in coeliac disease feels doughy. Hyposplenism is also found but only in adults [31]; its exact cause is unknown. Of skin lesions, dermatitis herpetiformis is the classical dermal manifestation [74] though a number of other skin complaints are seen, including vasculitis [45].

Laboratory findings

Table 30.3 shows the findings in 90 adult patients with coeliac disease at presentation to our unit. Mild anaemia was frequent, with iron deficiency in most cases. In contrast, vitamin B_{12} deficiency was uncommon, being

Table 30.3 Laboratory findings in 90 patients with adult coeliac disease at presentation.

Parameter	Mean	SD	Reference range
Haemoglobin	11.8	2.83	Male 14–18 g/dl Female 12–16 g/dl
Packed cell volume	0.37	0.08	Male 0.42–0.52 Female 0.37–0.47
Mean corpuscular volume	89.6	13.4	80–100 fl
Iron	12.9	8.96	14–29 mmol/l
Iron-binding capacity	70.3	14.7	45–75 mmol/l
B_{12}	216	133	150–800 ng/l
Folic acid	2.68	2.55	2.5–18.0 µg/l
Red cell folate	114	82.7	160–600 µg/l
Albumin	39	7.4	35–45 g/l
Calcium	2.21	0.19	2.33–2.60 mmol/l
Faecal fat	39.5	24.4	<17.0 mmol/day
Xylose absorption	0.50	0.31	0.65–1.33 mmol/l
Lactose absorption	0.9	0.7	>1.2 mmol rise
Immunoglobulin G	11.78	4.36	6.0–16 g/l
Immunoglobulin A	3.64	2.39	0.75–4 g/l
Immunoglobulin M	1.15	0.74	0.25–2.0 g/l
Reticulin antibody	49%	–	–

found in only 5 patients. As a group though, serum folic acid was at the lower limit of normal. However, red cell folate, representing body stores of folic acid, was almost invariably subnormal (85 out of 90 patients) and was the best single predictor of the presence of coeliac disease. Mild hypocalcaemia was also commonplace, though frank osteomalacia was only found in five patients.

A moderate steatorrhoea of approximately 40 mmol of fat daily was very typical of untreated coeliac disease. Xylose absorption, as assessed by the 1 hour serum xylose absorption test, was moderately impaired in the untreated coeliacs, as was lactose absorption.

Overall, the quantitative immunoglobulin levels were normal for the group, though six patients had selective IgA deficiency, raised levels of IgA were fairly typical otherwise. Half of the patients had antireticulin antibodies.

Small intestinal barium studies typically show a 'malabsorption pattern' with dilatation of the lumen, thickening of the mucosal folds and loss of the normal feathery pattern. More recently, using the technique of small bowel enema, a more specific lesion, jejunalization of

the ileum [26] has been described. A typical example is shown in Fig. 30.3, with a decrease in the jejunal fold pattern, and an increase in the ileal folds.

Jejunal morphology

By definition, there is an abnormal jejunal mucosa in coeliac disease, which improves morphologically when treated with a gluten-free diet [22]. The histological appearance of the jejunum can, however, be variable [34]; in contrast to finger-like villi seen in the normal jejunal mucosa, the classic appearance of untreated coeliac disease is a flat jejunal mucosa, with a mosaic pattern under the dissecting microscope (Figs. 30.4 and 30.5), though a ridged and/or convoluted appearance with partial villus atrophy may also be seen. The characteristic cellular infiltrate in the mucosa is taken as indicative of immunological events in the jejunum. The numbers of intraepithelial lymphocytes are increased in untreated coeliac disease (Fig. 30.6), and decrease on a gluten-free diet [64, 82]. In healthy individuals, these intraepithelial lymphocytes are found below the enterocyte nuclei, whereas in untreated

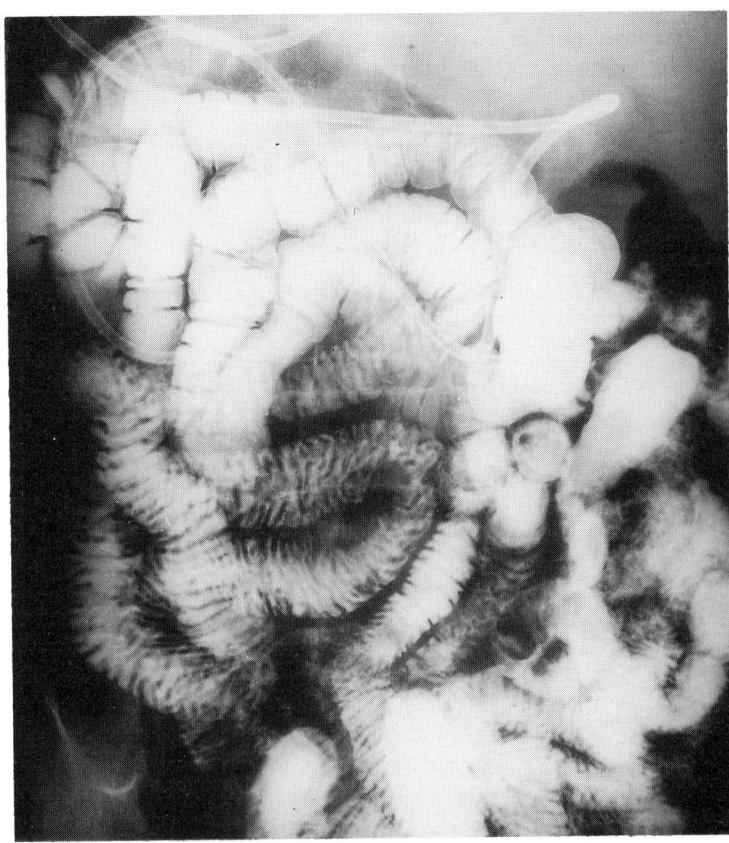

Fig. 30.3 Small bowel enema showing reversal of normal anatomical pattern with jejunalization of the ileum.

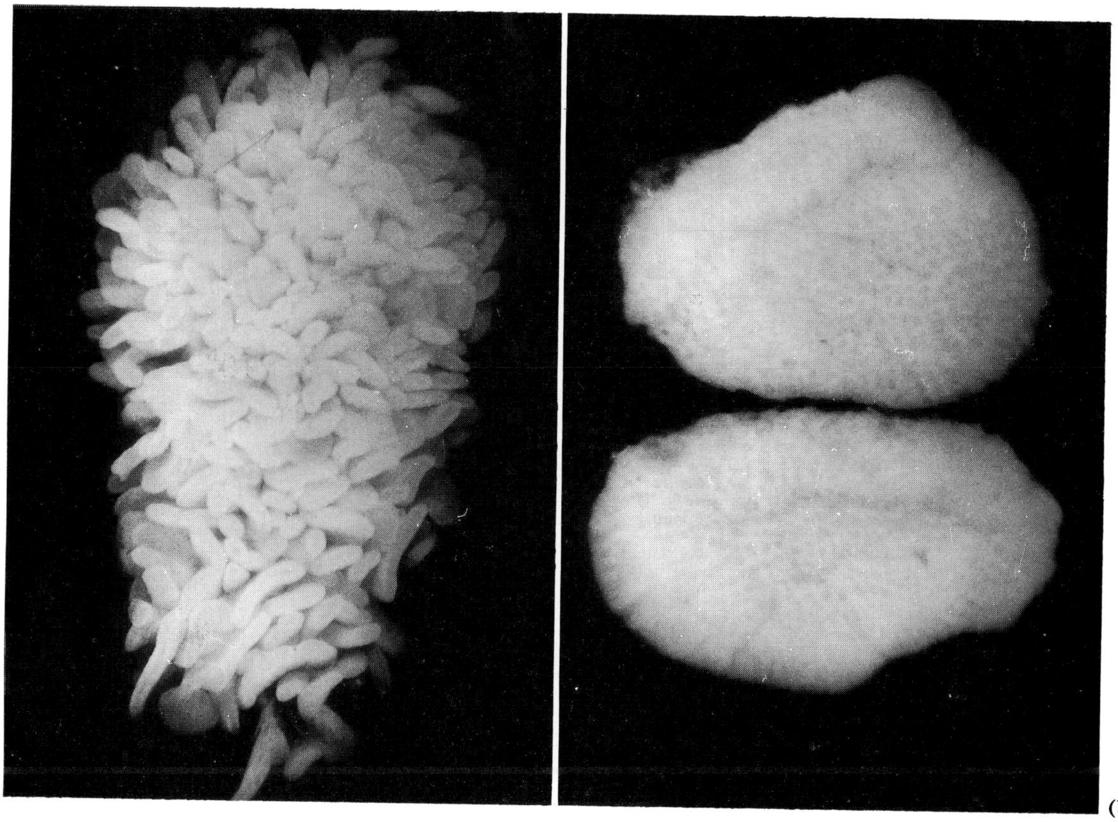

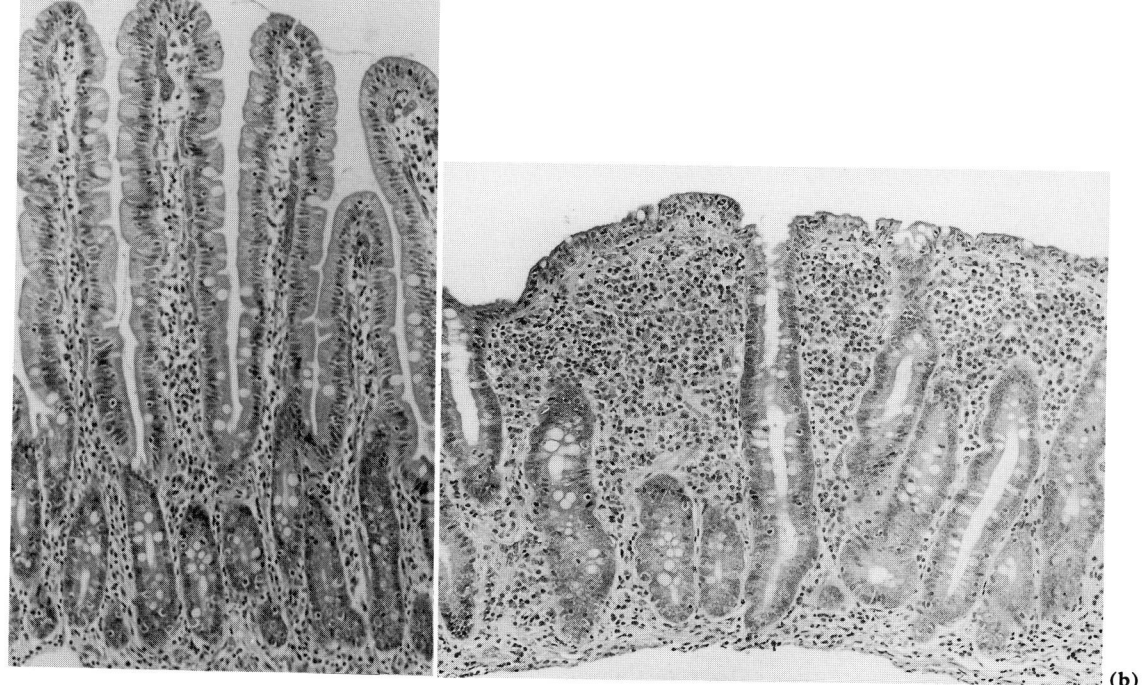

Fig. 30.4 Dissecting microscope appearance of (a) normal jejunal biopsy, with finger-like villi, and (b) a flat 'mosaic' jejunal biopsy from a patient with untreated coeliac disease.

Fig. 30.5 Histology of jejunal biopsy. (a) Normal villus pattern. (b) Subtotal villus atrophy in untreated coeliac disease.

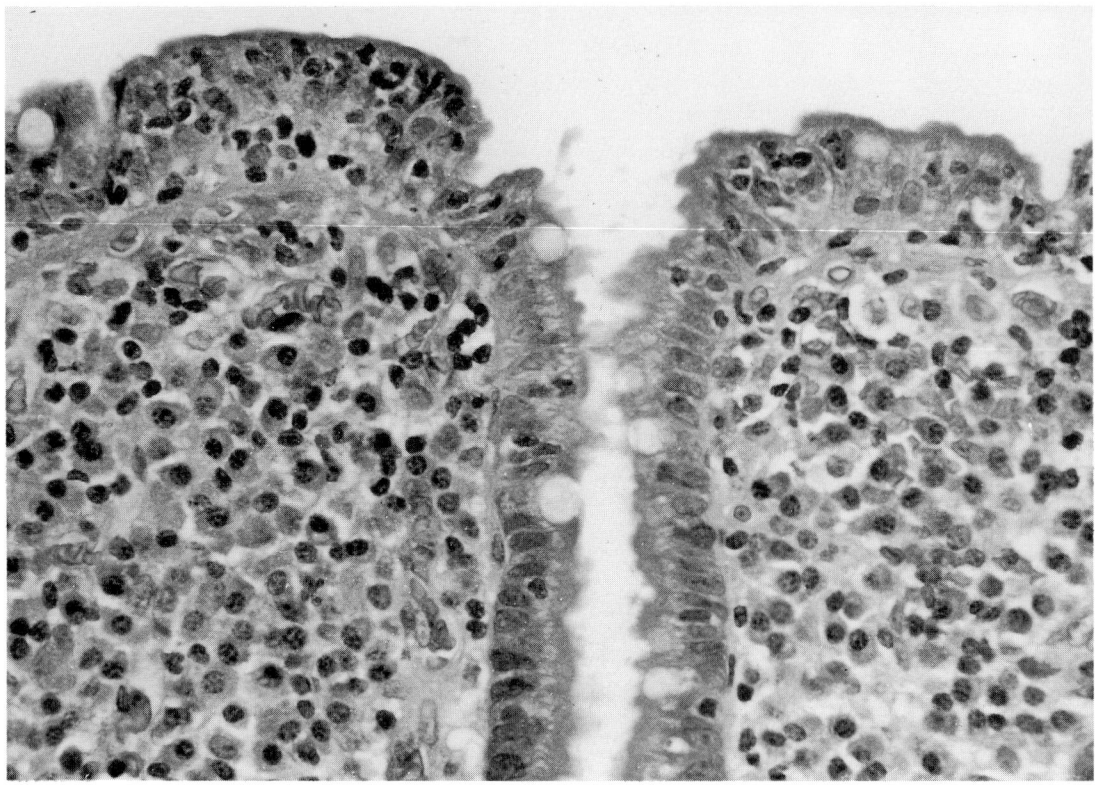

Fig. 30.6 High-power view of jejunal biopsy in coeliac disease demonstrating the increased numbers of intra-epithelial lymphocytes.

coeliac disease, they occur throughout the epithelium, suggesting they may be attracted there by gluten [74]. After oral gluten challenge these intraepithelial lymphocytes increase in number [102]. They are predominantly cytotoxic/suppressor T cells [68, 148] suggesting that cell-mediated immune responses are important at the mucosal level.

Further evidence for localized cell-mediated immunity comes from the morphological studies of Marsh, who has shown that in untreated coeliac jejunal mucosa, the intraepithelial lymphocytes are blast-transformed and highly mitotic (Fig. 30.7) [117, 118, 120]. A raised mitotic index is found only in untreated coeliac disease [119]; on a gluten-free diet the index falls to normal and it is quite likely that these immunoblasts are sensitized to gluten.

A further characteristic feature of untreated coeliac disease is villus atrophy with crypt hyperplasia (Fig. 30.8) A similar appearance is seen when local cell-mediated immunity is induced experimentally; for example, rats infested with *Nippostrongylus brasiliensis* develop a similar mucosal appearance [63]. Similar changes are also seen in allograft rejection and graft-versus-host disease [111, 112] both of

which are T lymphocyte induced. This again suggests that local cellular hypersensitivity is an important feature of untreated coeliac disease. However, the appearances in coeliac disease are not exactly like those in the animal models, in particular the enterocytes were normal in the animal studies, whereas they are always abnormal in coeliacs.

Further experimental data favouring altered cellular immunity in coeliac disease were provided by Ferguson et al [66] who showed that jejunal mucosa from coeliac patients, when cultured with α-gliadin in vitro, produces the lymphokine macrophage migration inhibition factor. This indicates the presence of a population of lymphocytes sensitized to α-gliadin in the jejunal mucosa and is more direct evidence of local cell-mediated immunity.

Effects of gluten challenge in coeliac disease in vivo

Gastrointestinal effects

If a patient with coeliac disease on a gluten-free diet and in remission ingests gluten regularly, the jejunal mucosa again becomes

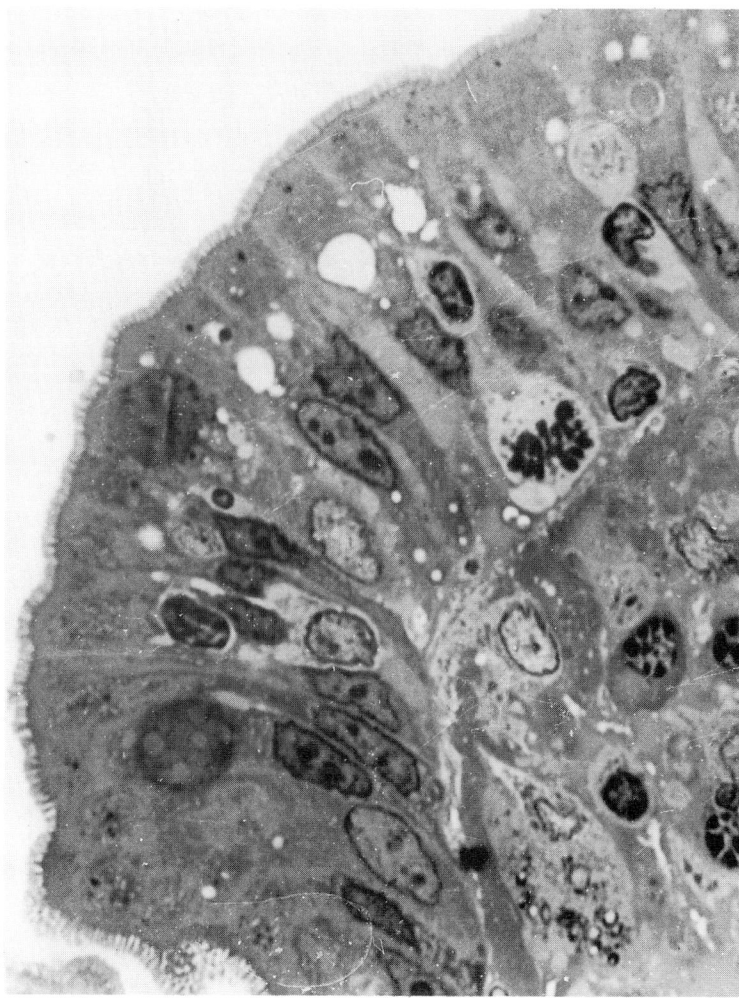

Fig. 30.7 High-power view of untreated coeliac jejunal epithelial cell layer showing gluten-dependent mitotic activity of intraepithelial lymphocytes. Reproduced from Marsh and Haeney [120], with permission from the editor of the *Journal of the Royal College of Physicians*.

flat. This usually happens soon after ingesting gluten, though in exceptional cases the jejunal abnormality may take months, or years, to develop [52]. Many data have accumulated on the early changes which occur in the intestinal mucosa after such gluten ingestion. Thus Booth et al [24] found slight oedema in the biopsy at 4 hours with infiltration of the lamina propria by polymorphs at 12 hours. After 24 hours there was a mononuclear infiltrate into the lamina propria with villus atrophy and enterocyte damage. This feature recovered within 48 hours.

In a further study of 10 coeliac patients in remission, Bramble et al [27] instilled 25 g of Frazer's gluten fraction III into the duodenum. Four control subjects in whom there was no significant change in any parameter were also studied. In the coeliac patients the levels of brush border enzymes alkaline phosphatase and lactase fell significantly by 4 hours, and began to recover by 24 hours. In

this study there were no significant changes in villus height or crypt depth at 1, 2, 3, 4, 8 or 24 hours. The number of cells in each villus fell significantly at 4 and 8 hours, whereas the number of cells in the crypts increased over 24 hours. This increase in crypt cells concomitant with the fall in villus cells, induced by gluten, suggests a negative feedback effect.

Degree of damage. The degree of gluten damage induced is dose and subfraction dependent. Thus, Dissanayake et al [44] using gluten fraction B, found more marked abnormalities after acute challenge, with partial villus atrophy, an increase in intraepithelial lymphocytes and decrease in the disaccharidases, maximal at 24 hours. Ferguson [61] also found an increase in intraepithelial lymphocytes within 4 hours of a challenge with 30 g of gluten. These changes persisted to 48 hours, with an increase in lymphocytes and plasma cells in the lamina propria [102].

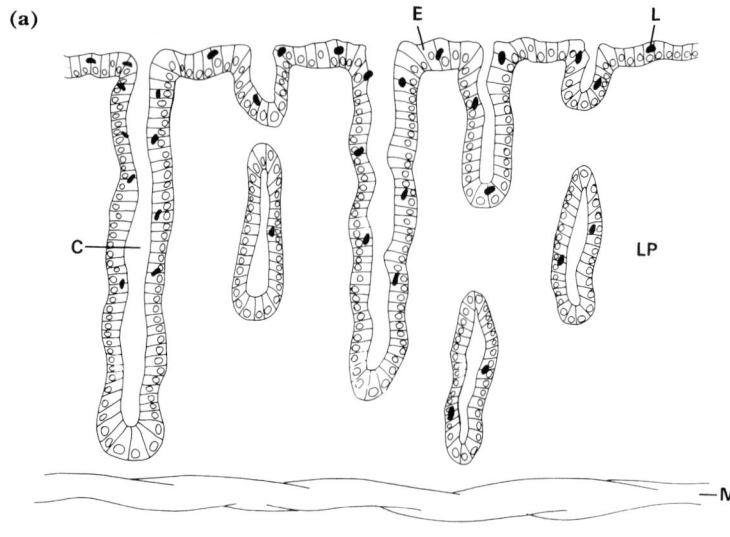

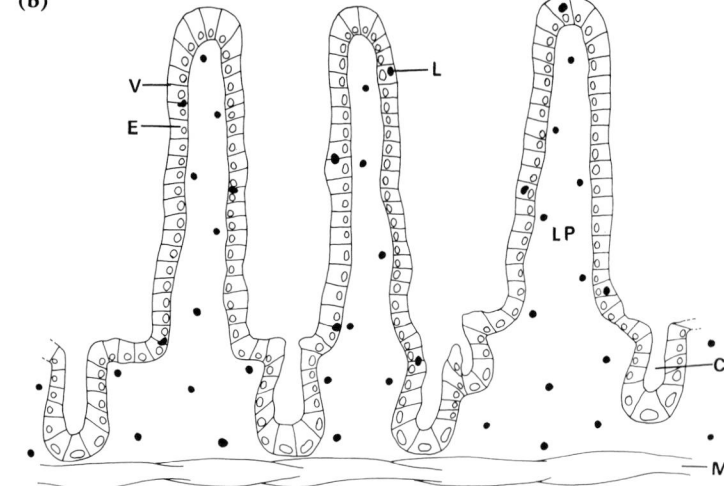

Fig. 30.8 Diagrammatic representation of (a) normal jejunal mucosa, and (b) jejunal mucosa in coeliac disease to illustrate jejunal villus atrophy and crypt hyperplasia. V = villus, E = enterocyte, L = intraepithelial lymphocyte, LP = lamina propria, C = crypt, M = muscularis mucosae.

Immunoglobulin production. Lancaster-Smith and colleagues [101] have also shown that after an acute gluten challenge, IgA- and IgM-producing cells increase in the lamina propria; interestingly IgE-producing cells also multiply [127]. In the study of Dissanayake et al [44] there was an increase in IgA- and IgM-producing cells, which peaked at 3-6 hours after challenge suggesting that a Type III hypersensitivity reaction was taking place. The early changes in Bramble et al's study [27] would also suggest a Type III immune complex-mediated reaction though direct gluten toxicity to the coeliac enterocytes is also a possibility.

Of related interest is the conclusive demonstration by Leonard et al [104] that patients with dermatitis herpetiformis whose rash is controlled with a gluten-free diet will relapse after prolonged challenge with gluten. Even when skin biopsies had been normal on a gluten-free diet, there was a recurrence of skin basement membrane IgA deposition following gluten challenge, indicating that dermatitis herpetiformis is indeed gluten-dependent, and does not remit spontaneously (see Chapter 36).

Skin tests

Intradermal skin testing to detect hypersensitivity to gluten has not been very successful in coeliac disease. Using Frazer's gluten fraction III, Asquith [7] found no macroscopic abnormality in 20 of 21 coeliacs at 48 hours. However, biopsies showed a delayed mononuclear cell infiltrate (48 hours) suggestive of delayed hypersensitivity. Unfortunately, a similar response was found in the non-coeliac controls and so must be non-specific. On the other hand, Baker and Read [12] also using gluten fraction III detected positive responses in 52% of untreated coeliacs and 33% of coeliacs on a gluten-free diet. In these patients, the timing of the response, and its histology, favoured an Arthus reaction. Additionally, Anand et al [2], using the B2 fraction (an ultrafiltrate of fraction III) found a positive Arthus-type response in 10 coeliacs and no reaction in 20 controls. However, Rawcliffe et al [140] using the same B2 antigen, though finding positive responses in all coeliacs tested, also found a high percentage of positives in patients with inflammatory bowel disease, and controls. To date, no antigenic fraction has been identified which will specifically react in coeliac patients only.

The effects of gluten withdrawal in coeliac disease

The improvement in general health occurring in many coeliacs on gluten withdrawal is striking; appetite improves, weight increases and diarrhoea ceases whilst other complications such as iron or folate deficiency, and osteomalacia take longer (the changes in laboratory parameters following gluten withdrawal are shown in Table 30.4), the recovery time varying from patient to patient.

Histological changes

In serial biopsies from patients on gluten

withdrawal, Yardley et al [177], demonstrated improvement in epithelial cell height within 6-10 days. However, the improvement in overall crypt height takes months or even years to occur. In general, clinical improvement correlates with the increase in epithelial cell height. McDonald et al [113] confirmed the degree of jejunal mucosal improvement was variable, and could be complete, or there could be no apparent response, even though the patient may have made a good clinical recovery on a gluten-free diet. These authors were also able to show that in some of these latter patients the failure of histological improvement was due to the coexistence of a small bowel lymphoma.

Intestinal permeability

Intestinal permeability is abnormal in coeliac disease, with a reduced absorption of small hydrophilic molecules, and an increase in absorption of larger molecules. Using a cellobiose-mannitol 'probe', Hamilton et al [77] were able to show that this abnormal permeability rapidly reverses on gluten withdrawal and occurs at a time when early morphological improvement is apparent, i.e. an increase in epithelial cell height with a reduction in the mitotic index.

The ^{51}Cr-labelled EDTA probe is a much more sensitive indicator of intestinal permeability than sugar solutions or polyethylene glycol [19]. As shown in Fig. 30.9 there is increased permeability to this small molecular weight probe in patients with untreated coeliac disease. In contrast to Hamilton et al's [77]

Table 30.4 The effect of gluten withdrawal on laboratory findings in 90 patients with adult coeliac disease.

	Normal diet	Gluten-free diet	Reference range
Haemoglobin	11.8	14.2	Male 14–18 g/dl
			Female 12–16 g/dl
Packed cell volume	0.37	0.422	Male 0.42–0.52
			Female 0.37–0.47
Mean corpuscular volume	89.6	90	80–100 fl
Iron	12.9	18.3	14–29 nmol/l
Iron-binding capacity	70.3	65.9	45–75 μmol/l
B$_{12}$	216	357	150–800 ng/l
Folic acid	2.68	5.5	2.5–18.0 μg/l
Red cell folate	114	250	160–600 μg/l
Albumin	39	37	35–45 g/l
Calcium	2.21	2.33	2.33–2.60 mmol/l
Faecal fat	39.5	15.8	17 mmol/day
Xylose absorption	0.50	0.97	0.65–1.33 nmol/l
Lactose absorption	0.9	1.6	71.2 nmol increase
Immunoglobulin G	11.78	11.55	6–16 g/l
Immunoglobulin A	3.64	2.14	0.75–4 g/l
Immunoglobulin M	1.15	1.3	0.25–2.0 g/l

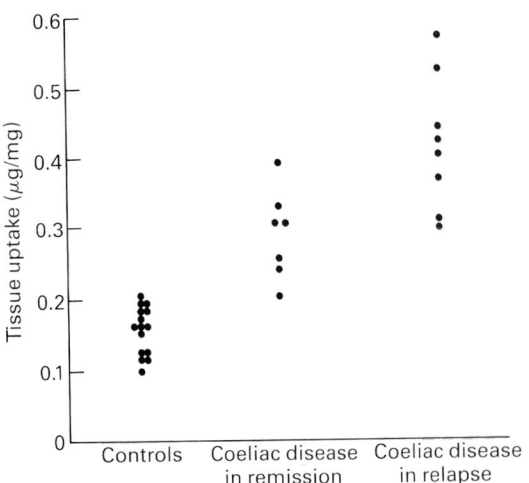

Fig. 30.9 Tissue uptake of ^{51}Cr-EDTA by controls and patients with coeliac disease. From Bjarnason and Peters [19], with permission of the authors and the editor of *Gut*.

study, the abnormal permeability persisted in the majority of patients with coeliac disease after treatment with a gluten-free diet. This study was based on in vitro uptake by samples of jejunal biopsy tissue. In vivo studies [20] gave very similar findings, with the most marked abnormality of permeability being found in coeliac patients in relapse, but persisting when in clinical and histological remission. In a later and more extensive study [21] with larger numbers of patients with both coeliac disease and dermatitis herpetiformis, the persistent abnormal permeability to ^{51}Cr-EDTA was confirmed. Furthermore, in those patients who had shown histological improvement on a gluten-free diet, with normal mucosal height to crypt depth ratio, and normal numbers of intraepithelial lymphocytes, the abnormal permeability persisted. This suggests that a persistent defect in permeability might be a primary factor in coeliac disease, allowing the entry of toxic fragments of gluten to the lamina propria. These interesting findings have not as yet been confirmed by other centres.

Mechanisms of gluten toxicity

Peptidase deficiency

It was suggested by Frazer [70] that coeliac disease was due to a deficient peptidase, which allowed toxic metabolites of gluten to accumulate, resulting in cellular damage. Thus, wheat protein was no longer harmful to coeliacs following incubation with hog's intestinal mu-

cosa; also, severely reduced jejunal brush border enzymes were found in untreated coeliac disease. However, gluten toxicity resides in large peptides, and therefore a jejunal peptidase deficiency is unlikely. More importantly, formal studies of peptidases [49, 69] have been unable to identify a defect or deficiency, and this theory seems increasingly less tenable.

Immune response

There is much evidence to suggest that an immune response to gluten is involved in coeliac disease. As described previously, increased numbers of lymphocytes are found at all levels of the epithelium [61] possibly attracted there by the presence of gluten in the intestinal lumen. Their numbers increase after gluten challenge [102] and fall on a gluten-free diet to nearly normal levels [82]. Furthermore, most of these intraepithelial lymphocytes are T cells [5, 65].

In the lamina propria in untreated coeliacs the number of lymphocytes is decreased, with a concomitant increase in the number of plasma cells [82]. It is thought that sensitized lymphocytes, in the presence of gluten, transform to plasma cells, thus accounting for this observation.

A number of other non-specific features also suggest that immunological mechanisms are important in coeliac disease, including the common findings of splenic atrophy, enlargement of the mesenteric nodes, peripheral nodes, and the increased incidence of malignancy [7]. Furthermore it is well recognized that steroids ameliorate the adverse effects of gluten [35], and can induce a clinical remission [169]. Cortisol halves the quantity of immunoglobulin secreted by coeliac jejunal mucosa in vitro [57] and additionally it ablates the toxic effects of gluten in coeliac jejunal mucosa in organ culture [93].

Humoral immunity

Immunoglobulins in serum and intestinal juice

There are alterations in generalized humoral immunity in untreated coeliac disease with serum levels of IgA elevated [9], and IgM reduced [79]. These return towards the normal on gluten withdrawal. Additionally, significantly higher levels of serum secretory IgA are found in untreated patients, compared with those on a gluten-free diet or patients with inflammatory bowel disease [159]. In the lamina propria of the small intestine there is a polyclonal increase in plasma cells with the most marked rise being in IgA and IgM cells [13] whilst in the intestinal juice, increased levels of IgA, IgM and IgG are found [8].

Intestinal permeability and antibody response

Because of the mucosal damage in coeliac disease, intestinal permeability is increased with enhanced non-specific macromolecular absorption. In consequence, antibodies to wheat protein and gluten are found in such patients, but this is a non-specific finding, since these antibodies are also detected in inflammatory bowel disease, and even in healthy controls [62, 96]. Antibodies to a number of other dietary antigens are also commonly found for the same reasons. In contrast, the finding of antibodies to gluten fraction III in the upper intestinal secretions was initially thought to be specific for the condition, but these have also been described rarely in children with other diarrhoeal illnesses [62].

Antibodies to crude gliadin fractions are invariably found in children with untreated coeliac disease, but again are non-specific, being detected in 50% of children with other upper gastrointestinal diseases [142, 155]. These antibodies were of the IgG class, whereas IgA antigliadin antibodies are perhaps more specific for coeliacs [163]. The presence of food antibodies in the serum is in any case not necessarily of pathological significance. Paganelli et al [132] suggested that food antigens are absorbed across the normal gastrointestinal tract and cleared via the formation of immune complexes.

Antibody to α-gliadin. The more purified wheat protein, α-gliadin, is more toxic to coeliac jejunal mucosa both in vivo and in vitro than the more crude gliadin extracts [85, 95]. There is also an increased (cellular) reactivity to this antigen in coeliac disease [75]. Using an enzyme-linked immunosorbent assay (ELISA), O'Farrelly and colleagues [131] found IgG antibodies to gliadin were significantly raised in untreated patients when compared with other individuals, and appeared disease specific (Fig. 30.10). Keiffer et al [94] also found antibodies to gliadin in most untreated coeliacs, but the antibodies were also found—though at a lower titre—in patients with other gastrointestinal diseases. Keiffer used a mixed reverse solid phase passive antiglobulin haemabsorption technique, and it is

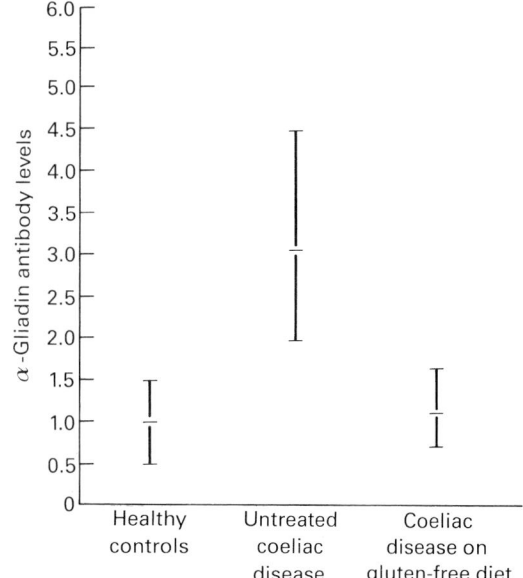

Fig. 30.10 Antibody to α-gliadin in controls; and patients with coeliac disease on a gluten-free diet and normal diet. The mean and standard deviation of ELISA indices are shown. From O'Farrelly et al [131], with permission of the authors and the editor of the *British Medical Journal*.

possible that the ELISA is a more sensitive and specific technique. Of great importance was the additional finding by O'Farrelly et al [131], that α-gliadin antibody titres fell to normal in those patients who adhered strictly to a gluten-free diet and therefore this can be used to monitor the progress of the disease and check strictness of diet. O'Farrelly et al [130] have subsequently also shown that peripheral blood mononuclear cells from coeliac patients but not controls bind with a monoclonal antibody to α-gliadin.

Antibody to gluten. Scott et al [145] using an ELISA technique have also found antibodies to gluten in coeliac patients. IgA antibodies to gluten were disease specific and the test could detect 94% of children and 80% of adults at presentation. IgA antibodies to other food antigens such as casein, ovalbumin and β-lactoglobulin were also found in such patients, again the levels falling on gluten withdrawal.

Antireticulin antibodies. Concerning non-dietary antibodies, an IgG antibody to reticulin was found in 36% of patients with coeliac disease by Seah et al [146] and at the time provoked considerable interest but reticulin antibody was subsequently also found in patients with other gastrointestinal diseases [147]. IgA-class antireticulin antibodies are in con-

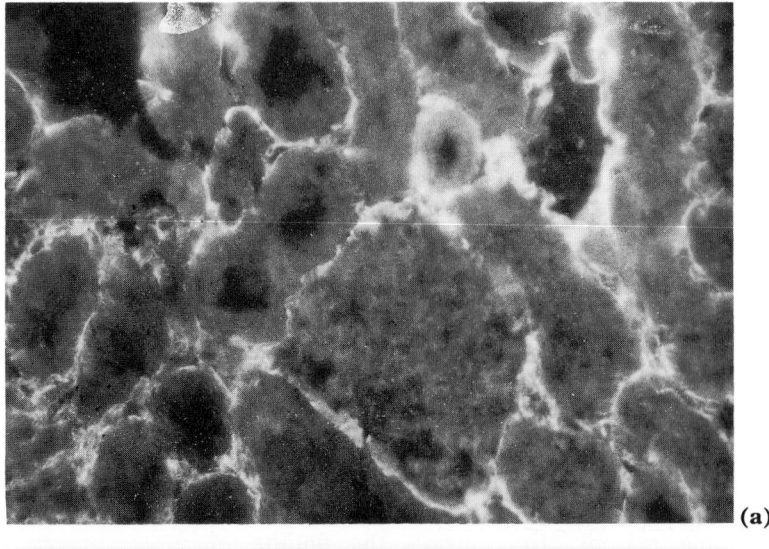

(a)

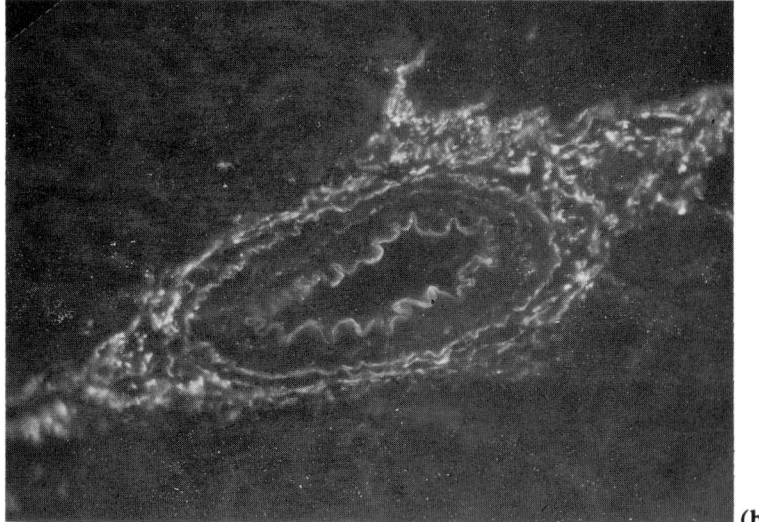

(b)

Fig. 30.11 (a) Type 1: antireticulin antibody directed against gastric mucosa. (b) Type 2: antireticulin antibody directed against glomerular basement membrane.

trast more specific, being found in 79% of coeliacs and only 13% of controls [51]. This IgA antibody is also found in the jejunal secretions, particularly of untreated coeliac patients [122]. The antireticulin antibody is directed against components of connective tissue, such as endothelial basement membrane, perivascular connective tissue, epithelial basement membrane and the glomerulus (Fig. 30.11) [175]. It does not react with type III collagen, fibronectin or the non-collagenous reticulin component of Pras and Glynn [164]. Nevertheless, the putative role of this reticulin antibody remains unknown.

Local humoral immunity following gluten challenge

Type I hypersensitivity. Immediate hypersen-

sitivity, Type I, reactions may have a role at the mucosal level. Strobel et al [157] have described an expanded population of mast cells in the jejunal mucosa in untreated patients. Following gluten challenge, jejunal mast-cell degranulation is an early finding and IgE plasma cells are also increased in untreated coeliac jejunal mucosa, falling to normal on treatment [144]. In addition, coeliac jejunal mucosa challenged with α-gliadin in vitro releases histamine [114]. It seems likely that this reaginic hypersensitivity, following exposure to gluten, causes damage to the mucosa and hence increased permeability, thus facilitating subsequent Type III and IV reactions.

Type III hypersensitivity. Following challenge of treated coeliacs with gluten, the jejunal mucosa secretes an increased amount of IgM and

IgA [106]. Much of this is specific gluten antibody [60]. Specific antigluten antibody is also secreted [28], whereas complement-fixing IgA complexes are also found along the jejunal basement membrane [151] and are thought to be involved in enterocyte cytotoxicity [150]. The time course of gluten challenge studies is compatible with an immune complex-mediated reaction [27,44]. It has therefore been postulated that, following gluten challenge, immune complexes are formed over 4–6 hours; these are then ingested by neutrophils with subsequent cell disruption and lysosomal release. Whether the antigen within the complex is gluten, or a fraction thereof, is not known.

Cell-mediated immunity

Non-specific reactions

Delayed hypersensitivity is thought to be of major importance in the pathogenesis of coeliac disease, and this is indicated by the fact that coeliac disease can, and does, occur in antibody deficiency states. Coeliac disease is found in the presence of selective IgA deficiency and this condition is 10 times more prevalent in coeliac disease than in the general population. More significantly, gluten-responsive coeliac disease has been described in a patient with common variable immunodeficiency [120, 172].

Depressed cellular activity. In non-specific cell-mediated immunity there is an overall depression of cellular reactivity which is manifested by depressed lymphocyte transformation in vitro [143] and by lymphoreticular atrophy [110]. The absolute numbers of T cells, and their proportion, are reduced in untreated coeliac patients [128], returning to normal after gluten withdrawal. Additionally, when challenged against tumour cells in vitro, lymphocytes from coeliac patients show a reduced proliferative and cytotoxic capacity [115]. O'Farrelly et al [130] further confirmed that lymphocyte proliferation in the presence of plant mitogens is depressed in such patients, both treated and untreated, and also demonstrated increased T suppressor cell activity, and it was suggested that this disturbance in immune regulation is the basis of the overall depressed cell-mediated immunity.

Specific cell-mediated immunity to gluten: leukocyte migration inhibition

Specific cellular hypersensitivity to gluten in coeliac disease has been most intensively studied by the leukocyte migration inhibition test, an in vitro correlate of cell-mediated immunity. Douwes [50] found that 12 patients with coeliac disease had inhibition of leukocyte migration in the presence of a gluten subfraction. This was not found in healthy controls or in patients with a variety of other gastrointestinal diseases. In a study by Haeney and

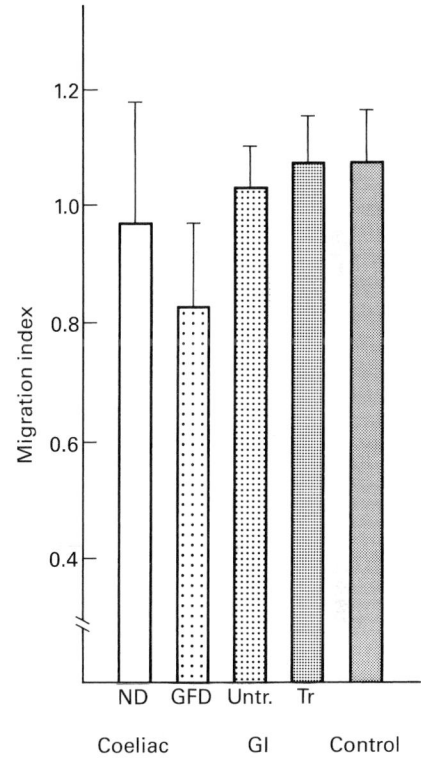

Fig. 30.12 Leukocyte migration inhibition by α-gliadin: comparison of responses (± SD) in untreated (ND) and treated (GFD) coeliacs, untreated (UN) and treated (Tr) gastrointestinal patients and healthy controls.

Asquith [75], using α-gliadin as the antigen, leukocyte migration inhibition occurred in 80% of coeliacs on a gluten-free diet, 37.5% of coeliacs on a 'normal' diet and in only 3.7% of non-coeliacs (Figs. 30.12 and 30.13). The most likely explanation for the higher reactivity in coeliacs on a gluten-free diet is that in patients on a 'normal' (i.e. containing gluten) diet, activated T lymphocytes are concentrated in the bowel mucosa at the site of the antigen stimulus, and are therefore not detected in peripheral blood. This suggestion was con-

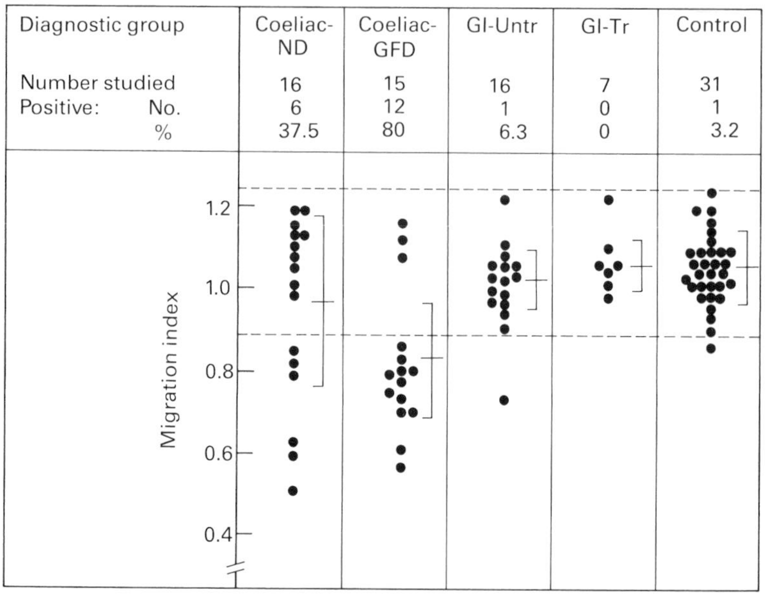

Diagnostic group	Coeliac-ND	Coeliac-GFD	GI-Untr	GI-Tr	Control
Number studied	16	15	16	7	31
Positive: No.	6	12	1	0	1
%	37.5	80	6.3	0	3.2

Fig. 30.13 Leukocyte migration inhibition by α-gliadin. Individual results in untreated (ND) and treated (GFD) coeliacs, untreated (UN) and treated (Tr) gastrointestinal (GI) patients and healthy controls. Vertical bar lines represent mean ± SD. Horizontal dashed lines indicate normal range.

firmed by Bullen and Losowsky [30] who used Frazer's gluten fraction III as the antigen, and found significant inhibition of leukocyte migration in 13% of coeliacs on a normal diet, and 54% on a gluten-free diet. When gluten was withdrawn from coeliac patients, migration indices fell into the sensitized range, suggesting that sensitized lymphocytes had indeed migrated from the gut to the blood compartment.

Increased specificity in children. As with many immunological techniques in coeliac disease, these tests have a higher specificity in children. Thus, Ashkenazi et al [6] found that overall, 94% of coeliac children demonstrate leukocyte migration inhibition in the presence of gluten subfraction. Of interest, and contrary to what occurs in adult coeliacs, a percentage of these children became negative in the test following prolonged gluten withdrawal.

Lymphokine production. The leukocyte migration inhibition test assesses lymphokine production (leukocyte inhibitory factor) in the presence of gluten. O'Farrelly et al [129], using a modification of the test with direct assay of lymphokine production, found positive results in the presence of α-gliadin in all eight untreated coeliacs studied, in 14 of 15 treated coeliacs but in only two of 28 controls. However, other studies have cast doubt on the disease specificity; Simpson et al [152] whilst confirming gluten inhibition of leukocyte migration in coeliacs noted a similar degree of migration was found in those non-coeliac con-

trols who possessed the HLA-B8 antigen. As more than 80% of coeliacs are HLA-B8 positive, a positive migration test could be merely an indicator of the presence of this HLA antigen. Furthermore, Simpson and co-workers [153] have also produced evidence that the leukocyte inhibition test, as used to assess gluten sensitivity in coeliac disease, may be measuring the effects of cytophilic antibody rather than lymphokine production.

Lymphocyte transformation. The other test of cell-mediated immunity to gluten employed in coeliac disease has been the lymphocyte transformation test. This is technically a more difficult and time-consuming test, and the results have been rather variable. Thus Ansaldi et al [4] and Morgenroth et al [125] found no evidence of lymphocyte blast transformation when coeliac lymphocytes were cultured with gluten. Holmes et al [81], however, found positive responses in 29% of coeliacs on a normal diet, and 52% of those on a gluten-free diet (Fig. 30.14). They felt that this difference in results was because they had used a higher, more appropriate, concentration of gluten in their studies.

The evidence that cell-mediated immunity to gluten is occurring in the small intestinal mucosa has already been mentioned. The best direct evidence of this comes from the study by Ferguson et al [66] who showed that coeliac jejunal mucosa, cultured in vitro with gliadin produced lymphokine. The cell type involved was not identified, however, and surprisingly these studies have not been extended.

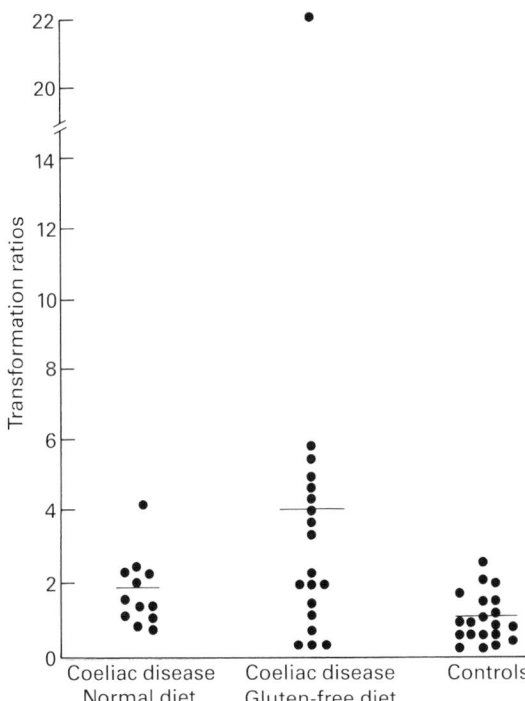

Fig. 30.14 Lymphocyte transformation ratios after 5 days of culture in 4 mg of gluten fraction III. From Holmes et al [81], with permission of Blackwell Scientific Publications Ltd.

GENETIC STUDIES
IN COELIAC DISEASE

It has been known for some time that coeliac disease is strongly associated with the histocompatibility antigens HLA-A1 and B8 [156]. The DR3 antigen, which is in linkage disequilibrium with A1 and B8 is found in an even higher proportion i.e. in 80% of coeliacs [97]. The allele DR7 is also increased [18], and if a patient possesses DR3 and DR7, the chances of having coeliac disease are even higher.

In addition to HLA-DR, two other loci, known as BR and DC, control alloantigenic specificities. The specific allele DC3 is in strong linkage disequilibrium with DR3 and DR7. In a study by Tosi et al [160], the DC3 allele was found in all 60 coeliac patients whilst Elliott et al [53] also found the DC3 allele in all the coeliac children they studied. This suggests that DC3 is the HLA specificity primarily associated with coeliac disease, and the association with DR3 and DR7 is because of their linkage disequilibrium with DC3.

These HLA antigens alone cannot, however, account for the susceptibility to coeliac disease as they are present in about 20% of the population, most of whom do not have the disease. Mann et al [116] described a gluten-sensitive enteropathy (GSE) B cell antigen in 75–80% of coeliacs (and 6–18% healthy controls). This B lymphocyte marker was found in 100% of parents of patients with coeliac disease. Coeliac disease occurred when a person was homozygous for this B cell antigen, and in addition possessed HLA-DR3 or one of its associated antigens. This GSE-associated B cell antigen is inherited separately and is distinct from the HLA antigens [134]. It is suggested that these two genes control coeliac disease, and act in cooperation to code for proteins which make up a single structure on the surface of the lymphoid cells.

PATHOGENESIS
OF COELIAC DISEASE

The exact mechanisms which forms the basis of hypersensitivity to gluten in coeliac disease is unknown. Three major concepts have been proposed (Table 30.5). The missing enzyme hypothesis is no longer tenable, for the reasons given previously.

Table 30.5 Major concepts of the aetiology of coeliac disease.

1	Missing enzyme hypothesis
2	Immune response to gluten
3	Lectin hypothesis

Immune response theory

Over the last two decades, most attention has been directed to the immune response theory. Tissue culture studies have shown that gluten activates an effector mechanism to cause mucosal damage in coeliac disease, and furthermore that the jejunal mucosa of patients with untreated coeliac disease produces humoral factors, or sensitized cells, which can mediate tissue damage [158]. Gluten has been demonstrated to bind to the epithelial cells [48] and immunocytes in the lamina propria [154] of coeliac mucosa. Furthermore, antibody to gluten is produced by the jejunal mucosa [32, 33, 58] and this antigluten antibody binds to epithelial cells [130].

Antibody, cells and HLA. These humoral factors work in cooperation with local cellular mechanisms, and the histocompatibility system is thought to play a central role in this. The HLA-B8 and DR3 antigens are associated with generalized immune hyperresponsiveness, in addition to an increase in the immune response to specific antigens. For instance, HLA-B8 positive healthy controls have a more marked immune response to wheat antigens than HLA-B8 negative subjects, as assessed in vitro by the lymphocyte transformation test [42]. A similar situation is seen with the leukocyte migration inhibition test, in which HLA-B8 positive control subjects showed a similar degree of reactivity to gluten as did patients with coeliac disease [152].

It is suggested that a specific immune response gene, linked to HLA-B8 and/or DR3 underlies the immune response to gluten seen in coeliac disease. More specifically, Falchuk [56] has suggested that in such patients who possess the HLA-B8/DR3 antigen and the GSE-associated B cell antigen, this codes for the production of cell-surface proteins on the enterocyte or intestinal lymphocyte which therefore act as receptors for gluten. When gluten binds to this cell-surface receptor, it becomes a target for the local immune responses (both humoral and cellular) with the production of antibodies and lymphokines resulting in tissue damage.

HLA-DC3. An alternative approach involves the HLA-DC3 antigen which is in strong linkage disequilibrium with B8, DR3 and DR7. The DC locus is thought to control the induction of T cell specific killing, and DC3 is presumably of prime importance in initiating cellular cytotoxicity. However DC3 is found in 30% of healthy subjects, and therefore in coeliac disease it is likely to be acting in cooperation with other effectors, such as the GSE-associated B cell antigen, or an immunoglobulin heavy chain marker.

The lectin hypothesis

It was first suggested by Weiser and Douglas [173] that gluten is acting as a toxic lectin in coeliac disease. This idea has been further assessed and extended in the last few years. Lectins are molecules that bind with high affinity to specific carbohydrate receptors. They are naturally occurring proteins and glycoproteins, which agglutinate erythrocytes and certain other cells. When plant lectins bind to exposed, reactive sites on the cell surface, they cause changes resulting in cell death (see Chapter 21).

The gluten fraction, Glyc-Gli, had been shown by Douglas [48] to bind to a crude membrane fraction of coeliac intestinal mucosa. Weiser and Douglas [173] suggested that in coeliac disease there is an increase in incomplete glycoproteins on the small intestinal cell-surface membrane, and that gluten (or one of its subfractions) could bind to these altered, exposed glycoproteins. The gluten would act as a toxic lectin, altering cell function, resulting in earlier death and increased cell turnover.

Animal studies. Animal studies add some support to this hypothesis. Thus it has been demonstrated that wheat germ lectin causes enterocyte damage with villus atrophy and crypt hyperplasia [108]. Kottgen et al [98] confirmed that gluten has lectin-like properties and also showed that glycoproteins from immature small intestinal crypt cells are more reactive than those from the mature villus zone. They suggested that in coeliac disease there is a genetically determined deficiency of the growth-dependent *N*-acetylglucosaminyl transferase I, leading to the presence of a high proportion of oligomannosyl glycoproteins in the brush border membrane to which gluten binds.

Also of importance in this respect is the fact that once lectins are bound to a cell, they can alter its antigenic composition. Furthermore, once bound these lectins could interfere directly with the immune response mounted against them; they particularly interfere with suppressor T lymphocytes [29].

This lectin hypothesis is compatible with both the enzyme deficiency theory, and the immune response in coeliac disease, and could act as a central unifying concept. Future developments are awaited with great interest.

NON-RESPONSIVE COELIAC DISEASE

Despite the fact that hypersensitivity to gluten is the hallmark of coeliac disease, and that a response to gluten withdrawal is a sine qua non for the diagnosis, a proportion of patients with jejunal villus atrophy either do not respond to a gluten-free diet or show only a partial response. There are a number of other causes of jejunal villus atrophy, as shown in Table 30.6, but, nonetheless, when these have been excluded, up to 10% of patients with coeliac disease show a suboptimal response to dietary treatment [135]. This condition has been given a number of names, including un-

Table 30.6 Causes of jejunal villus atrophy.

1	Coeliac disease
2	Postinfective malabsorption
3	Tropical sprue
4	Stasis syndrome
5	Milk protein enteropathy
6	Kwashiorkor
7	Intestinal lymphoma
8	Gastric surgery
9	Crohn's disease
10	Soya protein enteropathy
11	Fish, rice and chicken enteropathy
12	Radiation enteritis
13	Hypogammaglobulinaemia
14	Giardiasis
15	Zollinger–Ellison syndrome
16	Ulcerative colitis

responsive or non-responsive coeliac disease, collagenous sprue, unclassified sprue, ulcerative jejunitis, fatal malabsorption syndrome and refractory sprue.

Proportion of non-responders

The number of patients affected varies in different series (Table 30.7). French et al [72]

Table 30.7 The incidence of non-responsive coeliac disease.

Author(s)	Number of cases	Percentage with non-responsive coeliac disease
French and Hawkins [72]	6/26	23
Shiner [149]	4/17	23
Benson et al [16]	1/32	3
Pink and Creamer [138]	16/54	30
Douglas [47]	5/21	24
Holmes et al [83]	17/134	13
Mike and Asquith [122]	12/84	14
Total	61/368	17

treated 22 patients with malabsorption with a gluten-free diet. Six patients did not respond, of whom four died from complications of their illness. Shiner [149] in a study of biopsy-proven jejunal villus atrophy found four of 17 patients unresponsive, one of whom died. Benson et al [16], however, found only one of 32 patients unaffected by the gluten-free diet. In a large series, Pink and Creamer [138] studied 54 patients with coeliac disease in great detail. Sixteen did not respond to a gluten-free diet and these non-responders were further categorized into three groups. Firstly, patients with extensive, severe small intestinal lesions, with diminished mucosal thickness, crypt hypoplasia and epithelial dysplasia. These patients all had a deficiency of paneth cells.

Radiological studies showed a tubular appearance of the small intestine (moulage sign). This group of patients improved with steroids and dietary supplements. The second group had associated pancreatic hypofunction with no improvement on a gluten-free diet, steroids or pancreatic supplements. The third group showed some benefit from gluten withdrawal with improvement in their biopsy appearance, but they remained highly symptomatic.

Douglas [47] described unresponsive patients who continued to have malabsorption and abnormal jejunal histology. They were maintained in moderate health by enteral nutrition, medium chain triglycerides and corticosteroids. Finally in a large series from Birmingham [81, 83] a poor response was found in 13% of patients.

Causes of non-responsive coeliac disease

A number of factors have been suggested to account for this poor response to a gluten-free diet (Table 30.8). The most common explan-

Table 30.8 Causes of non-responsive coeliac disease.

1	Continued ingestion of gluten
2	Paneth cell deficiency
3	Intestinal lymphoma
4	Vasculitis
5	Subepithelial collagen deposition
6	Zinc deficiency
7	Pancreatic hypofunction
8	Hypersensitivity to foods other than gluten

ation is that the patient is not keeping to a strict diet, and is still ingesting gluten either accidentally or deliberately. If there is any question of this, then the detection of antibodies to gliadin by an ELISA technique should be very helpful [131]. Nevertheless, a significant proportion of patients are found to be keeping to their diets strictly, and other causes must be sought (Tables 30.6 and 30.8).

Paneth cell deficiency is commonly found but is nowadays considered to be an effect, rather than a cause of poor responsiveness [41, 170]. If the patient has developed an intestinal lymphoma, the jejunal villus atrophy often does not respond to gluten withdrawal. Vasculitis is a rare cause [22] and may require treatment with steroids. In some patients the response to a gluten-free diet is delayed because of a slowly reversible intestinal change due to subepithelial collagen deposition [25], or to an associated zinc deficiency [109]. Coexistent pancreatic hypofunction is found in some patients with coeliac disease [41] and requires treatment with pancreatic supplements.

Finally, hypersensitivity to foods other than gluten can cause jejunal villus atrophy. In this respect milk protein [171], soya protein [1], fish, rice and chicken [166] have all been implicated in individual cases (Table 30.9).

Table 30.9 Foods causing jejunal villus atrophy.

Gluten
Milk
Soya protein
Fish
Rice
Chicken

Epithelial turnover

Patients who do not respond to gluten restriction have decreased epithelial turnover [14]. In a number of studies, Jones and Peters [86, 87] have shown that non-responsive coeliacs have a lower rate of DNA synthesis than untreated coeliacs suggesting crypt hypoplasia. Endoplasmic reticulum activity, the activity of mitchondrial enzymes, and lysosomal activity, are all reduced in this group. In consequence mucosal protein synthesis is also reduced in such non-responsive coeliacs.

Soya protein hypersensitivity

Studies from Birmingham (UK) indicate that coexistent hypersensitivity to soya protein may be the cause of a poor response to a gluten-free diet alone in a significant number of

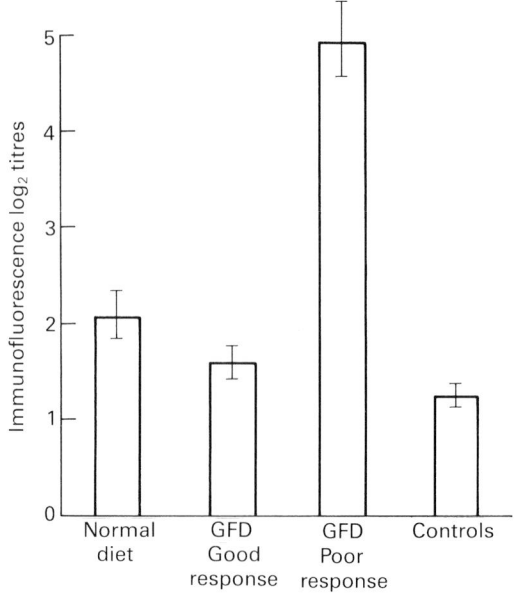

Fig. 30.15 Immunofluorescent antibodies to soya protein (group mean ± SEM) in healthy controls and patients with coeliac disease.

patients with coeliac disease. Of 84 adult patients with coeliac disease, 12 were identified who showed a suboptimal response to gluten withdrawal [122]. These patients remained symptomatic and had persisting malabsorption after 2 years or more on a gluten-free diet. They were found to have significant levels of antibody to soya protein, when compared with patients with other gastrointestinal diseases, or healthy controls (Fig. 30.15) [76]. The non-responsive coeliacs also had evidence of cell-mediated immunity to soya protein [124] as

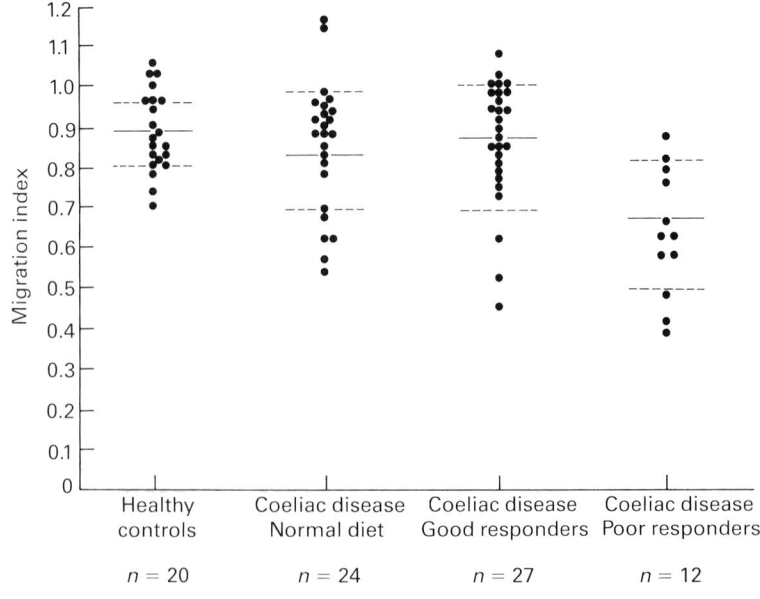

30.16 Leukocyte migration inhibition in patients with coeliac disease and controls in the presence of soya protein.

assessed by the leukocyte migration inhibition test (Fig. 30.16). Nine of the 10 patients who were placed on a diet excluding soya and gluten protein improved significantly, with normal haematological and biochemical parameters and no evidence of malabsorption. Jejunal histology, which had been significantly abnormal, now improved to a state in which it was indistinguishable from that in patients who had shown a good response to gluten withdrawal.

Soya protein is ubiquitous in the Western diet, but is particularly found in the diet of coeliac patients, as it is commonly used as a substitute for gluten in gluten-free products. In our experience, it appears that 10–15% of coeliacs have a coexistent immunological hypersensitivity to soya protein which impairs response to the gluten withdrawal. It seems likely that the soya is acting as a toxic lectin in these patients.

Transient gluten intolerance

Transient gluten intolerance is an uncommon condition of childhood, in which children with gastrointestinal symptoms have an abnormal jejunal biopsy. This responds to gluten withdrawal, but the child is subsequently able to tolerate a normal gluten-containing diet without relapsing [167] after at least 2 years.

The condition may be found in children who are also intolerant of other foods, such as milk and eggs, or following gastroenteritis. The pathogenesis of the condition is unknown, though it may be due to a temporary peptidase deficiency consequent on mucosal damage (e.g. in gastroenteritis), or it could represent a transient state of immunological hypersensitivity. The diagnosis rests on finding a normal jejunal biopsy after 2 years on a normal gluten-containing diet, partial or subtotal villus atrophy having previously been present in association with the initial illness. In a long-term follow-up study, Walker-Smith et al [168] found that 10 of 11 children with this diagnosis remained well, one having relapsed after 7 years on a normal diet (and therefore having coeliac disease). Further follow-up is in progress to see if any of the other 10 will relapse. It is noteworthy that this condition, which was not uncommon in the 1970s, is now rare. This may be because of the recent change in infant feeding practices, such that gluten is now introduced into the diet at a much later stage when the intestine is no longer so functionally immature.

GLUTEN AND ATOPIC DISEASE

The role of immediate hypersensitivity Type I reactions in the pathogenesis of coeliac disease remains a contentious subject, and there is as yet only limited information available. It is felt by some that immediate hypersensitivity to gluten increases intestinal permeability, making the gut more 'leaky' and thereby predisposing to the other, better characterized Type III and IV responses in the mucosa.

Gliadin shock

On the other hand, a number of reports over the years have confirmed the association between coeliac disease and atopic disease. One of the most striking manifestations is the development of 'gliadin shock' [100]. This is occasionally seen in children on a gluten-free diet, who after ingesting small quantities of gluten, rapidly develop anaphylaxis. This suggests an immediate hypersensitivity response, though the presence of specific IgE antibodies to gliadin in these children has not yet been demonstrated.

Asthma and eczema

An association between coeliac disease and asthma, eczema and urticaria has been well established over the last 20 years. Thus, Friedman and Hare [73] found an increased incidence of atopic eczema in patients with coeliac disease, and in some this could be ameliorated or cured by gluten withdrawal. Hodgson et al [80] found a significantly increased incidence of atopic disease in patients with coeliac disease (29%) compared with controls (5%). There was also a stronger family history of atopy in the coeliac population (51% versus 22%). In a much larger study of 314 adults with coeliac disease, Cooper et al [37] found the incidence of asthma and eczema to be only 7%. Of their 22 atopic patients, two showed dramatic improvements in their skin disease on gluten withdrawal. In contrast, Rossipal [141] found a very high incidence of allergic disease (43.6%) in a population of coeliac children, though it is noteworthy that he found allergic disease in 35% of the controls. There was a higher incidence of atopic disease in the siblings and parents of coeliac children than in their healthy counterparts. Finally Williams et al [174] in a study of 76 adult patients with coeliac disease, found 20% with asthma, compared with 5% in controls. Positive skin prick tests to foods and environmental allergens were more common in coeliac patients than controls (45% versus 27%).

Total and specific IgE

Total IgE concentrations were similar in coeliacs to controls [174]. Bahna et al [11] also found normal levels of total IgE in coeliac patients and more significantly they did not find specific IgE antibodies to wheat in coeliacs. Likewise, in the skin test studies coeliac patients did not show immediate hypersensitivity reactions to gluten subfractions [12]. Interestingly, Bahna et al [11] found normal levels of total IgD in coeliac disease, but significantly increased levels of specific IgD antibodies to wheat. The significance of this finding remains to be determined.

The mechanism of the increased incidence of atopy

The mechanism underlying the increased incidence of atopy in coeliac disease is unclear. Hodgson et al [80] suggest that it may be due to the abnormally leaky gut allowing entry of various antigens but this would not account for the high frequency of atopy in first degree relatives of coeliacs however. Alternatively, they postulate that abnormal IgA responses may be important; atopy is associated with selective IgA deficiency, which in turn is not uncommon in coeliac disease. Furthermore, in mucosal IgA deficiency, there is a compensatory increase in local IgE production and both of these may predispose to atopy.

The other possible explanation lies in the genetic link through HLA genes [37,80]. HLA-B8 is found in over 80% of coeliacs. This is also associated with asthma to some degree, and also with a generalized hyperimmune responsiveness, and could underlie the increase in atopy.

NON-COELIAC GLUTEN SENSITIVITY

This is a condition in which the person is sensitive to gluten, but does not have coeliac disease or wheat allergy. The syndrome in infants and young children consists of diarrhoea and vomiting after ingestion of food. Occasionally there is an enterocolitis with blood and mucus

in the stool [126]. Symptoms also occur outside the gastrointestinal tract, such as bronchitis, rhinitis and skin rashes. It should be stressed a normal jejunal biopsy is found in these children (unlike in transient gluten intolerance).

The condition has also been described in adults [38,54]. These patients suffered with abdominal pain, vomiting and diarrhoea, and recurrent mouth ulcers and headaches were common. Jejunal biopsy was normal or showed a mild increase in cellularity only. There was no evidence of malabsorption or immunological abnormality, such as is found in coeliac disease. Nonetheless, the patients improved on a gluten-free diet, and relapsed when re-exposed to gluten.

These patients do not satisfy the diagnostic criteria for coeliac disease, and nor do they have a 'patchy' lesion, as multiple biopsies from the same patient have all been normal. From our own studies [123] these patients do not have an allergy to wheat, nor does the illness appear to be psychological in nature. Whether the condition could be due to a peptidase deficiency, or a lectin effect from gluten, is presently being investigated.

Effect of gluten-free diet on oral ulceration

The association between coeliac disease and mouth ulcers is well recognized, with the incidence of coeliac disease in patients with recurrent oral aphthae probably being about 2–4% [15,103] though 24% was reported in one study [67]. Conversely, Wray [176] has shown that patients with recurrent oral aphthae who do not have coeliac disease may improve on a gluten-free diet. Twenty patients with recurrent aphthous stomatitis were studied, all of whom had a normal jejunal biopsy, and no symptoms of malabsorption. Five of the 20 patients had complete remission for prolonged periods of time on gluten withdrawal with relapse on reintroduction of dietrary gluten. Wray suggested that the basis for the oral ulceration was that sensitized basophils in the oral mucosa release histamine on exposure to gluten. This was a highly selected series of patients. In our own studies on unselected patients with recurrent mouth ulcers, we see the condition much less commonly, but nonetheless the response to a gluten-free diet can be dramatic. Whether the ulceration is due to a direct toxic effect of gluten on the buccal mucosa, or whether gluten is absorbed from the intestinal tract, and the damage results from circulating immune complexes, is one of the problems currently being tackled.

Behçet's disease

In preliminary results on patients with Behçet's disease, we have identified three out of 15 patients who have improved dramatically on a gluten-free diet in whom coeliac disease was excluded. Following the diet, it has been possible to discontinue steroids and immune suppressants, with no relapses on follow-up from 2 to 5 years. The mechanism in these patients is completely unknown, and, in particular, none possessed the HLA-B8, DR3 antigens.

Toxic effects of gluten in healthy subjects

It is assumed that in otherwise healthy people, the ingestion of gluten will have no adverse consequences, and this was confirmed by a study by Levine et al [105] who could find no deleterious effect in jejunal histology following prolonged gluten administration. However, Docherty and Barry [46] found that, after gluten challenge some first degree relatives of coeliac patients and also patients with 'immune deficiency' syndromes developed jejunal villus atrophy. In the careful histological study by Bramble et al [27] there was no detectable change in jejunal morphometry or brush border enzymes after gluten challenge in healthy controls.

Absorption of ingested carbohydrate

It is thought that ingested carbohydrate is completely absorbed in the small intestine. In a very interesting study by Anderson et al [3], 18 healthy subjects ingested test meals containing white wheat, macaroni, low gluten bread and rice bread. Breath hydrogen was measured to assess the absorption of carbohydrate. In this study 17 of the 18 subjects, after ingesting 100 g of wheat starch in the form of macaroni or bread made from all-purpose white flour, had increases in breath

hydrogen, indicative of incomplete absorption. In contrast, sucrose, low gluten wheat flour and rice flour were completely absorbed. The all-purpose wheat flour was composed of a protein–starch complex, in which 85% of the protein was gluten. The low gluten and rice (no gluten) flours were completely absorbed, suggesting that gluten caused the malabsorption of wheat starch.

Malabsorption of wheat flour. Malabsorption of wheat flour, in this context, could cause flatulence, abdominal distension and diarrhoea, as occurs in the irritable bowel syndrome. In this respect Long and O'Donoghue [107], using a similar technique, confirmed that starch is incompletely absorbed in normal subjects. Destruction of the amylase inhibitor in starch did not improve absorption. In this study elimination of gluten from the wheat did not improve carbohydrate absorption.

These two studies indicate that gluten, or wheat, can cause symptoms in otherwise healthy people, which mimic the irritable bowel syndrome. In this respect, Pock-Steen [139] found significant improvement in patients with colicky abdominal pain and diarrhoea on a gluten-free diet. Unfortunately these patients had minor villus abnormalities and a low-grade malabsorption, and therefore may have had patchy coeliac disease. However, there is no doubt that the occasional patient with irritable bowel syndrome does improve on a gluten-free diet, and formal trials are now in progress to assess this objectively (see Chapter 32). Despite these findings the great majority of people can, and do, ingest gluten without any symptoms.

Acknowledgments

We are very grateful to the following for their assistance: Dr Salli Muller for the photographs and illustrations of the jejunal mucosa; Dr Jaime Ferrando for the radiological studies; Dr Mansel Heaney and Dr Michael Marsh for permission to reproduce the photomicrograph illustrating mitotic indices; Dr R. Thompson for the photographs of reticulin antibodies; and to Miss Helen Sanders and Miss Gillian McDonald for typing the manuscript.

REFERENCES

1 Ament ME, Rubin CE: Soya protein: another cause of the flat intestinal lesion. Gastroenterology 1972; 62:227–34.

2 Anand BS, Truelove SC, Offord RE: Skin test for coeliac disease using a subfraction of gluten. Lancet 1977; i:118–20.

3 Anderson IH, Levine AS, Levitt MD: Incomplete absorption of the carbohydrate in all purpose wheat flour. N Eng J Med 1981; 304:891–2.

4 Ansaldi N, De Sanctis C, Fabris C, Ponzone A: Blastiz-zone linfocitaria in-vitro con fitoemoglutinina E con glutine in bambina effeti da morbo celiaco. Minerva Pediatr 1970; 22:1907.

5 Arnaud-Battandier F, Bundy NB, O'Neill M et al:

Cytotoxic activities of gut mucosal lymphoid cells in guinea pigs. J Immunol 1978; 121:1059.

6 Ashkenazi A, Idar D, Barzitai N et al: Effect of gluten free diet on an immunological assay for coeliac disease. Lancet 1981; 914–6.

7 Asquith P: Immunology of coeliac disease. Clin Gastroenterol 1974; 3:213–34.

8 Asquith P, Houseley J, Cooke WT: Serum and intestinal immunoglobulins in adult coeliac disease. In: Booth CC, Dowling RH, eds. Coeliac disease. Edinburgh: Churchill Livingstone, 1970; 151:61.

9 Asquith P, Thompson RA, Cooke WT: Serum immunoglobulins in adult coeliac disease. Lancet 1969; ii:129–31.

10 Auricchio S, De Ritis G, De Vincenzi M et al: Effects of gliadin derived peptides from bread and durum wheats on small intestine cultures from rat foetus and coeliac children. Pediatr Res 1982; 16:1004–10.

11 Bahna SL, Tateno K, Heiner DC: Elevated IgD antibodies to wheat in coeliac disease. Ann Allergy 1980; 44:146–151.

12 Baker PG, Read AE: Positive skin reactions to gluten in coeliac disease. Q J Med 1976; 45:603–10.

13 Baklien K, Brandtzaeg P, Fausa O: Immunoglobulins in jejunal mucosa and serum from patients with adult coeliac disease. Scand J Gastroenterol 1977; 12:149–59.

14 Barry RE, Read AE: Coeliac disease and malignancy. Q J Med 1973; 42:665–75.

15 Bateman R, Potts J, Frame J et al: Clinical features in unselected patients with recurrent aphthous oral ulceration. Clin Sci 1981; 63:23.

16 Benson GD, Kowlessar OD, Sleisenger MH: Adult coeliac disease with emphasis on response to the gluten free diet. Medicine 1964; 43:1–40.

17 Bernardin JE, Saunders RM, Kasarda DD: Absence of carbohydrate in coeliac-toxic A-gliadin. Cereal Chem 1976; 56:612.

18 Betuel H, Gebuhrer L, Descos L et al: Adult coeliac disease associated with HLA-DRW3 and -DRW7. Tissue Antigens 1980; 15:231–8.

19 Bjarnason I, Peters TJ: In-vitro determination of small intestinal permeability: a demonstration of persistent defect in patients with coeliac disease. Gut 1984; 25:145–50.

20 Bjarnason I, Peters TJ, Neall N: A persistent defect in intestinal permeability in coeliac disease demonstrated by a ^{51}Cr-labelled EDTA adsorption test. Lancet 1983; 323–5.

21 Bjarnason I, Marsh MN, Price A et al: Intestinal permeability in patients with coeliac disease and dermatitis herpetiformis. Gut 1985; 26:1214–9.

22 Booth CC: Definition of adult coeliac disease. In: Hekkens WTJM, Pena AS, eds. Coeliac disease. Leiden: Stenfert-Kroese, 1974; 17–22.

23 Booth CC: Proc Second Int Coeliac Symp. Hekkens WTJM, Pena AS, eds. Leiden: Stenfert-Kroese, 1974; 18.

24 Booth CC, Peters TJ, Doe WF: Immunopathology of coeliac disease. In: Immunology of the gut. CIBA Found Symp. North-Holland, Amsterdam: Elsevier Excerpta Medica, 1977; 46:329–41.

25 Bossart R, Henry K, Booth CC, Doe WF: Collagenous basement membrane thickening in jejunal biopsies from patients with adult coeliac disease. Gut 1975; 15:338.

26 Bova JG, Friedman AC, Weser E et al: Adaptation of the ileum in non-tropical sprue: reversal of the jejuno-ileal fold pattern. Am J Radiol 1985; 144: 299–302.

27 Bramble MG, Zucoloto S, Wright NA, Record CO: Acute gluten challenge in treated adult coeliac disease: a morphometric and enzymatic study. Gut 1985; 26:169–74.

28 Brandtzaeg P, Baklien K: Immunohistochemical studies of the formation of epithelial transport of immunoglobulins in normal and diseased human intestinal mucosa. Scand J Gastroenterol 1976; 11:36.

29 Brauer R, Henzgen S, Thoss K, Waldmann G: Biphasic changes of the immunological reactivity in the course of experimental lectin induced arthritis of rabbits. Exp pathol 1983; 24:117–31.

30 Bullen AW, Losowsky MS: Cell mediated immunity to gluten fraction III in adult coeliac disease. Gut 1978; 19:126–31.

31 Bullen AW, Hall R, Gowland G et al: Hyposplenism, adult coeliac disease and autoimmunity. Gut 1981; 22: 28–33.

32 Ciclitira PJ, Ellis HJ, Fagg NLK: Evaluation of a gluten free product containing wheat gliadin in patients with coeliac disease. Br Med J 1984; 289:83.

33 Ciclitira PJ, Evans DJ, Fagg NLK et al: Clinical testing of gliadin fractions in coeliac patients. Clin Sci 1984; 66:357–64.

34 Cluysenaer OJJ, Van Tongeren JHM: Morphology of the small intestine under normal conditions and in coeliac sprue. In: Malabsorption in coeliac sprue. The Hague: Martinus Nijhoff, 1977; 18–29.

35 Cooke WT: The effect of corticotrophin in idiopathic steatorrhoa. Lancet 1953; ii: 425–8.

36 Cooke WT, Holmes GKT: Coeliac disease. London: Churchill Livingstone, 1984; 81–105.

37 Cooper BT, Holmes GKT, Cooke WT: Coeliac disease and immunological disorders. Br Med J 1978; 1:537–9.

38 Cooper BT, Holmes GKT, Ferguson R et al: Gluten sensitive diarrhoea without evidence of coeliac disease. Gastroenterology 1980; 79:801–6.

39 Cornell HJ: Gliadin degradation and fractionation. In: Hekkens WTJM, Pena AS, eds. Coeliac disease. Leiden: Stenfert-Kroese, 1974; 74–5.

40 Cornell HJ, Rolles CJ: Further evidence of a primary mucosal defect in coeliac disease. In-vitro mucosal digestion studies in coeliac patients in remission, their relatives and control subjects. Gut 1978; 19:253–9.

41 Creamer B, Pink IJ: Paneth cell deficiency. Lancet 1967; i: 304–6.

42 Cunningham-Rundles S, Cunningham-Rundles C et al: Response to wheat antigen in in-vitro lymphocyte transformation among HLA-B8 positive normal donors. Transplantation Proc 1978; 10:977.

43 Dicke WK, Weijers HA, Van De Kamer JH: The presence in wheat of a factor having a deleterious effect in cases of coeliac disease. Acta Paediatr 1953; 42:34–42.

44 Dissanayake AS, Jerrome DW, Offord RE et al: Identifying toxic fractions of wheat gluten and their effect on the jejunal mucosa in coeliac disease. Gut 1974; 15:931–46.

45 Doe WF, Evans D, Hobbs JR, Booth CC: Coeliac disease, vasculitis and cryoglobulinaemia. Gut 1972; 13:112–3.

46 Doherty M, Barry RE: Gluten induced mucosal changes in subjects without overt small bowel disease. Lancet 1981; i:517–20.

47 Douglas AP: Long term prognosis and relation to diet. In: Hekkens WTJM, Pena AS, eds. Coeliac disease. Leiden: Stenfert-Kroese, 1974; 399–405.

48 Douglas AP: The binding of a glycopeptide compo-

nent of wheat gluten to intestinal mucosa of normal and coeliac human subjects. Clin Chim Acta 1976; 73:357–61.

49 Douglas AP, Peters TJ, Hoffrand AV, Booth CC: Studies of intestinal peptidases with special reference to coeliac disease. In: Booth CC, Dowling RH, eds. Coeliac disease. Edinburgh: Churchill Livingstone, 1970; 115–22.

50 Douwes FR: Gluten and lymphocyte sensitisation in coeliac disease. Lancet 1976; ii:1353.

51 Eade OE, Lloyd RS, Lang C, Wright R: IgA and IgG reticulin antibodies in coeliac disease and non-coeliac patients. Gut 18 1977; 991–3.

52 Egan-Mitchell B, Fottrell PF, McNicholl B: Prolonged gluten tolerance in treated coeliac disease. In: McNicholl B, Fottrell PF, McCarthy CF, eds. Perspectives in coeliac disease. Lancaster: MTP Press 1978; 251–7.

53 Elliott EJ, Sachs JA, Awad J et al: Histocompatibility antigens and clinical features in coeliac disease. Gut 1984; 25:10,F58.

54 Ellis A, Linaker BD: Non-coeliac gluten sensitivity. Lancet 1978; i:1358–9.

55 Ewart JAD: SDS—Electrophoresis of wheat gliadins. J Sci Food Agric 1973; 24:685.

56 Falchuk ZM: Gluten sensitive enteropathy. In: Sleisenger MH, ed. Malabsorption and nutritional support. London: WB Saunders, 1983; 475–94.

57 Falchuk ZM, Katz AJ: Organ culture model of gluten sensitive enteropathy. In: McNicholl B, McCarthy CF, Fottrell PF, eds. Perspectives in coeliac disease. Lancaster: MTP Press, 1978; 65–72.

58 Falchuk ZM, Strober W: Gluten sensitive enteropathy: synthesis of antigliadin antibody in-vitro. Gut 1974; 15:947.

59 Falchuk ZM, Gebhard RL, Strober W: The pathogenesis of gluten sensitive enteropathy (coeliac sprue): organ culture studies. In: Hekkens WTJM, Pena AS, eds. Coeliac disease. Leiden: Stenfert-Kroese, 1974; 107–17.

60 Falchuk ZM, Gebhard RL, Sessoms C, Strober W: An in-vitro model of gluten sensitive enteropathy. Effect of gliadin on intestinal epithelial cells of patients with gluten sensitive enteropathy in organ culture. J Clin Invest 1974; 53:487–500.

61 Ferguson A: Lymphocytes in coeliac disease. In: Hekkens WTJM, Pena AS, eds. Coeliac disease. Leiden: Stenfert-Kroese, 1974; 265–76.

62 Ferguson A, Caswell F: Precipitins to dietary proteins in serum and upper intestinal secretions of coeliac children. Br Med J 1972; 1:75–7.

63 Ferguson A, Jarrett EEE: Hypersensitivity reactions in the small intestine. I. Thymus dependence of experimental partial villous atrophy. Gut 1965; 16:114–7.

64 Ferguson A, Murray D: Quantitation of intraepithelial lymphocytes in human jejunum. Gut 1971 12:988–94.

65 Ferguson A, Parrott DMV: The effect of antigen deprivation on thymus dependent and thymus independent lymphocytes in the small intestine of the mouse. Clin Exp Immunol 1972; 12:477.

66 Ferguson A, McClure JP, MacDonald TT, Holden RJ: Cell mediated immunity to gliadin within the small intestinal mucosa in coeliac disease. Lancet 1975; i:895–7.

67 Ferguson R, Basu MK, Asquith P, Cooke WT: Jejunal mucosal abnormalities in patients with recurrent aphthous ulceration. Br Med J 1976; i:11–13.

68 Flores AF, Winter HS, Bhan AK: In-vitro model to assess immunoregulatory T lymphocyte sub-populations in gluten sensitive enteropathy. Gastroenterology 1982; 82:1058.

69 Fottrell PF, Dolly JO, Dillon A et al: Multiple forms of peptidases in intestinal mucosa of children with coeliac disease. In: Booth CC, Dowling RH, eds. Coeliac disease. Edinburgh: Churchill Livingstone, 1970; 124–33.

70 Frazer AC: Discussion on some problems of steatorrhoea and reduced stature. Proc R Soc Med 1956; 49:1009–13.

71 Frazer AC, Fletcher RF, Ross CAC et al: Gluten induced enteropathy: the effect of partially digested gluten. Lancet 1959; ii:252–5.

72 French JM, Hawkins CF: The gluten free diet in 1957; idiopathic steatorrhoea. Med Clin North Am 1957; 41:1585–96.

73 Friedman M, Hare PF: Gluten sensitive enteropathy and eczema. Lancet 1965; i:521–4.

74 Fry L, Seah PP, Harper PG et al: The small intestine in dermatitis herpetiformis. Clin Pathol 1974; 27:817–24.

75 Haeney MR, Asquith P: Inhibition of leucocyte migration by alpha gliadin in patients with gastrointestinal disease: its specificity with respect to coeliac disease and alpha gliadin. In: McNicholl B, McCarthy CF, Fottrell PF, eds. Perspectives in coeliac disease. Lancaster: MTP Press, 1978; 229.

76 Haeney MR, Goodwin BJF, Barratt MEJ et al: Soya protein antibodies in man: their occurrence and possible relevance in coeliac disease. J Clin Pathol 1982; 35:319–22.

77 Hamilton J, Cobden I, Rothwell J, Axon ATR: Intestinal permeability in coeliac disease. The response to gluten withdrawal and single-dose gluten challenge. Gut 1982; 23:202–10.

78 Hauri HP, Kedinger M, Haffen K et al: Re-evaluation of the technique of organ culture for studying gluten toxicity in coeliac disease. Gut 1978; 19:1090–8.

79 Hobbs JR, Hepner GW: Deficiency of γM globulin in coeliac disease. Lancet 1968; i:217–20.

80 Hodgson HJF, Davies RJ, Gent AE, Hodson ME: Atopic disorders and adult coeliac disease. Lancet 1976; i:115–7.

81 Holmes GKT, Asquith P, Cooke WT: Cell mediated immunity to gluten fraction III in adult coeliac disease. Clin Exp Immunol 1976; 24:259–65.

82 Holmes GKT, Asquith P, Stokes PL, Cooke WT: Cellular infiltrate of jejunal biopsies in adult coeliac disease in relation to gluten withdrawal. Gut 1974; 15:278–83.

83 Holmes GKT, Stokes PL, Sorahan TM et al: Coeliac disease, gluten free diet and malignancy. Gut 1976; 17:612–9.

84 Howdle PD, Ciclitira PJ, Simpson FG, Losowssky MS: Are all gliadins toxic in coeliac diseae? Gut 1981; 22:A874.

85 Howdle PD, Corazza GR, Bullen AW, Losowsky MS: Gluten sensitivity of small intestinal mucosa in-vitro. Quantitative assessment of histologic change. Gastroenterology 1981; 80:442–50.

86 Jones PE, Peters TJ: DNA synthesis by jejunal mucosa in responsive and non-responsive coeliac disease. Br Med J 1977; 1:1130–1.

87 Jones PE, Peters TJ: Oral zinc supplements in non-responsive coeliac syndrome: effect on jejunal morphology, enterocyte production and brush border disaccharidase activities. Gut 1981; 22:194–8.

88 Jones PE, L'Hirondel CL, Peters TJ: Protein

synthesis by cultured jejunal mucosa from control subjects and patients with coeliac disease. Gut 1981; 22:623–7.

89 Jos J, Lenoir G, De Ritis G, Rey J: In-vitro culturing of biopsies from children. In: Hekkens WTJM, Pena AS, eds. Coeliac disease. Leiden: Stenfert-Kroese 1974; 91–105.

90 Kasarda DD, Nimmo CC, Bernadin JE: Structural aspects and genetic relationships of gliadins. In: Hekkens WTJM, Pena AS, eds. Coeliac disease. Leiden: Stenfert-Kroese, 1974; 25–36.

91 Kasarda DD, Nimmo CC, Kohlerg O: Proteins and the amino acid composition of wheat fractions. Wheat Chem Technol AACA 1971; 227.

92 Katz AJ, Falchuk ZM: Definitive diagnosis of gluten sensitive enteropathy. Use of an in-vitro organ culutre model. Gastroenterology 1978; 75:695–700.

93 Katz AJ, Falchuk ZM, Strober W, Shwachman H: Gluten sensitive enteropathy. Inhibition by cortisol of the effect of gluten protein in-vitro. N Engl J Med 1976; 295:131–5.

94 Keiffer M, Frazier PJ, Daniels NWR, Coombs RRA: Wheat gliadin fractions and other cereal antigens reactive with antibodies in the sera of coeliac patients. Clin Immunol 1982; 50:651–60.

95 Kendall MJ, Cox PS, Schneider R, Hawkins CF: Gluten subfractions in coeliac disease. Lancet 1972; ii: 1065–7.

96 Kendrick KG, Walker-Smith JA: Immunoglobulins and dietary protein antibodies in childhood coeliac disease. Gut 1970; 11:635–40.

97 Keuning JJ, Pena AS, Van Leeuwen A et al: HLA-DW3 associated with coeliac disease. Lancet 1976; i: 506–8.

98 Kottgen E, Volk B, Kluge F, Gerok W: Gluten, a lectin with oligomannosyl specificity and the causative agent of gluten sensitive enteropathy. Biochem Biophys Res Commun 1982; 109:168–73.

99 Krainick HG, Mohn G, Fischer HH: Further studies on the harmful effects of wheat flour in coeliacs. II. The action of the enzymatic breakdown products of gliadin. Helv Paediatr Acta 1959; 14:124–40.

100 Krainick HG, Debatin F, Gauter E et al: Additional research on the injurious effect of wheat flour in coeliac disease. I. Acute gliadin reaction—gliadin shock. Helv Paediatr Acta 1958; 13:432–54.

101 Lancaster-Smith M, Kumar PJ, Clark ML: Immunological phenomena following gluten challenge in the jejunum of patients with adult coeliac disease and dermatitis herpetiformis. In: Hekkens WTJM, Pena AS, eds. Coeliac disease. Leiden: Stenfert-Kroese, 1974; 173–4.

102 Lancaster-Smith M, Kumar PJ, Dawson AM: The cellular infiltrate of the jejunum in adult coeliac disease, and dermatitis herpetiformis following the reintroduction of dietary gluten. Gut 1975; 16:683–8.

103 Lehner T: Oral ulceration and Behçets syndrome. Gut 1977; 8:491–511.

104 Leonard J, Haffenden G, Tucker W et al: Gluten challenge in dermatitis herpetiformis. N Engl J Med 1983; 816–19.

105 Levine RA, Briggs GW, Harding RS, Nolte LB: Prolonged gluten administration in normal subjects. N Engl J Med 1966; 274:1109–14.

106 Loeb PM, Strober W, Falchuk ZM et al: Incorporation of Leucine-14C into immunoglobulins by jejunal biopsies of the patients with coeliac sprue and other gastrointestinal diseases. J Clin Invest 1971; 50:559.

107 Long A, O'Donoghue D: Incomplete absorption of carbohydrate in normal subjects. Presented to Midlands Gastroenterological Society, June 1984.

108 Lorenzsonn V, Olsen WA: In-vivo responses of rat intestinal epithelium to intraluminal dietry lectins. Gastroenterology 1982; 82:838–48.

109 Love AHG, Elmes M, Golden MK, McMaster D: Zinc deficiency and coeliac disease. In: McNicholl B, McCarthy CF, Fottrell PF, eds. Perspectives in coeliac disease. Lancaster: MTP Press, 1978; 335–42.

110 McCarthy CF, Frazer ID, Evans KT, Read AE: Lymphoreticular dysfunction in idiopathic steatorrhoea. Gut 1966; 7:140–8.

111 MacDonald TT, Ferguson A: Effects of allograft rejection on mucosal architecture and lymphoid cell infiltrate Gut 1976; 17:81–91.

112 MacDonald TT, Ferguson A: The effects of allograft rejection and graft-versus-host disease on epithelial cell kinetics. Cell Tissue Kinet 1977; 10:301–12.

113 McDonald WC, Brandborg LL, Flick AL et al: Studies of coeliac sprue. IV. The response of the whole length of the small bowel to a gluten free diet. Gastroenterology 1964; 47:573–89.

114 McLaughlin P, Hunter JO, Easter GB et al: Histamine release, in-vitro, from the jejunal mucosa following challenge with gliadin and also anti-IgE. In: Proc Second Fisons Food Allergy Workshop. Oxford: Medicine Publishing Foundation, 1983; 7–9.

115 MacLaurin BP, Cooke WT, Ling NR: Impaired lymphocyte reactivity against tumour cells in patients with coeliac disease. Gut 1971; 12:794–800.

116 Mann DL, Katz SI, Nelson DL et al: Specific B-cell antigens associated with gluten sensitive enteropathy and dermatitis herpetiformis. Lancet 1976; i:110–11.

117 Marsh MN: Studies of the intestinal lymphoid tissue. III. Quantitative analyses of the epithelial lymphocytes in the small intestine of human control subjects and of patients with coeliac sprue. Gastroenterology 1980; 79:481–92.

118 Marsh MN: Studies of intestinal lymphoid tissue. V. The cytology and electron microscopy of gluten sensitive enteropathy with particular reference to its immunopathology. Scand J Gastroenterol [Suppl 70] 1981; 16:87–106.

119 Marsh MN: Immunocytes enterocytes and the lamina propria: an immunopathological framework of coeliac disease. J Roy Coll Physicians 1983; 17:205–12

120 Marsh MN, Haeney MR: Studies of intestinal lymphoid tissue. VI. Proliferative response of small intestinal epithelial lymphocytes distinguishes gluten from non-gluten induced enteropathy. J Clin Pathol 1983; 36:149–60.

121 Mawhinney H, Love AHG: Antireticulin antibody in jejunal juice in coeliac disease. Clin Exp Immunol 1975; 21:394–8.

122 Mike N, Asquith P: Soya protein hypersensitivity in non-responsive coeliac disease. Gut 1984; 25:10,F149.

123 Mike N, Chesner IM, Asquith: Non-coeliac gluten sensitivity: the role of abnormal intestinal permeability. (In preparation.)

124 Mike N, Haeney Mr, Asquith P: Cell mediated immunity to soya protein in coeliac disease. Gut 1983; 24:10,732.

125 Morgenroth J, Watson DW, French AB: Cellular and humoral sensitivity to gluten fractions in patients with treated non-tropical sprue. Am J Dig Dis 1972; 17:205–12.

126 Nussle D, Bozil C, Cox J et al: Non-coeliac gluten intolerance in infancy. In: McNicholl B, McCarthy CF, Fottrell PF, eds. Perspectives in coeliac disease. Lancaster: MTP Press, 1978; 277–86.

127 O'Donoghue DR, Swarbrick ET, Kumar PJ: Type I hypersensitivity reactions in coeliac disease. Gastroenterology 1979; 76:1211.

128 O'Donoghue DP, Lancaster-Smith M, Laviniere P, Kumar PJ: T-cell depletion in untreated coeliac disease. Gut 1976; 17:328–31.

129 O'Farrelly C, Feigherty C, Greally JF, Weir DG: Cellular response to alpha gliadin in untreated coeliac disease. Gut 1982; 23:83–7.

130 O'Farrelly C, Whelan CA, Feighery CF, Weir DG: Coeliac mononuclear cells bind alpha gliadin monoclonal antibody. Presented at Midland Gastroenterological Society, June 1984. (In press.)

131 O'Farrelly C, Kelly J, Hekkens W et al: Alpha gliadin antibody levels: a serological test for coeliac disease. Br Med J 1983; 286:2007–10.

132 Paganelli R, Levinsky RJ, Brostoff J,. Wraith DG: Immune complexes containing food proteins in normal and atopic subjects after oral challenge and effect of sodium cromoglycate on antigen absorption. Lancet 1979; i:1270–2.

133 Patey AL: The chemistry of gliadin. In: Hemmings WA, ed. Antigen absorption by the gut. Lancaster: MTP Press, 1978; 161–6.

134 Pena AS, Mann DL, Hague NE et al: Genetic basis of gluten sensitive enteropathy. Gastroenterology 1978; 75:230–5.

135 Peters TJ, Jones PE, Wells G: Analytical subcellular fractionation of jejunal biopsy specimens. Enzyme activities, organelle pathology and response to gluten withdrawal in patients with coeliac disease. Clin Sci Molec Med 1978; 55:285–92.

136 Phelan JJ, McCarthy CF, Stevens FM et al: The nature of gliadin toxicity in coeliac disease: a new concept. In: Hekkens WTJM, Pena AS, eds. Coeliac disease. Leiden: Stenfert-Kroese, 1974; 60–70.

137 Phelan JJ, Stevens FM, McNicholl B et al: Coeliac disease: the abolition of gliadin toxicity by enzymes from *Aspergillus niger*. Clin Sci Molec Med 1977; 53:35–43.

138 Pink IJ, Creamer B: Response to a gluten free diet of patients with the coeliac syndrome. Lancet 1967; i:300–4.

139 Pock-Steen OC: The role of gluten, milk and other dietary proteins in chronic or intermittent dyspepsia. Clin Allergy 1973; 3:373–83.

140 Rawcliffe PM, Anand BS, Offord RE et al: A skin test for coeliac disease. In: McNicholl B, McCarthy CF, Fottrell PF, eds. Perspectives in coeliac disease. Lancaster: MTP Press, 1978; 347–9.

141 Rossipal E: On the association of coeliac disease with allergic disorders. A study of family histories of 110 families with one or two children with coeliac disease. In: McConnel RB, ed. The genetics of coeliac disease. Lancaster: MTP Press, 1981; 85–93.

142 Savilahti E, Perkkio M, Kalimo K et al: IgA antigliadin antibodies: a marker of mucosal damage in childhood coeliac disease. Lancet 1983; i:320–2.

143 Scott BB, Losowsky MS: Cell mediated autoimmunity in coeliac disease. Clin Exp Immunol 1976; 26:243–6.

144 Scott BB, Goodall A, Stephenson PM, Jenkins D: Is reaginic hypersensitivity involved in coeliac disease? Gut 1983; 24:733.

145 Scott H, Fausa V, Ek J, Brandtzaeg P: Immune response patterns in coeliac disease: serum antibodies to dietary antigens measured by an enzyme linked immunosorbent assay (ELISA). Clin Exp Immunol 1984; 57:25–32.

146 Seah PP, Fry L, Hoffbrand AV, Holborow EJ: Tissue antibodies in dermatitis herpetiformis and adult coeliac disease. Lancet 1977; i:834–6.

147 Seah PP, Fry L, Holborow EJ et al: Antireticulin antibody: incidence and diagnostic significance. Gut 1973; 14: 311–15.

148 Selby WS, Janossy G, Bofill M, Jewell DP: Lymphocyte subpopulations in the human small intestine. The findings in normal mucosa and in the mucosa of patients with adult coeliac disease. Clin Exp Immunol 1983; 52:219.

149 Shiner M: Effect of a gluten free diet in 17 patients with idiopathic steatorrhoea. Am J Dig Dis 1963; 8:969–83.

150 Shiner M: Ultrastructural changes suggestive of immune reactions in the jejunal mucosa of coeliac children following gluten challenge. Gut 1973; 14:1–12.

151 Shiner M, Ballard J: Antigen-antibody reactions in jejunal mucosa in childhood coeliac disease after gluten challenge. Lancet 1972; i:1202.

152 Simpson FG, Bullen AW, Robertson DAF, Losowsky MF: HLA B8 and cell mediated immunity to gluten. Gut 1981; 22:633–6.

153 Simpson FG, Field HP, Howdle PD et al: Leucocyte migration inhibition test in coeliac disease—a reappraisal. Gut 1983; 311–17.

154 Stern M, Dietrich R, Gruttner R: Gliadin binding immunocytes in small intestinal lamina propria of children with coeliac disease. Pediatr Res 1981; 15:1196.

155 Stern M, Fischer K, Gruttner R: Immunofluorescent serum gliadin antibodies in children with coeliac disease and various malabsorptive disorders. Eur J Pediatr 1979; 130:155–64.

156 Stokes PL, Asquith P, Holmes GKT et al: Histocompatibility antigens associated with adult coeliac disease. Lancet 1972; ii: 162–4.

157 Strobel S, Busuttil A, Ferguson A: Human intestinal mucosal mast cells: expanded population in untreated coeliac disease. Gut 1983; 24:222–7.

158 Strober RW, Falchuk ZM, Rogentine GN et al: The pathogenesis of gluten sensitive enteropathy. Ann Intern Med 1975; 83:242–56.

159 Thompson RA, Asquith P, Cooke WT: Secretory IgA in the serum. Lancet 1969; ii:517–19.

160 Tosi R, Vismara D, Tan Gaki N et al: Evidence that coeliac disease is primarily associated with a DC locus allelic specificity. Clin Immuno Immunopathol 1983; 28:395–404.

161 Townley RRW, Bhathal PS, Cornell HJ, Mitchell JD: Toxicity of wheat gliadin fraction in coeliac disease. Lancet 1973; i:1363–4.

162 Trier JS: Organ culture of intestinal mucosa. In: Hekkins WTJM, Pena AS, eds. Coeliac disease. Leiden: Stenfert-Kroese, 1974; 81–8.

163 Unsworth DJ, Kieffer M, Holborrow EJ et al: IgA antigliadin antibodies in coeliac disease. Clin Exp Immunol 1981; 46:286–93.

164 Unsworth DJ, Scott DL, Walton KW et al: Failure of RI type anti-reticulin antibody to react with fibronectin, collagen, type III or the non-collagenous reticulin component (NCRC). Clin Exp Immunol 1984; 57:609–13.

165 Van De Kamer JH, Weijers HA: Coeliac disease: some experiments on the cause of the harmful effect of wheat gliadin. Acta Paediatr 1955; 44:465–9.

166 Vitoria JC, Camareru C, Sojo A et al: Enteropathy related to fish, rice and chicken. Arch Dis Child 1982; 57:44–8.

167 Walker-Smith JA: Transient gluten intolerance. Arch Dis Child 1970; 45:523–6.

168 Walker-Smith JA, Phillips AD, Rossiter M, Wharton BA: Transient gluten intolerance. Gut 1984; 25:10,F150.

169 Wall AJ, Douglas AP, Booth CC, Pearse AGE: Response of the jejunal mucosa in adult coeliac disease to oral Prednisolone. Gut 1970; 11:7-14.

170 Ward M, Ferguson A, Eastwood MA: Jejunal lysozyme activity and the paneth cell in coeliac disease. Gut 1979; 20: 55-8.

171 Watt J, Pincott JR, Harries JT: Combined cows milk protein and gluten induced enteropathy: common or rare? Gut 1983; 24:165-70.

172 Webster ADB, Slavin G, Shiner M et al: Coeliac disease and severe hypogammaglobulinaemia. Gut 1981; 22:153-7.

173 Weiser MM, Douglas AP: An alternative mechanism for gluten toxicity in coeliac disease. Lancet 1976; 1:567-9.

174 Williams A, Asquith P, Stableforth DE: Asthma, eczema, seasonal rhinitis and skin atopy in adult coeliac disease. Gut 1984; 25:10,F151.

175 Williamson N, Asquith P, Stokes PL et al: Anticonnective tissue and other antitissue 'antibodies' in the sera of patients with coeliac disease compared with the findings in a mixed hospital population. J Clin Pathol 1976; 29:484-94.

176 Wray D: Gluten-sensitive recurrent aphthous stomatitis. Dig Dis Sci 1981; 26:737-40.

177 Yardley JH, Bayless TM, Norton JH, Hendrix TR: Coeliac disease: a study of the jejunal epithelium before and after a gluten free diet. N Engl J Med 1962; 267:1173-9.

Chapter 31
Idiopathic Inflammatory Bowel Disease: A Form of Food Allergy?

Roy G. Shorter

Introduction

Although the term idiopathic inflammatory bowel disease (IBD) is widely used to embrace both chronic ulcerative colitis (CUC) and Crohn's disease (CD), it is uncertain whether these are separate entities which happen to share many clinical and laboratory features, or are parts of the spectrum of a single disease process. This doubt will remain until their aetiology is understood [32].

Epidemiology

IBD is worldwide in its distribution, its incidence is approximately equal in males and females and it is more common in Western countries, particularly in Jewish members of these populations, regardless of their degree of Orthodoxy [42]. In the United States and in Great Britain the incidence of IBD is of the order of 8-10 per 100 000 population per annum [42], and in the past two decades a real increase in the incidence of Crohn's disease has occurred in some regions of the Western world [40], while that of CUC has remained unchanged. However, this increase has 'levelled out' and, indeed, the incidence now may be on the decline [27].

Genetics

Although no simple Mendelian genetic mechanism is at work in the aetiology of IBD, there are definite familial aggregations, even among family members widely separated geographically, and CUC and CD are often intermingled in these susceptible groups [32]. Genetic theories have been put forward to explain this familial predilection, particularly by McConnell [38]. However, no HLA markers have been found which can be related clearly either to susceptibility or resistance to IBD.

Age of onset

Although the onset of CUC or CD may occur at any age, the peak is between 20 and 40 years, with a second, much smaller peak in the fifth to sixth decades of life [32, 42].

Primary target

Both CUC and CD are chronic diseases and while the 'primary target' in CUC is the mucosa of the large intestine [43], the lesions of CD may involve the gastrointestinal tract from mouth to anus [16-18, 20]. Also, approximately 60% of patients with Crohn's disease show non-caseating granulomas in the inflamed bowel [47]. Either form of IBD may give rise to extraintestinal complications, the onset of which sometimes precedes that of the intestinal disease [30, 32]. In addition, IBD may be associated with certain other diseases, such as ankylosing spondylitis [30, 32].

CHRONIC ULCERATIVE COLITIS (CUC)

Clinical features and diagnosis

In most instances, the diagnosis of CUC is first suggested by the development of persistent or recurrent bloody diarrhoea, with urgency, tenesmus and cramping abdominal pain. These signs and symptoms may be associated with fever, weight loss and in some cases with vomiting [30]. The incidence of the symptoms and signs is shown in Table 31.1.

Table 31.1 Clinical features of ulcerative colitis.

	Percentage
Bloody diarrhoea	90
Urgency, tenesmus	40
Cramping abdominal pain	65
Fever	10–40
Weight loss	20–60
Vomiting	15–25

The course of the disease is very variable: for example, a mild to moderately active colitis may persist but either does not worsen significantly or 'waxes and wanes' in activity, while in other cases (2–3%) the activity becomes fulminant with life-threatening toxic dilatation of the colon. In some the attack may resolve completely in weeks or months without sequelae. As Janowitz and Sachar [30] have emphasized, if the disease presents only as a protosigmoiditis it is impossible to predict whether it will extend proximally and thus become a total colitis, or whether it will remain confined to the distal large bowel as a more benign process. However, as a working rule, if the inflammation has not spread to the proximal colon by about six months from the clinical onset of disease it is relatively unlikely so to do, since late proximal extension only occurs in about 1 in 10 such patients.

Investigations important to establishing a diagnosis of CUC are summarized in Table 31.2. These include the need for appropriate microbiological and parasitological studies since certain specific infections (e.g. *Campylobacter enterocolitis*) or infestations may pro-

Table 31.2 Diagnostic studies in IBD.

1 History.

2 Physical examination and chest X-ray.

3 Endoscopy and biopsy when possible.

4 Barium enema (conventional and/or double contrast).

5 Small bowel X-ray.

6 Laboratory tests:
   (a) Complete blood count and ESR.
   (b) Urinalysis.
   (c) Serum creatinine.
   (d) Serum protein electrophoresis.
   (e) Serum alkaline phosphatase.
   (f) Stool for blood; stool microscopy for fat.
   (g)★ Cultures of stool or mucosa for microbia: e.g. *Shigella*, *Campylobacter* (*fetus* subsp. *jejuni*), *Clostridium difficile*, *Neisseria gonorrhoeae*, *Yersinia enterocolitis*, *Chlamydia*, etc.
   (h)★ Examination of stool for parasites, e.g. *Entamoeba histolytica*, *Giardia lamblia*, *Strongyloides stercoralis*, *Cryptosporidium*, etc.
   (i)★ In a few instances, serological testing for amoebiasis, histoplasmosis, lymphogranuloma venereum, cytomegalovirus, etc.
   (j) In some cases, PPD skin testing.

★ The extent of such studies can be adjusted to the clinical situation (see text).

duce clinical, endoscopic, histological and radiological features which closely resemble CUC, and these may be chronic, particularly in patients with immunodeficiency states [8, 13, 21]. However, the extent of such microbiologic and parasitological studies can be 'tailored', using good judgement, to fit the clinical setting.

CROHN'S DISEASE (CD)

Clinical features

Although ultrastructurally CD is a diffuse disease of the entire gastrointestinal tract, in the majority of patients (70–75%) the first clinical manifestations of active disease occur in the ileum, together with variable degrees of proximal colonic involvement. However, in about 20% of cases the initial, gross lesions are restricted to the colon, while in approximately 4% the presenting disease is limited to the stomach, duodenum, jejunum or anal region [41]. Thus, in most individuals with CD the presenting symptoms and signs are those of lower abdominal pain (which may awaken the patient at night), frequent loose stools (usually *not* bloody), fever, anorexia and weight loss. However, in children a 'failure to grow' and other extraintestinal problems may dominate the clinical presentation.

As a general rule, ileal disease is associated with 'obstructive' qualities, while patients with Crohn's colitis may have gross bleeding and perianal fistulae as prominent features. About 75% of individuals with ileocolic CD eventually require surgical therapy, as do 50% of those in whom the gross disease is confined either to the small bowel or to the colon [22, 29, 36]. Studies important to establishing a diagnosis of Crohn's disease are summarized in Table 31.2.

EXTRAINTESTINAL COMPLICATIONS AND OTHER DISEASES ASSOCIATED WITH IBD

Pragmatically, Janowitz and Sachar [30] have classified the motley collection of extraintestinal complications of IBD into two groups:
1 Those which seem to relate to the extent and degree of activity of the bowel (which they termed '*colitic*' complications).
2 Those which result from pathophysiologic changes in the small bowel induced either by the disease or by therapeutic surgical resection(s).

The components of these groups and the other diseases which may be associated with IBD are summarized in Table 31.3. The mechanisms involved in causing the 'colitic' complications are as ill-understood as those of the aetiopathogenesis of CUC or CD, but the observation that certain of these extraintestinal problems (e.g. arthritis) may also complicate jejunoileal bypass for morbid obesity [14, 54], has suggested to some that, for these patients at least, intestinal anaerobic microbial overgrowth may be important [51]. No clues exist as to why IBD and certain other diseases may be associated but speculation is rife, often involving a *hysteron proteron*.

Cancer risk in IBD

In the United States of America and the United Kingdom, patients with total colonic involvement by CUC and longstanding (> 10 years) disease are at considerably increased risk (5–30 times) of colorectal cancer compared to the general population [50], and the risk is also increased in those with chronic left-sided colitis, but to a lesser extent [23]. Furthermore, in these countries, individuals with longstanding Crohn's colitis are also at significantly (up to 20-fold) increased risk of such a cancer [45]. However, the degree of risk of these tumours to IBD patients elsewhere in

Table 31.3 Extraintestinal complications and diseases associated with IBD.

Extraintestinal complications of IBD		Diseases associated with IBD
'Colitic'	Problems due to small bowel pathophysiology	
Various nutritional deficiencies (e.g. protein and mineral losses).	Malabsorption of vitamin B12, folic acid, fat and fat-soluble vitamins (in Crohn's disease).	Sclerosing cholangitis.
Aphthous stomatitis.	Lactase deficiency (Crohn's disease).	Ankylosing spondylitis.
Erythema nodosum.		Takayusu's arteritis (with Crohn's disease).
Pyoderma gangrenosum.	Diminished bile salt pool and resulting gallstones (Crohn's disease).	Psoriasis (with Crohn's disease).
Conjunctivitis; episcleritis; iritis.		
Peripheral arthritis.	Renal calculi in CD, or following ileostomy (uric acid, oxalate).	
Finger clubbing.		
Pericholangitis.	Growth retardation in children.*	
Obstructive hydronephrosis (with Crohn's disease).		
Extraintestinal granulomas (Crohn's disease).		
Thrombocytosis.		
Amyloidosis (particularly renal) in Crohn's disease.		

* It is uncertain how to classify this complication.

the world is not well defined, and the mechanisms involved in producing the increased risk are not understood. Whether Crohn's disease is associated with a greater risk of primary adenocarcinoma of the small gut is unknown, although there is anecdotal evidence to suggest that this is so [30, 45, 50]. There are no data which show that in IBD there is any increased incidence of primary cancers outside the gastrointestinal tract.

AETIOLOGY OF IBD: IS THERE EVIDENCE FOR A ROLE FOR FOOD ALLERGY?

The aetiopathogenesis of IBD is unknown but the many theories put forward to explain it have been reviewed recently [32]. A popular working hypothesis involves three factors:
1　An external agent(s), either microbial or non-microbial.
2　Immunological responses in the host to the external agent(s).
3　Genetic influences on host immune responses.

Immunological reaction to food antigens

Pertinent to this brief review is the suggestion that IBD is a manifestation of immunologic reactions to food antigens [2], a concept which has derived indirect support from claims for a greater frequency of atopic disorders in patients with IBD than in controls [24, 31, 44]. Of the many suggested foodstuffs, that which has received the most attention is cow's milk, particularly since its withdrawal from the diet was shown in one controlled study to have a favourable effect on the course of CUC [56]. In another study, patients with CUC also had a higher incidence of positive skin tests to purified cow's milk proteins compared to controls [31]. In addition, some workers found a greater incidence and higher titres of circulating antibodies to cow's milk proteins in CUC, compared to controls [49]. However, others did not confirm this [31, 37], and even when such antibodies are present in the serum of patients with IBD [37] there is no correlation between their titres and disease activity, the course of the disease or the clinical response to a milk-free diet [31, 33, 56]. Furthermore, Jewell and Truelove [31] concluded that a reagin–IgE response to cow's milk proteins is *not* involved in the aetiopathogenesis of CUC or CD, and in many cases the beneficial effect

of withdrawing cow's milk from the diet is due to complicating lactase deficiency [3].

Early weaning: cow's milk

Although it appears that a history of early weaning on to cow's milk is more common in IBD patients than in controls [1, 5], there is no evidence that these and other observations [55] argue specifically in favour of allergy to cow's milk proteins as an aetiopathogenic factor in the diseases [46]. Indeed, it seems likely that the findings relate more to influences of early weaning on the maturation of the gut-associated lymphoid tissues and on the intestinal microbial flora, and possibly to sensitization by other antigens present in cow's milk or other components of a mixed diet, particularly those of microbial origin [10, 53]. Thus, while a role for cow's milk proteins in the aetiopathogenesis of IBD has not been completely excluded, from existing data it seems unlikely that these are involved.

Other food antigens

Attempts to implicate other food antigens in the aetiopathogenesis of IBD have been equally unsuccessful [3, 30, 32]. As a result, the only points that can be advanced to support an hypothesis that such antigens are important in this context are indirect and include:

1　Reports of increased numbers of eosinophil leukocytes and mast cells and an increased content of histamine in the rectal mucosa in CUC [4, 6, 25, 35, 57].
2　The presence of increased numbers of degranulated mast cells in Crohn's tissues [34].

However, such findings have been inconsistent, the number of IgE immunocytes in the mucosae of the small and large bowel seems to be normal in IBD [3, 32] and earlier reports of favourable responses by some patients with IBD either to the local application or the oral administration of disodium cromoglycate [26, 28, 39] were refuted by subsequent trials [7, 9, 15]. The significance of these 'negative' therapeutic findings is emphasized by Zanussi's [58] conclusions, from the available data, that the clinical and histological manifestations of food allergy respond in *all* instances, at least to some degree, to the action of this agent [11, 12, 19, 48, 52] (see Chapter 58).

SUMMARY

There is currently no evidence that allergic responses to food antigens have any relationship to the aetiopathogenesis of CUC or CD. However, future, more sophisticated studies may prove this false (but see Chapter 32).

REFERENCES

1 Acheson ED, Truelove SC: Early weaning in the aetiology of ulcerative colitis. Br Med J 1961; 2:929-33.

2 Andresen AFR: Ulcerative colitis—An allergic phenomenon. Am J Dig Dis 1942; 9:91-8.

3 Bartnik W, Shorter RG: Inflammatory bowel disease: immunologic developments. In: J Edward Berk, ed. Developments in digestive diseases. Philadelphia: Lea and Febiger, 1980; 109-27.

4 Bercovitz ZT, Sommers SC: Altered inflammatory reaction in nonspecific ulcerative colitis. Arch Intern Med 1966; 117(4):504-10.

5 Bergstrand O, Hellers G: Breast-feeding during infancy in patients who later develop Crohn's disease. Scand J Gastroenterol 1983; 18:903-6.

6 Binder V, Hvidberg E: Histamine content of rectal mucosa in ulcerative colitis. Gut 1967; 8:24-8.

7 Binder V, Elsborg L, Greibe J et al: Disodium cromoglycate in the treatment of ulcerative colitis and Crohn's disease. Gut 1981; 22:55-60.

8 Boyd WP Jr, Bachman BA: Gastrointestinal infections in the compromised host. Med Clin North Am 1982; 66:743-53.

9 Buckell NA, Gould SR, Day DW et al: Controlled trial of disodium cromoglycate in chronic persistent ulcerative colitis. Gut 1978; 19:1140-3.

10 Bullen CL, Tearle PV, Steward MG: The effect of 'humanized' milks and supplemented breast feeding on the faecal flora of infants. J Med Microbiol 1977; 10(4):403-13.

11 Byars NE, Ferraresi RW: Intestinal anaphylaxis in the rat as a model of food allergy. Clin Exp Immunol 1976; 24:352-6.

12 Dahl R, Zetterstrom O: The effect of orally administered sodium cromoglycate on allergic reactions caused by food allergens. Clin Allergy 1978; 7:109-15.

13 Doe WF: Immunodeficiency and the gastrointestinal tract. Clin Gastroenterol 1983; 12:839-53.

14 Drenick EJ, Ament ME, Finegold SM et al: Bypass enteropathy: an inflammatory process in the excluded segment with systemic complications. Am J Clin Nutr 1977; 30:76-89.

15 Dronfield MW, Langman MJ: Comparative trial of Suphasalazine and oral disodium cromoglycate in the maintenance of remission of ulcerative colitis. Gut 1978; 19:1136-9.

16 Dunne WT, Cooke WT, Allan RN: Enzymatic and morphometric evidence for Crohn's disease as a diffuse lesion of the gastrointestinal tract. Gut 1977; 18:290-4.

17 Dvorak AM, Dickersin GR: Crohn's disease: Transmission electron microscopic studies. I. Barrier function: possible changes related to alterations of cell coat, mucous coat, epithelial cells and paneth cells. Hum Pathol 1980; 11:561-71.

18 Dvorak AM, Connell AB, Dickersin GR: Crohn's disease: a scanning electron microscopic study. Hum Pathol 1979; 10:165-77.

19 Gerrard JW: Oral cromoglycate: its value in the treatment of adverse reactions to food. Ann Allergy 1979; 42:135-8.

20 Goodman MJ, Skinner JM, Truelove SC: Abnormalities in apparently normal bowel mucosa in Crohn's disease. Lancet 1976; 1:275-8.

21 Gottlieb MS, Groopman JE, Weinstein WM et al: The acquired immunodeficiency syndrome. Ann Int Med 1983; 99:208-20.

22 Greenstein AJ, Meyres S, Sher L et al: Surgery and its sequelae in Crohn's colitis and ileocolitis. Arch Surg 1981; 116:285-8.

23 Greenstein AJ, Sachar DB, Smith H et al: Cancer in universal and left-sided ulcerative colitis: factors determining risk. Gastroenterology 1979; 77:290-4.

24 Hammer B, Ashurst P, Naish J: Diseases associated with ulcerative colitis and Crohn's disease. Gut 1968; 9:17-21.

25 Heatley RV, James PD: Eosinophils in the rectal mucosa. A simple method of predicting the outcome of ulcerative proctocolitis? Gut 1978; 20:787-91.

26 Heatley RV, Calcraft BJ, Rhodes J et al: Disodium cromoglycate in the treatment of chronic proctitis. Gut 1975; 16:559-63.

27 Hellers G: Some epidemiological aspects of Crohn's disease in Stockholm county 1955-1979. In: Peña AS, Weterman IT, Booth CC, Strober W, eds. Recent advances in Crohn's disease. Boston: Martinus Nijhoff, 1981: 158-62.

28 Henderson A, Hishon S: Crohn's disease responding to oral disodium cromoglycate. Lancet 1978; 1:109-10.

29 Higgens CS, Allan RN: Crohn's disease of the distal ileum. Gut 1980; 21:933-40.

30 Janowitz HD, Sachar DB: Inflammatory bowel disease. In: Stollerman GH, ed. Advances in internal medicine, Vol. 27. Chicago: Year Book Medical Publishers, 1982; 205-46.

31 Jewell DP, Truelove SC: Reaginic hypersensitivity in ulcerative colitis. Gut 1972; 13:903-6.

32 Kirsner JB, Shorter RG: Recent developments in 'nonspecific' inflammatory bowel disease. N Engl J Med 1982; 306:775-848.

33 Kraft SC, Kirsner JB: The immunology of ulcerative colitis and Crohn's disease: clinical and humoral aspects. In: Kirsner JB, Shorter RG, eds. Inflammatory bowel disease. Philadelphia: Lea and Febiger, 1980 2nd Ed; 86-120.

34 Levo Y, Livni N: Mast-cell degranulation in Crohn's disease. Lancet 1978; 1:1262.

35 Lloyd G, Green FHY, Fox H et al: Mast cells and immunoglobulin E in inflammatory bowel disease. Gut 1975; 16:861-5.

36 Lock MR, Farmer RG, Fazio UW et al: Recurrence and reoperation for Crohn's disease: the role of disease location in prognosis. N Engl J Med 1981; 304:1586-8.

37 McCaffery TD, Kraft SC, Rothburg RM: The influence of different techniques in characterizing human antibodies to cow's milk proteins. Clin Exp Immunol 1972; 11:225-34.

38 McConnell RB: Inflammatory bowel disease: newer views of genetic influence. In: Berk JE, ed. Developments in digestive diseases. Philadelphia: Lea and Febiger, 1980; 129–37.

39 Mani V, Green FHY, Lloyd G et al: Treatment of ulcerative colitis with oral disodium cromoglycate. A double-blind controlled trial. Lancet 1976: 1:439–41.

40 Mayberry JF, Rhodes J: Studies on the incidence, prevalence, mortality and dietary history of patients with Crohn's disease. In: Peña AS, Weterman IT, Booth CC, Strober W, eds. Recent advances in Crohn's disease. Boston: Martinus Nijhoff, 1981; 163–7.

41 Mekhjian HS, Switz DM, Melnyk CS et al; Clinical features and natural history of Crohn's disease. Gastroenterology 1979; 77:898–906.

42 Mendeloff AI: The epidemiology of idiopathic inflammatory bowel disease. In: Kirsner JB, Shorter RG, etc. Inflammatory bowel disease. Philadelphia: Lea and Febiger, 1980 2nd ed; 5–22.

43 Morson BC: Pathology of ulcerative colitis. In: Kirsner JB, Shorter RG, eds. Inflammatory bowel disease. Philadelphia: Lea and Febiger, 1980 2nd ed; 281–95.

44 Roberts DL et al: Atopic features in ulcerative colitis. Lancet 1978; 1:1262.

45 Shorter RG: Risks of intestinal cancer in Crohn's disease. Dis Colon Rectum 1983; 26:686–9.

46 Soothill JF: Prevention of food allergy. In: Brostoff J, Challacombe SJ, eds. Vol. 2. Food allergy. London: WB Saunders, 1982; 243–4.

47 Surawicz CM, Meisel JL, Ylvisaker J et al: Rectal biopsy in the diagnosis of Crohn's disease: value of multiple biopsies and serial sectioning. Gastroenterology 1981; 80:66–71.

48 Syme J: Investigation and treatment of multiple intestinal food allergy in childhood. In: Pepys J, Edwards AM, eds. The mast cell. Tunbridge Wells, England: Pitman Medical, 1979; 438–42.

49 Taylor KB, Truelove SC: Circulating antibodies to milk proteins in ulcerative colitis. Br Med J 1961; 2:924–9.

50 Thayer WR Jr: Malignancy in inflammatory bowel disease. In: Kirsner JB, Shorter RG, eds. Inflammatory bowel disease. Philadelphia: Lea and Febiger, 1980 2nd ed; 265–78.

51 Thayer WR Jr, Kirsner JB: Enteric and extra-enteric complications of intestinal bypass and inflammatory bowel disease: are there some clues? Gastroenterology 1980; 78:1097–100.

52 Vaz GA, Tan LKT, Gerrard JW: Oral cromoglycate treatment of adverse reactions to food. Lancet 1978; 1:1066–8.

53 Walker WA: Mechanisms of antigen handling by the gut. In: Brostoff J, Challacombe SJ, eds. Vol. 2. Food allergy. London: WB Saunders, 1982; 15–40.

54 Walport MH, Parke AL, Hughes GRV: Food and the connective tissue diseases. In: Brostoff J, Challacombe SJ, eds. Vol. 2. Food allergy. London, WB Saunders, 1982; 113–20.

55 Whorwell PJ, Holdstock G, Whorwell GM, Wright R: Bottle feeding, early gastroenteritis, and inflammatory bowel disease. Br Med J 1979; 1:382.

56 Wright R, Truelove SC: A controlled therapeutic trial of various diets in ulcerative colitis. Br Med J 1965; 2:138–41.

57 Wright R, Truelove SC: Circulating and tissue eosinophils in ulcerative colitis. Am J Dig Dis 1966; 11:831–46.

58 Zanussi C: Food allergy treatment. In: Brostoff J, Challacombe SJ, eds. Vol. 2. Food allergy. London: WB Saunders, 1982; 221–40.

Chapter 32
Irritable Bowel Syndrome and Crohn's Disease

V. Alun Jones and J. O. Hunter

Introduction

The large surface area of the gut and its direct contact with food and food residues makes it entirely unsurprising that it should suffer the consequences of food intolerance. Indeed the first disease to be linked scientifically to a particular food was coeliac disease. Research in this field has recently been thoroughly reviewed [11, 13], as have paediatric gastrointestinal conditions associated with diet [65]. This chapter will concentrate on the evidence for a relationship between diet and the pathogenesis of irritable bowel syndrome and Crohn's disease.

IRRITABLE BOWEL SYNDROME

Epidemiology

Irritable bowel syndrome (IBS) is a common condition which has been estimated to account for between 33 and 70% of gastrointestinal consultations [18, 29]. It occurs approximately twice as frequently in women as in men. The point at which people choose to seek advice about gut symptoms varies, so that Thompson and Heaton [64] found that 30% of uncomplaining and apparently healthy British adults admitted to bowel disturbances. Affected patients complain of diarrhoea, constipation or an alternation between the two, and abdominal pain. IBS never produces rectal bleeding. There are no abnormalities detected radiologically or histologically [30], and biochemical tests are normal. Patients with IBS frequently suffer symptoms for many years, but never develop serious complications.

Clinical definition

Many gastroenterologists reserve the term for those patients who clearly have an abnormality of gut motility, which can be recognized readily from the spasm of the bowel apparent at sigmoidoscopy or colonoscopy. The abnormality of motility can be demonstrated in the small bowel and oesophagus as well as in the colon [1, 12, 15, 67], and this suggests that gut hormones might be important in the pathogenesis of IBS, though this has yet to be demonstrated [9, 34]. Thus the cause remains unclear; antispasmodic drugs such as mebeverine and peppermint oil sometimes give temporary relief.

Differential diagnosis

The differential diagnosis of IBS is wide, encompassing inflammatory bowel disease, colonic carcinoma, coeliac disease, alactasia, ulcer diathesis, biliary pathology and musculoskeletal pain. As no specific tests are available, IBS remains a diagnosis of exclusion and thus is probably a collection of disparate conditions which will gradually be clarified.

IBS has been considered a psychosomatic disorder [69] but treatment along these lines rarely produces dramatic improvements [63] and other workers have found no higher level of anxiety in patients with IBS than in sufferers of other gut diseases causing similar symptoms [55].

Many cases of IBS follow attacks of gastroenteritis, but enteropathogenic bacteria have not been identified in this condition.

The role of diet in the pathogenesis of IBS remains controversial.

Clinical experience of dietary management

Numerous reports exist in the older literature of patients with abdominal symptoms finding relief by modification of their diet. As early as 1771 Sir George Baker presented to the Royal College of Physicians a patient, Thomas Wood ('A Miller of Billericay') whose abdominal symptoms were improved by a diet of 'sea biscuits and salt meat' [19]. Although many reports of abdominal pain and diarrhoea responding to dietary modification were made in the United States in the first half of the twen-

tieth century (e.g. [20, 21, 57]), this work was largely ignored by mainstream gastroenterologists on both sides of the Atlantic.

It was recognized nearly 20 years ago that alactasia was responsible for a number of cases of IBS [26, 44, 66]. A recent study, however, suggested that the incidence of alactasia in White Gentiles with IBS was no higher than in symptom-free controls from a similar background [51] and alactasia is generally now considered to be a separate entity.

High-fibre diet

Initial enthusiasm for a high-fibre diet in IBS [46, 61] was not justified by later reports [41] and this diet is now usually reserved for patients whose predominant problem is constipation, and for patients with diverticular disease. In 1980 Cooper et al [14] presented seven cases of idiopathic diarrhoea which improved on a gluten-free diet but in which the jejunal mucosa was normal on biopsy. Perhaps in view of the enthusiasm at that time for high-fibre diets it was not surprising that the paper was greeted with considerable scepticism; indeed three years elapsed between its submission and its publication.

Table 32.1 Percentage of IBS patients intolerant to particular foods.

Food	%	Food	%	Food	%
Cereals		*Fruit*		*Vegetables (cont.)*	
Wheat	60	Citrus	24	Mushrooms	12
Corn	44	Apples	12	Parsnips	12
Oats	34	Rhubarb	12	Tomatoes	11
Rye	30	Banana	11	Cauliflower	11
Barley	24	Strawberries	8	Celery	11
Rice	15	Pineapple	8	Green beans	10
		Pears	8	Cucumber	10
Dairy products		Grapes	7	Turnip/swede	10
Milk	44	Melon	5	Marrow	8
Cheese	39	Avocado pear	5	Beetroot	8
Butter	25	Raspberries	4	Peppers	6
Yogurt	24				
		Vegetables		*Miscellaneous*	
Fish		Onions	22	Coffee	33
White fish	10	Potatoes	20	Eggs	26
Shell fish	10	Cabbage	19	Tea	25
Smoked fish	7	Sprouts	18	Chocolate	22
		Peas	17	Nuts	22
Meat		Carrots	15	Preservatives	20
Beef	16	Lettuce	15	Yeast	12
Pork	14	Leeks	15	Sugar-beet	12
Chicken	13	Broccoli	14	Sugar-cane	12
Lamb	11	Soya beans	13	Alcohol	12
Turkey	8	Spinach	13	Tap water	10
				Saccharin	9
				Honey	2

Data from Hunter et al [35], with permission.

Food intolerance: initial study

Our initial study [6] was a search for food intolerance in 25 successive patients diagnosed on clinical grounds as having IBS. Twenty-one agreed to follow a highly restrictive diet of lamb, pears and water for one week before reintroducing foods singly. Fourteen found subjective evidence of food intolerances and were able to control their symptoms by avoiding the foods in question. Of these, 11 agreed to undergo objective challenges. In six patients challenged double-blind on four occasions using nasogastric tubes with two test and two control foods, 21 out of 24 challenges were correctly identified. In the other five, test soups flavoured to disguise their constituents were given for four successive days on two occasions a month apart, and all were correctly identified.

Foods implicated. We have since extended our experience of food intolerance in IBS [35]. The foods that produced symptoms in 122 patients are listed in Table 32.1. The number of foods concerned in each patient varies from very few to more than 20 (Table 32.2), and

Table 32.2 Frequency of multiple food intolerances.

Intolerance of one food alone	5%
2–5 foods	28%
6–10 foods	35%
11–20 foods	17%
More than 20 foods	15%

Data from Hunter et al [35], with permission.

those patients with multiple food intolerances are difficult to manage. However, the benefits of the successful identification of food intolerance in patients is considerable, for follow up reveals that the great majority remain well for long periods of time (Table 32.3).

Proportion of patients who respond to diet

There is still considerable dispute over the relative proportion of patients with IBS who have food intolerance. Our experience suggests that approximately 70% of those with abdominal pain and diarrhoea may be successfully managed by diet, but other groups [8, 22, 60] have suggested lower prevalence rates for food intolerance in irritable bowel syndrome. These differences may reflect genuine geographical differences in the incidence of the condition, such as are seen for coeliac disease. Bentley et al [8] and Farah et al [22] found only three patients out of a total of 19, and three out of 49, respectively, to have food intolerances which could be objectively confirmed. This anomaly is likely to be related to differences in selection from a very heterogeneous group of patients. Furthermore we consider that the diets used by these teams were insufficiently rigorous since the patients were allowed to continue eating wheat and citrus fruits which we have found to cause symptoms in significant proportions of our patients. The challenge techniques were inadequate as capsules were used to administer food in double-blind challenges and thus gave a very small dose. Bentley's group did not use a prolonged challenge period, and it seems possible that these protocols revealed subjects with immunologically mediated food allergies, but failed to identify non-atopic patients with food intolerance.

These differences between the experiences of other research workers and ours should not be allowed to cloud the major point at issue which is that their results, like those of Lessof et al [40] Cooper et al [14] and Gerrard [27], confirmed objectively that patients exist whose abdominal symptoms may be reliably ascribed to food intolerance. With increasing experience, the true prevalence will be determined,

Table 32.3 Results of follow-up questionnaires.

	May 81	July 82	Dec 82
Date sent	May 81	July 82	Dec 82
Date patients started diet	Oct 79–March 81	April 81–May 82	Oct 79–March 81
Length of follow-up	2–20 months	2–16 months	22–39 months
No. of patients	80	42	71
Replies	71 (89%)	41 (98%)	61 (86%)
No. patients still on diet and			
improved	71 (100%)	41 (100%)	53 (87%)
Intolerance changed			
More foods	8 (11%)	2 (5%)	13 (25%)
Fewer foods	14 (20%)	10 (24%)	11 (21%)
Disappeared	0	0	3

Data from Hunter et al [35], with permission.

and it is to be hoped that this process will be aided by the development of diagnostic tests which allow a positive identification.

CROHN'S DISEASE

Crohn's disease is a chronic granulomatous inflammation which may affect any part of the gut from mouth to anus, but predominantly affects the terminal ileum and the colon. Extraintestinal manifestations such as anaemia, arthritis, uveitis and abscesses are common, and medical treatment involving corticosteroids, immunosuppressive drugs and antibiotics is often ineffective. Many patients require extensive gastrointestinal surgery. Although it may affect any age group, Crohn's disease is commonest in young adults, and its cause is unknown [59].

Link between diet and Crohn's disease

Reports of links between Crohn's disease and diet (e.g. [58]) have been regarded by gastroenterologists as curiosities rather than as a basis for the rational management of the disease [37], despite reports published in the 1970s of improvement of patients with Crohn's disease following total parenteral nutrition (TPN) [16, 17, 25, 49, 56]. The mechanism for this improvement was unknown and was generally ascribed to 'total bowel rest' rather than to any beneficial effect of avoiding specific foods.

Case report. Our interest in the role of diet arose with the case of a girl of 18 who presented with persistent diarrhoea and who was in good general health. Examination including sigmoidoscopy was normal and as it was thought that she had irritable bowel syndrome she was started on the elimination diet which was then our standard management [6]. A routine rectal biopsy, however, showed changes characteristic of Crohn's disease. She was recalled to the clinic, but reported that the diarrhoea had abated and that she wished to continue to explore diet as a means of controlling her symptoms. She discovered that wheat provoked her symptoms, and has now been well on a wheat-free diet for over five years. A further biopsy confirmed the diagnosis of Crohn's disease, which was limited to her rectum as radiological studies were normal. An objective challenge was made with wheat; this confirmed the association of this food with her diarrhoea and a subsequent jejunal biopsy

showed that she did not have coeliac disease. Food intolerances were then identified in 20 of 28 subsequent patients who were offered dietary management [36], and it became our standard approach [68].

Methods of inducing remission

In some patients with fairly mild Crohn's disease it may be possible to achieve remission of symptoms by means of exclusion diets based on those used in the management of irritable bowel syndrome. Most patients with Crohn's disease, however, are severely undernourished, and restricted oral diets are not suitable.

Total parenteral nutrition (TPN)

TPN is of proven value in the management of active Crohn's disease [16, 17, 25, 56] but has the disadvantages that it is invasive and highly expensive. It also requires supervision by a specialist nutrition team to ensure the meticulous care which is required to prevent complications such as infection.

Elemental diets. Elemental diets have the advantage of being simple, safe and comparatively cheap (at one-tenth of the cost of TPN). A number of reports have now appeared claiming excellent results for elemental diets in gaining remission in active Crohn's disease [48, 52, 53].

Randomized controlled trial:
Elemental diet compared with TPN

We have performed a randomized controlled trial to assess the relative efficacies of the two methods (TPN: standard preparations of Addenbrooke's Hospital Sterile Pharmacy and Travenol Ltd, Thetford; elemental diet: EO28, Scientific Hospital Supplies Ltd, Liverpool). Clinical details of the 36 successive patients recruited are given in Table 32.4 and the results in Table 32.5. All medication for Crohn's disease was tailed off and stopped during the period of induction of remission. No significant difference was found between the two treatments, both of which were highly successful. In view of the greater simplicity, safety and cheapness of elemental diet we now consider this to be the treatment of choice although patients who failed to go into remission may still be considered for subsequent TPN.

Table 32.4 Clinical details of patients in controlled trial of total parenteral nutrition (TPN) and elemental diet (ED).

Age (years)	<20	21–30	31–40	41–50	>50
TPN	6	6	4	1	2
ED	2	5	5	4	1

Sex	Male		Female	
TPN	4		15	
ED	5		12	

Length of history (months)	<12	13–24	25–36	37–48	49–60	>61
TPN	9	2	3	1	0	4
ED	3	3	0	1	0	10

Area of disease	Ileal	Colonic	Ileocolonic	Old colectomy
TPN	6	5	8	3
Ed	7	5	5	1

Data from Hunter [33], with permission.

Table 32.5 Results of controlled trial total parenteral nutrition (TPN) and elemental diet (ED).

	TPN ($\bar{x} \pm$ SD)	ED ($\bar{x} \pm$ SD)
No. recruited	19	17
Withdrawals	3	1
Unable to comply	0	3
Failure of method to induce remission in 14 days	2	2(NS)
Days to remission	9.0 ± 3.08	8.8 ± 2.56 (NS)
	($n = 16$)	($n = 13$)
Mean pre-trial CDAI	267.2 ± 94.2	247.7 ± 59.0 (NS)
Mean pre-trial albumin (g/l)	28.3 ± 6.99	29.3 ± 6.25 (NS)
Mean pre-trial orosomucoid (%)	213 ± 79	180 ± 68 (NS)
Mean post-trial CDAI	114.9 ± 84.9	118.7 ± 82.7 (NS)
Mean post-trial albumin (g/l)	28.5 ± 6.93	31.2 ± 4.84 (NS)
Mean post-trial orosomucoid (%)	205 ± 74	162 ± 50 (NS)

CDAI = Crohn's Disease Activity Index; NS = not significant.
Data from Hunter [33], with permission.

Maintenance of remission

Controlled trial of diets

Although most reports have suggested that the majority of patients in remission on TPN or elemental diet relapse promptly when they restart normal eating and require continuing corticosteroids [28, 54], a number of patients with Crohn's disease are known to enjoy spontaneous remissions [50]. We were concerned that the benefit apparent in our patients might possibly be a long-term effect of the previous artificial feeding and not necessarily the consequence of the search for food intolerances. A controlled trial was therefore set up using patients who had settled satisfactorily after either TPN or elemental diet. They were randomly assigned to follow the regime for the detection of food intolerances which has been outlined above (FI), or the unrefined carbohydrate, fibre-rich diet (UCFR) which has been suggested as an adjunct to conventional

medical management of Crohn's patients who have undergone gastrointestinal surgery [31]. Patients were followed up in the out-patients clinic for six months, and were seen by the dietitian as often as was thought necessary to provide adequate guidance and encouragement in following their diets. They were also seen each month by a separate physician who objectively assessed the activity of their disease without knowing which dietary regime they were following. Patients whose Crohn's disease activity index (CDAI) rose above 150 were considered treatment failures.

Clinical results. Clinical details of the patients are given in Table 32.6. Eight patients on the fibre-rich diet relapsed within the first two months—some within a few days of restarting normal eating (Fig. 32.1). Two remained well for longer but all had relapsed by six months. Although two patients in the other group failed to grasp the principles of the search for food intolerances and never achieved a diet on

Table 32.6 Clinical details of patients in controlled trial of unrefined carbohydrate, fibre-rich diet and exclusion diet.

	UCFR* diet	Exclusion diet
M:F ratio	1:9	1:9
Age (years)		
< 19	1	2
20–29	3	4
30–39	3	2
40–49	3	2
> 50	0	0
Length of history (months)		
< 12	2	3
13–24	2	0
25–36	2	3
37–48	0	1
49–60	1	2
> 60	3	1
Size of disease		
Ileum	2	4
Terminal ileum	10	7
Colon	4	10
Rectum	0	2
Previous management		
New patient	1	4
Steroids	9	5
Sulphasalazine	7	4
Surgery	3	1
Azathioprine	2	0
Antibiotics	2	1
Mean pre-trial ESR (mm/h)	26 ± 24.0 (SD)	37.9 ± 21.7 (SD)
Mean pre-trial orosomucoid (%)	232.5 ± 68.2 (SD)	236 ± 89.9 (SD)

Results given as numbers of patients except where indicated.
* UCFR = unrefined carbohydrate, fibre-rich.
† Normal range for orosomucoid 62.5–125%
Data from Alun Jones et al [4], with permission.

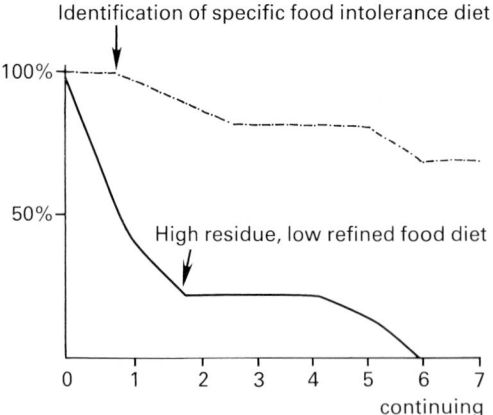

Fig. 32.1 Length of remission, in months, of patients in controlled trial of unrefined carbohydrate, fibre-rich diet and exclusion diet. $P < 0.05$, Fisher's exact test. From Alun Jones et al [4], with permision.

which they were symptom free, seven remained well after six months. The difference between the two groups is significant ($P < 0.05$, Fisher's exact test). Detailed results are given in Table 32.7.

Thus the prolonged remission seen in these patients is a consequence of the discovery and avoidance of foods of which the patient is intolerant and not merely a prolonged benefit of artificial feeding [4].

Overall clinical experience of diet in Crohn's disease

These dietary manipulations form the basis of a therapeutic strategy for the long-term management of Crohn's disease. Remission is at first achieved by elemental diet or occasionally TPN; it is then prolonged by the avoidance of specific foods which vary from patient to patient. This technique has become the standard management of patients with active Crohn's disease presenting at our clinic. Only those in whom the disease is inactive or those who suffer surgical complications are considered unsuitable for dietary treatment although it is clearly necessary that patients should be able and willing to cooperate with the regime.

Table 32.7 Results of controlled trial of unrefined carbohydrate, fibre-rich diet and exclusion diet.

	UCFR ($\bar{x} \pm$ SD)	FI ($\bar{x} \pm$ SD)
No. recruited	10	10
Withdrawals	0	0
Relapsing before	10	3
six months	($P < 0.05$, Fisher's exact test)	
Mean pre-trial ESR	26 ± 24.0	37.9 ± 21.7 (NS)
Mean pre-trial orosomucoid (%)	232.5 ± 68.2	236.1 ± 89.9 (NS)
Mean time to relapse (months)	1.375 ± 1.74	2.75 ± 1.98
Mean ESR at relapse	30.8 ± 25.7	41.3 ± 28.04
Mean orosomucoid at relapse (%)	220.5 ± 66.9	230 ± 124.89

FI patients in remission for 6 months

	Initial	3 months	6 months
ESR	37.9 ± 21.7	$16.1 \pm 8.8^\star$	$16.2 \pm 12.5^\star$
Orosomucoid (%)	232.5 ± 68.2	$138.3 \pm 36.6^\star$	$140 \pm 41.5^\star$

$^\star P < 0.05$, Student's t test.
Date from Hunter [33], with permission.

The results in 77 patients

Up to the end of September 1984, a total of 77 patients had been started on this management. These patients comprised a broad spectrum of Crohn's disease whose clinical features, including the duration of the disease and the extent of involvement of the gut, are well representative of the condition (Table 32.8).

nation diets. As perhaps might be foreseen, the diet has had no effect on pre-existing rectovaginal and enteric fistulae, nor on fibrous intestinal strictures, although narrowing of the terminal ileum produced by inflammation and oedema has been seen to resolve on radiographs (Fig. 32.2). In all cases an adequate state of nutrition has been achieved. Indicators of systemic inflammation such as the erythro-

Table 32.8 Clinical details of patients with Crohn's disease managed by diet.

M:F ratio	24:53	Previous treatment	
Age range (years)	16–65	Corticosteroids	47
	(Mean 35.5)	Sulphasalazine	31
Length of history (years)	0–20	Azathioprine	10
	(Mean 6)	Long-term antibiotics	10
Extent of disease		Surgery	29
Oral	1	New patient	17
Jejunal	6		
Ileal	20		
Terminal ileal	53		
Colonic	48		
Rectum	11		

Data from Alun Jones et al [4], with permission.

Successful food testing and dietary management. Sixty-four patients have successfully completed the food testing and have remained well on diet alone. The numbers of foods to which they were intolerant and the foods involved are shown in Table 32.9. These figures include patients with extensive Crohn's disease of the colon and the small intestine including the terminal ileum. We have had little experience of patients with severe anal disease. Extraintestinal problems such as arthritis, uveitis and oral ulceration have also cleared on the elimi-

cyte sedimentation rate (ESR) and serum orosomucoid level have returned to normal in most patients (Table 32.10) and repeat radiographs have often shown striking improvements (Figs. 32.2, 32.3).

Relapse rate. Nine of the 64 patients have since relapsed. In two, pre-existing terminal ileal strictures caused subacute obstruction and were resected. In retrospect, early surgery might have been a more appropriate treatment than diet. A further two patients found the

Table 32.9 Subjective food intolerances of 64 patients with Crohn's disease controlled by diet.

No. of provoking foods	No. of patients	Food	No. intolerant
0	5	Wheat	28
1	11	Dairy products	24
2	6	Brassicas	16
3	10	Maize (corn)	12
4	8	Yeast	11 each
5	3	Tomatoes	
6	5	Citrus fruits	10 each
7	5	Eggs	
8	3	Tap water	
9	3	Coffee	8 each
>10	5	Banana	
		Potatoes	
		Lamb	7 each
		Pork	
		Beef	5 each
		Rice	
		Tea	4
		Fish	3
		Onions	2
		Chicken	
		Barley	
		Rye	
		Turkey	
		Additives	1 each
		Alcohol	
		Chocolate	
		Shellfish	
		Swede	

Data from Alun Jones et al [4], with permission

Table 32.10 ESR and orosomucoid values of 64 patients with Crohn's disease controlled by diet.

Time	ESR (mean $\pm$ SD, mm/h)	Orosomucoid (mean $\pm$ SD, %)
Before start of dietary management	34.8 $\pm$ 25.6 *(43)*	215.7 $\pm$ 86.0★ *(41)*
After induction of remission	31.6 $\pm$ 24.6 *(33)*	185 $\pm$ 77.2 *(35)*
0.6 months	24.8 $\pm$ 18.7† *(52)*	156.3 $\pm$ 55.7★ *(51)*
7–12 months	19.1 $\pm$ 13.1★ *(29)*	147 $\pm$ 62.8★ *(25)*
13–18 months	14.4 $\pm$ 12.6★ *(15)*	135 $\pm$ 39.9★ *(15)*
19–24 months	15.9 $\pm$ 15.8† *(12)*	139 $\pm$ 44.4★ *(2)*

Numbers in parentheses refer to number of patients tested; results are of tests done towards the end of the time interval stated.
★$P < 0.01$; †$P < 0.02$; ‡$P < 0.05$ compared with value before start of dietary management (Student's *t* test).
Data from Alun Jones et al [4], with permission.

restrictions of the diet irksome and asked to restart corticosteroids in order to eat freely. One patient with wheat intolerance suffered a severe relapse after remaining well for 36 months and it was later discovered that his bakery had started to include wheat flour in its rye bread. Although he previously had terminal ileal disease, he developed a total Crohn's colitis and a rectal abscess which only settled with prolonged TPN, corticosteroids and surgical drainage. Three patients relapsed for no obvious reason although in two this followed a bout of gastroenteritis. One man developed cardiac arrhythmias and proved to have myocardial sarcoidosis requiring corticosteroids.

Failure to complete the dietary regime. Thirteen patients were unable satisfactorily to complete the regime for the detection of food intoler-

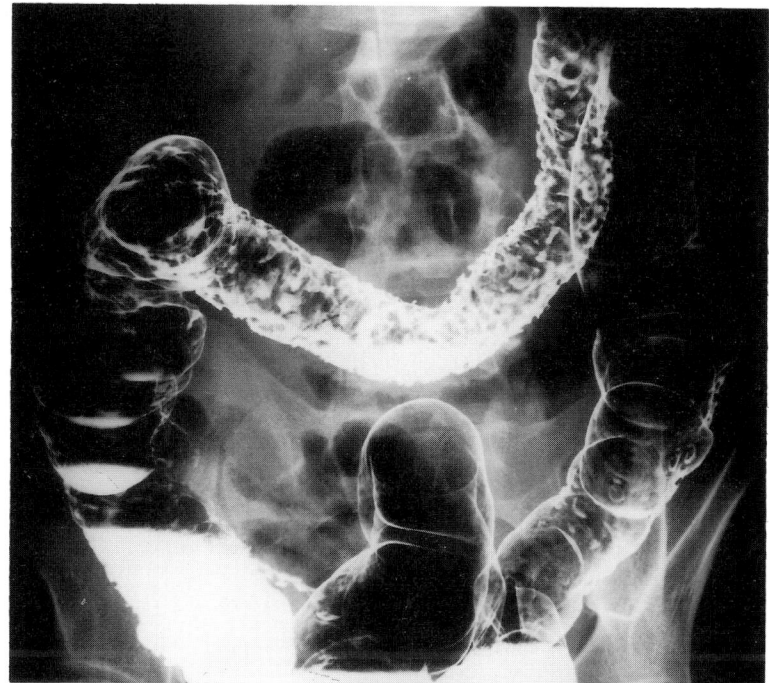

(a)

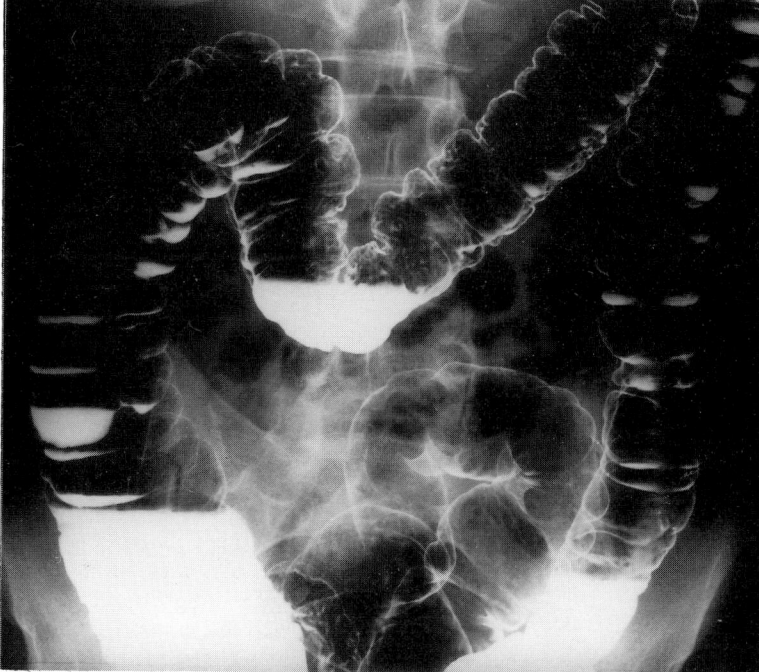

(b)

Fig. 32.2 Barium enema: (a) August 8, 1980, showing classic changes of severe ulcerating Crohn's colitis in the transverse colon with individual ulcers in the descending colon: (b) January 27, 1981, showing healed stage with asymmetrical fibrosis and pseudopolypoid change. From Alun Jones et al [4], with permission.

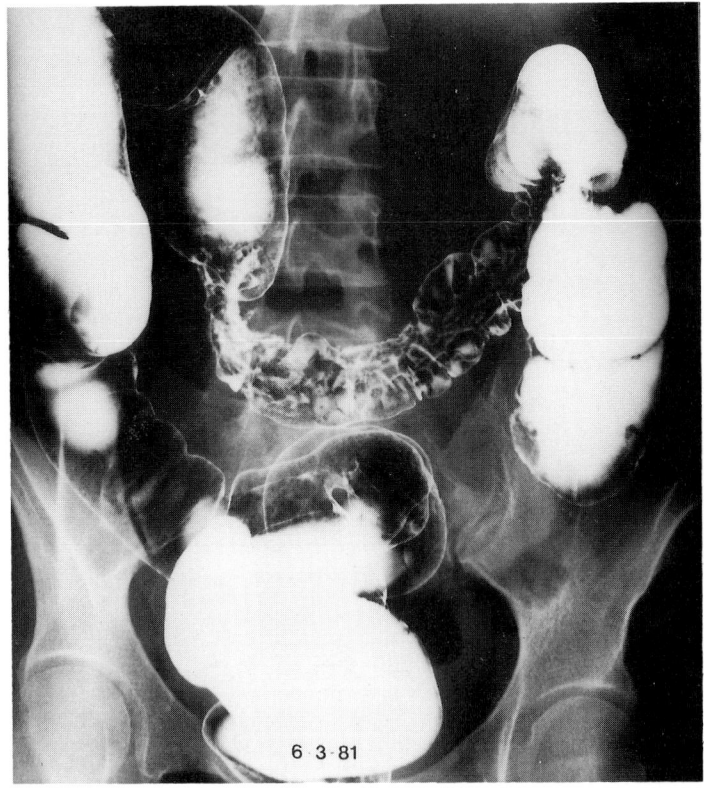

(a)

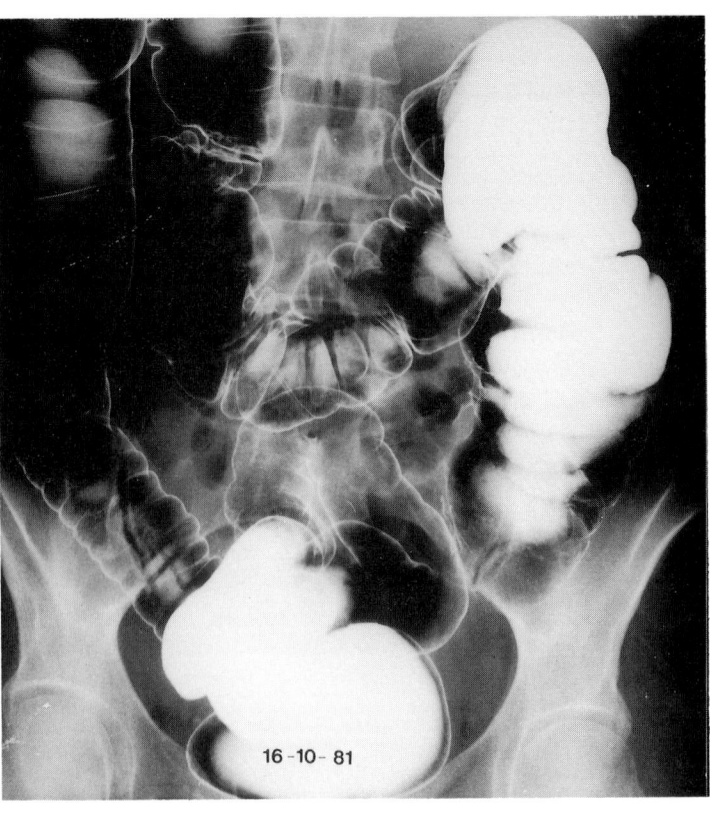

Fig. 32.3 Barium enema: (a) March 6, 1981, showing transverse colon affect by narrowing, ulceration, obliteration of the haustra and skip lesions; (b) October 16, 1981, showing no ulceration and a normally distensible colon, with puckering and pseudodiverticulum formation due to fibrosis from burnt-out Crohn's disease. From Alun Jones et al [4], with permission.

(b)

ances and were thus unable to establish a diet on which they remained symptom free. Inability or unwillingness to persevere with diet was not the only cause of failure to complete the regime although seven patients did come into that category, usually because of pressure from sceptical members of their families. Three patients found so many foods to provoke symptoms that the resulting diet was nutritionally inadequate. Despite a return to conventional medical management all three have since undergone major colonic surgery. Finally, three men relapsed dramatically in the early stages of food reintroduction and all underwent emergency surgery. Because of this we now ask patients with severe Crohn's disease to reintroduce the first few foods under close observation in the hospital, and delay the introduction of foods known to cause difficulty until late in the food reintroduction phase.

Overall results. As four patients have been lost to follow up (who were well up to 9, 11, 19 and 22 months, respectively), 51 remain in remission on diet alone, 15 for more than two years and the longest for 51 months. Three have succeeded in becoming pregnant and numerous patients with long experience of the orthodox management of Crohn's disease and its side effects have emphasized how well they feel on the diets [4].

Effects of diet on relapse rate. The most informative assessment of the value of diet in these patients is provided by the overall relapse rates (Table 32.11). Patients who are successful in establishing a diet have an average relapse rate

of less than 10% per annum over the next three years. This is comparable with the recurrence rate after successful surgery [24, 38]. It would be wrong to draw firm conclusions from a comparison between this work and other reports of the treatment of Crohn's disease, as patient selection may vary and the enthusiasm with which they are treated may influence their progress. However, it helps to put results of dietary management into perspective to realize that in the European Co-operative Crohn's Study [45] the percentage of patients with acute Crohn's who remained in remission after two years treatment with corticosteroids was less than 40%. The two-year percentage for *all* our patients is nearly 65%. If we consider only patients who were successful in establishing a diet the percentage still in remission at two years is much higher at 80%.

It is possible of course that patients who are successful in dietary studies suffer a less severe form of the disease and certainly the overall figures for subsequent surgery in our series (10 out of 13 in those who failed to establish a diet; three out of 64 in those who succeeded) would fit with such an interpretation. However, it could equally be argued that the benefits of the diet are such that they are the cause of the reduction in the need for surgery. Clearly a controlled trial of diet and orthodox management is necessary to establish its true place amongst the various options available.

Table 32.11 Life assurance table of overall relapse rates in 77 patients with Crohn's disease managed by diet.

Interval since treatment (months)	Number well at beginning of interval	Number lost to follow up during interval	Number well observed for only part of interval	Number exposed to risk of relapse during interval	Number relapsing during interval	Proportion relapsing during interval	Proportion remaining well during interval	Proportion remaining well from start of treatment to end of each interval
0–6	77 (64)	0	19	67.5 (54.5)	15 (2)	0.222 (0.036)	0.778 (0.964)	0.778 (0.964)
7–12	43	2	9	37.5	5	0.135	0.865	0.673 (0.834)
14–18	27	0	5	24.5	1	0.041	0.959	0.645 (0.800)
19–24	21	2	6	17	0	0.00	1.0	0.645 (0.800)
25–30	13	0	2	12	0	0.00	1.0	0.645 (0.800)
31–36	11	0	2	10	1	0.1	0.9	0.581 (0.72)
37–42	8	0	4	6	0	0.00	1.0	0.581 (0.72)
43–48	4	0	3	2.5	0	0.00	1.0	0.581 (0.72)
49–54	1	0	0	1	0	0.00	1.0	0.581 (0.72)

Figures in parentheses represent patients who found a suitable diet without difficulty.
Data from Alun Jones et al [4], with permission.

MECHANISMS OF FOOD INTOLERANCE

The objective demonstration of food intolerance in many patients with IBS and our clinical data on Crohn's disease has led to increased interest in the mechanisms linking food to disease. In popular parlance this is clearly an example of 'food allergy' but in detailed studies of patients with food-related IBS before and after challenge, we have yet to succeed in demonstrating a convincing immunological abnormality. Although all three of Bentley et al's [8] patients suffered from atopy, as did 60% of those reported by Smith et al [60], our experience in a much larger series [35] has been that this is true of only 11% of patients, a figure similar to that in the general population. Many workers have found that skin testing whether by prick test or intradermal testing is unreliable in diagnosing food intolerances in these patients [39].

Laboratory studies

Laboratory studies have been largely negative. Lessof et al [40] found that, in contrast to patients with asthma, rhinitis and urticaria, most patients with diarrhoea caused by food intolerances had normal levels of IgE. We have confirmed this finding [6]. In double-blind challenge studies we found no difference between test and control days in the eosinophil count, concentrations of plasma histamine or in immune complexes in the serum. Incubation of basophils with food antigens including milk proteins and gliadin led to no increased release of histamine [42]. We routinely perform jejunal biopsies on patients with wheat intolerance to exclude coeliac disease. However, incubation of the biopsy with gliadin did lead to an increased release of histamine in subjects with wheat intolerance and coeliac disease when compared to controls [43].

Local mucosal immune response

These results raise the possibility of the existence of a previously unrecognized type of local immune response in the jejunum of patients with food-intolerant IBS. However, molecules other than those recognized as messengers of the immune system may occupy the receptor sites on immune effector cells, causing them to release the mediators of the immune response, e.g. histamine [47]. Plant lectins have been shown to be capable of doing this [32], and it is possible that this is the role of gliadin in these patients.

Prostaglandins

The role of prostaglandins in food-intolerant IBS has attracted attention. Buisseret et al [10] reported the case of a woman who suffered diarrhoea after eating mussels but who found that she could prevent this reaction by taking the prostaglandin synthetase inhibitor ibuprofen. Objective challenge confirmed that the ingestion of mussels produced both diarrhoea and an increase in the prostaglandins E_2 and $F_{2\alpha}$ measurable in both blood and faeces, and that ibuprofen could block these effects. A number of similar patients were also described.

Rectal PGE₂. In the light of this report we studied PGE_2 production in the rectum in

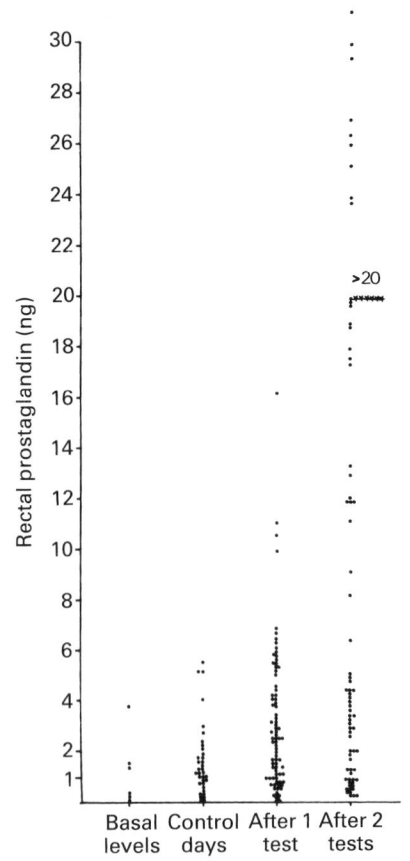

Fig. 32.4 Rectal prostaglandin level in response to food challenge. * For technical reasons, in six patients concentrations > 20 ng could not be determined more accurately. In all these patients the level was > 20 ng but was taken as 20 ng in subsequent analyses. From Alun Jones et al [6], with permission.

patients with food-intolerant IBS [6]. A dialysis bag made of Visking tubing and mounted on a catheter was passed into the rectum of patients undergoing objective double-blind food challenges, and replaced at hourly intervals. PGE_2 was measured by radioimmunoassay. A significant increase in PGE_2 production was seen after food challenge (Fig. 32.4) and in another study PGE_2 production was shown to correlate significantly with faecal weight (Fig. 32.5). Control studies indicated that the

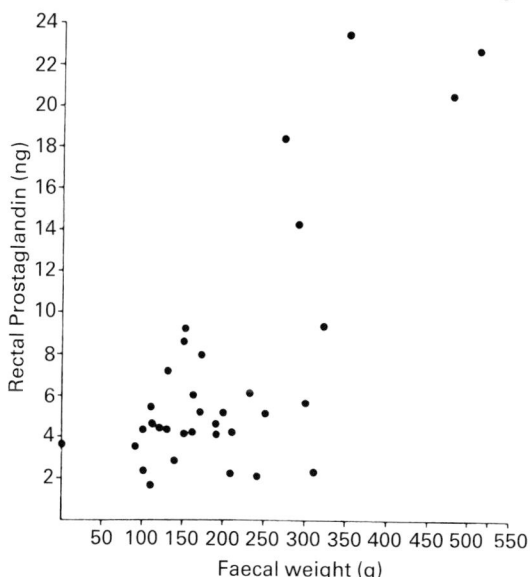

Fig. 32.5 Relation between prostaglandin level and wet faecal weight. From Alun Jones et al [6], with permission.

rise in prostaglandins was not a consequence of the insertion of the dialysis bags [5]. However, although increased PGE_2 production is usual in patients with diarrhoea, it is not universal amongst patients, and those with abdominal pain alone frequently show very little change in PGE_2 after food challenges. What is more, it is our experience that many patients derive little benefit from prostaglandin inhibitors. Thus we believe that the release of prostaglandins is likely to be a secondary phenomenon rather than the true cause of the condition.

Hysterectomy and IBS

Many women with IBS have undergone gynaecological operations [23] and we performed a study to assess prospectively the importance of hysterectomy in the pathogenesis of IBS [3]. In an initial study the course of 113 patients who underwent hysterectomy with or without prophylactic metronidazole was followed. All had been free of gut symptoms preoperatively, but 13 had developed the symptoms of IBS when reviewed six to eight weeks later. Twelve of these were from the 74 who had received prophylactic metronidazole, while only one was from the 39 who had not.

Metronidazole and IBS

A double-blind trial was then set up using metronidazole or placebo suppositories as prophylaxis at the time of hysterectomy. If infection occurred it was treated appropriately by other antibiotics. An analysis of 100 patients (Table 32.12) again supported the aetiological

Table 32.12 Postoperative irritable bowel syndrome in previously asymptomatic patients having metronidazole prophylaxis or placebo with hysterectomy, and those having other antibiotics in addition.

	Patients	Irritable bowel syndrome
Metronidazole alone	26	2
Placebo alone	20	0
Metronidazole + other antibiotics	14	1
Placebo + other antibiotics	22	4

Data from Alun Jones et al [3], with permission.

role of antibiotic usage in the development of IBS. Seven out of the 62 who had received antibiotics developed the syndrome while none did so amongst the 20 who did not receive antibiotics.

Antibiotics and gastrointestinal flora

In view of this relationship between antibiotics and surgery we have undertaken studies on the gastrointestinal flora of patients with IBS [7]. Six patients who were well on a wheat-free diet were found to have high faecal counts of aerobic bacteria compared to age- and sex-matched controls (Table 32.13). In two

Table 32.13 Excretion of aerobic bacteria in faeces.

	n	Samples	Viable bacteria/g dry weight faeces	
			Mean	Range
Patients	6	30	2.2×10^9	$2.9 \times 10^7 - 1.1 \times 10^{10}$
Controls	6	6	9.8×10^7	$3.9 \times 10^6 - 2.7 \times 10^8$

Data from Bayliss et al [7], with permission of authors and Cambridge University Press.

patients, increases of two orders of magnitude in the aerobic count were seen after food challenge (Fig. 32.6). Anaerobic counts did not change and were comparable to those of the controls. Clearly this is an area justifying further investigation.

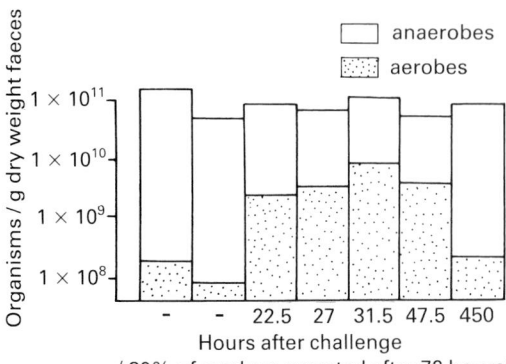

Fig. 32.6 Effect of wheat challenge on faecal flora. From Bayliss et al [7], with permission of the authors and Cambridge University Press.

CONCLUSIONS

Objective food intolerances have been shown by a number of independent workers to occur in some patients with IBS, and the trial of an exclusion diet should be considered in all patients with unexplained colonic pain or diarrhoea. Dietary manipulation represents a therapeutic strategy for the long-term management of Crohn's disease and the results would seen to compare favourably with orthodox treatment without carrying the same risk of side effects. Further controlled trials are necessary finally to establish its value in relationship to other established lines of treatment. Food intolerance may be a factor in the aetiology of Crohn's disease or could be a consequence. The mechanisms of this food intolerance remain obscure, and as yet no definite immunological abnormality has been found.

REFERENCES

1 Almy TP, Tulin M: Alterations in colonic function in man under stress: experimental production of changes simulating irritable colon. Gastroenterology 1947; 8:616–26.

2 Alun Jones V: Irritable bowel syndrome In: Alun Jones V, Hunter JO; eds: Food and the gut. Eastbourne: Baillière Tindall 1985: 208–20.

3 Alun Jones V, Wilson AJ, Hunter JO, Robinson RE: The aetiological role of antibiotic prophylaxis with hysterectomy in irritable bowel syndrome. Obstet Gynaecol 1984; 5 (Supplement 1): S22–S23.

4 Alun Jones V, Dickinson RJ, Workman E et al: Crohn's disease: maintenence of remission by diet. Lancet 1985; ii:177–80.

5 Alun Jones V, McLaughlan P, Shorthouse M et al: Food intolerance, prostaglandins and irritable bowel syndrome. Lancet 1983; i:124.

6 Alun Jones V, Shorthouse M, McLaughlan P et al: Food intolerance: a major factor in the pathogenesis of irritable bowel syndrome. Lancet 1982; ii:1115–17.

7 Bayliss CE, Houston AP, Alun Jones V et al: Microbiological studies on food intolerance. Proc Nutr Soc 1984; 43:16a.

8 Bentley SJ, Pearson DJ, Rix KJB: Food hypersensitivity in IBS. Lancet 1983; ii:295–6.

9 Besterman HS, Sarson DL, Rambaud JC et al: Gut hormone responses in the irritable bowel syndrome. Digestion 1981; 21: 219–24.

10 Buisseret PD, Youlten LJF, Heinzelman DI, Lessof MH: Prostaglandin-synthesis inhibitors in prophylaxis of food intolerance. Lancet 1978; i:906–8.

11 Bullen A: Mechanisms of gluten toxicity in coeliac disease. In: Alun Jones V, Hunter JO, eds: Food and the gut. Eastbourne: Baillière Tindall, 1985: 187–207.

12 Burns TW: Colonic motility in the irritable bowel syndrome. Arch Intern Med 1980; 140: 247–51.

13 Cooke WT, Holmes GKT: Coeliac disease. Edinburgh: Churchill Livingstone, 1984.

14 Cooper BT, Holmes GKT, Ferguson R et al: Gluten sensitive diarrhoea without evidence of coeliac disease. Gastroenterology 1980; 79: 801–6.

15 Corbett CL, Thomas S, Read NW et al: Electrochemical detector for breath hydrogen determination. Measurement of small bowel transit time in normal subjects and patients with IBS. Gut 1981; 22:836–40.

16 Dickinson RJ, Ashton MG, Axon AT et al: Controlled trial of intravenous hyperalimentation and total bowel rest as an adjunct to the routine therapy of acute colitis. Gastroenterology 1980; 79:1199–204.

17 Driscoll RH Jr, Rosenberg IH: Total parenteral nutrition in inflammatory bowel disease. Med Clin North Am 1978; 62:185–201.

18 Drossman DA, Powell DW, Sessions JT: The irritable bowel syndrome. Gastroenterology 1977:73 811–22.

19 Drummond JC, Wilbraham A: The Englishman's food. London: Jonathan Cape, 1959: 254.

20 Duke WD: Food allergy as a cause of abdominal pain. Arch Intern Med 1921; 28:151–65.

21 Duke WD: Food allergy as a cause of illness. J Am Med Assoc 1923; 81:886–9.

22 Farah DA, Calder I, Benson L, Mackenzie JF: Specific food intolerance: its place as a cause of gastrointestinal symptoms. Gut 1985; 26:164–8.

23 Fielding JF: The irritable bowel syndrome. 1; Clinical spectrum. Clin. Gastroenterol 1977; 6:607–22.

24 Fielding JF, Cooke WT, Williams JA: The incidence of recurrence in Crohn's disease. Surg Gynecol Obstet 1972; 134:467.

25 Fischer JE, Foster JS, Abel RM et al: Hyperalimentation as primary therapy for inflammatory bowel disease. Am J Surg 1973; 125: 165–73.

26 Fung W-P, Kho KM: The importance of milk intolerance in patients presenting with chronic (nervous) diarrhoea. Aust NZ J Med 1971; 1:374–6.

27 Gerrard JW: Food intolerance. Lancet 1984; ii:83–99.

28 Hanauer SB, Sitrin MD, Bengoa JM et al: Long term

follow-up of patients with Crohn's disease treated by supportive TPN. Gastroenterology, 1984; 86:1106.

29 Harvey RF, Salih SY, Read AW: Organic and functional disorders in 2000 gastroenterology out-patients. Lancet 1983; i:632-4.

30 Heaton KW: IBS: still in search of its identity. Br Med J 1983; 287:852-3.

31 Heaton KW, Thornton JR, Emmett PM: Treatments of Crohn's disease with an unrefined-carbohydrate, fibre-rich diet. Br Med J 1979; ii:764-6.

32 Helm RM, Froese A: Binding of the receptors for IgE by various lectins. Int Arch Allergy Appl Immunol 1981; 65:81-4.

33 Hunter JO: The dietary management of Crohn's disease. In: Alun Jones V, Hunter JO; eds: Food and the gut. Eastbourne: Baillière Tindall, 1985; 221-37.

34 Hunter JO, Alun Jones V: Studies in the pathogenesis of irritable bowel syndrome produced by food intolerance. In: Read NW; ed: The irritable bowel syndrome. New York: Grune and Stratton, 1985; 185-90.

35 Hunter JO, Workman E, Alun Jones V: Dietary studies. In: Gibson PR, Jewell DP, eds: Topics in gastroenterology, 12. Oxford: Blackwell Scientific, 1985: 305-13.

36 Hunter JO, Alun Jones V, Freeman AH et al: Food intolerance in gastrointestinal disorders. In: Second Fisons Food Allergy Workshop. Oxford: Medicine Publishing Foundation, 1983: 69-72.

37 Korelitz BI: Therapy of inflammatory bowel disease including use of immunosuppressive agents. Clin Gastroenterol 1980; 9:331-49.

38 Lee ECG, Papaionnou N: Recurrences following surgery for Crohn's disease. Clin Gastroenterol 1980; 9:419-38.

39 Lehmann CW: A double blind study of sub-lingual provocation food testing: a study of its efficacy. The leukocytic food allergy test: a study of its reliability and reproducibility. Effect of diet and sub-lingual food drops on this test. Ann Allergy 1980; 45:144.

40 Lessof MH, Wraight DG, Merrett TG et al: Food allergy and intolerance in 100 patients. Q J Med 1980; 195:259-71.

41 Longstretch GF, Fox DD, Youkeles L et al: Psyllium therapy in the irritable bowel syndrome: a double blind trial. Ann Int Med 1981; 95:53-6.

42 McLaughlan P, Easter GB, Hunter JO, Coombs RRA: Histamine release from blood basophils. In: The Second Fisons Food Allergy Workshop. Oxford: Medicine Publishing Foundation, 1983; 52-3.

43 McLaughlan P, Hunter JO, Easter GB et al: Histamine release *in vitro* from the jejunal mucosa following challenge with gliadin and also anti-IgE. In: The Second Fisons Food Allergy Workshop. Oxford: Medicine Publishing Foundation, 1983; 7-9.

44 McMichael HB, Webb J, Dawson AM: Lactose deficiency in adults: a cause of 'functional diarrhoea'. Lancet 1965; i:717-20.

45 Malchow H, Ewe K, Brandes JW et al: European co-operative Crohn's disease study: results of drug treatment. Gastroenterology 1984; 86:249-66.

46 Manning AP, Heaton KW, Uglow P, Harvey RF: Wheat fibre and the irritable bowel syndrome: a controlled trial. Lancet 1977; ii:417-18.

47 Moneret-Vautrin DA: False food allergies: non-specific reactions of foodstuffs. In: Lessof MH, ed: Clinical reactions to food. Chichester: John Wiley, 1983: 135-53.

48 Morin CL, Roulet M, Roy CC et al: Continuous elementaı enteral alimentation in the treatment of children and adolescents with Crohn's disease. J Parenter Nutr 1982; 6:194-9.

49 Mullen JL, Clark Hargrove W, Dudrick SJ et al: Ten years experience with intravenous hyperalimentation and inflammatory bowel disease. Ann Surgery 1978; 187:523-9.

50 The National Co-operative Crohn's Disease Study. Gastroenterology 1979; 77:825-944.

51 Newcomber AD, McGill DB: Irritable bowel syndrome. Role of lactose deficiency. Mayo Clin Proc 1983; 58:339-41.

52 O'Morain C, Segal AW, Levi AJ: Elemental diets in the treatment of acute Crohn's disease. Br Med J 1980; 281:1173-5.

53 O'Morain C, Segal AW, Levi AJ: Elemental diet as primary therapy of acute Crohn's disease; a controlled trial. Br Med J 1984; 288:1859-62.

54 Ostro MJ, Greenberg GR, Jeejeebhoy KN: TPN and complete bowel rest in the management of Crohn's disease. Gastroenterology 1984; 86:1203.

55 Raymer D, Weininger O, Hamilton JR: Psychological problems in children with abdominal pain. Lancet 1984; i:439-40.

56 Reilly J, Ryan JA, Strole W, Fishcer JE: Hyperalimentation in inflammatory bowel disease. Am J Surg 1976; 131:192-200.

57 Rowe AH: Food allergy. Its manifestations, diagnosis and treatment. J Am Med Assoc 1928; 91:1623-31.

58 Rowe A Jr, Uyeyama K: Regional enteritis—its allergic aspects. Gastroenterology 1953; 23:554-71.

59 Sachar DB, Auslander MO, Walfish JS: Aetiological theories of inflammatory bowel disease. Clin Gastroenterology 1980; 9:231-57.

60 Smith MA, Youngs GR, Barnes RMR, Finn R: Food intolerance and atopic status in the irritable bowel syndrome. Abstracts of the British Society of Gastroenterology Spring Meeting 1985: F67.

61 Soltoff J, Krag B, Gudmand-Hoyer E et al: A double blind trial of the effects of wheat bran on symptoms of irritable bowel syndrome. Lancet 1976; i:270-2.

62 Stanworth DR: The scope for pseudo-allergic responses to foods. In: Alun Jones V, Hunter JO, eds: Food and the gut. Eastbourne: Baillière Tindall, 1985: 113-20.

63 Svedlund J, Sjodin I, Ottoson J-O, Dotevall G: Controlled study of psychotherapy in irritable bowel syndrome. Lancet 1983; ii:589-91.

64 Thompson WG, Heaton KW: Functional bowel disorders in apparently healthy people. Gastroenterology 1980; 79:283-8.

65 Walker Smith JA: Cow's milk intolerance and other related problems in infancy. In: Alun Jones V, Hunter JO, eds: Food and the gut. Eastbourne: Baillière Tindall, 1985.

66 Weser E, Rubin W, Ross L, Sleisenger MH: Lactose deficiency in patients with the 'irritable bowel syndrome'. N Engl J Med 1965; 273:1070-5.

67 Whorwell PJ, Clouter C, Smith CL: Oesophageal motility in the irritable bowel syndrome. Br Med J 1981; 282:1101-2.

68 Workman EM, Alun Jones V, Wilson AJ, Hunter JO: Diet in the management of Crohn's disease. Hum Nutr Appl Nutr 1984; 38A:469-73.

69 Young SJ, Alpers DH, Norland CC, Woodruff PA: Psychiatric illness and the irritable bowel syndrome. Gastroenterology 1976; 70:162-6.

Chapter 33
Paediatric Gastrointestinal Food-Allergic Disease

R. P. K. Ford and J. A. Walker-Smith

Introduction

Gastrointestinal food-allergic diseases may be defined as those clinical syndromes characterized by the onset of gastrointestinal symptoms following food ingestion, where the underlying mechanism is an immunologically mediated reaction within the gastrointestinal tract. These symptoms may be accompanied by other manifestations outside the alimentary tract such as in the skin or the respiratory tract.

Patterns of illness

The number of adverse reactions to foods claimed to effect the gastrointestinal tract is vast. They range from an acute anaphylactic reaction, even leading to death, to relatively minor symptoms which are difficult to distinguish from other disorders such as toddler's diarrhoea or psychological disorders with gastrointestinal symptoms.

Frequently more than one system is involved in an adverse reaction to a food and the observed patterns of system involvement vary considerably between authors. The overall clinical patterns of system involvement for milk sensitivity are shown in Table 33.1. Gastrointestinal manifestations have been re-ported in the majority of children in most studies and often gastrointestinal symptoms were seen alone. The large variations between observations can probably be explained by the differences in criteria used to establish the diagnosis, the preselection bias of the investigators, the age of the patients and perhaps the pattern of infant feeding in a particular community.

In infancy and early childhood the proteins of cow's milk and soya have been highlighted as the major causes of food-allergic syndromes, although wheat (in individuals in whom coeliac disease has been excluded), egg, rice, fish, chicken meat and corn, as well as tomatoes, oranges, bananas and chocolate have been reported to produce gastrointestinal symptoms in some individuals [4]. The adverse responses to some of these foods have been much better documented than others as causes of gastrointestinal allergic disease. There is not always a consistent association between an individual food and a particular symptom or symptom complex. While in some individuals a single food may cause an adverse response, in others there may be clinical intolerance to multiple foods. A clear example of this is the varied gastrointestinal responses that may be provoked by the ingestion of cow's milk protein as shown in Table 33.2.

Table 33.1 Patterns of system involvement in cow's milk hypersensitivity.

| Author(s) | Patients: number and age | Percentage of patients with system involved | | | |
		Cutaneous	Respiratory	Gastrointestinal	Gastrointestinal symptoms only
Clein [8]	140 0–1 year	43	10	51	17
Goldman et al [28]	89 0–11 years	45	46	65	17
Gerrard et al [27]	59 0–2 years	46	44	61	15
Buisseret [6]	79 1–16 years	82	93	84	0
Stintzing and Zetterstrom [74]	25 (ages not stated)	40	16	84	50
Hill et al [39]	17 0–5 years	41	12	59	47

Table 33.2 The range of gastrointestinal manifestations seen in cow's milk hypersensitivity.

Common, well-documented manifestations
  Anaphylaxis
  Vomiting
  Diarrhoea, malabsorption, failure to thrive
  Colic, abdominal pain, nausea

Less common, well-documented manifestations
  Occult intestinal haemorrhage
  Protein-losing enteropathy
  Milk-induced colitis
  Functional intestinal obstruction

Unsubstantiated manifestations
  Intussusception
  Constipation

Furthermore, in the case of cow's milk protein intolerance the symptoms may change with increasing age in the one individual. For example, a child who developed diarrhoea and lethargy in infancy might later develop abdominal pain and irritability, although eventually becoming completely tolerant to cow's milk.

Age of onset and duration

The incidence of gastrointestinal food-allergic diseases is greatest in the first months and years of life and decreases with age. The natural history of gastrointestinal food-allergic disease is best documented for reactions to cow's milk, with most such children developing their adverse symptoms to milk within the first three months of life (Table 33.3).

The reported ranges of age of onset extend

Table 33.3 Age of onset and resolution of cow's milk hypersensitivity.

Author(s)	Patients	Age of onset (range)	Age of resolution (range)
Gyrboski [32]	21	'Most' by 6 weeks (2 days to 4 months)	'Most' by 2 years (8 months to 5 years)
Visakorpi et al [78]	12	NS	90% by 1 year, 100% by 2 years
Kuitunen et al [53]	54	Mean 9 weeks (1 day to 22 weeks)	Mean 13 months (7 months to 2 years)
Harrison et al [37]	25	Mean 10 weeks (1 week to 15 months)	Mean 18.4 months (7 months to 4 years)
Walker-Smith et al [85]	5	Mean 2 weeks (1 week–3 weeks)	100% by 2 years
Verkasalo et al [77]	65	Mean 9 weeks	97% by 2 years 100% by 3 years

NS = not stated.

from one day to 15 months old. The age at which these children were first exposed to milk will of course influence this to some extent. Adverse symptoms to milk become less severe with increasing age [11], and most children have become fully tolerant of milk by two years of age. Adequate catch-up growth has usually occurred by this time if there has been a period of growth failure. Verkasalo et al [77] found that after clinical tolerance to cow's milk had developed, one-third of their patients had persistent minor symptoms that did not seem to be associated with drinking milk. These symptoms included occasional abdominal pains, a tendency to have loose stools or constipation, eczema and recurrent respiratory infections, particularly otitis media. It is not known if these symptoms are related to an underlying gastrointestinal food allergy.

CLINICAL SYNDROMES

The major adverse gastrointestinal reactions to cow's milk are vomiting, diarrhoea and abdominal pain. These symptoms are also frequently seen in many childhood illnesses such as generalized infections, gastroenteritis, parasitic infestation, sugar malabsorption and stress-related psychosomatic illnesses. Symptoms must therefore be accurately assessed in relation to milk ingestion, and careful guidelines used for the diagnostic differentiation of gastrointestinal food-allergic disease from other conditions.

Time of onset of symptoms

Broadly, gastrointestinal reactions to food may be divided into those which manifest quickly—within minutes to an hour after taking the food—and those in which the onset is slower, taking several hours and even days to become manifest [22, 61]. The former syndromes are usually easy to diagnose on historical grounds and levels of food-specific IgE antibodies are usually raised. By contrast, the slow onset reactions are often difficult to diagnose clinically and the currently available diagnostic investigations may be impractical for general use.

An outline of the manifestations and clinical syndromes of gastrointestinal food-allergic disease is shown in Table 33.4.

Table 33.4 Manifestations and clinical syndromes seen in gastrointestinal food-allergic disease in children.

Quick onset reactions
    Anaphylaxis
    Vomiting, diarrhoea and abdominal pain

Slow onset reactions
    Vomiting, pallor and irritability
    Food-sensitive enteropathies
    Transient gluten intolerance

Other gastrointestinal reactions
    Milk-induced colitis
    Infantile colic
    Occult intestinal haemorrhage
    Protein-losing enteropathy
    Functional intestinal obstruction
    Oesophagitis
    Allergic gastroenteropathy
    Eosinophilic gastroenteritis
    Infantile colic

Quick onset reactions

Anaphylaxis

Acute anaphylaxis is the most serious of the quick onset gastrointestinal food reactions. Anaphylaxis results from a generalized immediate IgE-mediated reaction following the introduction of a sufficient amount of antigen into a previously sensitized individual which releases histamine and other biologically active mediators from sensitized mast cells. This phenomenon of an acute anaphylactic reaction to an ingested food represents the most severe extreme of the clinical spectrum of gastrointestinal food-allergic disease [12, 28] and may even result in death [19]. (Anaphylaxis is discussed in Chapter 25.)

Vomiting, diarrhoea and abdominal pain

Acute vomiting with or without diarrhoea and frequently accompanied by other system involvement is commonly the presenting feature of quick onset gastrointestinal reactions. These reactions occur within minutes to an hour of the food being ingested with often only small amounts of food needed to precipitate such a reaction. These reactions may occur at the first exposure to the food, the child having been previously sensitized via the breast milk [5] (see Chapter 18) or even in utero [58]. Many foods may produce such reactions.

Breast feeding and cow's milk allergy. Some entirely breast-fed infants are exquisitely sensitive to cow's milk. Small amounts of cow's milk given as a complement feed or in solids may lead to a rapid onset of vomiting which will cease when cow's milk is completely withdrawn from the diet. Often such vomiting may be accompanied by the onset of eczema. In some infants the lips and tongue may swell immediately upon contact with cow's milk and this oedema is sometimes associated with urticaria and angioedema which may in fact be the major presenting clinical problem. Characteristically these children have increased levels of total serum IgE and elevated milk-specific IgE antibodies [22] which can be demonstrated by skin prick test and RAST (radioallergosorbent test) responses. They also tend to have lower titres of IgG, IgA and IgM milk antibodies than do infants who develop cow's milk protein intolerance some months after they have been fed with cow's milk [20].

Egg hypersensitivity. Vomiting within a few minutes to an hour of egg ingestion is seen in about a quarter of children with egg hypersensitivity [56] (see Chapter 19). Diarrhoea, abdominal pain and nausea may also occur [21]. However, skin and respiratory manifestations also frequently occur and are usually a more important part of the clinical presentation than gastrointestinal symptoms. Again, skin prick test and RAST responses to egg are usually positive.

Acute abdominal pain. Acute abdominal pain seems to be a particular feature of fish hypersensitivity [64], whilst peanuts often produce immediate reactions of the oral mucosa [88] as well as abdominal pain.

Multiple food sensitivities. Some individuals have gastrointestinal and other symptoms related to a wide variety of foods. Such patients characteristically have a number of quick onset symptoms such as vomiting, urticaria or wheezing upon exposure to multiple foods. They often have an individual and family history of atopy, peripheral eosinophilia, elevated total serum IgE and positive RAST and skin tests to specific foods. Diets involving the elimination of a number of foods may be impractical or ineffective on their own. However, treatment with sodium cromoglycate may be highly effective as has been shown in the group of children described by Syme [75], and also in older patients reported by Wraith et al [88] but the therapeutic dose is empirical at present [52]. Curiously, if oral sodium cromo-

glycate alleviates the symptoms then these may not relapse when the drug is subsequently discontinued. These patients need to be distinguished from those with eosinophilic gastroenteritis.

Slow onset reactions

Slow onset reactions are much more difficult to diagnose because of the difficulty of associating symptoms with a food taken hours or even days before. However, in general the pathology is more site-specific. The problem is usually one of establishing whether or not the observed gastrointestinal pathology is in fact caused by an adverse immunological reaction to a food. Here elimination of the suspected food or foods and their subsequent reintroduction into the diet as food challenge is at the heart of the diagnostic approach.

Food-sensitive small intestinal enteropathies

Changes in the structure of the small intestinal mucosa in response to the ingestion of particular foods provide clear objective evidence of food-sensitive disorders involving the small intestinal mucosa. The approach of using serial small intestinal mucosal biopsies combined with dietary elimination and challenge has been adapted from the Interlaken Criteria used to diagnose coeliac disease [60]. However, the time scale is compressed in these disorders which unlike coeliac disease are transient conditions. Using this approach a number of foods have now been shown to produce sensitive enteropathy (Table 33.5).

Table 33.5 Food-sensitive enteropathies so far described

Cow's milk [53, 85]
Wheat [84]
Soya [1]
Chicken [79]
Egg [42]
Fish [79]
Rice [79]

Mechanisms. From the studies reported by Ferguson [18] in the experimental animal it seems likely that the enteropathy may be caused by a Type IV or T cell [26] mediated reaction. A Type I reaction in the gut is associated with only minimal changes of mast-cell degranulation and some oedema, while

Type III reactions are associated with polymorph infiltration and do not cause crypt hyperplasia. Of course more than one type of allergic response may coexist within the mucosa at any one time.

Gastroenteritis. Sometimes it appears that acute gastroenteritis may precede the development of food sensitivity enteropathy. However, although there is an association between postenteritis enteropathy and food-sensitive enteropathy in early infancy [79, 83], which condition came first is often impossible to establish. Acute gastroenteritis causes damage to the small bowel mucosal epithelium [2] which may permit the entry of excess food antigen into the body with subsequent food protein sensitization. It is therefore possible that gastroenteritis may predispose to the development of food hypersensitivity. Clinical support for this concept has been given by two groups [33, 37] who have both implicated an IgA deficiency as an underlying factor. However, the relationship between gastroenteritis and milk hypersensitivity has not been found by others [35].

IgA deficiency. There is evidence that IgA deficiency is associated with the development of gastrointestinal food hypersensitivity. This may be due to inadequate immune exclusion in the early months of life allowing sensitization to inhaled and ingested antigens [73]. IgA in colostrum and breast milk may give passive mucosal protection in this vulnerable period [30]. IgA deficiency has been found associated with milk hypersensitivity [33, 37, 62], although a defect in the quality of the IgA produced is also possible [59].

Food antigen absorption. Food antigens can be absorbed unaltered through the intestinal mucosa [70, 81]. These antigenically active proteins are not absorbed in sufficient quantity to be of nutritional importance, but enough can be absorbed to stimulate antibody production [7]. The vast majority of individuals show no ill effects from this limited intestinal permeability to large molecules, so it seems likely that other factors must be involved before clinical food protein hypersensitivity occurs.

Premature and newborn infants have been shown to have increased gastrointestinal permeability to β-lactoglobulin compared with older children or adults [67] which seems to be related to gut immaturity. A similar pattern of intestinal permeability has been found using small inert sugars as permeability probes [3].

Increased levels of food antigen are found in patients with diseases that damage the gastrointestinal tract such as gastroenteritis [31], inflammatory bowel disease [72] and coeliac disease. Also increased gastrointestinal permeability to polyethylene glycol (PEG) has been found in children with eczema, whether or not they had any food protein hypersensitivity [46]. In addition, studies with horseradish peroxidase have established that there is increased antigen entry via damaged enterocytes in cases of postenteritis enteropathy [45]. However, so far there has been no clear relationship found between food protein hypersensitivity and altered gastrointestinal transport of macromolecules. An hypothesis incorporating these interrelationships is illustrated in Fig. 33.1. Sugar permeability in gastroenteritis is shown in Fig. 33.2

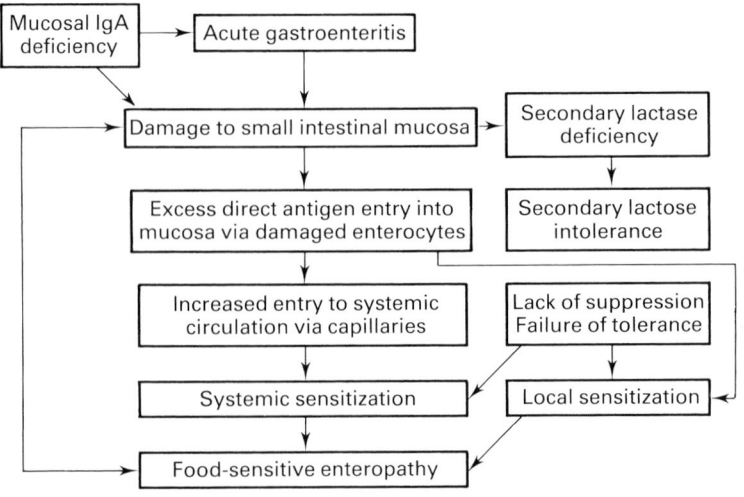

Fig. 33.1 Interrelationships between gastroenteritis, IgA deficiency and milk hypersensitivity. From Walker-Smith JA: Cow's milk intolerance and other related problems in infancy. In: Hunter JO, Alun Jones V eds: Food and the gut. Eastbourne: Baillière Tindall, 1985; 166–86, with permission.

MAJOR FOOD-SENSITIVE ENTEROPATHIES

Cow's milk sensitive enteropathy

Cow's milk sensitive enteropathy is a condition usually characterized by combinations of diarrhoea, vomiting, abdominal pain and failure to thrive following the ingestion of cow's milk protein in infancy. This reaction to milk is usually slow in onset, and not associated with atopic illness or positive specific IgE responses to milk [22]. Various tests to assess the integrity of the small bowel mucosa have been used to investigate this condition but often with conflicting reports of their diagnostic value.

Initially, the use of small bowel biopsy convincingly demonstrated that cow's milk protein could cause severe small bowel mucosal damage in young infants who had diarrhoea and were failing to thrive [53]. Once this

relationship between cow's milk protein and mucosal damage had been established, further studies performed before and after milk challenge documented mucosal changes after milk provocation [54]. Iyngkaran et al [43] subsequently suggested that evidence of mucosal damage should be necessary for the firm diagnosis of gastrointestinal milk hypersensitivity. However, not all children with gastrointestinal symptoms provoked by cow's milk protein have this recognizable mucosal damage [25, 39] and conversely histological damage has been observed in children who have developed no clinical symptoms with milk [69, 71]. Thus, unlike coeliac disease, this enteropathy is not necessarily an invariable finding on a single proximal biopsy from all such children. Nevertheless, when present, the enteropathy can be shown to be cow's milk sensitive by serial biopsies related to withdrawal and challenge with cow's milk (Fig. 33.3).

Pathology. Unlike the gluten-sensitive enteropathy of untreated coeliac disease, this cow's milk sensitive enteropathy is of variable severity on proximal mucosal biopsy, and patchy in its distribution. There is typically a thin mucosa [57], although a flat mucosa indistinguishable from the mucosal appearances found in coeliac disease may also occur. More often lesser degrees of mucosal abnormality are found. After a positive milk challenge, alteration in microvilli of the enterocyte may be seen in parallel with a fall in disaccharidase activity. In untreated cow's milk sensitive enteropathy, intraepithelial lymphocyte numbers are high, although not as high as found in coeliac disease. Subsequently these fall to a level below normal on a milk-free diet. Although the numbers of intraepithelial lymphocytes may rise again after a positive milk challenge, the level reached is usually within the normal range [66].

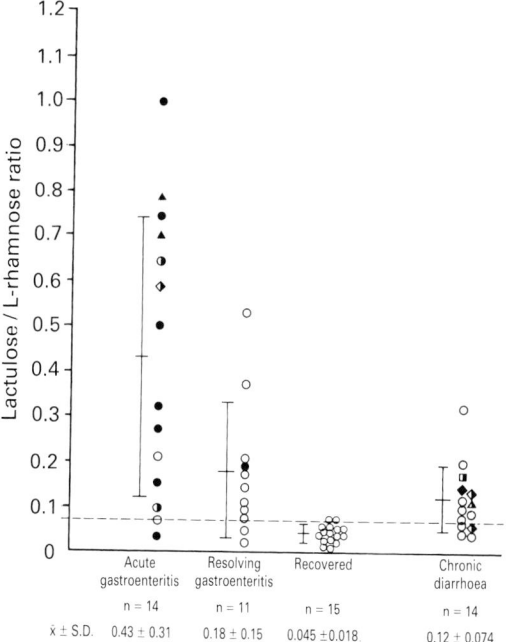

Fig. 33.2 Lactulose/L-rhamnose urinary excretion ratios expressed as percentage of the oral load, and pathogens detected in each clinical group. The dashed line represents the upper limit of normal. Horizontal bars with vertical lines denote mean and standard deviation of each group. Symbols: ○, none detected or no sample; ●, rotavirus; ▲, adenovirus; ◆, cornavirus; ◑, *Campylobacter*; ◈, *Cryptosporidia*; ◪, *Escherichia coli*; ▲, *Salmonella*; □, *Giardia*. From Ford RPK et al: Intestinal sugar permeability: relationship to diarrhoeal disease and small bowel morphology. J Pediatr Gastroenterol Nutr 1985; 4:568–74.

Clinical features. Most children with gastrointestinal symptoms due to cow's milk protein intolerance develop their sensitivity to milk within their first six months of life. In most of these children there is no family history of atopy or cow's milk protein intolerance. Symptoms may either present acutely or with the gradual onset of chronic diarrhoea.

Those with an acute presentation usually have sudden vomiting, with or without diarrhoea, occurring within one to four hours of drinking milk. This often follows their first known drink of milk. The vomiting may be

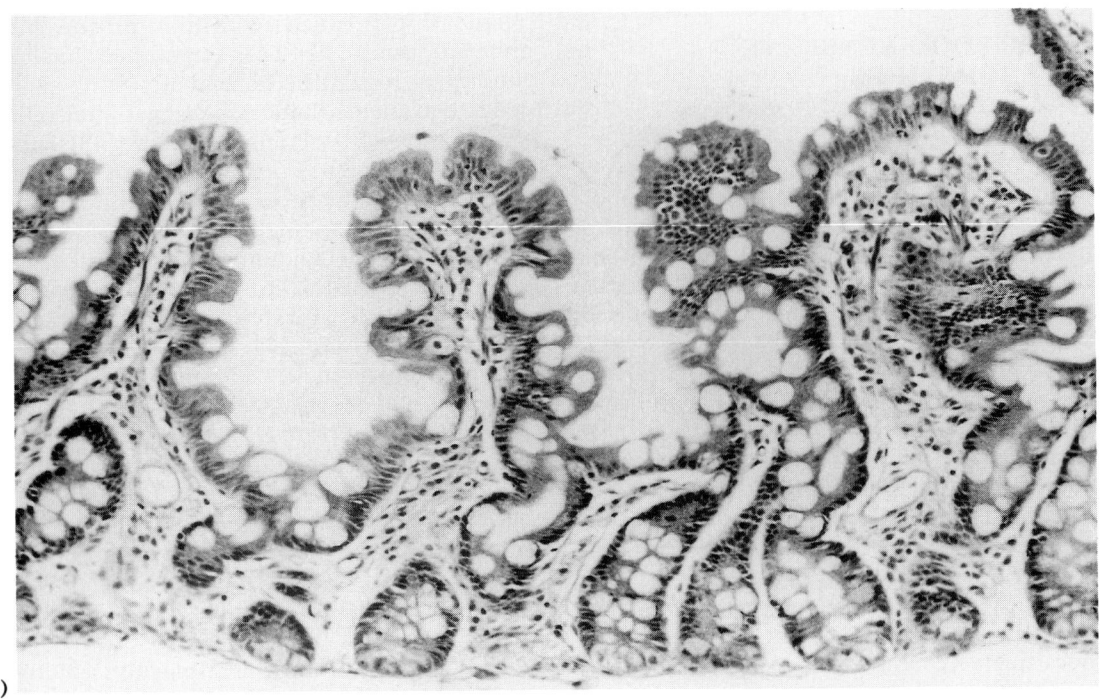

(a)

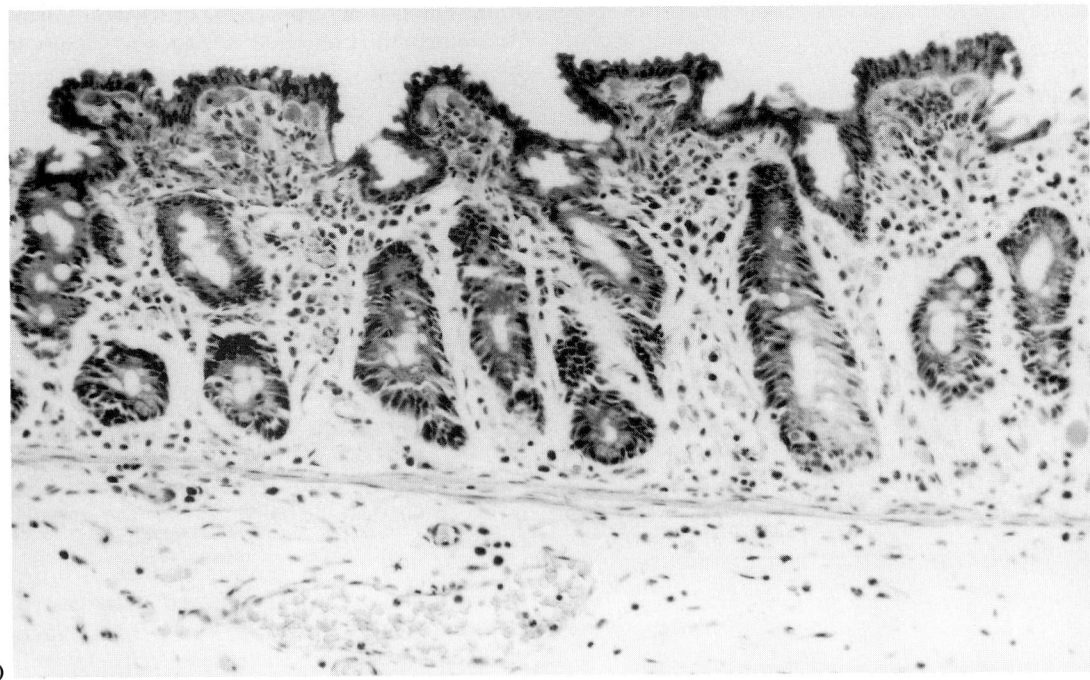

(b)

Fig. 33.3 Serial small intestinal biopsy before and after cow's milk challenge. (a) On a cow's milk free diet. (b) After a cow's milk challenge.

bile stained. It is frequently associated with pallor, lethargy, limpness and tachypnoea. The vomiting is usually short lived but can be protracted for several hours. If no further milk is given, the child will recover completely within four to six hours. This type of reaction is usually not associated with skin eruptions although in a child with eczema, existing lesions may transiently become red and itchy. If cow's milk continues to be given in the diet, the symptoms will persist but often with less intensity.

Differential diagnosis. It may be impossible at first to distinguish such symptoms from an acute episode of gastroenteritis, especially as it is not possible to detect a stool pathogen in most cases of acute gastroenteritis unless stool electron microscopy can be used to identify viral particles. Furthermore, cow's milk protein intolerance may itself be a sequel to gastroenteritis. Such infants may have been tolerating cow's milk feedings for several months up until this time. It is also important to recognize postenteritis lactose intolerance, but the two disorders may overlap [83].

Chronic symptomatology. The chronic presentation of cow's milk sensitive enteropathy usually manifests as chronic diarrhoea with failure to thrive. The clinical features are suggestive of coeliac disease except that the child may not be taking gluten. These children have usually been bottle fed from birth with their symptoms developing within the first six months of life. They often have a history of irritability and colic.

Soya-sensitive enteropathy

Ament and Rubin [1] have described damage of the small intestinal mucosa which improved with withdrawal of soya protein from the diet. The prevalence of soya-induced enteropathy is not known, but it is likely to increase if soya-based formulae are chosen more frequently as the feeding formulae for normal infants.

The events of soya enteropathy have been assumed to mirror those of cow's milk sensitive enteropathy. The close morphological similarity between cow's milk sensitive and soya-sensitive enteropathy has now been demonstrated in a thorough histological and immunological study by Perkkio et al [65]. Soya-sensitive enteropathy may occur on its own or as a sequel to cow's milk sensitive enteropathy.

Transient gluten intolerance

Transient gluten intolerance may be defined as the syndrome seen when a child with gastrointestinal symptoms and an abnormal small intestinal mucosa responds clinically and histopathologically to a gluten-free diet, but who subsequently thrives on a normal gluten-containing diet with the small intestinal mucosa remaining normal. Dicke in Holland, in 1952, described a transient wheat sensitivity

in preschool children after enteritis [13, 14]. Later, a similar state of transient gluten intolerance was described in 28 children, which in some cases was associated with cow's milk protein intolerance [78]. However, these reports did not include serial small intestinal biopsies. Children with transient gluten intolerance investigated by serial biopsies have subsequently been described [82, 84].

Pathology. The small intestinal mucosa is by definition abnormal with partial or total villus atrophy. Only long-term follow-up with serial small bowel biopsies can allow this retrospective diagnosis to be made in a child with a flat mucosa who earlier responded clinically to gluten withdrawal, but who subsequently has thrived on a gluten-containing diet.

Clinical features. In infants less than one year of age transient gluten intolerance should be considered as part of the differential diagnosis of an infant who develops gastrointestinal symptoms when he first encounters wheat protein, especially when intolerances to other food proteins such as milk and egg are present. This diagnosis should also be considered as a possibility in a child whose diet includes gluten and who fails to thrive following gastroenteritis in the presence of an abnormal small intestinal mucosa.

Other-food sensitive enteropathies

Recently infants have been described with food-sensitive enteropathies to fish, rice, chicken [79] and egg [42] diagnosed by serial small bowel biopsies in conjunction with dietary elimination and challenge. In all cases intolerance to these foods was preceded by cow's milk protein intolerance and was temporary. Thus present evidence indicates that a number of transient food-sensitive enteropathies do exist in infancy.

OTHER GASTROINTESTINAL REACTIONS

The following types of gastrointestinal reaction are for the most part probably related to the slow onset type pattern, and so are generally not associated with the presence of food-specific IgE antibodies.

Food-sensitive colitis

Rubin, in 1940, described rectal loss of fresh

blood which responded to cow's milk withdrawal [68]. Gryboski, in 1967, described eight children with cow's milk colitis established by elimination and challenge [32]. The main clinical features were explosive bloody diarrhoea, shock, pallor and colitis. This diagnosis was based upon evaluation of sigmoidoscopic appearances. No pathogens were isolated. The advent of safe colonoscopy and multiple mucosal biopsy even in early infancy has clearly established eosinophilic or allergic colitis as an important cause of chronic bloody diarrhoea in infancy [10, 49]. Colonoscopically there is erythema of the mucosa with aphthoid ulceration. Histopathologically, infiltration with eosinophils has been reported although Gryboski and Walker [34] describe a histopathological appearance not dissimilar to ulcerative colitis. Even breast-fed infants whose mothers drink much cow's milk may develop cow's milk colitis [55]. β-Lactoglobulin has been demonstrated in the breast milk of lactating mothers although the amounts are very small (see Chapter 18).

Differential diagnosis. This disorder needs to be distinguished from ulcerative colitis and Crohn's colitis. Ulcerative colitis has been observed to remit in a group of five children when on a milk-free diet, all having both symptomatic and histological relapse after milk was reintroduced [76]. It is possible that this was a secondary effect of increased antigen absorption through a diseased bowel mucosa with subsequent immune-complex deposition causing symptoms. Milk-specific antibodies were not measured in these children, although a later study [89] showed that children with high levels of specific antibodies to whole cow's milk relapsed more frequently than those with lower levels. These relapses were not necessarily caused by milk ingestion. It has also been suggested that proctitis may at times be caused by local IgE-mediated reaction to cow's milk protein [38].

Thus a response to cow's milk elimination may not accurately discriminate between these disorders and the diagnosis rests upon the histopathology demonstrated by mucosal biopsy and the subsequent clinical course. In food-sensitive colitis there is usually a dense infiltration of eosinophils in the mucosa with the lesion resolving on food elimination.

Occult intestinal haemorrhage

Occult gastrointestinal blood loss has been described in association with cow's milk inges-

tion. The first report [86] concerned 13 infants seen in a well-baby clinic aged 7–84 months who had iron-deficiency anaemia. Nine of these children had been fed with homogenized milk, of whom seven (78%) had precipitins to whole cow's milk compared with only two (17%) of 12 controls. These findings were later confirmed [87] with another 17 children who had occult gastrointestinal blood loss induced by whole cow's milk. In some children it was associated with hypoproteinaemia and oedema. Heat-labile cow's milk proteins, possibly bovine serum protein, were incriminated as aetiological agents. Occult blood loss was also observed after the ingestion of fresh goat's milk in some children, but was not seen with boiled cow's milk, proprietary heat-modified cow's milk formulae or soya-based formulae. When iron supplements were given while cow's milk ingestion was continued, the iron-deficiency anaemia improved in only 20% of the children, but improvement was seen in all children as soon as milk was withdrawn from the diet.

Others [63] have suggested that the increased milk precipitins and hypoproteinaemia may have resulted from altered gut permeability caused by iron deficiency rather than a primary hypersensitivity to milk. Holland et al [40] also observed an association between the presence of serum precipitins to cow's milk and the incidence of recurrent respiratory tract disease, iron-deficiency anaemia and failure to thrive. Precipitins to bovine serum albumin and bovine α-globulin were the most common. However, 17% of these children with increased precipitin to milk had no ill health despite continued milk ingestion.

Gastritis. Gastritis may also be a cause of gastrointestinal blood loss caused by cow's milk hypersensitivity. Four infants have been described [9] who had erosive gastritis or gastroduodenitis diagnosed by endoscopy. Vomiting, poor growth and iron-deficiency anaemia were the prominent clinical features associated with occult blood loss. One child had chronic diarrhoea. All children became asymptomatic on a milk-free diet with adequate weight gain and the endoscopic appearances of the upper gastrointestinal tract returned to normal. With later milk provocation, all children developed slow onset reactions.

Protein-losing enteropathy

Waldmann et al [80] described six children

presenting with peripheral oedema. This was associated with intermittent diarrhoea and vomiting, anaemia, hypoalbuminaemia, hypogammaglobulinaemia, eosinophilia and growth retardation. Loss of plasma proteins into the gastrointestinal tract was demonstrated in all patients. All of these children developed diarrhoea and vomiting after drinking milk. Three children had detailed studies with milk elimination and challenge which confirmed that the abnormal gastrointestinal protein loss was linked to the drinking of cow's milk.

Functional intestinal obstruction

Three children have been described who repeatedly developed functional intestinal obstruction with symptoms of vomiting and abdominal distension after milk ingestion [24]. No physical obstruction could be demonstrated by X-ray studies, and when milk was eliminated from the diet the symptoms disappeared and there was an improvement in weight gain, appetite and mood.

Intussusception

Two children have been described who developed ileocolic intussusceptions during a period of milk ingestion [32]. They had been diagnosed as being hypersensitive to milk by fulfilling Goldman's criteria [28]. At surgery they had enlarged mesenteric lymph nodes. There was good evidence given for implicating milk as the aetiological agent.

Constipation

In one study [8] chronic constipation was found in 5% of infants and children thought to have milk hypersensitivity. They developed normal stools when milk was removed from the diet. Another study [6] mentions constipation as a symptom of milk hypersensitivity but its frequency and severity were not mentioned. Weaning on to cow's milk is frequently associated with the faeces becoming firmer and less frequent. This change is probably due to differences in the physical nature of the diet. There is no evidence that constipation following cow's milk feeding is likely to be immunologically mediated.

Aphthous ulcers

Mouth, oesophageal and stomach aphthous ulcers have been reported in up to 20% of the population [29]. They may occur in association with coeliac disease and Crohn's disease. Dolby and Walker [15] have reported the successful use of sodium cromoglycate in a proportion of such ulcers, but whether they are truly food allergic in nature is uncertain. Forget et al [23] have described eosinophilic infiltration of the oesophagus which may be food related. Katz et al [51] have described eosinophilic infiltration of the stomach associated with a history of food intolerance, response to food avoidance and laboratory evidence of reaginic allergy (see Chapter 29).

Eosinophilic gastroenteritis

Eosinophilic gastroenteritis is characterized by protein-losing enteropathy, peripheral eosinophilia and iron-deficiency anaemia secondary to gastrointestinal blood loss. This condition must be distinguished from cow's milk sensitive enteropathy, although it merges with other disorders such as the 'allergic gastroenteropathy' described by Waldmann et al [80]. The pathological classification is confused [50] and not all reports clearly indicate that this is a definite food-allergic disorder. Some patients appear resistant to elimination diets and require treatment with corticosteroids, thus suggesting different pathogenesis.

Infantile colic

'Colic' is a ubiquitous part of infant behaviour in Westernized societies. It usually refers to a picture of episodes of restlessness due to presumed abdominal discomfort with eructation and flatulence. Many causes such as maternal anxiety or aerophagy distending the gut have been put forward. This behaviour pattern is so common that it is likely that many causes exist, but several studies have suggested that colic is frequently associated with milk ingestion [27, 28]. Although older children perhaps may also get abdominal pain or nausea, available data refer only to infants.

IgE plasma cells. Increased numbers of IgE-producing plasma cells have been found in the duodenal biopsy tissue of infants with colic after seven days of cow's milk feeding, suggesting that colic may be an IgE-mediated response to cow's milk protein [36]. However, most such children have negative skin prick responses to milk.

Milk-free diet. Relief from colic has been observed in breast-fed infants whose mothers have been put on a diet free of cow's milk and dairy products, the colic returning when maternal milk ingestion was recommenced [47]. On the other hand, a similar study [17] found no such association between milk ingestion by the mother and colic in the infant. Colic was not significantly more common on days when mothers drank cow's milk, but increased with increasing diversity of maternal diet. These studies also showed that cow's milk antigen could be found in mother's milk equally often in infants with or without colic.

Cow's milk intolerance. A prospective study by Jacobsson and Lindberg [48] in Sweden diagnosed, with two clinically positive challenges, 20 out of nearly 1000 infants as having cow's milk intolerance; all 20 had colic and seven had gastrointestinal symptoms only. Four of these infants were breast fed and suffered colic unless their mothers avoided cow's milk in their diet.

It seems that without a very clear clinical picture of relapse on challenge, or evidence of major atopy, that cow's milk avoidance as a treatment for so common a disorder as infantile colic may have little other than a placebo effect in the majority of babies for whom it might be considered. Thus although children with cow's milk protein intolerance frequently have colic, children with colic do not necessarily have cow's milk protein intolerance.

Irritable colon syndrome and Crohn's disease

In adults it has recently been reported that food elimination can induce a clinical remission in the irritable colon syndrome and also in some patients with Crohn's disease [41]. Whether this represents food-allergic disease has been discussed in Chapter 32.

Migraine-related gastrointestinal symptoms

Egger et al [16] reported a study investigating the effect of an oligoantigenic diet on 88 children with severe migraine. Two-thirds of these children had accompanying symptoms of abdominal pain, diarrhoea and flatulence. When treated for their migraine with the oligoantigenic diet, the majority (86%) also had alleviation of their gastrointestinal symptoms. The mechanism of these reactions was presumed to be of an allergic nature. That it was food causing these symptoms was confirmed by double-blind food provocation (see Chapter 38).

SUMMARY

The range of gastrointestinal manifestations caused by allergic food disease is vast. These can be broadly clinically categorized into quick and slow onset reactions. The quick onset reactions which occur within minutes to an hour of taking the food are usually associated with elevated specific food IgE antibodies, positive skin prick tests and atopy. Only small amounts of the foods are usually required to provoke such reactions. The slow onset reactions usually occur between one and four hours after food ingestion but may take days to manifest. These reactions are not associated with increased IgE-specific antibodies and often more of the food is required to produce any symptoms.

REFERENCES

1 Ament ME, Rubin CE: Soy protein—another cause of the flat intestinal lesion. Gastroenterology 1972; 62:227–34.

2 Barnes GL, Townley RRW: Duodenal mucosal damage in 31 infants with gastroenteritis. Arch Dis Child 1973; 48:343–9.

3 Beach RC, Menzies IS, Clayden GS, Scopes JW: Gastrointestinal permeability changes in the preterm neomate. Arch Dis Child 1982; 57:141–5.

4 Bleumink E: Allergies and toxic protein in food. In: Hekkens WTJM, Pena AS eds: Coeliac disease. Leyden: Kroese, 1975: 46–55.

5 Bjorksten F, Saarinen UM: IgE antibodies to cow's milk in infants fed breast milk and milk formulae. Lancet 1978; ii: 624–5.

6 Buisseret PD: Common manifestations of cow's milk allergy in children. Lancet 1978; i: 304–5.

7 Carswell F, Ferguson A: Food antibodies in serum—a screening test for coeliac disease. Arch Dis Child 1972; 47: 594–6.

8 Clein NW: Cow's milk allergy in infants. Ann Allergy 1951; 9: 195–204.

9 Coello-Ramirez P, Larraso-Haro A: Gastrointestinal occult hemorrhage and gastroduoderitis in cow's milk protein intolerance. J Pediatr Gastroenterol Nutr 1984; 3:215–18.

10 Cucchiara S, Guandalini S, Staiano A et al: Sigmoidoscopy, colonoscopy and radiology in the evaluation of children with rectal bleeding. J Pediatr Gastroenterol Nutr 1983; 2:667–71.

11 Dannaeus A, Johansson SGO: A follow-up of infants with adverse reactions to cow's milk. Acta Paediatr Scand 1979; 68:377–82.

12 de Peyer E, Walker-Smith JA: Cow's milk intolerance presenting as necrotizing enterotizing enterocolitis. Helv Paediatr Acta 1977; 32:509.

13 Dicke WK: De subacute, chronische en recidiverende darmstoornis van de kleuter. Ned Tijdschr Geneesk 1952; 96:860.

14 Dicke WK, Weijers HA, van de Kamer JH: Coeliac disease presence in wheat of a factor having a deleterious effect in coeliac disease. Acta Paediatr Scand 1953; 42:34–42.

15 Dolby AE, Walker DMA: Trial of cromoglycic acid in recurrent aphthous ulceration. Br J Oral Surg 1975; 12:292–5.

16 Egger J, Carter C, Wilson J et al: Is migraine food allergy? Lancet 1983; ii:865–8.

17 Evans RW, Fergusson DM, Allardyce RA, Taylor B: Maternal diet and infantile colic in breast fed infants. Lancet 1981; i:1340–2.

18 Ferguson A: Pathogenesis and mechanisms in the gastrointestinal tract. In: Proceedings of the First Fisons Food Allergy Workshop. Oxford: Medicine Publishing Foundation, 1980:28–38.

19 Finkelstein H: Kuhmilch als ursache akuter ernathrungstorungen bei sauglingen. Monatsschr Kinderheilkd 1905; 4:65–72.

20 Firer MA, Hosking CS, Hill DJ: Effect of antigen load on development of milk antibodies in infants allergic to milk. Br Med J 1981; 283:693–6.

21 Ford RPK, Taylor B: Natural history of egg hypersensitivity in childhood. Arch Dis Child 1982; 57:649–52.

22 Ford RPK, Hill DJ, Hosking CS: Cows milk hypersensitivity: immediate and delayed onset clinical patterns. Arch Dis Child 1983; 58:856–62.

23 Forget P, Eggermont E, Marchall G et al: Eosinophilic infiltration of the oesophagus in the infant. Acta Paediatr Belg 1978; 31:91–3.

24 Freier S: Paediatric gastrointestinal allergy. Clin Allergy (Suppl) 1973; 3:597–618.

25 Freier S, Kletter N, Gery I et al: Intolerance to milk protein. J Pediatr 1969; 75:623–31.

26 Gell PGH, Coombs RRA: Classification of allergic reactions. In: Gell RGH, Coombs RRA, eds: Clinical aspects of immunology. Oxford: Blackwell Scientific Publications.

27 Gerrard JW, MacKenzie JW, Goluboff N et al: Cow's milk allergy: prevalence and manifestations in an unselected series of newborns. Acta Paediatr Scand (Suppl), 1973; 234:1–21.

28 Goldman AS, Anderson DW, Sellers WA et al: Milk allergy. Pediatrics 1963; 32:425–43.

29 Graysowski EA, Barile MF, Lee WB, Stanley HR: Recurrent aphthous stomatitis; clinical, therapeutic, histopathologic, and hypersensitivity aspects. JAMA 1966; 196:637–44.

30 Gross SJ, Buckley RH, Wakil SS et al: Elevated IgA concentration in milk produced by mothers delivered of preterm infants. J Pediatr 1981; 99:389–93.

31 Gruskay FL, Cooke RE: The gastrointestinal absorption of unaltered protein in normal infants and in infants recovering from diarrhoea. Pediatrics 1965; 16:763–7.

32 Gryboski JD: Gastrointestinal milk allergy in infants. Pediatrics 1967; 40:354–62.

33 Gryboski JD, Kochoshis S: Immunoglobulin deficiency in gastrointestinal allergies. J Clin Gastroenterol 1980; 2:71–6.

34 Gryboski JD, Walker WA: The colon, rectum and anus. In: Gryboski JD, Walker WA eds. Gastrointestinal problems in the infant, 2nd ed. Philadelphia: WB Saunders, 1983:524.

35 Halliday K, Edmeades R, Shepherd R: Persistent post-enteritis diarrhoea in childhood. A prospective analysis of clinical features, predisposing factors and sequelae. Med J Aust 1982; 18:2.

36 Harris M, Petts V, Penny P: Cow's milk allergy as a cause of infantile colic: immunofluorescent studies on jejunal mucosa. Aust Paediatr J 1977; 13:276–81.

37 Harrison M, Kilby A, Walker-Smith JA et al: Cow's milk protein intolerance: a possible association with gastroenteritis, lactose intolerance, and IgA deficiency. Br Med J 1976; i:1501–4.

38 Heatley RV, Calcraft BJ, Fifield R: Immunoglobulins in rectal mucosa of patients with proctitis. Lancet 1975; ii:1010–12.

39 Hill DJ, Davidson GP, Cameron DJS, Barnes GL: The spectrum of cow's milk allergy in childhood. Acta Paediatr Scand 1979; 68:847–52.

40 Holland NH, Hong R, Davis NC, West CD: Significance of precipitating antibodies to milk proteins in the serum of infants and children. J Pediatr 1962; 61:181–95.

41 Hunter JO, Jones A, Freeman AH et al: Food intolerance in gastrointestinal disorders. In: Proceedings of Second Food Allergy Workshop. Oxford: Medicine Publishing Foundation, 1983:721.

42 Iyngkaran N, Abidain Z, Meng LL, Yadav M: Egg-protein-induced villous atrophy. J Pediatr Gastroenterol Nutr 1982; 1:29–35.

43 Iyngkaran N, Robinson MJ, Prathap K et al: Cow's milk protein sensitive enteropathy: combined clinical and histological criteria for diagnosis. Arch Dis Child 1978; 53:20.

44 Iyngkaran N, Robinson NJ, Sumithran E et al: Cow's milk protein-sensitive enteropathy. An important factor in prolonging diarrhoea in acute infective enteritis in early infancy. Arch Dis Child 1978; 53:150–3.

45 Jackson D, Walker-Smith JA, Phillips AD: Macromolecular absorption by histologically normal and abnormal small intestinal mucosa in childhood: an in vitro study using organ culture. J Pediatr Gastroenterol Nutr 2:235–48.

46 Jackson PG, Lessof MH, Baker RWR et al: Intestinal permeability in patients with eczema and food allergy. Lancet 1981; i:1285–6.

47 Jacobsson I, Lindberg T: Cow's milk as a cause of infantile colic in breast fed infants. Lancet 1978; ii:437–9.

48 Jacobsson I, Lindberg T: Prospective study of cow's milk protein intolerance in Swedish infants. Acta Paediatr Scand 1979; 68:853–9.

49 Jenkins HR, Milla PJ, Pincott TR et al: Food allergy: the major cause of infantile colitis. Pediatr Res 1983; 431 (Abstract).

50 Johnstone JM, Morson BC: Eosinophilic gastroenteritis. Histopathology 1978; 2:335–48.

51 Katz AJ, Goldman H, Grand RJ: Gastric mucosal biopsy in eosinophilic (allergic) gastroenteritis. Gastroenterology 1977; 73:705–9.

52 Kochoshis S, Gryboski JD: Use of cromolyn in combined gastrointestinal allergy. JAMA 1979; 242:1169–73.

53 Kuitunen P, Visakorpi JK, Hallman N: Histopathology of duodenal mucosa in malabsorption syndrome induced by cow's milk. Ann Paediat 1965; 205:54–63.

54 Kuitunen P, Rapola J, Savilahti E, Visakorpi JK: Light and electron microscopic changes in the small

intestinal mucosa in patients with cow's milk induced malabsorption syndrome. Acta Paediatr Scand 1972; 61:237.

55 Lake AM, Whitington PF, Hamilton SR: Dietary protein-induced colitis in breast fed infants. J Pediatr 1982; 101:906-10.

56 Langeland T: A clinical and immunological study of allergy to hen's egg white. Clin Allergy 1983; 13:371-82.

57 Maluenda C, Phillips AD, Briddon A, Walker-Smith JA: Quantitative analysis of small intestinal mucosa in cow's milk sensitive enteropathy. J Pediatr Gastroenterol Nutr 1984; 3:349-56.

58 Matsumura T, Kuroume T, Oguri M et al: Egg sensitivity and eczematous manifestations in breast-fed newborns with particular reference to intrauterine sensitization. Ann Allergy 1975; 35:221-9.

59 McDonald D, Habeshaw J, Malpas JS et al: Case report an unusual immune deficiency syndrome. Paediatric Research Society of Australia. Annual Meeting; 1983.

60 Meeuwisse G: Diagnostic criteria in coeliac disease. Acta Paediatr Scand 1970; 59:461-3.

61 Minford AMB, MacDonald A, Littlewood JM: Food intolerance and food allergy in children: a review of 68 cases. Arch Dis Child 1982; 57:742-7.

62 Minor JD, Tolber SG, Frick OL: Leukocyte inhibition factors in delayed-onset food allergy. J Pediatr 1980; 66:314-21.

63 Naiman JL, Oski EA, Diamond LK et al: The gastrointestinal effects of iron-deficiency anemia. Pediatrics 1964; 33:83-99.

64 Nizami RM, Lewin PK, Baloo MT: Oral cromolyn therapy in patients with food allergy: a preliminary report. Ann Allergy 1977; 39:102-5.

65 Perkkio M, Savilahti E, Kuitunen P: Morphometric and immunochemical study of jejunal biopsies from children with intestinal soy allergy. Eur J Pediatr 1981; 137:63-9.

66 Phillips AD, Rice SJ, France NE, Walker-Smith JA: Small intestinal lymphocyte levels in cow's milk protein intolerance. Gut 1979; 20:509-12.

67 Roberton DM, Paganelli R, Dinwiddie R, Levensky RJ: Milk antigen absorption in the preterm and term neonate. Arch Dis Child 1982; 57:369-72.

68 Rubin MI: Allergic intestinal bleeding in the newborn—a clinical syndrome. Am J Med Sci 1940; 200:385-90.

69 Savilanti E: Immunochemical study of the malabsorption syndrome with cow's milk intolerance. Gut 1973; 14:491-501.

70 Schloss OM, Warthen TW: The permeability of the gastroenteric tract of infants to undigested protein. Am J Dis Child 1916; 11:342-62.

71 Shiner M, Ballard J, Brook CGD, Herman S: Intestinal biopsy in the diagnosis of cow's milk protein intolerance without acture symptoms. Lancet 1975; ii:1060-3.

72 Shorter RG, Huizenga KA, Spencer RJ: A working hypothesis of the etiology and pathogenesis of non-specific inflammatory bowel disease. Am J Digest Dis 1972; 17:1024-32.

73 Soothill JF, Stokes CR, Turner MW et al. Predisposing factors and the development of reaginic allergy in infancy. Clin Allergy 1976; 6:305-19.

74 Stintzing G, Zetterstrom R: Cow's milk allergy, incidence and pathogenic role of early exposure to cow's milk formula. Acta Paediatr Scand 1979; 68:383-7.

75 Syme J: Investigation and treatment of multiple intestinal food allergy in childhood. In: Pepys J, Edwards AM, eds: The mast cell: its role in health and disease. Tunbridge Wells: Pitman Medical, 1979:438-42.

76 Truelove SC: Ulcerative colitis provoked by milk. Br Med J 1961; i:154-60.

77 Verkasalo M, Kuitunen P, Savilahti E, Tiilikainen A: Changing pattern of cow's milk intolerance. Acta Paediatr Scand 1981; 702:89-295.

78 Visakorpi JK, Immonen P: Intolerance to cow's milk and wheat gluten in the primary malabsorption syndrome in infancy. Acta Paediatr Scand 1967; 56:49-56.

79 Vitoria JC, Camarero C, Sojo A et al: Enteropathy related to fish, rice and chicken. Arch Dis Child 1982; 57:44-8.

80 Waldmann TA, Wochner RD, Laster L, Gordon RS Jr: Allergic gastroenteropathy. A cause of excessive gastrointestinal protein loss. N Engl J Med 1967; 276:761-9.

81 Walker WA, Isselbacher KJ: Progress in gastroenterology uptake and transport of macromolecules by the intestine. Possible role in clinical disorders. Gastroenterology 1974; 67:531-50.

82 Walker-Smith JA: Transient gluten intolerance. Arch Dis Child 1970; 45:523-6.

83 Walker-Smith JA: Cow's milk intolerance as a cause of post-enteritis diarrhoea. J Pediatr Gastroenterol Nutr 1982; 1:163-75.

84 Walker-Smith JA, Phillips AD: The pathology of gastrointestinal allergy. In: Pepys J, Edwards AM, eds: The mast cell: its role in health and disease. Tunbridge Wells: Pitman Medical, 1979:31-9.

85 Walker-Smith JA, Harrison M, Kilby A et al: Cow's milk sensitive enteropathy. Arch Dis Child 1978: 53:375-80.

86 Wilson JF, Heiner DC, Lahey ME: Studies on iron metabolism: I. Evidence of gastrointestinal dysfunction in infants with iron deficiency anaemia; A preliminary report. J Pediatr 1962; 60:787-800.

87 Wilson JF, Lahey ME, Heiner DC: Studies on iron metabolism: V. Further observations on cow's milk-induced gastrointestinal bleeding in infants with iron-deficiency anaemia. J Pediatr 1974; 84:335-44.

88 Wraith DG, Young GVW, Lee TH: The management of food allergy with diet and Nalcrom. In: Pepys J, Edwards AM, eds: The mast cell: its role in health and disease. Tunbridge Wells: Pitman Medical 1979; 443-6.

89 Wright R, Truelove SC: Circulating antibodies to dietary proteins in ulcerative colitis. Br Med J 1965; ii:142-4.

SECTION D
SKIN

Chapter 34
Atopic Eczema

Michael Pike and David J. Atherton

Clinical presentation

'Eczema' is a distinctive cutaneous response to a variety of traumatic stimuli. A number of fairly characteristic subtypes of eczema can be identified on clinical grounds, of which one of the most important is atopic eczema, the subject of this chapter.

Atopic eczema is largely a disease of children, especially of young children, and is therefore often referred to as 'infantile' eczema. This is a term best avoided, since other types of eczema also occur in infants, notably primary irritant eczema of the napkin area, and also because the disease frequently starts after infancy, occasionally even appearing for the first time in adult life. Nevertheless, the onset is usually early in infancy with 50% of cases developing the disease by six months of age and 75% by 12 months. The overall incidence in childhood is now 10–15%, and there is evidence that this is steadily increasing [90]. Highly irritating lesions generally appear first on the convexities of the face, soon spreading to those of the limbs. Subsequently the face clears and the disease tends to settle in the limb flexures, though in the more severely affected its distribution can be more or less universal (Fig. 34.1). The disease characteristically fluctuates in severity, with a trend to

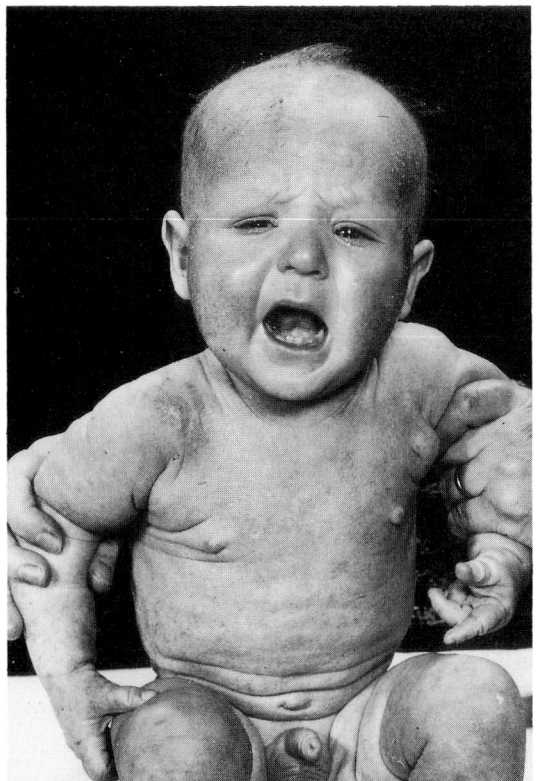

Fig. 34.1 Generalized atopic eczema in a severely affected 10-month-old boy.

spontaneous resolution. Remission occurs within five years of onset in 90% of children [99] and only in about 5% of cases does the disease persist into adult life. It also appears generally true that the later the onset, the worse the prognosis for long-term recovery.

Atopic eczema and IgE

This distinctive pattern of eczema occurs almost exclusively in atopics. However, a closely similar, if not identical, form of eczema has been described in hypogammaglobulinaemic boys [74, 105]. Furthermore, some patients appear to have normal serum IgE levels [46, 69]. Nevertheless, these exceptions aside, it remains true that in the vast majority of cases, this is a disease of atopics, and it is frequently accompanied or succeeded by asthma and/or hayfever. In infants, the development of elevated serum IgE levels precedes and tends to predict the appearance of atopic eczema [52, 62], and the relation between the atopy and the skin disease is clearly a close one. However, the precise nature of this relationship remains obscure and it should be borne in mind that the characteristic cutaneous mani-

festation of an IgE-mediated hypersensitivity reaction in the skin is urticaria, and not eczema.

FOOD ALLERGY AND ATOPIC ECZEMA: THE BACKGROUND

Introduction

There is now a body of literature relating foods and atopic eczema which stretches back over 60 years. Much of it can be justifiably described as anecdotal, consisting of descriptions of open and uncontrolled studies. Furthermore, the literature is bedevilled by a number of preconceptions, particularly that of the central role of IgE antibodies, which have led to confusions that are only now being clarified. These reports are nevertheless worthy of careful review and can be separated into four major categories:
1 Those concerned with evidence of immediate hypersensitivity to food in patients with atopic eczema;
2 Those in which specific foods have been shown to provoke atopic eczema;
3 Those in which elimination diets have been shown to be therapeutically effective;
4 Those in which manipulation of the diet in early infancy has been shown to influence subsequent incidence of atopic eczema.

Evidence of immediate hypersensitivity to food in patients with atopic eczema

Patients with atopic eczema differ from those with asthma and hayfever in having a much higher frequency of positive immediate skin tests to foods [6] and much greater levels of circulating food-specific IgE as measured by the RAST (radioallergosorbent test) [95]. They are also particularly liable to food-induced hypersensitivity reactions of rapid onset, most commonly contact urticaria (see Fig. 34.2), generalized acute urticaria and vomiting. It is thought likely that the underlying mechanism in such reactions is classical Type I hypersensitivity. Sampson used double-blind, placebo-controlled food challenges to demonstrate the frequency of this kind of reaction in patients with atopic eczema [79], their association with a concurrent rise in plasma histamine [81] and their close correlation with positive skin prick tests and IgE antibody measurements [80].

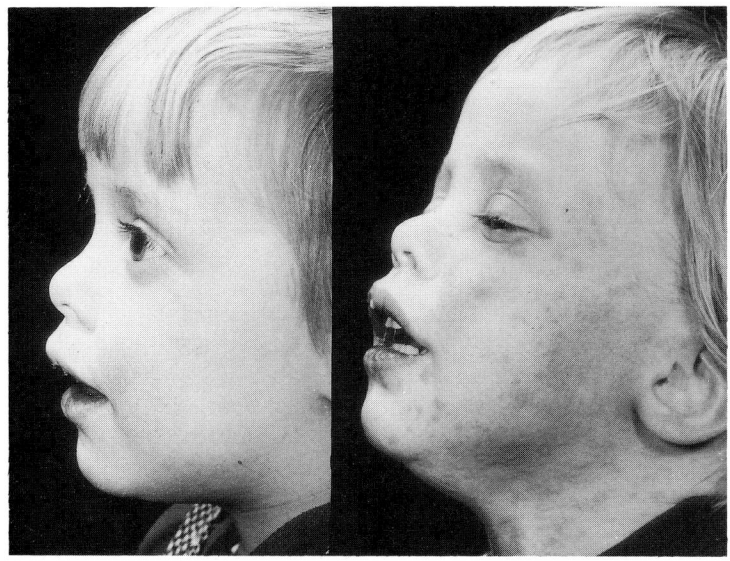

Fig. 34.2 Contact urticaria to egg. This three-year-old boy, with atopic eczema, was photographed before, and 15 minutes after, the application of raw egg-white to his cheek.

Role of IgE

However, although such clinical reactions are themselves assumed to be IgE-mediated, the role IgE antibody plays in the pathogenesis of the associated atopic eczema remains unclear. It appears that skin test reactivity to foods tends to precede reactivity to airborne antigens and is usually transient [97] and the association of the former with atopic eczema, which usually antedates other atopic disease, may not be a causal one. The hypothesis that the scratching precipitated by cutaneous immediate hypersensitivity reactions itself induces eczema [79] is an interesting but as yet unproven one.

Provocation of atopic eczema by foods

Several workers have reported results of studies in which specific foods were administered to eczematous atopic subjects as a 'challenge', in an attempt to elucidate the aetiological role of foods (Table 34.1). One of the first of these was Meara [63], who first eliminated egg from the diet of 29 eczematous children showing positive prick tests to egg only, which resulted in clinical improvement in 11 cases. When egg was subsequently reintroduced, exacerbation of the eczema itself was detected in only two, though eight developed urticarial lesions within minutes of eating egg. Freedman [24] found that 14 out of 48 children with eczema had positive immediate skin tests to cow's milk. The parents reported that milk was responsible for aggravation of the disease in 12 of the 48 cases, and

seven of the positive skin tests occurred in these 12. However, milk challenge was not considered to cause reproducible provocation of the eczema in any child.

Goldman et al [25] challenged 37 children with eczema which was considered by their parents to be aggravated by milk ingestion, and reported that convincing exacerbations followed each of three challenges with milk in 31 of these. Stifler [87] challenged 27 children with a variety of foods to which they had demonstrated positive immediate skin tests, and reported definite exacerbations in four, with equivocal exacerbations in a further six. The author implies that urticarial reactions were frequently present, often being followed later by worsening of the eczema. Sedlis [83] performed similar challenges and found that five out of 27 children who were skin-test positive to egg showed provocation of eczema on challenge. This author similarly noted a high incidence of urticarial reactions on challenge; these were observed in 16 of the 27 children challenged with egg, and in four of the five children who experienced exacerbation of eczema. More recently, Hammar [33] studied 81 unselected children with atopic eczema, all under five years of age. The parents suspected aggravation by cow's milk in seven cases, and in six of these the author reported exacerbation of eczema on challenge with milk in hospital. Of the 73 children with no history of milk aggravation, eight were considered to experience exacerbation of eczema on challenge.

Bonifazi et al [9] studied 134 adults and children with atopic eczema. In this group only three patients out of the total of 24 sub-

Table 34.1 Food challenge studies in atopic eczema.

Author(s)	No. of subjects	Food	Skin tests or RAST		History of provocation		Response to dietary elimination	Skin lesions on challenge		
			+ve	−ve	+ve	−ve		Eczema	Urticaria	All
Meara [63]	112	Egg	29(26%)	83(74%)	—	—	11/29(38%)	2(7%)	8(28%)	8(28%)
Freedman [24]	48	Milk	14(29%)	34(71%)	12(25%)	36(75%)	1(2%)	—	0	0
Goldman et al [25]	37	Milk	—	—	37(100%)	0	—	31(84%)	—	—
Stifler [87]	40	Various	27(68%)	13(32%)	—	—	10/27(37%)	10(25%)	—	—
Sedlis [83]	38	Egg	27(71%)	11(29%)	—	—	—	5/27(19%)	16/27(59%)	17/27(63%)
							—	2/11(18%)	4/11(36%)	4/11(36%)
Hammar [33]	81	Milk	—	—	7(9%)	74(91%)	—	6/7(86%)	—	—
							—	8/74(11%)	—	—
Bonifazi et al [9]	134	Egg and milk	Egg: 37(28%)	—	24(18%)	110(82%)	—	3/24(13%)	—	—
			Milk: 28(21%)				—			
Bonifazi et al [10]	541	Various	—	—	42(8%)	500(92%)	—	13/42(31%)	—	—
Juto et al [47]	20	Milk	—	—	—	—	7/20(35%)	12/19(63%)	—	—
Bock et al [8]	7	Various	7(100%)	0	7(100%)	0	—	4(57%)	3(43%)	5(71%)

jects who had reported aggravation by egg or milk showed exacerbation of eczema by appropriate challenge, though as in several of the other studies, urticarial reactions were relatively common. This study was subsequently extended to include a total of 541 patients, of whom 42 had a history of provocation of the eczema by particular foods [10]. It was reported that an exacerbation of eczema was observed following challenge in 13 of these individuals but not in the other 29. Challenge tests were reported to be positive in only five out of 253 individuals in whom high levels of food-specific IgE were detected in the absence of a history of provocation.

Juto et al [47] challenged 19 children with atopic eczema, all under two years of age, by repeated administration of cow's milk after a period of elimination; eczematous reactions were reported in 12 of the 19. Bock et al [8] used a double-blind challenge technique to study children with histories of a variety of reactions to foods. Amongst these were seven children with eczema whose parents had implicated particular foods, particularly peanuts, eggs and milk. The authors were able to demonstrate exacerbation of eczema on appropriate challenge in four of these seven children.

Conclusions from provocation tests

It is difficult to reach an overall conclusion from these studies since each used its own individual design and all contained what may be regarded as major flaws. Nevertheless, these data do provide evidence that, in at least some individuals with atopic eczema, ingestion of certain foods will provoke a reaction of some kind, be it eczematous or urticarial. They also indicate the need for certain fairly strict criteria, both of design and definition, if a coherent view of the precise role of foods in atopic eczema is to be made possible. Some of these criteria have been incorporated into more recent work and they will be discussed later at greater length.

Treatment of atopic eczema by elimination diets

Open studies

Successful treatment of atopic eczema by exclusion of particular foods from the diet has been reported by numerous authors [29, 33, 47, 50, 56, 77, 83, 87, 89, 98]. These reports describe the open evaluation of simple, empirical elimination diets in fairly large numbers of eczematous children. In spite of the uncontrolled nature of the data, it would be imprudent for the sceptical to reject them out of hand. These authors, all known for their special interest in atopic eczema, and practising in a variety of countries over a period of 60 years, have independently described the value of what has, throughout this period, been an unfashionable therapy.

Controlled studies

Nevertheless, the above reports are unquestionably of a highly subjective nature, and convincing demonstration of benefit from an elimination diet requires properly designed, placebo-controlled studies. The first such study was that of milk and egg exclusion in childhood eczema by Atherton et al [5]. In this study, a diet excluding milk and eggs was selected for trial, on an entirely empirical basis, because these were the foods most frequently implicated by other authors. The problem of a control diet was overcome by the use of a soya substitute, the patients being unaware of the constituents of either diet (it should be remembered that soya preparations were not in current use at that time). A double-blind crossover design was used, in which both diets were taken by every patient, each for a period of four weeks in random order, with an intervening 'washout' period. Neither of the two dermatologists who made the clinical evaluations had previously employed dietary therapy, and both were impressed and somewhat surprised by the unequivocal nature of the results of this study, despite the relatively small number of patients taking part. Over half of the children showed clear preference for, and worthwhile benefit from, the regime avoiding egg and milk.

A more recent study [68], using a similar design but including both children and adults, showed a less striking overall response rate of 25%, though this reached 35% if one considered only those subjects under eight years old. It is conceivable that this less striking response reflects an increased exposure of patients to soya in recent years, particularly in processed foodstuffs, which may render it a less satisfactory milk substitute for such studies than it used to be.

Poor predictive value of history, skin tests and RASTs. Of particular importance in the study by Atherton et al was the finding that many children benefited from egg and milk avoidance in the absence of any previous suspicion that these foods could aggravate the eczema. Also of interest was the lack of any association between response to diet and the presence or absence of positive immediate skin tests or raised serum levels of IgE antibodies to milk and egg antigens [2]. Therefore, neither these tests nor a careful history would have allowed reliable identification of individuals likely to benefit from dietary therapy.

Elemental and oligoantigenic dietary studies

As has been stated, the foods excluded in all the studies mentioned above were chosen empirically, probably because they are the foods most frequently reported by parents to provoke overt allergic reactions. More recently, the possibility that other foods—indeed any food—might be responsible has been pursued. In an open uncontrolled study, Hill and Lynch [39] used an elemental feed (Vivonex, Eaton) in 10 children with severe atopic eczema; they reported an improvement in eight, followed by deterioration when a normal diet was reintroduced. It was not stated whether the children had previously tried a simple milk- and egg-free diet.

Hathaway and Warner [35] described their experience with 40 children who all responded to dietary manipulation. If they were not helped by simple empirical elimination diets, they were given increasingly strict hypoallergenic diets until improvement occurred. Of these 40 children, seven responded to milk and egg exclusion alone. Of the remainder, who had not improved on this simple diet, 30 responded to strict hypoallergenic diets, and three improved only when placed on an elemental feed. The foods responsible for exacerbating the eczema were then identified in the whole group by serial reintroduction, and some of these were confirmed by double-blind challenges. In addition to cow's milk and egg, foods frequently implicated included citrus fruit, colouring and preservatives, nuts, fish, wheat, tomatoes, lamb, chicken and soya, demonstrating that unresponsiveness to a simple diet by no means excludes the possibility of an important provocative role for foods in a child with atopic eczema.

More recently, a placebo-controlled therapeutic trial of an elemental diet in adults with atopic eczema failed to demonstrate benefit [67]. This study raises the possibility that food

provocation of atopic eczema is less frequent in adults than in children. Furthermore, one worries that the possible benefits of such a harsh regime might at least to some degree be counterbalanced by associated deleterious psychological stress.

Breast feeding as prophylaxis for atopic eczema

This issue provides the basis for the fourth broad group of publications relating foods and atopic eczema. It now appears likely that eczema does develop rather more frequently in wholly bottle-fed infants than in wholly breast-fed infants [16, 27, 62, 78]. Nevertheless, conclusive proof is lacking, and several studies have failed to demonstrate this effect [32, 38, 54]. A number of problems are encountered in the design and execution of such studies which help to explain these inconsistencies. One problem is that it is very difficult to be certain that breast feeding has been truly exclusive. Another, and probably more important, problem is the difficulty of obtaining even approximately random allocation to breast or bottle feeding. It would clearly be unethical to allocate a feeding method against maternal preference. A belief that breast feeding may prevent allergic disease is now widespread in the community, so that mothers who themselves have allergic diseases, or whose husbands or children have them, will tend to elect to breast feed more frequently than other mothers [38]. Furthermore, this trend is likely to be particularly pronounced in mothers of higher socioeconomic class. Since a positive family history and high socioeconomic class are both associated with an increased risk of atopic eczema [90], this might easily introduce a bias towards more eczema in the breast-fed infants, which would in its turn tend to obscure any real protective effect.

Children 'at risk'

Careful review of the published data shows, however, that prospective studies that have considered infants genetically at risk as a separate group, and in which exclusive breast feeding has been continued for at least 12 weeks, have fairly consistently shown a protective effect. That this effect is only relative is underlined by the concurrent increasing rates both of breast feeding and of the incidence of the disease. How long the protection lasts is also not clear, though two of the studies demonstrating this effect appeared to show continuing protection many months after stopping exclusive breast feeding [62, 78]. A more recent study, however, suggests that delayed introduction of solids may be more important in prophylaxis than whether the infant was originally fed breast or cow's milk [48]. A further complication is provided by the growing suspicion that the atopic eczema occurring in at least some exclusively breast-fed infants may reflect the transmission, in human milk, of antigens derived from the mother's diet [3] (see Chapter 18).

Conclusions

Taking the data available from the literature as a whole, a strong case can be made for a link between atopic eczema and foods in at least a proportion of affected individuals. The precise nature of this link, and the proportion of patients affected, remain unclear. Nor, as yet, have any in vivo or in vitro characteristics been described that reliably identify these patients. If future studies are to help us answer these questions a number of guidelines need to be established.

Identification of patients. Patients for dietary treatment and foods for exclusion and challenge should *not* be identified solely on the basis of history or of IgE-based investigations such as skin prick tests and RASTs. Apart from doubts about the role of IgE antibodies in pathogenesis, the general relevance of currently available tests for such antibodies in food allergy is questionable, for a number of reasons. For example, important and unrecognized antigens could be inactivated during the preparation of extracts for prick testing or the RAST. Maibach [60] described a patient in whom immediate wealing reactions followed application of fresh foods to the skin, whereas prick tests to the same foods, using commercially prepared extracts, were negative.

It is also quite possible that some important antigens only appear during digestive degradation in the gastrointestinal tract. Spies et al [85, 86] demonstrated the production of potent new antigens by pepsin hydrolysis of a milk protein, β-lactoglobulin, and Haddad et al [28] have published preliminary data suggesting that some patients have IgE antibodies to digestion products of this protein in the absence of antibodies to the intact parent protein. More recently, however, Schwartz et al [82] studied patients with various symptoms apparently caused by allergy to cow's milk, and found that reactivity in the RAST to new antigens produced by pepsin hydrolysis was invariably accompanied by reactivity to the parent protein which was at least as great. Taking these data together it would seem that, for the time being, these tests must be regarded as unreliable predictors of food allergy.

Avoidance of food antigens. All relevant food antigens must be avoided for an adequate period of time to allow improvement to occur. As reported by Hathaway and Warner [35], this may mean excluding a large number of foods for several weeks. Clearly, food challenge studies are only relevant once adequate food elimination has produced an improvement. Diagnostic challenges, undertaken in an individual whose eczema is constantly being exacerbated by the foods which continue to be eaten, are clearly unlikely to produce identifiable changes in the condition.

Diagnostic challenges: double blind. Diagnostic challenges should be given double-blind, though obviously this can be exceedingly difficult. A particular problem in atopic eczema is that the quantity of food generally required to induce a reaction may be relatively large, so that concealment in a capsule is unlikely to be adequate. However, it is possible to conceal reasonable amounts of such foods as tomato, pork, beef and chicken in a fairly strongly flavoured savoury base comprising riceflour, carrots, sage, onion and some caramel to provide additional colour. The base alone can be used as the control material provided the patient has been shown not to react to any of its constituents. Other foods, such as cow's milk, egg and wheat, can more easily be concealed in a sweet base, containing banana, sugar, rice flour and citric acid. All these challenges are prepared in tins, giving a prolonged shelf life. (These products were supplied by courtesy of H. J. Heinz Co Ltd.)

Single challenges. Single diagnostic challenges are almost certainly inadequate. The evidence for this statement is largely anecdotal, but it has been our own experience that, while single challenges frequently fail to elicit an exacerbation of eczema, repeated challenges on successive days may succeed in doing so. Such challenges may need to be given for as many as seven consecutive days before one can conclude that no reaction has occurred.

Time of reactions. Eczematous reactions should be sought for at least 48 hours after the last challenge dose, especially if few test doses were given. Eczematous reactions are often slow to develop [33], and their onset may be delayed for as long as 72 hours after challenge.

Location of challenge. Ideally, diagnostic challenges should be undertaken in the patient's home. The studies mentioned above were largely conducted in hospital, an environment known to have a profound effect on the course of this disease.

THERAPEUTIC IMPLICATIONS

'Simple' empirical diets

All dietary manipulations are difficult if done properly, and it is therefore our view that dietary treatment of atopic eczema should only be proposed when other, less uncomfortable measures, such as emollients, mild topical corticosteroids and oral antihistamines have themselves failed to secure adequate improvement. If this is the case, and the patient and family (in the case of children) are suitable, then it is our practice in the first instance to recommend the empirical elimination from the diet of eggs, chicken—as this shares antigens with egg [55]—cow's milk and artificial colourings and preservatives. If there is a good history of adverse reactions of any kind to other foods, it is clearly wise to ensure that these are also eliminated. It is important that the relevant foods are excluded *totally*, which implies the careful identification and avoidance of any manufactured foods containing these products.

Duration of diet. An elimination diet should be maintained for a minimum of four weeks as benefit may not be apparent if it is any shorter than this. Then, if improvement has occurred, each of the excluded items should be reintroduced separately, allocating seven days for each item and starting with small quantities on the first day of each introduction (see note on anaphylaxis, below). From the second day, each food should be given in at least one normal serving for every day of the introductory week. A period when the child's eczema is fairly stable should be selected for food introductions, and any deterioration during the course of any week of reintroduction should signal the need to renew avoidance of the relevant food for a further period. Where one believes that deter-

ioration may have occurred for other reasons, reintroduction should be attempted again fairly soon afterwards.

Oligoantigenic (oligoallergenic; hypoallergenic) diets

In the individual who still has troublesome eczema in spite of adequate topical therapy and a thorough empirical diet, the possibility of a provocative role for other foods must be considered. However, in our hands, the response rate to more complex diets has been of the order of 25% where an empirical diet has already failed. Therefore, given the considerable difficulties involved, such manoeuvres should be reserved for carefully selected individuals and families in a setting of experienced medical and dietetic support.

The use of hypoallergenic or oligoantigenic diets, such as those in Table 34.2, represents

Table 34.2 Outline of two examples of oligoallergenic diets.

Diet 1	Diet 2
Duck	Rabbit
Potato and potato flour	Rice and rice flour
Carrots and parsnips and swedes	Brassica vegetables
Olive oil	Sunflower oil
Grapes and grape juice	Rhubarb and rhubarb juice
Calcium and vitamin supplement	Calcium and vitamin supplement

a compromise with the theoretically ideal but generally unacceptable option of an elemental diet. The individual is restricted for a period of three or four weeks to a limited diet comprising foods which appear to be infrequently involved in provoking eczema.

Principles for reintroduction of foods. If the patient shows an unequivocal clinical improvement during this period, then consecutive diagnostic reintroduction of all the excluded items can be undertaken. The principles are the same as those outlined above in relation to empirical elimination diets. The child and parents carefully identify those foods that appear to exacerbate the eczema during individual reintroduction over seven successive days. If no adverse reaction is noted, each food tested in this way can be added to the basic diet and subsequently eaten freely. If any reaction is noted, particularly a cutaneous reaction, the parents note the details in a special diary, and the food is not given again.

There are, of course, special problems with those foods containing several constituents, such as bread, in which the ingredients may include wheat, soya, yeast and often also milk and pork fat. With such foods, particular recipes or commercial brands with well-specified contents should be used and, if a reaction occurs, the constituents should subsequently be introduced individually. Similarly, with a number of infrequently implicated foods it may be reasonable to introduce two foods concurrently, with the proviso that both will need to be excluded and introduced individually should the eczema deteriorate.

If the child fails to improve during the initial phase, one may surmise either that foods are not the main aetiological factor in that child's case, or that the child is reacting to one or more of those foods which remain in the oligoantigenic regimen. The latter possibility might be overcome by utilizing a second diet, which comprises entirely different foods, as illustrated in Table 34.2.

Fluctuation of eczema. The identification of provoking foods may be hampered by unrelated fluctuations in the eczema and, if there is any doubt, a food should be excluded and tried a second time at a later date. At the end of several months, the patient will have identified a list of foods for which a provocative role is suspected.

PROBLEMS ASSOCIATED WITH DIETARY TREATMENT

Nutritional hazards

A recent report highlighted the risk of nutritional deficiencies, particularly of calcium, developing in children on exclusion diets for eczema [20]. This is a hazard of even the simplest dietary manipulation and is a special problem in young children in whom a few individual foods may play an essential nutritional role. For example, cow's milk contributes an increasingly large proportion of dietary protein and calcium the younger the child; 500 ml of cow's milk would supply a two-year-old with almost 100% of his daily calcium and riboflavin requirements, and about 50% of his protein and 25% of his calorie intake. Hence, if cow's milk is excluded for any length of time, an alternative source of these nutrients must be found; furthermore, this milk substitute must be of an appropriate constitution and osmolarity for the child's age, palatable and neither strongly sensitizing in its own right nor antigenically cross-reactive with cow's milk.

Milk substitutes: soya and casein hydrolysate formulae

Appropriately modified soya milk products such as Cow and Gate Formula S, Prosobee (Mead Johnson) and Wysoy (Wyeth) provide a nutritionally adequate alternative to cow's milk for all age groups. Although allergic sensitization to soya may occur, this seems to be less of a problem than in gastrointestinal disease. The casein hydrolysate formula, Pregestimil (Mead Johnson), is nutritionally suitable for all ages and Nutramigen (Mead Johnson) is appropriate for those over four months old. Studies by McLaughlan et al [58] on Pregestimil suggest that such casein hydrolysate-based formulae are both non-antigenic in themselves and only minimally cross-reactive with cow's milk.

Both soya formulae and casein hydrolysate-based formulae may be refused as unpalatable, particularly by older children. The use of a 'trainer' beaker or a straw rather than an open cup may help by minimizing the unpleasant aroma of these feeds.

Milk substitutes: goat's milk

Goat's milk provides a more palatable option but is associated with a number of other drawbacks which warrant consideration. Firstly, it is 'unmodified', and therefore inappropriate on any grounds for infants less than six months of age. Secondly, although liquid goat's milk is now widely available, it is almost invariably unpasteurized. Furthermore, the conditions under which goats are kept and milked are not subject to the controls mandatory in the dairy industry. Hence, goat's milk frequently contains potentially pathogenic bacteria, including *Salmonella* spp., *Staphylococcus aureus*, *Escherichia coli*, *Klebsiella* spp. and *Campylobacter jejuni*, derived from clinical and subclinical mastitis in goats, and from faecal contamination from both goats and herdsmen. Although reports of tuberculosis and brucellosis are very rare among British goats, the risk of contracting these infections from goat's milk remains a real one. For these reasons, goat's milk should be heat-treated to destroy such organisms before it is drunk particularly when it is to be given to young children. Since pasteurization is not a practical proposition in the home, this will mean boiling the milk. Unfortunately, this process reduces the nutritional value of the milk by decreasing the content of heat-labile vitamins, particularly folic acid [92]. Supplementary vitamins A, D, C, B$_{12}$ and folic acid may be required.

Antigenic cross-reactivity between milks. The third problem relates to the considerable antigenic cross-reactivity demonstrable between goat's and cow's milk. In guinea pigs anaphylactically sensitized to cow's milk, an intravenous challenge with raw goat's milk produced anaphylaxis in 70% of animals challenged [59]. However, the authors showed that boiling considerably reduced the antigenicity of both cow's and goat's milk, and this was particularly marked in the case of goat's milk. Thus boiling has two benefits, the one immunological and the other microbiological. Nevertheless, some cross-reactivity remains after boiling, which reduces the value of goat's milk as a substitute for cow's milk in these diets.

In the school-age child in whom none of these alternatives are acceptable for one reason or another, the option is to provide no milk substitute but to give supplementary calcium in tablet form. In any child on an elimination diet, a close watch will need to be kept on the nutritional value of what is eaten in relation to protein, calories, vitamins and calcium.

Social and emotional problems of elimination diets

The ubiquity of substances such as cow's milk, egg and artificial colours and preservatives in processed foods means that even the simplest elimination diet requires careful dietetic advice and will involve the family in extra time and expense when shopping or preparing food. The emotional consequences to the child must also be borne in mind. Not only is there a daily preoccupation with what he can and cannot eat, but he also may not be able to partake fully in social and festive occasions.

On a more disturbing note, Warner and Hathaway [104] have illustrated the susceptibility of the concept of food allergic disease to abuse by disturbed parents who may fabricate 'allergic' symptoms for their child, resulting in unnecessary investigation and dietary restriction (Meadow's syndrome or 'Munchausen syndrome by proxy').

Anaphylaxis

As has been discussed above, immediate IgE-mediated reactions to foods are relatively common in children with atopic eczema. The vast majority of these are not serious but David [19] has recently drawn attention to the small but worrying risk of anaphylaxis when previously eliminated foods are reintroduced, whether intentionally or inadvertently, to atopic children. In his series, this occurred in four of 1862 food introductions in 80 patients. Particularly disturbing was the apparent absence of any way of predicting these reactions in the individual case, though the possible value of skin prick test responses or the IgE RAST is not discussed. It is however worth noting that, in two patients, there was evidence of contact urticaria to the relevant food or to a closely related one. Another worrying finding was the development, in one patient, of the anaphylactic reaction as long as 10 hours after the food was first eaten.

'Test' doses

It is our practice to precede the reintroduction of any food with a very small 'test' dose, thus minimizing the risk of serious reaction, and to take special precautions with foods which have previously caused immediate-type reactions such as angioedema, contact urticaria and vomiting, and with any food associated with a strongly positive skin prick test response or a very high level of circulating IgE antibody. In such cases, a little of the relevant food should first be rubbed on to the lips. If the lips become swollen, the reintroduction is abandoned. After 90 minutes, if no swelling occurs, a minute test dose is given by mouth, 1 ml in the case of milk—diluted with a little water—and equivalent amounts in the case of other foods. If 1 ml is taken without ill-effect, 10 ml may be taken 90 minutes later, then 100 ml. However, as David points out, these measures may not obviate the very occasional severe reaction with a later onset.

NON-FOOD ALLERGENS AND THEIR ROUTE OF ENTRY

Though publications concerned with the role of food allergy in atopic eczema are numerous, relatively little attention has been paid to the possible relevance of common environmental non-food allergens. A number of cases have been reported in the literature in which atopic eczema appears to have been provoked by such allergens [15, 37, 45, 77, 94, 101] and there is evidence that at least some patients will benefit from house dust mite elimination procedures [1, 93], or from specific hyposensitization using non-food allergens [22, 23, 49, 108].

Airborne allergens

If an allergen entering the circulation can provoke atopic eczema, it seems unlikely that the route by which it does so would be of particular importance. Those who have treated patients by specific parenteral hyposensitization regularly comment on the marked provocation of eczema that may follow antigen injection [21, 23], and this has been our own experience. From the point of view of aeroallergen absorption, the gastrointestinal tract is likely to be more relevant than the lower respiratory tract. It should be remembered that airborne particulate matter is largely deposited in the oropharynx, from where it passes to the gastrointestinal tract, only a very small proportion entering the lower airways [106]. However, it seems possible that the nasal mucosa could be an important site of aeroallergen absorption, perhaps more important than the gastrointestinal tract by virtue of the absence of either intraluminal digestion or hepatic clearance of antigen.

Skin contact with allergens

There is, in addition, evidence that eczema can be aggravated by direct cutaneous contact with both food and non-food antigens to which immediate skin-test reactivity is present [15, 40, 60, 65, 88]. This may be the cause of much eczema that is localized to the perioral area and/or the hands. Under experimental conditions, atopic eczema cannot normally be provoked by direct antigen contact unless the skin is damaged [60, 65, 88] or has been the site of previous damage [40]. Therefore, although cutaneous antigen contact is able to exacerbate established eczema it probably does not initiate the disease. It seems likely that the most important factor is entry of antigen into the systemic circulation, for which the gastrointestinal tract is principally responsible in the case of foods and for which the nasal mucosa might also be important in the case of aeroallergens.

ANTI-ALLERGY DRUG TREATMENT

An alternative to dietary and environmental manipulation would be the pharmacological modification of allergic reactions. For this reason, sodium cromoglycate has been tried both topically and orally.

Topical sodium cromoglycate

The results of an initial controlled study did suggest that sodium cromoglycate was beneficial when applied topically to the skin in atopic eczema [30]. Unfortunately, others have failed to confirm this [91, 108], despite the development of formulations which allowed superior percutaneous absorption of the sodium cromoglycate [75].

Oral sodium cromoglycate

Molkhou and Waguet [66], in an open study, reported that orally administered sodium cromoglycate was effective in helping atopic eczema. If this compound were helpful, it seemed reasonable to suppose that it might reflect a local effect in the alimentary tract, as its systemic absorption is extremely limited [102]. It is possible that it could inhibit the enhancement of antigen absorption that appears to occur in at least some atopic individuals and which might reflect local allergic reactions in the gastrointestinal tract (see Chapter 33). Such an effect has been suggested both by animal experiments [102] and human studies [11, 18, 71].

A more recent controlled study [4] of oral sodium cromoglycate did not demonstrate effectiveness in an unselected group of children with atopic eczema. Graham et al [26], also in a controlled study, failed to show an additional effect from oral sodium cromoglycate when children were already benefiting from appropriate exclusion diets. However, Businco et al [12] did report usefulness of oral sodium cromoglycate in the prevention of allergic symptoms on reintroduction of foods previously identified as allergens by exclusion and provocation tests in patients with atopic eczema. More work is needed to establish the potential value of such a role for this agent.

HYPOTHESES FOR THE ROLE OF FOOD IN THE PATHOGENESIS OF ATOPIC ECZEMA

A metabolic effect?

That the link between food and atopic eczema has an exclusively immunological basis has not been established and, indeed, an underlying nutritional disturbance was suggested many years ago, in the form of a relative deficiency of unsaturated fatty acids [34]. Furthermore, sources rich in essential fatty acids (EFA) have been reported to be beneficial in atopic eczema [34, 107]. Wright and Burton [107] suggested that a deficiency of the enzyme Δ^6-desaturase might be present in patients with atopic eczema and support for this hypothesis is provided by the plasma EFA profiles demonstrated in some patients [61]. This enzyme is responsible for the conversion of linoleic to γ-linolenic acid, and it may be the γ-linolenic acid content that is the important constituent in evening primrose seed oil, the EFA source used by Wright and Burton [107]. Horrobin et al [42] have reported that prostaglandin E_1, a metabolite of γ-linolenic acid, is important for T lymphocyte function; thus one could speculate that defective EFA metabolism contributes to the T lymphocyte abnormalities which have been demonstrated in patients with atopic eczema [14].

An abnormality of food antigen handling?

Absorption of antigen from the gut. The absorption of intact antigens is a feature of normal gastrointestinal function [103]. The amounts which enter the circulation are nutritionally insignificant, but are undoubtedly sufficient to immunize, since antibodies to intact food proteins can be demonstrated in most healthy individuals [73]. It is assumed that the function of these antibodies is the safe elimination of those food antigens that succeed in gaining access to the circulation. It is likely that the complexes formed by the combination of antibody and food antigen are removed from the blood by phagocytic cells, this sequence of events occurring asymptomatically after each meal. It is possible that this system has broken down in the individual with atopic eczema, and that the eczema arises as a direct consequence of defective handling of normally harmless antigens which have entered the circulation by the gastrointestinal route (see Fig. 34.3).

Antigen elimination: role of mucosal immunity. Under normal circumstances, the safe elimination of antigenic proteins derived from food and airborne particulate matter is probably a function of serum IgA [31]. This protective IgA response is thought to arise as a consequence of intact antigen exposure via the gastrointestinal tract in early infancy. Genetically determined immunodeficiencies and/or a critical timing or dosage of antigen might lead to the development of a pathological immunological response to such antigens. A prominent IgE response is not the sole consequence of these immunodeficiencies, and many atopics also mount excessive IgG and IgM responses. Possibly the type and size of these abnormal antibody responses are crucial factors in deter-

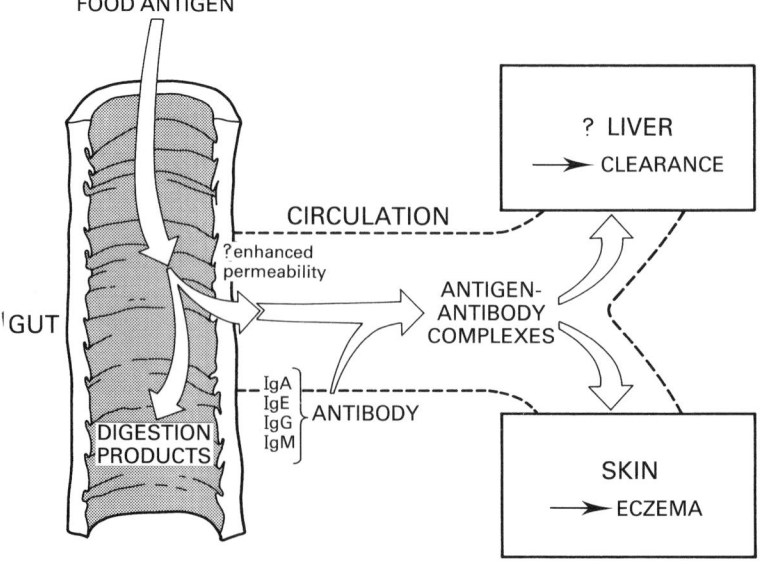

Fig. 34.3 A hypothetical pathway for the pathogenesis of atopic eczema. In normal individuals, food antigen–antibody complexes are formed in the circulation in small quantities after meals, and these appear to be rapidly cleared by the reticuloendothelial system. The evidence suggests that in individuals with atopic eczema such complexes may be formed in greater quantity, and that they have different properties. It seems possible that eczema results from their deposition in the cutaneous microvasculature. Reprinted from Atherton DJ: Atopic eczema. Clin Immunol Allergy 1982; 2: 77–100, with permission.

mining whether such individuals actually develop one of the atopic diseases, and maybe even which disease or diseases they develop.

In a child with atopic eczema, some food antigen will enter the circulation after a meal, as in normal children. Preliminary evidence indicates the possibility that the entry of such antigens may be greater in at least some atopics [18, 71].

Mucosal hypersensitivity and antigen absorption. Rats which have been reaginically sensitized against food antigens demonstrate enhanced gastrointestinal permeability to the same antigens subsequently given by mouth [13]. The increased permeability appears to be the consequence of an IgE-mediated hypersensitivity reaction, and in these rat experiments it could be blocked by parenteral cyproheptadine or by oral sodium cromoglycate. Bloch et al [7] demonstrated enhanced uptake into the circulation of orally administered bovine serum albumin in rats subjected to a mild degree of systemic anaphylaxis. Anaphylaxis was induced by intravenously injecting rats infected by the nematode *Nippostrongylus brasiliensis* with an extract of the same parasite. This result implies that antigen entry enhanced by this mechanism is enhanced in an antigen non-specific way. Support for this concept has also been provided by the interesting findings from experiments in preruminant calves made allergic to soya flour, in which simultaneous administration of soya enhanced the absorption of β-lactoglobulin [51].

Abnormal gastrointestinal mucosa. Minor morphological abnormalities of the small intestinal mucosa have been demonstrated in a proportion of children with atopic eczema [53, 57, 84], which might reflect the long-term impact of this type of allergic reaction. Occasionally atopic eczema is complicated by full-blown protein-losing enteropathy which is similarly assumed to have an allergic cause [44, 100].

Indirect evidence of more subtle mucosal damage is provided by reports of increased gastrointestinal permeability to inert molecules which are not normally subject to significant absorption from the gut lumen, including polyethylene glycol of mean molecular weight 4000 [43], and lactulose [72, 75a, 96].

Taken together, these findings suggest the possibility that the absorption of macromolecular antigens from the gastrointestinal tract is increased in at least some patients with atopic eczema, that this phenomenon is often associated with a mild degree of mucosal damage and that the mechanism in both cases may be an IgE-mediated hypersensitivity reaction in the gut wall. Though the initial hypersensitivity reaction would clearly be antigen-specific, the resulting enhancement of permeability is likely not to be.

Fate of absorbed food antigens. Most food antigens which gain access to the systemic circulation will become bound shortly afterwards by antibodies. Their subsequent fate probably largely depends upon the properties of the antigen–antibody complexes thus formed (see Fig. 34.3). The appearance of circulating antigen–antibody complexes following food challenge has been demonstrated in normal humans [11, 70]. The antibodies in these complexes appear to be predominantly of IgA class [11], and the formation of such complexes is not associated with the development of symptoms. The harmless nature of these complexes is almost certainly related to the relative biological inertness of IgA, which does not activate complement by the classical pathway [17]. Under the same conditions, it has been found that many patients with atopic eczema form not only IgA-containing complexes, but also complexes containing IgG and IgE, and complexes which bind C1q [11]. These complexes can be shown to contain food antigens [70]. Their fate is unknown, but it does not seem impossible that atopic eczema could result from the deposition of such complexes in the skin.

Eczema and urticaria: different manifestations of a similar pathological process?

Eczema and urticaria may be reflections of similar degrees of cutaneous microvascular damage affecting vessels at somewhat different levels in the skin. Is 'eczema' simply 'urticaria' occurring very superficially in the dermis? In urticaria, perivascular inflammation is typically seen at the level of the mid-dermis, sparing the finger-like dermal papillae which project up into the epidermis. On the other hand, in eczema the perivascular inflammation predominantly affects the upper dermis, and the papillary processes in particular. The resulting oedema and inflammatory cell infiltrate would be unable to escape in any direction other than into the epidermis, which effectively surrounds these dermal papillae (Fig. 34.4).

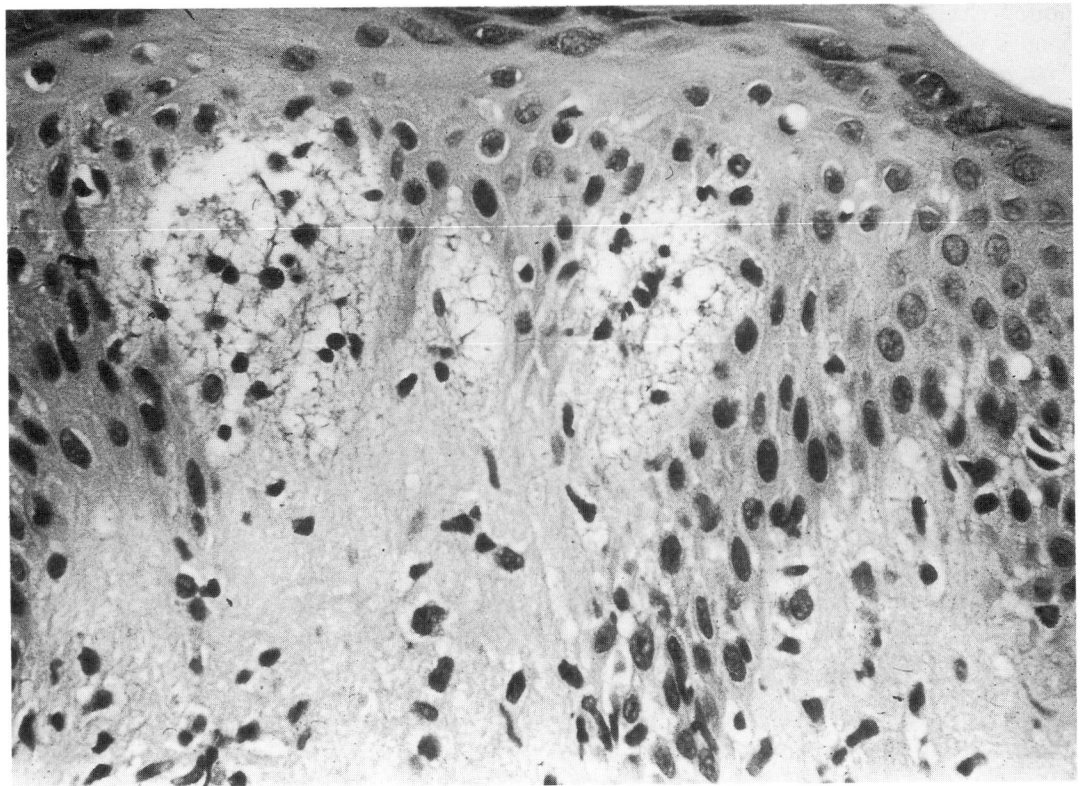

Fig. 34.4 Atopic eczema, showing intense oedema of the dermal papillae.

Though it might initially be contained by the structures comprising the basement membrane at the dermoepidermal junction, when the inflammation is intense, it would probably eventually 'burst' through into the epidermis (Fig. 34.5). Indeed, the presence of oedema ('spongiosis') and inflammatory cells (principally lymphocytes and monocyte-macrophages) within the epidermis are the histological hallmarks of acute eczema, whose clinical counterparts are vesiculation and exudation.

Some support for such a hypothetical sequence is provided by the observation of many parents that exacerbation of their children's eczema by foods is regularly preceded by widespread erythema, or even by frank urticaria. This pattern has been reported experimentally by Stifler [87] and by Sedlis [83].

Histological features of atopic eczema

The histological features observed in atopic eczema are perfectly consistent with such a sequence of events. Mihm et al [64] reported fairly prominent changes in the vessel walls of the superficial dermal venular plexus that included endothelial cell hypertrophy and thick-ening and reduplication of the vascular basement membrane, changes that are entirely compatible with deposition of antigen–antibody complexes. As one would anticipate, these changes were also observed, albeit to a milder degree, in skin that appeared clinically uninvolved.

Proposed sequence of events

The sequence of events proposed is a complex one, which may involve hypersensitivity reactions of Types I, III and possibly also IV, at different stages. Although there is some evidence to support the existence of individual elements of this sequence, much of what we have suggested is unconfirmed and as a whole it must be regarded as entirely hypothetical. Nevertheless, it would seem important to have a working hypothesis to test experimentally. While many pages have been expended in the argument whether 'IgE causes atopic eczema', the situation is, in practice, likely to be so complex that such apparently simple questions become inappropriate.

Finally, mention should be made of the reports that immunoglobulin deposition can be demonstrated by direct immunofluorescence

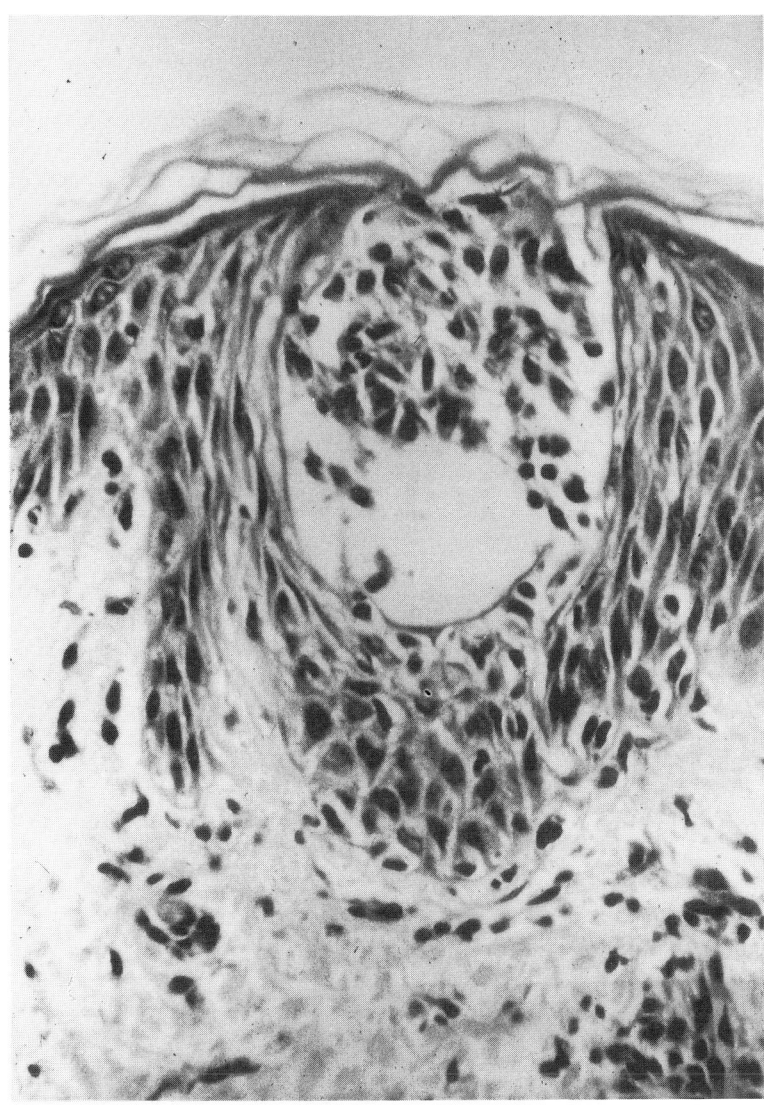

Fig. 34.5 Atopic eczema, showing intense epidermal intercellular oedema ('spongiosis') with an intraepidermal vesicle.

in the basement membrane zone at the dermoepidermal junction [41, 76]. Similar immunoglobulin deposition is also a feature of both systemic lupus erythematosus and allergic vasculitis, and it seems possible that the basement membrane zone in all these disorders is simply acting as a non-specific trap for antigen–antibody complexes that have escaped from vessels in the upper dermis.

SUMMARY

In this chapter, the relationship between foods and atopic eczema has been considered by posing three principal questions:

1 'What is the evidence that food allergy is an important aetiological factor in atopic eczema?' While a substantial amount has been written on this subject, it remains impossible to arrive at firm conclusions. Many of the available data are open to scientific criticism, but it is our view that overall a reasonable case has been made for a role for foods in the aetiology of atopic eczema in many patients, particularly children. The relative importance of foods vis-à-vis other aetiological factors is unclear, and in this context the possible contribution of non-food environmental allergens should perhaps not be underestimated. It is probably rare for foods alone to be responsible for an individual's atopic eczema.

2 'What are the therapeutic implications of what we know about food allergy in atopic eczema?' In our opinion, a case for a dietary approach to treatment has been made, though the best method is still to be established.

3 'What is the sequence of pathological

events by which foods induce eczema?' It is important to be aware that we are so far from answering this question that we are for the present only able to assume that the mechanisms are principally immunological rather than nutritional. However, that these two are *not* mutually exclusive is illustrated by the proposed link between essential fatty acid metabolism and T lymphocyte function.

We have postulated a hypothetical sequence of pathological events initiated by the absorption of intact food antigens from the alimentary tract (Fig. 34.3). Gastrointestinal absorption of food antigens is possibly increased in atopic eczema, and their handling subsequent to absorption may be abnormal. It is speculated that, while in normal subjects they become complexed predominantly with IgA, these IgA complexes being rapidly and safely cleared, possibly by the liver, in atopic eczema they may be complexed to a significant degree with antibodies of the IgG or IgE class, and a chain of events initiated that results in damage to the superficial dermal microvasculature, leading in its turn to oedema and infiltration of the dermal papillae by inflammatory cells.

The eruption of oedema and inflammatory cells into the epidermis is the final event and the hallmark of eczema.

We are often asked by sceptical colleagues, 'Do you really believe all this "food business"?' It remains one of the sadder aspects of mainstream medicine that we should see such an important problem as a question of 'belief' or 'non-belief'. What is actually needed is an open, enquiring attitude and careful, critical investigation. By failing to study the relationship between foods and atopic eczema scientifically, we might deny ourselves the opportunity of understanding and thus eventually overcoming this common and distressing disease.

Endnote

Copies of diet sheets for the 'simple' empirical diets (excluding egg, cow's milk, colourings, preservatives and chicken) used at The Hospital for Sick Children, London may be obtained from Ms D. E. M. Francis, Group Chief Dietitian, The Hospital for Sick Children, Great Ormond Street, London WC1 3JH.

REFERENCES

1 Alani M, Hjorth N: Sensitivity to house-dust mites in atopic dermatitis. Acta Allergol 1970; 25: 41–7.

2 Atherton DJ: Dietary antigen avoidance in the treatment of atopic eczema. Acta Derm Venereol (Stockh) 1980; (Suppl 92): 99–102.

3 Atherton DJ: Breast feeding and atopic eczema. Br Med J 1983; 287: 775–6.

4 Atherton DJ, Soothill JF, Elvidge J: A controlled trial of oral sodium cromoglycate in atopic eczema. Br J Dermatol 1982; 106: 681–5.

5 Atherton DJ, Sewell M, Soothill JF et al: A double-blind controlled crossover trial of an antigen avoidance diet in atopic eczema. Lancet 1978; 1: 401–3.

6 Barnetson RSTC: Hyperimmunoglobulinaemia E in atopic eczema (atopic dermatitis) is associated with 'food allergy'. Acta Derm Venereol (Stockh) 1980; (Suppl 92): 94–6.

7 Bloch KJ, Bloch DB, Stearns M, Walker WA: Intestinal uptake of macromolecules. VI. Uptake of protein antigen in vivo in normal rats and in rats infected with *Nippostrongylus brasiliensis* or subjected to mild systemic anaphylaxis. Gastroenterology 1979; 77: 1039–44.

8 Bock SA, Lee W-Y, Remigio LK, May CD: Studies of hypersensitivity reactions to foods in infants and children. J Allergy Clin Immunol 1978; 62: 327–34.

9 Bonifazi E, Garofalo L, Monterisi A, Meneghini CL: Food allergy in atopic dermatitis: experimental observations. Acta Derm Venereol (Stockh) 1978; 58: 349–52.

10 Bonifazi E, Garofalo L, Monterisi A, Meneghini CL: History of food allergy, RAST and challenge test in atopic dermatitis. Acta Derm Venereol (Stockh) 1980; (Suppl 92): 91–3.

11 Brostoff J, Carini C, Wraith DG et al: Immune complexes in atopy. In: Pepys J, Edwards AM, eds: The mast cell—its role in health and disease. London: Pitman, 1979; 380–93.

12 Businco L, Cantini A, Benincori N et al: Effectiveness of oral sodium cromoglycate (SCG) in preventing food allergy in children. Ann Allergy 1983; 51 (1): 47–50.

13 Byars NE, Ferraresi RW: Intestinal anaphylaxis in the rat as a model of food allergy. Clin Exp Immunol 1976; 24: 352–6.

14 Byrom NA, Timlin DM: Immune status in atopic eczema: a survey. Br J Dermatol 1979; 100: 491–8.

15 Champion RH: Atopic sensitivity to algae and lichens. Br J Dermatol 1971; 85: 551–7.

16 Chandra RK: Prospective studies of the effect of breast feeding on the incidence of infection and allergy. Acta Paediatr Scand 1979; 68: 691–4.

17 Colten HR, Bienenstock J: Lack of C3 activation through classical or alternate pathways by human secretory IgA antibody group A antibody. Adv Exp Med Biol 1974; 45: 305–13.

18 Dannaeus A, Inganaes M, Johansson SGO, Foucard T: Intestinal uptake of ovalbumin in malabsorption and food allergy in relation to serum IgG antibody and orally administrered sodium cromoglycate. Clin Allergy 1979; 9: 263–70.

19 David TJ: Anaphylactic shock during elimination diets for severe atopic eczema. Arch Dis Child 1984; 59: 983–6.

20 David TJ, Waddington E, Stanton RHJ: Nutritional hazards of elimination diets in children with atopic eczema. Arch Dis Child 1984; 59: 323-5.

21 Derbes VJ, Caro MR: Localised eczema induced by house dust extract injections. Arch Dermatol 1957; 74: 804-5.

22 Diamond HE: Atopic dermatitis caused by inhalant antigens and its immunologic therapy. Ann Allergy 1953; 11: 146-56.

23 Di Prisco de Fuenmayor MC, Champion RM: Specific hyposensitization in atopic dermatitis. Br J Dermatol 1979; 101: 697-700.

24 Freedman SS: Milk allergy in infantile atopic eczema. Am J Dis Child 1961; 102: 106-11.

25 Goldman AS, Anderson DW, Sellers WA et al: Milk allergy. 1. Oral challenge with milk and isolated milk proteins in allergic children. Pediatrics 1963; 32: 425-43.

26 Graham P, Hall-Smith SP, Harris JM, Price ML: A study of hypoallergenic diets and oral sodium cromoglycate in the management of atopic eczema. Br J Dermatol 1984; 110: 457-67.

27 Grulee CG, Sanford HN: The influence of breast and artificial feeding on infantile eczema. J Pediatr 1936; 9: 223-5.

28 Haddad ZH, Verma S, Kalra V: IgE antibodies to peptic and peptic-tryptic digests of beta-lactoglobulin: significance in food hypersensitivity. J Allergy Clin Immunol 1979; 63: 198.

29 Hagerman G: The importance of food factors in atopic dermatitis. Acta Derm Venereol (Stockh) 1966; (Sven Hellerström 65 years): 81-6.

30 Haider SA: Treatment of atopic eczema in children: clinical trial of 10 per cent sodium cromoglycate ointment. Br Med J 1977; 1: 1570-2.

31 Hall JG, Andrew E: Biliglobulin: a new look at IgA. Immunol Today 1980; 1(5): 100-4.

32 Halpern SR, Sellars WA, Johnson RB et al: Development of childhood allergy in infants fed breast, soy or cow milk. J Allergy Clin Immunol 1973; 51: 139-51.

33 Hammar H: Provocation with cow's milk and cereals in atopic dermatitis. Acta Derm Venereol (Stockh) 1977; 57: 159-63.

34 Hansen AE, Knott EM, Wiese HF et al: Eczema and essential fatty acids. Am J Dis Child 1947; 73: 1-16.

35 Hathaway MJ, Warner JO: Compliance problems in the dietary management of eczema. Arch Dis Child 1983; 58: 463-4.

37 Hewitt M, Barrow GI, Miller DL et al: Mites in the personal environment and their role in skin disorders. Br J Dermatol 1973; 89: 401-9.

38 Hide DW, Guyer BM: Clinical manifestations of allergy related to breast and cow's milk feeding. Arch Dis Child 1981; 56: 172-5.

39 Hill DJ, Lynch BC: Elemental diet in the management of severe eczema in childhood. Clin Allergy 1982; 12: 313-5.

40 Hjorth N, Roed-Petersen J: Occupational protein contact dermatitis in food handlers. Contact Dermatitis 1976; 2: 28-42.

41 Hodgkinson GI, Everall JD, Smith HV: Immunofluorescent patterns in the skin of Besnier's prurigo. Br J Dermatol 1977; 96: 357-66.

42 Horrobin DF, Manku MS, Oka M: The nutritional regulation of T-lymphocyte function. Med Hypotheses 1979; 5: 969-85.

43 Jackson PG, Lessof MH, Baker RWR et al: Intestinal permeability in patients with eczema and food allergy. Lancet 1981; 1: 1285-6.

44 Jenkins HR, Walker-Smith JA, Atherton DJ: Protein-losing enteropathy in atopic dermatitis. Pediatr Dermatol (in press).

45 Jillson OF, Adami M: Allergic dermatitis produced by inhalant moulds. Arch Dermatol 1955; 72: 411-9.

46 Johnson EE, Irons JS, Patterson R, Roberts M: Serum IgE concentration in atopic dermatitis. J Allergy Clin Immunol 1974; 54: 94-9.

47 Juto P, Engberg S, Winberg J: Treatment of infantile atopic eczema with a strict elimination diet. Clin Allergy 1978; 8: 493-500.

48 Kajosaari M, Saarinen UM: Prophylaxis of atopic disease by six months' total solid food elimination. Acta Paediatr Scand 1983; 72: 411-4.

49 Kaufman H, Roth HL: Hyposensitization with alum precipitated extracts in atopic dermatitis: a placebo controlled study. Ann Allergy 1974; 32: 321-30.

50 Kesten BM: Allergic eczema. NY State J Med 1954; 54: 2441-8.

51 Kilshaw PJ, Slade H: Passage of ingested protein into the blood during gastrointestinal hypersensitivity reactions: experiments in the preruminant calf. Clin Exp Immunol 1980; 41: 575-82.

52 Kjellman N-IM, Johansson SGO: IgE and atopic allergy in newborns and infants with a family history of atopic disease. Acta Paediatr Scand 1976; 65: 601-7.

53 Kokkonen J, Simila S, Herva R: Gastrointestinal findings in atopic children. Eur J Paediatr 1980; 134: 249-54.

54 Kramer DW, Moroz B: Do breast-feeding and delayed introduction of solid foods protect against subsequent atopic eczema? J Pediatr 1981; 98: 546-50.

55 Langeland T: A clinical and immunological study of allergy to hen's egg white. VI. Occurrence of proteins crossreacting with allergens in hen's egg white as studied in egg white from turkey, duck, goose, seagull and hen's egg yolk, and hen's and chicken's sera and flesh. Allergy 1983; 38: 399-412.

56 Longo G, Poli F: Trattamento dell'eczema atopico infantile con dieta de eliminazione. Rev Ital Pediatr 1980; 6: 41-9.

57 McCalla R, Savilahti E, Perkkiö M et al: Morphology of the jejunum in children with eczema due to food allergy. Allergy 1980; 35: 563-71.

58 McLaughlan P, Anderson KJ, Coombs RRA: An oral screening procedure to determine the sensitizing capacity of infant feeding formulae. Clin Allergy 1981; 11: 311-8.

59 McLaughlan P, Anderson KJ, Widdowson EM, Coombs RRA: Effect of heat on the anaphylactic sensitizing capacity of cow's milk, goat's milk and various infant formulae fed to guinea-pigs. Arch Dis Child 1981; 56: 165-71.

60 Maibach H: Immediate hypersensitivity in hand dermatitis. Arch Dermatol 1976; 112: 1289-91.

61 Manku MS, Horrobin DF, Morse NL et al: Essential fatty acids in the plasma phospholipids of patients with atopic eczema. Br J Dermatol 1984; 110: 643-8.

62 Matthew DJ, Taylor B, Norman AP et al: Prevention of eczema. Lancet 1977; 1: 321-4.

63 Meara RH: Skin reactions in atopic eczema. Br J Dermatol 1955; 67: 60-4.

64 Mihm MC, Soter NA, Dvorak HF, Austen KF: The structure of normal skin and the morphology of atopic eczema. J Invest Dermatol 1976; 67: 305-12.

65 Mitchell EB, Chapman MD, Pope FM et al: Basophils in allergen-induced patch test sites in atopic dermatitis. Lancet 1982; 1: 127-30.

66 Molkhou P, Waguet JC: Oral disodium cromoglycate

in the treatment of atopic eczema in children. In: Pepys J, Edwards AM, eds: The mast cell—its role in health and disease. London: Pitman, 1979; 617–9.

67 Munkvad M, Danielsen L, Høj L et al: Antigen-free diet in adult patients with atopic dermatitis. Acta Derm Venereol (Stockh) 1984; 64: 524–8.

68 Nield VS, Marsden RA, Bailes JA: A double-blind crossover trial of egg and milk exclusion diets in atopic eczema. Br J Dermatol 1984; III (Suppl 26): 33.

69 Ohman S, Johansson SGO: Immunoglobulins in atopic dermatitis—with special reference to IgE. Acta Derm Venereol (Stockh) 1974; 54: 193–202.

70 Paganelli R, Levinsky RJ, Atherton DJ: Detection of specific antigen within circulating immune complexes. Validation of the assay and its application to food antigen–antibody complexes found in healthy and food allergic subjects. Clin Exp Immunol 1981; 46: 44–53.

71 Paganelli R, Levinsky RJ, Brostoff J, Wraith DG: Immune complexes containing food proteins in normal and atopic subjects after oral challenge, and effect of sodium cromoglycate on antigen absorption. Lancet 1979; 1: 1270–2.

72 Parrilli G, Ayala F, Lembo G et al: Abnormal intestinal permeability to lactulose in patients with atopic dermatitis. In: MacDonald DM, ed: Immunodermatology. London: Butterworths, 1984; 21–2.

73 Peterson RDA, Good RA: Antibodies to cow's milk proteins—their presence and significance. Pediatrics 1963; 31: 209–21.

74 Peterson RDA, Page AR, Good RA: Wheal and erythema allergy in patients with agammaglobulinaemia. J Allergy 1962; 33: 406–11.

75 Pike MG, Gratton RJ, Atherton DJ: Trial of a new topical formulation of sodium cromoglycate in atopic eczema. Clin Exp Dermatol (in press).

75a Pike M, Heddle RJ, Boulton P et al: Increased intestinal permeability in atopic eczema. J Invest Dermatol 1986;86:101–4.

76 Ring J, Senter T, Cornell RC et al: Complement and immunoglobulin deposits in the skin of patients with atopic dermatitis. Br J Dermatol 1978; 99: 495–501.

77 Rowe A, Rowe AH: Atopic dermatitis in infants and children. J Pediatr 1951; 39: 80–6.

78 Saarinen UM, Kajosaari M, Backman A, Siimes MA: Prolonged breast feeding as prophylaxis for atopic disease. Lancet 1979; 2: 163–6.

79 Sampson HA: Role of immediate food hypersensitivity in the pathogenesis of atopic dermatitis. J Allergy Clin Immunol 1983; 71(5): 473–80.

80 Sampson HA, Albergo R: Comparison of results of skin tests, RAST, and double-blind, placebo-controlled food challenges in children with atopic dermatitis. J Allergy Clin Immunol 1984; 74(1): 26–33.

81 Sampson HA, Jolie PL: Increased plasma histamine concentrations after food challenges in children with atopic dermatitis. N Engl J Med 1984; 311: 372–6.

82 Schwartz HR, Nerurka LS, Spies JR et al: Milk hypersensitivity: RAST studies using new antigens generated by pepsin hydrolysis of beta-lactoglobulin. Ann Allergy 1980; 45: 242.

83 Sedlis E: Conference on infantile atopic eczema: some challenge studies with foods. J Pediatr 1965; 66 (Suppl): 235–41.

84 Sloper KS, Brook CGD, Kingston D et al: Eczema and atopy in early childhood; low IgA plasma cell counts in the jejunal mucosa. Arch Dis Child 1981; 56: 939–42.

85 Spies JR, Stevan MA, Stein WJ: A method for esti-

mation of the relative antigenic potencies of preparations containing common new antigens derived from a precursor protein (β-lactoglobulin). J Immunol Methods 1972; 2: 35–43.

86 Spies JR, Stevan MA, Stein WJ: The chemistry of allergens. XXI. Eight new antigens generated by successive pepsin hydrolysis of bovine β-lactoglobulin. J Allergy Clin Immunol 1972; 50: 82–91.

87 Stifler WC: Conference on infantile atopic eczema: some challenge studies with foods. J Pediatr 1965; 66 (Suppl): 235–41.

88 Strauss JS, Kligman AM: The relationship of atopic allergy and dermatitis. Arch Dermatol 1957; 75: 806–11.

89 Talbot FB: Eczema in childhood. Med Clin North Am 1918; 1: 985–96.

90 Taylor B, Wadsworth J, Wadsworth M, Peckham C: Changes in the reported prevalence of childhood eczema since the 1939–45 war. Lancet 1984; 2: 1255–7.

91 Thirumoorthy T, Greaves MW: Disodium cromoglycate ointment in atopic eczema. Br Med J 1978; 2: 500–1.

92 Tripp JH, Francis DEM, Knight JA, Harries JT: Infant feeding practices: a cause for concern. Br Med J 1979; 2: 707–9.

93 Tuft LA: The importance of inhalant allergens in atopic dermatitis. J Invest Dermatol 1949; 12: 211–9.

94 Tuft L, Tuft HS, Heck VM: Atopic dermatitis. I. An experimental clinical study of the role of inhalant allergens. J Allergy 1950; 21: 181–6.

95 Turner MW, Brostoff J, Mowbray JF, Skelton A: The atopic syndrome: in vitro immunological characteristics of clinically defined subgroups of atopic subjects. Clin Allergy 1980; 10: 575–84.

96 Ukabam SO, Mann RJ, Cooper BT: Small intestinal permeability to sugars in patients with atopic eczema. Br J Dermatol 1984; 110: 649–52.

97 Van Asperen PP, Kemp AS, Mellis CM: Skin reactivity and clinical allergen sensitivity in infancy. J Allergy Clin Immunol 1984; 73(3): 381–6.

98 Van Asperen PP, Lewis M, Rogers M et al: Experience with an elimination diet in children with atopic dermatitis. Clin Allergy 1983; 13: 479–85.

99 Vickers CFH: The natural history of atopic eczema. Acta Derm Venereol (Stockh) 1980 (Suppl 92): 113–5.

100 Waldmann TA, Wochner RD, Laster L, Gordon RS: Allergic gastroenteropathy. N Engl J Med 1967; 276: 761–7.

101 Walker C: Causation of eczema, urticaria and angioneurotic oedema by proteins other than those derived from food. JAMA 1918; 70: 897–900.

102 Walker SR, Evans ME, Richards AJ, Paterson JW: The fate of (^{14}C) disodium cromoglycate in man. J Pharm Pharmacol 1972; 24: 525–31.

103 Walker WA, Isselbacher KJ: Uptake and transport of macromolecules by the intestine. Gastroenterology 1974; 67: 531–50.

104 Warner JO, Hathaway MJ: Allergic form of Meadow's syndrome (Munchausen by proxy). Arch Dis Child 1984; 59: 151–6.

105 Webster ADB, Wood CBS: Skin disorders in immunodeficiency. In: Verbov J, ed: Modern topics in paediatric dermatology. London: Heinemann, 1979; 179–200.

106 Wilson AF, Novey HS, Berke RA, Surprenant EL: Deposition of inhaled pollen and pollen extract in human airways. N Engl J Med 1973; 288: 1056–8.

107 Wright S, Burton JL: Oral evening primrose seed oil improves atopic eczema. Lancet 1982; 2: 1120–2.

108 Zachariae H, Thestrup-Pedersen K, Thulin H et al: Experimental treatment in atopic dermatitis: immunological background and preliminary results. Acta Derm Venereol (Stockh) 1980 (Suppl. 92): 121–7.

Chapter 35
Food Sensitivity and Urticaria or Vasculitis

R. K. Winkelmann

ACUTE URTICARIA

Clinical features

Urticaria (hives) is the pruritic, localized oedema of the skin expressed as white or pink papules or plaques (wheals) with surrounding axon flare. These lesions are typical of histamine wheals and occur within minutes, often fade in four to six hours and are gone in 24 hours. The lesions may develop variable erythema or coalesce to form large plaques. They may fade spontaneously or with antihistamine therapy to resistant red papules, usually with a white halo of longer duration, which have a relationship to kinin or prostaglandin formation [119]. About half the patients with urticaria develop angioedema—a deep, less defined swelling of the subcutaneous and soft tissue. Angioedema often occurs by itself and so is maintained as an independent clinical entity of immediate hypersensitivity and histamine release. The lesions are slow to develop and to fade, and usually no skin colour or dermal tissue changes are observed.

Histology of urticaria

The microscopic pattern of urticaria has generally been considered to be non-specific in nature. There may be scattered perivascular and dermal inflammatory cells which may include polymorphonuclear leukocytes, lymphocytes, eosinophils and monocytes. Acute urticarial lesions are characterized by dilated dermal lymphatics, and the content of the lymphatics may be periodic acid–Schiff positive. Pressure urticaria is noted for its content of eosinophils (Fig. 35.1). Physical urticarial lesions may show an acute phase of perivenular neutrophils as well as dilated lymphatics. Late lesions of all forms of urticaria most frequently show perivascular lymphocytosis with varying numbers of eosinophils. Chronic urticaria biopsies invariably show perivascular lymphocytosis with the cells recognized as T cells by monoclonal antibody studies. No

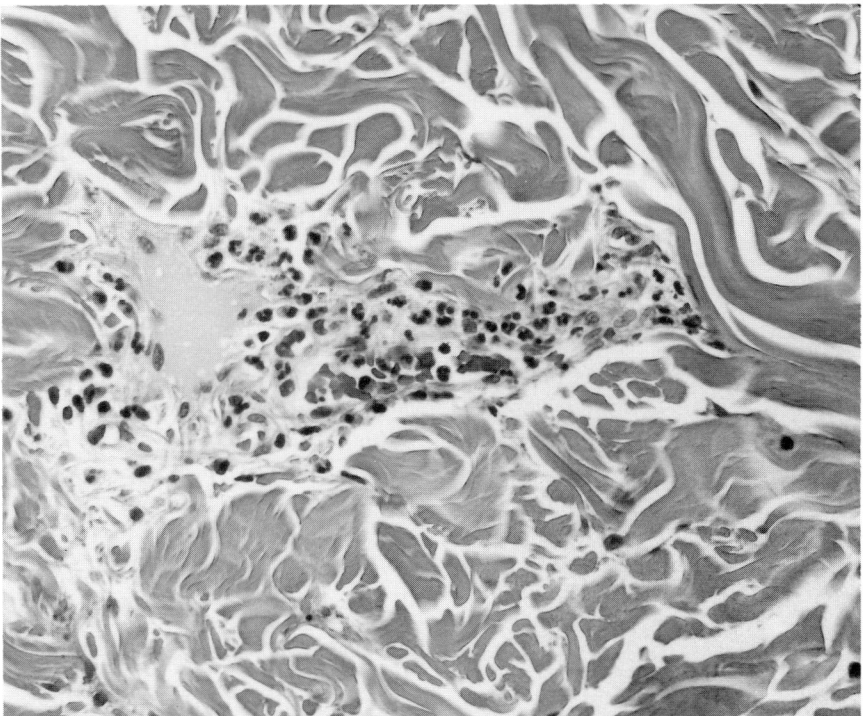

Fig. 35.1 Perivascular inflammation of the deep dermis in a case of pressure urticaria. Over 20% of the cells are eosinophils. Note the dilated lymphatic vessel. H&E × 400.

known histologic studies of acute food urticaria have been reported. Urticarial vasculitis has the histology of leukocytoclastic or necrotizing vasculitis (Fig. 35.2). The dermal venules are surrounded and invaded by inflammatory cells, particularly neutrophils. The neutrophils undergo destruction and neutrophil globules or nuclear dust characterize the pathology. Fibrinoid deposition about the vessel accompanies the haemorrhage. Endothelial cell necrosis may be seen.

At times the histology is not specific due to

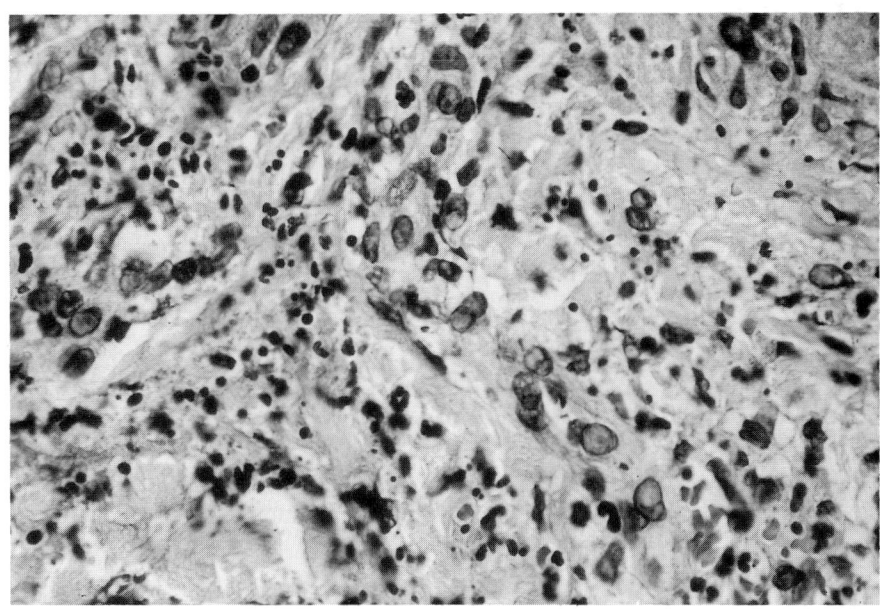

Fig. 35.2 Perivascular and dermal leukocytoclastic vasculitis from skin of a patient with urticarial vasculitis. H&E × 640.

biopsy site or time and the use of direct im-munofluorescence may help. Skin biopsies frozen in liquid nitrogen and stained with fluorescent isothiocyanate-labelled antibodies to immunoglobulins, fibrinogen and comple-ment may demonstrate angiocentric inflam-mation consistent with vasculitis (Fig. 35.3).

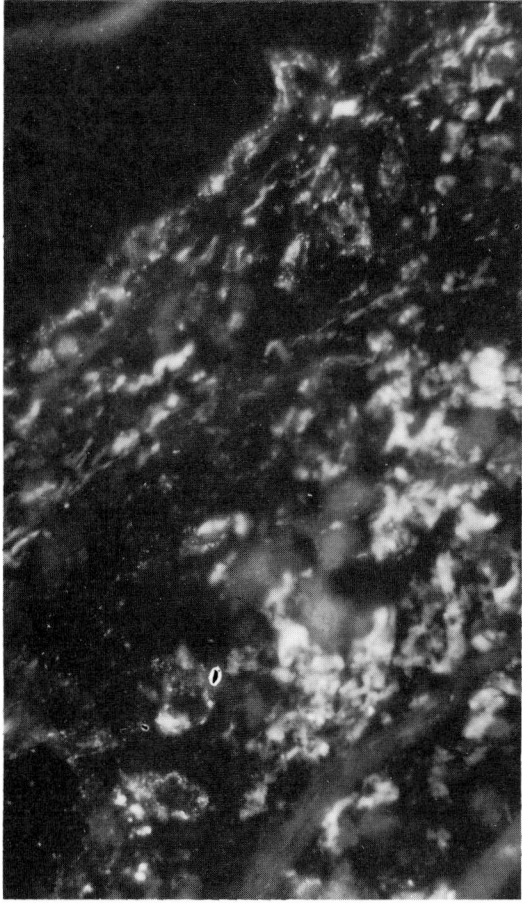

Fig. 35.3 Perivascular fibrinogen deposition in urticarial vasculitis. Isothiocyanate antibody method × 250.

Incidence

Mathews [74] states that 15% of students re-late a history of at least one episode of urti-caria. Others suggest that 20% of the general population gives a history of urticaria [98]. These estimates differ from data obtained from dermatology and allergy clinics where 2–3% of admissions are for urticaria. The true incidence is between these figures. Urticaria can occur about equally in both sexes and at all ages. Chronic urticaria occurs more often in adult female patients.

FOOD-INDUCED URTICARIA

Food may cause urticaria by pharmacological or by immunological means. Food intolerance has been used synonymously with hyper-sensitivity but as has been pointed out it may carry the connotation of aversion or emotional reaction to multiple foods and not of an im-munological hypersensitivity response [68]. The diagnosis of food allergy rests on the de-monstration of an immunological mechanism. The patterns of food sensitivity related to ur-ticaria are outlined in Table 35.1. The physi-

Table 35.1 Urticaria and foods

Type		Mechanism
I	Acute	IgE mediated
II	Chronic	Immunological, pharmacological
III	Contact	Immunological, pharmacological
IV	Postprandial exercise	Physiological
V	Idiosyncrasy	Unknown

cal urticarias do not have any significant rela-tionship to food sensitivity and so are omitted. This does not mean that a chemical contained in a food might not aggravate a physical urti-caria but solar, heat and cold urticaria as well as demographism are forms of whealing where foods have not been found to be related to primary aetiology.

Mechanisms

The majority of food-related urticarial re-actions are IgE Type I immediate hypersen-sitivity reactions (Table 35.2). Type II re-

Table 35.2 Mechanism of food urticarial reactions.

Immunological
    Type I—immediate hypersensitivity—IgE
    Type II—cytotoxic—antibody
    Type III—antigen—antibody
Non-immunological
    Mast cell—histamine-releasing agents
    Vasoactive agents—vasodilators

actions of histamine release urticaria are exemplified by the complement-mediated cy-totoxic reactions as in mismatched ABO blood transfusion urticaria. There is no specific ex-ample of a food producing urticaria by this mechanism but it will probably be found occurring via the cross-reactivity of food anti-gens and natural cellular antigens. Type III

Table 35.3 Percentage of patients showing urticarial reactions to different foods.

Food	Michailov [82] (%)	Galant et al [39] (%)	Wraith [121] (%)
Milk	24	28	0
Fish	22	28	6
Meat	19	ND	ND
Egg	18	21	10
Beans	13	ND	ND
Nuts	ND	28	80

ND = not done.

reactions, producing antigen–antibody immune complex urticaria, are discussed in the section of this chapter entitled 'Vasculitis'.

IgE-mediated reactions

IgE-sensitized mast cells may be triggered by food allergens to produce urticaria by histamine release. Type I reactions usually occur within minutes of exposure and this makes it possible for the patient to recognize the offending food. IgE antibody formation is a genetically linked response of the atopic individual. It follows, then, that many patients with acute IgE-mediated urticarial responses to food allergens are also atopic. Although dermatitis and respiratory symptoms occur frequently with food challenge [66], urticaria is an uncommon expression of food allergy [69, 106]. It is accepted that egg, milk and fish are the most common food allergens in atopic patients. Milk and fish are also important in producing urticarial rashes [3, 48].

History and skin tests. The study of food sensitivities and food challenges that produce signs and symptoms of immediate hypersensitivity has developed a relatively stable list of relevant food allergens in spite of variations in testing material, test methods and interpretation of results. Investigation by skin prick test yields a similar list of reaginic responses. Since many of these patients fall within clinical and laboratory definitions of atopy it is not surprising that many authors have noted that responses to many foods are common [39, 82, 121].

Certain food materials which have been identified in various studies as commonly causing urticarial reactions are shown in Table 35.3. The simple food avoidance list used by the Dermatology Department at the Mayo Clinic (Table 35.4) may be helpful for the patient who does not have an idea as to

Table 35.4 Food elimination diet useful in the identification and treatment of patients with food-associated urticaria.

The foods to eliminate are:
Beverages —coffee, cola
Cheese —fermented and cheese spreads
Chocolate
Meat —fresh pork, corned beef
Fish —fish, shellfish
Eggs
Fruit —fresh apples, cherries, berries, fresh or cooked bananas, grapes, mangos, melon, pineapple, rhubarb and raisins

whether a food may be significant in his urticarial reaction. Remarkably, when skin testing and radioallergosorbent tests (RAST) were developed they only confirmed the strong antigenicity of those food stuffs recognized previously by clinical experience. Hannuksela [48] divided the allergens by peak age of food intolerance as can be seen in Table 35.5.

Table 35.5 Allergens relative to peak age of food intolerance.

Years	
0–2	Egg, milk, fish, soya, pea, banana
2–7	Egg, fish, apple, pear, plum, carrot, celery, tomato, nuts, spices
Over 7	Fish, nuts, spices, fruits and vegetables as above

Cross-reactivity between natural allergens

Cross-reactivity between natural allergens, particularly in atopic individuals, demonstrates a link with inhalant food sensitivity. The correlation between ragweed inhalant sensitivity and reactions to melon and banana originally seemed to be only a connection via general atopic sensitivity [10]. However, in northern Europe where birch pollen sensitivity is frequent, immediate positive skin test reactions to fresh foods are also frequent [49]. In Scandinavia, one-quarter of the patients with asthma or allergic rhinitis gave a history of food sensitivity [36]. Hazelnut, apple and shellfish were the most common allergens but sensitivity to nuts, apple, peach, cherry, plum, pear, carrot and potato also significantly increased ($P < 0.001$). Nearly one-half of these asthma or rhinitis patients were birch pollen sensitive. Part of the major allergen of birch pollen occurs in hazelnut [15] and it is assumed that similar antigen determinants may exist in a variety of foodstuffs. Clinical cross-reactions can be seen in Table 35.6.

Table 35.6 Associated food sensitivities in patients with rhinitis, asthma or due to silver birch sensitivity ($n = 230$).

Food	Frequency (%)
Parsnip	27
Apple	26
Potato	23
Carrot	20
Celery	18
Parsley	14
Onion	13
Tomato	11

A control group of patients ($n = 158$) not sensitive to silver birch pollen showed 0–4% sensitivity.

Handling fresh food can also produce signs and symptoms. Although common antigens have not been demonstrated, the similarity of plant groups suggests such relationships may exist.

Silver birch pollen and apple

The relationship between silver birch sensitivity and apple intolerance has been well recognized [62]. Of patients allergic to silver birch pollen, 30% develop tingling of the lips and tongue after eating apple; however, urticaria and angioedema are rare following ingestion of apple. It was suggested that this could be due to contact urticaria caused by either an allergen or a plant lectin [62]. IgE antibodies may recognize a common carbohydrate determinant in many natural substances including silver birch and apple as well as hymenoptera venom, thus accounting for the clinical and RAST cross-reactivity [1]. Another form of exposure is emphasized by the angioedema and systemic symptoms reported in a compositae-sensitive beekeeper who ate Mexican honey [18] Honey contains varying amounts of compositae pollen.

Emergency room problems. Golbert et al [42] described 15 patients who appeared as emergency cases with urticaria and angioedema problems. Ten of 13 antigens involved proved to be foods: pinto beans, rice, halibut, potato, Brazil nut, shrimp, milk, cereal, garbanzo bean and tangerine. Eight of their 10 patients also had a history of allergic rhinitis or asthma. This relationship of acute urticaria from food to atopy in general is repeated throughout the literature, and the higher the IgE antibody level to inhalant allergens the more a food sensitivity is likely to occur, particularly to milk, fish and egg [66]. The converse was noted by Speer [106]; that is, of those patients who react on skin testing to three or more foods, 85% also react to inhalants. This emphasizes the relationship between inhalant and food-induced IgE responsiveness of the atopic.

Food sensitivity and complement consumption

IgG antibodies to food protein have been found in 69% of patients with immediate sensitivity reactions [39]. This response may be explained in part by the short-term sensitizing (STS) IgG antibodies described by Parish [87]. This type of antibody has been found in patients with shellfish allergy [46] as well as in 24% of patients 'suspected' of food hypersensitivity due to milk. This was four times the incidence found due to other allergens. Berrens et al [16] reported a case of egg white sensitivity and a case of fish sensitivity with normal IgE values where the serum showed complement fixation and consumption at high dilution due to IgG antibody, possibly of the IgG4 subclass.

Anaphylatoxin

Both the classical and alternative pathways of complement activation produce anaphylatoxin which is a histamine-releasing component of the complement system. Thus the effect of C5a on mast cells could produce urticaria, and undoubtedly more cases of food intolerance with complement consumption will be ascribed in the future.

CHRONIC URTICARIA

Clinical features

Recurrent or persistent urticaria lasting beyond six to 12 weeks is termed chronic or recurrent urticaria. The process occurs at all ages but is most common in adult women. The individual lesions often show persistent erythema and a white halo. The typical histamine release features may not be present. Angioedema occurs intermittently in most patients. Atopy may not be an important factor but is found in about one-third of the cases [50, 56, 77, 115]. IgE levels are usually normal in patients with chronic urticaria but when elevated, and in association with eosinophilia, indicate the presence of atopy. A history of an early episode of food-related urticaria is often found in adults with chronic urticaria, and while atopy is not the major cause of chronic hives it should not be overlooked. The most significant fact about chronic urticaria is how infrequently a single specific aetiology is discovered; in only 21% of one series [26] and 30% of another was a cause found. Where the success rate is high, the authors have usually included acute urticaria [108].

Drug sensitivity

Drug sensitivity is a relatively unimportant cause of chronic urticaria [26, 43], although Miller reported 28% of urticaria cases with drug sensitivity, an example of a rare high correlation [83]. Urticaria and angioedema are more related to salicylate sensitivity than is asthma [107].

Aspirin. The incidence of acetylsalicylic acid sensitivity varies widely in the reported series of chronic urticaria patients, from 10% [56], 18% [48] and 41% [41] to 54% [116]. The frequency of aspirin intolerance was 20 times greater in individuals with chronic urticaria (6.5%) than in normal controls (0.3%) [100].

Penicillin. These variations found in the frequency of salicylate sensitivity are also found in penicillin sensitivity. In Juhlin's 330 chronic urticaria patients, 11% did not tolerate penicillin [56]. In another series of 245 patients with chronic urticaria, 24% had positive skin tests and 12% positive penicillin RAST tests [17]. Patients in this latter study who showed positive responses to penicillin improved on a dairy product-free diet (22 of 45). However, challenging patients who gave positive skin tests with penicillin-containing meat showed no positive responses [70]. Most American dairies have been testing milk for penicillin for 20 years and, now that a rapid ^{14}C biochemical method (15 minutes) is avail-

able, it is unlikely that sensitivity to penicillin in milk is a significant factor in chronic urticaria in the USA.

The role of food in chronic urticaria

The role of food in causing acute urticaria is clearly defined, but in chronic urticaria foods are not commonly recognized as important aetiological factors [85]. In one series, food was found to be important in 30% of 330 cases of chronic urticaria [56]. The types of food believed by the patients to provoke their urticaria were almost identical to those shown in the lists in Tables 35.1 and 35.4. However, the history given by patients is an unreliable indicator. In a study of 94 children which included 21% whose history indicated foods as aetiologic factors, in only two cases could this be confirmed by testing and elimination diet [50]. Others have confirmed the low frequency of single foods as a cause of chronic urticaria. One case (of mustard sensitivity) was found in a study of 150 patients [79], and some patients sensitive to milk and fish have been reported [69]. Confirmation by skin tests and RAST tests was possible in only a few cases. Castellain et al [25] studied 100 cases of chronic urticaria and found 17 cases which they believed were alimentary in origin. A variety of foods were implicated but no confirmation by challenge tests was noted.

Yeast sensitivity

Sensitivity to yeast as expressed by immediate Type I skin intradermal test reactions was noted in 10–15% of normal individuals by Holti [54]. In a classic study, James and Warin found a positive prick test to *Candida* in 36 of 100 chronic urticaria patients [55], although they could find no other differences between the skin test positive and negative groups. However, they did note that 47% of the skin test positive group had personal atopy compared to 17% in the negative group. This was confirmed by a fivefold greater incidence of positive skin prick tests to other allergens. At a clinical level, 30 of the 33 skin test positive patients gave a positive response to administration of food yeast and/or *Candida albicans*. On this basis a yeast-free diet was prescribed as outlined in Table 35.7. No oral yeast tablets were permitted. Treatment with Mycostatin (nystatin) led to the clearing of symptoms in 16 of 28 patients. A more recent study by the same authors [116] showed that only 14% re-

Table 35.7 Yeast-free diet—foods to be eliminated.

Bread, buns
Wine, beer, cider
Grapes, raisins
Cheese
Marmite
Vinegar, ketchup, pickles
Canned foods containing yeast

sponded to yeast challenge but these cases did respond to the low yeast diet. This last figure is closer to those obtained by Juhlin (16%) [56] and Gibson and Clancy (12%) [41]. Atopic patients with chronic urticaria may have exacerbations with food yeast but the elimination diet also restricts other preservatives and chemicals (see also Chapter 49).

Additives to food

Food chemicals

The multiple mixtures of chemicals, both organic and inorganic, that the omnivorous human eats with relish are partly to blame for the confusion about food allergy or food toxicity and it is difficult to establish the constituents of a particular foodstuff (Table 35.8).

The recognition of lectins (see Chapter 21) and carcinogens as natural components of plants was one step towards the development of understanding by clinicians that food plants may be toxic as well as allergenic. Bacterial and mould action on food may produce toxins such as aflatoxin [7], and histamine-releasing agents extracted from crustacea and similar materials may be found in strawberries [88, 89, 97]. Histamine-releasing agents, most

Table 35.8 Constituents of foods and additives in foods which may cause urticarial reactions.

Food chemicals
  Protein allergens
  Lectins
  Toxins
  Carcinogens
  Histamine-releasing agents
  Vasoactive agents—amines
  Salicylates, benzoates

Prepared foods
  Aldehydes—osmylogenic urticaria
  Carcinogens, benzpyrene

Food additives
  Food colouring—azo dyes
  Food flavouring—salicylates
  Food preservatives—benzoate, nitrite, sorbic acid
  Antioxidant—hydroxytoluene, sulphite, gallate
  Emulsifiers, stabilizers—polysorbate, gums

of which are found in food, can be divided into categories that can be related to clinical urticaria: proteolytic agents, surface active agents and histamine liberators including amines [117]. Phenylethylamine in chocolate and tyramine in cheese or wine may cause aggravation of vasopermeability disease by their capacity to act on vessels as well as mast cells. A number of pharmacologically active chemicals (Table 35.9) are present in food and can

Table 35.9 Food vasoactive agents.

Nitrites—sausage, 'hot dogs'
Glutamate—soya sauce, oriental food
Tyramine—cheese, wine
Phenylethylamine—chocolate, cheese, wine
Histamine—wine

cause vasodilator headaches and erythema and/or aggravation of an urticarial state [91] (see Chapter 23). Tyramine activity is particularly reinforced if the patient is taking monoamine oxidase inhibitors. Nitrites, which are preservatives, and food colourings, which can cause a flush and headache, will exacerbate urticaria. Moneret-Vautrin et al [84] found positive provocation tests with sodium nitrite in 4 of 76 patients with urticaria. Salicylates, to which many chronic urticaria patients are sensitive, are found naturally in berries, bananas, green peas, apples, rhubarb, almonds and liquorice. Benzoates are also found in many of the same foods in smaller amounts (see also Chapter 49).

Food colours

Azo dyes, in particular tartrazine, occur in many packaged and prepared foods. Tartrazine sensitivity has been calculated as occurring in 0.1% of the population [73]. Patients with urticaria may react on challenge to yellow, red or blue azo dyes. Tartrazine (F.D. & C. Yellow No. 5) was the first food dye reported to be related to urticaria in 1959 [71]. Such patients may also be sensitive to aspirin, as was shown by Samter and Beers who demonstrated tartrazine sensitivity in 30 of 40 aspirin-sensitive individuals [95]. Since that time a variable incidence of tartrazine sensitivity has been reported, from 54% [80] to 18% [57]. Various authors have noted a lower incidence, as illustrated in Table 35.10. A strict double-blind oral test procedure produced a value of 8% (3 of 38) of chronic urticaria patients sensitive to tartrazine challenge [101]. Two of the three positive patients were also

Table 35.10 Food additives and chronic urticaria (percentages of positive reactions)

	Number of cases	Aspirin	Penicillin	Benzoic acid	Sorbic acid	Azo dye	BHT	Yeast
Warin and Smith [116]	111	41	15	10	–	13	–	14
Gibson and Clancy [41]	76	54	18	34	–	26	–	12
Juhlin et al [57]	330	10	11	11	9	18	15	16
Hannuksela [48]	137	18	0	4	0	1	–	0

BHT = butylated hydroxytoluene.
– = Not recorded.

sensitive to aspirin. Other double-blind investigations showed a cross reactivity to tartrazine in aspirin-sensitive patients of up to 20% [34, 99]. Non-azo dyes and the reduction product of azo dyes, sulphanilic acid, give no responses.

Food-flavouring agents

A broad range of salicylic acid esters is used to flavour foods such as cake mixes, puddings, ice cream, chewing gum and soft drinks and both benzyl- and methylsalicylate are known allergens for Type IV contact-mediated reactions. The mechanism of action of these agents on urticaria might be similar to that of aspirin. Other flavouring agents such as cinnamon, benzoic acid and vanilla may cross-react with each other. Balsam of Peru, a strong allergen, contains cinnamates and benzoates. The menthol and oil of wintergreen flavours have been associated with exacerbations of urticaria. The menthol in cigarettes can also be related to exacerbation of urticaria.

Food preservatives

Benzoates. Benzoates and benzoic acid are used as food and medicine preservatives and are the most common ones used. The incidence of reactions is said to be less than 1%. The frequency of positive challenges with benzoate in patients with chronic urticaria varies from 4 to 34% (Table 35.10). Doeglas [35] showed that benzoate as a preservative occurred frequently in fish and shrimp in quantities up to 1000 mg/kg which is 2 to 20 times the amount needed to produce an exacerbation of urticaria. The variable content of benzoate in shrimps may account for the erratic response on challenge.

Antioxidants. Food antioxidants are a special type of preservative calculated to reduce oxidation of chemicals in food. The gallate esters are trihydroxybenzoic acid derivatives widely

present in nature. These compounds sensitize and are responsible for contact dermatitis. The synthetic agents butylated hydroxytoluene (BHT) and butylated hydroxyanisol (BHA) are the principal agents used; as may be seen in Table 35.10, these compounds may cause flares of urticaria after oral challenge in approximately 15% of patients [56, 113]. Prepared and packaged foods contain these substances.

Sodium sulphite–sulphur dioxide antioxidants and similar compounds are found in processed food, dried food, potato chips and beverages such as fruit juices, soft drinks, wines, beer, cider and vinegar. These are antibrowning agents and so they are used to maintain fresh food such as lettuce, seafoods such as shrimp, fruits and vegetables. Ingestion of sulphites may cause asthma, urticaria and angioedema [60, 90]. The source may be as varied as lettuce or wine or medications [29]. It is estimated that 100 mg of bisulphite may be ingested in a restaurant meal.

Emulsifying and stabilizing agents

Commercial foods often need materials to ensure that solids do not settle out or separate. Vegetable gums such as acacia, gum arabic, tragacanth, quince, carob seed or carageenin have been known as urticarial allergens for many years. Polysorbates are common modern materials for producing these effects. Urticaria to polysorbate in ice cream has been reported [24]. All of the foods containing these agents are mixtures, and usually preservatives, dyes and antioxidants are also present.

Mechanism of action

The mechanism of action of food additives as an aggravating or causative factor in urticaria is not clear. The IgE and complement levels of the chronic urticaria patients are normal and do not change during salicylate or other provocation. Antibody formation has been reported in response to tartrazine but no evidence of its relation to the urticaria has been provided [8]. Repeated studies to show the immunological mechanism of salicylate and other food additives in urticaria have been largely inconclusive [32, 44, 122]. It appears logical therefore to assume that there may be a direct effect of the salicylates and similar food additives on the complement, kinin or lipooxygenase–cyclooxygenase systems. It is also possible that the effect is on the blood vessels at a time when chronic vasopermeability already exists. The dose–effect response to these chemicals of chronic urticaria patients is a reason to believe in the non-immunological mechanism. There is no clear antigenic type or structural relationship common to the food additives that exacerbate urticaria. No sensitizing episode is observed. Most important, the regression of salicylate and additive responsiveness can occur when the urticaria regresses.

Desensitization

It is possible to desensitize patients with urticaria and salicylate sensitivity [11] by giving the patients 650 mg of aspirin daily for three weeks. Following this regime, foods which had previously caused signs and symptoms no longer did so. The patients gave a history of reaction to pineapple, milk, eggs, cheese, fish, chocolate, pork, strawberries and plums, but when tested after salicylate exposure did not give a reaction. Resting plasma $PGF_{2\alpha}$ was $24.89 \pm pg/ml$ in the patients compared to control subjects with $6.7 \pm 1.1 \, pg/ml$ $(P < 0.01)$. This could be a direct effect of salicylate on the prostaglandin pathway and could show the way for measurement of the effects of other food additives. Others have confirmed that aspirin tolerance could be induced in aspirin-sensitive patients but found that it returned within nine days of stopping the treatment [61].

CONTACT URTICARIA

The immediate wheal and flare response elicited within 30–60 minutes by normal skin exposure to certain agents is called contact urticaria. A less well-defined four to six hour delayed contact urticaria also exists. Recent reviews of this subject indicate how important foods and food additives are in the expression of contact urticaria [63].

Classification

Krogh and Maibach [63] classified contact urticaria as
Stage I: localized wheal and flare restricted to area of contact,
Stage II: generalize urticaria including angioedema,
Stage III: urticaria combined with asthma, and
Stage IV: urticaria and anaphylaxis.

Approximately 15% of patients have associated systemic signs and symptoms of rhino-conjunctivitis, oral, pharyngeal or gastrointestinal reactions and 10% react with widespread urticaria. Atopy is found in 10–20% of patients.

Immunological mechanisms

The mechanism of action of food in contact urticaria may be immunological or non-immunological. The IgE mechanism of histamine release is triggered by an antigen in contact with the skin producing a wheal. The milk-sensitive patient of Golbert et al [42] (case 6) is an example of an IgE-mediated reaction. Milk poured over the hands produced wheals. Contact urticaria to proteins has been shown in food handlers [52] Obviously, food proteins can create a markedly increased reaction when tested through scratch test sites. RAST often correlate with contact testing and the Prausnitz–Küstner response may also be positive.

The presence and significance of contact urticaria in atopic disease may have been underestimated [78]. Perhaps this is the basis of the itching, tingling and/or oedema of the lips and oral tissue experienced by birch pollen sensitive (atopic) individuals when eating raw apple, potato, carrot or tomato. Hannuksela and Lahti [49] noted that simple handling of these foods can also cause contact urticaria in such patients.

Penetration of the skin. Penetration of the allergen may be a factor in elicitation of the contact urticaria. Normal skin varies markedly in epidermal permeability in the various body areas. Permeability is increased in areas of healed but recently involved dermatitic skin. Krogh and Maibach [63] demonstrated contact urticaria in such areas to turkey, lamb and flour at a time when testing of comparable normal skin was negative. Vehicles are important, for an allergen in ethanol may show a wheal within 15 minutes while the same allergen in petrolatum produces a reaction at closer to one hour. The temperature of the skin (blood flow?) may influence the development of contact urticaria. Minimal reactions at 25°C may be urticarial responses at 45°C.

Foods inducing contact urticaria. The food allergens found to have the frequent capacity to produce contact urticaria are listed in Table 35.11. This is almost identical to the list of foods that commonly cause acute urticaria [38,67,75]. Some cases of acute urticaria may actually be acute contact urticaria. Some of the gastrointestinal signs and symptoms associated may be the direct reaction of the allergen on the intestinal wall, as in cutaneous contact urticaria.

Non-immunological mechanisms

An excellent argument for the existence of non-immunological urticaria is the whealing produced by first contact with a low molecular weight chemical. Table 35.11 lists the food ad-

Table 35.11 Foodstuffs related to contact urticaria

Food
　Seafood—fish, lobster, shrimp, cod liver oil
　Meat—chicken, turkey, lamb, beef, liver
　Vegetables—potato, tomato, lettuce, endive, celery
　Miscellaneous—egg, milk, cheese, flour, malt, peanut butter
　Spices—cinnamon, vanilla, mustard, cassia and caraway oil, paprika

Additives
　Aspirin
　Benzoic acid—parabens
　Sorbic acid
　Sulphur dioxide
　Polyethylene glycol

ditives which may produce histamine release, prostaglandin alterations or react by unknown mechanisms. Sorbic acid and benzoic acid in salad dressing were noted to cause contact urticaria [30]. Such reactions are not blocked by antihistamines. Lahti [65] found that the local site could be exhausted by repeated application and a local dose–response effect could be shown. The ability of the chemical additives to produce local contact urticaria and to exacerbate chronic urticaria could be caused by the same mechanism.

Post-prandial exercise urticaria

The influence of blood flow on the activity of clinical urticaria is not doubted by physicians who have observed a well-regulated urticarial treatment programme destroyed by a patient resuming a physical activity such as jogging. Those physiological changes that result in vasodilation and perspiration will aggravate urticarial lesions. The vasopermeability state will be exacerbated whether the influence is external heat or heat radiation from exercise.

The effect of increased vasopermeability on atopic reactivity has recently been characterized as exercise anaphylaxis [102] (see also Chapter 25). Pruritus was the first sign but urticarial lesions developed, as did asthma. A final state of anaphylaxis was present in some patients. Subsequently, it has been found that this occurred after a meal in some patients and that without the specific challenge contained in the meal the physiological response would produce minimal or no symptoms [76]. The patients have a history of multiple atopic diseases [59] although Novey et al [86] did not show histamine or complement changes in the blood during the reaction. Buchbinder et al [22] showed elevated plasma histamine levels in the patients during the general reaction. Allergens recognized include celery, shellfish, peach and at times simply multiple food exposures.

Exercise alone with heat-retaining clothing did not produce the reaction. It is possible that alcohol and vasodilating drugs will play a similar role to exercise. The effect of food additives plus exercise has not been studied.

DIAGNOSTIC TESTS

A major clinical problem in food-induced urticaria is the difficulty in confirming the diagnosis. It is not possible to reproduce in vitro the ingested food mixture and its effects, its change by digestion or bacterial action, its absorption or its eventual circulation to the shock organ—the dermal subpapillary venules. Multiple allergens may be found in a single food such as milk e.g. lactoglobulin, lactalbumin, casein, immunoglobulin as well as food additives and contaminants. Aas [2] notes that only a few allergens can reliably be used in skin testing and RAST. Isolating a single chemical allergen may be pure science but may also be irrelevant to a given patient's problem. The fact that many patients are sensitive to more than one food points to the area of usefulness of tests. Testing is useful if the reaction is IgE mediated, if the patient is atopic and if the sensitivity is to a strong antigen such as fish, milk, egg or nuts. Laboratory testing has not been of value for non-IgE-mediated urticaria to date.

Skin tests

Intradermal and scratch tests for immediate hypersensitivity. Intradermal or scratch tests identify the atopic patient by the multiple reactions to relevant antigens. While atopy is usually established by case history and examination, occasionally patients with urticaria who have atopic skin reactivity may not have previously demonstrated clinical disease. The cutaneous vascular and inflammatory responses of the atopic patient have their own unique reactivities and these may modulate the urticarial response [118]. The positive skin test to a food allergen will often correlate with a history of immediate food hypersensitivity. The higher the IgE value the larger may be the cutaneous wheal and flare skin test. This relationship is most apparent in other atopic disease but may also be observed in urticaria. In chronic urticaria patients there is rarely a correlation between history, skin test and RAST [43, 69]. In acute urticaria immediate skin hypersensitivity reactions are more common to the expected allergens, i.e. fish, nuts, shellfish, egg, milk and chocolate [42, 45]. The presence of positive skin tests may be relevant in cases of recurrent urticaria particularly if the skin reaction is large and the patient is atopic.

Patch tests for delayed hypersensitivity. Patch tests using common antigens have been studied by the International Contact Dermatitis Group in chronic urticaria patients. Surprisingly, 22% of positive reactions were recorded in one series [20]. Formaldehyde, nickel and balsam of Peru gave the highest percentage positive reactions. Balsam of Peru is important because it contains cinnamate and benzoate and may cross-react with vanilla.

Specific IgE

RAST. The radioallergosorbent (RAST) method of testing for IgE antibody to food antigens has had some success in confirming food sensitivity diagnosis. Wraith et al [121] found 79% of foods causing signs and symptoms gave positive RAST results. It must be emphasized that where the food reaction was immediate the patient was usually aware of the offending food and there was 100% correlation

with the RAST. These authors state 'We found the RAST method a useful and safe guide upon which to base a clinical investigation for food allergy ...' However, this is by no means a universal experience and indeed only one patient with urticaria in their series (2.5%) had a positive RAST, 11 giving negative results. This experience echoes the results of others [27, 28, 53]. The RAST is invariably negative when the clinical history and skin prick tests are negative. Aas [2] believes it is best to use the skin tests and RAST together and best also when the allergen is a strong one, such as fish, egg or nut.

ELISA. The enzyme-linked immunosorbent assay (ELISA) has been used to measure food-specific IgE to 12 common foods [12]. Six patients had urticaria as their presenting sign and atopic and non-atopic patients were compared. Atopic patients had significantly higher ELISA values. However, ELISA values to egg white did not correlate with RAST results. The RAST and ELISA tests depend on high values of specific IgE and correlate with history and skin test results. For these reasons they are not of much use in blind testing for food sensitivity in chronic urticaria. The few positive responses obtained are not usually worth the expense of the test.

Histamine release. Tests involving histamine release from in vivo and in vitro sources have been used successfully to confirm food allergy. In most instances the reactions have been positive in patients with acute urticaria and usually with an atopic history. Plasma histamine was increased in the blood of two patients with urticaria given an oral challenge with chocolate and with aspirin, respectively [51]. The rise in plasma histamine correlated with the onset of urticaria. Plasma histamine changes following aspirin challenge in asthma patients have shown conflicting results, with some groups showing no change [51] and some an elevation [92, 109]. The contrasting study of food dyes and sodium benzoate effects on rat mast cells showed no degranulation or histamine release, supporting a non-immunological mechanism for the effects of these substances in food [19].

Skin window and blast transformation. Examination of other cells may be useful in the diagnosis of food allergy. Eosinophils may migrate to a skin window treated with food antigen [23]. It has also been reported but not confirmed that food antigens will cause blast transformation in lymphocytes of susceptible individuals with urticaria [114]. It is harder to explain a similar response produced by food additives.

VASCULITIS

The clinical usage of the term vasculitis commonly means leukocytoclastic or allergic vasculitis. This is a Type III antigen–antibody complex reaction producing local perivascular inflammation and purpura [96, 104, 105]. Purpura predominates in most clinical lesions but gradually in the past decade it has been recognized that a form of chronic urticaria has been caused by this specific mechanism. Clinical, histological and laboratory evaluation can readily distinguish between Type I and Type III urticarial lesions.

Clinical features

The lesions begin as indistinct macules which gradually become mottled pink and white macules or plaques. Itching is common. The lesions may last 24–96 hours. On occasion faint petechiae may be observed, particularly after diascopy. Residual scaling or pigmentation may follow the lesions. Angiodema is less common. The patients are usually ill, presenting with a low-grade fever, arthralgia or joint swelling as well as myalgia and malaise.

Histopathology

The microscopic picture should be of a necrotizing or leukocytoclastic vasculitis or venulitis. Most series of cases rely on the histopathology of the skin for diagnosis. At times this may be confirmed by direct immunofluorescence study of the skin biopsy. Occasionally the immunofluorescence study is positive and the histopathology is not characteristic. Injections of epinephrine or histamine into the normal skin may induce a purpuric papule. Direct immunofluorescence of the normal skin may be positive in systemic small vessel vasculitis.

Laboratory tests

Laboratory evaluation of these patients has revealed decreased complement [72], elevated sedimentation rate, abnormal proteins such as cryoglobulins and positive antinuclear anti-

bodies and rheumatoid factor in some cases. While hypocomplementaemia in chronic urticaria is important in indicating Type III disease it is only one of many laboratory tests that are useful. Circulating immune complexes are found in this type of chronic urticaria [41, 103]. These serological results reflect a Type III mechanism and may indicate a relationship to the more severe systemic illness.

Systemic disease

Patients with urticarial vasculitis are often found to have a significant infectious disease such as hepatitis, systemic connective tissue disease, e.g. lupus erythematosus, or other immunoreactivity such as mixed cryoglobulinaemia. The exhaustive literature reviews of urticarial vasculitis do not reveal food as an important factor in this syndrome.

Food-related purpura

Much of the literature on the relation of food to purpura/vasculitis consists of anecdotal case reports [4].

For 50 years occasional cases of food-related purpura have been reported (Table 35.12). It was not until the 1960s, however, that skin biopsy confirmation of vasculitis was utilized. It is an interesting side-light that Galloway's case [40] from 1903 and the case listed in 1964 [120] both occurred with blackberry ingestion. Review of all these cases leads to the conclusion that vasculitis may indeed be the proper diagnosis even if microscopical and immunological confirmation are not present. Most of these cases were reported because multiple exposures to the listed food correlated with repeated episodes of purpura, arthralgia, melaena or haematuria.

Tartrazine sensitivity. The case reported by Criep [31] of a 22-year-old female with repeated butter and margarine sensitivity giving rise to purpura is the first instance of tartrazine sensitivity and vasculitis. Clinically, the patient demonstrated inflammatory purpura but the biopsy was not confirmatory. Subsequently vasculitis cases have been reported who showed positive azo dye oral provocation tests [81]. The patients improved on an additive-free diet. Juhlin's group have suggested that nicotinate would increase the ease of diagnosis but this treatment of the skin by itself will produce vasculitis in the skin of patients with systemic vasculitis.

Table 35.12 Reported cases of food-related purpura.

Author	Date	Age	Sex	Foods	Signs of disease			
					Purpura	Gastro-intestinal	Renal	Joint
Galloway [40]	1903	—	F	Blackberries, nuts	+	+	+	
Sachs [94]	1916	—	—	Anchovy	+			
Alexander and Eyermann [5]	1927	32	F	Milk	+	+	+	
		4	M	Egg	+			+
Alexander and Eyermann [6]	1929	50	M	Milk	+	+		
		5	M	Egg, potato, wheat	+	+		
		532	F	Egg, chicken, beans	+	+		
		14	M	Plums	+	+		
		50	F	Wheat	+	+		
		52	F	Pork, strawberries	+			
Kahn [58]	1929	49	F	Wheat, fish	+			
Barthelme [13]	1930	22	F	Wheat	+			
Eyermann [37]	1935	30	F	Egg, chicken, beans	+	+		
		19	F	Milk	+			
Diamond [33]	1936	10	F	Milk	+			
		4	F	Tomato, chocolate	+			
		3	M	Popcorn	+			
		11	F	Chocolate	+			
		4	F	Chocolate	+			
		5	M	Oats, chocolate	+			
Hampton [47]	1941	15	F	Milk	+	+		+
		20	F	Milk, wheat, apple, prune, orange, bean	+	+		
Brown [21]	1946	9	M	Tomato	+	+	+	+
Acona et al [9]	1951	30	M	Shellfish	+		+	
Winkelmann [120]	1964	47	F	Blackberries	+	+	+	+

Another case of tartrazine sensitivity has been reported in a 49-year-old female with a one-year history of recurrent purpura of the lower legs and arthritis [64]. No biopsy was reported but after provocation by tartrazine a biopsy showed leukocytoclastic vasculitis. The patient also had a positive reaction to benzoate. A diet free of additives was of help. This patient also had a long history of asthma and review of the individual cases reported to date shows a frequent incidence of a personal and family history of atopic diseases. A simple listing of the antigens reported to cause food-related purpura/vasculitis shows a similarity to the foods commonly related to acute Type I atopic urticaria. Milk, fish, eggs, chocolate and berries are common antigens that have been related as causative factors. It appears that a background of atopy is closely correlated with vasculitis where foods have been isolated as provoking agents.

Iodine. Iodine is among the food materials that may produce allergic reactivity and exacerbation of vaculitis. The tendency to use 'natural' foods has created a demand for seaweed and kelp pills containing iodides. Alfalfa pills have caused exacerbation of lupus erythematosus and probably vasculitis.

Vitamins. Various health cults have been suggesting megavitamin doses for many illnesses. These large pharmacological doses of vitamins are toxic and cause aggravated vasculitis. Bear et al [14] report a patient who took 40 vitamin tablets per day with coincident exacerbation of vasculitis. This could have been due to iodide content. Ruzicka et al [93] reported the case of a 68-year-old woman who gave a three-week history of oedema and purpuric papulopustules of the feet. Biopsy was consistent with leukocytoclastic vasculitis and testing revealed immediate and delayed hypersensitivity to vitamin B_6 or pyridoxine and to sulphinpyrasone. Avoidance of the pyridoxine produced a remission.

p-Aminobenzoate. Another component of the B vitamin complex is *p*-aminobenzoate. Recently a case of chronic urticaria related to taking of aminobenzoic acid was reported [112] The patient had a chronic urticaria resistant to treatment and diet. When her multivitamin was stopped her hives ceased. Oral provocation test with the vitamin product and with aminobenzoic acid resulted in urticaria. This same relationship should be sought in vasculitis.

Pharmacological agents. The demonstration that histamine and catecholamines will induce vasculitis lesions may tell us how foods are able to produce aggravation of purpuric and vasculitis reactions. The systemic use of pressor amines as a recreational drug can lead directly to vasculitis. These agents also act as trigger factors for established necrotizing vasculitis. The pattern of reactions between food and vasculitis may be due to an atopic sensitivity to food which releases histamine. The histamine in turn may then provoke the lesions of a latent or ongoing vasculitis. Food additives will provide the same stimulus capable of inducing vasculitis, perhaps by a non-immunological mechanism of histamine or mediator release [110]. The patients who show a food additive reaction are also frequently atopic individuals. A study of food-related vasculitis patients with new methodology to show a relation between histamine release, antibodies, complement levels and lesion production may confirm this hypothesis.

REFERENCES

1 Aalberse RC, Koshte V, Clemens JG: Immunoglobulin E antibodies that cross react with vegetable, foods, pollen, and *Hymenoptera* venom. J Allergy Clin Immunol 1981; 68:356-64.

2 Aas K: Diagnosis of hypersensitivity to ingested food. Clin Allergy 1978; 8:39-50.

3 Aas K, Lundquist V: The radioallergosorbent test with a purified allergen from cod. Clin Allergy 1973; 3:255-61.

4 Ackroyd JF: Allergic purpura including purpura due to foods, drugs, and infections. Am J Med 1953; 14:605-32.

5 Alexander HL, Eyermann CH: Food allergy in Henoch's syndrome. Arch Dermatol Syph 1927; 16: 322-7.

6 Alexander HL, Eyermann CH: Allergic purpura. J Am Med Assoc 1929; 92:2092-4.

7 Ames BN: Dietary carcinogens and anticarcinogens. Science 1983; 221:1256-64.

8 Amos HE, Drake JJP: Problems posed by food additives. J Hum Nutr 1976; 30:165-78.

9 Ancona GR, Ellerhorn MJ, Falconer EH: Purpura due to food sensitivity. J Allergy 1951; 22:487-93.

10 Anderson L, Dreyfuss E, Logan J et al: Melon and banana sensitivity coincident with ragweed pollinosis. J Allergy 1970; 54:310-18.

11 Asad SI, Youlten LJF, Lessof MH: Specific desensitization in aspirin sensitive urticaria. Clin Allergy 1983; 13:459-66.

12 Bambdad S, Goodwin BFJ, Hill JE: IgE antibodies to food allergies detected by ELISA, RAST, and money PCA. Clin Allergy 1983; 13:96-7.

13 Barthelme FL: Allergic purpura. J Allergy 1930; 1:170-1.

14 Bear RA, Lang AP, Garvey MB: Vasculitis and vitamin abuse. Arch Pathol Lab Med 1982; 103:48.

15 Belin L: Immunological analysis of birch pollen antigens with special reference to the allergenic components. Int Arch Allergy Appl Immunol 1972; 42:300-22.

16 Berrens L, Dyk AG, van Weemaes CMP: Complement consumption in egg white and fish sensitivity. Clin Allergy 1981; 11:101-9.

17 Boonk WJ, van Ketel WG: The role of penicillin in the pathogenesis of chronic urticaria. Br J Dermatol 1982; 106:183-8.

18 Bousquet J, Campos J, Michel FB: Food intolerance to honey. Allergy 1984; 39:73-5.

19 Breindler JJ, Slutsky J, Haddad ZH: The effect of food colors and sodium benzoate on rat peritoneal mast cells. Ann Allergy 1980; 44:76-81.

20 Bronk WJ, van Ketel WG: Skin testing in chronic urticaria. Dermatologica 1981; 163:151-9.

21 Brown A: Henoch-Schöenlein purpura and acute nephritis due to food allergy. Glasgow Med J 1946; 27:84-7.

22 Buchbinder EM, Bloch KJ, Moss J, Guiney TG: Food dependent exercise-induced anaphylaxis. JAMA 1983; 250:2973-4.

23 Bullock JD, Bodenbender JG: A simple laboratory aid in diagnosing food allergy. Ann Allergy 1970; 28:127-32.

24 Camarassa JM: Acute contact urticaria. Contact Dermatitis 1982; 8:347-8.

25 Castellain P-Y, Bonniol P, Saint-Andre P, Varenne E: New research on the etiology and therapy of chronic urticaria. Bull Soc Fr Dermatol Syph 1971; 78:578-84.

26 Champion RH, Roberts SOB, Carpenter RG, Roger JW: Urticaria and angioedema. A review of 554 patients. Br J Dermatol 1969; 81:588.

27 Chua YY, Bremner K, Kaldawalla N et al: In vivo and in vitro correlates of food allergy. J Allergy Clin Immunol 1976; 58:299-308.

28 Chua YY, Bremner K, Llobet JK et al: Diagnosis of food allergy by the radioallergosorbent test. J Allergy Clin Immunol 1976; 58:477-82.

29 Clayton DE, Busse W: Anaphylaxis to wine. Clin Allergy 1980; 10:341-3.

30 Clemmensen O, Hjorth N: Perioral contact urticaria from sorbic acid and benzoic acid in salad dressing. Contact Dermatitis 1982; 8:1-6.

31 Criep LH: Allergic vascular purpura. J Allergy Clin Immunol 1971; 48:7-12.

32 De Weck AL: Immunological effects of aspirin anhydride. Int Arch Allergy Appl Immunol 1971; 41:393-408.

33 Diamond J: Anaphylactoid or allergic purpura. J Pediatr 1936; 8:697-703.

34 Doeglas HMG: Reactions to aspirin and food additives in patients with chronic urticaria. Br J Dermatol 1975; 93:135-44.

35 Doeglas HMG: Dietary treatment of patients with chronic urticaria and intolerance to aspirin and food additives. Dermatologica 1977; 154:308-10.

36 Ericksson NE: Food sensitivity reported by patients with asthma and hay fever. Allergy 1978; 33:189-96.

37 Eyermann CH: Allergic purpura. South Med J 1935; 28:341-5.

38 Fisher AA: Contact urticaria due to medicaments, chemicals, and foods. Cutis 1982; 30:168-74.

39 Galant SP, Bullock J, Frick OL: An immunological approach to the diagnosis of food sensitivity. Clin Allergy 1973; 3:363-72.

40 Galloway J: An address on the erythemata as indicators of disease. Brit Med J 1903; 2:12-123.

41 Gibson A, Clancy R: Management of chronic idiopathic urticaria by the identification and exclusion of dietary factors. Clin Allergy 1980; 10:699-704.

42 Golbert TM, Patterson R, Pruzansky JJ: Systemic allergic reactions to ingested antigens. J Allergy 1969; 44:96-107.

43 Green GR, Koelsche GA, Kierland RR: Etiology and pathogenesis of chronic urticaria. Ann Allergy 1965; 23:30-48.

44 Guinaldo B, Blumenthal MN, Spink WW: Aspirin intolerance and asthma. Ann Intern Med 1969; 71:479-86.

45 Haddad ZH, Korotzer JL: Immediate hypersensitivity reactions to food antigens. J Allergy Clin Immunol 1972; 49:210-18.

46 Halpern GM: Sensitization to shellfish. Nouv Presse Med 1977; 6:3111-13.

47 Hampton SF: Henoch's purpura based on food allergy. J Allergy 1941; 12:579-89.

48 Hannuksela M: Food allergy and skin diseases. Ann Allergy 1983; 51:269-72.

49 Hannuksela M, Lahti A: Immediate reactions to fruits and vegetables. Contact Dermatitis 1977; 3:79-84.

50 Harris A, Twarog FJ, Geha RS: Chronic urticaria in childhood: natural course and etiology. Ann Allergy 1983; 51:161-5.

51 Harris MG, O'Brien IM, Burge PS, Pepys J: Effects of orally administered sodium chromoglycate in asthma and urticaria due to foods. Clin Allergy 1978; 8:423-7.

52 Hjorth N, Roed-Petersen J: Occupational protein contact dermatitis in food handlers. Contact Dermatitis 1976; 2:28-42.

53 Hoffman DR, Haddad ZH: Diagnosis of IgE mediated reactions to food antigens by radioimmunoassay. J Allergy Clin Immunol 1974; 54:165-72.

54 Holti G: Candida allergy. In: Winner HI, Hurley R, eds. Symposium on Candida infections, 1966; Edinburgh: Churchill Livingstone.

55 James J, Warin RP: An assessment of the role of Candida albicans and food yeasts in chronic urticaria. Br J Dermatol 1971; 84:227-37.

56 Juhlin L: Recurrent urticaria. Br J Dermatol 1981; 104:369-81.

57 Juhlin L, Michaelsson G, Zetterstrom O: Urticaria and asthma induced by food and drug additives in patients with aspirin hypersensitivity. J Allergy Clin Immunol 1972; 50:92-104.

58 Kahn IS: Henoch's purpura due to food allergy. J Lab Clin Med 1929; 14:835-6.

59 Kidd JM, Cohen SH, Sosman AJ et al: Food dependent exercise-induced anaphylaxis. Allergy Clin Immunol 1983; 71:407-11.

60 Koepke JW, Christopher KL, Chai H, Selner JC: Dose-dependent bronchospasm from sulfites in isoetharine. J Am Med Assoc 1984; 251:2982-4.

61 Kowalski ML, Grzelewski-Ryzmowska I, Rozniecki J, Szmidt M: Aspirin-induced tolerance in aspirin sensitive asthmatics. Allergy 1984; 39:171-8.

62 Kresmer M, Lindemayr W: The frequency of the so-called 'apple allergy' (apple contact urticaria syndrome) in patients with birch pollinosis. Z Hautkr 1983; 58:543-52.

63 Krogh GJ, Maibach H: The contact urticaria syndrome: an updated review. J Am Acad Dermatol 1980; 5:328-42.

64 Kubba R, Champion RH: Anaphylactoid purpura caused by tartrazine and benzoate. Br J Dermatol [Suppl 11] 1975; 93:61-2.

65 Lahti A: Nonimmunologic contact urticaria. Acta Derm Venereol [Suppl 91] (Stock) 1980; 60:8-49.

66 Langeland T: A clinical and immunological study of allergy to hen's egg white. Clin Allergy 1983; 13:371-82.

67 Larko O, Lindstedt G, Lundberg PA, Mobacken H: Biochemical and clinical studies in a case of contact urticaria to potato. Contact Dermatitis 1983; 9:108-14.

68 Lessof MH: Food and allergy—a review. Q J Med 1983; 206:111-19.

69 Lessof MH, Wraith DG, Merrett TG et al: Food allergy and intolerance in 100 patients—local and systemic effects. Q J Med 1980; 195:259-71.

70 Lindemayr H, Knobler R, Kraft D, Baumgartner W: Challenge of penicillin-allergic volunteers with penicillin-containing meat. Allergy 1981; 36:471-88.

71 Lockey SD Sr: Allergic reactions due to F, D & C yellow No. 5, tartrazine, an aniline dye used as a coloring and identifying agent in various steroids. Ann Allergy 1959; 17:719-21.

72 McDuffie FC, Sams WM, Maldonado JE: Hypocomplementemia with cutaneous vasculitis and arthritis. Mayo Clin Proc 1973; 48:340-8.

73 MacGibbon B: Adverse reactions to food additives. Proc Nutr Soc 1983; 42:233-340.

74 Mathews KP: Urticaria and angioedema. J Allergy Clin Immunol 1983; 72:1-14.

75 Mathias GG: Contact urticaria from peanut butter. Contact Dermatitis 1983; 9:66-8.

76 Maulitz RM, Pratt DS, Shocket AL: Exercise-induced anaphylactic reaction to shellfish. Allergy Clin Immunol 1979; 63:433-4.

77 Meynadier J, Guilhou JJ, Levanture N: Chronic urticaria. Ann Dermatol Venereol 1979; 106:153-8.

78 Meynadier J, Meynadier JM, Guilhou JJ: Contact urticaria in atopic patients. Ann Dermatol Venereol 1982; 109:871-4.

79 Meynadier J, Guilhou JJ, Meynadier J, Levanture N: Chronic urticaria. Ann Dermatol Venereol (Paris) 1979; 106:153-64.

80 Michaelsson G, Juhlin L: Urticaria induced by preservatives and dye additives to food and drugs. Br J Dermatol 1973; 88:525-34.

81 Michaelsson G, Petterson L, Juhlin L: Purpura caused by food and drug additives. Arch Dermatol 1974; 109:49-52.

82 Michailov P, Berova N: Gastrointestinal disorders in the pathogenesis of urticaria. Z Haut Geschlechtskr 1971; 46:609-12.

83 Miller DA, Freeman GL, Akers WA: Chronic urticaria. Am J Med 1968; 44:68-79.

84 Moneret-Vautrin DA, Einhorn C, Tisserand J: The role of sodium nitrite in histamine urticaria of dietary origin. Ann Nutr Alim 1980; 34:1125-32.

85 Monroe EW, Jones HE: Urticaria. Arch Dermatol 1977; 113:80-90.

86 Novey HS, Fairshter RD, Selness K et al: Postprandial exercise-induced anaphylaxis. J Allergy Clin Immunol 1983; 71:498-504.

87 Parish W: Short term anaphylactic IgG antibody in human serum. Lancet 1970; ii:591-2.

88 Paton WDM: Histamine liberation and lymphogogue. J Physiol 1954; 123.

89 Paton WDM: The mechanism of histamine release in

histamine. Ciba Foundation Symposium. Boston Mass: Little, Brown Co, 1956; 59–73.

90 Prenner BM, Stevens JJ: Anaphylaxis after ingestion of sodium bisulfite. Ann Allergy 1976; 37:180–2.

91 Raskin NH: Chemical headaches. Ann Rev Med 1981; 32:63–71.

92 Reimann HJ, Ultsch B, Wendt P et al: Release of gastric histamine in patients with urticaria and food allergy. Agents Actions 1982; 12:111–13.

93 Ruzicka T, Ring J, Braun-Falco O: Vasculitis allergica through vitamin B-6. Hautarzt 1984; 35:197–9.

94 Sachs O: Uber eine noch nicht beschriebeue Purpura Form nach Genuss von sadellen Butter. Arch Dermatol Syph 1916; 123:835–7.

95 Samter M, Beers RF: Concerning the nature of intolerance to aspirin. J Allergy 1967; 40:281–91.

96 Sanchez NP, Winkelmann RK, Schroeter Al, Dicken CH: The clinical and histopathological spectrum of urticarial vasculitis. J Am Acad Dermatol 1982; 7:595–605.

97 Schachter M: Histamine release and the angioedema reaction in histamine. Ciba Foundation Symposium. Boston Mass: Little, Brown Co. 1956; 167–9.

98 Schneider SB, Atkinson JP: Urticaria and angioedema. In: Fitzpatrick TB, ed. Update dermatology in general medicine. New York: McGraw-Hill, 1983; 61–79.

99 Settipane GA, Pudupakkam RK: Aspirin intolerance. III. Subtypes, familial occurrence and cross reactivity with tartrazine. J Allergy Clin Immunol 1975; 56:215–21.

100 Settipane RA, Constantine HP, Settipane GA: Aspirin intolerance and recurrent urticaria in adults. Allergy 1980; 35:149–54.

101 Settipane GA, Chafee FH, Postman MI et al: Significance of tartrazine sensitivity in chronic urticaria of unknown etiology. J Allergy Clin Immunol 1976; 57:541–9.

102 Sheffer AL, Austen KF: Exercise-induced anaphylaxis. J Allergy Clin Immunol 1980; 66:106–11.

103 Small P, Barrett D, Biskin N, Champlin E: Chronic urticaria and angioedema. Clin Allergy 1982; 12: 131–6.

104 Soter NA: Urticarial vasculitis. In: Wolff K, Winkelmann RK, eds. Vasculitis. London: Lloyd-Luke, 1980; 183–7.

105 Soter NA, Austen FR, Gigli J: Urticaria and arthraligias as manifestations of necrotizing vasculitis. J Invest Dermatol 1974; 63:485–90.

106 Speer F: Multiple food allergy. Ann Allergy 1975; 34:71–6.

107 Speer F, Dennison TR, Baptist JE: Aspirin allergy. Ann Allergy 1981; 49:123–9.

108 Steinhardt MJ: Urticaria and angioedema: a statistical study of five hundred cases. Ann Allergy 1954; 12:241.

109 Stevenson DD, Arroyave CM, Ghat KN, Tan EM: Oral aspirin challenges in asthmatic patients: a study of plasma histamine. Clin Allergy 1976; 6:493–507.

110 Theorell H, Blomback M, Klockum C: Demonstration of reactivity to airborne and food allergens in cutaneous vasculitis by variations in fibrinopeptide A and other blood coagulation, fibrinolysis and complement parameters. Thromb Haemost 1976; 36:593–604.

111 Thiel CL, Fuchs E: Spice and vegetable allergies in pollen allergic individuals. 2nd International Symposium on Immunological and Clinical Problems of Food Allergy, Milan, Italy, October 25–26, 1982. Abstract, P96.

112 Thomas DR, Pursley TV, Jorizzo JL: Chronic urticaria secondary to aminobenzoic acid. Arch Dermatol 1984; 120:961–2.

113 Thune P, Granhold A: Provocation tests with antiphlogistic and food additives in recurrent urticaria. Dermatologica 1975; 151:360–72.

114 Valverde E, Vich JM, Garcia-Calderon JV, Garcia-Calderon PA: In vitro stimulation of lymphocytes in patients with chronic urticaria induced by additives and food. Clin Allergy 1980; 10:691–8.

115 Warin RP, Champion RH: Urticaria. London: WB Saunders, 1974.

116 Warin RP, Smith RJ: Challenge test battery in chronic urticaria. Br J Dermatol 1976; 94:401–10.

117 Winkelmann RK: Chronic urticaria. Proc Staff Mayo Clin 1957; 32:329–34.

118 Winkelmann RK: Nonallergic factors in atopic dermatitis. J Allergy 1966; 37:29–37.

119 Winkelmann RK: Molecular inflammation of the skin. J Invest Dermatol 1971; 57:197–208.

120 Winkelmann RK, Ditto WB: Cutaneous and visceral syndromes of necrotizing or 'allergic' angiitis. A study of 38 cases. Medicine 1964; 43:59–89.

121 Wraith DG, Merrett J, Roth A et al: Recognition of food allergic patients and their allergens by the RAST technique and clinical investigation. Clin Allergy 1975; 9:25–36.

122 Yurchak AM, Wicher K, Arbesman CJ: Immunologic studies on aspirin. J Allergy 1970; 46:245–53.

Chapter 36
Dermatitis Herpetiformis

Jonathan Leonard and Lionel Fry

Introduction

Dermatitis herpetiformis (DH) is a specific disease entity. Although the clinical and histological features of the rash are not diagnostic, the demonstration by immuno-fluorescence of IgA deposits in the papillary dermis of uninvolved skin leaves little doubt over the diagnosis. Following the discovery that patients with DH have an associated gluten-sensitive enteropathy, overwhelming evidence has been presented during the past 15 years that gluten, a protein found in many cereals, is causally related to the development of both the rash and the enteropathy of DH in genetically predisposed individuals. Over 80% of patients with DH have the histocompatibility antigens HLA-B8 and DR3. The exact mechanisms by which gluten causes the lesions are not clear though there is evidence of disordered immunity. This chapter will present a background to the disease and review the evidence that gluten is responsible for the rash. It will also discuss mechanisms that have been proposed to explain the pathogenesis of the rash.

BACKGROUND

Clinical features of dermatitis herpetiformis

DH is a rare disease. Precise estimates as to its prevalence are not possible but it appears to be about one-fifth as common as coelic disease (CD)—its aetiological counterpart. Gawkrodger et al [28] estimated the incidence of DH in the Lothian region of Scotland as 11 per 100 000 but there is wide variation in different regions of the United Kingdom.

DH may present at any time from weaning to old age, but in our experience, onset before the age of 10 is rare. The usual age of onset is in early adult life with a peak in the mid-thirties. Men are affected about twice as often as women. The incidence of spontaneous remission is low—between 5% and 15% [22, 28]. In the majority of patients the illness, once acquired, persists for life.

DH presents clinically as an itchy, blistering rash. The lesions consist of herpetiform clusters of vesicles on an urticarial background. Because the lesions are so itchy, most patients with DH scratch the tops off the vesicles at an

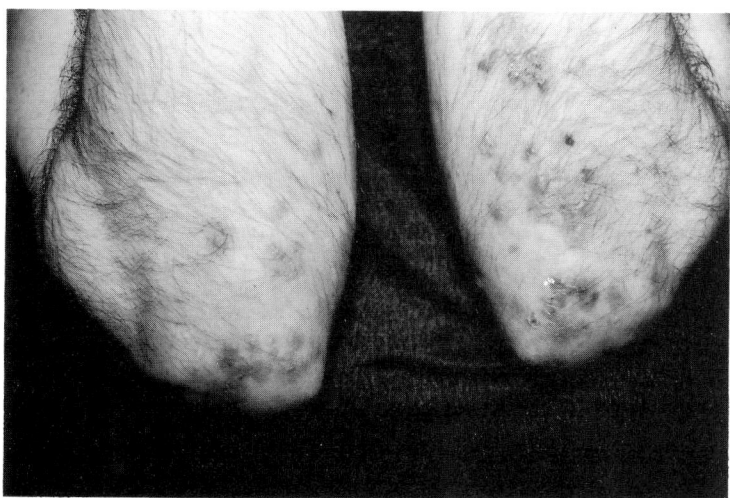

Fig. 36.1 Vesicles and excoriated papules distributed symmetrically over the extensor aspects of the elbows and forearms.

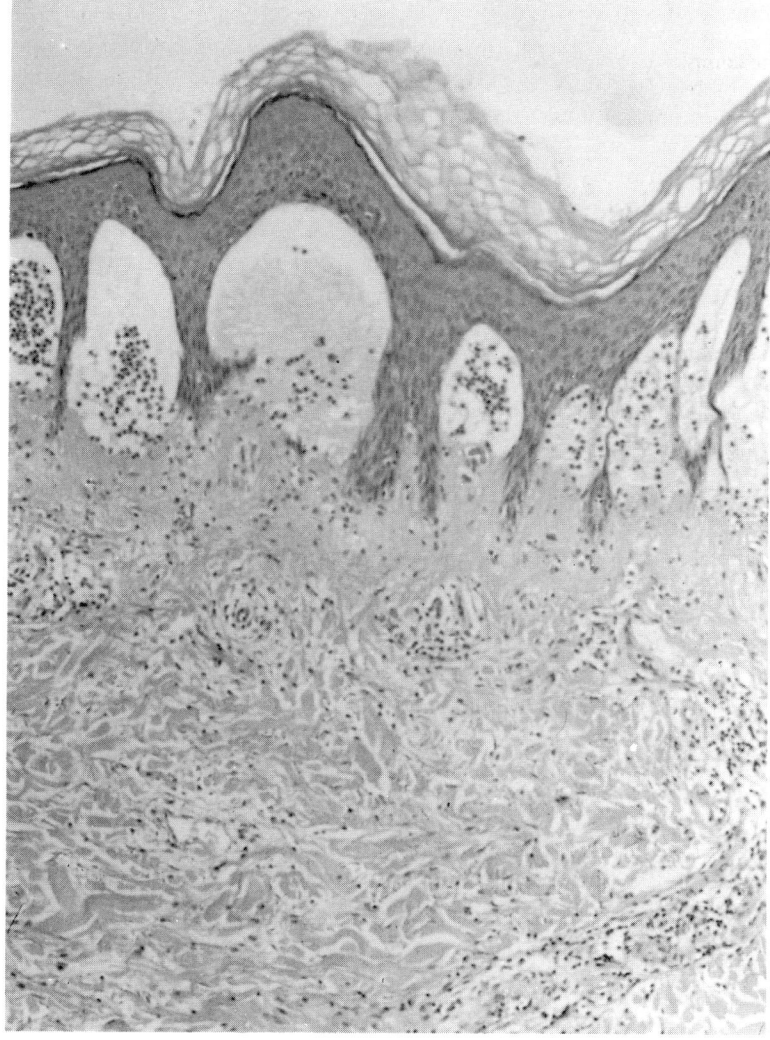

Fig. 36.2 Low-power view of the histology of dermatitis herpetiformis showing papillary microabscesses adjacent to the main bulla.

early stage. The predominant morphological feature, therefore, is of excoriated papules on an urticarial base (Fig. 36.1). The characteristic distribution of the rash is over the extensor aspects of the elbows and proximal forearms, knees and buttocks, though the lesions may occur anywhere on the skin.

Histology of the lesions

The site of vesicle formation is subepidermal. There is an intense polymorphonuclear infiltrate in the mature lesion with a variable amount of eosinophilia. Collections of polymorphs in the dermal papillae are the most characteristic feature. These are seen in an early lesion or adjacent to the main blister of a mature lesion and are termed papillary microabscesses (Fig. 36.2). They are not diagnostic of DH, however, and may be found in other subepidermal bullous dermatoses such as pemphigoid [4].

Response to drug therapy

The response of the rash of DH to therapy with sulphones (e.g. dapsone) and some sulphonamides (e.g. sulphapyridine) is impressive. Itching subsides within 24 hours of commencement of therapy and new lesions stop appearing after 48 hours. Cessation of therapy leads to rapid recurrence of the rash. For many years the therapeutic response of the rash to these drugs was considered to be diagnostic for DH. Since the early 1970s, however, the demonstration of IgA deposits in the uninvolved skin has become the diagnostic criterion for DH.

Dapsone. Dapsone is of help in a variety of skin diseases that are characterized histologically by a polymorphonuclear infiltrate. Evidence has been presented that dapsone acts by inhibition of polymorph migration towards chemotactic agents released into the skin by complement activation [37]. Alternative explanations for its action include inhibition of polymorphonuclear myeloperoxidase activity, suppression of complement activity and suppression of the Arthus reaction [57, 79, 82].

Side-effects of dapsone. The use of dapsone is limited by its side-effects. It is a powerful oxidizing agent. In therapeutic dosages of about 100 mg daily, it causes a chemical haemolysis. This may be severe in some patients—especially in those with glucose-6-phosphates

dehydrogenase deficiency. Elderly atherosclerotic patients tolerate poorly even moderate degrees of haemolysis. Dapsone also has idiosyncratic side-effect such as headache and lethargy. The combined effect of all of these unwanted actions of dapsone leads to withdrawal of dapsone therapy in about 25% of patients in whom it is prescribed [22]. Substitution with sulphonamides such as sulphapyridine or sulphamethoxypyridazine will usually bring about adequate therapeutic control without causing haemolysis and many centres now prefer to use these drugs as a first line of therapy.

Effects of iodides on the rash of dermatitis herpetiformis

The deleterious effect of iodides on the rash of DH has been known for many years. Oral ingestion of iodides causes a generalized outbreak of the rash whilst topical application leads to a local lesion that is histologically indistinguishable from a spontaneous one [1, 33]. The mechanism by which iodides cause this reaction is not known. It is inhibited by sulphone therapy and cannot be elicited in patients whose rash is controlled by a gluten-free diet (GFD).

IMMUNOGLOBULIN DEPOSITION IN THE SKIN

The advent of immunofluorescence techniques in the early 1960s gave dermatologists an invaluable tool for distinguishing between the bullous dermatoses. The first report on immunoglobulins in the skin of patients with DH was by Cormane [9] who found immunoglobulins in both the involved and uninvolved skin though no mention was made of their class. In 1969 van der Meer [91] reported IgA deposits in the uninvolved skin in 10 out of 12 patients with a previous diagnosis of DH. Van der Meer had shown that DH had an immunological basis and one that was distinct from other bullous dermatoses. The presence of IgA in the dermal papillae of uninvolved skin in patients with DH is now the major laboratory criterion for diagnosing the disease. Fry and Seah [18] considered that the diagnosis should not be made without it.

Patterns of IgA deposition

Chorzelski et al [7] were the first to recognize the different sites of IgA deposition in the bul-

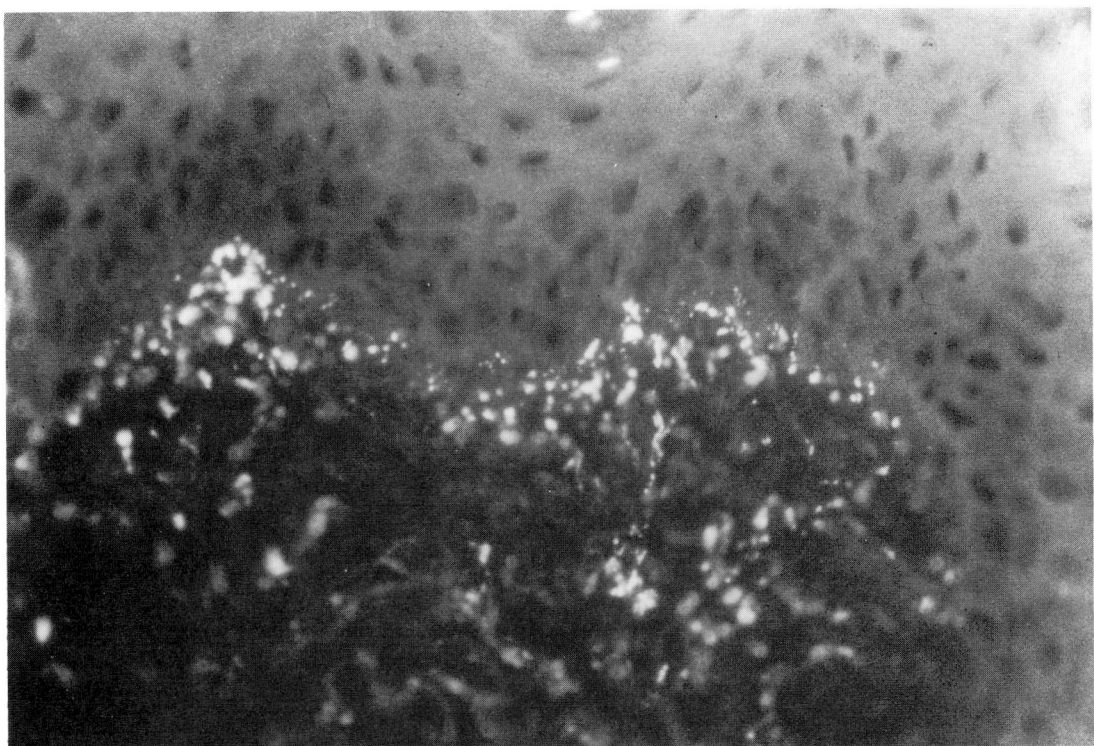

Fig. 36.3 Direct immunofluorescence of uninvolved skin showing the papillary pattern of deposition of IgA in dermatitis herpetiformis (courtesy GP Haffenden).

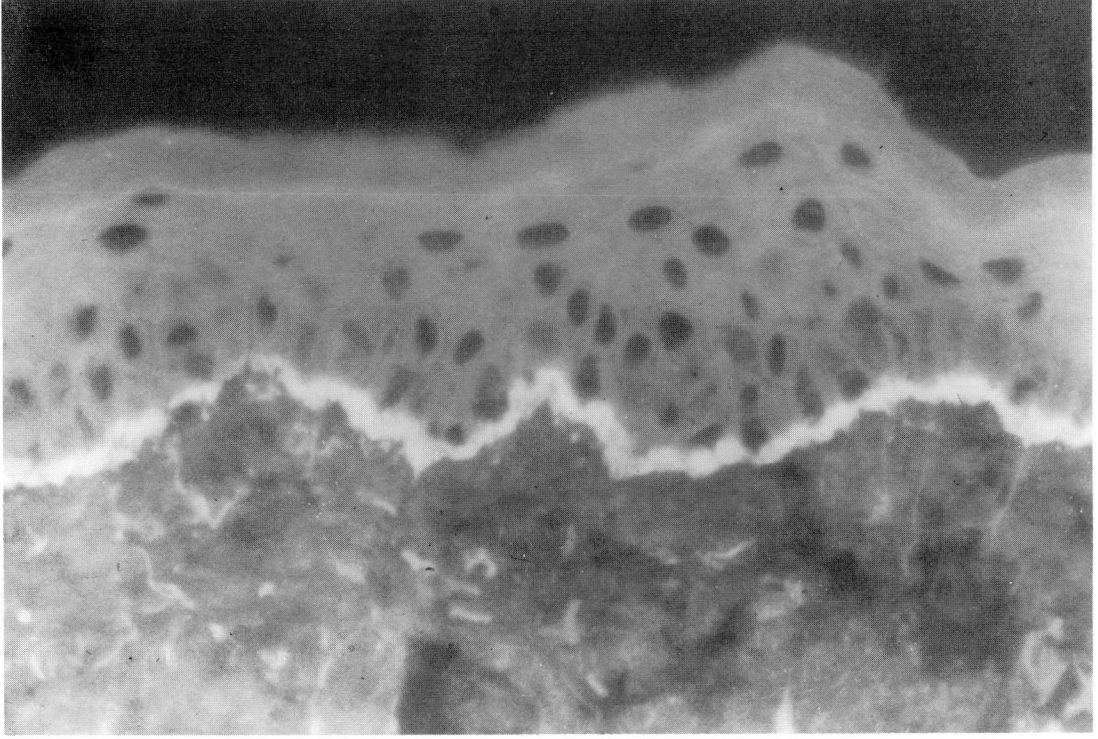

Fig. 36.4 Direct immunofluorescence of uninvolved skin showing the linear pattern of deposition of IgA in linear IgA bullous dermatosis (courtesy GP Haffenden).

lous diseases. They described two patterns of fluorescence—one in the dermal papillae (Fig. 36.3) and the other in a homogeneous line along the dermoepidermal junction (Fig. 36.4). Other groups of workers have confirmed these initial findings [43, 71] and shown that the papillary pattern is the more common, occurring in 84–90% of patients with IgA deposits. The nosological classification of patients with the linear IgA pattern of deposition has caused much argument over recent years. The current view of most workers in the field is that the linear pattern represents a distinct disease entity from DH and is now termed linear IgA bullous dermatosis [8]. The term DH should only refer to those with IgA deposited in the papillary dermis.

Site of attachment of the IgA in dermatitis herpetiformis

Initial studies, comparing the pattern of IgA fluorescence with that produced by silver stains, suggested that the IgA was bound to reticulin in the papillary dermis [70]. More recently, immunoelectron microscopy has shown the IgA to be bound within clumps in the dermal papillae, closely associated either with anchoring fibrils [97] or with the microfibrillar component of elastic dermal microfibrillar bundles [80]. Haffenden and Ring reported that the IgA was localized in large aggregates in the papillary dermis and in small deposits lying in the bundles of collagen fibres [31].

Diagnostic specificity of papillary IgA deposits

IgA deposits in the uninvolved skin of patients with DH have diagnostic value [6, 18, 43, 51], although this has been questioned by the finding that IgA was present in four out of 15 patients with CD [67]. It is likely that these patients had latent DH.

In a study of the clinically normal skin of 22 patients with established CD, two were found to have immunoglobulins deposited in the skin, one patient having IgM and the other IgA in the papillary dermis [77]. It was apparent on further study of the second patient that she had had an itchy rash on the elbows and knees which had cleared on the gluten-free diet given for the coeliac disease. In another group of 16 patients in whom IgA was not found in the skin, but who had a rash clinically consistent with DH (and which responded to dapsone), an alternative diag-nosis could be made in 13 of these patients [27].

Origin of the IgA

The association of DH with a gluten-sensitive enteropathy suggests that the IgA is of gut origin. This view was supported by Unsworth et al [90] who showed that the IgA in the skin of patients with DH contained J chain and was able to bind secretory component in vitro. The IgA therefore was predominantly dimeric and probably of mucosal origin. However, Hall and his colleagues [34], using monoclonal antibodies against IgA1 and IgA2, found that all 22 patients tested had IgA1 whereas none had IgA2. They came to the opposite conclusion about the origin of the IgA deposits. These techniques are at the limit of our current investigative capability and the results, though interesting, should be interpreted with caution for the time being.

Other classes of immunoglobulins in the skin of patients with dermatitis herpetiformis

Although all patients with DH have IgA deposition, IgG and IgM are sometimes found in addition. Chorzelski et al [7] found IgG in six of their 19 patients and IgM in five. Seah and Fry [71] found IgG in three of their 78 biopsies and IgM in eight. Of the nine patients who had IgG or IgM in addition to the IgA, the pattern of immunofluorescence was the same in eight of them. In the one biopsy in which there was a difference, IgA was present in the homogeneous-linear pattern and IgM in the papillary pattern. (This patient would now be classified as having linear IgA bullous dermatosis.) In the single biopsy in which all three classes of immunoglobulins were found, IgA was present in the papillary pattern and IgG and IgM in the homogeneous-linear pattern. There appears to be no correlation between the presence of immunoglobulins other than IgA and any clinical or prognostic factor in patients with DH. Repeat biopsies taken over a period of time from any given patient with DH consistently show papillary IgA but the presence of other immunoglobulin classes is variable. It is possible that these other immunoglobulins represent secondary antibodies following damage to the basement membrane. Alternatively they may just represent the deposition of immune complexes of different classes with different affinity for the various structures of the basement membrane zone [17].

Complement in the skin

The C3 component of complement has been found in the uninvolved skin of patients with DH by a number of workers [20,32,39, 65,91]. However, IgA is not thought to be able to activate complement by the classical pathway, and it has to be explained how complement can be deposited in the absence of IgG or IgM. In 1971 it was shown that aggregated IgA was capable of activating complement by the alternative pathway [30]. A study of C3 and C1q deposition in relation to immunoglobulin deposition in both the involved and the uninvolved skin in 34 biopsies from 19 patients showed that IgA was present in all these biopsies, IgG in three and IgM in nine [75]. C3 was found in 16 (47%) of the specimens. The highest frequency was found in the subgroup of biopsies taken from an early lesion (eight out of nine). However, C3 was also found in the uninvolved skin in three out of nine patients whose rash was controlled by diet. C1q was present in only three of the 34 biopsies; in one IgG was present and in two IgM was also present.

These results were taken to imply that complement fixation in the skin of patients with DH occurred through the alternative rather than the classical pathway and could be attributed to the IgA. This view was supported by the work of Provost and Tomasi [63] who found properdin and Factor B—evidence of alternative pathway activation—in the skin of patients with DH. These studies demonstrated that complement is present in the skin of patients with DH and is likely to play some part in the pathogenesis of the skin lesion. In a recent evaluation of the influence of a gluten-free diet (GFD) in DH [20], C3 was found in the skin in 12 out of 18 patients who were taking a normal diet and requiring dapsone to suppress their rash, but in only three out of 19 patients whose rash was controlled by a strict GFD alone.

The immunogenetics of dermatitis herpetiformis

The suggestion that genetic factors play a role in the pathogenesis of the disease was supported by the finding that DH, in common with CD [13,81], is accompanied by a high incidence of certain histocompatibility anti-

gens. Before precise diagnostic techniques became available for DH, reports showed between 58% and 78% of patients to have HLA-B8 [29,44]. When the presence of papillary IgA in uninvolved skin became the absolute diagnostic criterion for DH, the true incidence of HLA-B8 rose to over 80% [66,74]. Pehamberger et al [60] reported an increased incidence of the Class II histocompatibility antigen—DR3—in patients with DH. The incidence of this antigen was found to be in excess of 90%—a finding similar to that previously reported in CD [45].

EVIDENCE THAT GLUTEN IS RESPONSIBLE FOR DERMATITIS HERPETIFORMIS

The first indications that gluten was implicated in the pathogenesis of DH came in the late 1960s. Although some of the earlier descriptions of DH mentioned ill health, loss of weight and mental symptoms occurring in patients, these were attributed to the effects of chronic skin irritation which is a major feature of the disease. In 1966 and 1967 there were three reports of a high prevalence of structural changes of the jejunal mucosa in patients with DH. The changes resembled those of idiopathic steatorrhoea [15,58,92]. The finding of abnormalities in small intestinal structure and function as well as haematological changes in 12 patients with DH suggested that gluten was the cause of the disease [21]. In addition to the enteropathy, a high incidence of increased faecal fat excretion, reduced serum levels of folate and iron and low serum IgM levels with evidence of splenic atrophy were also seen. The analogy was made with CD where the enteropathy had been clearly shown to be caused by gluten [68].

Specificity of gluten

Further conclusive evidence of the association between DH and CD was provided when it was shown that there was an improvement in the small intestinal mucosa, a reduction in faecal fat excretion and restoration of normal serum levels of folate and iron with treatment by a GFD. On reintroduction of gluten into the diet, these changes were reversed, demonstrating the specificity of gluten in the pathogenesis of DH [24,26].

Incidence of enteropathy

The incidence of enteropathy in patients with DH was initially thought to be 70% [15,21]. However, further studies have shown that a gluten-sensitive enteropathy occurs in all patients with DH but to varying degrees. Firstly, multiple biopsies of the small intestine have shown the enteropathy to be patchy, so that if only one biopsy had been taken it would have been possible to have missed a morphologically abnormal area of small intestine [5]. When eight biopsies were taken simultaneously from the upper small intestine, the incidence of morphological abnormality rose to 95%. Secondly, Weinstein [93] was able to induce structural changes in a previously normal-looking small intestine by giving patients with DH an increased amount of gluten in the diet. This response to gluten loading does not generally occur in normal individuals but there has been a recent report of its occurrence in relatives of patients with CD and in normal individuals with HLA-B8 [11]. Thirdly, it has been shown that, irrespective of the morphological change in the small intestine, a histological abnormality can be demonstrated in the majority of DH patients.

Histological evidence

The most useful marker is the increased infiltration of the epithelium with lymphocytes as this can be easily quantitated. The intraepithelial lymphocyte count is expressed as the number of lymphocytes per 1000 epithelial cells [25]. There is also an increase in the number of lymphocytes in the lamina propria but the cells here are more difficult to count reliably. The lymphocytes are presumably attracted to the mucosal surface as part of the immunological response to gluten. Although the number of lymphocytes infiltrating the epithelium is increased in patients with DH, the predominance of T suppressor cells seen in the normal gut is maintained [52].

It is possible that there is an increased permeability of the small intestine to large molecules in patients with DH who have a morphologically normal-looking small intestine. Recently described techniques using probe molecules such as polyethylene glycol [41] or using a ^{51}Cr-labelled absorption test [3] may help to demonstrate a physiological abnormality in this group.

Effect of a gluten-free diet on the rash of dermatitis herpetiformis

It has now been established beyond all reasonable doubt that the skin lesions of DH are associated with gluten sensitivity. Within two years of the initial report of structural changes in the small intestine in DH, the beneficial effect of a six month gluten-free period on the skin lesions of seven patients was described [23,24]. It was found that two patients were able to stop taking dapsone and another three showed a significant reduction in the dose of dapsone required to suppress the rash. There was a correlation between the fall in dapsone requirements and the improvement in small intestinal structure; i.e. both the skin and the intestinal lesions improved on the GFD. The same group of workers showed that the skin lesions of patients who had been on a GFD for a year would reappear when gluten was added back to the diet. The dapsone had to be reintroduced or increased in dosage to suppress the rash.

The intestinal abnormalities paralleled the dapsone requirements in that there was a deterioration in the structure and function of the small intestine on reintroduction of the gluten. It was suggested that the skin lesions, as well as the intestinal lesions, were related to gluten and that there was a direct relationship between the two [24]. The fall in dapsone requirement on treatment with a GFD could not simply be attributed to improved intestinal absorption of the drug since some patients were able to stop taking dapsone altogether yet the rash relapsed on gluten challenge.

Failures on diet

A number of other reports [78,83,94] stated that the rash did not improve with a GFD and that the relationship between the skin and small intestine was indirect. However, it has to be stressed that the diet has to be strict to be successful and has to be taken for many months before the rash can be controlled by diet alone [26]. It was evident from the reports by Shuster et al [78] and Weinstein et al [94] that in the reported cases of failure the diet had not been adhered to for long enough to be effective (only one patient had taken the diet for over nine months), or that it had not been strict enough (the enteropathy was still present in some patients on repeat biopsy whilst the patient was allegedly adhering to the diet). Support for the efficacy of a strict GFD in the treatment of DH has now come from many sources [16, 28, 36, 38, 43, 51, 59, 65].

Long-term follow-up

The long-term follow-up of patients with DH with and without treatment by a GFD has been reviewed [22]. Seventy-eight patients were included in the study of whom 42 opted for a GFD whilst 36 took a normal diet and controlled their rash with drugs alone. Thirty of the 42 patients (71%) taking a GFD were able to discontinue the drugs previously required to control the rash compared with five of the 36 patients (14%) taking a normal diet. The mean time taken to reduce drug requirements for patients taking a GFD was eight months (range 4–30) and for stopping the drugs 29 months (range 6–108). The incidence of morphological abnormality of the small intestine decreased from 69% to 15% and there was a significant reduction in the mean intraepithelial lymphocyte count in those patients controlled by diet alone. The improvement in the skin and intestinal lesions was related to the strictness of the GFD. Twenty-three of the 42 patients who opted for a GFD were considered by the dietician to be strictly adhering to the diet; 22 of these patients (96%) were able to stop drug therapy.

Gawkrodger et al [28] found that 27 out of 51 patients (53%) on a strict diet were able to stop taking dapsone, and in 12 others (23.5%) the drug requirements were reduced by at least half. The remaining 12 patients were not able to reduce their drug dosage but four of these had been on the diet for less than 12 months. The mean time for cessation of drug therapy in the 27 patients eventually controlled by a GFD alone was 25 months (range 1–91), which is similar to the figure of Fry and his colleagues [22].

Central role of gluten

Conclusive evidence for the central role of gluten in the pathogenesis of DH is now available [50]. Twelve patients with DH whose rash had been controlled with a strict GFD alone for an average period of 7.6 years were challenged. The rash returned in 11 of the 12 patients after an average interval of 11.9 weeks from the start of the challenge. Biopsies of the small intestine performed before the challenge and again at reappearance of the rash showed a deterioration of the mucosa in seven of the 11

patients. The patient who failed to relapse on challenge probably represents the 10% of patients with DH who enter spontaneous remission [22, 28].

The question remains as to why all patients with DH do not respond to a GFD. The success rate of the diet depends on how strictly it has been adhered to [22] (Table 36.1). It

Table 36.1 Relationship of the strictness of a gluten-free diet and ability to stop medication.

GFD grade*	Number of patients	Number who stopped drugs
1	23	22 (96%)
2	17	8 (47%)
3	2	0

* The GFD was graded by a dietician: Grade 1 = strict with no gluten intake; grade 2 = very occasional gluten intake, and usually unintentional; grade 3 = small quantities of gluten taken intentionally but not more than once a week (From Fry et al [22]).

should be noted that not all patients with CD respond to a strict GFD [35] and the same may be true for DH. There has been a report that a milk-free diet in addition to a GFD may be necessary to control the rash in some patients with DH but this remains to be substantiated [62]. However, the most likely reason for failure of a GFD is that it has not been adhered to strictly.

Effect of gluten on the intensity of IgA fluorescence

Harrington and Read [36] reported a series of 10 patients with DH treated with a GFD. They found that two patients no longer required dapsone after six months on the diet and that IgA was no longer demonstrable in the skin biopsies once the rash had been controlled by diet alone. Others have not been able to demonstrate such a rapid disappearance of the IgA but have found that the intensity of the fluorescence was slowly reduced. It disappeared from the skin in only four out of the 23 patients who had been on a strict GFD for a minimum of seven years [22]. Similarly, Reunala and Salo found that only six out of 42 patients on a strict GFD lost the IgA from the skin, and then only after a number of years [64]. Another interesting observation is that IgA can still be demonstrated in the skin of patients who have entered spontaneous remission [49].

Gluten challenge of GFD-controlled patients.
Twelve patients with DH (three of whom had
lost their IgA staining), whose rash had been
controlled with a strict GFD alone for a number of years were challenged [50]. One month
later, IgA deposits were demonstrated in the
skin of all three of the patients who had previously lost their staining. Two of these
patients relapsed clinically although the other
has still not relapsed three years after challenge commenced. In the other nine patients
there was no detectable increase in the intensity of the IgA fluorescence at the time of relapse of the rash compared with that prior to
challenge.

MECHANISMS BY WHICH GLUTEN MAY CAUSE THE RASH

Serum immunoglobulins

Although some changes in the serum levels of
immunoglobulins have been reported, they
occur only in a minority of patients. Only a
small proportion of patients have raised serum
IgA levels [21]. Low serum IgM levels are
present in one-third of patients with DH taking a normal diet [14]; this is possibly due to
the lymphoreticular dysfunction and splenic
atrophy that are known to occur in patients
with DH [61].

Evidence for a Type I hypersensitivity reaction

Although an urticarial background to the
vesicles is characteristic of DH, and although
there is an increased incidence of atopy in
patients with DH [10], no evidence has been
submitted that convincingly implicates a Type
I, IgE-mediated hypersensitivity mechanism
in the pathogenesis of the rash. In our experience, neither H_1 nor H_2 antagonists have any
influence on the rash. Oral disodium cromoglycate does not influence either the enteropathy or the dapsone requirements of patients
with DH [19]. Furthermore, the 28 months
that it takes following gluten withdrawal for
the rash to be controlled by diet alone [22], is
too long to readily support a Type I hypersensitivity reaction as being responsible.

Circulating antibodies in dermatitis herpetiformis

Auto-antibodies

A high incidence of tissue reactive auto-antibodies occurs in the serum of patients with
DH [10,72]. Gastric parietal cell antibodies,
thyroid antibodies and antinuclear antibodies
are the most common. The incidence of circulating auto-antibodies in DH is higher than
that found in CD which suggests that there
may be a more widespread immunological disturbance in DH than CD [72].

Ljunghall et al [53] found that auto-antibodies were present in 29 of 43 patients with
DH and that 12 of these patients had more
than one auto-antibody. Antinuclear antibodies were the most commonly found in their
series. Zone et al [98] found an increased prevalence of thyroid antibodies in DH.

Of 50 patients studied, two were hyper-
thyroid, five were hypothyroid, three had thyroid nodules requiring thyroidectomy and five
had symptomatic goitres. Microsomal thyroid
antibodies were found in 38% of patients with
DH compared with 12% of age- and sex-, but
not HLA-matched, controls. The incidence of
thyroglobulin antibodies was lower, occurring
in 12% of the patients. Gawkrodger et al [28]
found gastric parietal or thyroid antibodies in
38% of 76 patients with DH; two cases of pernicious anaemia and three of thyroid disease
were detected.

Antireticulin antibodies

In 1971 an auto-antibody in the serum of
children with CD was described which
appeared to be directed against a component
of connective tissue [76]. It could be demonstrated by indirect immunofluorescence on a
composite block of rat tissues (Fig. 36.5). The
staining was not abolished by pretreatment of
the sections with collagenases but was absorbed by treatment of the serum with adult
human spleen reticulin. The pattern of staining was similar to that obtained with silver
[73] and it was concluded that the antibody
was directed against reticulin.

Incidence of antireticulin antibodies. The incidence of the antireticulin antibody (ARA) in
patients with DH is approximately 20%
[47,73] but it is higher in adults with CD at
approximately 40% [2,47,73]. The highest incidence of ARA is found in childhood CD
where it lies between 30% and 70%
[72,73,76]. It seems that the incidence of
ARA is related to the severity of the gluten-
sensitive enteropathy which is most severe in
childhood CD and least severe in DH. In
addition, in patients with DH or CD, the in-

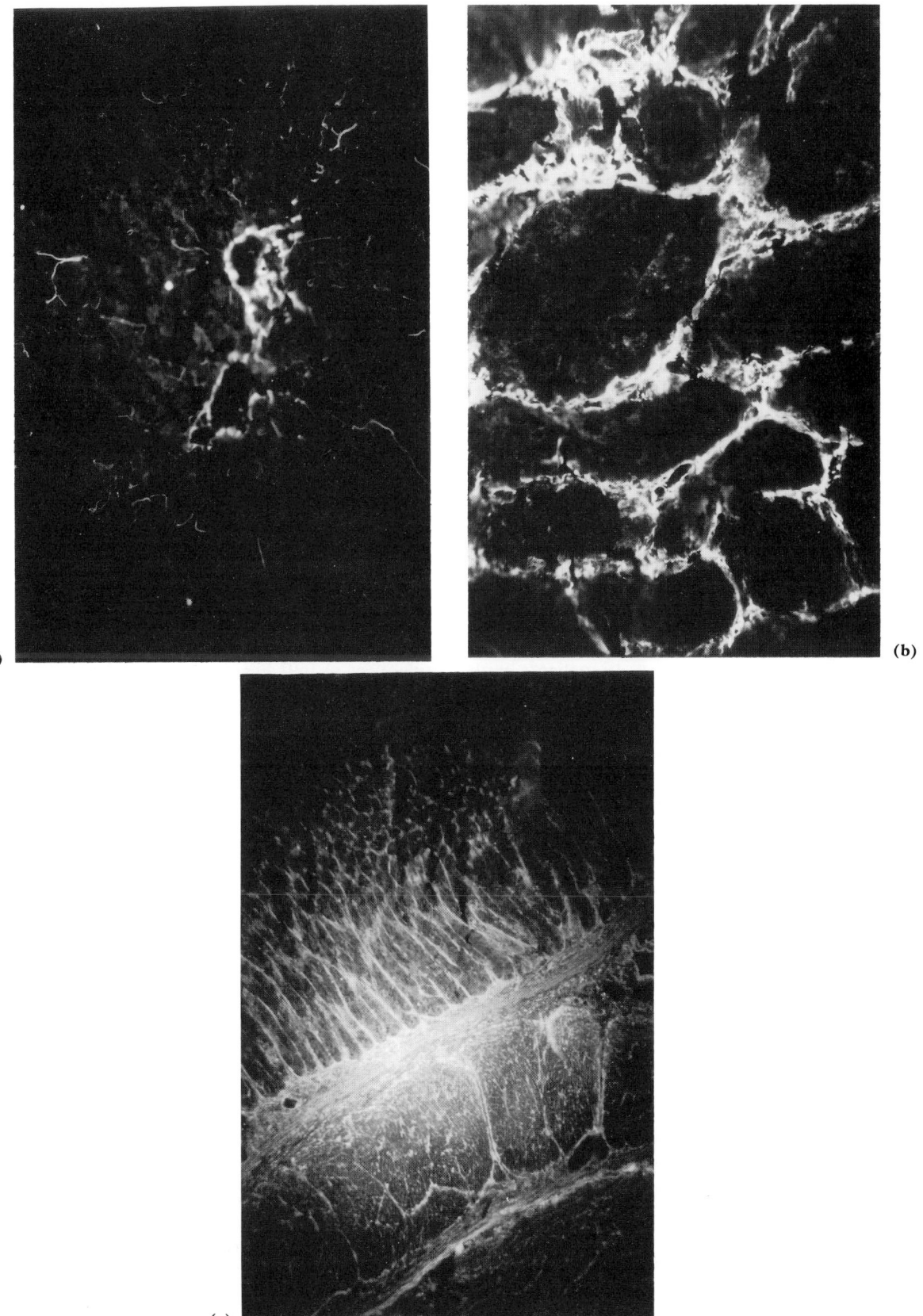

Fig. 36.5 Indirect immunofluorescence showing R1 pattern of antireticulin antibody using a composite block of rat tissue as the substrate: (a) liver; (b) kidney; (c) stomach (courtesy DJ Unsworth).

cidence of ARA was related to the severity of the enteropathy on jejunal biopsy [47]. In patients who have ARA present in their serum, a GFD results in a gradual fall and eventual disappearance of the antibody [54, 73].

Significance of antireticulin antibodies. The true significance of the ARA has yet to be determined. The recent observation by Unsworth et al [85] that gliadin binds in vitro to reticulin is of interest (Fig. 36.6), particularly in view of the higher incidence of ARA in patients with a severe enteropathy. It is possible that gluten in some way damages the reticulin of patients with a gluten-sensitive enteropathy and renders it immunogenic leading to the production of the antibody. Although the IgA in the skin of patients with DH is thought to be attached to reticulin, there is little evidence for implicating the ARA in the pathogenesis of the rash. Firstly, the incidence of ARA is much higher in patients with CD and, secondly, the majority of reports show the class of ARA to be IgG rather than IgA. An exception was the report of Ljunghall and her colleagues [53] who found that 12 out of 15 patients with positive sera had ARA of IgA class.

Antigliadin antibodies

The associated gluten-sensitive enteropathy has given rise to speculation that antibodies against gluten may play a pathogenic role in DH. Previous studies, however, have shown only 20% of patients with DH to have anti-gluten antibodies in the serum [12, 40, 46, 56]. In contrast, a newly developed immuno-fluorescence technique [84, 89] and a modification of the ELISA method have allowed the detection of antibodies to gliadin (the alcohol-soluble component of gluten) in the serum of 46% of adults with DH [87]. The presence of antigliadin antibodies (AGA) correlated well with the severity of the gluten-sensitive enteropathy.

Using similar techniques on the sera of patients with CD, Unsworth et al [86] found that *all* untreated children had AGA and that the titre of antibody fell on treatment with a GFD. Patients with gluten-sensitive enteropathy, whether caused by CD or associated with DH, tended to have AGA of the IgG class with or without those of IgA class. Although IgG AGA were more common, Salvilahti et al [69] have shown that IgA AGA, when present, are a better indicator of

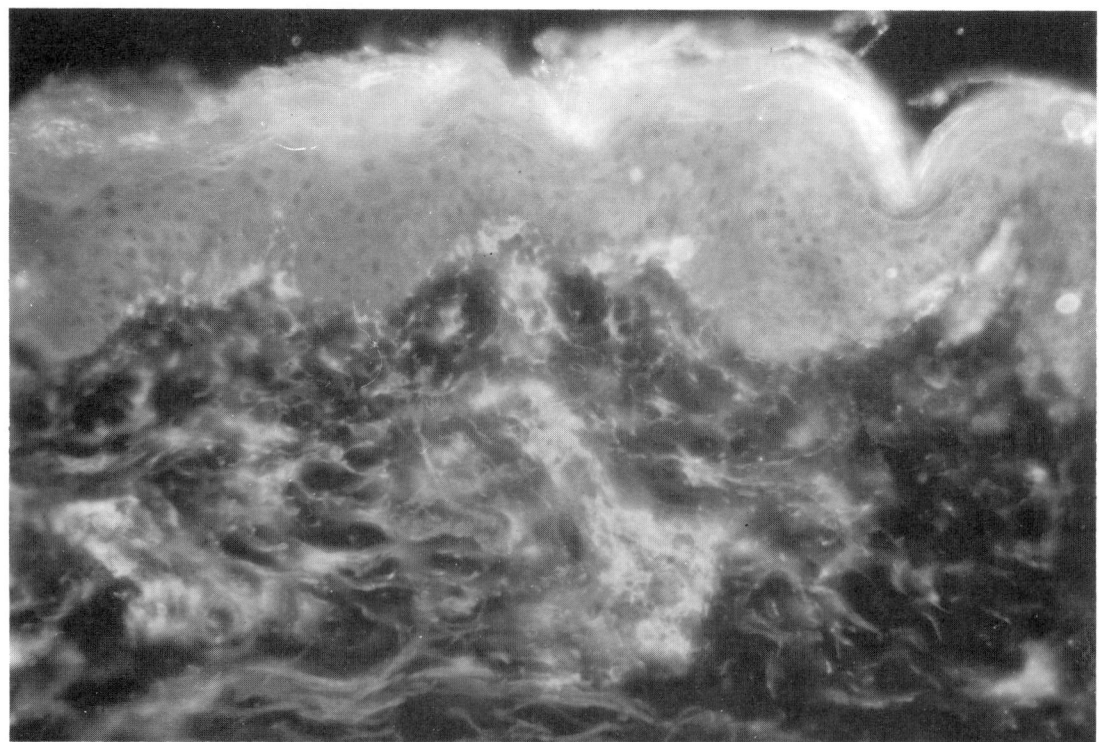

Fig. 36.6 Gliadin binding in vitro to reticulin of normal human skin. The cryostat section was incubated with gliadin prior to indirect immunofluorescence using a rabbit antigliadin antibody and fluoresceinated antirabbit antiserum (courtesy DJ Unsworth).

gluten-sensitive enteropathy. The titres fell with time on a GFD in keeping with the clinical improvement of the patients and the morphological improvement of the gut whereas IgG AGA persisted for longer.

Diagnostic value of antigliadin antibodies

The value of AGA in screening tests for gluten-sensitive enteropathy associated with DH is limited by an unacceptably high incidence of false positives (IgG class) and false negatives (IgA class). IgG AGA are found in other skin and gut diseases that are unrelated to gluten sensitivity [84]. Their presence in these diseases has not yet been satisfactorily explained. IgA AGA are more specific [84, 89] but they are not very sensitive as a screening test as not all patients with biopsy-proven gluten-sensitive enteropathy have them. Nevertheless, the fall in the titre of IgA AGA when present is a useful guide to the response of the enteropathy to a GFD.

AGA have not fulfilled their initial promise. The observation that gliadin bound in vitro to reticulin [85] suggested that an immune complex consisting of gliadin and IgA AGA might be produced in the small intestine and circulate to the skin where it could bind to dermal reticulin through the gliadin. However, the inability to demonstrate gliadin in the skin of patients with DH and the finding that there is a high incidence of AGA in patients with CD make this suggestion untenable. Similarly the possibility that AGA cross-react with the reticulin in the papillary dermis of patients with DH but not those with CD seems unlikely.

Circulating immune complexes

The regular finding of IgA and C3 in the skin of patients with DH has led to the suggestion that these individuals have circulating immune complexes that give rise to the cutaneous deposition of immune reactants in the skin. Circulating immune complexes have been reported in a variable proportion of patients with DH ranging from 20% to 30% in the majority of studies [43, 95]. Most of the assays used in these studies, however, were only able to detect IgG- and IgM-containing complexes. Zone et al [99] described an immunofluorescence assay for the detection of immune complexes of IgA class and found them to be present in 30% of their patients.

Methods of detection

Katz and his co-workers [42] used three methods to detect immune complexes: the ^{125}I-C1q binding assay which is able to detect IgG- or IgM-containing complexes; the conventional Raji cell assay which detected IgG-containing immune complexes; and a modified Raji cell assay which detected IgA-containing immune complexes. They found IgA-containing complexes to be present in 26% of patients with DH whereas IgG- and IgM-containing complexes were found in only 13%. They also found that the presence of immune complexes did not correlate with disease activity or mode of treatment and they concluded that IgA-containing immune complexes were not a primary factor in the pathogenesis of DH. Their test of IgA-containing complexes relied on the ability of IgA to fix complement in the fluid phase which is an assumption that may not be valid.

Role of immune complexes

The role of circulating immune complexes in the pathogenesis of DH is uncertain. A major problem is the lack of satisfactory methods for the detection of IgA-containing immune complexes. The finding of Lane et al [48] that patients with DH and CD have gluten in their sera and the knowledge that these groups of patients have AGA indicates that such complexes should exist. However, the inability to demonstrate gluten in the skin of patients with DH indicates that such complexes, if they do exist, may not be pathogenic. Zone and his colleagues [100] were able to induce immune complexes in patients with DH by feeding them gluten. Conversely, Yancey et al [96] demonstrated that gluten challenge does not influence the levels of circulating immune complexes in patients with DH.

A further failing of the current methods for detecting immune complexes is that they do not allow for detailed analysis of the components of the complex. Unsworth et al [88] recently applied sucrose density centrifugation techniques to enable both the demonstration and analysis of immune complexes in patients with DH and CD but with disappointing results. Although there was evidence for complexes containing AGA these were present in only 30% of patients and were of the IgG class.

The current situation with immune complexes in DH is that there is no good evidence to implicate their role in the pathogenesis of the disease. It is worthwhile remembering at this stage that the clinical observations argue against DH being an immune complex disorder. It takes an average of 28 months for the skin lesions to clear on a GFD and an average of three months for relapse after gluten challenge.

Evidence for a Type IV hypersensitivity reaction

Very little work has been reported on the role of Type IV hypersensitivity mechanisms in the pathogenesis of DH. The poor solubility of gliadin in reagents other than alcohol makes the preparation of materials suitable for skin testing containing this antigen impracticable.

CONCLUSIONS

There is overwhelming evidence that gluten is the cause of both the rash and enteropathy of patients with DH. The precise details of the pathogenic pathways have not yet been elucidated, but Type I hypersensitivity mechanisms have not been shown to be responsible. They are undoubtedly complicated and multifactorial involving genetic and environmental agents. There is good evidence for disordered immunity in these patients and the presence of IgA in the skin supports an immune basis for the disease.

REFERENCES

1 Alexander JO'D: Dermatitis herpetiformis. London: WB Saunders, 1979; 318-21.

2 Alp MH, Wright R: Autoantibodies to reticulin in patients with idiopathic steatorrhoea, coeliac disease and Crohn's disease and their relationship to immunoglobulins and dietary antibodies. Lancet 1971; ii: 682-5.

3 Bjarnasson I, Peters TJ, Veall N: A persistent defect in intestinal permeability in coeliac disease demonstrated by a ^{51}Cr-labelled EDTA absorption test. Lancet 1983; i: 323-5.

4 Blenkinsopp WK, Fry L, Haffenden GP, Leonard JN: Histology of linear IgA disease, dermatitis herpetiformis and bullous pemphigoid. Am J Dermatopathol 1983; 5:547-54.

5 Brow JR, Parker F, Weinstein WE et al: The small intestinal mucosa in dermatitis herpetiformis. II. Relationship of the small intestinal lesion to gluten. Gastroenterology 1971; 60:355-61.

6 Chorzelski TP, Jablonska S: Diagnostic significance of the immunofluorescent pattern in dermatitis herpetiformis. Int J Dermatol 1975; 14:429-34.

7 Chorzelski TP, Beutner EH, Jablonska S et al: Immunofluorescence studies in the diagnosis of dermatitis herpetiformis and its differentiation from bullous pemphigoid. J Invest Dermatol 1971; 56:373-80.

8 Chorzelski TP, Jablonska S, Beutner EH: Adult form of linear IgA bullous dermatosis. In: Beutner EH, Chorzelski TP, Bean SF, eds. Immunopathology of the skin, 2nd ed. New York: John Wiley and Sons 1979; 316-9.

9 Cormane RH: Immunofluorescent studies of the skin in lupus erythematosus and other diseases. Pathol Eur 1967; 2:170-5.

10 Davies MG, Marks R, Nuki G: Dermatitis herpetiformis—a skin manifestation of a generalised disturbance in immunity. Q J Med 1978; 47:221-48.

11 Doherty M, Barry RE: Gluten induced mucosal changes in subjects without overt small bowel disease. Lancet 1981; i:517-20.

12 Eterman PK, Feltkamp TEW: Antibodies to gluten and reticulin in gastrointestinal disease. Clin Exp Immunol 1978; 31:92-9.

13 Falchuk ZM, Strober W: HLA antigens and adult coeliac disease. Lancet 1972; ii:1310.

14 Fraser NG, Dick HM, Crickson WB: Immunoglobulins in dermatitis herpetiformis and various other skin diseases. Br J Dermatol 1969; 71:89-95.

15 Fraser NG, Murray D, Alexander JO'D: Structure and function of the small intestine in dermatitis herpetiformis. Br J Dermatol 1967; 76:509-18.

16 Frodin T, Gotthard R, Hed J et al: Gluten free diet for dermatitis herpetiformis. The long term effect on cutaneous, immunological and jejunal manifestations. Acta Derm Venereol (Stockh) 1981; 61:405-11.

17 Fry L: Dermatitis herpetiformis—basic findings. In: Beutner EH, Chorzelski TP, Bean SF, eds. Immunopathology of the skin, 2nd ed. New York; John Wiley and Sons, 1979; 283-301.

18 Fry L, Seah PP: Dermatitis herpetiformis. An evaluation of diagnostic criteria. Br J Dermatol 1974; 90:137-46.

19 Fry L, Swain AF, Leonard J, McMinn RMH: Disodium cromoglycate in dermatitis herpetiformis. Br J Dermatol 1981; 105:83-6.

20 Fry L, Haffenden GP, Wojnarowska F et al: IgA and C3 component of complement in the uninvolved skin in dermatitis herpetiformis after gluten withdrawal. Br J Dermatol 1978; 99:31-7.

21 Fry L, Kier P, McMinn RMH et al: Small intestinal structure and function and haematological changes in dermatitis herpetiformis. Lancet 1967; ii:729-33.

22 Fry L, Leonard JN, Swain AF et al: Long term follow up of dermatitis herpetiformis with and without dietary gluten withdrawal. Br J Dermatol 1982; 107:631-41.

23 Fry L, McMinn RMH, Cowan JD et al: Effects of a gluten free diet on dermatological, intestinal and haematological manifestations of dermatitis herpetiformis. Lancet 1968; i:557-61.

24 Fry L, McMinn RMH, Cowan JD et al: Gluten free diet and reintroduction of gluten in dermatitis herpetiformis. Arch Dermatol 1969; 100:129-35.

25 Fry L, Seah PP, Harper PG et al: The small intestine in dermatitis herpetiformis. J Clin Pathol 1974; 27:817-24.

26 Fry L, Seah PP, Riches DJ et al: Clearance of skin lesions in dermatitis herpetiformis after gluten withdrawal. Lancet 1973; i:288–91.

27 Fry L, Walkden V, Wojnarowska F et al: A comparison of IgA positive and IgA negative dapsone responsive dermatoses. Br J Dermatol 1980; 102:371–82.

28 Gawkrodger DJ, Blackwell JN, Gilmour HM et al: Dermatitis herpetiformis: diagnosis, diet and demography. Gut 1984; 25:151–7.

29 Gebherd R L, Katz SI, Marks JM et al: HLA antigen type and small intestinal disease in dermatitis herpetiformis. Lancet 1973; ii:760–2.

30 Gotze O, Muller-Eberhard HJ: The C3 activator system. An alternative pathway of complement activation. J Exp Med [Suppl] 1971; 134:905.

31 Haffenden GP, Ring NP: Immuno-electron microscopy studies. In: Kukita A, Seiji M, eds. Proceedings of the XVIth International Congress of Dermatology. University of Tokyo Press, 1983; 408–11.

32 Haffenden GP, Wojnarowska F, Fry L: Comparison of immunoglobulin and complement deposition in multiple biopsies from the uninvolved skin in dermatitis herpetiformis. Br J Dermatol 1979; 101:39–45.

33 Haffenden GP, Blenkinsopp WK, Ring NP et al: The potassium iodide patch test in dermatitis herpetiformis in relation to treatment with a gluten free diet and dapsone. Br J Dermatol 1980; 103:313–17.

34 Hall RP, Nelson DL, Lawley TJ: Identification of IgA subclasses in the skin of patients with dermatitis herpetiformis. J Invest Dermatol 1983; 80:364 (Abstract).

35 Hamilton JD, Chambers RA, WynneWilliams A: Role of gluten, prednisolone and azathioprine in non-responsive coeliac disease. Lancet 1976; i:1213–16.

36 Harrington CI, Read NW: Dermatitis herpetiformis: effect of a gluten free diet on skin and jejunal structure and function. Br Med J 1977; 1,2:872–5.

37 Harvath L, Yancey KB, Katz SI: Selective inhibition of neutrophil chemotaxis by sulfones. J Invest Dermatol 1983; 80:321 (Abstract).

38 Heading RC, Patterson WD, McClelland DBL et al: Clinical response of dermatitis herpetiformis skin lesions to a gluten free diet. Br J Dermatol 1976; 94:509–14.

39 Holubar K, Doralt M, Eggerth G: Immunofluorescent patterns in dermatitis herpetiformis. Investigations on skin and intestinal mucosa. J Br Dermatol 1971; 85:505–10.

40 Huff JC, Weston WL, Zirker DK: Wheat protein antibodies in dermatitis herpetiformis. J Invest Dermatol 1979; 73:570–4.

41 Jackson PG, Lessoff MH, Baker RWR et al: Intestinal permeability in patients with eczema and food allergy. Lancet 1981; i:1285–6.

42 Katz SI: Dermatitis herpetiformis—the skin and the gut. Ann Intern Med 1980; 93:857–74.

43 Katz SI, Strober W: The pathogenesis of dermatitis herpetiformis. J Invest Dermatol 1978; 70:63–75.

44 Katz SI, Falchuk ZM, Dahl MV et al: A genetic link between dermatitis herpetiformis and gluten sensitive enteropathy. J Clin Invest 1972; 51:2977–80.

45 Keuning JJ, Pena AS, van Leuven A et al: HLA-Dw3 associated with coeliac disease. Lancet 1976; i:506–7.

46 Kumar P, Ferguson A, Lancaster-Smith M et al: Food antibodies in patients with dermatitis herpetiformis and adult coeliac disease—relationship to

jejunal morphology. Scand J Gastroenterol 1976; 11:5–10.

47 Lancaster-Smith M, Kumar PJ, Clark ML et al: Antireticulin antibodies in dermatitis herpetiformis and adult coeliac disease. Their relationship to a gluten free diet and jejunal morphology. Br J Dermatol 1975; 92:37–42.

48 Lane AF, Huff JC, Weston WL: Detection of gluten in human sera by an enzyme linked immunoassay: Comparison of dermatitis herpetiformis and celiac disease patients with normal controls. J Invest Dermatol 1982; 79:186–8.

49 Leonard JN, Haffenden GP, Ring NP et al: Linear IgA disease in adults. Br J Dermatol 1982; 107:301–16.

50 Leonard JN, Haffenden GP, Tucker WFG et al: Gluten challenge in dermatitis herpetiformis. N Engl J Med 1983; 308:816–19.

51 Ljunghall K, Tjerlund U: Dermatitis herpetiformis—effect of gluten restricted and gluten free diet on dapsone requirement and on IgA and C3 deposits in uninvolved skin. Acta Derm Venereol (Stockh) 1983; 63:129–36.

52 Ljunghall K, Loof L, Forsum U: T lymphocyte subsets in the duodenal epithelium in dermatitis herpetiformis. Acta Derm Venereol (Stockh) 1982; 62:485–9.

53 Ljunghall K, Scheynius A, Forsum U: Circulating reticulin autoantibodies of IgA class in dermatitis herpetiformis. Br J Dermatol 1979; 100:173–6.

54 Ljunghall K, Scheynius A, Jonsson T et al: Gluten free diet in patients with dermatitis herpetiformis. Effect on the occurrence of antibodies to reticulin and gluten. Arch Dermatol 1983; 119:970–4.

55 Marks JM: Dogma and dermatitis herpetiformis. Clin Exp Dermatol 1977; 2:189–207.

56 Menzell EJ, Pehamberger H, Holubar K: Demonstration of antibodies to wheat gliadin in dermatitis herpetiformis using ^{14}C-radioimmune assay. Clin Immunol Immunopathol 1978; 10:193–201.

57 Millikan LE, Conway FR: Effect of drugs on Pillemer pathway—dapsone. J Invest Dermatol 1974; 62:541 (Abstract).

58 Marks JM, Shuster S, Watson AJ: Small bowel changes in dermatitis herpetiformis. Lancet 1966; ii:1280–2.

59 Marks R, Whittle MW: Results of treatment of dermatitis herpetiformis with a gluten free diet after one year. Br Med J 1969; ii:772–5.

60 Pehamberger H, Holubar K, Mayr WR: HLA-antigens in dermatitis herpetiformis. Br J Dermatol 1981; 104:321–4.

61 Petit JE, Hoffbrand AV, Seah PP et al: Splenic strophy in dermatitis herpetiformis. Br Med J 1972; 28:438–41.

62 Pock-Steen OC, Niorsson AM: Milk sensitivity in dermatitis herpetiformis. Br J Dermatol 1970; 83:614–19.

63 Provost TT, Tomasi TB: Evidence for activation of complement via the alternate pathway in skin disease. II. Dermatitis herpetiformis. Clin Immunol Immunopathol 1974; 3:178–86.

64 Reunala T, Salo OP: Effects of long term gluten free diet in dermatitis herpetiformis. In: Kukita A, Seiji M, eds. Proceedings of the XVIth International Congress of Dermatology. University of Tokyo Press, 1983; 411–13.

65 Reunala T, Blomquist K, Tarpilla S et al: Gluten free diet in dermatitis herpetiformis. Br J Dermatol 1977; 97:473–80.

66 Reunala T, Salo OP, Tillikainen A et al: Histocompatibility antigens and dermatitis herpetiformis with special reference to jejunal abnormalities and acetylator phenotype. Br J Dermatol 1976; 94:139–43.

67 Ross IN, Thompson RA, Montgommery RD et al: Immunoglobulin staining in the skin of patients with gastrointestinal disease. Specificity and significance of IgA deposition in dermatitis herpetiformis. In: McNicholl B, McCarthy CF, Fottrell PF, eds. Perspectives in coeliac disease. Lancaster: MTP Press, 1978; 217.

68 Rubin CE, Brandborg LL, Flick AL et al: Studies of coeliac sprue. III. The effects of repeated wheat instillation into the proximal jejunum of patients on a gluten free diet. Gastroenterology 1962; 43:621–41.

69 Salvilahti E, Vilander M, Perkkio M et al: IgA antigliadin antibodies—a marker of mucosal damage in childhood coeliac disease. Lancet 1983; i:320–2.

70 Seah PP: Immunological studies in dermatitis herpetiformis. University of London, 1975. Doctoral thesis.

71 Seah PP, Fry L: Immunoglobulins in the skin in dermatitis herpetiformis and their relevance in diagnosis. Br J Dermatol 1975; 92:157–66.

72 Seah PP, Fry L, Hoffbrand AV et al: Tissue antibodies in dermatitis herpetiformis and adult coeliac disease. Lancet 1971; i:834–6.

73 Seah PP, Fry L, Holborow EJ et al: Antireticulin antibody: incidence and diagnostic significance. Gut 1973; 14:311–15.

74 Seah PP, Fry L, Kearney JW et al: A comparison of histocompatibility antigens in dermatitis herpetiformis and coeliac disease. Br J Dermatol 1976; 94: 131–8.

75 Seah PP, Fry L, Mazaheri MR et al: Alternate pathway complement fixation by IgA in the skin in dermatitis herpetiformis. Lancet 1973; ii:175–7.

76 Seah PP, Fry L, Rossiter MA et al: Antireticulin antibodies in childhood coeliac disease. Lancet 1971; ii:681–2.

77 Seah PP, Fry L, Stewart JS et al: Immunoglobulins in the skin in dermatitis herpetiformis and coeliac disease. Lancet 1972; i:611–14.

78 Shuster S, Watson A, Marks JM: Coeliac syndrome in dermatitis herpetiformis. Lancet 1968; i:1101–6.

79 Stendahl O, Molin L, Dahlgreen C et al: The inhibition of polymorphonuclear leucocyte cytotoxicity in the treatment of dermatitis herpetiformis. J Clin Invest 1978; 62:214–20.

80 Stingl G, Honigsmann H, Holubar K et al: Ultrastructural localisation of immunoglobulins in the skin of patients with dermatitis herpetiformis. J Invest Dermatol 1976; 67:507–12.

81 Stokes PJ, Asquith P, Holmes GKT et al: Histocompatibility antigen associated with adult coeliac disease. Lancet 1972; ii:162–4.

82 Thompson DM, Souhami RL: Suppression of the Arthus reaction in the guinea pig by dapsone. Proc R Soc Med 1975; 68:273 (Abstract).

83 Trier JS; Dermatitis herpetiformis and coeliac sprue. Gastroenterology 1971; 60:468–9.

84 Unsworth DJ: Humoral immunity in gluten sensitive enteropathy. University of London, 1982. 278pp. Doctoral thesis.

85 Unsworth DJ, Johnson GD, Haffenden GP et al: Binding of wheat gliadin in vitro to reticulin in normal and dermatitis herpetiformis skin. J Invest Dermatol 1981; 76:88–93.

86 Unsworth DJ, Kieffer M, Holborow EJ et al: IgA antigliadin antibodies in coeliac disease. Clin Exp Immunol 1981; 46:286–93.

87 Unsworth DJ, Leonard JN, McMinn RMH et al: Antigliadin antibodies and small intestinal mucosal damage in dermatitis herpetiformis. Br J Dermatol 1981; 105:653–8.

88 Unsworth DJ, McCarthy DA, Leonard JN et al: Circulating immune complexes containing IgG antigliadin antibody in dermatitis herpetiformis detected by sucrose density centrifugation and subsequent serological analysis. In: MacDonald DM, ed. Proceedings of the First Immunodermatology Symposium. Cambridge: Cambridge University Press, 1984; 231–5.

89 Unsworth DJ, Manuel PD, Walker-Smith JA et al: A new immunofluorescent test for gluten sensitivity. Arch Dis Child 1981; 56:864–71.

90 Unsworth DJ, Payne AW, Leonard JN et al: The IgA in dermatitis herpetiformis skin is dimeric. Lancet 1982; i:478–9.

91 van der Meer JH: Granular deposits of immunoglobulins in the skin of patients with dermatitis herpetiformis—an immunofluorescent study. Br J Dermatol 1969; 81:493–503.

92 von Tongren JHM, van der Staak WJBM, Schilling PHM: Small bowel changes in dermatitis herpetiformis. Dermatologica 1967; 140:231–4.

93 Weinstein WM: Latent coeliac sprue. Gastroenterology 1973; 64:819 (Abstract).

94 Weinstein WM, Brow JR, Parker F et al: The small intestinal mucosa in dermatitis herpetiformis. II. Relationship of the small intestinal lesions to gluten. Gastroenterology 1971; 60:362–9.

95 Yancey KB, Lawley TJ: Circulating immune complexes: their immunocytochemistry, biology and detection in selected dermatologic and systemic diseases. J Am Acad Dermatol 1984; 10:711–32.

96 Yancey KB, Cason JC, Hall RP et al: Dietary gluten challenge does not influence the levels of circulating immune complexes in patients with dermatitis herpetiformis. J Invest Dermatol 1983; 80:468–71.

97 Yaoita H, Katz SI: Immuno-electron microscopic localisation of IgA in the skin of patients with dermatitis herpetiformis. J Invest Dermatol 1976; 67:502–6.

98 Zone JJ, Cunningham MC: An increased prevalence of thyroid abnormalities in dermatitis herpetiformis patients. J Invest Dermatol 1983; 80:363 (Abstract).

99 Zone JJ, LaSalle BS, Provost TT: Circulating immune complexes of IgA type in dermatitis herpetiformis. J Invest Dermatol 1980; 75:152–5.

100 Zone JJ, LaSalle BS, Provost TT: Induction of IgA circulating immune complexes after wheat feeding in dermatitis herpetiformis patients. J Invest Dermatol 1982; 78:375–80.

SECTION E
CENTRAL NERVOUS SYSTEM

Chapter 37
Food-induced Migraine

Jean Monro

Introduction

Migraine has in the past been regarded as a minor condition since it is not usually organ destructive. However, migraineurs comprise the largest group attending neurological clinics—up to 30% in some centres. Some estimates have placed the incidence of migraine in the population as high as 30%, and according to a statement from a national charitable organization concerned with migraine there are more working days lost through headache than through any other single category of complaint in the UK. Even so, some migraineurs work with a headache and therefore less efficiently. This puts the problem into a totally different perspective, as the complaint becomes one of serious economic importance.

Apart from economic factors, the quality of life of people subject to such headaches is diminished. Many feel they cannot plan their working and social lives well for fear of attacks of headaches and consequently do not fulfil their whole potential. Migraine must therefore be regarded as a major complaint.

Definition

The Ad Hoc Committee for the Classification of Headache defined migraine as 'recurrent attacks of headache widely varied in intensity, frequency and duration, being commonly unilateral in onset, usually associated with anorexia, sometimes associated with nausea and vomiting, preceded by or associated with conspicuous sensory motor and motor disturbances and often familial'. Migraine headaches were divided into classic, common and cluster headache, hemiplegic and ophthalmoplegic migraine and lower half headache.

In *common migraine*, periodic headaches occur in association with nausea and dizziness. *Classical migraine* is characterized by severe unilateral headache preceded by teichopsia or scotomata. Following the headache, nausea and vomiting, constipation or diarrhoea, diuresis or urinary retention, alterations in temperature control with associated pallor or sometimes hyperaemia and some sensory phenomena such as heightened perception of sound and photophobia may occur.

Hemiplegic migraine is again unilateral with sensory disturbances, paraesthesiae and motor associations, hemiplegic limb weakness or disturbances of speech which are generally fleeting but may occasionally become permanent. Similarly, ocular palsies may be temporary or permanent in *ophthalmoplegic migraine*. The third cranial nerve is most commonly affected.

Lower half headache is a headache of possibly vascular origin centred primarily in the lower face; there may be some patients with atypical facial neuralgia and sphenopalatine ganglion neuralgia.

Basilar migraine is heralded by paraesthesiae around mouth and lips, bilateral paraesthesiae of the hands and feet and sometimes the sensation of a rushing feeling in the epigastrium and chest. The ensuing headache is bilateral. Often with this form of headache there may be an associated feeling of fear, panic and doom and strong emotional sensations which are difficult to dispel, though short-lived.

DIET AND MIGRAINE

Review of the literature

'One man's meat is another man's poison' is a very well-known phrase. Hippocrates himself was amongst the first to recognize that food can provoke symptoms; in his writings he described headaches affecting one side of the head.

Historically it has been well recognized that dietary provocants can induce migraine. A review of the literature since 1873 is given in Appendix 37.1. It can be seen that in those reports where any significant number of patients have been studied about 75% of patients have been helped by elimination diets.

It is significant that in many studies the value of prick testing has varied; in many studies it was negative, in others some positive correlation has been noted.

Dietary elimination and challenge

Elimination and challenge has remained the cornerstone of diagnosis. Rowe was amongst the first to record a numerically large group of patients responding to elimination diets in 1928 and 1931. Others followed suit (see Appendix 37.1). In 1938 Rowe corroborated foods implicated by elimination followed by challenge and again others investigated similar elimination and challenge regimens.

Recent work has included that by Grant [26] who reported 60 patients on elimination diets who reacted to an average of ten common foods each, diagnosed from a combination of symptoms and pulse responses. Instigation of elimination diets resulted in 65% of the patients becoming headache-free for the following 3 months. The monthly incidence of migraine in the group was reduced from 402 to 6, and headache incidence from 533 to 22. Monro et al [46] found that, of a group of severe migraineurs attending the National Hospital for Nervous Diseases, London, two-thirds had allergy to certain foods as shown by dietary exclusion and subsequent challenge. These studies were undertaken double-blind and confirmed incontrovertibly that allergy to food can cause migraine.

Double-blind trial of food elimination

Egger et al [20] showed by a double-blind trial of oligoantigenic diets that migraine is likely to be due to food allergy in a majority of cases. Of 88 children with severe frequent migraine 93% recovered on these dietary elimination regimens. The diet consisted of one meat (lamb or chicken), one carbohydrate (rice or potato), and one fruit (banana or apple), one vegetable (brassica), water and vitamin supplements for 3–4 weeks. Those who did not improve were offered a different combination of foods. Thereafter one food was reintroduced at a time. If no reaction occurred, the patient was advised to eat the food regularly. Foods that provoked symptoms were withdrawn at the end of the week. A double-blind placebo-controlled cross-over trial, which tested the response to one of the foods which had provoked symptoms in the reintroduction phase, was then instituted using a savoury base and a sweet base in turn.

Many foods were found to be provocants, and the researchers concluded that the metabolic process involved was therefore more likely to be allergenic rather than idiosyncratic. Other associated symptoms also improved, including abdominal pain, behavioural disorders, fits, asthma and eczema (see Chapter 38).

Immune complexes, intestinal hypersensitivity and the effect of sodium cromoglycate. We and others have shown that migraine can be relieved by dietary elimination and that symptoms are provoked after food challenge. We have also shown that immune complexes containing IgE appear in the circulation following such a challenge, associated with migraine headache. Both the symptoms and the immune complexes can be prevented by pretreatment with oral sodium cromoglycate.

In a further formal study we have shown that sodium cromoglycate orally, and not placebo, protects a patient from the effect of food challenge. As sodium cromoglycate is not absorbed from the gut and acts locally on the intestinal mucosa, it suggests that a local mucosal hypersensitivity reaction is being blocked which then fails to trigger the absorption of immune complexes and possibly mediators. If the sensitivity is limited to the mucosa, this would explain the efficacy of sodium cromoglycate and also the lack of specific antibodies in the circulation [46].

STUDIES TO HELP DEFINE THE CAUSES OF MIGRAINE

In any condition in which there is no sign or objective clinical measurement that can be documented, assessment of the condition is extremely difficult. Attack rates can be recorded, although in conditions where there may be a gradation of symptoms from a mild headache through to a full-blown attack with teichopsia, nausea and vomiting, some patients may tend to record only the latter whilst others may register every nuance in the continuum from mild to severe.

A study of patients with migraine was undertaken to attempt to quantify these subjective responses. The patients for this study were ones who had severe recurrent migraine. Being clinical, the diagnostic criteria did not depend on mechanism or aetiology; they were those described by the Ad Hoc Committee on Headache.

Study 1: Effect of diet

Patients. A total of 300 patients were asked to fill in a medical questionnaire (Appendix 37.2) and tick symptoms that had recurred regularly over the past year. The patients were also asked to complete a diet questionnaire (Appendix 37.3). Groups of patients were then put on different diets: for example, a basic allergy diet in which tea, coffee, colourings and additives, sugar and alcohol were forbidden (Appendix 37.4), a milk-free diet (instructions were included) (Appendix 37.5). A further group were put on a wheat-free diet (Appendix 37.6). Some patients were put on to combinations of the basic allergy diet and milk-free diet, or basic allergy diet and wheat-free diet.

Migraine attacks. The frequency, duration and severity of their migraine attacks were recorded by the patients. The period over which the trial took place varied from 1.5 to 21 months. No data were included if the period of the trial was less than 1 month. The majority covered a period of 6 months (mean 6.5 months). At the end of the survey patients were asked to complete another questionnaire.

Symptom scores. Patients were asked to score the frequency, duration and severity of their migraine symptoms on a chart. The severity was calculated on a score of 1–4 as shown in Table 37.1.

Table 37.1 Symptom scoring in migraine.

Score:	
1	mild—no analgesic required
2	moderate—analgesics required
3	severe—unable to work or carry out activities of daily living
4	prostrating—bedridden

A graph was drawn comparing frequencies of attacks before diet against attacks afterwards. The frequency of attacks was divided into high (more than 250 attacks per year), medium (100–250 attacks per year), and low (fewer than 100 attacks per year).

The percentage reduction of frequency was divided into bands as follows: 100% (totally free); 90–100%; 75–100%; 50–75%; 1–50%; 0% (no change).

The results show that:

1. No-one became worse.
2. Less than 10% of the patients showed no improvement.
3. More than 80% of the subjects showed a reduction of 75% or more in their frequency of attack.
4. 35% of the group became totally free of symptoms.
5. Although about 80% of the patients on any diet had at least a 75% reduction in attacks, those following the basic allergy diet included a much smaller proportion who became totally symptom free.

Relation of diet to symptoms. The relation of diet to specific medical symptoms was then analysed. All patients who had completed a questionnaire were tabulated in groups according to diet, together with the symptoms to which they gave a positive response.

Those symptoms to which at least half the diet group gave a positive response were considered. There was no clear relationship between symptoms and original diet choice. In general a relationship between wheat and problems associated with digestion, water retention, skin symptoms and sleep seem to be apparent, and those who had skin symptoms and eating disorders seemed to respond better to the basic allergy diet; there was not enough evidence for these to be statistically significant.

Selection of diet. In general, the choice of a diet for a patient was made mainly by assessing that patient's eating habits. If these were poor and a large proportion of foods containing colourings, additives, tea, coffee and sugar were being consumed, the elimination of these

as a first line was selected. If, however, the diet was good with plenty of fresh food and no preponderance of foods containing many colourings or additives, tea, coffee or sugar, then either the wheat-free diet or the milk-free diet was selected.

There was a very clear association of milk and wheat, in particular, with migraine. Unfortunately, it has not been possible to classify the degree of improvement of a wide variety of other symptoms as well as the migraine.

The conclusions from this study were:

1. The patient's dietary history can give positive guidance as to which foods to eliminate. Those foods eaten either very frequently or infrequently were amongst the commonest culprits for any individual.
2. There were many symptoms associated with the migraine attacks, in particular fatigue, arthralgia and rhinitis (see also Table 37.2).

Table 37.2 Common symptoms associated with migraine.

Conjunctivitis and rhinitis	approx. 15%
Angioedema	approx. 15–20%
Irritable bowel syndrome (abdominal bloating, flatulence and diarrhoea)	approx. 20–23%
Aching muscles and joints	approx. 20%
Severe fatigue	approx. 30%
Depression	approx. 23%
Skin itching	approx. 17%
Seasonal symptoms/diurnal symptoms were worse first thing in the morning	approx. 17%

Study 2: The incidence of associated symptoms

A further study of migrainous patients was undertaken to quantify associations with other conditions. A group of patients with migraine completed questionnaires (Appendix 37.2) which were then analysed. The results show that migraineurs have many symptoms other than headache. Conversely, patients with other major complaints may also have migraine. Migraine is one of a constellation of conditions, most of which will respond to allergy management.

Common symptoms in various categories which are associated with migraine are shown in Table 37.2.

Study 3: The value of RAST and diet

A group of 286 patients with migraine was studied using the radioallergosorbent test

(RAST) for some common foods [47]. They were also tested by intradermal injections of allergens using the Miller provocation-neutralization technique and by dietary manipulation, elimination and challenge. This study revealed an association between migraine and foods in the majority of these patients (Table 37.3).

A strong association with foods was found in the majority of patients, suggesting that food allergy is causative in provoking migraine in migraineurs. Most patients were found to be allergic to more than one food group, often to as many as three. The high levels of specific IgE to food in some of these patients suggested that Type I hypersensitivity may play

Table 37.3 Foods associated with migraine by RAST, diet or desensitization in 286 patients.

Food	RAST and desensitization	RAST alone	RAST and diet	Diet alone	Diet and desensitization	Desensitization alone	RAST, desensitization, diet	Total
Grain	12	38	44	30	28	46	21	219
Apple and orange	7	62	15	1	0	20	5	110
Dairy products	23	46	39	28	22	53	13	224
Rice	12	91	1	1	1	20	0	126
Fish	8	94	6	3	0	12	0	123
Wheat	12	58	16	18	25	52	18	199
Maize/oats	0	0	0	1	15	38	0	54
Egg	15	77	10	10	4	38	8	162
Tomatoes	11	94	6	1	1	13	0	126
Tea	7	59	25	11	3	13	4	122
Cheese	16	75	15	18	3	29	5	161

Study 4: Effect of immunotherapy

A group of 11 migrainous patients, difficult to manage on a complex elimination diet, have been treated with immunotherapy using the provocation-neutralization method described by Lee and modified by Miller [42]. The efficacy of their treatment was tested by double-blind assessment of immunotherapy versus placebo. The results indicated a marked preference for immunotherapy in protecting them from challenge with relevant food and inhalant allergens and chemicals which they met during the 1-month period of the study (Table 37.4).

INVESTIGATIONS INTO MIGRAINE

Value of RAST

The diagnostic methods for the identification of allergens in migraine have relied primarily upon elimination and challenge to identify food provocants. However, the RAST has been used to corroborate the relevance of foods found to be allergenic and, secondarily, has been used prospectively in the diagnosis of food allergens [47]. In each case the specific IgE level was assayed using the technique of Wide et al [69], and the total IgE was measured by the method of Kjellman et al [36].

a part in the production of symptoms. High total IgE levels were not found in these patients.

Control data. In assessing the value of RAST, each patient had to be their own control. Analysis of the specific IgE titres to a variety of foods revealed RAST values that were higher than the background levels for those foods that had been associated clinically with migraine.

Food intake and RAST. The degree of detectable food allergy was found to be changeable in individual patients; thus the RAST profiles varied according to each patient's exposure to particular foods. The specific IgE to allergenic foods was found to drop with avoidance of these foods, whereas other frequently taken foods could become allergenic. False negative RAST results may occur in patients who have been avoiding their trigger foods for some time (Fig. 37.1).

Sodium cromoglycate

Sodium cromoglycate prevents antigen-induced mast cell histamine release. Taken orally it can be used to protect patients exposed to food challenges. Preliminary results of one study [46] show that of 10 patients taking sodium cromoglycate one had complete pro-

Table 37.4 Clinical details of patients.

Patient	Age/sex (years)	Challenge	Order of treatment	Symptoms	Choice of treatment
1	60 F	Wheat milk egg	Active 2	Slight headache at 4 h grade 1	Active
			Placebo 1	Headache at 24 h grade 3	
2	55 F	Milk egg wheat	Active 1	No headache	Active
			Placebo 2	Headache at 24 h grade 4	
3	30 F	Milk	Active 2	No headache	Active
			Placebo 1	Headache grade 4	
4	64 M	Milk wheat	Active 2	No headache, flatulence	
			Placebo 1	No headache, flatulence	Placebo
5	52 M	Milk wheat	Active 1	Headache grade 1	Active
			Placebo 2	Headache grade 1, diarrhoea	
6	38 F	Milk wheat	Active 2	Diarrhoea	Active
			Placebo 1	Diarrhoea, nausea, and headache	
7	31 F	Wheat milk	Active 1	No headache	Active
			Placebo 2	Headache at 24 h grade 2, nausea	
8	45 M	Milk wheat	Active 1	No headache	Active
			Placebo 2	Headache at 48 h grade 1–3 next day	
9	37 F	Milk wheat	Active 2	No headache	Active
			Placebo 1	Abdominal symptoms, nausea, teichopsia, no headache	

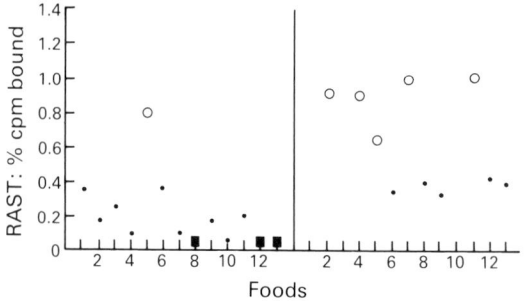

Fig. 37.1 RAST profile in migraine patient with food allergy. (Left) One positive RAST was obtained (tea) and avoidance of this gave complete relief from headaches. (Right) Avoidance of milk and milk products, chocolate, tea, coffee, fish, and wheat gave complete relief from headaches. (Foods: milk (1), cheese (2), egg (3), chocolate (4), tea (5), tomato (6), coffee (7), shellfish (8), orange (9), fish (10), wheat grain (11), rice (12), apples (13), ○, clinically relevant foods.) From Monro et al [47], with permission.

tection when taking 400 mg of sodium cromoglycate daily for 7 days before challenge with those foods that had previously provoked migraine when taken in similar amounts. Another eight patients showed partial or complete protection when taking 800 or 1600 mg, and only one showed no protection; he had probably not kept to his elimination diet between challenges. In each of these patients elimination diets were being followed, and the challenges with antigenic foods were sporadic. If a normal diet was resumed, sodium cromoglycate did not offer sufficient protection, perhaps because in these individuals there were multiple sensitivities, particularly to common foods, and also because the volume of antigen taken on a normal diet would have been larger.

Optimum dosage. A further trial of sodium cromoglycate has confirmed the optimum daily dosage as 1600 mg in divided doses before meals. This is effective with a partial elimination diet such as, one, perhaps, which allows the use of butter and cream and small amounts of milk in beverages in a milk-sensitive patient, but not the resumption of a large volume of milk, as would be taken, for example, with cereals and in milk puddings.

Conclusions

Formal food challenge can provoke migraine, and pretreatment with oral sodium cromoglycate exerts a protective effect. Food allergy is responsible for migraine in these patients. As sodium cromoglycate is poorly absorbed from the gastrointestinal tract the protection it affords suggests that the drug acts locally on the gut mucosa to block an immunological 'trigger' for the absorption of antigen, immune complexes, and possibly mediators.

The platelet is known to have Fc receptors for IgE. Patients with migraine show platelet hyperaggregability, which may result from the presence of immune complexes containing IgE and IgG. There are several ways in which immune complexes containing IgE could produce migraine. The complexes may aggregate platelets, producing small microthrombi, or allow the release of platelet mediators. They may also react with mast cells in the cerebral vasculature.

The observation that these patients are protected by oral sodium cromoglycate does suggest that an allergic mechanism in the gut triggers the production of symptoms, with immune complexes acting as a messenger. In general we have found that sodium cromoglycate is not useful as a primary treatment, but when used as an adjunct to diet it is helpful.

BIOCHEMICAL FACTORS IN MIGRAINE

Pressor amines

The association of migraine with food allergy is not the only evidence linking food to migraine. There are many publications suggesting other aetiological relationships. Hanington et al [29] reported that approximately one-third of the patients attending a migraine clinic stated that some of their headaches were related to specific foods; Table 37.5 lists those cited most frequently. These workers noted the close similarity between this list and those foods that depressive patients on monoamine oxidase inhibitors have to avoid, such as alcohol, cheese, fish, beans, milk and dairy products, and chocolate.

Tyramine metabolism

The severe headache which can be induced by these foods in depressive patients on monoam-

Table 37.5 Foods considered to be migraine precipitants and thus excluded from the diet of 500 patients.

Food	Percentage
Chocolate	74
Dairy products (cheese)	46
Fruits (citrus)	30
Alcohol	25
Fatty fried foods	18
Vegetables (onions)	17
Meat (pork)	14
Tea and coffee	14
Seafood	10

From Monro [44], with permission.

ine oxidase inhibitors led Hanington to consider that pressor amines may have aetiological significance in the production of both migraine and the iatrogenic headaches occurring in depressive patients, since monoamine oxidase inhibitors make available more monoamines, one of the main ones being tyramine. (The tyramine content of various foods is listed in Table 37.6.) It was therefore considered that mig-

Table 37.6 Foods containing tyramine and other pressor amines.

	Content $\mu g/g$
Cheese in varying amounts	50–1415
Alcoholic drinks	0.4–25.4
Banana	7
Red plum	6
Tomato	4
Avocado	23
Potato	1
Spinach	1
Orange pulp	10
Eggplant	3
Raspberry	55
Pickled herring	3030
Marmite	1600

Other pressor amines are: phenylethylamine, present in chocolate; octopamine, in citrus fruits; dihydrophenylalanine (a precursor of dopamine), in broad beans; 5-hydroxytryptamine, in tomatoes, pineapple and bananas.

raine could be caused by faulty metabolism of tyramine in particular, thus a controlled trial of challenge with oral tyramine was conducted. Capsules of 125 mg of tyramine hydrochloride were given to patients, or dummy tablets containing lactose; the results are shown in Table 37.7.

Platelet monoamine oxidase

Other writers, however, have not confirmed the association between tyramine and the provocation of migraine. Chocolate, which is

Table 37.7 Results of administration of tyramine and control lactose in 50 dietary migraine patients.

	Total no. of challenges	No effect	Migraine attack
Lactose	66	60	6
Tyramine	100	20	80

From Monro [44], with permission.

one of the most commonly cited migraine provocants, does not contain tyramine, but does contain phenylethylamine. Sandler et al [58] proposed that migraine is due to a deficit of phenylethylamine and tyramine oxidation and that one of the forms of monoamine oxidase on platelets is defective. Phenylethylamine is thought to stimulate alpha receptors and thus produce migraine. This gives a rationale to some of the drugs used prophylactically to protect migraineurs which block alpha receptors.

Other associations. There have been sporadic reports about other food associations with headache such as 'ice-cream headache' which is possibly stimulated by temperature change. Kwok's disease, in which pressor reactions to the monosodium glutamate in Chinese food result in headache, is also well recognized. Histamine headache has been recorded but raised levels are not present in all forms of migraine.

Changes in serotonin, 5-hydroxytryptamine (5-HT), metabolism during migraine attacks have been demonstrated. Plasma 5-HT has been found to rise just prior to the onset of headache in classical migraine and to fall during the headache phase. 5-Hydroxyindole-acetic acid (5-HIAA) excretion increases during attacks, indicating, as it is a metabolite of 5-HT, that more 5-HT is being released and utilized. Ninety-eight per cent of the 5-HT in blood is contained in platelets. Hence, release of 5-HT is likely to be from platelets when they aggregate. An increase in platelet aggregation has been described by Hilton and Cumings [31], and Hanington [30] has hypothesized that migraine is a blood disorder caused by abnormal platelet function.

A 5-HT-releasing factor has been demonstrated by Lance and colleagues to be active during the vasoconstrictor phase of migraine. This releases 5-HT from platelets. In the subsequent painful vasodilator phase of a migraine attack, low levels of 5-HT are found. Increased platelet aggregability has been shown in patients with migraine with a fall in

platelet 5-HT and monoamine oxidase levels during migraine attacks.

An increase in β-thromboglobulin during migraine attacks is reported by Gawel et al [24]. This is regarded as an index of the platelet release reaction. Other aggregating agents have also been considered, including adrenaline, noradrenaline and adenosine diphosphate.

When platelets aggregate, arachidonic acid is released by the action of platelet phospholipase A_2 via the cyclooxygenase pathway. Prostaglandins and thromboxane A_2 are synthesized. Thromboxane A_2 is a potent vasoconstrictor and may be involved in the aetiology of migraine.

Phenolic compounds in foods

Consistent with the concept that a potential unifying link between migraine and foods may be the content of pressor amine in the latter, is the evidence from Gardiner that major 'cross-reactions' between foods may be because of their common phenolic constituents and not the relationship associated with botanical families, or even their tyramine content.

This concept, that there are some biochemical constituents in foods which are common and to which a susceptibility may arise, has been accepted with regard to salicylates. A representative group of foods is shown in Appendix 37.7 showing their content of 14 different phenolic compounds. Highly represented are gallic acid and rutin/quercetin. Desensitization has been attempted with these chemicals with encouraging results (Appendix 37.6) (see also Chapter 24).

Chemicals

Apart from foods many patients have reactions to chemicals as shown in Table 37.8 and no

Table 37.8 Chemicals that may provoke migraine.

Chlorine
Perfume and other toiletries
Gas
Cleaning agents, e.g. containing phenol
Exhaust fumes
Diesel fumes
Formaldehyde
Solvents
Tobacco smoke
Paint fumes
Ammoniacal odours
Smoke from coal or bonfires
Laboratory chemicals

enquiry into migraine provocants is complete without a consideration of these items.

It is very well known that many migraineurs may be triggered into attacks by the slightest whiff of perfume or other odour. The mechanism of this may be immunological as in many patients the use of sodium cromoglycate as an inhalant aerosol (Intal) or nasal instillation (Rynacrom) can prevent the provocation when used prior to unavoidable social exposure. Prevention of encounter with these items may have to be rigorous.

MANAGEMENT OF MIGRAINE

History

The patient's history of migraine is recorded, with notes on the type, frequency, duration and severity of attack. Since many conditions that are due to allergy can be polysymptomatic, a symptom questionnaire (Appendix 37.1) is answered and a diary of the patient's normal diet maintained. If a patient is sure that particular foods may provoke migraine, he is informed of other related foods and may avoid all members of that food family, or take

other members only sporadically. The dietary regimen is instituted. Initially, a diet excluding tea, coffee, sugar, colourings and additives is recommended, leaving fresh food only. Records of diet and symptoms for 2–4 weeks are analysed and those foods that provoke headaches may be pinpointed. On withdrawal of a food, symptoms can be transiently worse. The patient may crave that food and find that it alleviates the withdrawal symptoms. This may be the explanation of the observation that most migraineurs have headaches when they miss a meal.

Food groupings

Foods are grouped not only into botanical families, but also into zoological families (see Chapter 17) and those related to each other must be considered together. Examples of this are that some egg-sensitive people will react to chicken and some milk-sensitive people will react to beef. Likewise, cane sugar, which is derived from the grass family, must be grouped with wheat, rye, barley, millet, maize, oats and rice. Not only must corn oil, margarine and vegetable oils which may contain corn oil be considered with this family, but so also

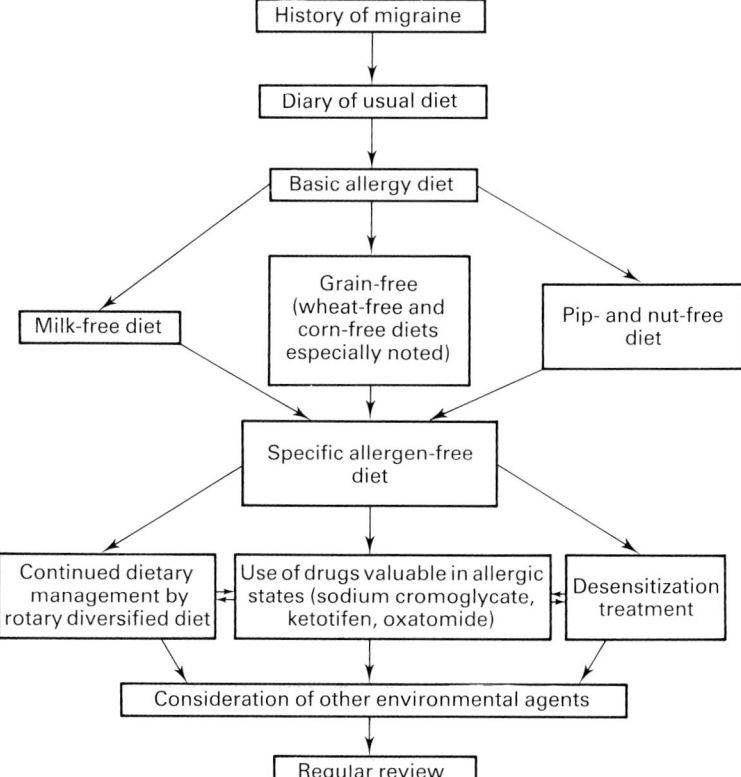

Fig. 37.2 Flow chart of management of migrainous patients. From Monro [44], with permission.

must corn syrup, glucose syrup, dextrose and glucose (all of which come from maize) be grouped with the grain family.

Block elimination diets. Subsequent to the intial basic allergy diets, block elimination diets are used for 2–4 weeks. The elimination of milk and milk products is recommended, followed by the elimination of all grains, and subsequently the elimination of pips and nuts. During each exclusion period the principles of the basic allergy diet are maintained. In some patients elimination of combinations of these food groups may be necessary. All other foods are taken not more frequently than once in 4 days or once a week, this being known as a diversified rotation diet (see Chapter 17). Records are kept for each subject and the foods which provoke reactions are identified. Patients will need advice about which foods to avoid and also what may be eaten; for example, when grains are to be eliminated suitable substitutes such as soya and other legume flours, or sago, tapioca, buckwheat or potato flour are suggested.

Confirmation by challenge. The results of elimination dieting in identifying provoking foods must be confirmed by challenges. Once on an elimination diet some individuals may become less sensitive quite quickly. The optimum time for a challenge is after five days' avoidance, and the food should be taken on an empty stomach. Specific allergen-free diets are then maintained and, to minimize the risk of further sensitivities developing, a diversified rotation diet is maintained.

Drug therapy

To treat an acute attack one should minimize exposure to the trigger and to any other triggers, including chemicals. Fresh air is important. A simple solution of a teaspoonful of a mixture of alkali salts (e.g. two parts of sodium bicarbonate to one part potassium bicarbonate in pure water) may alleviate the headache but gastric stasis may be a problem. Simple analgesics taken early are best. Ergotamine derivatives may help if taken early but they are not without immediate side-effects of hypertension, muscle cramps and nausea, and long-term effects of addiction and, paradoxically, withdrawal headaches. Prolonged use or even a single overdose may provoke gangrene.

Drugs used prophylactically include:

Propranolol and other β-blockers. The side-effects may include hypotension and asthma.

Pizotifen which may act as an anti-5-HT drug. The side-effects are weight gain and drowsiness.

Methysergide. Again may act as an anti-5-HT agent but has serious side-effects of retroperitoneal fibrosis and vasoconstriction.

Clonidine, an α-adrenoceptor agonist. Side-effects include hypotension and depression.

A vaccine containing the specific trigger or triggers prepared by the provocation–neutralization technique can be used both preventatively and therapeutically, and can be most effective.

Treatment summary

Prevention is better than cure, for once the migraine attack is in progress it is difficult to abort. Investigation of the causative factors and their avoidance is at present the most promising remedy.

One of the main preventative measures is to minimize the 'load' the patient faces by excluding the worst offenders or minimizing the lesser offenders. There is a threshold beyond which a migraine attack is triggered; to lower the load so that the threshold is never reached enables the individual to maintain health rather than to have to treat an illness.

Exposure to chemicals should be minimized. This includes avoidance of oral contraceptives which may increase the frequency of migraine. Permanent neurological sequelae to migraine are rare, but the risk is greater in subjects taking oral contraceptives. Other drugs which can provoke attacks are reserpine, viloxazine and dipyridamole.

Ketotifen

Like sodium cromoglycate, ketotifen has been stated to have an inhibitory effect on the release of mast cell mediators by allergens. It is also reputed to act on neutrophils. Ketotifen has been shown to be protective in patients with food allergy. In particular, a preliminary report by Borge [7] of a double-blind trial of ketotifen has shown that patients with multiple sensitivities are protected. One of the patients detailed had attacks of migraine whose incidence was 47 in 3 months when taking a placebo and 11 during treatment with ketotifen 1 mg b.d.

In an open trial of ketotifen we have found that the frequency, duration and severity of migraine attacks before and after treatment was considerably reduced, with an average improvement in all 'scores' of 72%.

The results of the trial are shown in Fig. 37.3. Eleven of the 13 patients improved, whereas only two remained the same or got

response. This evidence comes from a number of sources.

(1) A large variety of foods can be shown to provoke migraine, suggesting multiple allergenic causes. A caveat here is the possibility of cross-reacting chemicals providing a common denominator between foods.

(2) Sodium cromoglycate will protect a patient from a food challenge. This drug acts locally on the mucosa and is not absorbed systemically, and leads to the suggestion that a

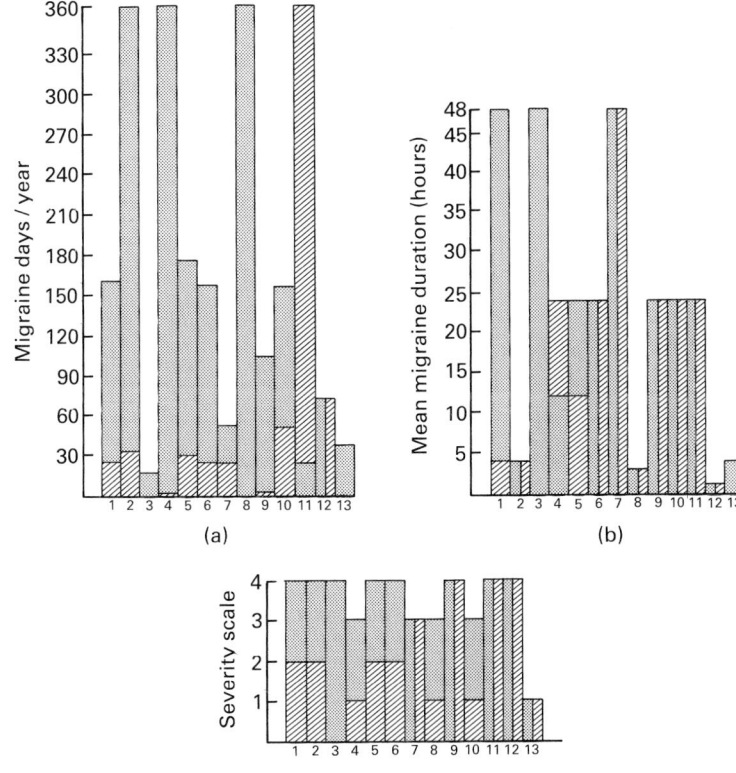

Fig. 37.3 The frequency (a), duration (b) and severity (c) of attacks in 13 respondents before (▫) and after (▨) treatment with ketotifen. From Monro [44], with permission.

worse. The results of the trials of these two antiallergy drugs (ketotifen and sodium cromoglycate) support the view from clinical observations that most cases of migraine are due to food allergy.

CONCLUSIONS

It must be emphasized that the patients we have studied are a selected group with attacks of migraine weekly and not just an occasional attack once or twice a year. The evidence that migraine in these patients can be provoked by food is now overwhelming and there is increasing evidence that this is due to an allergic

local mucosal hypersensitivity reaction triggers the events which lead to the migraine attack.

(3) Not only are the clinical effects of the food challenge prevented by pretreatment with sodium cromoglycate, but so is the appearance of immune complexes containing IgE. This further supports the concept of chronic migraine being due to allergic mechanisms triggered by primary events in the gut.

Our aim must be to restore these patients to health rather than just treating the symptoms of their disease. We can achieve this by searching diligently for the causes of their symptoms.

APPENDICES

Appendix 37.1 Review of dietary regimens in migraine.

Date	Author	Details	Food implicated	Number of patients	Method of Diagnosis	Success rate
1873	Liveing	In his renowned treatise *On Megrim, Sick Headaches and some Allied Disorders* Liveing describes the migrainous syndrome well—its periodic recurrence, unilateral and bilateral attacks of headache, disturbance in sight, tactile sensations, speech, psychic functions, giddiness, nausea and vomiting, its familial nature and its associations with other conditions. He states that 'certain articles of diet occasionally act as exciting causes of the seizures.' He reported a case in which headaches had occurred for 30 years from the smallest amount of wine or from burnt pastry.	Wine Burnt pastry	4		
1913	Leone and Richet	Migraine considered to be due to milk or egg allergy in young suspects.	Milk Egg			
1918	Pagniez, et al	Allergy believed to be a cause of migraine.	Chocolate			
1920	Brown, R. C.	Cylindrical headaches were thought to be caused by 'protein poisoning' after the ingestion of some foods. (Diet trial was suggested with polished rice, butter, toast and a few green vegetables and water.)	Cow's milk Eggs Fruit Tomato Mushrooms Rhubarb Coffee Tea Chocolate		Elimination diets Skin tests negative	
1921	Brown, T. R.	Migraine subjects were treated with a dietary regimen in the belief that carbohydrate metabolism was at fault. A diet of vegetables and fats was recommended, or a vegetarian diet, and on this regimen alleviation of headache in some cases was reported.	Cereals Animal protein		Elimination diets	
1923	Minot	Limitation of starch proved beneficial in some cases of migraine. In others elimination of a specific meat or meats as a whole was an effective remedy. In particular cereals were eliminated in these regimens as they were a source of starch.	Grains and other carbohydrate foods Some meat, or all meats		Skin tests negative Elimination diets	
1923	Miller and Raulston	Allergy was believed to be the basis of migraine. Peptone injections were used.		25	Peptone injections	84% migraine alleviation

Date	Author	Details	Food implicated	Number of patients	Method of Diagnosis	Success rate
1922–1935	Vaughan	Many case reports.	Wheat Milk Peanuts Chocolate Pork pie Bean Onion Egg Banana (in this order)		Elimination diets 62 different foods implicated in several studies	50.8% to 70%
1925	Van Leeuwen	Eggs and chocolate were reported to provoke headache which was attributed to allergy.	Eggs Chocolate			
1927	Ball	Of 1000 randon family histories migraine occurred in 26.1% of the families, asthma in 16.2%, hayfever in 9.1%, urticaria in 19.9%, epilepsy in 2.7% and eczema in 6.1%.		20	Peptone injections	50%
1927	Diamond	Food idiosyncrasies in migrainous subjects were reported but the condition was accorded to liver dysfunction.				
1927	McClure and Huntsinger	Of 8 patients with migraine 4 had positive skin scratch tests to food. These items (milk, meat and eggs in particular) were eliminated and the patients improved.	Milk Meat Eggs	8	Skin test	50%
1928	Rowe, A. H.	Rowe first reported on 48 patients with migraine all of whom had complete or almost complete relief from migraine with elimination diets.	Cereals predominantly	48	Elimination diets	100%
1931	Rowe, A. H.	Rowe further reported on 86 cases similarly managed; 139 cases were analysed. Good results were obtained in 73.1%, fair in 6.9% and poor in 20%. However, 21% did not cooperate well; 14 patients who had cooperated well did not benefit. Skin reactions were absent in 58%. He reported the following associations with migraine from family history:		86	Elimination diets (i) Cereal free (ii) Fruit free, cereal free (iii) Minimal elimination diets (vi) Rotary diversified diets	73.1% good 6.9% fair 20% poor

	Migraine as a major complaint	Migraine as a minor complaint	Total		
Number of cases	46	40	86		
Male	16	7	23	(27%)	
Female	30	33	63	(73%)	
Age	38.4	41	39.6 (average)		
Positive family history	39	25	64	(74%)	
Associated allergic conditions:					
asthma	3	7	10	(12%)	
hayfever	4	11	15	(17%)	
cutaneous allergy	18	19	37	(43%)	
abdominal allergy	22	33	55	(64%)	

Date	Author	Details	Food implicated	Number of patients	Method of Diagnosis	Success rate
1931	Eyermann			63	Skin tests then elimination diets	69% good results
1931	Balyeat and Rinkel	Skin tests were used to detect allergy. Milk was the most prevalent allergenic food found.	Milk especially	202	Skin tests	22% excellent 38% good
1932	DeGowin	Treatment—elimination diets.		60	Skin test negative Elimination diets	78% relief
1933	Todd			12	Elimination diets	83% improved
1935	Sheldon and Randolph			127	Elimination diets	60.8% benefited
1937	Rowe	Data on 247 patients with headache as a major complaint was presented as follows:	Cereals principally	247	Skin tests. Hypoallergenic diet for 2–3 weeks. Then the addition of one food at a time. Challenge with foods followed. The allergenic foods were then eliminated	63.5% good 19.5% fair 17% failure

	No. of cases		No. of cases %	
Age:		Personal history:		
1–15 years	3	nasal congestion	80	
15–35 years	72	hay fever	35	
35–55 years	135	asthma	25	
55 years up	37	chronic indigestion	98	
Male	66	nausea	130	
Female	181	vomiting	91	
Duration of symptoms:		abdominal pain	47	
0.5–1 year	23	constipation	142	
1–5 years	40	diarrhoea	24	
>5 years	184	eczema	40	
Family history:		Results:		
headaches	113	failure	43	17.0
asthma	50	fair	49	19.5
hayfever	39	good	155	63.5
eczema	8			
urticaria	12	Cooperation:		
chronic indigestion	42	none	6 ⎫	
Skin reactions:		poor	15 ⎬ 19	
foods	68	fair	26 ⎭	
inhalants	45	good	200	81
miscellaneous	26			

Date	Author	Details	Food implicated	Number of patients	Method of Diagnosis	Success rate
1948	Meyer	The detection of reactions to food by noting a relative tachycardia after its ingestion was reported.		13	Challenge	13
1948	Unger and Unger	After 14 days' avoidance of the food patients were challenged with individual foods and their response noted. Those patients	33% milk 31% chocolate 22% wheat 18% pork	55	Elimination diets Challenge	64% excellent 16% good

Date	Author	Details	Food implicated	Number of patients	Method of Diagnosis	Success rate
		whose attacks occurred more frequently than once in 6 weeks were usually sensitive to foods eaten almost daily in some form.				
1965	Shapiro and Eisenberg	100 patients with migraine and headache were skin tested; 13 had migrainous symptoms such as teichopsia, and 88 had nausea, vomiting vertigo, nasal disturbance, photophobia or other symptoms. These patients showed positive skin tests for foods. Elimination diets and desensitization treatments were used. 36 became headache-free and 40 improved greatly.		100	Skin tests Elimination diets	36% headache free 40% great improvement
1977	Speer	Milk, chocolate, cola and corn were responsible for causing symptoms on challenge in 31%, 24% and 17% respectively.	Milk Chocolate Cola Corn		Elimination diets Skin tests Challenge	
1977	Grant	A combination of elimination diets and relative tachycardia were used. In 60 patients 10 common foods provoked reactions (wheat 78%, Orange 65%, egg 45%, tea 40%, coffee 40%, chocolate 37%, milk 37%). When cheese, chocolate, citrus fruit and alcohol were avoided only 13% of patients became headache-free; whereas 85% of the remainder became headache-free for 3 months with avoidance of the specific foods responsible for their headache. Furthermore the monthly incidence of migraine was reduced from 402 to 6, and the headache incidence from 533 to 22. IgE levels to specific foods were raised in some patients.	Wheat Orange Egg Tea Coffee Chocolate Milk	60	Elimination diets Challenge with assessment of relative tachycardia	85%
1980	Monro et al		Wheat Rice Milk Egg Chocolate Tea Coffee Tomato Shellfish Cheese Orange Fish Apple	Two groups: (a) 47, 33 intensively. (b) 26	(a) Dietary elimination followed by RAST corroboration (b) RAST used diagnostically followed by elimination diets	70% 88%
1983	Egger et al	'Is migraine food allergy?' A double-blind trial of oligoantigenic diet treatment.	Many	88	Elimination and challenge	93%

Date	Author	Details	Food implicated	Number of patients	Method of Diagnosis	Success rate
1984	Monro et al	Foods which provoked migraine in 9 patients with severe migraine refractory to drug therapy were identified. The patients were then given either sodium cromoglycate of placebo orally in a double-blind manner, with foods previously identified as provocants. Sodium cromoglycate exerted a protective effect, thus confirming that it can prevent a hypersensitivity mechanism as well as the symptoms of migraine. Immune complexes were not produced in those patients who were protected by sodium cromoglycate. These observations confirm that a food-allergic reaction is the cause of migraine in this group of patients.		9	(a) Elimination and challenge (b) Prick testing (c) Intradermal testing (d) Exhibition of sodium (e) IgE (f) Sucrose/ polyethylene glycol gradient (g) Isokinetic ultracentrifugation gradient	89%

From Monro [44], with permission.

Appendix 37.2 Medical questionnaire.

Name ....   Date ....

Address ....

....   Tel ....   **MAIN SYMPTOM**

Occupation   Age: Height: Weight: B/P

Pulse (first thing before eating):   Do you live in town or country: Near main road:

Is there gas   Coal fires: Do you smoke: Any smokers   Where do
  in the house: in the family: you shop:

─────────────── MEDICAL QUESTIONNAIRE ───────────────

☐ (tick those which have occurred
  regularly over the past year)

1 ☐ Overweight	109 ☐ Mouth ulcers	111 ☐ Cramp	86 ☐ After meals
2 ☐ underweight	33 ☐ Cold	61 ☐ inability to	87 ☐ After shopping
3 ☐ fluctuating weight	34 ☐ hot	concentrate	88 ☐ In heavy traffic
4 ☐ Skin: itching	35 ☐ sweating	62 ☐ forgetfulness	89 ☐ All the time
5 ☐ burning	36 ☐ Pulse: fast	63 ☐ depression	90 ☐ Have you ever taken
6 ☐ eczema	37 ☐ slow	64 ☐ anxiety state	cortisone
7 ☐ urticaria	38 ☐ breathlessness	65 ☐ irritability	
8 ☐ itching scalp	39 ☐ Frequency	66 ☐ aggressiveness	**LADIES ONLY**
9 ☐ dandruff	micturition	67 ☐ Cannot miss or be	91 ☐ Menopause
10 ☐ Abdominal cramps	40 ☐ water retention	late for a meal	Menstrual cycle:
11 ☐ nausea	41 ☐ Dark puffy circles	68 ☐ Obsessional eating	92 ☐ Regular
12 ☐ diarrhoea	under the eyes	69 ☐ Eating for comfort	93 ☐ Irregular
13 ☐ constipation	42 ☐ Aching: Muscles	70 ☐ Craving for a	94 ☐ Amenorrhoea
14 ☐ bloating after meal	43 ☐ joints	specific food	95 ☐ Painful
15 ☐ Flatulence	44 ☐ back	71 ☐ Poor appetite	96 ☐ Cysts: Breast
16 ☐ colitis	45 ☐ Fibrositis	72 ☐ High blood	97 ☐ ovarian
17 ☐ Weeping eyes	46 ☐ Fatigue for no	pressure	98 ☐ Toxaemia
18 ☐ itching eyes	reason	73 ☐ Low blood	pregnancy
19 ☐ visual problems	47 ☐ drowsiness	pressure	
20 ☐ Sneezing	48 ☐ especially after	74 ☐ Were you ever	Contraceptive pill
21 ☐ sinusitis	meals	bottle fed	dates:-
22 ☐ itching nose	49 ☐ waking up tired	When are you worse:	
23 ☐ runny nose	50 ☐ Clumsiness	75 ☐ Spring	Pregnancy dates:
24 ☐ post-nasal drip	51 ☐ floating feeling	76 ☐ Summer	
25 ☐ Sore throat	52 ☐ tenseness	77 ☐ Autumn	Miscarriage dates:
26 ☐ hoarseness	53 ☐ headaches	78 ☐ Winter	
27 ☐ cough	(tension)	79 ☐ At home	
28 ☐ catarrh	54 ☐ Nervousness	80 ☐ At work	
29 ☐ wheezing	55 ☐ insomnia	81 ☐ On holiday	
30 ☐ bronchitis	56 ☐ waking during	82 ☐ First thing in	
31 ☐ Ears: ringing	night	morning	
32 ☐ aching	57 ☐ hypoactive	83 ☐ Daytime	
	58 ☐ hyperactive	84 ☐ Night	
	59 ☐ hysterical	85 ☐ Before meals	
	60 ☐ mental confusion		
	110 ☐ Tingling lips		

Operations:

Brief history of past illnesses:
  (other than normal childhood)

Family history:

What drugs/medicine
  are you taking now:

Diagnoses: 99 ☐ Migraine   100 ☐ Myxoedema
101 ☐ Ulcerative colitis   102 ☐ Thyrotoxicosis
103 ☐ Multiple sclerosis   104 ☐ Agoraphobia
105 ☐ Osteoarthritis   106 ☐ Schizophrenia
107 ☐ Rheumatoid arthritis   others:
108 ☐ Asthma

List of known allergies:
  (including drugs)

Name of your Doctor ....

Address ....

....

....   Tel. No.......

Appendix 37.3 Diet questionnaire.

Describe a typical day's diet	How often, if at all, do you consume the following:					
Breakfast		never	infrequently	sometimes	regularly or daily	more frequently
	1. bread					
	2. coffee					
	3. tea					
	4. alcoholic drinks					
	5. chocolate					
Lunch	6. sugar (cane) brown					
	7. oranges					
	8. corn and corn products					
	9. pork/bacon					
	10. preserved meats					
	11. milk					
	12. cheese					
Tea	13. cakes or biscuits					
	14. eggs					
	15. potatoes					
	16. beetroot or beet sugar (white)					
	17. tomatoes					
	18. cereals/breakfast foods					
	19. fish					
Dinner	20. beef					
	21. lamb					
	22. salt					
	23. nuts					
	24. soft drinks					
	25. root vegetables					

Space left for food not listed above.

26 What medicines do you take?

27 Is there any food that you eat at least one a day (or crave for)?

28 Since your symptoms started, have you increased your intake of any food?

29 Do you eat regularly, and how many times a day?

30 Is there any food you dislike?

31 Is there any food that you avoid because it disagrees with you?

32 How often, if at all, do you eat out?

33 When you were a child were there any foods you disliked, or felt ill after eating?

34 Do traffic fumes upset you?

35 Do crop sprays or pesticides affect you?

36 Do gas fumes upset you?

37 Do enclosed shopping areas affect you?

Appendix 37.4 Basic allergy diet.

(1) Record daily, in duplicate, your diet and any symptoms. Also note if any drugs are taken.
(2) Record your pulse: (1) before a meal; (2) 20 minutes after a meal) (3) 40 minutes after that. This should be done in the following manner: sit quietly for 5 minutes before taking the pulse, then count the pulse for half a minute, and multiply this figure by 2.
(3) Do NOT eat between meals, and drink only spring water if you are thirsty. (Three main meals and three snacks have been allowed for.)
(4) Take PLAIN FRESH FOOD and sea salt only. Vary your diet, eating only reasonable quantities as too much of anything is bad for you. Read all labels carefully. Have a high protein breakfast, and fruit and nuts at snacktimes.
(5) Take no ALCOHOL or CIGARETTES.
(6) Take no flavourings, colourings or additives (junk foods).
      Take no processed foods, white flour, preserved, smoked, salted, canned or pickled foods (e.g. bacon, beef stock cubes, ham, pickled herrings, smoked haddock, kippers, sausages, etc).
(7) Take no caffeine, tannin, chocolate, instant drinks.
(8) Limit yourself to only 4 eggs and 4 oz of cheese per week.
(9) Take cold pressed unrefined oils—sunflower, safflower, sesame and apricot kernels. Use these sparingly: 3 consecutive days on, 4 consecutive days off.
(10) Take no white sugar (beet), brown sugar (cane), honey, treacle, molasses, syrups; instead use fructose.
(11) When possible, try to avoid unnatural chemical air pollutants, avoid fumes from : paint, hairdressers, nail varnish, perfumes, soft plastics, glue, aerosol sprays, tar, chlorine (bleach), tobacco and heavy traffic.

IMPORTANT
DO NOT FAST, ELIMINATE FOOD FROM YOUR DIET, OR TAKE VITAMIN SUPPLEMENTS, UNLESS YOU CONTACT YOUR DOCTOR FIRST

ANTIDOTES
You will have to find out which of the following suits you:
Potassium bicarbonate (1 teaspoon) + Soda-bicarbonate (2 teaspoons) in a glass of warm water.
OR
Milk of magnesia 1 dessert spoonful.
OR
Vitamin C (1 gram) in a glass of water. Redoxon, or Cantassium.
Again—plenty of fresh spring water and exercise.
Most allergic reactions will gradually pass over a period of 4 days.
If you come off your allergic food you will have 'withdrawal' symptoms. If you take back an allergic food having eliminated it from your diet you may have a rise in pulse, 20–60 minutes after eating, and an allergic reaction, usually within 4 hours.
The above antidotes may be used.

NO INSTANT DRINKS—COFFEE, TEA, CHOCOLATE

WHAT TO DRINK

All natural tolerated FRUIT JUICES unsweetened.
Instead of coffee (Caffeine):
   Chicory ROOTS.
   Dandelion ROOTS.
   Decaffeinated GROUND COFFEE BEANS (HAG) **not** instant.
Instead of tea (caffeine, tannin):
   A wide range of herb teas—find out which ones suit you, note that some contain fruit.
   Rooibosch tea (low tannin only) Test after 14 days.
   Green tea (low tannin) test after 14 days (also contains low caffeine).
Instead of chocolate try plain Carob powder.

ALL DRINKS STRICTLY ON A 3 DAY ON, 4 DAY OFF ROTATION

NO CHLORINE

Stay away from fumes, swimming baths, taps, bleach.
Drink bottled spring waters, glass bottles preferable.
'Sparkling' Perrier, Evian.
'Still' Volvic, Malvern, Evian, Highland Spring, etc.
   or Boil tap water vigorously for 5 minutes
   or Stand tap water in refrigerator for 36 hours.
Get someone else to run your bath and leave to settle for 10 minutes.
Better still, add photographer's hypo solution (sodium thiosulphate) 4-6 teaspoons to bath water.
Water filters: Royal Doulton, Elga Spectrum, Norwegian Mayrei, Botan Limited, Culligan Safari.

CHICORY ROOTS (make as coffee) filter, percolate, etc. 1 dessertspoon—1 teaspoon per pint of water to taste.

DANDELION ROOTS percolate or simmer 10 minutes. 1 small teaspoon—1 cup water—beware of making too strong.

DECAFFEINATED GROUND COFFEE BEANS (HAG) (make as coffee).
filter, percolate, etc. 1 dessertspoon to 1 tablespoon per pint.

HERB TEAS treat as tea bags.
Place tea bag in a tea cup, cover with boiling water and allow to infuse 5 minutes, squeeze bag and remove.

ROOIBOSCH TEA
1 teaspoon tea into warmed pot.
Add just enough boiling water to cover.
Leave 30 seconds.
Then strain and discard liquid, putting strained tea leaves back into pot.
Then add enough boiling water for one cup of tea.
Steep for 4 minutes.
Then pour out cup of tea, straining again.
These strained leaves can be used time and time again for several cups of tea.

CAROB POWDER (make as chocolate)
1-2 teaspoons per cup, dissolve in a little liquid and add boiling water, milk or milk substitute to taste.

SHOPPING LIST   (Read all labels carefully)

Dandelion roots
Chicory roots
Decaffeinated ground coffee beans (not instant or freeze dried)
Assorted herb teas—Alfonal Ltd, Pompadour
Rooibosch tea
Carob powder
Fructose (Cantassium)
Sparkling spring water, Perrier, etc. (glass bottle)
Spring still water: Volvic, Evian, Highland Ashe Parke, Wells
          Some people cannot tolerate the plastic bottles
          Malvern & Highland Spring in glass bottles
Cold pressed unrefined oils: sesame, sunflower, safflower, olive oil, apricot kernel
Coconut oil (excellent if fats are difficult to digest)
(Cold pressed unrefined corn and soya oil used only if you have desensitizing drops for corn and soya)
Margarines: Golden Rose (coconut oil, soya), Telma (corn), unsalted butter for clarifying. Vitaquel (wheat, maize (corn), sunflower)

Nut milk, coconut, almond, cashew, etc
Soya milks: Be-mil Pro Sorbe (powdered only) (Granose contains raw sugar, permission to use)
(Do not have soya milks containing beet (white) or cane (brown sugar))
Peanut, cashew nut, sesame seed, sunflower seed spreads: pure, nothing added, no salt
Sago, potato flour (pure)
Sweet potato balls—tapioca flour (Chinese)
Burdalls gravy browning (caramel)
Sea salt
Cider vinegar
Morga, stock cubes and vegetable broth mix (Blue label only)
Pareve-Mate, Coffeemate (formulated for Israel only, milk free)
Whole Earth jams and marmalades

These vitamins and minerals only:

Complete B & C (Cantassium)
Cantassium Dri Fill range
Halibut oil capsules
Calcium carbonate (pure only)
Redoxon Effervescent Vitamin C

BRITA water filter
MAYREI 2000 water filter

Appendix 37.5 Milk-free diet.

Basic Allergy Diet
REMEMBER TO READ ALL LABELS CAREFULLY
BE AWARE—lactose, lactic acid, whey, casein, sodium caseinate, are all extracted from milk.
NO MILK MEANS no cream, fresh, dried or skimmed milk, goat's or sheep's milk, butter, cheese, yoghurt, batter.

MOST COMMERCIALLY MADE FOOD contains MILK in some form:
Bread, biscuits, cakes, sweets, chocolates, salad creams and dressings, pickles, sauces, instant food (potato), soups, cereals, baby foods, instant drinks (Bournvita, Horlicks, dandelion coffee, Ovaltine, etc.), margarines, artificial sweeteners, food covered in breadcrumbs.

INSTEAD

HOMEMADE—the best, you know what you have put in it.
HOWEVER—Most large food manufacturers, e.g. Sainsburys, Marks and Spencer, Waitrose, etc., will supply you with lists of their milk-free products. Apply direct to firm you are interested in.
A liquidizer is a good investment.

MILK SUBSTITUTES:
Soya milks—Be-mil Pro Sorbee (powdered only).
Do not have soya milks containing beet (white) or cane (brown) sugar.
Nut milks—coconut cream, almond milk.
Magic milk—if you can tolerate eggs:
  Recipe: 3 lightly poached eggs or 3 egg yolks
            ¼ cup water   ½ cup oil
            1 cup oil   3–4 cups water
      Liquidize eggs and oil and add water gradually.
      Pour into jug and make up to 2 pints with water.
      Keeps the same time as milk in refrigerator, but whisk up before use.
        Excellent for a milk substitute in cooking.
Evaporated milk SOMETIMES can be tolerated, but please consult your doctor or dietician before testing it.

BUTTER SUBSTITUTES:
Margarines: Kosher (Tomor), Waitrose and Superfine low fat spread contain corn and other oils, artificial flavouring and colouring, and therefore do not suit everyone.
Vitaquel is cold pressed, unrefined, wheat, maize (corn), sunflower.
Cold pressed unrefined oils for cooking, sunflower, safflower and sesame, grapenut, olive oil.
Coconut oil
Cashew nut, peanut, sesame seed, sunflower seed spreads.
Lamb, beef and pork lard can be used.
Ghee—available Indian stores.

Clarified butter is usually tolerated:
> Recipe: Bring unsalted butter to the boil and skim off curds. Then strain hot fat through cotton sieve. When nearly set, add a little sea salt to taste. Keep in refrigerator.

ALL THE ABOVE SUBSTITUTES MUST BE USED SPARINGLY AND ON A STRICT 3 DAY ON 4 DAY OFF ROTATION

Beef cannot be tolerated by some milk allergic people.

Vitamin supplements: Calcium carbonate—1 teaspoon per day.
1 teaspoon cold pressed oils or margarines per day.
Halibut oil capsule—2 per week.

Appendix 37.6 Wheat-free diet

If you are allergic to wheat you will probably be allergic to, or easily become allergic to, the other grains, i.e. rice, rye oats, barley, millet. These grains must be eliminated from your diet and tested. Corn must be eliminated from the diet. Once a week you may have a grain day.

'Starch' usually means wheat or corn (Chinese food—it will refer to rice).
Hydrolysed vegetable protein—wheat. Monosodium glutamate—wheat or soya.
Lecithin—soya or egg. Gluten—wheat. Malt—barley.

Foods you cannot have:
All breads contain wheat—whole wheat, brown, processed white, gluten free, rolls, muffins, crumpets, dumplings, doughnuts; rye, rice potato and soya bean breads unless made at home, sauces, binders, fillers, cereals, cakes, pastries, crackers, sweets, ice cream, spaghetti, macaroni, ravioli (pastas); salad dressings, soups, semolina, farina, rusks, alcohol; stock cubes.

Instead:
Sago and tapioca flours the best alternatives (see recipes). Buckwheat flour. Thickeners for sauces—arrowroot, agar agar, tomato puree, pureed pulses, nuts. Salt-free baking powder (Cantassium) potato base. OR Soda bicarbonate ($\frac{1}{2}$ teaspoon) + cream of tartar (1 teaspoon) to half a pound of permitted flour.
Sago and tapioca can be ground down to flour in a coffee grinder, but it must be dried (not browned) in the oven first—otherwise the grinder blades will snap.
Cantassium—Trufree cantabread and bread mix may suit you.
Potato, yams, sweet potatoes, mashed parsnips are good as alternative fillers.
Burdalls gravy browning may be used.
PLEASE DON'T TAKE YOURSELF OFF ANY PRESCRIBED MEDICINES WITHOUT DISCUSSING THE SITUATION FIRST WITH YOUR DOCTOR.

Appendix 37.7   Allergenic chemicals in foods.

	Acetaldehyde	Acetone	Adenine*	Aflatoxins	Aminobenzoic acid (PABA)*	Aminobutyric acid (GABA)*	Amygdalin	Anethole	Anisole	Apiol	Asparagine	Benzaldehyde	Benzoic acid	Benzyl alcohol	Butylated hydroxyanisole	Butylated hydroxytoluene	Butyric acid	Caffeic acid*	Caffeine	Camphor*	Capsaicin	Carotene*	Caryophyllene	Chalcone	Choline*	Chlorogenic acid*	Cineol	Cinnamaldehyde	Cinnamic acid
Albumin, cow's milk				●	●					●	●		●																●
Allspice																											●	●	
Almond							●			●		●					●												
Anise seed	●	●						●		●																			
Apple	●	●										●						●								●			●
Apricot							●					●	●					●								●			●
Artichoke																		●											
Asparagus											●																		
Avocado	●																												●
Banana	●										●																		●
Barley											●																		
Basil																											●		
Bass, black																													
Bay leaf											●																		
Bean, lima																		●											
Bean, navy																		●											
Bean, pinto																		●											
Bean, red																		●											
Bean, soya											●	●																	
Bean, string																		●											
Beef											●	●																	
Beer													●				●												
Beet																													●
Beet, sugar																	●												●
Blackberry	●											●	●																●
Blueberry	●											●	●																●
Boysenberry													●																●
Broccoli	●											●																	
Brussels sprouts																													
Buckwheat																													
Cabbage																													
Cantaloupe																													
Caraway seed																													
Carrot											●							●											
Casein, cow's milk																													
Cashew nut																													
Catfish																													
Cauliflower																		●											
Celery											●																		
Cheese, American											●	●	●																
Cheese, Cheddar											●	●																	
Cheese, cottage											●																		
Cherry												●	●													●			●
Chicken											●																		
Chili powder	●			●																●	●								
Cinnamon																				●			●						
Clam											●																		
Clove																							●						●
Cocoa				●											●	●	●		●				●				●		
Coconut												●																	●

* Chemicals which are considered to be ubiquitous to nature. As such, marks in those columns are restricted to those foods containing unusually large amounts

Appendix 37.7   (cont.)

	Coniferyl, alcohol/coniferin	Coumarin	L-DOPA	Dopamine	Ellagic acid	Eugenol	FD & C Blue No. 1	FD & C Blue No. 2	FD & C Green No. 3	FD & C Red No. 40	FD & C Red No. 3	FD & C Red No. 2	FD & C Violet No. 1	FD & C Yellow No. 5	FD & C Yellow No. 6	Folic acid*	Formaldehyde	Furfural	Gallic acid	Genistein (biochanin A)	Glutamic acid/Glutamine*	Hesperetin	Histamine	Indole*	Isoascorbic acid*	Limonene	Linalool	Malvin (anthocyanidins)	Menadione (naphthoquinones)
Albumin, cow's milk		●	●														●											●	●
Allspice						●																							
Almond						●																							
Anise seed						●																							
Apple		●															●	●	●	●								●	●
Apricot																			●							●	●	●	
Artichoke																													●
Asparagus	●																●												●
Avocado			●	●													●											●	●
Banana		●	●	●															●									●	
Barley		●																	●										
Basil																			●								●		
Bass, black																							●						
Bay leaf																													
Bean, Lima			●																●										
Bean, navy			●																●										
Bean, pinto			●																●										
Bean, red			●																●										
Bean, soya			●																●	●									
Bean, string			●																●										
Beef		●																											
Beer		●																	●				●						
Beet	●	●								●	●	●																●	
Beet, sugar	●	●																										●	
Blackberry																		●	●									●	
Blueberry																		●	●									●	
Boysenberry																												●	
Brocoli																													
Brussels sprouts																			●										
Buckwheat																													
Cabbage																												●	
Cantaloupe																			●										
Caraway seed																													
Carrot						●																						●	
Casein, cow's milk																			●		●			●					
Cashew nut																			●									●	
Catfish																							●						
Cauliflower																			●										
Celery		●																											●
Cheese, American		●												●	●				●										
Cheese, Cheddar		●												●					●										
Cheese, cottage		●																	●										
Cherry											●	●					●									●		●	
Chicken		●																						●					
Chili powder																													
Cinnamon		●																									●		
Clam																													
Clove						●												●											
Cocoa		●																	●					●					●
Coconut																	●												

* Chemicals which are considered to be ubiquitous to nature. As such, marks in those columns are restricted to those foods containing unusually large amounts

Appendix 37.7   *(cont.)*

	Menthol	Methyl salicylate(s)	Naringenin	Nicotine	Noradrenaline	Octopamine	Oestrogenic compounds	Phenylalanine*	Phenyl isothiocyanate	Phloridzin	Pinene*	Piperine	Piperonal	Progesterone	Putrescine	Pyridine	Pyrrole	Rutin/Quercetin	Safrole	Serotonin (5-hydroxytryptamine)	Thujone*	Thymol	Thymine*	Tryptamine	Tyramine	Tyrosine	Uric acid	Vanillin	Vanillylamine	Xanthine
Albumin, cow's milk							●		●					●				●					●	●	●	●	●			●
Allspice																					●									
Almond																		●												
Anise seed							●				●								●										●	
Apple										●								●												
Apricot																		●											●	
Artichoke																														
Asparagus																		●												
Avocado																				●										
Banana				●	●															●				●	●				●	
Barley									●									●												
Basil																														
Bass, black																							●	●	●	●				
Bay leaf																			●											
Bean, Lima								●										●												
Bean, navy								●										●												
Bean, pinto								●										●												
Bean, red								●										●												
Bean, soya								●										●							●					
Bean, string																														
Beef		●					●							●				●							●		●			●
Beer							●							●				●	●						●					
Beet																		●												
Beet, sugar																														
Blackberry		●																●												
Blueberry		●																●												
Boysenberry		●																●												
Broccoli									●																					
Brussels sprouts		●							●																					
Buckwheat																		●												
Cabbage																		●											●	
Cantaloupes																		●												
Caraway seed																		●												
Carrot																		●												
Casein, cow's milk									●																				●	
Cashew nut																													●	
Catfish															●								●	●	●	●	●			
Cauliflower																		●												
Celery																														
Cheese, American				●					●					●				●							●					
Cheese, Cheddar				●					●					●				●							●					
Cheese, cottage				●					●					●				●							●					
Cherry																														
Chicken																		●							●		●			
Chili powder											●																			
Cinnamon													●						●										●	
Clam																														
Clove		●											●															●	●	
Cocoa				●			●	●										●	●	●					●	●		●	●	
Coconut																														

*Chemicals which are considered to be ubiquitous to nature. As such, marks in those columns are restricted to those foods containing unusually large amounts

Appendix 37.7 (cont.)

	Acetaldehyde	Acetone	Adenine*	Aflatoxins	Aminobenzoic acid (PABA)*	Aminobutyric acid (GABA)*	Amygdalin	Anethole	Anisole	Apiol	Asparagine	Benzaldehyde	Benzoic acid	Benzyl alcohol	Butylated hydroxyanisole	Butylated hydroxytoluene	Butyric acid	Caffeic acid*	Caffeine	Camphor*	Capsaicin	Carotene*	Caryophyllene	Chalcone	Choline*	Chlorogenic acid*	Cineol	Cinnamaldehyde	Cinnamic acid
Codfish											•																		
Coffee																			•							•	•		
Corn	•			•																									
Crabmeat											•																		
Cranberry												•	•	•															
Cucumber	•																												
Curry																													
Date																													•
Dill										•																			
Egg, white											•																		
Egg, whole											•																		
Egg, yolk											•																		
Eggplant	•																												
Fig																													
Flounder											•																		
Garlic																													
Gelatin																													
Ginger																											•		
Grape (red & green)	•											•	•					•											•
Grapefruit	•												•																•
Haddock	•										•																		
Halibut	•										•																		
Ham											•																		
Honey	•																												•
Hops	•			•																									
Horseradish																													•
Lemon										•			•																•
Lettuce										•										•									
Lime													•																•
Liver																													
Lobster											•											•							
Malt, barley											•																		
Mango													•																•
Milk, cow			•							•	•		•			•									•				•
Milk, goat			•							•	•		•												•				•
Milk human			•								•		•												•				•
Mushroom	•																												
Mustard seed						•																							
Mutton											•																		
Nutmeg										•																			
Oat																													
Okra																													
Olive, green																		•								•			•
Olive, ripe																		•								•			•
Onion																													
Orange	•	•								•			•															•	
Oregano																													
Oyster											•														•				
Papaya																													
Paprika																					•								

* Chemicals which are considered to be ubiquitous to nature. As such, marks in those columns are restricted to those foods containing unusually large amounts

Appendix 37.7 (*cont.*)

Food	Coniferyl, alcohol/coniferin	Coumarin	L-DOPA	Dopamine	Ellagic acid	Eugenol	FD & C Blue No. 1	FD & C Blue No. 2	FD & C Green No. 3	FD & C Red No. 40	FD & C Red No. 3	FD & C Red No. 2	FD & C Violet No. 1	FD & C Yellow No. 5	FD & C Yellow No. 6	Folic acid*	Formaldehyde	Furfural	Gallic acid	Genistein (biochanin A)	Glutamic acid/Glutamine*	Hesperetin	Histamine	Indole*	Isoascorbic acid*	Limonene	Linalool	Malvin (anthocyanidins)	Menadione (naphthoquinones)
Codfish																							●						
Coffee																	●												
Corn		●																										●	
Crabmeat																			●				●					●	
Cranberry						●				●																		●	
Cucumber																			●										
Curry																													
Date																													
Dill																													
Egg, white																			●										
Egg, whole																			●										
Egg, yolk		●																	●										
Eggplant																												●	
Fig																												●	
Flounder																							●						
Garlic																			●										
Gelatin							●	●	●	●	●	●	●	●	●					●									
Ginger																			●										
Grape (red & green)																			●							●		●	●
Grapefruit											●							●				●				●	●		
Haddock																							●						
Halibut																							●						
Ham						●																	●						
Honey																	●											●	
Hops																			●										
Horseradish																									●				
Lemon		●				●													●							●	●		
Lettuce		●														●													●
Lime		●																								●			
Liver																													
Lobster																							●						
Malt, barley																													
Mango										●																			
Milk, cow		●				●										●	●						●						●
Milk, goat		●				●										●	●						●						●
Milk, human		●				●										●	●						●						●
Mushroom																	●												
Mustard seed																										●			
Mutton		●				●																	●						
Nutmeg						●																							
Oat		●																											
Okra																●													●
Olive, green																			●									●	
Olive, ripe																			●									●	
Onion																												●	
Orange						●					●							●				●				●	●		
Oregano																													
Oyster																							●						
Papaya																			●									●	
Paprika																													

* Chemicals which are considered to be ubiquitous to nature. As such, marks in those columns are restricted to those foods containing unusually large amounts

Appendix 37.7   (*cont.*)

Food	Menthol	Methyl salicylate(s)	Naringenin	Nicotine	Noradrenaline	Octopamine	Oestrogenic compounds	Phenylalanine*	Phenyl isothiocyanate	Phloridzin	Pinene*	Piperine	Piperonal	Progesterone	Putrescine	Pyridine	Pyrrole	Rutin/Quercetin	Safrole	Serotonin (5-hydroxytryptamine)	Thujone*	Thymol	Thymine*	Tryptamine	Tyramine	Tyrosine	Uric acid	Vanillin	Vanillylamine	Xanthine
Codfish								●																						
Coffee																		●												●
Corn																		●												
Crabmeat								●																						
Cranberry																		●												
Cucumber												●	●																	
Curry																														
Date						●																								
Dill																														
Egg, white								●									●													
Egg, whole								●										●						●		●	●			
Egg, yolk								●										●												
Eggplant																		●												
Fig																														
Flounder																														
Garlic																													●	
Gelatin								●																						
Ginger																			●											
Grape (red & green)								●										●											●	
Grapefruit			●																											
Haddock																														
Halibut																														
Ham					●													●									●			
Honey													●					●												
Hops								●																						
Horseradish									●									●												
Lemon		●									●																		●	
Lettuce																		●				●							●	
Lime		●									●																		●	
Liver																														●
Lobster						●																								
Malt, barley			●															●											●	
Mango		●																●												
Milk, cow			●		●	●		●					●	●				●									●		●	●
Milk, goat						●								●				●									●			●
Milk, human				●				●						●				●									●		●	●
Mushroom																														
Mustard seed									●				●																	
Mutton						●			●				●					●											●	●
Nutmeg											●								●											
Oat																		●												
Okra																		●												
Olive, green																														
Olive, ripe																														
Onion									●																				●	
Orange			●		●						●										●		●							
Oregano																		●												
Oyster																									●	●	●			●
Papaya																		●												
Paprika																														●

* Chemicals which are considered to be ubiquitous to nature. As such, marks in those columns are restricted to those foods containing unusually large amounts

Appendix 37.7 (*cont.*)

	Acetaldehyde	Acetone	Adenine*	Aflatoxins	Aminobenzoic acid (PABA)*	Aminobutyric acid (GABA)*	Amygdalin	Anethole	Anisole	Apiol	Asparagine	Benzaldehyde	Benzoic acid	Benzyl alcohol	Butylated hydroxyanisole	Butylated hydroxytoluene	Butyric acid	Caffeic acid*	Caffeine	Camphor*	Capsaicin	Carotene*	Caryophyllene	Chalcone	Choline*	Chlorogenic acid*	Cineol	Cinnamaldehyde	Cinnamic acid
Parsley										●																			
Parsnip																													
Pea, blackeyed																													
Pea, green										●																			
Peach	●						●					●														●			●
Peanut			●																									●	
Pear	●											●	●																●
Pecan																													
Pepper, black										●											●	●							
Pepper, green & red										●											●	●							
Perch											●																		
Pimento																													
Pineapple	●												●																
Plum													●																●
Poppy seed																							●						
Pork										●																			
Potato																					●					●	●		
Potato, sweet																													
Prune													●																●
Pumpkin																						●							
Quince													●																●
Radish																													
Raisin													●																●
Rhubarb													●																●
Rice																													
Rye																													
Sage																											●		
Salmon											●									●					●				
Scallop																													
Sesame, seed																													
Shrimp											●									●					●				
Spearmint																											●		●
Spinach																													
Squash, yellow																													
Strawberry	●	●										●	●	●												●			●
Sunflower seed																													
Tea																			●										
Thyme																													
Tomato	●	●								●		●									●							●	●
Trout											●																		
Tuna fish											●																		
Turkey											●																		
Turnip																													
Vanilla																													
Walnut										●																			
Watermelon	●																												●
Wheat bran																													
Wheat, whole																											●		
Whey, cow's milk											●																		
Yeast mix	●			●							●																		●

* Chemicals which are considered to be ubiquitous to nature. As such, marks in those columns are restricted to those foods containing unusually large amounts

Appendix 37.7   (cont.)

	Coniferyl, alcohol/coniferin	Coumarin	L-DOPA	Dopamine	Ellagic acid	Eugenol	FD & C Blue No. 1	FD & C Blue No. 2	FD & C Green No. 3	FD & C Red No. 40	FD & C Red No. 3	FD & C Red No. 2	FD & C Violet No. 1	FD & C Yellow No. 5	FD & C Yellow No. 6	Folic acid*	Formaldehyde	Furfural	Gallic acid	Genistein (biochanin A)	Glutamic acid/Glutamine*	Hesperetin	Histamine	Indole*	Isoascorbic acid*	Limonene	Linalool	Malvin (anthocyanidins)	Menadione (naphthoquinones)
Parsley																													
Parsnip																													
Pea, blackeyed		•																										•	
Pea, green		•																										•	•
Peach																		•	•									•	
Peanut		•																	•										
Pear																			•									•	•
Pecan																													
Pepper, black		•																								•			
Pepper, green & red																										•			
Perch																							•						
Pimento						•																						•	
Pineapple																	•	•	•										
Plum																			•									•	
Poppy seed																													
Pork																													
Potato																			•									•	
Potato, sweet		•																	•										
Prune																			•										
Pumpkin																			•										
Quince																			•									•	
Radish																												•	
Raisin																			•										
Rhubarb																			•									•	
Rice			•																										
Rye																													
Sage	•	•																											
Salmon																							•						
Scallop																							•						
Sesame, seed																													
Shrimp																							•						
Spearmint																										•	•		
Spinach																													
Squash, yellow																													•
Strawberry																	•	•	•							•		•	•
Sunflower seed																													
Tea																			•										
Thyme																													
Tomato		•				•													•							•			
Trout																							•						
Tuna fish		•																					•						
Turkey		•																					•						
Turnip																												•	•
Vanilla		•																	•										
Walnut					•	•													•									•	
Watermelon																			•									•	
Wheat bran		•																											
Wheat, whole		•																	•										
Whey, cow's milk		•																											
Yeast mix	•	•															•		•		•		•						

* Chemicals which are considered to be ubiquitous to nature. As such, marks in those columns are restricted to those foods containing unusually large amounts

Appendix 37.7 *(cont.)*

	Menthol	Methyl salicylate(s)	Naringenin	Nicotine	Noradrenaline	Octopamine	Oestrogenic compounds	Phenylalanine*	Phenyl isothiocyanate	Phloridzin	Pinene*	Piperine	Piperonal	Progesterone	Putrescine	Pyridine	Pyrrole	Rutin/Quercetin	Safrole	Serotonin (5-hydroxytryptamine)	Thujone*	Thymol	Thymine*	Tryptamine	Tyramine	Tyrosine	Uric acid	Vanillin	Vanillylamine	Xanthine
Parsley																		●												
Parsnip																		●												
Pea, blackeyed								●										●												
Pea, green								●										●							●					
Peach													●					●										●		
Peanut																		●										●		
Pear																		●												
Pecan																		●										●		
Pepper, black								●			●	●	●					●	●									●		●
Pepper, green & red											●	●	●					●												
Perch																									●					
Pimento																														
Pineapple			●										●					●		●					●					
Plum		●		●														●		●					●					
Poppy seed																		●										●	●	●
Pork						●												●							●		●			
Potato				●	●		●											●							●	●		●		
Potato, sweet					●		●											●							●	●				
Prune																		●							●					
Pumpkin																		●												
Quince																		●												
Radish									●																					
Raisin																		●							●					
Rhubarb																		●												
Rice																														
Rye																		●												
Sage											●										●	●								
Salmon																														
Scallop																														
Sesame seed																		●												
Shrimp																														
Spearmint	●																				●	●								
Spinach																		●							●					
Squash, yellow																		●												
Strawberry				●														●												
Sunflower seed																		●												
Tea																					●	●								
Thyme																		●				●								
Tomato				●					●		●							●		●				●	●					
Trout																														
Tuna fish																														
Turkey																		●										●		
Turnip									●									●												
Vanilla											●							●	●									●	●	●
Walnut													●					●							●					●
Watermelon							●											●												
Wheat bran																		●												
Wheat, whole																		●												
Whey, cow's milk																														
Yeast mix				●			●	●			●	●						●		●				●	●	●		●	●	

* Chemicals which are considered to be ubiquitous to nature. As such, marks in those columns are restricted to those foods containing unusually large amounts

REFERENCES

1 Anthony M, Serotonin in migraine. In: Pearce JMS, ed. Topics in migraine. London: Heinemann, 1975.

2 Anthony M, Hinterberger H, Lance JW: Total plasma serotonin migraine and stress. Arch Neurol 1967; 16:544-52.

3 Ball FE: Migraine, its treatment with peptone and its familial relation to sensitisation diseases. Am J Med Sci 1927; 173:781.

4 Balyeat RM, Rinkel HJ: Further studies in allergic migraine. Int Med 1931; 5:713-28.

5 Bills TK, Smith JB, Silver MJ: Metabolism of (^{14}C) arachidonic acid by human platelets. Biochim Biophys Acta 1976; 424:303-14.

6 Blau JN: Towards a definition of migraine headache. Lancet 1984; i:444-5.

7 Borge P: Ketotifen in multiple allergies. Res Clin Forums 1982; 4(1):79-83.

8 Breneman J: Food allergy. New York: Marcel Dekker, in press.

9 Brostoff J, Carini C, Wraith DG: Food allergy: an IgE immune complex disorder. Theoretical and clinical aspects of allergic diseases. Stockholm: Almquist & Wiksell International, 1983.

10 Brostoff J, Carini C, Wraith DG, Johns P: Production of IgE complexes by allergen challenge in atopic patients and the effect of sodium cromoglycate. Lancet 1979; i:1268-70.

11 Brostoff J, Carini C, Wraith DG et al: Immune complexes in atopy. In: Pepys J, Edwards AM, eds. The mast cell. Tunbridge Wells: Pitman Medical; 1979; 380-93.

12 Brown RC: The protein of foodstuffs as a factor in the cause of headache. Wisconsin Med J 1920; 19:337.

13 Brown TR: Role of diet in etiology and treatment of migraine and other types of headache. J Am Med Assoc 1921; 77:1396.

14 Couch JR, Hassanein RS: Platelet aggregability in migraine. Neurology 1977; 27:843-8.

15 Curran DA, Hinterberger H, Lance JW: Total plasma serotonin, 5-hydroxyindolacetic acid and *p*-hydroxy-*m*-methoxymandelic acid excretion in normal and migrainous subjects. Brain 1965; 88:997-1010.

16 DeGowin EL: Allergic migraine review of 60 cases. J Allergy 1932; 3:557.

17 Deshmukh SV, Meyer JS: Cyclic changes in platelet dynamics and the pathogenesis and prophylaxis of migraine. Headache 1977; 17:101-8.

18 Diamond JS: Liver function in migraine, with report of 35 cases. Am J Med Sci 1927; 174:695.

19 Edmeads J: Headache 1977; 17:48.

20 Egger J, Carter CM, Wilson J et al: Is migraine food allergy? A double blind trial of oligoantigenic diet treatment. Lancet 1983; ii:865.

21 Enderssen G, Farre O: Studies on the binding of immunoglobulins and immune complexes to the surface of human platelets: IgG molecules react with platelet Fc receptors with cH3 domain. Int Arch Allergy Appl Immunol 1982; 67:33-9.

22 Eyerman CH: Allergic headache. J Allergy 1931; 2:106.

23 Friedman AP: Ad Hoc Committee on Classification of Headache. J Am Med Assoc 1962; 179:717-18.

24 Gawel MJ, Burkitt M, Rose FC: The platelet release reaction during migraine attacks. Headache 1979; 19:323-7.

25 Goltman MA: J Allergy 1936; 7:351.

26 Grant EEC: Food allergies and migraine. Lancet 1979; i:966-9.

27 Hamberg M, Svensson J, Samuelson B: Thromboxane, a new group of biologically active compounds derived from prostaglandin endoperoxides. Proc Natl Acad Sci (USA) 1975; 72:2994-8.

28 Hanington E: Further observations on platelet behaviour in migraine. In: Rose FC, Zilkha J, eds. Progress in migraine research. Vol. I. London: Pitman, 1981; 80-4.

29 Hanington E, Horn M, Wilkinson M: In Cochrane AL, ed. Proceedings of the third migraine symposium, 1969. London: Heinemann, 1969; Chapter 2.

30 Hanington E, Jones RJ, Amess JAL, Wachowicz B: Migraine: a platelet disorder. Lancet 1981; ii:720-3.

31 Hilton BP, Cumings JN: An assessment of platelet aggregation induced by 5-hydroxytryptamine. J Clin Pathol 1971; 24:250-8.

32 Holmsen H: Biochemistry of the platelet release action. Ciba Found Symp 1975; 35:175-205.

33 Humphrey J, Jacques R: The release of histamine and 5-hydroxytryptamine (serotonin) from platelets by antigen-antibody reactions (in vitro). J Physiol 1955; 128:9-27.

34 Hungerford GD, du Boulay GH, Zilkha KJ: Computerised tomography in patients with severe migraine. J Neurol Neurosurg Psychiatry 1976; 39:990-4.

35 Joseph M, Auriault C, Capron A et al: A new function for platelets: IgE-dependent killing of schistosomes. Nature 1983; 303:810-12.

36 Kjellman N, Johansson SGO, Roth A: Serum IgE levels in healthy children quantified by a sandwich technique (PRIST). Clin Allergy 1976; 6:51-9.

37 Laroche G, Richet C, Saint Girons E: Alimentary anaphylaxis. Paris, 1919; translated by Rowe. University of California Press, 1930.

38 Little CH, Stewart AG, Fennessy MR: Platelet serotonin release in rheumatoid arthritis: a study in food-intolerant patients. Lancet 1983; ii:297-9.

39 Liveing E: On megrim, sick headaches and some allied disorders. London: J and A Churchill, 1873.

40 McClure CW, Huntsinger ME, Observations on migraine. Boston Med Surg J 1927; 196:270.

41 Meyer MG: Non-reaginic allergy. Ann Allergy 1948; 6:417-27.

42 Miller JL, Raulston BO: Treatment of migraine with peptone. J Am Med Assoc 1923; 80:1894.

43 Minot GR: The role of a low carbohydrate diet in the treatment of migraine and headache. Med Clin North Am 1923; 7:715.

44 Monro JA: Food allergy and migraine. Clin Immunol Allergy 1982; 2:137-63.

45 Monro JA: Food allergy in migraine. Proc Nutr Soc 1983; 42:241.

46 Monro J, Carini C, Brostoff J: Migraine is a food-allergic disease. Lancet 1984; ii:719-21.

47 Monro JA, Brostoff J, Carini C, Zilkha KJ: Food allergy in migraine. Lancet 1980; ii:1-4.

48 Moore S, Pepper DS, Cash JD: The isolation and characterisation of platelet specific globulin. Biochim Biophys Acta, 1975; 379:360-69.

49 Neligan P, Harriman DGF, Pearce JMS: Respiratory Arrest in familial hemiplegic migraine: a clinical and neuropathological study. Br Med J 1977; ii:732-734.

50 Olesan J, Larsen B, Lauritzen M: Focal hyperaemia followed by spreading oligaemia and impaired activa-

tion of CBF in classic migraine. Ann Neurol 1981; 9:344–52.

51 Olesan J, Tfelt-Hansen P, Henriksen L, Larsen B: The common migraine attack may not be initiated by cerebral ischaemia. Lancet 1981; ii:438–40.

52 Pagniez P, Vallery-Raddt P, Nast A: Therapeutique preventative de certaines migraine. Presse Med 1919; 27:172.

53 Pearce JMS, Migraine, mechanisms and management. Springfield, Illinois: Charles C Thomas, 1969;1–9.

54 Penttinen K, Myila G, Makela O, Vaheri A: Soluble antigen–antibody complexes and platelet aggregation. Acta Pathol Microbiol Scand 1969; 77:309–17.

55 Rowe AH: Abdominal food allergy. Its treatment with elimination diets. Calif West Med 1928; 29:5.

56 Rowe AH: Food allergy, its manifestations, diagnosis and treatment. Philadelphia: Lea and Febiger, 1931.

57 Rowe AH: Food allergy: its control by elimination diets. Westminster Hosp Nurses' Rev 1928; 13.

58 Sandler M, Youdim MBH, Hanington E: Conjugation defect in tyramine-sensitive migraine. Nature 1974; 250:335–7.

59 Shapiro RS, Eisenberg BC: Allergic headache. Ann Allergy 1965; 23:123–6.

60 Sheldon JM, Randolph TG: Allergy in migraine-like headaches. Am J Med Sci 1935; 190:232.

61 Sicuteri F, Testi A, Anselmi B: Biochemical investigations in headache: increase in hydroxyindolaecetic acid excretion during migraine attacks. Int Arch Allergy Appl Immunol 1961; 19:55–8.

62 Smith JB, Ingerman C, Kocik JJ, Silver MJ: Formation of prostaglandins during aggregation of human blood platelets. J Clin Invest 1973; 52:965–9.

63 Speer F: Migraine. Chicago: Nelson-Hall, 1977.

64 Todd LC: Food allergy with special reference to migraine. South Med J 1933; 95:587.

65 Unger AH, Unger L: Migraine is an allergic disease. J Allergy 1952; 23:429–40.

66 Vane JR: Inhibition of prostaglandin synthesis as a mechanism of action for aspirin-like drugs. Nature 1971; 231:232–5.

67 Van Leeuwen WS: Allergic diseases. Philadelphia: Lippincott, 1925.

68 Vaughan WT: Disease associated with protein sensitisation. Virginia Med Monthly, 1922.

69 Wide L, Bennich H, Johansson SGO: Diagnosis of allergy by an in vitro test for allergen antibodies. Lancet 1967; ii:1105.

Chapter 38a
Food Allergy and the Central Nervous System in Childhood

Joseph Egger

Introduction

Food allergy as a cause of disorders of the central nervous system (CNS) has been much neglected because it is not easy to diagnose and because a connection between the gut and the brain is not obvious. Moreover, emotional factors often appear to trigger symptoms and so relatively greater importance has been given to them. Food-allergic symptoms of the CNS rarely occur soon after eating: they usually appear gradually, hours or days afterwards. Thus, especially with common foods, the relationship between ingestion and symptoms may not be obvious. Diagnosis is difficult because there are no laboratory tests to identify provoking foods. The management of food allergy is equally difficult; provoking foods have to be avoided, sometimes only temporarily, but often the offending foods are those the patient likes most.

MIGRAINE IN CHILDHOOD

Headaches in childhood have been relatively neglected and have frequently been interpreted as a symptom of nervous tension. The work of Bille [4] was highly significant in call-ing attention to migraine as a frequent disorder in childhood.

As a single event headaches usually occur in the context of an intercurrent illness. Recurrent headaches are divided into vascular (usually migraine), psychogenic (to be distinguished from the Münchausen syndrome and Münchausen syndrome by proxy [46]) and organic (in which the headache is due to structural, metabolic or infectious disease). Often a new headache may be assigned to one of the three categories only with passage of time, pending re-examination for the development of possible neurological signs.

Diagnosis

Criteria for the diagnosis of migraine are outlined in Table 38a.1. The problem of a generally acceptable clinical definition of migraine versus psychogenic headaches is almost insurmountable. Most studies have been content to identify migraine and to leave the issue of psychogenic headaches ambiguous.

The principal variables that form the basis of the symptomatic diagnosis of headache are occurrence (periodic versus continuous), the quality of painful discomfort and associated symptoms. The chief clinical characteristic of

Table 38a.1 Criteria for the diagnosis of migraine.

Essential criteria	Necessary symptoms
Recurrent headaches with symptom-free intervals, plus	three of the following: abdominal pain or nausea or vomiting unilateral throbbing relief after sleep aura (visual, sensory, motor) family history

vascular headaches, in the majority of cases, is their periodic occurrence. In contrast the usual psychogenic headache is thought to be continuously present.

The quality of pain in vascular headaches varies from an aching sensation to sharp pain. Throbbing pain is more often reported by older children but rarely before puberty. In psychogenic headaches the more commonly used description is of sensations of frontal or occipital pressure or tightness.

Associated symptoms are important for the diagnosis of vascular headaches; during an episode of migraine, children are almost always pale and frequently mention photophobia and vertigo. Visual symptoms are not especially common in children, but abdominal symptoms are, and sometimes motor and sensory hemisyndromes occur. The symptoms thought to be associated with psychogenic headaches are those related to the psychiatric disorder and may consist of depression, irritability, apathy and outbursts of temper.

Association with underlying disease

Any headache in childhood may be symptomatic of underlying systemic, cranial or intracranial disease (Table 38a.2), and it must be

Table 38a.2 Causes of symptomatic headache.

Trauma	Congenital malformation and hydrocephalus
Tumour	
Arachnoid cyst	Paranasal sinusitis
Arteriovenous malformations	Epidural abscess
	Cerebral abscess
Berry aneurysm	Meningitis
Acute subarachnoid haemorrhage	Encephalitis
	Pheochromocytoma
Connective tissue disease	Hypoglycaemia
Hypertension and hypertensive encephalopathy	Ornithine transcarbamylase deficiency
Childhood stroke (haemorrhagic, embolic, thrombotic)	

remembered that brain tumours are more frequent in the first 6 years of life than at any time thereafter. History, clinical signs, CCT and other laboratory tests may be helpful in distinguishing migraine from symptomatic headaches.

More difficult is the separation of psychogenic headaches from migraine as there are no tests available. In my experience pschogenic headaches are overestimated and are uncommon under 12 or 13 years of age; probably many of the patients who are relegated to the psychogenic group have migraine and are likely to respond to similar treatments. However, juvenile migraine is often aggravated by psychological factors.

Classification

Different types of migraine are recognized (Table 38a.3). They reflect the involvement of different parts of the brain and do not differ in response to treatment [12], except alternating hemiplegic migraine, which is probably a different disorder [37].

Table 38a.3 Types of migraine.

Common migraine [17]
Classical migraine [35]
Complex and complicated migraine syndromes
    Hemiplegic migraine [9]
    Basilar artery migraine [3]
    Ophthalmoplegic migraine [16]
    Migrainic vertigo [34]
    Confusional migraine [18]
    Migraine and syncope [27]
    Migraine and epilepsy [39]
    Migraine and stroke [6]
    Migraine and fever [47]
    Migraine and cerebrospinal fluid (CSF) pleocytosis [36]
Cluster headaches [24]
Alternating hemiplegic migraine [37]

Epidemiology. Most epidemiological studies of headaches have been conducted on adult populations [7, 28]. The incidence varies considerably and has been reported as 23% in women and 15% in men. In children, the classic study is that of Bille [4], who analysed questionnaires given to 9059 schoolchildren between ages 7 and 15 in Uppsala, the results of which can be seen in Table 38a.4. Four percent had migraine as defined by the criteria ofVahlquist [44], i.e. paroxysmal headaches separated by free intervals and at least two of the following four: one-sided pain, nausea, visual aura and family heredity. Due to the restricted definition, Bille's data probably

Table 38a.4 Epidemiology of headache in children 7-15 years of age. $n = 9059$.

Never had headaches	4%
Infrequent non-migrainous headaches	48%
Frequent non-migrainous headaches	7%
Migraine	4%

underestimate the frequency of vascular headaches in childhood. However, using the same criteria, Sillanpää [40] obtained similar results.

Pathogenesis

The cause of migraine is not known. Perhaps it is best regarded as a neurovascular syndrome with a generalized vasomotor instability and vulnerability to multiple extraneous factors. The apparent precipitating factors (Table 38a.5) may be the final event leading to decompensation of the system.

Table 38a.5 Precipitating factors.

Emotional
Food
Trauma
Exertion
Upper respiratory tract infections
Hypoglycaemia
Lactose intolerance
Irregular sleep
Travel
Bright light
Hormonal

A number of humoral factors (Table 38a.6) have been incriminated as a cause of migraine. However, like platelet hyperaggregability [25] changes occur mainly during migraine attacks and are therefore likely to be effects rather than the cause of the disease.

Table 38a.6 Humoral factors suspected to be involved in the pathogenesis of migraine.

Serotonin
Histamine
Prostaglandins
Leukotrienes
Substance P
Peptide kinins
Catecholamines
Tyramine
Phenylethylamine

Genetic factors

There are a number of reports on the inheritance of childhood migraine [2, 10, 35]; the family incidence ranged from 72% to 89%. However, there are no series of comparable controls and it is my experience that almost everybody has relations with recurrent headaches. Controlled studies are urgently needed to establish whether there is really a genetic factor involved or not. In contrast there is a high familial incidence in hemiplegic migraine [5, 20].

Food idiosyncrasy and food allergy also play a role in the causation of migraine; these will be discussed below.

Abdominal migraine and the periodic syndrome

Wyllie and Schlesinger [47] created the concept of the periodic syndrome. Children with this condition usually present themselves with one or a combination of the following symptoms: cyclical vomiting, recurrent abdominal pains, recurrent headaches, dizzy spells, periodic attacks of fever and periodic limb and joint pains.

Recurrent central abdominal pains (abdominal migraine) occur in one of 10 children of school age [1]. Frequent associated symptoms are pallor, vomiting and headaches. Abdominal migraine has to be separated from recurring appendicitis, mesenteric enteritis, Meckel's diverticulum and school phobia. It is indistinguishable from the 'irritable bowel syndrome' which is largely provoked by foods [26] (see Chapter 32). Carbohydrate intolerance (enzyme deficiency) or protein intolerance (allergy) may be causatively involved, although often an infant may be both protein and carbohydrate intolerant [48]. It is perhaps not surprising that patients with the irritable bowel syndrome often have recurrent headaches (Hunter, personal communication).

The features of the periodic syndrome are reminiscent of juvenile migraine and, indeed, follow-up studies have shown that the incidence of later migraine and/or psychiatric disorders is considerably higher compared to control groups [22].

THERAPY

The aim of therapy is to interrupt a step in the pathogenesis of migraine. The measures consist of: reassurance, pharmacotherapy, behavioural modification, acupuncture and diet.

Reassurance

In double-blind studies of treatment of patients with migraine, 20-30%, and occa-

sionally more, responded to administered placebo. Reassurance of the benign nature of the
recurring syndrome may be all that is necessary, especially if the headaches are mild and
infrequent. Reassurance should be combined
with general advice about lifestyle, including
avoidance of trigger factors (Table 38a.5).

Pharmacotherapy

If the headaches are severe but infrequent
(<3 to 4 times per month) treatment may be
focused on the individual attacks and aspirin
is the first thing to try [31]. If the headaches
are of sufficient frequency (>3 times per
month) daily prophylactic pharmacotherapy
may be the treatment of choice. Derivatives of
ergot have a long history of successful use in
the treatment of migraine [17], but the risk of
side-effects such as retroperitoneal fibroplasia
[21], thrombophlebitis [8] and possibly stroke
due to the additional vasoconstriction have
to be considered. Propranolol, clonidine and
pizotifen have all been reported to be effective, but double-blind placebo-controlled
studies showed that in children the effect was
not superior to placebo [14,19,41]. A number
of other drugs have been reported to be effective [2].

Behavioural treatment

Behavioural modification techniques have become increasingly popular and useful for the
management of migraine as well as psychogenic headaches. The development of relaxation skills and the recognition of environmental influences are the basic issues and the
components of treatment involve training in
meditative relaxation, electromyographic biofeedback and assessment of headache occurrence [32].

Acupuncture

Acupuncture can remove headaches of organic
origin, at least temporarily. Its usefulness was
assessed by Loh et al [30] who undertook a
trial of acupuncture versus medical treatment
in 48 patients with severe migraine and other
types of headaches. A larger proportion preferred acupuncture to medical treatment. A
beneficial response to acupuncture was more
likely when the patient had local tender muscular points. The technique of acupuncture is
painful for the patient and time-consuming for
the doctor. Another disadvantage is that the

majority of patients need to come back for
more treatment at intervals of 2-6 months.
However, it is a safe and cheap method and its
use is undoubtedly justified in adults, but
children do not accept it easily because it is
painful.

DIET

Although the production and marketing of
headache remedies involves a major proportion of the modern pharmaceutical industry,
their value in childhood migraine is limited
[10,14,19,41] and in many cases their safety
is in question. Acupuncture is difficult to
adopt in children and often works only as long
as it is applied regularly [30]. Apart from behaviour modification programmes, whose
effects have as yet to be established by controlled trials, dietary treatment is a logical
approach to view of the evidence that food
intolerance is responsible for much migraine
(see Chapter 37). Publications concerning the
relationship between migraine and dietary factors can be separated into two major groups:
tyramine hypothesis, and food allergy hypothesis.

Tyramine hypothesis

Hannington [23] reported that foods containing tyramine, a vasoactive amine, may precipitate headaches, particularly in patients
who are treated with monoamine oxidase inhibitors (Table 38a.6). Foods rich in tyramine
include cheese, pickled herring, chicken
livers, canned figs and the pods of broad
beans. Other vasoactive amines too were suspected to cause migraine such as phenylethylamine present in chocolate and 5-hydroxy-
tryptamine present in bananas, pineapple
and tomatoes. A defect in the conjugation
of tyramine and phenylethylamine has been
incriminated by some authors [38] and others
proposed a deficiency of platelet phenolsulphotransferase [29]. However, these enzymes were
found to be reduced only during migraine
attacks and therefore seem to represent an
effect rather than the cause of migraine. Moreover, double-blind administration of tyramine
to patients who benefited from a low tyramine
diet did not provoke migraine [10].

Food allergy hypothesis

A role for food allergy in migraine has been
postulated since the second half of the last cen-

tury (for review see Chapter 37), and oral sodium cromoglycate was found to have a protective effect in some patients [12, 33]. The value of an oligoantigenic diet was demonstrated by a double-blind, placebo-controlled cross-over trial [12] where 93% of children with severe and frequent migraine (>once per week) were shown to benefit.

During the sequential reintroduction of food at weekly intervals, 90% of the responders relapsed with one or more foods (Tables 38a.7, 38a.8 and 38a.9) and recovered

Table 38a.7 Provoking foods in 88 patients treated by diet.

Food	Tested	Symptoms	%
Cow's milk	75	29	39
Chocolate	64	24	37
Benzoic acid	46	17	37
Eggs	71	26	36
Tartrazine	45	15	33
Wheat	71	22	31
Cheese	48	15	31
Citrus	72	22	30
Coffee	21	5	24
Fish	51	11	22
Maize	53	9	17
Grapes	23	4	17
Goat's milk	44	7	16
Tea	44	7	16
Pork	60	8	13
Beef	64	8	12
Beans	42	9	12
Malt	33	3	9
Lentils	21	2	9
Apples	74	6	8
Yeast	54	4	7
Pears	69	4	6
Apricots	48	3	6
Sugar	56	3	5
Potatoes	78	4	5
Peas	37	2	5
Banana	78	4	5
Carrots	76	3	4
Chicken	73	3	4
Peaches	51	2	4
Lamb	75	2	3
Rice	75	1	1
Brassica	76	1	1

again avoiding them. The interval between eating a provoking food and migraine varied between different patients and between different foods in the same patient (Table 38a.10). Forty-six children in whom a provoking food was identified entered a double-blind placebo-controlled cross-over trial of the provoking food and highly significantly more patients had headaches with active material ($P < 0.001$) than with placebo (Table 38a.11).

Table 38a.8 Results of specific food challenge in those of the 76 patients who reacted to antigenically related material.

Food	Tested	Symptoms
Reacted to cow's milk		
Soya	16	11
Sheep's milk	2	0
Pregestamil	1	0
Reacted to cow's cheese		
Sheep's cheese	3	0
Reacted to wheat		
Rye	27	12
Oats	22	8

Table 38a.9 Number of provoking foods in individual patients.

Patients	Foods
8	0
17	1
14	2
16	3
8	4
2	5
2	6
2	8
2	10
2	11
2	12
1	13
1	14
1	16
1	22
1	24

Table 38a.10 Intervals between eating the provoking food and symptoms.

<1 day	63 times
2 days	56 times
3 days	51 times
4 days	14 times
5 days	8 times
6 days	1 times
>7 days	14 times

Table 38a.11 Double-blind placebo-controlled cross-over trial: occurrence of headaches.

	AP	PA	Total
Neither food	2	6	8
Active food	14	12	26*
Placebo	0	2	2
Both foods	1	3	4
Total	17	23	40

* Difference between active and placebo; $P < 0.001$.
Data from Egger et al [12], with permission.

The oligoantigenic approach

Patients with migraine are not usually aware of foods that provoke migraine. Moreover, causative foods are as a rule favourite ones. Unfortunately, skin prick tests and other laboratory tests are not helpful in identifying provoking foods [12] and at present the only method of sorting them out is an oligantigenic diet, followed by sequential reintroduction of foods (see Chapter 38b for a discussion of the oligoantigenic approach in the hyperkinetic syndrome).

Who should be treated by diet?

Oligoantigenic diets are very demanding and potentially dangerous from the point of view of malnutrition [43] and anaphylaxis when foods are reintroduced [11]. Therefore only patients with severe and frequent attacks of migraine should be considered for such treatment. The patients reported in our trial [12] were selected because they had migraine at least once a week. Oligoantigenic diets should not be attempted in patients with fewer headaches, because the diet would be worse than the disease and because it would not be possible to gauge the progress.

Patients with migraine attacks at least four times a month should be considered for prophylactic pharmacotherapy. However, such treatment does not lead to improvement or recovery in 90%. Rotation diets (diets in which major items are eliminated one or two at a time) are sometimes used in patients with fewer attacks of migraine but their effect has yet to be studied.

Diet and associated symptoms

Migraine often affects other organs apart from the brain, causing a number of symptoms (Table 38a.12). Patients with and without such associated symptoms respond equally well to oligoantigenic diets [12] and usually the associated symptoms too resolve.

The incidence of gastrointestinal symptoms (nausea, abdominal pain, flatulence, vomiting and diarrhoea) is given as ranging from 70% to 100% in a compilation of eight reported series [35]. When provoking foods are given, abdominal symptoms usually recur first (the allergic reaction may therefore occur in the gut, and the other manifestations may result from released mediators or from circulating antigen or antigen–antibody complexes).

Table 38a.12 Associated symptoms and signs.

	Patients completing oligoantigenic diet ($n = 88$)	
	Before diet	On diet
Abdominal symptoms	61	8
Behaviour disorder	41	5
Aches in limbs	41	7
Rhinitis	34	15
Recurrent mouth ulcers	15	2
Epilepsy	14	2
Vaginal discharge	11	1
Enuresis	8	2
Asthma	7	3
Eczema	6	3

Other symptoms. Periodic limb pain of considerable severity [47], myalgia [42] and somnolence and lassitude alternating with irritability and restlessness are common complaints and enuresis nocturna [13], epilepsy [39] and fevers without infection [47] occur more frequently in a migraine population than one would expect. Although asthma and eczema may improve on diet, the frequency of atopy is not increased in migraineurs [12].

History of associated symptoms

A history of associated symptoms is not always given spontaneously by the patients, perhaps because they are mainly worried about the headaches, and only careful questioning will reveal the presence of other symptoms. Sometimes different symptoms are provoked by different foods in the same patient.

Diet and non-specific triggers

Rarely the expression of migraine only occurs with specific precipitating factors. More commonly, most migraine episodes are apparently spontaneous, and only occasionally may an identified trigger be responsible for an attack (Table 38a.5). In either circumstance recognition of such factors is of value because some of them can be avoided. Recognized trigger factors, however, fail to provoke migraine in patients who are on appropriate diets (Table 38a.13), which is important in migraine provoked by changes of climate or by other factors which cannot be avoided. On diet, only cigarette smoke, pollens, perfumes and other inhalants continue to trigger attacks of migraine which would suggest a causative role of inhaled antigens too.

Table 38a.13 Non-specific provokers of migraine in 38 patients.

	Before diet	On diet
Exercise	13	1
Trauma	11	1
Emotional	10	0
Perfumes, or cigarette smoke	10	9
Travel	9	0
Bright light	5	0
Heat	2	1
Noise	2	0

Data from Egger et al [12], with permission.

SUMMARY

Migraine is a common and sometimes disabling disorder in childhood. A number of factors are known to provoke migraine, but the mechanisms are not understood. Foods and synthetic additives can provoke migraine; more than 90% of children with severe and frequent attacks of migraine recover or improve on oligoantigenic diets. Provoking foods can be identified by elimination followed by sequential reintroduction.

All types of migraine as well as the associated symptoms may respond to diet. Other recognized trigger factors lose importance once provoking foods are avoided. Future work has to concentrate on the development of useful in vitro tests, by which provoking foods can be identified.

REFERENCES

1 Apley J, Naish N: Recurrent abdominal pains: a field survey of 1000 school children. Arch Dis Child 1958; 33:165–70.

2 Barlow CF: Headaches and migraine in childhood. Oxford: Blackwell Scientific Publications, Philadelphia: JB Lippincott, 1984.

3 Bickerstaff ER: Basilar artery migraine, Lancet 1961; i:15–17.

4 Bille B: Migraine in schoolchildren. Acta Paediatr [Suppl] 1962; 51:136–51.

5 Blau JN, Whitty CWM: Familial hemiplegic migraine. Lancet 1965; ii:1115–16.

6 Bousson MG, Baron JC, Chiras J: Ischaemic strokes and migraine. Neuroradiology 1985; 27:583.

7 Bruyn GW: Epidemiology of migraine: a personal view. Headache 1983; 23:127–33.

8 Carter ER: Bilateral thrombophlebitis after a single dose of ergotamine tartrate for migraine. Br Med J 1958; ii:1453.

9 Clarke JM: On recurrent motor paralysis in migraine, with a report in which recurrent hemiplegia accompanied the attacks. Br Med J 1910; i:1534–8.

10 Congdon PJ, Forsythe WI: Migraine in childhood: a study of 300 children. Dev Med Child Neurol 1979; 21:209–16.

11 David DJ: Anaphylactic shock during elimination diets for severe atopic eczema. Arch Dis Child 1984; 59:983–6.

12 Egger J. Carter CM, Wilson J et al: Is migraine food allergy? A double-blind controlled trial of oligoantigenic diet treatment. Lancet 1983; ii:865–9.

13 Filipowics A: Migraine in children with functional nocturnal enuresis—a long-term prospective study of 32 cases. Cephalalgia [Suppl]1985; 5:186.

14 Forsythe WI, Gilles D, Sills MA: Propranolol (inderal) in the treatment of childhood migraine. Dev Med Child Neurol 1984; 26:737–41.

15 Friedman AP, Merritt HH: Treatment of headache. J Am Med Assoc 1957; 163:1111.

16 Friedman AP, Harter DH, Merrit HH: Ophthalmoplegic migraine. Arch Neurol 1962; 7:320–7.

17 Friedman AP, Finley KH, Graham JR et al: Classification of headache. Arch Neurol 1962; 6:173–6.

18 Gascon G, Barlow CF: Juvenile migraine presenting as an acute confusional state. Pediatrics 1970; 45:628–35.

19 Gillies D, Sills M, Forsythe J: Pizotifen (Sanomigran) in childhood migraine. A double-blind controlled trial. Eur Neurol 1986; 25:32–5.

20 Glista GG, Mellinger JF, Rooke ED: Familial hemiplegic migraine. Mayo Clin Proc 1975; 50:307–11.

21 Graham JR, Suby HI, LeCompte PR, Sadovsky NL: Fibrotic disorders associated with methysergide therapy for headache. N Engl J Med 1966; 274:359–68.

22 Hammond J: The late sequelae of recurrent vomiting of childhood. Dev Med Child Neurol 1974; 16:15–22.

23 Hannington E: Preliminary report on tyramine headache. Br Med J 1967; ii:550–1.

24 Harris W: The facial neuralgias. London: Oxford Medical Publications, 1937.

25 Hilton BP, Cumings JM: 5-Hydroxytryptamine levels and platelet aggregation responses in subjects with acute migraine headache. J Neurol Neurosurg Psychiatry 1972; 35:505–9.

26 Jones A, McLaughlan P, Shorthouse M et al: Food intolerance: a major factor in the pathogenesis of irritable bowel syndrome. Lancet 1982; ii:1115–17.

27 Lance JW, Anthony M: Some clinical aspects of migraine. Arch Neurol 1966; 15:356–61.

28 Leviton A: Epidemiology of headache. Adv Neurol 1978; 19:341–51.

29 Littlewood J, Glover V, Sandler M: Platelet phenolsulphotransferase deficiency in dietary migraine. Lancet 1982; ii: 983–6.

30 Loh L, Nathan PW, Schott GD, Zilkha KJ: Acupuncture versus medical treatment for migraine and muscle tension headaches. J Neurol Neurosurg Psychiatry 1984; 47:333–7.

31 Majerus PW: Why aspirin? Circulation 1976; 54: 357–9.

32 Masek B, Russo DC, Varni JF: Behavioral approaches to the management of chronic pain in children. Pediatr Clin North Am 1984; 31:1113–32.

33 Monro J, Carini C, Brostoff J: Migraine is a food-allergic disease. Lancet 1984; ii:719–21.

34 Moretti G, Manzoni GC, Caffarra P, Parma M: Benign recurrent vertigo and its connection with migraine. Headache 1980; 20:344–6.

35 Prensky AL: Migraine and migrainous variants in pediatric patients. Pediatr Clin North Am 1976; 23:461–71.

36 Rossi LN, Vasella F, Bajc O et al: Benign migraine-like syndrome with CSF pleocytosis in children. Dev Med Child Neurol 1985; 27:192–8.

37 Salmon MA, Wilson J: Drugs for alternating hemiplegic migraine. Lancet 1984; ii:980.

38 Sandler MMBH, Hannington E: A phenyethyamine oxidizing defect in migraine. Nature 1974; 250:335.

39 Seshia SS, Reggin JD, Stanwick RS: Migraine and complex seizures in children. Epilepsia 1985; 26:232–6.

40 Sillanpää M: Changes in the prevalence of migraine and other headache during the first seven school years. Headache 1983; 23:15–19.

41 Sills M, Congdon P, Forsythe WI: Clonidine and childhood migraine. A pilot and double-blind study. Dev Med Child Neurol 1982; 24:837–41.

42 Simons DJE, Day E, Goodell H, Wolff HG: Experimental studies on headache: muscles of the scalp and neck as sources of pain. Assoc Res Nerv Dis Proc 1943; 23:228–44.

43 Tripp JH, Francis DE, Knight JA, Harries JT: Infant feeding practice: a cause for concern. Br Med J 1979; ii:707–9.

44 Vahlquist B: Migraine in children. Int Arch Allergy 1955; 7:348–55.

45 Walker-Smith JA: Cows milk intolerance as a cause of post-enteritic diarrhoea. J Pediatr Gastroenterol Nutr 1982; 1:163–75.

46 Warner JO, Hathaway MK: Allergic form of Meadow's syndrome (Münchhausen by proxy). Arch Dis Child 1984; 59:151–6.

47 Wyllie WG, Schlesinger B: The periodic group of disorders in childhood. Br J Child Dis 1933; 30:1–21.

Chapter 38b
The Hyperkinetic Syndrome

Joseph Egger

Introduction

The first recorded description of a hyperactive child that we know about was in a poem written in 1844 by a German physician named Hoffmann. The poem includes the following lines [28]:

> ... But Fidgety Phil,
> He won't sit still,
> He wiggles and giggles,
> And then, I declare,
> Swings backwards and forwards,
> And tilts up his chair,
> Just as a rocking-horse—
> 'Philip! I am getting cross!'
> See the naughty, restless child,
> Growing still more rude and wild,
> Till his chair falls over quite,
> Philip screams with all his might ...

This poem encapsulates in a colourful style the kind of child who is the subject of this chapter. The typical child with the hyperkinetic syndrome is generally brought to professional attention early in his elementary school years. However, careful questioning usually reveals symptoms present from early childhood. The clinical picture is that of overactivity, impulsivity, distractability and excitability [8]. Aggressive and antisocial be-

haviour, specific learning problems and emotional lability are often considered part of the syndrome [40]. However, careful clinical studies reveal that only a small but significant minority of hyperkinetic children present with antisocial behaviour when initially seen [52, 60]. Since antisocial behaviour is seen more frequently in older hyperkinetic children it may develop as a secondary reaction.

Comparison with conduct disorder

Hyperkinetic behaviour has to be distinguished from conduct disorder. This is a diagnostic category for children who are rebellious, defiant, cruel, bullying, aggressive, frequently fighting, disobedient and who also lie and steal. However, it is claimed that 75% of hyperkinetic children are antisocial and that about 40% of conduct-disordered children are hyperactive [8, 50].

Two-thirds of overactive children are reported by their parents to be underachieving at school and up to a half are rated as below average in school by their teachers [51]. Learning difficulties are evident not only in reading disability but also in spelling, language and conceptual areas and in mathematical skills. Attentional deficits are common in hyperkinetic children, consisting of distractability, poor concentration, short interest span and a flitting disorganized approach to task demands. These problems present particular difficulties in the classroom and contribute to the child's frequent learning delays.

Normal activity

We lack a standard of what is a normal level of activity on which to base comparisons. Activity measures such as actometers, wiggle chairs and stabilometric cushions have been largely unsuccessful since overactive and normal children do not differ greatly on such measures [4].

The same applies for other cardinal symptoms; there are no measurements of impulsivity and attention. Because of the frequency of attention deficits in overactive children many authors prefer the term attention deficit syndrome and distinguish attention deficits with and without overactivity. However, attention deficits do not as yet have any precise definition; the term is as broad as hyperactivity itself and equally heterogeneous, and not all overactive children have attention deficits.

Thus far, reliable and valid tests of overactivity are not possible. Moreover, the overactive child may behave quite reasonably in the clinician's room especially at the first visit. For practical purposes behaviour rating scales are used such as that of Conners [13], and classification is by the criteria of the *Diagnostic and Statistical Manual* [1] (Table 38b.1).

Prevalence

Prevalence estimations of the hyperkinetic syndrome range from 1.2% to 20% [6, 30, 31, 61] of all school children. There are more boys with diagnosed overactivity than girls with male to female ratios ranging from 4:1 to 6:1. However, the results of a recent study [5] suggest that girls with the syndrome may be underidentified because cognitive deficits have a more prominent role in girls whereas behavioural disturbances are more often seen in boys.

Follow-up studies have shown that the difficulties first evident in early childhood all too often have sequelae that persist into adult life. Overactivity per se diminishes with age [37, 38, 60], but psychotic and criminal behaviour often become major problems [36].

AETIOLOGY

Many causes of overactivity have been proposed (Table 38b.2). The simplistic equation of 'hyperactivity equals brain damage' has to be rejected as there is no evidence for it. Moreover overactivity does not seem to represent a single disease entity; 92 terms have been used to describe hyperactive children [55] reflecting a number of diagnostically distinctive subgroups. Less than 5% of hyperactive children show any signs of neurological impairment [48] and the presence of soft neurological signs such as deficiencies in motor coordination, reflex asymmetries, mild visual,

Table 38b.1 Conners' abbreviated rating scales.

Observation	Degree of activity			
	Not at all	Just a little	Pretty much	Very much
Restless or overactive				
Excitable, impulsive				
Disturbs other children				
Fails to finish things				
Short attention span				
Constantly fidgeting				
Inattentive, easily distracted				
Demands must be met immediately				
Easily frustrated				
Cries often and easily				
Mood changes quickly and drastically				
Temper outbursts				
Explosive and unpredictable behaviour				
Scoring:	0	1	2	3

Score > 15 Hyperactivity likely.

Table 38b.2 Suspected causes of overactivity.

Inherited hyperkinetic syndrome
Adverse psychosocial situations
Brain damage
Brain dysfunction
Epilepsy
Anticonvulsants
Lead poisoning
Maternal smoking and alcohol intake during pregnancy
Atopy
Sensitivity to salicylates and synthetic food additives
Food allergy

hearing or language impairment, general clumsiness, right–left discrimination difficulties, choreiform jerks and athetoid movements in some of the children with overactive behaviour do not justify the term 'minimal brain dysfunction' for all.

Family studies

A number of studies suggest a genetic link. There is a 100% concordance rate for the hyperkinetic syndrome in monozygotic twins [33] and a 50% concordance rate in full siblings compared to 14% in half sibs [49] and there was no increased prevalence for psychiatric illness or the hyperkinetic syndrome in the non-biological relatives of adopted hyperkinetic children [8]. Few of the studies have been able to disentangle genetic from environmental influences such as family problems [12] or problems at school [3], lead poisoning [27], maternal smoking and alcohol intake [2].

Effect of diet

Feingold reported that 70% of overactive children responded to a diet avoiding colourings, preservatives and salicylates [24], but controlled studies did not show such an effect [14, 26, 56, 57, 59, 62].

Randolph [44] proposed that any food could cause the trouble and this hypothesis was supported by a double-blind placebo-controlled cross-over trial [20].

The latter part of this chapter presents detailed outlines of the principles and practice of dietary therapy for hyperactive children.

THERAPY

Hyperactivity is not just a chemical defect that needs the right pill to correct it. A number of treatments have been used of which psycho-stimulant drugs, behavioural approaches and diet changes are the commonest.

Psychostimulant drugs

The major stimulant drugs are the amphetamines (e.g. amphetamine sulphate (Benzedrine); dexamphetamine sulphate (Dexedrine)) and methylphenidate (Ritalin). The beneficial effects are increased alertness and control of attentional processes and decreased socially inappropriate behaviour. Negative side-effects include insomnia, appetite suppression, increased heart rate, abdominal pain, weight loss, growth suppression, headaches and personality and mood changes [3]. Moreover, while there is agreement that stimulant medication may have positive effects on some aspects of the behaviour in the short term, the picture is disappointing in the long term. Medicated children show no long-term benefits in either social or academic areas [11] and, although drug treatment may increase the time spent focussing on a task, it does not necessarily improve task performance [25].

Behavioural approaches

A wide variety of target behaviours, settings and programmes have been used [34]. These aim at reduction of excess behaviours and of disruptive antisocial behaviour, together with increases in desirable behaviour such as improved on-task attention, more adaptive cognitive strategies and enhanced academic achievement [17]. These needs derive from the multifaceted nature of hyperactivity, which involves the difficulties children experience in dealing with their environment and the difficulties parents and teachers experience with the children's behaviour [43].

While there is little agreement that behavioural methods can be effective in modifying problem behaviour in the short term, there is no evidence of a long-term effect. In addition, behavioural therapy requires a high degree of consistent, sustained and often dedicated effort on the part of teachers and parents [43] and sometimes parents have so many adjustment difficulties of their own that they would not make good candidates for a successful behavioural programme [39].

Diet

Concern about the undesirable effects of drug treatment as well as the mounting evidence for the lack of long-term efficacy of both drug treatment and of behavioural methods has led to a focus on diets as treatment. Publications concerning the relationship between the hyperkinetic syndrome and food allergy can be broadly separated into two major groups: Feingold's hypothesis, and the food allergy hypothesis.

THE FEINGOLD HYPOTHESIS

In June 1973 a preliminary report was presented by Feingold in which it was proposed that hyperkinesis in childhood is associated with the ingestion of salicylates, of compounds which cross-react with salicylates and with common food additives such as artificial flavours and colours. Feingold noted that an adult patient with aspirin sensitivity showed remission of psychiatric disturbances when placed on a diet free of natural salicylates, food colours and artificial flavours. Because of the supposed cross-reactivity of salicylates and dyes, Feingold treated hyperactive children with a diet free of so-called natural salicylates and all artificial colours and flavours and claimed success in 70% of them [24].

Criticisms

A number of criticisms were immediately raised against his claims, and indeed his findings were impressionistic, anecdotal and lacking in objective evidence. Included among the criticisms were that the patients reported were not described by any standard methods, no controls were utilized, no objective measures of change were employed, the observer of change was not blind to the treatment being evaluated and alternative explanations based on commonly accepted placebo phenomena were not considered.

Double-blind trials

Subsequently a number of double-blind trials involving control diets and diets eliminating artificial colours, flavours and natural salicylates were conducted on children with well-defined hyperkinetic syndrome. Two groups of psychologists, Conners et al [14] and Harley et al [26], each carried out a similar investigation in which they carefully studied hyperactive children for a baseline period of 1 month before the children were placed on special diets. The children had several types

of psychological and other tests to determine their usual behaviour. They were then randomly and alternately placed on either the Feingold diet for 1 month or on a control diet which seemed equally difficult. After each diet, psychological tests and evaluations were repeated.

Results: Study 1. In Conner's study, both parents and teachers agreed that the Feingold diet reduced the children's activity compared to the baseline period. The teachers noted a few children who had highly significant reductions of symptoms on the Feingold diet but not on the control diet. The control diet ratings did not differ from the baseline period ratings for either parents or teachers.

It was concluded that there may be a small subgroup of hyperkinetic children who might benefit from the Feingold diet, although the final results were inconclusive partly because the few hyperactive children who improved were generally the ones who received the Feingold diet after the placebo diet.

Results: Study 2. In another study of Feingold's hypothesis [62] 26 children were randomly assigned to treatment conditions whereby they were given active or placebo medications in combination with challenge biscuits with artificial food colours or control biscuits without the additives. The children were crossed over into each of the four treatment conditions and double-blind assessments and behaviour checklists were completed by teachers and parents. Although stimulant medications were more effective than diet in reducing hyperactive behaviour, both parent and teacher ratings indicated that there was some reduction in symptoms in one-quarter of the children who received the Feingold diet.

Results: Study 3. Harley et al [26] studied 36 school-age hyperactive boys and 10 hyperactive preschool boys under experimental and control diet conditions. Parental ratings revealed positive behaviour changes for the experimental diet, but teacher ratings, objective classroom and laboratory observational data, attention–concentration and psychological measures yielded no support for Feingold's hypothesis.

Results: Study 4. Swanson et al [56] studied 40 children for 5 days on a diet free of artificial food dyes and other additives. Twenty of the children were hyperactive and the behaviour of the other 20 was normal. Oral challenges with large doses (100–150 mg) of synthetic food dyes or placebo were administered on days 4 and 5 of the experiment. The performance of the hyperactive children on paired associate learning tests on the day they received the colours was impaired relative to their performance after they received the placebo ($P < 0.01$). The performance of the non-hyperactive group was not affected by the challenge with the food dyes. The Conner's rating scale was also filled out twice daily, but no difference between the dye and placebo conditions was manifested on this measure of social behaviour.

Results: Study 5. Weiss et al [59] challenged 22 children, maintained on a diet excluding certain foods, with a blend of seven artificial colours in a double-blind placebo-controlled cross-over trial. Parents' observations provided the criteria of response. One child reacted mildly to the challenge and another one reacted dramatically. The doses of synthetic additives employed in this study were about 50 times lower than the maximum allowable daily intakes recommended by the Food and Drug Administration. The challenge was given once on each of 8 days randomly distributed among weeks 3 through 10 of the study period. It was concluded that Feingold's diet was effective in a small subgroup of hyperactive children.

Results: Study 6. In another study of Feingold's hypothesis [57] 10 institutionalized children were maintained on an additive-free diet for 2 weeks, followed by 2 weeks in which two high, consecutive doses of artificial food colours were administered orally in a placebo-masked, double-blind experimental design. For the three psychometric measures examined (Porteus mazes, paired-associate learning test, and actometer readings) the trend was in the direction hypothesized, i.e. group scores deteriorated under colour challenge. However, the results failed to reach statistical significance. The teachers' ratings changed in the opposite direction to that predicted. However, as with the psychometric tests, the behavioural rating measures did not reach statistical significance.

Conclusion

The results of the controlled studies of Feingold's hypothesis are all somewhat equivocal,

but the broad conclusions were that his claims were probably exaggerated. The reason for the uncertainty was the lack of comparability between studies because of the heterogeneity of subject groups used, differences in dietary manipulations and additive substances given and the diversity of dependent variables employed. Overriding all these problems were inadequate research designs; Conners et al [14] and Harley et al [28] used a control diet whose effects on behaviour were not studied before. Williams et al [62], Harley et al [28], Swanson and Kinsbourne [56], Weiss et al [59] and Thorley [57] did not insert washout periods in between the test periods, which were probably disturbed by carry-over effects. Williams et al [62], Swanson and Kinsbourne [56] and Thorley [57] disguised the active and placebo ingredients in chocolate and sugar-containing materials, although it was known that these substances are likely to have adverse effects on behaviour. Swanson and Kinsbourne [56] and Weiss et al [59] administered the challenges only for 1 or 2 days, thus not allowing the symptoms to develop. However, all studies showed that some hyperactive children or certain subgroups of them may benefit from an additive-free diet.

THE FOOD ALLERGY HYPOTHESIS

A role for food allergy in the hyperkinetic syndrome has been postulated since early this century [15, 16, 29, 44, 45, 46, 54]. Because of the lack of scientific documentation, this hypothesis was rejected until the highly significant results of a double-blind placebo-controlled cross-over trial were published [20]. During a previous double-blind, controlled trial of the effect of diet on migraine, it was noted that any combination of foods could cause symptoms in children [21]. What was also of interest was that many responders had also been overactive and that their overactivity usually improved with food avoidance, in some instances with avoidance of foods other than those causing migraine. We therefore undertook a trial of diet in hyperkinetic children, and, in those who responded, provoking foods were identified by sequential reintroduction and tested in a double-blind cross-over trial.

Double-blind trial

Clinical characteristics. Seventy-six children took part in the experiment. All were socially handicapped by their behaviour, and overactivity and inattention were prominent features. The children were selected for severe overactivity and may not be representative of hyperkinetic children in the general population. A surprisingly high proportion had associated symptoms such as headaches, abdominal pains and seizures and only 10 did not have any such symptoms. The study was criticized for the selection method, because headaches and recurrent abdominal pains are not usually recognized as part of the hyperkinetic syndrome. However, only a few patients and parents gave a history of associated symptoms because they were troubled more by the behaviour problems and only careful questioning revealed the presence of these other symptoms.

Results. Of all the children, 82% responded to an oligoantigenic diet. However, only 27% recovered completely (Table 38b.3). Most of the

Table 38b.3 Changes in severity of symptoms of hyperactivity with diet.

	Total	No improvement	Improved	Recovered
Mild	6	1 (17%)	0 (0%)	5 (83%)
Moderate	31	5 (16%)	16 (52%)	10 (32%)
Severe	39	8 (21%)	25 (64%)	6 (15%)

No improvement = grade unchanged; improved = 1 or 2 grades less severe; recovered = requires normal management only.

associated symptoms also improved with diet (Table 38b.4). During the subsequent reintroduction the commonest substances that caused problems were tartrazine and benzoic acid but no child reacted to these alone. Forty-six other provocative foods were also identified (Table 38b.5) and most patients reacted to several (Table 38b.6). The interval between eating the provoking food and reaction varied from a few minutes to more than 7 days, but was usually 2–3 days. There was no difference between synthetic additives and foods.

Reintroduction of provoking food. Altogether 28 patients completed the double-blind placebo-controlled cross-over trial of the effect of reintroduction of a provoking food. The parents kept daily Conner's scores and a paediatrician and a psychologist independently made an assessment of the children's behaviour for each arm of the double-blind trial. At the end of the second period parents also recorded preference based on difference of symptoms. The psychologist employed actometer readings,

Table 38b.4 Clinical features of 76 children with the hyperkinetic syndrome.

Feature	Start of study	On diet
Number of subjects	76	76
Age (years, mean and range)	7.3 (2–15)	—
Sex (male/female)	60/16	—
Adverse psychosocial factors in the family	37	—
Overactivity		
Normal	0	21
Mild	6	28
Moderate	31	19
Severe	39	8
Mean Conners' score	24	12
Antisocial behaviour	32	13
Emotional difficulties	7	0
Severe mental retardation	6	
Specific developmental delay	10	
Headaches	48	9
Fits	14	1
Abdominal discomfort	54	8
Chronic rhinitis	33	9
Aches in limbs	33	6
Skin rashes (eczema, etc.)	28	9
Mouth ulcers	15	5
Atopy	30	—

matching familiar figures tests and the Porteus Maze test. Parents, the paediatrician and the psychologist assessed the period in which the placebo material was administered as being linked more often with better behaviour (Table 38b.7). There was no significant order

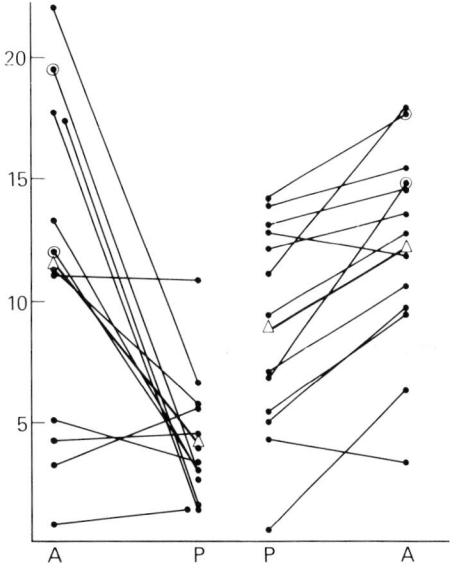

Fig. 38b.1 Mean Conners' abbreviated scale scores (closed circle) while patients were on placebo (P) and active (A) material. Means of each group are shown by open triangles. Those values which include assigned maximum scores for a part of the period, after withdrawal of the material because of severity of the symptoms are encircled. Reproduced with permission from the *Lancet* [20].

Table 38b.5 Reactions to foodstuffs.

Food	Number tested	Number reacted (%)	Food	Number tested	Number reacted
1 *Foods universally tested*			2 *Foods rarely‡ tested and positive*		
Colourant and preservatives	34	27 (79)	Plums	9	2
Soya*	15	11 (73)	Rabbit	6	3
Cow's milk	55	35 (64)	Sago	5	2
Chocolate	34	20 (59)	Duck	4	3
Grapes	18	9 (50)	3 *Foods tested*		
Wheat	53	28 (49)	*only in patients*		
Oranges	49	22 (45)	*who reacted to*		
Cow's cheese	15	6 (40)	*antigenically*		
Hen's eggs	50	20 (39)	*related foods*		
Peanuts	19	6 (32)	To cow's milk:		
Maize	38	11 (29)	Goat's milk	22	15
Fish	48	11 (23)	Ewe's milk	12	4
Oats	43	10 (23)	To wheat:		
Melons	29	6 (21)	Rye	29	15
Tomatoes	35	7 (20)	4 *Foods to which*		
Ham/bacon	20	4 (20)	*there was no*		
Pineapple	31	6 (19)	*reaction*		
Sugar†	55	9 (16)	Cabbages	54	
Beef	49	8 (16)	Lettuces	53	
Beans	34	5 (15)	Cauliflowers	50	
Peas	33	5 (15)	Celery	49	
Malt	20	3 (15)	Goat's cheese	4	
Apples	53	7 (13)	Duck eggs	2	
Pork	38	5 (13)			
Pears	41	5 (12)			
Chicken	56	6 (11)			
Potatoes	54	6 (11)			
Tea	19	2 (10)			
Coffee	10	1 (10)			
Other nuts	11	1 (10)			
Cucumbers	32	3 (9)			
Bananas	52	4 (8)			
Carrots	55	4 (7)			
Peaches	41	3 (7)			
Lamb	55	3 (5)			
Turkey	22	1 (5)			
Rice	51	2 (4)			
Yeast	28	1 (4)			
Apricots	34	1 (3)			
Onions	49	1 (2)			

* Given only to those who reacted to cow's milk.

† Five reacted to both beet and cane sugar, three to cane sugar only and one to beet sugar only. The parents of several other patients thought that large quantities of sugar provoked symptoms, without definite confirmation.

‡ Tested in < 10 patients.

effect. However, Conners' scales scored by the parents showed a significant but expected treatment order interaction (Fig. 38b.1).

Psychological tests. Except for the actometer readings, all the psychological tests showed a trend in favour of the placebo material. However, the differences between the active and placebo periods were not significant, possibly because they did not measure those skills most helped by dietary treatment or they were not sensitive enough to detect the deterioration induced by a brief challenge with a limited dose of the provoking food. The number of patients studied was also small.

The oligoantigenic approach

Lack of diagnostic tests

Questioning of the patient and parents to identify possible provoking foods is worthwhile,

Table 38b.6 Number of foods causing symptoms in the patients.

Number of foods	Number of patients
1	5
2	4
3	4
4	8
5	4
6	9
7	3
8	4
9	3
10	3
11	2
12	2
18	1
21	1
27	1
30	2

weeks. If improvement occurred this was followed by open sequential reintroduction of single foods. Response to a selected food was confirmed by double-blind food provocations where possible (Fig. 38b.2).

The oligoantigenic diet

All foods are potential allergens and an oligoantigenic diet should contain as few foods as possible. A typical oligoantigenic diet contains one meat, one carbohydrate source, a few vegetables (brassicas) and one fruit (Table 38b.8). Although the foods chosen may cause problems, they are less likely to do so than most others. Since adherence to such a strict and demanding diet is difficult, a modified oligoantigenic diet containing a greater variety of

Table 38b.7 Double-blind trial of assessment of behaviour in hyperactive children. Reproduced with permission from the *Lancet*.

	Overactivity									Any symptom		
	Paediatric neurologist			Parents			Psychologist			Parents		
	PA	AP	Both	PA	AP	Both	PA	AP	Both	PA	AP	Both
Behaviour better on:												
Neither	3	4	7	2	2	4	5	4	9	3	2	5
Placebo	12	8	20	13	10	23	7	6	13	12	11	23
Active	0	1	1	0	4	1	0	2	2	9	0	0
Total	15	13	28	15	13	28	12	12	24	15	13	28
P value												
PA *v.* AP		NS			NS			NS			NS	
A *v.* P		<0.001			<0.001			≃0.01			<0.001	

NS = not significant.

but most children and parents do not give such a history, and its presence or absence is not a good predictor of response to diet. Skin prick tests and IgE RASTS to food antigens are also unhelpful in this respect [21]. Identification of food antigens can be achieved by oligoantigenic diets and subsequent sequential reintroduction of foods [10].

This method was used to study the food allergy hypothesis of migraine and hyperkinetic behaviour (i.e. any food can cause the trouble). Each patient was first put on a very restricted oligoantigenic diet (few foods) for 4

Table 38b.8 Ideal oligoantigenic diet (A) and alternative oligoantigenic diet (B).

A	B
Turkey	Lamb
Cabbage, sprouts, cauliflower, broccoli	Carrots, parsnips
Potato, potato flour	Rice, rice flour
Banana	Pears
Soya oil, Tomor margarine	Sunflower oil
Water, salt	Water, salt
Calcium and vitamins	Calcium and vitamins

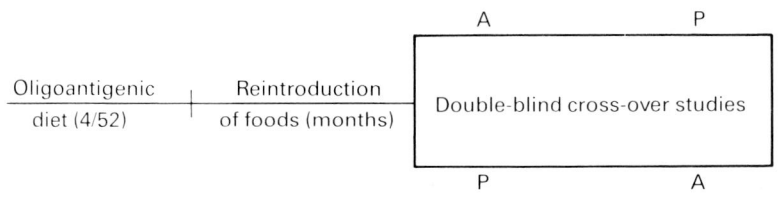

Fig. 38b.2 Method of the oligoantigenic approach to diagnosis of food-induced hyperactivity.

Table 38b.9 Modified oligoantigenic diet.

Meat	Include two meats, e.g. lamb and turkey. Also offal from these meats if liked
Carbohydrate	Rice, potatoes, arrowroot
Vegetables	Choose two of the following food families: Broccoli, cauliflower, cabbage, sprouts (brassicas) Carrots, parsnips, celery Cucumber, marrow, courgettes, melon Leeks, onions, asparagus
Fruit	Choose two of the following: apples, pears, bananas, peaches and apricots, pineapple
Fats	Milk-free margarine, e.g. Tomor—Van den Bergh (typical analysis, palm and palm kernel oil with soya or rape oils) Sunflower oil
Drinks	Pure fruit juice from included fruits, tap water, pure bottled water
Miscellaneous	Salt, pepper, pure herbs Plain potato crisps (preferably only one pack per day) Sugar and golden syrup and pure jam from included fruits Raising agents for baking A calcium (300 mg/day) and vitamin supplement is advisable: Calcium gluconate tablets (1 g) × 3 daily or calcium lactate tablets (300 mg) × 6 daily. Abidec (Parke Davis) 0.6 ml per day Avoid coloured toothpaste, medicines containing artificial colour and preservative and discourage chewing of chalks, etc.

foods was developed, including some more foods which had seldom provoked symptoms in the early patients (Table 38b.9). This diet can be altered to suit the individual. If medicines have to be given, preparations free of colours should be used.

Response to diet

If there is no improvement on the oligoantigenic diet it can be assumed that the patient is either intolerant to foods in the diet, or did not adhere to it or is not food intolerant. Unless adherence is suspect an alternative diet with no foods in common with the first can be tried (Table 38b.8).

Children are treated at home, since hospitals are not usually capable of providing a wide variety of meals from only a few foods.

Symptoms may worsen for a few days when the diet is started and some patients show withdrawal-like reactions. Improvement normally occurs during the second week, but may be seen almost immediately or only after 3 weeks.

Open sequential reintroduction of foods. If recovery or definite improvement occurs during the period of oligoantigenic diet, foods are reintroduced one by one at weekly intervals with the new food being given daily in normal quantities. If no adverse reaction occurs with the new food it is incorporated into the diet and the next food is introduced. If symptoms

occur with a certain food it is withdrawn and tested again at a later stage. After the child has recovered, another food is introduced. The order in which foods are introduced depends both on improving the nutritional adequacy and on the patients' preference (Table 38b.10). If alarming reactions such as anaphylaxis, angiodema or status epilepticus are expected with the reintroduction of certain foods the patient should be admitted to hospital for its reintroduction, which should begin with small quantities (e.g. 5 g).

Double-blind provocation. Diets have a powerful placebo effect, so double-blind provocations are a necessary step in most patients with suspected food allergy. This is also the only method to identify patients with the allergic Munchausen by proxy syndrome [58].

Concealing a food in the necessary quantities presents problems. It is mixed with other foods to which the patient is known not to react and whose flavour, smell and appearance will conceal the food to be tested. The disguising material is given as a placebo. For example, if cow's milk was a provoking food and the child could drink soya, goat's milk or sheep's milk without problems, blind cow's milk preparations could be made by mixing it with one of these [10]. Each active and placebo material should be given daily for at least 1 week with a washout period of at least a week in between.

Table 38b.10 Reintroduction of foods to diet of hyperactive children following oligoantigenic diet.

Chicken	Fresh or frozen chicken and chicken liver
Oats	Porridge oats, Scottish oatcakes, home-made flapjacks etc. if sugar is already allowed
Beef	Fresh or frozen beef, any cut or offal
Wheat	Wholemeal or unbleached white flour for baking, spaghetti and pasta (egg-free), shredded wheat, puffed wheat
Yeast	Give homemade wholemeal bread, or buy wholemeal bread from a local baker or health food shop after checking there is no soya or preservative Wholemeal pitta bread
Cow's milk	Pasteurized cow's milk. If no symptoms arise, cream, pure plain yoghurt, pale uncoloured butter may be given
Cow's milk substitute	If cow's milk is not tolerated, substitutes can be tried one by one, diluted ewe's milk if available or goat's milk (boiled or pasteurized), or soya milk, e.g. Cow and Gate S Formula, or bovine casein hydrolysate, e.g. Nutramigen (Mead Johnson). Non-dairy or imitation cream, e.g. Sainsbury's 2 oz diluted to 1 pint (this contains some additives and is not a nutritional substitute for milk but it is a good vehicle for breakfast cereal etc)
Eggs	Use whole fresh eggs e.g. 1 per day (a few who react will tolerate duck eggs)
Fish	Use fresh or frozen fish (not smoked, processed or battered etc) e.g. cod, herring. Try shellfish separately later
Orange	Pure natural unsweetened orange juice, oranges, satsumas etc. If oranges are tolerated all citrus fruit probably is too
Tomatoes	Fresh tomatoes, additive-free canned and puréed tomatoes, and additive-free ketchup, e.g. Heinz
Pork	Fresh or frozen pork, any cuts or offal
Sugar	Use ordinary sugar (brown or white) on cereal, in puddings, drinks and in baking etc. If sugar is not tolerated try cane and beet sugars separately. Tate and Lyle's sugar and syrup is of cane origin. Silver Spoon sugar and syrup is largely of beet origin but may contain some cane. If this is not tolerated try glucose, fructose or glucose polymer
Chocolate	Try only if sugar is tolerated. If diet is milk-free, use milk-free chocolate, e.g. Terry's Bitter Chocolate and plain continental chocolate, e.g. Côte d'Or. If milk is taken milk chocolate may be used. Cocoa powder may be used in cooking.
Peas and beans	These include peas, runner beans, kidney beans, lentils. Also additive-free backed beans in tomato sauce if tomatoes are tolerated, e.g. Heinz
Rye	This is particularly worth trying if wheat is not tolerated e.g. Ryvita—the original rye crispbread, or Ryking (blue pack)
Malt	Rice Krispies if rice is tolerated, Weetabix and Shreddies if wheat is tolerated
Corn	Sweetcorn, homemade popcorn, cornflour, maize flour, corn oil, cornflakes if malt is tolerated
White flour	Use white flour in cooking and for homemade white bread. White pitta bread (white flour contains a bleaching agent)
Soya and propionate preservative	Supermarket white bread contains both these. Its introduction tests for both, but a reaction necessitates distinguishing them
Tea	Add milk and sugar only if these are already in the diet
Coffee	
Colours and benzoic acid	Orange squash, e.g. Robinson's, usually contains tartrazine and benzoate preservative and can be tried if oranges and sugar are tolerated. Other items such as jelly, fruit gums, boiled fruit sweets etc contain colours but not benzoate preservative. Tartrazine and benzoic acid can also be tested using tartrazine or benzoic acid in capsules, e.g. 5 to 50 mg per day
Nitrites	These are preservatives in cooked or cured meats. Use ham and bacon if pork is tolerated, and corned beef if beef is tolerated.
Sodium glutamate	Use stock cubes, e.g. Knorr cubes, or gravy mixes, e.g. Gravy Mate made by Bovril Ltd. provided their other ingredients are tolerated
Peanuts	Use plain or salted peanuts and peanut butter
Other nuts	These may be tried singly or mixed as preferred, e.g. almonds, walnuts etc

Other foods, e.g. fruits and vegetables, and manufactured foods such as ice cream, biscuits etc can be introduced weekly taking into account avoidance of foods to which the patient is sensitive. If cereals or grains have to be avoided or restricted, buckwheat flour, wheatstarch, soya flour, grain (chickpea) flour and some of the special dietary products made for gluten-free and low protein diets may be tried but always check that the other ingredients are suitable for the individual.

At present the oligoantigenic approach is the only method of identifying provoking foods. The provoking foods are not usually the ones the patient dislikes or the ones expected to be responsible, but are often frequently eaten or even craved. Therefore if only foods suspected by the patient are avoided, no response to diet will be seen, this being clearly shown by such an experiment [42].

WHO SHOULD BE TREATED BY DIET?

Diets are socially disruptive, expensive and dangerous if not properly supervised, and are justified only in patients with severe disease. The patients selected for dietary treatment by Egger et al [20] were handicapped by their behaviour problems and made life difficult for families and schools; patients less severely affected are not suitable for the dietary approach.

Associated symptoms

Children with severe hyperkinetic behaviour often suffer from a number of associated symptoms (Table 38b.4) although these are rarely the presenting ones.

Fatigue. Fatigue or the feeling that the child is 'rundown' is often a major complaint. The parents are concerned about his sluggishness, drowsiness and lack of interest in both school-work and play, although most of the time the child is restless, impulsive and highly irritable. This combination of behaviour pattern was seen in one-third of severely hyperkinetic children [20].

Abdominal symptoms and headache. Recurrent abdominal pains and headaches are the most common associated symptoms. However, only a quarter of patients mentioned them spontaneously, whereas careful questioning revealed their presence in more than half. Some had been investigated previously by gastroenterologists and/or neurologists.

Less frequently seen but not uncommon are aching limbs, excessive thirst, enuresis and fever.

Most of these symptoms are relieved on oligoantigenic diets and can be reproduced with provoking foods. Sometimes the foods causing associated symptoms differ from those which cause hyperkinetic behaviour. Of the 76

patients reported by Egger et al [20], 66 had associated symptoms relieved and reproduced on several occasions by avoiding and reintroducing certain foods and only 10 were hyperkinetic alone. Of the latter, nine responded to diet.

Hyperactivity combined with other symptoms has been reported by a number of authors [16, 44, 45, 46, 54] but was not mentioned by others [5, 14, 26, 56, 57, 59, 62]. No indication is given by the latter authors as to whether the children gave such a history or simply did not have the symptoms. It is my experience that only a minority of severely hyperactive children do not have associated symptoms if a careful history is taken.

The combination of symptoms often would suggest an underlying psychosomatic illness. Despite such an association patients should not be excluded from a dietary experiment; it is possible that some so-called psychosomatic illnesses in fact are caused by food allergy and polysymptomatic patients responded to diet as well as those with single symptoms. [20]

Family pressures

There is impressive evidence in support of 'family system' influences in the development of child behaviour problems, in particular the negative effects of marital discord, and continuous negative parent–child interactions have been incriminated [12, 41]. Children in such unfavourable situations should not be regarded as unsuitable for dietary treatment since the disturbances within the family might have arisen from food allergy in other family members, as food allergy is familial. Of the 72 families reported by Egger et al [20] 35 had adverse psychosocial backgrounds. Although response to diet was less common in those families than in families not exposed to adverse psychosocial situations, such factors were present in more than 40% of the responders. Moreover some family members with psychosocial problems, who underwent dietary treatment together with the children reported relief of their symptoms. Others commented that the family life had improved simultaneously with the child's improvement.

PROGNOSIS

Some of our patients [20] ceased to react to provoking foods when they were tested again after about 1 year on the oligoantigenic diet.

Others realized that their child was no longer intolerant to a particular food after mistakes had been made in the diet with no ill-effects. On the other hand, foods previously shown not to cause problems sometimes started to provoke symptoms and this sometimes coincided with viral infections. The majority of children however continued to have problems when provoking foods were given.

Being on an acceptable diet did seem to make a remarkable difference to family life and schoolwork improved in a number of children. Many of the patients however continued to have some behavioural problems and needed alternative management in addition to the diet.

Growing out of hyperactivity?

Early investigators thought that the hyperkinetic syndrome was a time-limited condition which disappeared as the child grew older [22, 32]. It is now recognized that, although hyperactivity may diminish with age, antisocial behaviour, educational retardation, depression and psychosis are prevalent in grown-up hyperkinetic children [35, 36, 60]. It is too early to speculate whether dietary management will influence the prognosis of hyperkinetic children. However, there are reports suggesting that antisocial behaviour in young delinquents was often related to certain foods or food additives [53], and that schizophrenics on a milk- and cereal-free diet were released from hospital twice as fast as those given the regular hospital diet [18]. More recently Dohan et al [19] tested this hypothesis by comparing the incidence of schizophrenia in a New Guinea population that consumes little or no grain or milk with one that consumes grain but no milk. They found that schizophrenia is infrequent in tribal populations where grains and milk are rare and more frequent in similar populations that do consume grains but no milk.

Prospective studies of the effect of dietary management into adulthood are urgently needed and the reports on dietary treatment of antisocial behaviour and psychiatric disorder in adults must be tested by double-blind placebo-controlled trials.

SUMMARY

The hyperkinetic syndrome can be provoked by foods. There is no evidence as to which mechanism(s) is (are) involved, but the diversity of foods and the fact that children grow out of reactivity suggests allergy rather than idiosyncrasy. At present the only method of identifying provoking foods is an oligoantigenic diet followed by sequential reintroduction of foods. Food-allergic reactions may be immediate or slow (more than 7 days), therefore each food has to be tested for at least 1 week. Double-blind studies are essential, since diets have a powerful placebo effect. Only severe disease should be treated by diet and careful supervision by experienced doctors and dieticians is essential, because of the danger of malnutrition and the fact that diets are expensive and socially disruptive.

REFERENCES

1 American Psychiatric Association: Diagnostic and statistical manual of mental disorders. 3rd edn. Washington DC: American Psychiatric Association, 1980; 42-4.

2 Barkley RA: Hyperactive children: a handbook for diagnosis and treatment. New York: Guilford Press, 1981.

3 Barkley RA, Cunningham CE: Do stimulant drugs improve the academic performance of hyperkinetic children? A review of outcome studies. Clin Pediatr 1978; 17:85-92.

4 Barkley RA, Ullman DG: A comparison of objective measures of activity and distractibility in hyperactive and nonhyperactive children. J Abnorm Child Psychol 1975; 3:231-44.

5 Berry CA, Shaywitz SE, Shaywitz BA: Girls with attention deficit disorder: a silent minority? A report on behavioural and cognitive characteristics. Pediatrics 1985; 76:801-9.

6 Bosco JJ, Robin SS: Hyperkinesis: prevalence and treatment. In: Whalen C, Henker B, eds. Hyperactive children: the social ecology of identification and treatment. New York: Academic Press, 1980: 173.

7 Cantwell D: A critical review of therapeutic modalities with hyperactive children. In: Cantwell D, ed. The hyperactive child: diagnosis, management and current research. New York: Spectrum Publications, 1975.

8 Cantwell D: Genetic studies of hyperactive children: psychiatric illness in biologic and adopting parents. In: Fieve R, Rosenthal D, Brill H, eds. Genetic research in psychiatry. Baltimore: Johns Hopkins University Press, 1975.

9 Cantwell D: Hyperkinetic syndrome. In: Rutter M, Hersov L, eds. Child psychiatry: modern approaches. Oxford: Blackwell, 1976; 524-55.

10 Carter CM, Egger J, Soothill JF: A dietary management of severe childhood migraine. Hum Nutr Appl Nutr 1985; 39A: 294-303.

11 Charles L, Schain R: A four-year follow-up study of the effects of methylphenidate on the behavior and

academic achievement of hyperactive children. J Abnorm Child Psychol 1981; 9:495–505.

12 Christensen A, Phillips S, Glasgow R, Johnson S: Parental characteristics and interactional dysfunction in families with child behavior problems: a preliminary investigation. J Abnorm Child Psychol 1983; 11:153–66.

13 Conners CK: Rating scales for use in drug studies with children. Psychopharmacol Bull [Special Issue—Pharmacotherapy with children] 1973; 24–84.

14 Conners CK, Goyette CH, Southwick DA et al: Food additives and hyperkinesis: a controlled double-blind experiment. Pediatrics 1976; 58:154–66.

15 Cooke RA: Studies in specific hypersensitiveness. On the phenomenon of hyposensitization (the clinically lessened sensitiveness of allergy). J Immunol 1922; 7:219.

16 Crook WG, Harrison WW, Crawford SE, Emerson BS: Systemic manifestations due to allergy. Pediatrics 1961; 27:790–9.

17 Cunningham CE, Barkley RA: The role of academic failure in hyperactive behavior. J Learn Disabil 1978; 11:274–80.

18 Dohan FC, Grasberger FJ: Relapsed schizophrenics: earlier discharge from the hospital after cereal-free, milk-free diet. Am J Psychiatry 1973; 130:685–8.

19 Dohan FC, Harper EH, Clark MH et al: Is schizophrenia rare if grain is rare? Biol Psychiatry 1984; 19:385–99.

20 Egger J, Carter CM, Graham PJ et al: Controlled trial of oligoantigenic diet treatment in the hyperkinetic syndrome. Lancet 1985; i: 540–5.

21 Egger J, Carter CM, Wilson J et al: Is migraine food allergy? A double-blind controlled trial of oligoantigenic diet treatment. Lancet 1983; ii:865–9.

22 Eisenberg L: The management of the hyperkinetic child. Dev Med Child Neurol 1966; 8:593–8.

23 Feingold BP: Introduction to clinical allergy. Springfield, Illinois: Charles C Thomas, 1973.

24 Feingold BF: Hyperkinesis and learning disabilities linked to artificial food flavours and colors. Am J Nurs 1975; 75:797–803.

25 Flintoff MM, Barron RW, Swanson JM et al: Methylphenidate increases selectivity of visual scanning in children referred for hyperactivity. J Abnorm Child Psychol 1982; 10:145–63.

26 Harley JP, Ray RS, Tomasi L et al: Hyperkinesis and food additives: testing the Feingold hypothesis. Pediatrics 1978; 61:818–28.

27 Harvey PG: Lead and children's health: recent research and future questions. J Child Psychol Psychiatry 1984; 25:517–22.

28 Hoffmann H: Der Struwelpeter: oder lustige Geschichten und drollige Bilder. Leipzig: Insel Verlag, 1845.

29 Hoobler BR: Some early symptoms suggesting protein sensitization in infancy. Am J Dis Child 1916; 12:129.

30 Huessy H: Study of the prevalence and therapy of the choreatiform syndrome or hyperkinesis in rural Vermont. Acta Paedopsychiatr (Basel) 1967; 34:130–5.

31 Lambert NM, Sandoval J, Sassone D: Prevalence of hyperactivity in elementary school children as a function of social system definers. Am J Orthopsychiatry 1977; 48:446.

32 Laufer M, Denhoff E: Hyperkinetic behavior syndrome in children. J Pediatr 1957; 50:463–74.

33 Lopez R: Hyperactivity in twins. Can Psychiatr Assoc J 1965; 10:421–6.

34 Mash EJ, Dalby JT: Behavioral interventions for hyperactivity. In: Trites RL, ed. Hyperactivity in children: etiology, measurement and treatment implications. Baltimore: University Park Press, 1978.

35 Mendelson W, Johnson N, Stewart M: Hyperactive children as teenagers: a follow-up study. J Nerv Ment Dis 1971; 153:237–9.

36 Menkes MM, Rowe JS, Menkes JH: A twenty-five year follow-up study on the hyperkinetic child with minimal brain dysfunction. Pediatrics 1967; 39:393–9.

37 Minde K, Weiss G, Mendelson N: A five-year follow-up study of 91 hyperactive school children. J Am Acad Child Psychiatry 1972; 11:595–610.

38 Minde K, Weiss G, Lavigueuer H et al: The hyperactive child in elementary school: a 5 year, controlled follow-up. Except Child 1971; 38:215–22.

39 O'Leary K, O'Leary S: Classroom management: the successful use of behavior modification. 2nd edn. New York: Pergamon, 1977.

40 O'Malley JE, Eisenberg L: The hyperkinetic syndrome. Semin Psychiatry 1973; 5:5–17.

41 Patterson G, Jones R, Whittier J, Wright M: A behaviour modification technique for the hyperactive child. Behav Res Ther 1965; 2:217–26.

42 Pearson DJ, Rix KJB, Benley SJ: Food allergy: how much in the mind? Lancet 1983; i:1259–61.

43 Prior M, Griffin M: Hyperactivity. Diagnosis and management. London: William Heinemann Medical Books, 1965.

44 Randolph TG: Allergy as a causative factor of fatigue, irritability, and behavior problems of children. J Pediatr 1947; 31:560–72.

45 Rapp DJ: Allergies and the hyperactive child. Cornerstone Library, 1979.

46 Rowe AH: Allergic toxemia and fatigue. Ann Allergy 1950; 8:72.

47 Rutter ML: Relationships between child and adult psychiatric disorders. Acta Psychiatr Scand 1972: 48:3–21.

48 Rutter ML: Brain damage syndromes in childhood: concepts and findings. J Child Psychol Psychiatry 1977; 18:1–21.

49 Safer DJ: A familial factor in minimal brain dysfunction. Behav Genet 1973; 3:175–86.

50 Safer DJ, Allen RP: Hyperactive children: diagnosis and management. Baltimore, Maryland: University Park Press, 1976.

51 Sanson AV: Sub-classification of hyperactive children. Victoria, Australia: La Trobe University, 1984.

52 Satterfield JH, Hoppe CM, Schell AM: A prospective study of delinquency in 110 adolescent boys with attention deficit disorder and 88 normal adolescent boys. Am J Psychiatry 1982; 139:795–8.

53 Schoenthaler SJ: Diet and delinquency: a multi-state replication. Int J Biosoc Res 1983; 5:70–117.

54 Speer F: Allergy of the nervous system. Springfield, Illinois: Charles C Thomas, 1970.

55 Sulzbacher SJ: The learning-disabled or hyperactive child: diagnosis and treatment. J Am Med Assoc 1976; 234:939–41.

56 Swanson JM, Kinsbourne M: Food dyes impair performance of hyperactive children on a laboratory learning test. Science 1980; 207:1485–7.

57 Thorley G: Pilot study to assess behavioural and cognitive effects of artificial food colours in a group of retarded children. Dev Med Child Neurol 1984; 26:56–61.

58 Warner JO, Hathaway MJ: Allergic form of Meadow's syndrome (Munchausen by proxy). Arch Dis Child 1984; 59:151–6.

59 Weiss B, Williams JH, Margen S et al: Behavioral response to artificial food colors. Science 1980; 207:1487-9.

60 Weiss G, Minde K, Werry JS et al: Studies on the hyperactive child. VIII 5-year follow-up. Arch Gen Psychiatry 1971; 24:409-14.

61 Wender PH: Minimal brain dysfunction in children. New York: Wiley-Interscience, 1971.

62 Williams JJ, Cram DM, Tausig FT, Webster E: Relative effects of drugs and diet on hyperactive behaviors: an experimental study. Pediatrics 1978; 61:811-17.

Chapter 39
Psychological Effects of Food Allergy

D. J. Pearson and K. J. B. Rix

Introduction

The idea that what one eats influences how one feels and behaves is not new. In the seventeenth century Richard Burton proclaimed in *The Anatomy of Melancholy* that 'Milk and all that comes from milk increase melancholy.' The anaphylactic nature of some responses to foods was only recognized at the beginning of the present century, and from 1922 reports began to appear of psychological symptoms caused by food allergy. Since then, abundant evidence has demonstrated clear associations between allergic disorders and mental changes. However, the significance of that evidence has been a repeated source of controversy. Modern advances in clinical immunology, psychology and psychiatry now provide a basis for a reinterpretation and a much clearer understanding of this important area.

Interactions between psyche and soma are complex, and nowhere is this better demonstrated than in atopy. Allergies, like any other physical disease, can lead to difficulties in psychosocial functioning and secondary psychological distress. Psychological factors can also affect bodily functions and influence the perception of sensations arising from normal or diseased organs. In some cases these 'somatopsychic' and 'psychosomatic' influences interact leading to a vicious circle of mutual exacerbation. As in other branches of medicine, proper treatment of the allergic patient demands an understanding, not only of the pathological process and the physical factors which influence it, but of the patient's personality and coping resources, relationships, work adjustment, social adjustment and emotional life (Fig. 39.1).

Particularly in young children, apparent emotional problems or behavioural abnormalities may be the main presenting complaints of food-allergic states associated with physical changes and may be controlled by treatment of the allergy. It has been inferred that the psychological changes are primary allergic

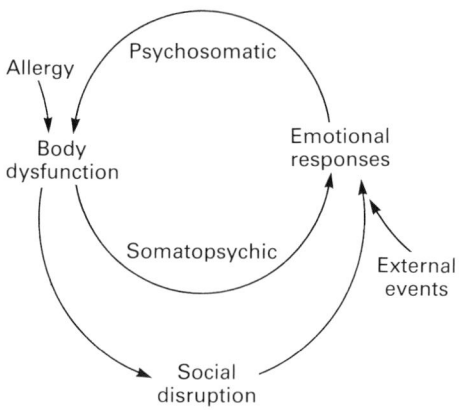

Fig. 39.1 Somatopsychic and psychosomatic arcs.

phenomena and claims have been made that they can occur in the absences of physical manifestations of allergy. Indeed, recently it has been suggested that food allergy is a common (if not the usual) cause of various psychiatric disorders. There has been a tendency to dismiss these latter claims out of hand because of the way they have been presented in popular media and obscure publications. However, they demand the closest objective scrutiny, both because of their implications for our view of psychiatric disorders and because they have become accepted as verified scientific fact by many lay people.

Regardless of the truth concerning the direct role of food allergy in the generation of psychological dysfunctions, examination of many of the arguments and the evidence on which they are based, reveals that the subject is bedevilled by the same errors which have plagued the whole area of food intolerance for more than 50 years. As pointed out by May [69], these include overconfidence in clinical impressions and the veracity of previous 'authorities'; failure to improve the accuracy of observations by procedures for the elimination of placebo effects and observer bias; theoretical concepts based on false assumptions; and faulty performance and interpretation of diagnostic tests.

Arguments concerning relationships between allergy and psychological changes have also often contained basic errors in logic, particularly the confusion of evidence of association with proof of causation, and unjustified extrapolation. At different times the same psychological observations in allergic disease have been interpreted as evidence that allergies are the result of psychosocial problems, the converse, and that both share common aetiological mechanisms. Questionable

deductions have also been used as justification for the use of controversial diagnostic techniques and for failure to apply acceptable objective criteria. For example, it has been argued that since some patients giving positive responses to particular diagnostic tests can be shown to have reproducible reactions on blind feeding, then other patients with similar test results would also react if subjected to such provocations, and therefore that the test is itself adequate proof of organic intolerance. Systematic use of double-blind feeding throws considerable doubt on these contentions.

Allergy or intolerance

Perhaps the two most important areas of confusion in any of these discussions are the distinction between direct and indirect effects of allergic processes, and the meaning given to the word *allergy*. Although it may appear a purely academic point, the former is crucial. If it can be shown that psychological changes in atopic disease are due to a direct effect of immunological responses to food then there is good reason for seeking allergic factors in psychiatric disorders in general. But if they are purely secondary to the other physical effects of the disease process, then many of the arguments involving extrapolation from atopic to non-atopic states are invalid.

Most clinical immunologists prefer to restrict the term *allergy* to immunologically mediated intolerances, and some to only IgE (reaginic) reactions. Others put forward several reasons for applying it as a more general term for adverse reactions, the most persuasive of which is that this is the usage given to it by most patients. Although both positions have valid points, it is almost certain that the wider application and failure to distinguish between immunological, pharmacological and toxic responses has been the origin of some problems, particularly the inappropriate application of allergological tests and therapies to non-immunological disorders. For this reason *allergy* will be used in this chapter to imply adverse responses of immunological aetiology, but not restricted to IgE-mediated reactions.

Fair appraisal of the evidence demands a sense of historical perspective. Many statements concerning an allergic aetiology of psychological disorder are based on conclusions drawn by workers such as Rowe [95], Rinkel [90] and Randolph [83] in the 1930s and 1940s when diagnoses of food allergy were often based on techniques of very dubious val-

Table 39.1 Possible explanations for apparent associations between psychological changes and physical manifestations in allergic diseases.

Causal Associations
Physical responses to psychological events
CNS involvement by immunological processes
Indirect psychological effects of allergy
  (i) Emotional and behavioural reactions to illness
  (ii) Secondary non-immunologic organic brain syndromes, e.g. due to hypoxaemia in asthma

Non-causal Associations
CNS side-effects of antiallergic medication

Fictitious Associations
Coincidental occurrence of common disorders
Confusion between allergic and pharmacological, toxic and metabolic non-immunological organic reactions
Application of inappropriate techniques and criteria in the absence of organic intolerance and in the presence of:
  (i) Fictitious 'allergy' in psychiatric illness
  (ii) Power of suggestion to produce physical and mental symptoms

idity, when allergy was a fashionable explanation for virtually all unexplained conditions and when the understanding of psychosomatic relationships was in its infancy. Although a large amount of data concerning psychological, atopic and other organic diseases were collected in the 1950s and 1960s, the interpretation of much of this was heavily influenced by contemporary, and now largely discredited, psychoanalytic concepts.

In order to achieve an up-to-date, objective and balanced view of psychological effects of food allergy it is first necessary to consider non-immunological organic syndromes whose features may be confused with those of allergic processes and, secondly, psychological influences which can either induce the physical manifestations of allergic disease or lead to other difficulties in diagnosis. Then, having established that allergic diseases can induce mental changes, the indirect organic and psychological processes which may be responsible for these will be examined. Finally, consideration will be given to the evidence that food allergy has a direct effect on brain function and is involved more generally in psychiatric disorders (Table 39.1).

ORGANIC BRAIN SYNDROMES WHICH MAY BE MISATTRIBUTED TO ALLERGY

The features of organic brain syndromes include a wide range of effects on higher intellectual functions, emotional state and behaviour. In some cases, such as toxicity of antiallergic medication, association of such symptoms with atopic manifestations may lead to drug effects being blamed on the underlying disease process. Other non-immunological

syndromes, which bear little or no resemblance to classical atopic disease, are described as 'allergy' because of their clear relationship to food ingestion. A third group, which may or may not be associated with food, come to be attributed to allergic processes because some of their features have superficial similarities with genuine allergic responses. An aetiological classification of organic syndromes with psychological features which may be misattributed to allergy is shown in Table 39.2.

Table 39.2 Organic brain syndromes which may be misattributed to allergy.

Central Nervous System Effects of Medication
Adrenaline
Alcohol*
Antihistamines
Corticosteroids
Ephedrine and pseudoephedrine
Theophylline

Non-immunological Reactions to Food
Pharmacological, e.g. caffeinism
Metabolic, e.g. hypoglycaemia
Toxic, e.g. fungal contaminants

Hyperventilation syndrome

* As an ingredient of some preparations.

Pharmacological

The pharmacological effects of substances cross-reacting with aspirin, food dyes and sulphur dioxide have been a major source of confusion in the study of allergic reactions to foods. In relation to psychological changes, the most important naturally occurring pharmacoactive agents are the methyl xanthines (Table 39.3).

Many drugs which have been used to treat allergic disorders have significant CNS (cen-

Table 39.3 Pharmacological effects of caffeine and other methyl xanthines.

Valued CNS Effects
Promotion of speed and clarity of thought, intellectual effort and acuity
Decreased drowsiness, fatigue and reaction time

Other Somatic Effects
Stimulation of medullary respiratory, vasomotor and vagal centres
Dilatation of coronary, pulmonary, cerebral and systemic blood vessels
Direct stimulation of heart rate and force of contraction
Bronchodilation, diuresis, increased gastrointestinal secretion

Toxic Symptoms
Insomnia: delayed onset and broken sleep
Nervousness, irritability, agitation, tremulousness, reflex hyperexcitability and muscle twitching
Headache, hyperaesthesia, ringing in the ears, visual flashes of light
Flushing, tachypnoea
Palpitations, extrasystoles, tachycardias, arrhythmias
Nausea, vomiting, diarrhoea, epigastric pain
Occasional reports of circulatory failure, collapse, dehydration, fever and oedema

tral nervous system) side-effects. Apart from the common emotional side effects of steroid treatment and the less frequent steroid psychoses, the importance of these cerebral effects is not always appreciated.

The naturally occurring agent ephedrine has CNS side-effects similar to those produced by the amphetamines and often causes anxiety, restlessness and insomnia. More severe side-effects include euphoria, toxic confusional states and psychoses [46, 96]. It was the main oral sympathomimetic agent until the development of more selective adrenergic drugs and was often prescribed in combination with a barbiturate. It is still contained in a few proprietary mixtures.

Ephedrine is now prescribed rarely, but pseudoephedrine continues to be used widely in nose drops and in proprietary oral cough and decongestant preparations, many of which can be obtained without prescription in the UK. Although pseudoephedrine is stated to have fewer CNS and cardiovascular side-effects than ephedrine, euphoria [19] and chronic hallucinatory and delusional states [29, 55] have been reported after oral and intranasal overdosages. There are suggestions of an increased incidence of nightmares and behaviour problems in children taking normal doses, and hallucinatory states have also been described [98].

The sympathomimetics oxymetazoline [7] and phenylephrine [101] have also been implicated in psychotic states related to the abuse of nasal sprays.

The xanthine derivatives theophylline, theobromine and caffeine have stimulatory effects on the heart and CNS. Caffeine is found in coffee, tea, cocoa and the cola nut as well as being contained in a number of analgesic preparations. Moderate doses stimulate mental activity, reduce fatigue and inhibit sleep. Toxic CNS symptoms include nervousness, irritability, agitation and headache in addition to tachypnoea, tremulousness, reflex hyperexcitability and muscle twitchings. Other effects can include cardiac dysrhythmias, nausea, vomiting, abdominal pain and diarrhoea [81].

Caffeinism

'Caffeinism' can induce hyperactive behaviour in children and simulate anxiety states in patients of all ages [39]. It is the true explanation for symptoms in many cases of self-reported tea or coffee 'allergy'. It is also the more probable explanation in some case reports (e.g. [31]) purporting to demonstrate the role of food allergy in non-atopic and psychological symptoms. Potentially toxic doses above 250 mg can be easily ingested in everyday life. Children are more sensitive to the CNS effects of caffeine and are often prevented from drinking coffee because of this but cola drinks, which may contain up to 60 mg of caffeine per glass, irrationally escape this prohibition.

There is also a well-described, but less commonly recognized, caffeine withdrawal syndrome [27, 39] (Table 39.4). Irritability,

Table 39.4 Caffeine withdrawal syndrome.

Headache
Disinclination to work, poor concentration, lethargy, depression, drowsiness
Irritability, nervousness
Yawning, nausea, rhinorrhoea

nervousness, restlessness, nausea and headache are features of both caffeine toxicity and withdrawal. Drowsiness, lethargy, a disinclination to work and inability to concentrate effectively are typical complaints of regular coffee drinkers who omit their morning cup [36]. Headache is a very common feature of more prolonged abstinence and may be associated with yawning, depression and somatic symptoms, some of which are also features of allergic states. Caffeine has a direct effect on the nasal mucosa and withdrawal leads to local hyperaemia, congestion and hyperresponsiveness with complaints of rhinorrhoea, nasal blockage and occasionally sneezing. Many of the features ascribed to 'masked food allergy' are identical with those of caffeine toxicity/withdrawal.

Theophylline has generally similar effects but it is a more potent bronchodilator [3]. CNS effects, apart from insomnia, are not usually seen with therapeutic levels in adults although there may be increased toxicity of coincident coffee or tea ingestion because of shared metabolic pathways. Theophylline may have greater psychotoxicity in children than is generally suspected. In a double-blind study, behavioural or school problems were reported in 5% of children taking theophylline for the control of their asthma, but in none of those taking disodium cromoglycate. A follow-up study of a small number of these children provided strong evidence that the intellectual, mood and behavioural disturbances were indeed related to theophylline therapy [33].

Until recently, proprietary teething and cough medicines commonly contained significant amounts of alcohol and even opiates. Several paediatric preparations prescribed for the treatment of allergic diseases have also been formulated with alcohol. It is possible that some children may have been ingesting enough alcohol to have had a significant effect on behaviour and intellectual function.

Work, school and particularly exam performance can also be affected adversely by the sedative action of antihistamines. Inadequate cognisance is given to this well-recognized side-effect when antihistamines are used as the first line treatment of skin and nasal allergies. Drug-induced sedation may be one of several reasons for the underachievement of atopic children compared with non-atopic children of similar intelligence [38]. Virtually none of the published studies in which psychological changes have been attributed to allergy have addressed the possibility that any of the observations could have been the result of drug effects.

Food-related metabolic and toxic responses

A number of symptom complexes which include psychological features depend on the calorific value, protein and carbohydrate content or availability, total bulk or osmotic load of the meal. Some are now well recognized, others are only just being elucidated. It is quite common for patients with unrelated psychiatric problems to interpret these metabolic responses as evidence that they suffer from allergies to specific foods. In addition, the features of several of these syndromes bear striking similarities to what have been described as the symptoms of 'masked allergy'.

Hypoglycaemia

Hypoglycaemia is associated with both physical and psychological symptoms. Fatigue, clouding of consciousness, amnesia and aggressive or bizarre behaviour can be attributed to neuroglycopenia, whereas anxiety, irritability, hunger, palpitations and tremor are the result of compensatory adrenergic activity. Even falls in blood glucose to levels above those defined as hypoglycaemic may result in minor but measurable reductions in intellectual function [40].

Many individuals given large doses of glucose after fasting will develop rebound chemical hypoglycaemia without significant symptomatology. Although there has been considerable controversy concerning the subject, the evidence suggests that genuine symptomatic essential reactive hypoglycaemia is rare in individuals with a normal lifestyle and diet [48]. However, alcohol-induced reactive hypoglycaemia occurs in about 20% of healthy, non-obese subjects a few hours after a carbohydrate meal taken with alcohol (the 'pub lunch', for example) and drowsiness with impairment of higher mental processes may follow [91]. Furthermore, late postprandial symptoms including severe hunger and irritability, without overt hypoglycaemia, are relatively common in individuals with abnormal diets containing a very high refined carbohydrate intake. This pattern may reflect successful compensation of blood glucose levels by adrenergic mechanisms in patients with defective gluconeogenic responses secondary to their obesity.

A wide range of symptoms is also seen in the various well-documented 'dumping syndromes'. Even in normal individuals the ingestion of very large meals, particularly those with a high carbohydrate content, regularly produces somnolence and torpor. Despite the universality of this experience, some hypochondriacal patients interpret it as evidence of disease. This may be particularly common in depressed patients, in whom feelings of general anergia are usual, and who may react with distress to postprandial exaggerations of their tiredness.

Amino acids

Research into affective disorders and Parkinson's disease has highlighted the importance of amino acid-derived neurotransmitters in the regulation of brain function and has shown that brain levels can be affected by dietary precursors. Several of the opposing CNS effects of carbohydrate-rich and protein-rich carbohydrate-poor meals, including those on appetite regulation, may be mediated by alterations in the availability of the serotonin precursor tryptophan relative to that of other competing neutral amino acids [113]. In addition to influencing mood, experimental tryptophan feeding reduces total calorie intake and the proportion of carbohydrate taken in a free diet. Depressed serotonin synthesis may be responsible for the carbohydrate craving of obese dieters eating low carbohydrate meals with a high amino acid content but a relative paucity of tryptophan [113]—a feature occasionally attributed to the 'addiction' phase of masked food allergy.

Peptides with activities similar to those of opiates in in vitro systems have been derived from several food proteins (including milk and wheat) by partial enzymic hydrolysis [114]. Although the postulation that such 'exorphins' could account for food-induced mental changes is intriguing, there is yet no objective evidence that such substances are produced, absorbed, cross the blood-brain barrier or have any significant biological effect after feeding, in intact animals or man.

Hyperventilation

The syndrome of chronic hyperventilation (reviewed in [60, 67]) can mimic several other physical and psychiatric disorders, and its features (Table 39.5) bear striking similarities to those sometimes attributed to food allergy.

Table 39.5 Some symptoms of chronic hyperventilation.

General
Fatigue, exhaustion

Neurological
Central: dizziness, headache
Peripheral: numbness, paraesthesiae

Cardiovascular
Chest pains, palpitations, Raynaud's phenomenon

Respiratory
Shortness of breath

Gastrointestinal
Bloating, heartburn, gas, epigastric pain

Musculoskeletal
Muscle pains, cramps

Psychiatric
Anxiety or depression, panic attacks

However, it is often not recognized, its frequency is generally underestimated and it is often misdiagnosed. For example, failure to seek objective evidence of bronchoconstriction in patients with recurrent episodes of dyspnoea may lead to it being labelled as asthma. Chronic hyperventilation is the true explanation of symptoms in many patients who become convinced falsely that they suffer from allergic disease [61, 78].

The causes of hyperventilation have been categorized into organic, physiological, emotional and habit [57]. The last includes a tendency to thoracic rather than abdominal breathing even at rest. However, most authorities are agreed that, regardless of initial precipitating factors, anxiety and fear created by the symptoms of hyperventilation, and failure of physicians to recognize their true origin, are major causes of their maintenance.

Hyperventilation produces hypocapnia and a rapid fall in serum inorganic phosphorus which is out of proportion to the degree of respiratory alkalosis. Acute hypophosphataemia produces malaise, dizziness, paraesthesias and mental changes including disorientation. Other neurological, cardiac and muscular symptoms are caused by the alkalosis; cerebral hypoxia, resulting in lightheadedness, dizziness, blurring of vision and occasionally syncope, follows cerebral vasoconstriction associated with a shift to the left of the oxyhaemoglobin dissociation curve.

Persistent hypocapnia produces a down-setting of the sensitivity of the respiratory centre to $P_a CO_2$ with the sensation of dyspnoea at normal $P_a O_2$ and $P_a CO_2$ levels. This may be an important factor in the tendency of hyperventilation to become self-perpetuating. Once established, the metabolic abnormalities can be maintained with only an occasional deep breath superimposed on a normal respiratory rate. In this state, small increases in the depth or rate of respiration with minimal exertion or mild stress can induce acute symptoms. Sufferers are typically unable to re-establish a normal pattern of breathing when asked to do so even if the hyperventilatory response has been triggered by voluntary deep breathing.

Signs and symptoms of hyperventilation

Signs and symptoms encountered in the chronic hyperventilation syndrome are shown in Table 39.5. Although chronic and early fatiguability, paraesthesias, dyspnoea and light-headedness or dizziness are very common, the patient may not complain of them spontaneously, being more concerned about the significance of symptoms referable to specific organ systems. Although genuine cardiac dysrhythmias can be triggered by hyperventilation, chest pain more usually arises from the intercostal muscles. Unfortunately misinterpretation of hyperventilatory 'pseudo-ischaemic' ST segment ECG changes may lead to patients being told that they do have organic heart disease. Abdominal symptoms are also common presenting complaints. However, most patients are polysymptomatic and on direct questioning admit to other symptoms suggestive of the syndrome.

The symptoms of chronic hyperventilation syndrome can become associated with food by physical or psychological processes. First, gastric distension induced by the ingestion of a significant volume of solid, fluid or gas may lead to exaggeration of the abnormal thoracic breathing pattern through diaphragmatic splinting or interference with abdominal wall movements. This may act synergistically with the aerophagy which is commonly seen with hyperventilation and which may be secondary to the drying effects of oral breathing or be an associated nervous habit. Secondly, once patients suspect any particular food of being related to their distressing symptoms, the apprehension and adrenergic activity associated with its ingestion may be adequate to trigger a hyperventilatory episode. Every further recurrence after that food reinforces the apprehension associated with it and increases the likelihood of more severe symptoms on re-exposure. Typical blood-gas changes following open wheat ingestion in a patient who believed she was wheat allergic, but who did not react to it on double-blind provocation, are shown in Fig. 39.2.

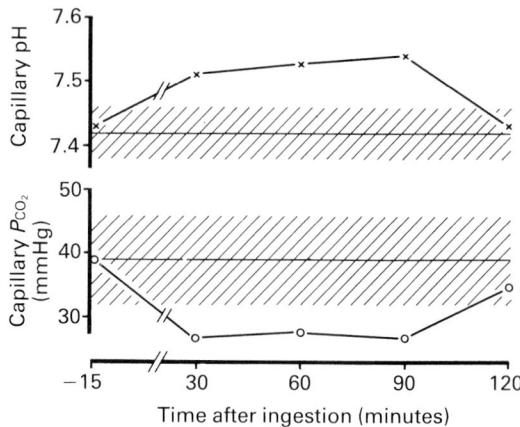

Fig. 39.2 Hyperventilation in psychogenic wheat intolerance. Multiple symptoms and hyperventilatory blood-gas changes induced by open wheat provocation in a 43-year-old woman who believed she was allergic to wheat. Symptoms relieved by bag rebreathing or by 5% CO_2 in air; reproduced by voluntary hyperventilation. No consistent reaction to blind wheat administration.

Hyperventilation often occurs against a background of seemingly complex medical and psychological problems but many patients respond rapidly to simple explanation and supportive therapy. A provisional diagnosis can be made after a test of voluntary hyperventilation although some patients who previously blamed food require blind provocation studies before they will accept that their symptoms were not due to an organic intolerance.

PSYCHOLOGICAL DETERMINANTS OF ATOPIC AND OTHER SOMATIC SYMPTOMS

It is not possible to make a realistic appraisal of food allergy-induced mental changes without recognition of psychological influences on physical function. Many misconceptions concerning the whole area of food allergy have derived from a failure to appreciate the power of suggestion and from misinterpretation of the significance of the somatic manifestations of psychiatric disorder.

Psychologically determined atopic symptoms

Many valid observations have demonstrated that atopic manifestations can be produced or modified by emotional changes. Hippocrates warned the asthmatic to guard against anger. Modern information concerning biochemical abnormalities [108] and bronchial hyperreactivity [41,62] in atopy provides a rational and organic explanation of how any physical or mental stimulus to autonomic activity can influence atopic symptoms. Thus several forms of psychosomatic change in atopic individuals can be considered an imbalanced response to non-specific autonomic arousal, which can occur against a background of completely normal psychological functioning.

In humans and experimental animals allergic changes may become a conditioned reflex after repeated allergen exposure [17,49]. In 1885 John MacKenzie of Baltimore described how he was able to induce rhinitis and asthma in an allergic subject by showing her an artificial rose. Even patients who are aware that they no longer react physically can have a lifelong aversion to foods which produced severe allergic reactions during their childhood. However, suggestion can also induce organic and psychological changes without preceding organic sensitization. Under hypnosis the bronchi can be made to constrict or dilate by suggestion alone and hypnosis can also affect the response to physical bronchoconstrictor stimuli such as exercise [5]. Inhibition of suggestion-induced asthmatic changes by atropine [63] indicates that these are indeed mediated by parasympathetic neural pathways.

Clear evidence of the role of psychological factors in some subjective and objective food-related changes (Fig. 39.3) was provided by the classical studies of Wolff and his colleagues, who were the first to utilize blind food provocations in 1950 [37]. They showed that discussion of stressful events, or conditions associated with previous attacks, could induce urticaria, measurable changes in skin blood flow, nasal secretion and eosinophilia. They also demonstrated the lack of organic basis in the responses of several patients who attributed asthmatic, gastrointestinal, skin and other more subjective symptoms to specific food allergies, when blind administration of these foods elicited no reaction. The fact that the attacks could be induced by misleading patients into believing that they had been given the relevant food provided positive evidence of the power of suggestion. Subsequent experience with both ingested and inhaled antigens has confirmed the frequency of such psychogenic responses. These findings are underlined by discussions with patients which reveal that a surprisingly high proportion of atopic children are well aware of how to manipulate their environment by consciously causing exacerbations of their skin or chest disease.

Somatic manifestations of psychological disorder wrongly attributed to food

A number of psychologically determined eating disorders are now well recognized. These include anorexia nervosa and its variant bulimia nervosa, as well as neurotic food fads. Food avoidance in such patients may sometimes be justified as an 'allergy'. Patients have been described who have deliberately produced, or simulated anaphylactic reactions to foods in themselves (Munchausen's syndrome) [44] as has the allergic form of Meadow's syndrome (Munchausen by proxy) [111].

Patients with a wide variety of other common neuroses and personality disorders can become falsely convinced that they suffer from food allergies, often with potentially hazardous repercussions on their physical health when

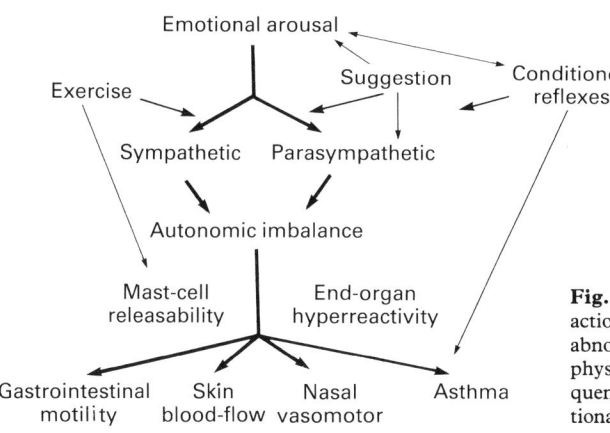

Fig. 39.3 Neural pathways in psychogenic physical reactions in atopy. In the presence of the pharmacological abnormalities of the atopic syndrome most psychogenic physical responses can be viewed as idiosyncratic consequences of the autonomic nervous system activity of emotional arousal.

they impose severe dietary restrictions on themselves [79]. Several factors may operate in producing this situation [79, 92]. First, somatic features occur in anxiety and depressive states (Table 39.6) and commonly lead to fears of a serious disease. Some patients go further and assume that their more overtly psychological symptoms are also a direct result of physical changes. Similar misinterpretations of the significance of physical symptoms in psychological disorders have almost certainly been responsible for some earlier medical statements concerning the role of food allergy in non-atopic disorders, particularly when psychological changes and associated somatic complaints have occurred as a reaction to the physical disability of severe chronic atopic disorders.

Secondly, many patients who falsely attri-

they have received, these psychologically disturbed patients accept the presence of any of the features in Tables 39.3–39.6 or the occurrence of any of the pharmacological or metabolic responses discussed earlier as proof that they are indeed 'food allergics'. Some continue to remain convinced of this despite being unable to discover any food which elicits their symptoms. A proportion of patients claim relief on diets excluding specific foods, but review of symptom diaries reveals no actual change in symptom frequency or severity. Others explain failure to respond to exclusion diets by inadvertent non-compliance, or by presuming food adulteration. A proportion of patients do show consistent exacerbations on open food reintroductions, which are not repeatable under double-blind conditions and which are associated with high placebo re-

Table 39.6 Some common symptoms in psychiatric disorders.

Common symptoms in depression	*Somatic symptoms of anxiety*[*]
Lowered mood	Palpitations
Lack of confidence	Breathlessness
Depersonalization	Chest pain
Tiredness, etc.	Headache
Sleep disturbance	Paraesthaesia
Breathing difficulty	Trembling
Dizziness	Fatigue
Headaches	Sweating
Appetite disturbance	Flushes
Excessive perspiration	Dry mouth
Disturbed sexual function	Urinary frequency

[*]From Wheeler PD, Reed EW, Cohen ME: Neurocirculatory asthenia (anxiety neurosis, effort syndrome, neurasthenia). J Am Med Assoc 1950; 142:878, with permission.

bute psychological symptoms to food are highly suggestible and have been exposed to considerable publicity regarding allergy. Most of our own series of such patients had read popular books [65, 87] claiming that many non-atopic physical conditions and psychological symptoms are often caused by allergy. Very many had had this conviction reinforced by practitioners of 'alternative medicine'.

Thirdly, perhaps as a result of the stigma of psychiatric illness, these patients prefer an organic to a 'psychological' label for their problems and grasp gratefully at any explanation they find less threatening than a psychiatric diagnosis. A similar ignorance of mind–body relationships was demonstrated by an ecology clinic publicity leaflet which many of our patients carried. It declared that the medical use of the term psychosomatic 'is the crime of accusing patients of suffering imaginary illnesses'.

In keeping with the written and oral advice

sponse rates [79]. Such reactions are often associated with the blood-gas changes of hyperventilation.

Since the 1950s experience in all branches of medicine has confirmed the ability of the 'placebo' to produce virtually any subjective symptom and to improve many symptoms as well. More recent double-blind feeding studies have shown the unreliability of clear histories of reactions to foods and open food exclusion–reintroduction, as well as of all other presently available ancillary tests, in the diagnosis of organic food intolerance [4, 6, 8, 68, 79, 97].

Since we have very clear evidence that psychosomatic changes are not figments of the patient's or the doctor's imagination, that psychogenic food intolerances are common and that dietary avoidance regimes have very significant hazards, it is essential that the diagnosis of organic food sensitivity is only accepted on the basis of the strongest evidence. At the present time the only valid proof of such a diagnosis is double-blind feeding (see Chapters 46–49).

INDIRECT PSYCHOLOGICAL EFFECTS OF ALLERGY

Food allergy can cause a number of psychological symptoms and behavioural changes secondary to the physical effects of allergy (Tables 39.7–39.8). Most are common consequences of particular physical changes whether produced by food or inhalant allergens, or by non-allergic mechanisms.

In addition to drug side-effects, two main mechanisms can be distinguished: first, mental symptoms and signs which are features of organic brain syndromes; secondly, the mental symptoms and signs which are understandable, although occasionally exaggerated, psychological reactions to physical symptoms or their effects on life adjustment.

Cases of sleep deprivation are difficult to classify according to these mechanisms since some cases will begin with insomnia which results from worrying or is a feature of a depressive disorder and others are due to organic symptoms interrupting sleep. Either may lead to a form of organic brain syndrome termed 'sleep deprivation' [58]. However, with the exception of 'sleep deprivation', the final pathway common to most of the organic brain syndromes related to allergic disorders is cerebral hypoxia.

Physical distress can lead directly to changes in observed behaviour in young children and disease affects many of the influences on personality development in childhood and adolescence. Anxiety or depression severe enough to be classified as pathological is an understandable response to crippling disorders at any age.

Cerebral hypoxia

Generalized cerebral hypoxia may result from deficient oxygenation of the arterial blood in asthma and angioedema (anoxic anoxia), or from reduced perfusion pressure in shocked

Table 39.7 Indirect influences on mental function in allergy.

Organic Cerebral Dysfunction
Acute cerebral hypoxia, secondary to asthma, anaphylactic shock, etc.
Permanent neurological/psychological sequelae of anoxic episodes
Sleep deprivation syndrome
Drug side-effects

Psychological Reactions to Somatic Dysfunction
Anxiety
Depressive reactions
Personality developments secondary to influences on parent–child relationships, socialization, etc.
Secondary effects of educational underachievement, restricted activity, etc.

Table 39.8 Secondary psychological effects of physical manifestations of allergic disease.

Reduced Intellectual Functioning
Due to cerebral hypoxia, sleep disorder, drug effects

Anxiety
Concerning life-threatening events, effects of chronic disease on work, personal life, etc.

Dysphoria
Secondary to drugs, cerebral hypoxia or depressive reactions to disabilities

Temper Tantrums, Screaming, Hyperactive and other Disturbed Behaviours
As the presentation of pain, itching or general distress in young children

Alterations in Parent-Child Relationships
Especially overprotective behaviour leading to emotional immaturity, overdependency

Other Influences on Personality Development
Including effects secondary to decreased socialization with peers, exclusion from physical activity, educational underachievement, etc.

Sexual Dysfunctions
Including 'sexercise-induced asthma', rejection of disfigurement and drug-induced prolactinaemia

states (stagnant anoxia). The cause of coma associated with cyanosis or absent blood pressure is obvious, but the ubiquity of less severe cerebral changes due to minor degrees of hypoxia in asthma receives little attention in standard texts.

The brain is uniquely sensitive to oxygen deficit and cerebral features tend to dominate the clinical picture of hypoxia. In the normal adult, brain respiration accounts for about 25% of total body oxygen uptake and in the young child this requirement may be up to 50%. A reduction of 10 to 20% in inspired oxygen concentration can normally be accommodated, mainly through a compensatory increase in cerebral blood flow. It is possible that cerebral hypoxic symptoms occur in asthma at levels of arterial Po_2 higher than would otherwise be expected due to interference with this mechanism by the effects of hypocapnia and respiratory alkalosis discussed earlier. Hypoxia may also potentiate CNS drug side-effects.

Under conditions of acute, marginally reduced cerebral oxygen uptake there may be varying degrees of impairment of consciousness. Minor degrees of impairment of consciousness may be manifest in mental slowing with diminished alertness, reduced attention span, difficulty in judging the passage of time, difficulty thinking and memory difficulties in the area of new learning. There may also be emotional symptoms such as depression, anxiety and irritability. With more severe degrees there may be drowsiness, apathy, slowing of movement, evident mental fatigue, incoherence of speech, impaired grasp of what is happening, perceptual disturbances such as illusions, hallucinations and delusions, disorientation for place and person as well as time, and emotional indifference. There may also be muscular twitching, tremor or epileptic fits. Coma may progress to death.

Permanent sequelae of cerebral anoxia are not common in survivors and recovery usually leaves behind only a dense amnesia for the period of impairment of consciousness. If permanent sequelae do result they range from relatively circumscribed memory disorders such as a Korsakoff state to more global impairment of higher intellectual functions such as a dementia. Hyperkinetic states and focal brain disturbances including apraxias and aphasias may also be seen. Degree and rate of recovery are very variable and may be related to the severity and length of anoxia.

Long-standing mild hypoxia may reveal itself in a picture closely resembling severe fatigue with tiredness, apathy, inattentiveness and delayed responding. Alternatively there may be relatively few obvious organic features and instead merely an exaggeration of characteristic personality traits.

Food-related mental changes

There are multiple case reports in the older literature of mental symptoms, usually with focal neurological signs, which have been associated with severe generalized allergic reactions to foods [51, 52, 77, 104, 110]. Although still sometimes quoted as evidence for a direct influence of allergy on the brain, it seems at least equally likely that many of these cases had suffered anoxic cerebral injury. Identical changes can follow any state producing severe hypoxaemia or circulatory collapse.

Some descriptions of food-related mental changes associated with focal neurological signs are highly suggestive of variants of migraine. The cortical ischaemia secondary to arterial spasm can lead to a wide variety of focal symptoms and signs including paralyses, paraesthesias and aphasias and also mental symptoms [58]. In the prodrome of an attack there may be feelings of anxiety or irritability. Exceptionally hypomanic features occur in the prodrome with increased energy, elevation of mood, overactivity and pressure of speech. Similar hypomanic symptoms may occur after an attack. During attacks there may be a prominent amnesia either on its own or along with visual aura, delirious states characterized by clouding of consciousness with hallucinations and delusions often of a persecutory nature, complex visual and auditory hallucinations occurring in clear consciousness, body image disturbances and severe affective symptoms such as profound anxiety and depression. Although these symptoms sometimes accompany the headaches, there are some reports of these symptoms occurring as so-called migraine equivalents.

Foods are responsible for only a proportion of migraine attacks. Although there is good evidence [28] to incriminate food allergy in children with severe migraine (who are atypical of migraineurs as a whole) and in occasional adult sufferers, the bulk of the evidence suggests that most food-related migraine is due to pharmacological rather than immunological processes [34, 59, 70]. Even in that small proportion in whom IgE-mediated responses do appear to trigger attacks, there is

no evidence that this is due to central involvement of allergic mechanisms rather than an
influence on the permeability of the gut allowing increased ingress of vasoactive molecules.
It is therefore unwise to accept reports concerning migraine as valid proof of direct
nervous system effects of food allergy.

Psychological and behavioural reactions to allergy

Many of the reports concerning psychological
aspects of allergic diseases were published in
the 1950s and 1960s. Most were purely anecdotal, concerned only severely affected hospitalized patients and were heavily influenced by
contemporary psychoanalytical and psycho-
dynamic theories, now regarded as impressionistic and unscientific. Many studies
attempted to identify the typical personality or
abnormality of parent–child relationships
which were assumed to be of aetiological significance. A review of 65 such studies from
this period reveals considerable disagreement
concerning supposedly characteristic traits
[45]. However, allergic children have been
most commonly described as emotionally insecure with an intense need of parental love
and protection and having a tendency to cling
to their either rejecting or overprotective
mother. Certain characteristics in later life
have been seen as a development of this basic
childhood pattern. These include emotional
immaturity, lack of self-confidence, feelings of
inadequacy, compensatory aggression and
sometimes repressed hostility. In eczema, evidence of sexual difficulties has been taken as
evidence that the rash is due to 'cutaneous
eroticization'. Such views of psychosomatic
causation are now regarded as of little more
than historical interest.

More modern objective studies do confirm
that some of the above characteristics, and
other behavioural and emotional responses,
are relatively common in atopic population
(Table 39.8). However, they also indicate that
these are often understandable consequences
of the physical changes, or of the social disruption, which follows from them [1, 35, 38,
73, 76, 112]. The results vary with age and, in
children, are also influenced by parental attitudes and responses.

It is very difficult to assess the subjective
experiences of young children and disturbed
behaviour may be the only outward manifestation of any form of distress. All children become 'difficult' when they are ill, whatever the
cause. In a child unable to communicate its
feelings, hyperactivity might reflect frustration, pain, generalized itching or a toxic
response to a drug such as theophylline.
Abdominal pain is a common feature of
gastrointestinal allergic reaction to foods and
in infancy this commonly presents as irritability, screaming or temper tantrums.

Effects on child

Allergic diseases can also have less direct
effects on psychological development and
function. Recurrent absences from school are
probably the major cause of the recorded underachievement, for their intellectual ability,
of atopic children. But intellectual function at
school and work may also be affected by hypoxia, sleep loss and medication. Exercise-
induced asthma can have a number of secondary effects, from a child's exclusion from play
with its peers leading to difficulty in establishing social contacts, through general restrictions on sporting activities which may affect
development of self-esteem and influence the
adoption of more passive hobbies such as reading, to interference with sexual activity. Responses to eczema on the part of others often
include horror and revulsion. These are not
only likely to decrease self-esteem and impede
social integration but they can be the origin of
sexual difficulties leading to yet further problems in self-esteem and interpersonal adjustment.

Effects on parents

The effects of a child's disease on the parents
can also produce disturbances within the
family resulting in further indirect influences
on the child's psychological and social development. Exaggeration of normal parental
concern and anxiety often leads to overprotec-
tion with increased social isolation and emotional dependency on the parents. Family out-
ings and holidays may be restricted by the
need to avoid environments with a high risk of
exposure to allergens such as house dust mite
and animal dander. Special diets for food allergy produce further social problems as well
as being a very real financial burden on many
families. Doubt concerning their ability to
cope with the child's illness can lead to further
parental anxieties, guilt and resentment.
Sometimes children may deliberately induce
or aggravate asthmatic symptoms or scratch
eczematous lesions to avoid certain undesir-

able situations or to increase levels of parental anxiety or protectiveness.

With regret one also has to admit that occasionally, supposedly pathological psychological responses have been a direct result of medical attitudes: in particular the now mercifully rare overemphasis on psychosomatic aetiology to the exclusion of proper physical treatment. For example, treatment of acute asthma with invitations to 'pull yourself together', more professional psychotherapy, or by administration of barbiturates or benzodiazepines to patient and/or parent, not only may have had no long-term beneficial effect on anxiety, but may well have been responsible for increased mortality and much of the anger and hostility sometimes reported in asthmatics and their families.

Asthma as an example

Objective comparisons of atopic patients with healthy individuals of the same age and other disease groups are entirely compatible with the above factors being responsible for the observed differences. Most have concentrated on asthma. Studies of children and adults with only mild disease, or whose symptoms are adequately suppressed by medical treatment, reveal no or only trivial differences in personality from controls[1]. As a group, children with persistent asthma score significantly more maladjusted or neurotic on psychological tests than do their own healthy siblings or age-matched controls, showing traits of anxiety, insecurity and dependency [73]. However, they do not differ significantly from children restricted by heart disease [73]. Observations of acute psychological changes with exacerbations of asthma have demonstrated only increased anxiety, fatigue and changes typical of cerebral hypoxia [112]. However, children growing up with asthma seem to adapt remarkably well to their disease and become less frightened in acute attacks provided previous episodes have responded rapidly to treatment. Adult asthmatics also show a tendency to anxiety, neuroticism and introversion, but these are if anything rather less marked than in patients with breathlessness due to chronic bronchitis [76]. In both groups levels of anxiety and neuroticism are related to the degree of respiratory difficulty [76].

Behavioural disturbances are not prominent in older allergic children. A large prospective study [66] of 7- to 14-year-old asthmatics found no differences in behaviour between patients with mild to moderate disease and controls. The small subgroup with severe and persisting asthma were found to be less socially mature and demonstrated an increased frequency of anxious, demanding and aggressive behaviours.

Food sensitivity and behaviour

No published studies have compared the frequency of abnormal 'behaviours' in very young children with proven food sensitivity to that in non-allergic states. Buisseret [11] reported that 84% of milk-intolerant children between 11 months and 17 years of age had had milk-induced abdominal pain or colic and that a third had at some time received medical advice for apparent psychological disturbance. Malingering had often been suspected if abdominal pain was the major symptom occurring before departure for school after a milk and cereal breakfast. In another recent series of 68 children with various food allergies [71] 24 babies had had prolonged screaming or colic and this was the main presenting complaint in 12. Eight had mood alterations in association with their physical symptoms and two had hyperactivity unrelated to food.

Considering the difficulties facing them it is perhaps surprising that overt psychological problems do not occur more commonly in allergic individuals. Reports of psychiatric disorder in allergic disease mainly involve severely affected hospitalized individuals, but epidemiological studies reveal no or only a slightly increased frequency in general atopic populations. A randomly selected sample of 10- to 15-year-old asthmatic children from Scotland showed a similar rate of psychiatric disorders to the general population [72]. A survey of all handicapped children on the Isle of Wight showed a slight, but not statistically significant, increased frequency of psychiatric disorder amongst asthmatics compared to the general population, but the rate was almost identical to that in children with other (non-brain) physical handicaps [38]. The increase in the asthmatic group as a whole could be accounted for by the increase in the most severely physically handicapped individuals. It is worth noting that there was no correlation of psychiatric problems with either personal or family history of eczema and therefore, presumptively, with increased risk of food sensitivity.

Any association of childhood depression and atopy might be due simply to the fact that atopic diseases are the commonest cause of chronic and recurrent physical problems in childhood. In one series, 45% of children diagnosed as being depressed had associated allergies [75]. Given the known prevalence of atopy and an overall frequency of childhood depressive disorders of 1–2% [50], this would represent an incidence of depression of 1.5 to 3% in atopic children. Reports in this field need to be interpreted with caution since many of the features said to be indicative of depression in young children (irritability, easy frustration, short attention span, difficulty in sleeping, abdominal pain, temper tantrums, etc.) are also common results of cerebral hypoxia and other indirect allergic effects and also may be manifestations of drug toxicity.

FOOD ALLERGY AS A DIRECT CAUSE OF PSYCHOLOGICAL SYMPTOMS

It has been suggested that food allergy is directly responsible for a wide range of somatic symptoms, psychological changes and psychiatric disorders. Recent years have seen claims that food allergy is commonly, or even usually, the cause of such phenomena even if they occur in the absence of classical atopy [65, 82].

Many claims are based directly on conclusions drawn earlier this century from anecdotal clinical observations subject to the several criticisms listed in the introduction to this chapter. In many earlier reports these changes came to be attributed to food allergy because of their association with classical atopic manifestations and the most usual non-atopic symptoms observed could now be interpreted as being due to cerebral hypoxia, or as the psychological and somatic features of the anxiety or depressive states which may be secondary to physical symptomatology.

Most of the present claims concerning the importance of food allergy in apparently neurotic and psychotic states come from the school of 'clinical ecology', which has diverged from mainstream allergology by adopting a wider concept of maladaption to the general environment, and in some cases an active rejection of the techniques and philosophy of orthodox medical science [85].

While accepting that not all reactions described by themselves as 'allergy' are immunologically mediated, some clinical ecologists continue to view features of several different types of response as common to all 'allergies'. Many accept as proven Randolph's [84] theoretical developments of Rinkel's [90] hypotheses of masked and cyclical allergy. According to these, frequent exposure to an allergen leads to 'addiction'; withdrawal results in worsening of physical symptoms and mental depression; re-exposure not only does not produce acute worsening of physical symptoms but alleviates the withdrawal syndrome and actually produces mental stimulation. The extremes of this spectrum are described as severe depression with disturbed consciousness and mania with or without convulsions [86].

Several independent lines of evidence have been taken together as circumstantial indications of a more general role for food allergy in the production of mental symptoms (Table 39.9). These include the occurrence of food-induced migraine and the various reported associations of personality features and emotional reactions with atopic diseases, evidence concerning behaviour disorders in children (particularly hyperkinesis and the allergic tension–fatigue syndrome) and purported links between gluten sensitivity and schizophrenia.

The evidence concerning the role of foods in migraine has been considered in a prior section and in Chapter 37. We have also already seen that classical atopic conditions can cer-

Table 39.9 Main circumstantial evidence for the general role of food allergy in the generation of mental disorders.

Cases of anxiety or depression associated with severe atopic disease
Impressions of characteristic allergic personality
Symptoms of lethargy, mental clouding or disorientation in acute asthma
Behaviour of children with physical symptoms due to allergy
Neurological features in some severe anaphylactic reactions
Food-induced migraine
Neurological features in immune-complex vasculitides (serum sickness, lupus)
Pharmacological and metabolic responses (e.g. caffeinism) considered as allergy
Claims of salicylate and dye hypersensitivity in childhood hyperactivity
Reported associations between gluten sensitivity and schizophrenia
Clinical impressions from open food exclusions and reintroductions
Evidence derived from the use of controversial diagnostic techniques

tainly have psychological consequences. However, there is no evidence that these are other than the indirect effects of cerebral hypoxia, medication or the secondary psychological processes considered in the preceding section.

The allergic tension–fatigue syndrome

Irritability, restlessness, fretfulness and sleeplessness had been reported as features of anaphylactic food sensitivity in children in 1916 [47]. Emotional and behavioural disturbances in children which responded to food elimination were attributed to 'allergic toxaemia' by Rowe in 1930 [94] and designated the 'fatigue syndrome of allergic origin' by Randolph in the 1940s [82]. Originally two forms were recognized: one in which chronic weakness and sluggishness predominated; in the other motor and sensory hyperexcitability.

By 1950 collections of such anecdotal reports were considered to have removed any possible doubt that these symptoms must be considered the direct results of allergic reactions in the nervous system [15]. Believing this to be the case, Speer considered both over- and underactivity to be aspects of a single abnormality which he described as the 'allergic tension–fatigue syndrome' in 1954 [102]. In expanding this concept, he later came to attribute virtually every personality, emotional and behavioural abnormality ever described in atopic individuals to this putative primary abnormality, which he considered characteristic of the allergic state [103].

In all early and subsequent published case reports of this condition, the behavioural and emotional symptoms have been associated with physical features of allergy. The five cardinal signs of the allergic tension–fatigue syndrome have been described [14] as fatigue, irritability, other mental and emotional symptoms (including sluggishness, drowsiness, lack of interest in school or play, peevishness and unpredictable behaviour), circles under the eyes and nasal congestion. The same authors have emphasized the frequency of abdominal pain and other physical symptoms. Several reports have been published in which cases described as having this syndrome have reacted to blind or double-blind food provocation [14, 88]. In each, the description of the mental features is entirely compatible with their having been secondary to the associated physical changes.

Several recent series of children with well-documented organic food intolerance have included significant numbers with abdominal pain, colic, screaming attacks and hyperactive and other disturbed behaviours. None have recorded any case in which such 'emotional' food-related changes have occurred in the absence of physical symptoms.

Hyperactivity in children

Hyperactivity is considered more fully in Chapter 38. However, several points are germane to the wider discussion of food-related mental changes. It is clear that the various terms used to describe pathologically overactive behaviour (hyperactivity, hyperkinesis and hyperkinetic syndrome) have been used very loosely. Also that the threshold for viewing such behaviour as pathological, or as a specific syndrome, varies very markedly between countries, between parents and between different physicians within countries. Traits attributed to hyperactivity as a syndrome include not only overactive, but impulsive and disruptive behaviours, resistance to discipline, poor concentration, short attention span and resultant underachievement at school.

The features described above can be the result of numerous processes, from neurological deficits to sociocultural factors. Many also complicate the course of asthma and other atopic conditions, as well as severe childhood migraine, and can be produced by theophylline, caffeine and other drugs. Although most authorities put the incidence very much lower, Feingold [30] has suggested that the incidence of hyperactivity may be up to 25% in some schools, and that 30 to 50% of hyperactive children achieve a complete remission on a salicylate- and additive-free diet.

Feingold's highly publicized claims have been used as a major argument in support of the importance of allergy in other psychological disorders. However, it has been noted that his only data are uncontrolled anecdotes and these claims have been received with scepticism [109]. Most controlled studies designed to test his hypothesis have failed to find a significant effect of diet on behaviour in the majority of hyperactive children. However, a few studies have found that performance on laboratory learning tests, or behaviour, can be adversely affected by food dyes in a small minority of children considered hyperactive. Unfortunately, these studies did not record whether or not these changes were associated with physical symptomatology. Salicylates and food dyes are relatively common causes of chronic urticaria and a proportion of children presented as hyperactive can be observed to be suffering from abdominal pain or itching, which have gone unrecognized by the parents. No case has been documented in which it has been recorded that double-blind administration of salicylate, or food dye or preservative, has led to hyperactive or other pathological behaviour in the absence of physical symptoms.

Gluten sensitivity in schizophrenia

In the last 20 years the putative role of allergic reactions to foods as a cause of mental illness has become intertwined with the hypothesis that schizophrenia may be caused by gluten intolerance. Although often cited in the 'food allergy' literature, Dohan [22, 23] has pointed out that it is inaccurate to regard his work as concerned with 'allergy' when his hypothesis is that the basic biological defect in schizophrenia is a genetic impairment of the gut and other barrier systems which permits the passage of food-derived neuroactive peptides from the gut lumen to the brain cells [23].

Dohan's claim that there is a relationship between schizophrenia and coeliac disease is based upon his belief that schizophrenics have small intestinal abnormalities characteristic of coeliac disease; that the two conditions occur in the same person more commonly than would be expected by chance; and that the ingestion of gluten by coeliac patients can result in psychosis [22].

However, two large studies have failed to find evidence of coeliac disease in schizophrenics [16, 105]; three out of four of the studies regarded by Dohan as demonstrating a more than coincidental association of coeliac disease and schizophrenia concern childhood psychosis rather than schizophrenia; and none of the studies quoted by him contains a convincing account of schizophrenia occurring in a patient with coeliac disease.

Circumstantial immunopathological evidence for the gluten hypothesis is the finding that 17–20% of schizophrenics have antibodies to wheat gliadin detected by enzyme-linked and latex agglutination techniques [26, 42]; that antibodies to whole wheat and rye detected by indirect immunofluorescence are more common in schizophrenics than controls [43]; and that 50% of schizophrenics have lymphocyte reactivity to gluten similar to that found in coeliac disease [2]. However, other studies have failed to confirm a relationship between schizophrenia as a diagnosis, or schizophrenic symptoms, and antibodies to wheat or gluten [54, 64, 93].

A number of dietary studies have been carried out. Three have appeared to find minor and more rapid improvements in schizophrenics fed gluten-free diets [24, 25, 99]. One has been criticized in several respects [56, 100]. Three other published dietary trials have provided no support for the gluten hypothesis [74, 80, 106] but one has provided some support in that one of 16 patients improved on the gluten-free diet and deteriorated on gluten challenge [89].

For the time being Dohan's hypothesis of a toxic effect of cereal-derived peptides in the genesis of schizophrenia must remain a hypothesis. The evidence in favour of it is not convincing and the fairest judgement is the Scottish legal verdict of 'Not Proven'. The only data which can be taken as supporting the hypothesis are circumstantial and do not provide any direct evidence to incriminate a role for allergic mechanisms in the generation of mental symptoms or psychosis.

Other psychological changes and psychiatric disorders

Several publications on food allergy contain statements that mania, depression and other unspecified 'neurotic' and 'psychotic' changes can be induced by food. A small number of cases are cited where these contentions are said to have been confirmed by blind feeding experiments, but virtually none of these provide enough detail of experimental procedure to allow an objective appraisal of the conclusions.

Suggestion can produce virtually any subjective symptom, as well as many measurable organic changes. Experience with double-blind feeding tests has shown clearly the unreliability of histories of previous reactions to foods, of open reintroduction and of most commonly used ancillary tests for the diagnosis of organic food intolerance, even in patients with classical physical allergic states. However, despite this, many of those who attribute mania, depression and other psychological symptoms to food deny the possible relevance of the placebo effect to their findings, or the necessity to prove their claims by double-blind feeding.

In a high proportion of the reports under discussion the main evidence to support the involvement of foods, other than subjective impressions, has been the results of controversial techniques such as the pulse test and variations of sublingual and subcutaneous provocation tests (e.g. [53, 65]). Although the administration of antigen extracts by any route can induce a wide range of changes, including anaphylaxis, in patients with genuine IgE-mediated allergy, these tests are not accepted as reliable indicators of clinically relevant sensitization by most scientific workers. Reviews of the evidence concerning them by committees of eminent bodies in both Britain [32] and the USA [9, 12] have concluded that their efficacy is highly doubtful even in atopic disease.

The most important evidence quoted as supporting the validity of these controversial techniques in psychological disorders is the double-blind study of King [53]. Thirty patients attending a Center for Bio-ecologic Disease were selected for study on the basis of their inclusion of at least one psychological symptom (such as anxiety, depression, confusion, difficulty in concentrating) among their presenting complaints. The group scored highly on a standard personality inventory (MMPI) for 'depression', 'hysteria', 'hypochondriasis' and 'schizophrenia'. Acute changes were assessed after sublingual administrations of four individually selected antigens and two placebos given at 10-minute intervals.

King found no significant differences in mean pulse-rate changes after allergen or placebo challenges, but mean 'cognitive–emotional' symptom scores were greater after allergen than placebo administrations. However, these symptoms did occur after placebo in a significant number of patients, in some of whom mean post-placebo 'cognitive–emotional' symptom scores were greater than those postallergen. The study can be criticized on the grounds that it is doubtful that it remained truly double-blind: the placebo was triple-distilled water, whereas the allergens were standard extracts which taste of phenol. Data within the report indicate that the subjects virtually always distinguished allergen extracts from water and that they identified more than half of the placebo administrations as water or saline. In addition, by interacting with the kinin system, phenols may themselves induce symptoms such as fatigue, lethargy and irritability [107] (see also Chapter 40 for discussion).

At the present time, no test, other than double-blind feeding, can be accepted as adequate proof that any response to food is due to organic sensitivity. To the best of our knowledge, apart from the studies already considered in this chapter, there are only three other sufficiently detailed reports in which it has been suggested that psychological symptoms have been produced in this manner: that of Finn and Cohen [31], that of Brown and colleagues [10] and that of Denman [18].

Clinical cases

In 1978 Finn and Cohen [31] reported six cases of patients with severe physical symptoms and either social or psychological problems which resolved on dietary exclusion and in three of whom physical symptoms were produced by food provocation through a nasogastric tube. Tea and coffee were the most important foods held responsible. Five of the cases had symptoms compatible with caffeinism and three were recorded as usually ingesting unusually large doses of caffeine-containing drinks. One self-professed 'tea-fiend' suffered from anxiety and agoraphobia whilst having recurrent supraventricular tachycardias, but returned to a normal social life when these settled with tea and coffee avoidance.

Few clinical details of their 12 subjects were given by Brown et al [10] except that they had multiple symptoms and were similar to those studied by Finn and Cohen. It was stated that eight had depression, eight had headache or migraine and seven bowel disturbances. The most commonly incriminated foods were grain, milk, egg, coffee and tea. Unspecified symptoms followed double-blind provocation with the incriminated foods, more commonly than with placebo, in the group as a whole. However, only three patients reacted to each antigen preparation without reacting to any of the placebos and it is not clear if any of the depressed patients were in this group. The diagnosis of organic intolerance cannot be considered to have been confirmed in the six patients in this series who apparently responded to 50% or more of the control challenges. This casts some doubt on any conclusion that depression was a direct consequence of the foods themselves, since at least two of the patients with this complaint must have been included in the latter group.

Denman [18] briefly described the case of a 14-year-old girl who had a history of gastrointestinal symptoms in childhood which were related to milk intolerance. When she lapsed from her milk-free diet she developed 'mental disturbance' which took the form of irrational bouts of crying and 'hysteria' and episodes when she would withdraw, 'hear voices' and develop 'similar illusions'. When provoked double-blind only milk was said to lead to a recurrence of her physical and psychological symptoms and they were blocked by sodium cromoglycate. It was also stated that milk provocation led to complement activation and an increase in serum IgE levels. Although the latter observations would suggest that this was a case of food *allergic* disease, the approach to the description of the psychopathology raises doubts, perhaps unjustifiably, concerning this aspect of the case. (See Table 39.10.)

caffeinism and toxic responses to some less common food contaminants, there is no convincing scientifically acceptable evidence that demonstrates that foods are directly responsible for any form of psychological disorder whether occurring in the presence or absence of physical features of allergy.

There is growing evidence that large numbers of people may wrongly attribute psychological symptoms and signs to 'food allergy' when they are actually suffering with common minor psychiatric disorders for which they prefer an organic to a psychologi-

Table 39.10 Evidence for and against direct involvement of allergic mechanisms in psychological disorders.

For	Against
1 General associations of certain personality characteristics and neurotic symptoms with atopic diseases	Explicable as psychological responses to physical disorder and its consequent social disturbances
2 Case reports of acute neurological and psychological changes associated with shock or severe asthma	Explicable as features of cerebral hypoxia
3 Psychological changes of 'allergic tension–fatigue' syndrome and other behavioural changes in children	Not confirmed to occur in the absence of distressing physical symptoms
4 Gluten hypothesis of schizophrenia	Evidence is circumstantial and contested
5 Occurrence of food-induced migraine	Anatomical site of immunological reaction uncertain. Many cases may be pharmacological or toxic rather than immunological
6 Small number of studies utilizing double-blind food provocation in non-atopic conditions	Most fail to show evidence of acute psychological responses during allergic reactions. Some psychological responses may be pharmacological

CONCLUSIONS

People with allergic diseases, and especially children with food intolerances, can experience psychological distress and display behavioural abnormalities which are secondary to the physical symptoms from which they are suffering. In very young children these behavioural features may be the reason for their presentation, particularly if the underlying physical symptoms are overlooked.

The presence of any disease in childhood interacts with the other influences on personality and social development. Anxiety and depressive reactions are understandable responses to physical disability at any age. In addition hypoxia caused by even relatively mild asthma can have significant effects on cerebral function and there is inadequate appreciation of the central nervous system side-effects of many of the drugs used to treat allergic disorders.

Apart from mental changes associated with

cal explanation, and that these false beliefs are derived ultimately from medical workers having failed to apply objective criteria to their study of putative allergic phenomena.

Whether or not the diagnosis of food allergy can be confirmed objectively, there is no doubt that dietary treatment carries significant risks of malnutrition and deficiency diseases in both children and adults. Considering the risk, particularly in psychologically unstable individuals, there is presently no justification for applying exclusion diets to patients who do not have classical atopic disorders except as part of a properly controlled research project.

When it comes to the prevention and relief of human suffering there is likely to be more to gain from the adoption of a truly holistic approach to patients with classical physical allergic diseases than searching for rare cases of psychosis or neurosis directly attributable to food allergy. In atopic disease allergic and non-allergic external physical factors often interact with somatic and psychological responses to the social environment. Adequate treatment of the physical features of the condition may also have both short- and long-term psychological and social benefits. However, in some cases proper treatment of co-incident psychiatric or social problems will have a beneficial effect on somatic symptomatology. Effective drugs for the treatment of allergic symptoms often have unwanted physical and psychological side-effects, but allergen-avoidance regimes can be socially disruptive and, in the case of foods, are not without hazards to physical health. In every case the potential benefit of each form of therapy must be balanced against its risks.

REFERENCES

1 Aitken RCB, Zealley AK, Rosenthal SV: Psychological and physiological measures of emotion in chronic asthmatic patients. J. Psychosom Res 1969; 13:289-97.

2 Ashkenazi A, Krasilowsky D, Levin S, et al: Immunologic reaction of psychotic patients to fractions of gluten. Am J Psychiatry 1979; 136:1306-9.

3 Becker AB, Simons KJ, Gillespie CA, Simons FE: The bronchodilator effects and pharmacokinetics of caffeine in asthma. N Engl J Med 1984; 310:743-6.

4 Bentley SJ, Pearson DJ, Rix KJB: Food hypersensitivity in irritable bowel syndrome. Lancet 1983; ii:295-7.

5 Ben-Zvi Z, Spohn WA, Young SH, Kattan M: Hypnosis for exercise-induced asthma. Am Rev Respir Dis 1982; 125:392-5.

6 Bernstein M, Day JH, Welsh A: Double-blind food challenge in the diagnosis of food sensitivity in the adult. J Allergy Clin Immunol 1982; 70:205-10.

7 Blackwood GW: Severe psychological disturbance resulting from abuse of nasal decongestants. Scott Med J 1982; 27: 175-6.

8 Bock SA, Lee W-Y, Remigio L, et al: Appraisal of skin tests with food extracts for diagnosis of food hypersensitivity. Clin Allergy 1978; 8:559-64.

9 Breneman JC, Hurst A, Heiner D, et al: Final report of the Food Allergy Committee of the American College of Allergists on the clinical evaluation of sublingual provocative testing method for diagnosis of food allergy. Ann Allergy 1974; 33:164-6.

10 Brown M, Gibney M, Husband PR, Radcliffe M: Food allergy in polysymptomatic patients. Practitioner 1981; 225:1651-4.

11 Buisseret PD: Common manifestations of cow's milk allergy in children. Lancet 1978; i:304-5.

12 Committee on Provocative Food Testing. Ann Allergy 1973; 31:375-81.

13 Cooper B: Epidemiology. In: Wing JK, ed. Schizophrenia: towards a new synthesis. London: Academic Press, 1978; 31-51.

14 Crook WG, Harrison WW, Crawford SE, Emerson BS: Systemic manifestations due to allergy. Report of 50 patients and a review of the literature on the subject (sometimes referred to as allergic toxaemia and the allergic-tension-fatigue syndrome). Pediatrics 1961; 27:790-9.

15 Davison HM: In discussion of paper by Clarke TW. The relation of allergy to character problems in children: a survey. Ann Allergy 1950; 8:175.

16 Dean G, Hanniffy L, Stevens F, et al: Schizophrenia and coeliac disease. J Irish Med Assoc 1975; 68: 545-6.

17 Dekker E, Pelser HE, Grosen J: Conditioning as a cause of asthmatic attacks: a laboratory study. J Psychosom Res 1957; 2:97-108.

18 Denman AM: The relevance of immunopathology to research into schizophrenia. In: Hemmings G, ed. Biochemistry of schizophrenia and addiction. Lancaster: MTP Press, 1980; 97-109.

19 Diaz MA, Wise TN, Semchyshyn GO: Self-medication with pseudoephedrine in a chronically depressed patient. Am J Psychiatry 1979; 136: 1217-8.

20 Dohan FC: Wartime changes in hospital admissions for schizophrenia. Acta Psychiatr Scand 1966; 42:1-23.

21 Dohan FC: Cereals and schizophrenia. Data and hypothesis. Acta Psychiatr Scand 1966; 42:125-52.

22 Dohan FC: The possible pathogenic effect of cereal grains in schizophrenia. Celiac disease as a model. Acta Neurol (Napoli) 1976; 31:195-205.

23 Dohan FC: Schizophrenia and neuroactive peptides from food. Lancet 1979; i:1031.

24 Dohan FC, Grasberger JC: Relapsed schizophrenics: earlier discharge from the hospital after cereal-free, milk-free diet. Am J Psychiatry 1973; 130:685-8.

25 Dohan FC, Grasberger JC, Lowell FM, et al: Relapsed schizophrenics: more rapid improvements on a milk- and cereal-free diet. Br J Psychiatry 1969; 115:595-6.

26 Dohan FC, Martin L, Grasberger JC et al: Antibodies to wheat gliadin in blood of psychiatric patients: possible role of emotional factors. Biol Psychiatry 1972; 5:127-37.

27 Dreisbach RH, Pfeiffer C: Caffeine-withdrawal headache. J Lab Clin Med 1943; 28:1212-9.

28 Egger J, Carter CM, Wilson J, et al: Is migraine food allergy? A double-blind controlled trial of oligoantigenic diet treatment. Lancet 1984; ii:865-9.

29 Escobar JI, Karno M: Chronic hallucinosis from nasal drops. J Am Med Assoc 1983; 247:1859-60.

30 Feingold B: Why your child is hyperactive. New York: Random, 1975.

31 Finn R, Cohen NH: 'Food allergy': fact or fiction? Lancet 1978; i:426-8.

32 Food intolerance and food aversion. Joint report of the Royal College of Physicians and the British Nutrition Foundation. J R Coll Physicians Lond 1984; 18:83-123.

33 Furukawa CT, Shapiro GG, DuHamel T, et al: Learning and behaviour problems associated with theophylline therapy. Lancet 1984; i:621.

34 Glover V, Peatfield R, Zammit-Pace R, et al: Platelet monoamine oxidase activity and headache. J Neurol Neurosurg Psychiatry 1981; 44:786-90.

35 Golbert TM, Patterson R, Slavin RG: Psychiatric aspects of allergic diseases. In: Patterson R, ed. Allergic diseases: diagnosis and treatment. Philadelphia and Toronto: Lippincott 1972; 547-58.

36 Goldstein A, Kaizer S: Psychotropic effects of coffee in man, IIIA. Questionnaire survey of coffee drinkers

and its effects in a group of housewives. Clin Pharmacol Ther 1969; 10:477–88.

37 Graham DT, Wolf S, Wolff HG: Changes in tissue sensitivity associated with varying life situations and emotions: their relevance to allergy. J Allergy 1950; 21:478–86.

38 Graham PJ, Rutter ML, Yule W, Pless IB: Childhood asthma: a psychosomatic disorder? Some epidemiological considerations. Br J Prev Soc Med 1967; 21:78–85.

39 Greden JF: Anxiety or caffeinism: a diagnostic dilemma. Am J Psychiatry 1974; 131:1089–92.

40 Hale F, Margen S, Rabak D: Postprandial hypoglycaemia and 'psychological' symptoms. Biol Psychiatry 1982; 17:125–30.

41 Hargreave FE, Ryan G, Thomson NC, et al: Bronchial responsiveness to histamine or methacholine in asthma: measurement and clinical significance. J Allergy Clin Immunol 1981; 68:347–55.

42 Hekkens WThJM: Antibodies to gliadin in serum of normals, coeliac patients and schizophrenics. In: Hemming GW, Hemmings WA, eds. The biological basis of schizophrenia. Lancaster: MTP Press, 1978; 259–61.

43 Hekkens WThJM, Schipperijn AJM, Freed DLJ: Antibodies to wheat proteins in schizophrenia: relationship or coincidence? In: Hemmings G, ed. Biochemistry of schizophrenia and addiction. Lancaster: MTP Press, 1980; 125–33.

44 Hendrix S, Sale S, Zeiss CR, et al: Factitious Hymenoptera allergic emergency: a report of a new variant of Munchausen's syndrome. J Allergy Clin Immunol 1981; 67:8–13.

45 Herbert M: Personality factors and bronchial asthma. A study of South African Indian children. J Psychosom Res 1965; 8:353–64.

46 Herridge CF, A'Brook MF: Ephedrine psychosis. Br Med J 1968; ii:160.

47 Hoobler BR: Some early symptoms suggesting protein sensitization in infancy. Am J Dis Child 1916; 12:129–35.

48 Johnson DD, Dorr KE, Swenson WM, Service FJ: Reactive hypoglycaemia. J Am Med Assoc 1980; 243:1151–5.

49 Justesen DR, Braun EW, Garrison RG, Pendleton RB: Pharmacological differentiation of allergic and classically conditioned asthma in the guinea pig. Science 1970; 170:864–6.

50 Kashani J, Simonds JF: The incidence of depression in children. Am J Psychiatry 1979; 136:1203–5.

51 Kennedy F: Cerebral symptoms induced by angioneurotic oedema. Arch Neurol Psychiatry 1926; 15:28–33.

52 Kennedy F: Certain nervous complications following the use of therapeutic and prophylactic sera. Am J Med Sci 1929; 177:555–9.

53 King DS: Can allergic exposure provoke psychological symptoms? A double-blind test. Biol Psychiatry 1981; 16:3–19.

54 Kinnell HG, Kirkwood E, Lewis C: Food antibodies in schizophrenia. Psychol Med 1982; 12:85–9.

55 Leighton KM: Paranoid psychosis after abuse of Actifed. Br Med J 1982; 284:789–90.

56 Levy DL, Weinreb HJ: Wheat-gluten schizophrenia findings. Science 1976; 194:448.

57 Lewis BI: Hyperventilation syndromes: clinical and physiological observations. Postgrad Med 1957; 21:259–71.

58 Lishman WA: Organic psychiatry: the psychological consequences of cerebral disorder. Oxford: Blackwell, 1978.

59 Littlewood J, Glover V, Sandler M, et al: Platelet phenolsulphotransferase deficiency in dietary migraine. Lancet 1982; ii:983–6.

60 Lum LC: The syndrome of chronic habitual ventilation. In: Hill OW, ed. Modern trends in psychosomatic medicine. Vol 3. London: Butterworth, 1976;196–230.

61 Lum LC: Total allergy. Br Med J 1982; 284:1044.

62 McFadden ER Jr: Pathogenesis of asthma. J Allergy Clin Immunol 1984; 73:413–28.

63 McFadden ER Jr, Luparella T, Lyons HA, Bleecker ER:The mechanism of action of suggestion in the induction of acute asthma attacks. Psychosom Med 1969; 31:134–43.

64 McGuffin P, Gardiner P, Swinburne LM: Schizophrenia, celiac disease and antibodies to food. Biol Psychiatry 1981; 16:281–5.

65 Mackarness R: Not all in the mind. London: Pan, 1976.

66 McNichol KN, Williams HL, Allan J, McAndrew I: Spectrum of asthma in children. III. Psychological and social components. Br Med J 1973; iv:16–20.

67 Magarian GJ: Hyperventilation syndromes: infrequently recognized common expressions of anxiety and stress. Medicine (Baltimore) 1982; 67:219–36.

68 May CD: Objective clinical and laboratory studies of immediate hypersensitivity reactions to foods in asthmatic children. J Allergy Clin Immunol 1976; 58:500–15.

69 May CD: Food allergy: lessons from the past. J Allergy Clin Immunol 1982; 69:255–9.

70 Merrett J, Peatfield RC, Clifford Rose F, Merrett TG: Food related antibodies in headache patients. J Neurol Neurosurg Psychiatry 1983; 46:738–42.

71 Minford AMB, MacDonald A, Littlewood JM: Food intolerance and food allergy in children: a review of 68 cases. Arch Dis Child 1982; 57:742–7.

72 Mitchell RG, Dawson B: Educational and social characteristics of children with asthma. Arch Dis Child 1973; 48:467–71.

73 Neuhaus EC: A personality study of asthmatic and cardiac children. Psychosom Med 1957; 20:181–6.

74 Osborne M, Crayton JW, Javaid J, Davis JM:Lack of effect of a gluten-free diet on neuroleptic blood levels in schizophrenic patients. Biol Psychiatry 1982; 17:627–9.

75 Ossofsky HJ: Endogenous depression in infancy and childhood. Compr Psychiatry 1974; 15:19–25.

76 Oswald NC, Walker RE, Drinkwater J: Relationship between breathlessness and anxiety in asthma and bronchitis: a comparative study. Br Med J 1970; ii:14–7.

77 Pardee I: Two cases demonstrating allergic reactions in the nervous system. J Nerv Ment Dis 1938; 88:88–91.

78 Pearson DJ, Rix KJB: Allergomimetic reactions to food and pseudo-food allergy. In: Dikor P, Kallos P, Schumberger HD, West GB, eds. Pseudo-allergic reactions. Vol 4. Basel: Karger, 1985; 59–105.

79 Pearson DJ, Rix KJB, Bentley SJ: Food allergy: how much in the mind? A clinical and psychiatric study of suspected food hypersensitivity. Lancet 1983; i:1259–61.

80 Potkin SG, Weinberger D, Kleinman J, et al: Wheat gluten challenge in schizophrenic patients. Am J Psychiatry 1981; 138:1208–11.

81 Rall TW: Central nervous system stimulants, The

xanthines. In: Gilman AG, Goodman LS, Gilman A, eds. Goodman and Gilman's pharmacological basis of therapeutics. 6th edn. New York: Macmillan, 1980; 592–607.

82 Randolph TG: Fatigue and weakness of allergic origin (allergic toxaemia) to be differentiated from nervous fatigue and neurasthenia. Ann Allergy 1945; 3:418–30.

83 Randolph TG: Allergy as a causative factor of fatigue, irritability and behaviour problems of children. J Pediatr 1947; 31:560–72.

84 Randolph TG: Concepts of food allergy important in specific diagnosis. J Allergy 1950; 21:471–7.

85 Randolph TG: Adaptation to specific environmental exposures enhanced by individual susceptibility. In: Dickey LD, ed. Clinical ecology. Springfield: Charles C Thomas, 1976; 46–66.

86 Randolph TG: Stimulatory and withdrawal levels and the alternations of allergic manifestations. In: Dickey LD, ed. Clinical ecology. Springfield: Charles C Thomas, 1976; 156–75.

87 Randolph TG, Moss RW: Allergies: your hidden enemy. How the new science of clinical ecology is unravelling the causes of mental and physical illness. Wellingborough: Turnstone Press, 1981.

88 Rapp DJ: Double-blind confirmation and treatment of milk sensitivity. Med J Aust 1978; 1:571–2.

89 Rice JR, Ham CH, Gore WE: Another look at gluten in schizophrenia. Am J Psychiatry 1978; 135:1417–8.

90 Rinkel HJ: Food allergy: the role of food allergy in internal medicine. Ann Allergy 1944; 2:115–24.

91 Rix KJB, Lumsden Rix EM: Alcohol problems. Bristol: Wright PSG, 1983:81.

92 Rix KJB, Pearson DJ, Bentley SJ: A psychiatric study of patients with supposed food allergy. Br J Psychiatry 1984; 145:121–6.

93 Rix KJB, Ditchfield J, Freed DLJ, et al: Food antibodies in acute psychoses. Psychol Med 1985; 15:347–54.

94 Rowe AH: Allergic toxaemia and migraine due to food allergy. Calif West Med 1930; 33:785–93.

95 Rowe AH: Food allergy: its manifestations, diagnosis and treatment with a general discussion of bronchial asthma. London: Baillière, Tindall and Cox, 1931.

96 Roxanas MG, Spalding J: Ephedrine abuse psychosis. Med J Aust 1977; 2:639–40.

97 Sampson HA: Role of immediate food hypersensitivity in the pathogenesis of atopic dermatitis. J Allergy Clin Immunol 1983; 71:473–80.

98 Sankey RJ, Nunn AJ, Sills JA: Visual hallucinations in children receiving decongestants. Br Med J 1984; 288:1369.

99 Singh MM, Kay SR: Wheat gluten as a pathogenic factor in schizophrenia. Science 1976; 191:401–2.

100 Smith JM: Wheat-gluten schizophrenia findings. Science 1976; 194:448.

101 Snow S, Logan T, Hollender M: Nasal spray addiction and psychosis: a case report. Br J Psychiatry 1980; 136:297–9.

102 Speer F: The allergic-tension-fatigue syndrome. Pediatr Clin North Am 1954; 1:1029–37.

103 Speer F: Allergy of the nervous system. Springfield: Charles C Thomas, 1970.

104 Staffiere D, Bentolila L, Levit L: Hemiplegia and allergic symptoms following ingestion of certain foods. Ann Allergy 1952; 10:38–9.

105 Stevens FM, Lloyd RS, Gerachty SMJ, et al: Schizophrenia and coeliac disease—the nature of the relationship. Psychol Med 1977; 7:259–63.

106 Storms LH, Clopton JM, Wright C: Effects of gluten on schizophrenics. Arch Gen Psychiatry 1982; 39:323–7.

107 Streeten DHP, Kerr LP, Kerr CB, et al: Hyperbradykinism: a new orthostatic syndrome. Lancet 1972; ii:1048–53.

108 Szentivanyi A, Fishel CW: The beta-adrenergic theory and cyclic AMP-mediated control mechanisms in human asthma. In: Weiss EB, Segal MS, eds. Bronchial asthma, mechanisms and therapeutics. Boston: Little, Brown and Co, 1976; 137–53.

109 Taylor E: Annotation: food additives, allergy and hyperkinesis. J Child Psychol Psychiatry 1979; 20:357–63.

110 Vaughan WT, Hawke IK: Angioneurotic oedema with some unusual manifestations. J Allergy 1931; 2:125–9.

111 Warner JO, Hathaway MJ: Allergic form of Meadow's syndrome (Munchausen by proxy). Arch Dis Child 1984; 59:151–6.

112 Weiss JH: Mood states associated with asthma in children. J Psychosom Res 1966; 10:267–73.

113 Wurtman RJ: Behavioural effects of nutrients. Lancet 1983; i:1145–7.

114 Zioudrou C, Streaty RA, Klee WA: Opioid peptides derived from food proteins: the exorphins. J Biol Chem 1979; 254:2446–9.

Chapter 40
Effects of Food Allergy on the Central Nervous System

Iris R. Bell

Introduction

The purpose of this chapter is to discuss the effects of adverse food reactions, allergies and intolerances on the central nervous system (CNS) that have not been covered elsewhere in this volume. Such areas include (a) neurological disorders, e.g. seizures and sleep disorders, and (b) psychiatric disorders, e.g. schizophrenia, depression, bulimia, anxiety and somatization disorder. A systems perspective with the biopsychosocial model will provide the framework for evaluation of theory and methodology of the relevant studies.

The debate over the existence of adverse food reactions with CNS symptoms has raged for many years [12, 71, 79, 96]. As the review of the literature below will suggest, definitive conclusions are still not justified from the available data. Overall the evidence suggests that some, but not all, patients with certain neurological and psychiatric diagnoses may react adversely to foods. Such reactions generally do not meet strict criteria for Type I, reaginic allergy, but rather occur due to other immunological and non-immunological mechanisms.

Foods and central nervous system function: non-immunological

Table 40.1 [71] lists ways in which foods may alter central nervous system function. These include biological mechanisms—metabolic, pharmacological, toxic or immunological—and psychological mechanisms—expectation, suggestion or classical conditioning. The diet provides the precursors with which the brain makes neurotransmitters and neuromodulators. These are the endogenous chemicals with which brain cells communicate with each other [23]. Furthermore, the gastrointestinal system releases various endogenous and food-derived hormones during digestion that are themselves neuromodulators [32, 39]. Finally, immunological reactions also release various mediators such as histamine, kinins and prostaglandins that can modify nervous tissue function.

When brain chemistry changes, the behaviours that the affected parts of the brain control may also change [41, 91]. An assumption behind much of the work on adverse CNS reactions to foods is that the foods induce dysfunctional changes in brain chemistry. Dysfunction of the central nervous system can present with either neurological or psychiatric symptoms [61]. The nature of the symptoms

Table 40.1 Examples of food intolerance due to non-immunological mechanisms.

1 Contaminants
  (a) Dyes
     Tartrazine
  (b) Flavourings and preservatives
     Nitrites and nitrates
     Monosodium glutamate
     Sulphiting agents
     Antibiotics
  (c) Toxins
    (i) Bacterial
      Botulism
    (ii) Endogenous
      Certain mushrooms
      Shellfish
  (d) Insect parts
  (e) Moulds
2 Gastrointestinal disease
  (a) Structural abnormalities
     Hiatal hernia
     Intestinal obstruction
  (b) Enzyme deficiencies
     Lactase deficiency
     G-6-PD deficiency
     Galactosaemia
     Favism
  (c) Malignancy
  (d) Other
     Peptic ulcer disease
     Gall bladder disease
     Parasites
     Cystic fibrosis
3 Pharmacological agents
  (a) Endogenous
     Histamine
     Tyramine
     Phenylethylamine
  (b) Exogenous
     Alcohol
     Caffeine
4 Psychological reactions
5 Other
  (a) Collagen vascular diseases
  (b) Endocrine disorders

Reprinted from Metcalfe [71], with permission.
G-6-PD = glucose-6-phosphate dehydrogenase.

depends on the location of the affected areas in the brain.

Systems theory and adverse food reactions in the CNS

A diverse body of scientific evidence suggests that foods can affect brain function by both biological and psychological means [7]. Furthermore, such mechanisms are likely to interact in any given patient. Systems theory and its multilevelled corollary, the biopsychosocial model, can accommodate simultaneous causes at multiple, interacting levels for a net disease or disorder [37, 38, 59, 89, 90, 98, 106]. The dictionary defines a system as 'a

regularly interacting or interdependent group of items forming a unified whole' [109]. Any system may be itself a component of a larger system or a synthesis of a group of smaller systems (Fig. 40.1). Disorder in a system at

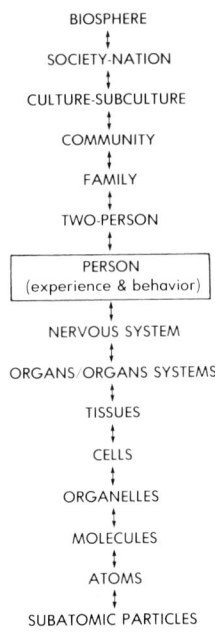

Fig. 40.1 Hierarchy of natural systems. Reprinted from Engel [38], with permission.

any level of organization implies disorder in systems above and/or below the identified system of the hierarchy.

The recent description of exercise-induced anaphylaxis to foods is an example of interactive factors in clinical allergy. In this phenomenon, patients are tolerant to specific food ingestion alone or to exercise alone, but not to the combination [50, 69, 92]. Other research, on interactive effects of psychological and biological stressors, has produced similar findings [48, 57, 93]. Hence, the psychological and physical environment in which a subject receives a substance can alter the biological impact of that substance. These considerations may be useful to apply in evaluating the clinical and research studies on adverse CNS effects of foods.

NEUROLOGICAL DISORDERS AND ADVERSE FOOD REACTIONS

Seizure disorders

Throughout this century, various clinical observers have reported the provocation of epileptic convulsions by specific foods and/or other allergens (see [16, 27, 96, 104] for reviews). Some have examined populations of epileptics and found an unusually high prevalence of allergic disorders or eosinophilia [1, 18, 26, 28, 29, 95, 107, 108]. Others have considered groups of allergic patients and noted a high prevalence of neurological and electroencephalographic (EEG) abnormalities, including seizure disorders [5, 17, 20, 30, 43, 99, 103]. Dees [28-30] observed increased prevalence of occipital dysrhythmias in allergic-convulsive patients. Campbell [18] has commented that the types of seizures reported in association with allergic reactions range from rare cases of grand mal and petit mal to, more commonly, focal seizures, including temporal lobe patterns. Some clinical studies have not

not chicken (placebo) ingestion (Fig. 40.2). A criticism that could be levelled at this study is possible contamination, by order effects, of the results. That is, the patient received a timed sequence of placebo-active-placebo-active. It can be argued that different results might follow from a reversed order, i.e. active-placebo-active-placebo, or from a larger number of trials. The number of trials in this protocol was too low to rule out accurate guessing of the identity of the test items by the patient.

Nonetheless, the systematic approach of this controlled case study is an important contribution to clinical research in this area and essential to any future studies on larger population of epileptics. In protocols such as that of Egger and associates [35], for example, follow-up research on the reported reduction

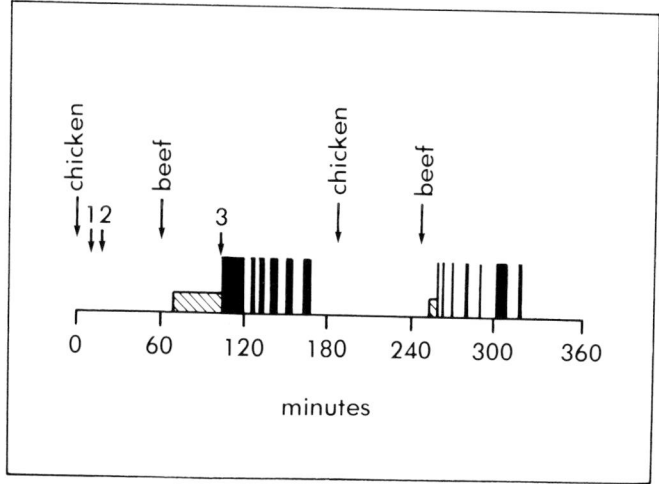

Fig. 40.2 Sequence of double-blind challenges. Capsules containing 6 g of chicken or beef were given at the indicated times. There was no response to the chicken. Within 15 minutes of beef ingestion, the patient became unresponsive (hatched area). The patient then had a series of grand mal seizures (solid bars). Numbers 1, 2 and 3 locate points where EEG illustrations were recorded. Reprinted from Crayton et al [25], with permission.

found an association between epilepsy and allergy [10, 40].

The concomitant occurrence of allergic and epileptic phenomena in the same patient at best implies a correlative, not necessarily a causative, relationship between the disorders. In addition, the majority of reports in the literature on foods and seizures lack rigour in their methodology and omit appropriate statistical analyses of their results. They are therefore open to alternative hypotheses to explain the reported 'seizures' in their patients, such as patient expectation, psychogenic seizures and psychologically conditioned triggering of seizures with awareness of test-food identity [25].

However, Crayton and colleagues [25] have documented a single case study with double-blind, placebo-controlled methodology. They demonstrated provocation of tonic-clonic, grand mal convulsions after beef (active) but

of fits on oligoantigenic diets might utilize EEG laboratory studies of double-blind, controlled challenge feedings.

Cerebral transient ischaemic attacks (TIAs)

One case report in the literature [36] claimed that a 58-year-old patient with TIAs experienced a marked decrease in frequency of attacks on reduction of egg ingestion. The patient was skin test negative for egg allergy. He exhibited a correlated drop in blood cholesterol levels with reduced egg intake. This study is suggestive, but not convincing. The investigators relied on subjective reports by the patient of TIA frequency rather than on any objective measure of neurological or cerebrovascular function. Improvement with expectation alone and with attention from the physicians might have led to biased and selective reporting of episodes by the patient.

Furthermore, the authors concluded that acute increases in cholesterol were the mechanism of their patient's TIAs. However, they failed to address a wide range of other possible mechanisms, including non-reaginic immunological events and non-immunological mediator release leading to vascular spasm. Although this case report raises the issue of adverse food reactions in transient ischaemic attacks, the area remains unexplored in larger groups of patients.

Sleep disorders

Disorders of sleep include the insomnias and the hypersomnias [46]. Direct or indirect effects of adverse food reactions may play a key role in certain subtypes of the sleep disorders. These phenomena may also link certain types of psychopathology to abnormalities of sleep.

Sleep apnoea. For example, sleep apnoea is a syndrome characterized by repetitive cessations of breathing during the sleep state. The apnoeas can be central (triggered by CNS respiratory drive failure) and/or obstructive (triggered by local tissue blockage of the upper airway with naso-oropharyngeal muscle relaxation in sleep) [47]. Many cases of sleep apnoea involve mixed central and obstructive factors. Symptoms and signs associated with sleep apnoeas include frequent nocturnal awakenings, complaints of insomnia, daytime fatigue and hypersomnolence and hypertension [47, 58].

Using a within-subjects design, researchers found that experimentally induced, complete nasal obstruction in normal men caused a significant increase in sleep disturbance as well as in mixed and central apnoeas as compared with unobstructed control sleep nights [111]. Another group investigated male and female patients with partial nasal occlusion due to seasonal allergic rhinitis [66]. They found a greater number and longer duration of obstructive apnoeas during the rhinitis period than during a subsequent, unobstructed period.

It is also relevant that investigators have noted a greater prevalence of depression in sleep apnoeics than in normals [11, 81]. Hypotheses that would follow from these data are that: (a) adverse reactions to foods cause rhinitis, with nasal and oropharyngeal oedema and local obstructive occlusion, in some individuals; (b) such individuals might therefore experience varying degrees of sleep apnoea; and (c) the psychobiological sequelae of sleep apnoea in some rhinitis patients might account in part for major depressive disorders—and perhaps for symptoms of the allergic tension-fatigue syndrome (see discussion below and [11, 96]. Research on these potential, indirect CNS effects of food reactions remains to be done.

Restless legs syndrome. A more direct, pharmacological factor from the diet in another type of sleep disorder may be caffeine. Restless legs is a syndrome characterized by severe discomfort in the extremities at rest that often leads to insomnia with a need to move the limbs. Lutz [63] concluded that excessive caffeine intake in his case series of 62 patients was the aetiological agent for restless legs syndrome. However, he presented no group data on his sample and failed to study control subjects. He mixed caffeine avoidance with diazepam treatment in some cases. He apparently based his conclusions on these clinical observations alone. While his comments pose the hypothesis that caffeine ingestion induces restless legs in susceptible individuals, he presently lacks systematic, controlled data to support his position. Furthermore, various clinicians have claimed benefit from other nutritional, as well as pharmacological, treatments for this condition [46].

Hypersomnia. Non-pharmacological dietary constituents may play a role in the hypersomnic sleep disorders. Some clinical observers in the fields of allergy and neurology have reported cases of idiopathic hypersomnia associated with specific food ingestion [8, 27, 70, 102]. Again, no systematic work on such patients has yet been completed.

Narcolepsy. Narcolepsy is a type of hypersomnia with irresistible sleep attacks, cataplexy, sleep paralysis and hypnogogic hallucinations [47]. Bell and colleagues [6, 9] have compared diet and symptom histories of narcoleptic patients versus normals and food-allergic patients (diagnosed by history and clinical testing). They found that the narcoleptics were significantly more overweight than were the other two groups. In addition, the narcoleptics reported significantly higher prevalence (71%) of sleepiness after meals as compared with normals (9%) and food allergics (20%). Both patient groups craved sweets more than did the normals.

Diet and sleep. The narcoleptics anecdotally observed a worsening of their condition on high-carbohydrate diets and a lessening of symptoms on high-protein diets. Systematic laboratory study of this subjective observation is also lacking in narcoleptics. Nevertheless, extensive research in other areas of the neurosciences is consistent with the narcoleptics' reports of carbohydrate versus protein effects.

This latter observation may relate to the narcoleptics' exaggerated response to a normal physiological mechanism. Recently Fernstrom and Wurtman [22, 41, 110] completed a series of animal and human studies on the effects of varying dietary constituents on brain chemistry and behaviour. They discovered that ingestion of a high-carbohydrate diet leads to increases in brain uptake of the precursor amino acid tryptophan and thereby to more synthesis of the neurotransmitter serotonin. Serotonin is one the key transmitters in the induction of normal sleep. Indeed, sleep researchers have found in EEG studies that nutritional supplements of L-tryptophan will produce improvement in the sleep of certain insomniacs [60].

Diet changes and sleep in non-allergic subjects. Spring et al [97] have expanded on this work and examined the effects of high-carbohydrate (non-dairy sherbet) and high-protein (turkey meat) meals on normal human subjects at different times of day. Female subjects reported greater sleepiness and male subjects more calmness after the high-carbohydrate versus the protein meals. Older subjects also showed some cognitive impairment with attentional deficits after a high-carbohydrate meal at lunchtime, but not at breakfast time.

Taken together, such data suggest that the general composition of the diet, age and sex of the subjects and time of day may recruit specific physiological mechanisms for regulation of neurological and behavioural functioning.

Some narcoleptics and hypersomniacs may suffer adverse food reactions via an exaggerated response to these normal fluctuations in brain chemistry in susceptible neural pathways. In such situations, allergic or immunological mechanisms would not necessarily mediate the food effects. The food reactions would constitute a necessary but not sufficient condition for expression of the sleep syndrome. Dietary changes might nonetheless alter the course of the sleep disorder. An alternative hypothesis, even in the Spring study,

of course, is that a physiological and/or psychological variable other than serotonin synthesis mediated the food effects on the subjects. No effort was made in that particular experiment to blind the identity of the foods, despite a systematic between-group design.

PSYCHIATRIC DISORDERS AND ADVERSE FOOD REACTIONS

Schizophrenia

Various observers have reported dietary factors in chronic schizophrenia [33, 34, 65, 94]. The most prominent hypothesis recently has been Dohan's assertion [34] that wheat gluten exacerbates and a cereal-free, milk-free diet lessens psychiatric symptoms in hospitalized schizophrenics. Dohan based his approach on epidemiological evidence for an association between coeliac disease, wheat consumption and schizophrenic symptoms. Singh and Kay [94] also studied the effects of blind administration of wheat gluten on hospitalized schizophrenics. They found worsening of multiple psychopathological symptoms with the 4-week gluten-containing diet.

Subsequent researchers reported attempts to replicate these findings without success [72, 74, 100]. Another group of investigators [82] found that only two out of 16 schizophrenics in their sample suffered adverse psychiatric effects of gluten ingestion. Important differences in methodology may explain some of the discrepancies between the positive and negative gluten experiments.

The importance of correct statistics

Notably, King [53] has pointed out a relationship between the statistical power and the outcome of these various studies (Table 40.2). Statistical power reflects the probability of detecting an effect that is present in a population. As his table suggests, gluten studies with smaller sample sizes and lower power had negative outcomes while those with larger samples and higher power had positive findings. Overall his observations suggest that researchers may fail to find an effect that is actually present if they sample too few patients for a factor (e.g. gluten or other food sensitivity) from which only some of the total population of patients with the same diagnosis may suffer.

These considerations make it important to avoid confusing two hypotheses in the same

Table 40.2 Sample size, power and experimental outcome.

Study	Sample size	Power		Statistically significant?
Between-group design				
Dohan and Grasberger, 1973	115	0.75		Yes
Dohan et al, 1969	102	0.71		Yes
Storms et al, 1982	26	0.23		No
Within-group design		$r=0.6$	$r=0.8$	
Singh and Kay, 1976	14	0.52	0.80	Yes
Potkin et al, 1981	8	0.30	0.54	No
Osborne et al, 1982	5	<0.30	<0.54	No

Reprinted from King [53], with permission.

study. One question is: do adverse food reactions trigger psychiatric symptoms in *some* patients (responders)? Subject selection in this situation requires limiting the sample to identified food responders. A separate question is: How many responders exist in the total population of patients with a given diagnosis? Subject selection in the latter case involves sampling the population of responders and non-responders. Such issues pertain to future research on any of the CNS effects of foods that clinicians have reported.

Lymphocyte studies. Another approach to the possible role of food factors is the study of immunological variables in schizophrenics. Ashkenazi's group [3] reported that the lymphocytes of a subgroup of schizophrenics and other psychotics responded to gluten with increased production of leukocyte migration inhibition factor similar to that of coeliac patients. The cells of the remainder of the sampled schizophrenics showed no such responses. They also found no evidence for gastrointestinal malabsorption in the schizophrenics, in contrast to that seen in coeliacs. Other workers have noted the presence of B-type atypical lymphocytes in some schizophrenics [49], as well as decreased numbers of T cells [21].

Antibody studies. Apart from cellular immunity, between-group investigations of humoral immunity in schizophrenics have also yielded mixed outcomes. McGuffin et al [64] found no significant difference in food antibody titres to milk, egg white or gluten extract in schizophrenics, affective disorder patients and normal controls. Their sample size was roughly 30 per group, and they did not preselect subjects as food responders. A subsequent study by Kinnell et al [55] compared food antibody titres to oats, chicken, gluten, calf and milk in 98 schizophrenics with those of 90 psychiatrically normal relatives of the patients. This latter study found antibodies in only a small fraction of the patient group.

At best, studies of immune system status and food responsiveness suggest that some, but not most, schizophrenics may experience adverse CNS reactions to particular foods. Immune mechanisms may not play a key role in such reactions. An alternative physiological mechanism is peptide effects of specific foods. For example, some researchers have discovered that digestion of wheat gluten generates exorphins—peptides with opiate-like actions in the body [56]. Once absorbed, these substances could act as neuromodulators of brain chemistry and thereby alter behaviour [23]. Direct evidence for a role of exorphins in schizophrenic psychopathology is still needed.

Affective disorders

Randolph [78, 79] and other allergists [96] have reported clinical observations that adverse food reactions can trigger both unipolar and bipolar affective disorders. Surprisingly few systematic studies are available on this issue. Crayton's group (Crayton, JW, personal communication, 1984) has recently completed a double-blind, placebo-controlled study of capsule food challenges in a group of 40 depressed and schizophrenic patients compared with 20 control subjects. Their preliminary analyses suggest that a subgroup of the patients experienced significant provocation of their psychiatric symptoms and activation of the early components of complement with specific food challenges [24]. More detailed evaluation of this research must await a fuller presentation of the work in the literature.

Depression

Psychoimmunologists have also turned their attention to patients with major depressive disorders. One group [101] has found positive allergen-specific IgE tests to a wide range of inhalant substances and foods such as egg white in a greater percentage of depressives than control. As the authors themselves emphasize, these data can suggest a correlative, but not necessarily causative relationship between reaginic allergy and the psychiatric symptoms in their particular sample of patients. Another report [68] examined differences in the prevalence of typical allergic disorders (e.g. hay fever, eczema, asthma, urticaria) in different subgroups of depressed patients. In this survey, unipolar depressed women had the highest frequency of allergic disorders. However, these researchers made no effort to investigate the possible role of food versus other allergens in the allergies. In any event, coexistence of depression and allergies in the same patients may reflect correlation and not cause–effect.

Pearson and Rix discuss their work [73, 83] in Chapter 39. They found that a number of patients in whom food sensitivity was not confirmed had neurotic depressive disorders. Although they sampled the population of individuals who believed that they suffered psychological symptoms from food, their sample size was small ($n = 23$) and may have overlooked true responders.

Capsule challenges. An additional point about their work and that of Crayton is that the double-blind testing relied on capsule challenge feedings. It is possible that this means of administration in the experimental situation could not approximate meal-sized portions of test foods. For example, an adult would have to swallow approximately 12–13 No. 1 size capsules to achieve the small total dose of one tablespoon (8 g) of wheat flour. While this criticism may be irrelevant in true reaginic allergy reactions, a threshold effect for quantity may have led to false-negative tests in some patients with non-reaginic food intolerance.

T and B lymphocytes. Rea [80], in an uncontrolled study, has reported decreased absolute counts of T and B cells in patients with adverse food and chemical reactions. He observed both chronically low counts and acute T cell drops with psychological—often depressive—and somatic symptom provoca-

tion by foods. It is important to note, however, that many researchers in this area hypothesize that depressed mood per se induces the immune dysfunction. For instance, Schleifer's group [88] found a reduction in mitogen responsiveness and in absolute T and B cell counts in patients with major depressive disorders, compared with controls.

Their work followed the prospective study that documented a decrease in mitogen responsiveness in lymphocytes of bereaved spouses within weeks after the deaths [4]. Depressed affect often accompanies the grieving process. There was no report of adverse food reactions in the bereaved spouses before or after the deaths, and their immune defects emerged only after the specific psychosocial stressor. These data suggest that emotional distress could have been a primary trigger for these particular findings.

Some might argue that adverse food reactions trigger both the depression and the immunological abnormalities. Others might insist that foods trigger immune disorder that then causes depression by immunological mechanisms. However, psychoimmunologists might argue with equal force at this stage that psychosocial life stressors induce the depression, which in turn induces immune disturbances [2, 13, 48, 62] and perhaps even food intolerances in certain individuals. Further research on the biopsychosocial dimensions may elucidate the undoubtedly complex interactions among these different variables.

Eating disorders

Randolph [77, 79] proposes that many individuals with non-reaginic, chronic adverse food reactions become addicted to the offending foods. He states that such addictions develop as a manifestation of an adaptational process to the repeated insults with substances to which the patient has become intolerant. As a result, he suggests that these individuals suffer specific food cravings, withdrawal syndromes with increased symptoms on extended periods between ingestion of the offending items and temporary symptom relief on ingestion. Randolph also postulates that obesity is a consequence of food addiction in some patients. The discovery of opiate-like peptides in milk [15] and in digestion products of wheat [56] does make a food addiction hypothesis plausible, but no other data on this issue are available.

Some of Randolph's clinical cases [78] suggest histories of binge eating that might meet current criteria for bulimic eating patterns [31]. However, neither clinical case reports nor controlled research efforts to date have specifically addressed the question of bulimia or even food cravings in selected groups of food-sensitive or food-intolerant patients. The literature also lacks formal hypotheses on any possible links between adverse food reactions and anorexia nervosa.

Anxiety and somatoform disorders

Many clinical allergists, including Rowe [84], Randolph [76,78], Speer [96] and Finn and Cohen [42] have reported anxiety and panic states in association with adverse reactions to a range of foods, relieved by avoidance. Psychologists and psychiatrists have focused more specifically on adverse effects of caffeine-containing beverages such as coffee, tea and colas [14, 19, 44, 45, 67, 75, 86, 105]. The data on the adverse effects of caffeine are complex.

Caffeine

Caffeine is a xanthine derivative that millions of people ingest on a daily basis for its mild stimulant effect on the CNS. Controlled studies (see [86] for review) on the effects of caffeine have generated findings of headaches, anxiety, insomnia, irritability, muscle twitching, increased release of adrenaline (epinephrine) and/or noradrenaline (norepineph-rine), elevated respiratory and cardiac rates, ventricular premature contractions [75] and decreased cerebral blood flow [67] in normal adults. The caffeine withdrawal syndrome on abrupt cessation of intake reportedly includes severe headache, fatigue, myalgias and a flu-like syndrome.

Correlational studies between self-reported caffeine intake and psychological scale measurements have found a positive association between greater caffeine intake and greater levels of anxiety in psychiatric patients with anxiety and panic disorders [14, 44, 45]. Table 40.3, for example, summarizes psychological characteristics for 83 psychiatric inpatients with differing levels of chronic caffeine ingestion [45]. Higher caffeine users had greater anxiety and depression scores than did low users. This correlational data, however, cannot address the question of cause–effect. Experimental investigations with known amounts of the xanthine in normal adults have also shown acute increases in measures of anxiety with increasing doses of caffeine [105].

Variability in study results. However, a number of researchers in this area have pointed out variability in the specific outcomes of the different studies. They have suggested that individual differences in usage and tolerance to caffeine at the time of study, in susceptibility to its acute effects and in reliability of self-reports may all contribute to these inconsistencies. Moreover, the correlational studies

Table 40.3 Rating scale scores and selected clinical symptoms of caffeine users.

| Subgroup | State–Trait anxiety index scores | | | | Beck Depression Scale Score (percentage of patients) | | Response to caffeine (% of patients) | |
| | Trait items | | State items | | >16 (moderate depression) | >23 (serious depression) | Impaired sleep if consumed before bedtime | Headache if omitted in morning |
	Mean	Median	Mean	Median				
Low users, 0–249 mg/day (n = 30)	45	44	42	40	40	17	53	7
Moderate users, 250–749 mg/ day (n = 35)	52	52	48	48	59	34	43	14
High users, 750 mg/day or more (n = 18)	51	52	48	51	83	50	22	11
Total (n = 83)	49	50	46	47	57	31	42	11
Significance	<0.05*	<0.05†	<0.10*	<0.05†	<0.02‡	<0.05‡	<0.05‡	NS‡

* Univariate one-way analysis of variance.
† K-sample comparison of medians.
‡ Chi-square, d.f. = 2, NS = not significant.
Reprinted from Greden et al [45], with permission.

relied on patients' retrospective reporting of caffeine intake rather than on direct measurement.

The experimental studies may be hampered by difficulty in finding an appropriate physiological placebo. As some psychologists have argued, awareness of bodily arousal due to adrenaline alone may or may not lead to changes in psychological state, depending on the cognitive labels available to the subject [87]. Subjects in a research study are aware that they receive caffeine and thereby may mobilize their previous expectations and cognitive sets about the psychological effects of the substance on them whenever they detect the physiological arousal. Such considerations are important because they pertain as well to any non-blind or inappropriately blinded studies on adverse effects of foods and other food-related substances.

Tension–fatigue syndrome

Certain allergists have claimed that food-allergic patients in particular experience a polysymptomatic disorder called the 'tension-fatigue syndrome' [76, 84, 96]. Table 40.4 summarizes Rowe's reported frequencies of patient complaints in this syndrome [7, 84]. It is notable that a large number of such patients might also meet criteria for a psychiatric diagnosis—i.e. the polysymptomatic somatization disorder [31]. In fact, intolerance to a variety of foods is listed as one criterion of this latter diagnosis, which must include at least 14 symptoms for women and 12 for men out of a possible 37 total. Similar to the tension-fatigue syndrome, somatization disorder patients report a sickly state, pain problems, gastrointestinal complaints, pseudoneurological symptoms, menstrual dysfunction, sexual apathy and/or difficulties and cardiopulmonary symptoms.

As with other aspects of this field, careful investigation of the population of somatization disorder patients for a subgroup of responders with adverse food reactions remains to be undertaken. King [51, 52] has looked at provocation of psychological and 'psychosomatic' symptoms in a within-subjects, placebo-con-

Table 40.4 Symptoms of allergic tension–fatigue syndrome.

Symptom	Percentage of patients ($n = 70$) (no control group reported)
Fatigue	94
Food sensitivities	91
Gastrointestinal symptoms	63
Headache	50
Arthralgias	47
Drowsiness	37
Myalgias	36
Nervous tension	34
Nasal symptoms	34
Depression	30
Difficulty concentrating	27
Irritability	20
Confusion	17
Hives	16
Insomnia	11
Aching in chest	10
Fever	10
Eczema	10
Tachycardia	10

Patient sample reportedly included 72% female and 28% male patients, with mean age of 42 years (range 10–70).
Reprinted from Bell [7], with permission.

trolled, double-blind study of a group of adult patients who presented with suspected food sensitivities. He utilized sublingual administration of diluted food extracts and a distilled water placebo. Some of his results appear in Table 40.5. He found significantly greater provocation of cognitive and emotional symptoms and of mixed psychosomatic symptoms in this subject sample on food versus placebo trials, as well as greater heart rate variability on food versus placebo trials.

Rix et al [83] have discounted King's findings with doubts about his blinding procedure. However, his data included manipulation checks for subject awareness. Any trials with awareness were removed and separately analysed.

Moreover, the same worker (King, DS, unpublished observations, 1984; [54]) has recently found validity for his modified sublingual blinding procedures using prune juice concentrate as the base in a related study on children. He again found significant behavioural, heart rate and heart rate variability effects of foods versus placebo.

the presence of an interactive psychological component in the clinical situation.

On the other hand, psychological diagnoses such as somatization disorder are always diagnoses of exclusion of organic factors. If a double-blind study is inadequately designed (see schizophrenia section above), researchers might miss a true biological effect and mistakenly conclude a psychogenic basis for the presenting complaints. In addition, the finding of psychological factors does not rule out biological components to a phenomenon.

For example, the demonstration that guinea-pigs can learn by classical conditioning to release histamine to previously neutral odours [85] does not disprove the ability of allergens and non-immunological agents (e.g. peptides, toxins) to release histamine biologically as well. Rather, these findings emphasize the need for a biopsychosocial assessment and acceptance of multiple possible causes for clinical phenomena. Data suggest a two-way communication between mind and body, as well as between CNS and the immune system [2].

Table 40.5 Statistical analyses of number of symptoms by experimental condition for all categories of symptoms (double-blind trials only).

	Cognitive–emotional	Mixed	Somatic	Overall
Over trials	Al > Pl* $Pl_{unaware} = Pl_{aware}$	Al > Pl† $Pl_{aware} > Pl_{unaware}$†	Al > Pl* $Pl_{unaware} = Pl_{aware}$	Al > Pl† $Pl_{unaware} = Pl_{aware}$
Over subjects	Al > Pl† Pl = BR 1	Al > Pl* Pl > BR* BR = Scr	Al = Pl Pl > BR* BR = Scr	Al = Pl Pl > BR* BR = Scr

Abbreviations used: $1 = n$ too small, symptom too infrequent; Al = allergen, Pl = placebo, BR = base rate, Scr = screening. $Pl_{unaware}$ = trials on which the patient received a placebo and was scored as *unaware* of the placebo; Pl_{aware} = trials on which the patient received a placebo and was scored as *aware* of the placebo.
* $0.01 \leqslant P < 0.05$.
† $P < 0.01$.
Reprinted from King [51], with permission.

CONCLUSIONS

Conflicting results and conclusions in the CNS literature must lead the reader to look closely at methodologies and analyses for explanations of discrepancies between studies. At this point the data are inadequate to conclude that the polysymptomatic syndrome of any given patient has a wholly biological aetiology (i.e. physiologically triggered food reactions) or a wholly psychological aetiology. On the one hand, well-controlled, double-blind studies can indicate the presence of a biological component, but would not rule out

Taken together, the available research suggests that particular types of adverse food reactions sometimes correlate with neurological, psychiatric and psychophysiological symptoms in certain patients. It is possible that a minority of food-responder patients with seizure disorders, sleep disturbances, schizophrenia, affective disorders, anxiety and somatoform syndromes suffer from biologically mediated (food-induced) difficulties. The adverse food effects on the CNS may cause, or perhaps only correlate with, immune dysfunction in the cellular and humoral branches of such patients. Further research in these areas is essential.

REFERENCES

1 Adamson WD, Sellers ED: Observations on the incidence of a hypersensitive state in 100 cases of epilepsy. J Allergy 1932; 4:315–23.

2 Ader R, ed.: Psychoneuroimmunology. New York: Academic Press, 1981.

3 Ashkenazi A, Krasilowsky D, Levin S et al: Immunologic reaction of psychotic patients to fractions of gluten. Am J Psychiatry 1979; 136:1306–9.

4 Bartrop RW, Luckhurst E, Lazarus L et al: Depressed lymphocyte function after bereavement. Lancet 1977; i:834–6.

5 Beauchemin JA: Allergic reactions in mental diseases. Am J Psychiatry 1935; 92:1190.

6 Bell IR: Diet histories in narcolepsy. In: Dement WC, Passouant P, eds. Narcolepsy. New York: Spectrum, 1976; 221–7.

7 Bell IR: Clinical ecology. A new medical approach to environmental illness. Bolinas, California: Common Knowledge Press, 1982.

8 Bell IR, Guilleminault C, Dement WC: Hypersomnia, multiple-system symptomatology, and selective IgA deficiency. Biol Psychiatry 1978; 13:751–7.

9 Bell IR, Hawley CD, Guilleminault C, Dement WC: Diet and symptom histories in food allergics versus narcoleptics and normals. Sleep Res 1976; 5:155.

10 Berman BA, Engel GL, Glaser J: The electroencephalogram in allergic children. Ann Allergy 1959; 17:188–93.

11 Beutler LE, Ware JC, Karacan I, Thornby JI: Differentiating psychological characteristics of patients with sleep apnea and narcolepsy. Sleep 1981; 4:39–47.

12 Bock SA: Food sensitivity. A critical review and practical approach. Am J Dis Child 1980; 134:973–82.

13 Borysenko J: Stress, coping and the immune system. In: Matarazzo JD, Weiss SM, Herd JA, Weiss SM, eds. Behavioral health. New York: John Wiley, 1984; 248–60.

14 Boulenger JP, Uhde TW, Wolff EA, Post RM: Increased sensitivity to caffeine in patients with panic disorders. Preliminary evidence. Arch Gen Psychiatry 1984; 41:1067–71.

15 Brantyl V, Teschemacher HA: A material with opioid activity in bovine milk and milk products. Naunyn-Schmiedebergs Arch Pharmacol 1979; 306:301–4.

16 Campbell MB: Allergy and epilepsy. In: Speer F, ed. Allergy of the nervous system. Springfield, Ill: C C Thomas, 1970; 59–78.

17 Campbell MB: Neurologic manifestations of allergic disease. Ann Allergy 1973; 31:485–98.

18 Campbell MB: Neurological and psychiatric aspects of allergy. Otolaryngol Clin North Am 1974; 7:805.

19 Cherek DR, Steinberg JL, Brauchi JT: Effects of caffeine on human aggressive behavior. Psychiat Res 1983; 8:137–45.

20 Chobot R, Dundy HD, Pacella BL: The incidence of abnormal electroencephalographic patterns in allergic children. J Allergy 1950; 21:334–8.

21 Coffey CE, Sullivan JL, Rice JR: T lymphocytes in schizophrenia. Biol Psychiatry 1983; 18:113–9.

22 Cohen EL, Wurtman RJ: Brain acetylcholine: control by dietary choline. Science 1976; 191:561–2.

23 Cooper JR, Bloom FE, Roth RH: The biochemical basis of neuropharmacology, 3rd edn. New York: Oxford University Press, 1978.

24 Crayton JW: Effects of food challenges on complement components in 'food-sensitive' psychiatric patients and controls. J Allergy Clin Immunol [Suppl] 1984; 73:134.

25 Crayton JW, Stone T, Stein G: Epilepsy precipitated by food sensitivity: report of a case with double-blind placebo-controlled assessment. Clin Electroencephalogr 1981; 12:192–8.

26 Cunningham AS: Allergy, immunodeficiency, and epilepsy. Lancet 1975; ii:975.

27 Davison HM: Allergy of the nervous system. Q Rev Allergy Immunol 1952; 6:157–88.

28 Dees SC: Electroencephalography in allergic epilepsy. South Med J 1953; 46:618–20.

29 Dees SC: Neurologic allergy in childhood. Pediatr Clin North Amer 1954; 1:1017–27.

30 Dees SC, Lowenbach H: Allergic epilepsy. Ann Allergy 1951; 9:446–58.

31 Diagnostic and statistical manual of mental disorders, 3rd edn. Washington, DC: American Psychiatric Association, 1980.

32 Dockray GJ: The physiology of cholecystokinin in brain and gut. Br Med Bull 1982; 38:253–8.

33 Dohan FC, Grasberger JC: Relapsed schizophrenics: earlier discharge from the hospital after cereal-free milk-free diet. Am J Psychiatry 1973; 130:685–8.

34 Dohan FC, Grasberger JC, Lowell FM et al: Relapsed schizophrenics: more rapid improvement on a milk- and cereal-free diet. Br J Psychiatry 1969; 115:595–6.

35 Egger J, Wilson J, Carter CM et al: Is migraine food allergy? A double-blind controlled trial of oligoantigenic diet treatment. Lancet 1983; ii:865–9.

36 Ellis ME, Stevens DL: Transient cerebral ischaemic attacks related to egg consumption. Postgrad Med J 1981; 57:642–4.

37 Engel GL: The need for a new medical model: a challenge for biomedicine. Science 1977; 196:129–36.

38 Engel GL: The clinical application of the biopsychosocial model. Am J Psychiatry 1980; 137:535–44.

39 Fargeas MJ, Fioramonti J, Bueno L: Prostaglandin E2: a neuromodulator in the central control of gastrointestinal motility and feeding behavior by calcitonin. Science 1984; 225:1050–1.

40 Fein BT, Kamin PB: Allergy, convulsive disorders, and epilepsy. Ann Allergy 1968; 26:241–7.

41 Fernstrom JD, Wurtman RJ: Brain serotonin content: increase following ingestion of carbohydrate diet. Science 1971; 174:1023–5.

42 Finn R, Cohen HN: Food allergy: fact or fiction? Lancet 1978; i:426–8.

43 Fowler WM, Heimlich EM, Walter RD et al: Electroencephalographic patterns in children with allergic convulsive and behavior disorders. Ann Allergy 1962; 20:1–14.

44 Greden JF: Anxiety or caffeinism: a diagnostic dilemma. Am J Psychiatry 1974; 131:1089–92.

45 Greden JF, Fontaine P, Lubetsky M, Chamberlin K: Anxiety and depression associated with caffeinism among psychiatric inpatients. Am J Psychiatry 1978; 135:963–6.

46 Guilleminault C, ed.: Sleeping and waking disorders: indications and techniques. Menlo Park, Calif: Addison-Wesley, 1982.

47 Guilleminault C, Tilkian A, Dement WC: The sleep apnea syndromes. Annu Rev Med 1976; 27:465–84.

48 Henry JP, Stephens PM: Caffeine as an intensifier of stress-induced hormonal and pathophysiologic

changes in mice. Pharmacol Biochem Behav 1980; 13:719–27.

49 Hirata-Hibi M, Higashi S, Tachibana T, Watanabe N: Stimulated lymphocytes in schizophrenia. Arch Gen Psychiatry 1982; 39:82–7.

50 Kidd JM, Cohen SH, Sosman AJ, Fink JN: Food-dependent exercise-induced anaphylaxis. J Allergy Clin Immunol 1983; 71:407–11.

51 King DS: Can allergic exposure provoke psychological symptoms? A double-blind test. Biol Psychiatry 1981; 16:3–19.

52 King DS: Food and chemical sensitivities can produce cognitive-emotional symptoms. In: Miller SA, ed. Nutrition and behavior. Philadelphia: Franklin Institute Press, 1981; 119–30.

53 King DS: Statistical power of the controlled research on wheat gluten and schizophrenia. Biol Psychiatry 1985; 20:785–7.

54 King DS, Margen S, Ogar D, Durkin N: Double blind food challenges affect sensitive children's behavior and heart rate. Presented at the 92nd Annual Convention of the American Psychological Association, Toronto, 1984.

55 Kinnell HG, Kirkwood E, Lewis C: Food antibodies in schizophrenia. Psychol Med 1982; 12:85–9.

56 Klee WA, Zioudrou, Streaty RA: Exorphins: peptides with opioid activity isolated from wheat gluten, and their possible role in the etiology of schizophrenia. In: Usdin E, Bunney WE, Kline NS, eds. Endorphins in mental health research. New York: Oxford University Press, 1979; 209–18.

57 Laudenslager ML, Ryan SM, Drugan RC et al: Coping and immunosuppression: inescapable but not escapable shock suppresses lymphocyte proliferation. Science 1983; 221:568–70.

58 Lavine P: Nasal obstructions, sleep, and mental function. Sleep 1983; 6:244–6.

59 Leigh H: Behavioral medicine: toward a comprehensive psychosomatic approach. Psychother Psychosom 1981; 36:151–8.

60 Lindsley G, Hartmann EL, Mitchell W: Selectivity in response to L-tryptophan among insomniac subjects: a preliminary report. Sleep 1983; 6:247–56.

61 Lishman WA, ed.: Organic psychiatry: the psychological consequences of cerebral disorder. Oxford: Blackwell Scientific, 1978.

62 Locke SE: Stress, adaptation, and immunity: studies in humans. Gen Hosp Psychiatry 1982; 4:49–58.

63 Lutz EG: Restless legs, anxiety, and caffeinism. J Clin Psychiatry 1978; 39:693–8.

64 McGuffin P, Gardiner P, Swinburne LM: Schizophrenia, celiac disease, and antibodies to food. Biol Psychiatry 1981; 16:281–5.

65 Mackarness R: Not all in the mind. Lond: Pan Books, 1976.

66 McNicholas WT, Tarlo S, Cole P et al: Obstructive apneas during sleep in patients with seasonal allergic rhinitis. Am Rev Respir Dis 1982; 126:625–8.

67 Mathew RJ, Barr DL, Weinman ML: Caffeine and cerebral blood flow. Br J Psychiatry 1983; 143: 604–8.

68 Matussek P, Agerer D, Seibt G: Allergic disorders in depressive patients. Compr Psychiatry 1983; 24:25–34.

69 Maulitz RM, Pratt DS, Schocket AL: Exercise-induced anaphylactic reaction to shellfish. J Allergy Clin Immunol 1979; 63:433–4.

70 May E: Attacks of unnatural somnolence of anaphylactic origin. Bull Soc Med Hosp Paris 1923; 47:704.

71 Metcalfe DD: Diagnostic procedures for immunologically-mediated food sensitivity. Nutr Rev 1984; 42:92–7.

72 Osborne M, Crayton JW, Javaid J, Davis JM: Lack of effect of a gluten-free diet on neuroleptic blood levels in schizophrenic patients. Biol Psychiatry 1982; 17:627–9.

73 Pearson DJ, Rix KJ, Bentley SJ: Food allergy: how much in the mind? A clinical and psychiatric study of suspected food hypersensitivity. Lancet 1983; i:1259–61.

74 Potkin SG, Weinberger D, Kleinman J et al: Wheat gluten challenge in schizophrenic patients. Am J Psychiatry 1981; 138:1208–11.

75 Prineas RJ, Jacobs DR, Crow RS, Blackburn H: Coffee, tea and VPB. J Chronic Dis 1980; 33:67–72.

76 Randolph TG: Fatigue and weakness of allergic origin (allergic toxemia); to be differentiated from 'nervous fatigue' or neurasthenia. Ann Allergy 1945; 3:418–30.

77 Randolph TG: The descriptive features of food addiction. Addictive eating and drinking. Q J Stud Alc 1956; 17:198–224.

78 Randolph TG: Clinical ecology as it affects the psychiatric patient. Int J Soc Psychiatry 1966; 12:245–54.

79 Randolph TG: Specific adaptation. Ann Allergy 1978; 40:333–45.

80 Rea WJ: Environmentally-triggered cardiac disease. Ann Allergy 1978; 40:243–51.

81 Reynolds CF, Kupfer DJ, McEachran AB, et al: Depressive psychopathology in male sleep apneics. J Clin Psychiatry 1984; 45:287–90.

82 Rice JR, Ham CH, Gore WE: Another look at gluten in schizophrenia. Am J Psychiatry 1978; 135:1417–8.

83 Rix KJB, Pearson DJ, Bentley SJ: A psychiatric study of patients with supposed food allergy. Br J Psychiatry 1984; 145:121–6.

84 Rowe AH, Rowe A Jr: Food allergy. Its manifestations and control and the elimination diets. Springfield, Illinois: C C Thomas, 1972.

85 Russell M, Dark KA, Cummins RW et al: Learned histamine release. Science 1984; 225:733–4.

86 Sawyer DA, Julia HL, Turin AC: Caffeine and human behavior: arousal, anxiety, and performance effects. J Behav Med 1982; 5:415–39.

87 Schacter S, Singer JE: Cognitive, social, and physiological determinants of emotional state. Psychol Rev 1962; 69:379–99.

88 Schleifer SJ, Keller SE, Meyerson AT et al: Lymphocyte function in major depressive disorder. Arch Gen Psychiatry 1984; 41:484–6.

89 Schwartz GE: A systems analysis of psychobiology and behavior therapy. Psychother Psychosom 1981; 36:159–84.

90 Schwartz GE: Testing the biopsychosocial model: the ultimate challenge facing behavioral medicine? J Consult Clin Psychol 1982; 50:1040–53.

91 Seltzer S, Dewart D, Pollack RL, Jackson E: The effects of dietary tryptophan on chronic maxillofacial pain and experimental pain tolerance. J Psychiatr Res 1983; 17:181–6.

92 Sheffer AL, Soter NA, McFadden ER, Austen KF: Exercise-induced anaphylaxis: a distinct form of physical allergy. J Allergy Clin Immunol 1983; 71:311–6.

93 Siegel S, Hinson RE, Kronk MD: Heroin 'overdose' death: contribution of drug-associated environmental cues. Science 1982; 216:436–7.

94 Singh MM, Kay SR: Wheat gluten as a pathogenic factor in schizophrenia. Science 1976; 191:401–2.

95 Spangler RH: Allergy and epilepsy. J Lab Clin Med 1927; 12:41–58.

96 Speer F, ed.: Allergy of the nervous system. Springfield, Ill: C C Thomas, 1970.

97 Spring B, Maller O, Wurtman J et al: Effects of protein and carbohydrate meals on mood and performance: interactions with sex and age. J Psychiatr Res 1983; 17:155–67.

98 Stein M: A biopsychosocial approach to immune function and medical disorders. Psychiatr Clin North 1981; 4:203–21.

99 Sternberg TH, Baldridge GD: Electroencephalographic abnormalities in patients with generalized neurodermatitis. J Invest Dermatol 1948; 11:401–3.

100 Storms LH, Clopton JM, Wright C: Effects of gluten on schizophrenics. Arch Gen Psychiatry 1982; 39:323–7.

101 Sugerman AA, Southern DL, Curran JF: A study of antibody levels in alcoholic, depressive, and schizophrenic patients. Ann Allergy 1982; 48:166–71.

102 Suwa K, Toru M: A case of periodic somnolence whose sleep was induced by glucose. Folia Psychiatr Neurol Jpn 1969; 23:253–62.

103 Terrell CO, Stephens WE, Morris R: Eosinophilia and neurological dysfunction—a preliminary report. Ann Allergy 1967; 25:673–7.

104 Thompson J: Clinical types of convulsive seizures in very young babies with a special consideration of so-called idiopathic convulsions of early infancy and their treatment. Br Med J 1921; ii:679–83.

105 Veleber DM, Templer DI: Effects of caffeine on anxiety and depression. J Abnorm Psychol 1984; 93:120–2.

106 von Bertanlanffy L: General systems theory. New York: Braziller, 1978.

107 Wallis RM, Nicol WD, Craig M: The importance of protein hypersensitivity in the diagnosis and treatment of a special group of epileptics. Lancet 1923; i: 741–3.

108 Ward JF, Peterson HA: Protein sensitization in epilepsy. Arch Neurol Psychiat 1927; 17:427–43.

109 Webster's new collegiate dictionary. Springfield, Mass: G and C Merriam, 1981: 1175.

110 Wurtman RJ, Hefti F, Melamed E: Precursor control of neurotransmitter synthesis. Pharmacol Rev 1981; 32:315–35.

111 Zwillich CW, Pickett C, Hanson FN, Weil JV: Disturbed sleep and prolonged apnea during nasal obstruction in normal men. Am Rev Respir Dis 1981; 124:158–60.

SECTION F
RHEUMATOLOGY

Chapter 41
Joints and Connective Tissue

J. A. Wojtulewski

Background

The role of diet and dietary factors in the management of arthritis and rheumatism remains controversial. There are numerous popular publications offering conflicting advice to the sufferer whilst usually claiming to possess good evidence, invariably anecdotal, that the disease can be alleviated or even cured by following a particular diet either by exclusion or enhancement.

A recent authoritative textbook of rheumatology [70] expresses a different view concerning the role of diet in this group of conditions. It stresses the importance of maintaining the rheumatoid patient in a good general state of nutrition by means of a diet liberal in calories and protein and high in vitamin and mineral content, and in cases of osteoarthritis the avoidance of obesity. By contrast, an equally large text [69] expressed the view of clinical ecologists by stating that, with rare exceptions, cases of rheumatoid arthritis respond favourably to the detection and avoidance of incriminating foods and chemical exposures, and extends these views to other painful musculoskeletal syndromes.

RHEUMATIC AND ARTHRITIC SYMPTOMS IN ALLERGIC DISEASE

That joint symptoms and signs do occur in patients who present with classical allergic syndromes has been well established.

Serum sickness

Serum sickness and drug allergies often manifest an arthritic component. When joint swelling is accompanied by urticaria and by local or generalized angioedema, the condition rarely demands further complex investigations in order to establish a diagnosis of serum sickness. Clear examples of this picture in relation to food allergy are described [20].

Henoch–Schönlein syndrome

Historically, the possibility that the Henoch–Schönlein syndrome could be related to food allergy was first suggested by Osler's comments in 1914 concerning the possible role of protein sensitivity in this disease [61]. A decade later, Alexander and Eyermann [1] produced good evidence, with case reports, that food allergy could be a key factor in this condition with the involvement of joints a prominent manifestation. Meanwhile, angioneural arthrosis was described [81] in 27 allergic patients where intermittent attacks of joint pains and swelling occurred with complete resolution between attacks. Dietary indiscretions were implicated as one of the provoking factors in this condition [12, 86].

Palindromic rheumatism

Hench and Rosenberg [35] had considered, but rejected, the possibility that palindromic rheumatism could be precipitated by dietary factors. Vaughan studied a somewhat different population of 1000 consecutive patients with asthma, hay fever, urticaria, angioneurotic oedema, gastrointestinal allergy or allergic dermatitis, and revived the possibility of such an association [88].

Of the 206 patients in the group who were found to have rheumatic complaints, 27 had definitely established that their intermittent joint flare-ups were caused by certain foods. In approximately half of this group, the diagnosis of palindromic rheumatism had been made. Criep [15] described four more cases which fall into this category and emphasized the allergic nature of the condition and co-existence with other general allergic features.

Features of food hypersensitivity-induced arthritis

The diagnostic features which differentiate food hypersensitivity arthritis associated with allergic disease from rheumatoid arthritis [72] are shown in Table 41.1 [98]. The association with other forms of allergy, the background of a positive family history and the poor correlation with skin tests must be stressed and also the value of Rowe's [74] elimination diet emphasized.

A number of recent publications, although

Table 41.1 Diagnostic features of food hypersensitivity arthritis as distinct from rheumatoid arthritis.

Association with other forms of allergy
Positive family history of allergy
Poor correlation with skin tests
Time relationship of symptoms to food intake not obvious
Value of elimination diets

From Zussman [98], with permission.

usually dealing primarily with a wide spectrum of allergic disease include comments which relate not only to musculoskeletal syndromes but also to arthritis. Wraith [95] described a series of 500 patients, the majority suffering from asthma and eczema, in whom articular symptoms and signs were present among other clinical features. In some patients, joint pains and swelling were much improved by the avoidance of specific foods, and returned when challenged with these foods. He pointed out that the majority of symptoms related to food may only appear gradually and the relationship between food intake and symptoms of arthralgia may not be immediately obvious.

Effect of disodium cromoglycate

Vaz and his colleagues [89] studied 20 patients with allergic symptoms due to food and found, in a double-blind controlled study, that disodium cromoglycate prevented reactions in 14 of the subjects (70%). They also found that complaints not usually attributed to allergy, such as joint symptoms, were both produced by ingestion of foods and prevented by prior use of disodium cromoglycate. One case with a clinical picture of juvenile rheumatoid arthritis responded quite dramatically to food elimination.

Limb pains in children

A controlled trial of dietary avoidance in childhood migraine showed that many associated symptoms which accompany migraine, including limb pains (in almost 50% of the patients), also respond to treatment with an oligoallergenic diet [25].

Few other studies of children with food intolerance and allergy mention any musculoskeletal problems [53]. In one study, only one case of joint complaints in 100 young patients was reported, and was a patient with joint pains after eating beef [43].

MYALGIA AND ARTHRALGIA

The idea that musculoskeletal pain might be related to diet has been recorded in some of the earliest medical writings, but, on closer scrutiny, it is gout that, in fact, features predominantly.

In recent years, considerable progress has been made in the definition and in the classification of rheumatic disorders. However, there is still a wide spectrum of symptomatology that defies proper diagnosis. These conditions provide us with a difficult task when attempting to judge response to a particular treatment because of lack of uniform diagnostic criteria.

'Allergic' toxaemia

Rowe described a syndrome of 'allergic tox-

pains. The challenges were made double-blind using a basic puréed vegetable soup supplemented by either allergen or placebo [10].

Gerrard described 33 patients suffering from a multiplicity of symptoms including a number with arthralgia [29]. The patients were treated by fasting followed by individual food challenge. Over half the patients were either cured of their symptoms or substantially improved and, of eight patients subjected to a double-blind challenge, seven identified the offending food correctly.

GASTROINTESTINAL DISEASE AND ARTHRITIS

Gastrointestinal infections

The strong relationship between gastrointestinal disease and arthritis (see Table 41.2)

Table 41.2 Relationship of gastrointestinal disease to arthritis

Gastrointestinal infection, e.g. *Salmonella, Shigella, Yersinia*
Spondyloarthritis, e.g. *Klebsiella* and HLA-B27
Gastrointestinal bypass, ?overgrowth of *Escherichia coli* and *Bacillus fragilis*
IgA deficiency, e.g. failure of immune exclusion and production of immune complexes
Coeliac disease, e.g. gluten sensitivity and increased gut permeability
Crohn's disease, e.g. response to food elimination

aemia' where prominent features of a polysymptomatic state were muscle aches and pains [73]. Other symptoms included fatigue, weakness, headaches, drowsiness, mental confusion, lack of initiative and slowness of thought. This syndrome has been reviewed by Randolph from an ecologically orientated point of view [68]. He included conditions such as Ekbom's, or restless leg, syndrome in this group and stressed the importance of avoiding incriminating foods as well as chemical exposure. Among his observations was a typical exacerbation of symptoms on the second or third day of the fast. He also mentioned the therapeutic value of a rotary diversified diet as a means of prophylaxis. More recently it was demonstrated that food challenge could induce rheumatic symptoms that were indistinguishable from the presenting complaints in 35 out of 40 polysymptomatic patients [47]. Brown and her associates obtained impressive results in a food challenge study involving 12 patients with multiple symptoms, including six with musculoskeletal

is exemplified by the association of gastrointestinal infection and arthritis. A reactive arthritis is well known to occur as a result of infection with *Salmonella, Shigella, Yersinia* and *Campylobacter* [8, 78]. Articular features have also been described in connection with giardiasis and amoebiasis. There are also strong reasons for considering that an infective organism plays a major role in the causation of Whipple's disease.

Ankylosing spondylitis

The association between bowel disease and ankylosing spondylitis has been accepted for many years. For example, HLA B27-positive patients are prone to arthritis following bowel infection. Much discussion has taken place concerning alteration in gut flora and the development of arthritis. There have been reports that an increased faecal carriage rate of *Klebsiella* correlates with disease activity in patients suffering from ankylosing spondylitis [23, 24]. However, in another study, an exclusion diet in patients with ankylosing spondylitis failed to influence *Klebsiella* excretion and no correlation was found between acquisition of *Klebsiella* and deterioration in disease symptoms [77].

Arthritis and intestinal bypass

The popularity of intestinal bypass procedures in the treatment of obesity a decade or two ago began to wane when the high rate of complications, including joint disease, became apparent [76]. The possibility that arthritis and other problems associated with the operation could result from increased dietary or bacterial antigen absorption was considered, and the hypothesis was strengthened when in one study antibodies against *Escherichia coli* and *Bacillus fragilis* were found in association with circulating cryoproteins in three out of five patients studied [90].

A review of over 100 patients following this operation puts the articular complication rate at 35%. The problems were independent of other postoperative complications. In a control group of patients who underwent rapid weight loss either by diet or by gastroplasty, no case of arthritis was documented, implying that weight loss as such was not a factor [18].

There have also been reports of a bowel-associated dermatosis–arthritis syndrome following gastric surgery without a bypass [21] or related simply to gastrointestinal disease with either the presence of diverticulae or inflammatory colitis. The same sequence of events in pathogenesis with bacterial proliferation and antigen absorption was suggested.

It is attractive to imagine that this relatively simple sequence of events provokes the arthritis. In reality, however, we do not have adequate evidence that this is indeed the case. The concept of direct involvement by bacterial or dietary antigens must be left in abeyance, although increased gut permeability in patients with rheumatoid arthritis does support the general concept.

IgA deficiency and arthritis

Immunoglobulin deficiency, particularly of IgA, is much more frequent in patients with atopy [39] and also in juvenile chronic polyarthritis [3]. One mechanism to be considered is the possible excess absorption of dietary proteins due to associated increase in gut permeability and failure of immune exclusion. When a group of 30 patients who were found

to have IgA deficiency was studied, six were found to have some form of autoimmune disease and three had arthritis. Precipitins to cow's milk were found and immune complexes were also demonstrated in half the cases [16].

Coeliac disease

Recent surveys leave us in no doubt that a strong link exists between coeliac disease and other autoimmune conditions, with one in five coeliacs having associated autoimmune disorders [41]. Scott and Losowsky [75] postulated that the high degree of association may have been as a result of deposition in other organs of immune complexes derived from the small intestinal mucosa. A further survey reported a figure of 20% with autoimmune disease and an overall 6% with connective tissue disease. Most of these disorders were found to develop while the patient was still on a normal diet [14]. A gluten-free diet did not prevent the associated conditions, but an occasional dramatic improvement in an atopic patient was seen.

In contrast to the above observations, there are reports of positive responses in non-atopic individuals. We presented the case of a young woman with a progressive polyarthropathy whose disease completely remitted following diagnosis of coeliac disease and the institution of a gluten-free diet [93].

A review of three cases of adult coeliac disease in association with arthritis described a positive response of the arthritis to diet in one of the patients [65]. Circulating immune complexes were detected on a number of occasions but this finding did not correlate with disease activity. Gut permeability studies in coeliac disease, rheumatoid arthritis and Sjögren's syndrome have shown abnormalities only in the untreated coeliac patients. The arthralgia in six cases of coeliac disease where joint symptoms preceded the diagnosis responded to a gluten-free diet [9]. However, subsequent gluten challenge failed to provoke arthritis. A survey of a further 160 coeliac patients failed to identify any cases of arthritis attributable to the disease (see also Chapter 30).

Crohn's disease and ulcerative colitis

The most common extraintestinal manifestations of these diseases involve the locomotor system [32]. The incidence of polyarthritis is more common than that of spondylitis, and articular disease is more frequent in cases of

Crohn's disease with colonic involvement. In ulcerative colitis especially, there may be a close relationship between activity of gut disease and flares of arthritis. There is considerable strength of opinion that the extraintestinal manifestations of these diseases must have an immunological basis, with an increased absorption of antigens related to changes in the bacterial colonization of the gut, or possibly affected by diet. Successful treatment of Crohn's disease by means of an elemental diet has been reported [60] (see Chapter 33). The arthritis of Crohn's disease in childhood has also been shown to respond to this form of treatment [20].

RHEUMATOID ARTHRITIS

Epidemiology

There is a considerable body of opinion that rheumatoid arthritis is one of the 'diseases of civilization' especially as early writings fail to provide us with adequate descriptions of the disease. This implies that the environmental changes of recent times play a major role in the pathogenesis. The first classical description of this condition is as late as 1800 [42].

Epidemiological studies have shown that the disease occurs worldwide but with a tendency towards reduced prevalence and milder disease amongst more primitive peoples [52, 56]. Two surveys in South Africa comparing rural and urban populations of similar genetic stock reveal rheumatoid arthritis to be more common and more severe in the urban population, raising the possibility that environmental factors including diet could be responsible for this difference [5, 82]. However, a more recent study in Lesotho found the condition to be common and described many cases of severe disease [54]. One of the grounds for recommending a recent popular 'arthritic' diet was the fact that it was based on the dietary habits and life style of mainland China and the supposed rarity of the disease in that country [22]. Evidence suggests that rheumatoid arthritis is quite common in China.

Gastrointestinal tract in rheumatoid arthritis

In recent years there has been considerable attention paid to the possible connection between either gastrointestinal infection or dietary factors in the pathogenesis and clinical course of rheumatoid arthritis. In 71 patients with a variety of connective tissue diseases but predominantly rheumatoid arthritis, a significant amount of gastritis was found compared to controls [79]. However, only minor abnormalities were found on small bowel biopsy in the rheumatoid patients. Further evidence of abnormal gastric function in rheumatoid arthritis is shown by reduced gastrin secretory volume [58] and raised serum immunoreactive gastrin [71]. Patients with raised gastrin levels had histologically normal mucosa. Gastric, colonic and rectal biopsies were performed with the conclusion that the various abnormalities found were merely a result of systemic rheumatoid disease [50]. Interestingly, villus abnormalities were more common in seronegative than in seropositive rheumatoid subjects and treatment of one case of total villus atrophy by gluten exclusion led to the disappearance of all signs of arthritis [28]. Gut permeability studies have been performed with varying results; one group reported no abnormalities in rheumatoid arthritis and Sjögren's syndrome [64] while another found reduced permeability to polyethylene glycols of smaller molecular weight but a possibility of paradoxical increase in larger molecular permeability [85].

The principal enzyme changes of the jejunal mucosa in arthritic patients were elevated levels of histidine methyl esterase [7]. The presumed disturbance in histidine metabolism was considered to be due to alteration in intestinal flora.

Gastrointestinal bacterial flora and rheumatoid arthritis

Investigations into intestinal anaerobic flora in cases of arthritis revealed abnormal flora in two-thirds of the patients with rheumatoid arthritis and this increase was related to disease activity [59]. The corollary is the evolution of porcine arthritis by dietary elimination and consequent changes in bacterial flora [49]. Bennett [6] has discussed the role of bacteria in the gastrointestinal tract, the release of bacterial debris and the consequent formation of immune complexes as the possible sequence of events leading to the clinical picture of rheumatoid arthritis. Drugs such as sulphasalazine (Salazopyrin), known to alter the gut flora, are effective in rheumatoid arthritis.

Animal studies

Pigs. Pigs fed on a diet rich in fish protein developed abnormal intestinal flora within 1 week [49]. The main feature was a significant increase in the number of atypical *Clostridium perfringens* type A. The animals then developed swollen joints, and in later months joint deformities, with clinical and histological characteristics of rheumatoid arthritis (Figs. 41.1 and 41.2). The arthritis was considered to be the result of a remote immunological reaction to altered intestinal flora [49] (see Chapter 16).

Rabbits. Infiltrative synovial lesions were induced in rabbits by feeding the animals between half and three-quarters of a pint of cow's milk per day for 12 weeks [13]. The induction of these lesions was thought to be due to small but repeated antigenic stimuli derived from intestinal absorption.

Linoleic acid. Ziff [97] has reviewed some of the effects of diet on experimental animals and stressed the possibly important role of linoleic acid, a precursor of arachidonic acid, which is in turn a precursor of prostaglandins and leukotrienes. Besides a possible pro- or antiinflammatory effect, a number of immunological functions could be influenced. Autoimmune disease could be affected by its effect

on cell membrane function. Kunkel and his colleagues [40] demonstrated that evening primrose oil, rich in linoleic acid, significantly inhibited the development of adjuvant arthritis in rats. However, treatment with *cis*-linoleic acid and γ-linolenic acid over 12 weeks appeared to have no effect upon the experimental arthritis [33]. On the other hand, the sicca syndrome is said to have been improved by the addition of highly saturated evening primrose oil to the diet [37].

Allergy

Although a substantial case has been made in favour of an increased incidence of joint complaints in allergic disorders, the evidence that immediate hypersensitivity reactions contribute to rheumatoid arthritis is sparse. The incidence of atopic disorders in juvenile chronic arthritis is no higher than in controls [66] and no increase in the prevalence of allergy was discovered in a sample of 50 rheumatoid patients [94].

IgE. Raised IgE in serum and synovial fluid has been found in rheumatoid arthritis [38] but with no relationship to the clinical severity

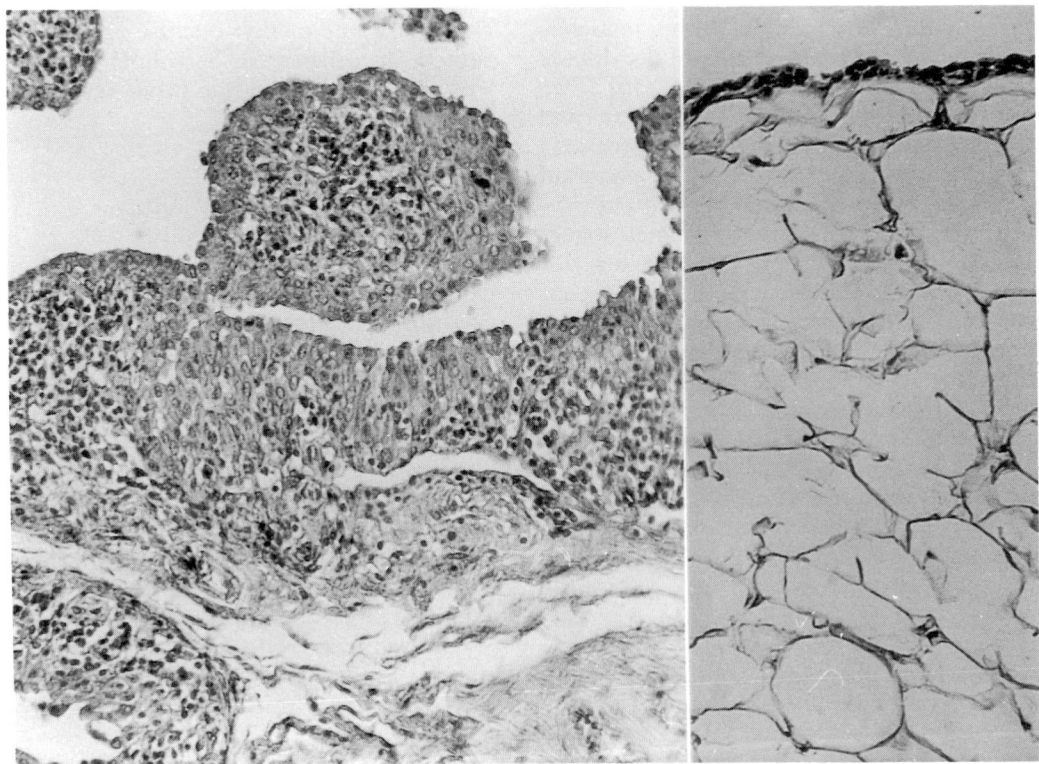

Fig. 41.1 Synovial membrane of pig. Hyperplasia and hypertrophy of synovial lining cells (left). Normal structure (right). From Mansson [49], with permission.

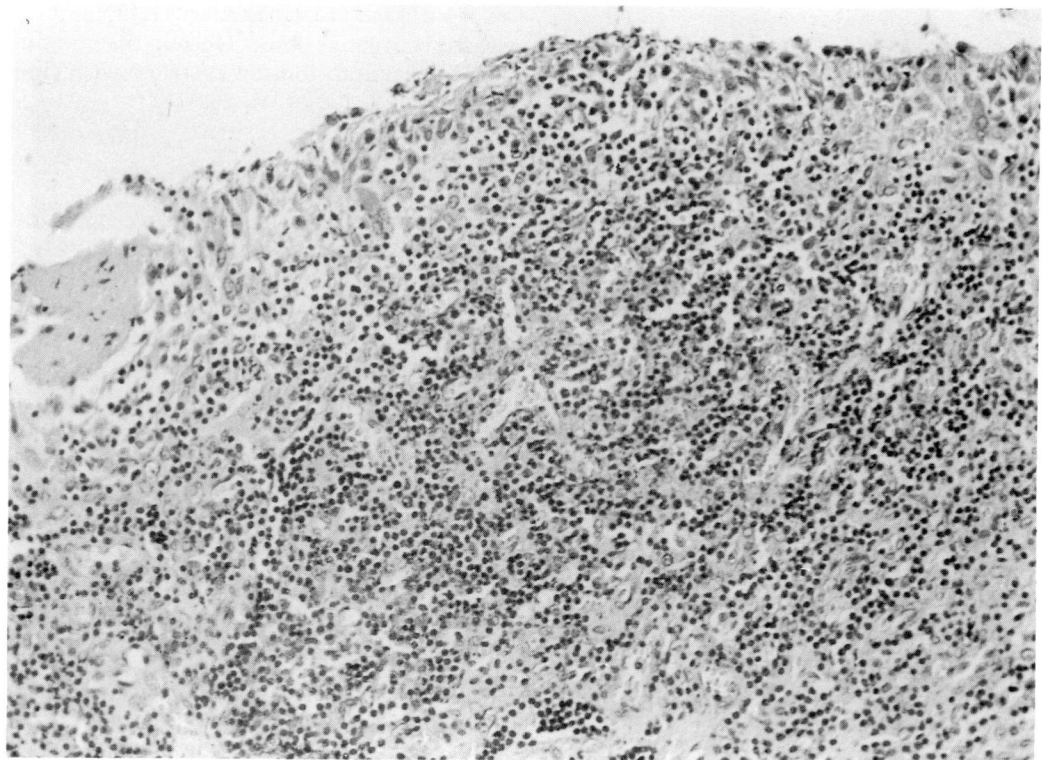

Fig. 41.2 Granulation tissue with proliferation of fibroblasts and profuse amounts of small lymphocytes, macrophages and plasma cells. From Mansson et al [49], with permission.

of the disease. There has also been doubt as to the clinical significance of IgE rheumatoid factor and IgE antinuclear antibodies. Patients with highly elevated radioallergosorbent tests (RAST) to milk and cheese did not improve clinically by exclusion of these products alone and RAST levels remained unaffected by the diet [94].

Platelets. Little and his colleagues [45] studied platelet serotonin release in patients with rheumatoid arthritis who had proven exacerbations of their disease within 4 hours of eating specific foods. A marked and sustained decrease in platelet serotonin took place in the patients in contrast to controls and was followed by a significant increase in 5-hydroxyindoleacetic acid (5-HIAA) (Fig. 41.3). The proposed mechanism was that serotonin release occurred as a result of cross linking of platelets by dietary immune complexes with the enhanced deposition of immune complexes in synovial membrane by 5-HIAA contributing to the inflammation in the rheumatoid joint.

ARE DIETS HELPFUL IN CHRONIC ARTHRITIS?

Links between nutrition and immunity have been thoroughly researched and are well established [11]. Nutritional assessments have been performed in rheumatoid arthritis with one report estimating the incidence of malnutrition at 26% [34]. The conclusion here was that the severity of disease adversely affected nutrition and not the reverse. In a controlled study of the relationship between anergy and malnutrition in rheumatoid arthritis, cutaneous anergy was present in 36% of patients but in none of the controls. Dietary assessment, however, revealed no evidence of malnutrition in the rheumatoid patients [26].

The question of whether a specific diet is effective in chronic arthritis was raised well over half a century ago. Bauer [4] reviewed a number of different dietary regimes, including the previously popular low carbohydrate diet, and came to the conclusion that no form of dietary manipulation had any effect in rheumatoid arthritis. The dietary habits of rheumatoid patients prior to onset of their disease have been analysed and found to be no differ-

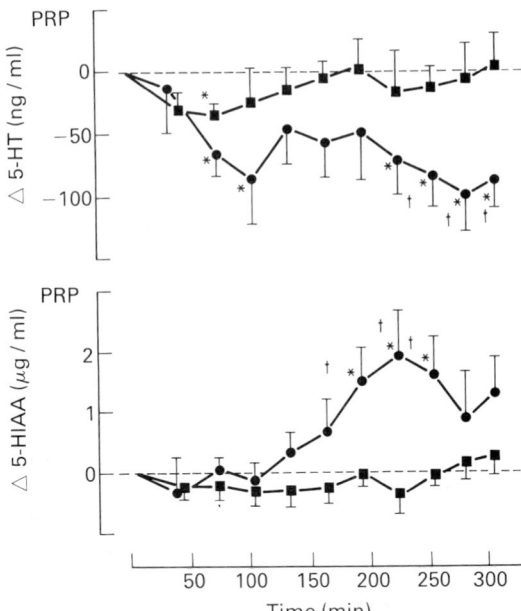

Fig. 41.3 Changes in 5-HT and 5-HIAA in platelet-rich (PRP) plasma after ingestion of positive foods in food intolerant patients (●) and healthy controls (■). Results are expressed as mean changes from control levels (average of two estimations on samples taken before food ingestion) and 1 SEM. There were seven subjects in each group. From Little et al [45], with permission.

*$P<0.05$. Student's paired t test, compared with control concentrations (broken lines).

†$P<0.05$. Student's unpaired t test indicates a difference in magnitude of mean changes from concentrations in controls compared with patients at certain times after food ingestion.

ent from controls. On the other hand, a prospective double-blind study has demonstrated that patients with rheumatoid arthritis improved on a diet high in polyunsaturated and low in saturated fats with a daily supplement of eicosapentaenoic acid [39a]. An effect on prostaglandin metabolism which influences the immune response was suggested as a reason for improvement.

Food allergy in rheumatoid arthritis

Zeller [96] in 1949 wrote enthusiastically about the role of food allergy in rheumatoid arthritis but admitted some failures. Most of his successfully treated patients appear to have had other allergies or a family history of allergy, similar to the patients described by Vaughan [88]. Randolph [67] has suggested that some of the apparently poor results obtained by Zeller could be improved by combining the detection of reactions to specific foods with those to environmental chemical

exposure. He described seven out of eight successfully treated cases. He felt that immunological reactions did not correlate with clinical findings.

Effect of fasting in rheumatoid arthritis

The beneficial effects of fasting upon rheumatoid arthritis have been conclusively demonstrated. Earlier impressions have been confirmed by subsequent controlled studies. A fast is known to have a number of systemic effects (see Table 41.3) including a generalized

Table 41.3 Effect of fasting in rheumatoid arthritis

Reduction of sympathomimetic activity
Depression of acute phase proteins
Decreased intestinal permeability
Impaired reticuloendothelial function
Improved neutrophil bactericidal activity
Short-term subjective and objective improvement in joint disease

reduction in sympathomimetic activity and depression of serum levels of acute phase reactants. A 7- to 10-day fast in rheumatoid patients compared with another rheumatoid group on a normal diet was shown to produce considerable subjective and objective improvement of a short-term duration [80]. It is interesting to note that, in addition, intestinal permeability was reduced during the period of fasting [84].

Other studies have confirmed the beneficial effects of fasting and found that there was in addition a positive association between clinical improvement and neutrophil bactericidal capacity [87]. As part of a study into the effect of comprehensive environmental control in predominantly seronegative rheumatoid arthritis [83], the positive effects of complete (water only) fasting were recorded but variations in individual response noted. Transient flares were encountered during the early period of fasting.

A reduced food antigen load and decreased intestinal permeability during fasting with consequent improvement in disease activity creates fertile ground for the hypothesis that diet-related circulating immune complexes play a significant role in rheumatoid disease activity.

At the conclusion of the 7- to 10-day fast, the patients in one of the above studies [80] went into a 9-week period of a lactovegetarian diet with the control group pursuing a normal diet. No difference was found between the two groups at the end of the study, suggesting that relevant foods were still included in the lacto-vegetarian regime. Intestinal permeabilty which was decreased during fasting returned to normal when on the diet [84].

Food sensitivities. Sensitivities to a variety of foods were reported in 22 patients with rheumatoid arthritis of whom 20 responded well to low allergen diets [36]. Improvement was noted within 18 days. The greatest number of reactions were reported with grain, pips/nuts and cheese. These observations were uncontrolled. A case study of a patient with seronegative rheumatoid arthritis with hypersensitivity to Elastoplast and detergents, whose disease was clearly exacerbated by eating dairy products, created considerable interest [63]. Dramatic improvement took place whilst on an exclusion diet, with severe exacerbations occurring on challenge (Fig. 41.4). This was

she was taking for control of her disease. Another patient with rheumatoid arthritis and a history suggestive of food sensitivity was virtually symptom-free whilst nourished on Vivonex but relapsed when subjected to a double-blind challenge with milk. Immunological hypersensitivity to milk related to exacerbation of arthritis [62a].

Elimination diet and challenge

We have studied 41 patients with rheumatoid arthritis who underwent a 4-week elimination diet. The 23 patients (56%) who improved on this regime then went through a 1-week challenge with four different food groups in random order. Ten patients were considered to have had positive reactions to challenge and rechallenge with reactions most common during the dairy product week. These patients were then treated double-blind with disodium

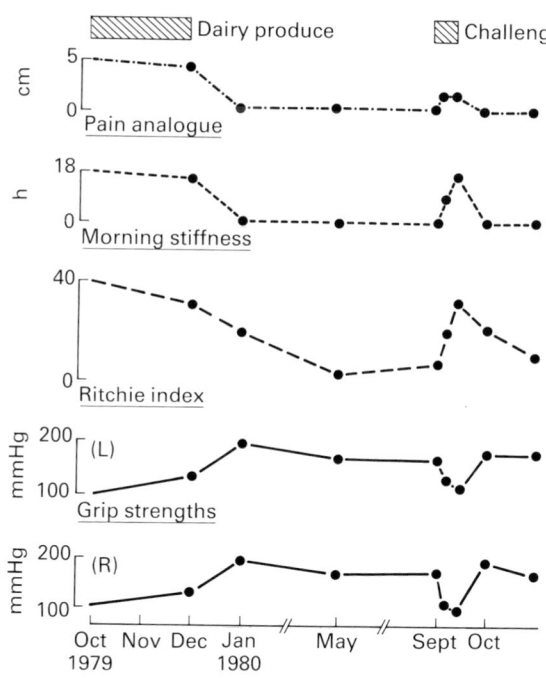

Fig. 41.4 The clinical effects of an exclusion diet and the results of oral challenge with dairy produce in a patient with rheumatoid arthritis. From Parke and Hughes [63], with permission.

associated with the appearance of IgE immune complexes with antibody specificate to milk and cheese. There was a 12-day impairment in clearance of autologous heat-damaged erythrocytes suggesting impairment of reticuloendothelial function.

An anecdotal report [92] involved a patient with severe progressive rheumatoid arthritis who dramatically improved on dietary and environmental exclusion of corn and corn products. This included the packing of the tablets

cromoglycate but with negative results [31].

A prospective pilot study investigating allergic reactions to food, inhalants and environmental chemicals in patients with rheumatoid arthritis by means of an elimination diet and end-point dilution skin testing revealed reactions to many foods [17]. Withdrawal of allergenic substances and desensitization to them produced a wide spectrum of responses ranging from complete remission to deterioration. Initial response of a double-blind placebo-controlled trial [48] seemed to confirm that a proportion of patients obtained significant relief. More recently the same group found dietary manipulation superior to placebo in a controlled study involving 53 patients with rheumatoid arthritis [17a].

Denman and his colleagues [19, 20] monitored 24 patients for periods of 1 to 6 months on an elimination diet which did not relate to food families. No short-term or long-term benefit was detected. Long-term properly controlled observations in this field are clearly needed.

The Dong diet

An attractive and widely publicized diet for arthritis, the Dong diet [22], prompted Panush and his co-workers to embark on a 10-week controlled double-blind randomized trial comparing the diet (see Table 41.4) with a placebo

Table 41.4 Foods eliminated from the Dong diet [22].

Additives
Preservatives
Alcohol
Red meat
Dairy products
Fruit
Herbs and spices

regime [62]. Meticulous care was taken to ensure compliance. Twenty-six of 33 patients completed the trial. No clinical, laboratory or nutritional difference was observed between patients on the experimental diet and those on the placebo diet. It was concluded that the experimental diet was of no more benefit than the placebo. However, two patients on the experimental diet did improve substantially. It is interesting to note that in the first patient there was a strong history of atopy and, in the second, a history of hypersensitivity was suspected.

OTHER CONNECTIVE TISSUE DISEASES

Intermittent arthritis

A variety of other connective tissue diseases have been implicated in association with food allergy, intolerance and dietary factors. This is particularly true of some of the intermittent and periodic syndromes. Palindromic rheumatism in association with allergic disorders has already been discussed [88]. Further case reports incriminating sodium nitrate and peppermint in palindromic attacks [27, 91] have been published. Intermittent hydroarthrosis due to ingestion of walnuts has been described [44] and walnuts have been implicated as the cause of exacerbation of Behçet's syndrome [51] with concomitant depression of lymphocyte activity.

Systemic lupus erythematosus

Alfalfa seeds, which reduce cholesterolaemia in man and prevent atherosclerosis in rabbits, when fed in large quantities to monkeys induced a systemic lupus erythematosus-like syndrome [46].

In contrast, NZB/W mice maintained on a low (1%) fat diet showed a greatly reduced incidence of immune complex nephritis [55]. It was therefore suggested that efforts should be made to treat autoimmune disease with such a diet [55].

A menhaden oil diet rich in eicosapentaenoic acid protected female NZB × NZW/F_1 mice from autoimmune nephritis [67]. One mode of action of the diet may be to reduce inflammation through the ability of eicosapentaenoic acid to alter prostaglandins and leukotrienes.

An investigation into allergic reactivity in systemic lupus erythematosus patients showed significant increases in only allergic rhinitis and drug allergy [30]. The prevalence of food allergy was not significantly different from controls. Reviews of the gastroenterological manifestations of systemic lupus erythematosus rarely mention food allergy or intolerance. IgE antinuclear antibodies have been reported to systemic lupus erythematosus and found to be non-organ specific but related to disease activity.

Scleroderma

Gastrointestinal involvement is a common accompaniment of generalized scleroderma. Another relationship between scleroderma and the gut lies in the development of scleroderma-like lesions as a manifestation of carcinoid lesions of the gut. It is thought that the effect of serotonin with increased vascular permeability, oedema and consequent fibrosis is the likely sequence of events.

Scleroderma-like changes have recently been described as a complication of the toxic oil syndrome following ingestion of adulterated cooking oil [2].

Kashin–Beck disease

Apart from obesity, no satisfactorily proven relationship exists between diet and osteoarthritis. A chronic disabling generalized osteoarthritic disease has been described in Eastern Siberia [57] and the cause found to be cereal grain which had been contaminated with the fungus *Fusaria sporotrichella*. Denaturation of bread grain proteins resulted in toxic amines being produced with consequent vasoconstriction which was thought to interfere with articular nutrition.

SUMMARY

There is justification for the current revival of interest in the association between dietary factors and arthritis, but on present published evidence, food allergy and food intolerance seem unlikely to exert any significant effect upon the course of the majority of rheumatic and arthritic disorders. Although it is clear that short-term improvement can be achieved by changes in diet, exemplified by the effect of fasting on rheumatoid arthritis, substantially more positive and controlled evidence needs to be presented to justify long-term dietary restriction in the majority of arthritic patients.

On the other hand it would be unwise to ignore totally the possibility of food factors when dealing with individual cases. The literature provides sufficient data to arouse our suspicions in cases where arthritis is associated with an allergic condition such as asthma and eczema or where a family history of hypersensitivity exists. The occasional cases of seronegative polyarthritis may prove to be the presenting manifestations of latent intestinal disorders, such as coeliac disease, and can be rewarding to treat. The few extra minutes spent in taking a detailed dietary history when faced with a patient with intermittent arthritis could in some instances be the key to successful diagnosis and management.

REFERENCES

1 Alexander HL, Eyermann CH: Food allergy in Henoch's purpura. Arch Dermatol Syphilatol 1927; 16: 322–7.

2 Alonso-Ruiz A, Zea-Mendoza AC, Gonzáles-Lanza M, Gómez-Catalán E: Digital tuft alterations in toxic oil syndrome. Lancet 1984; ii: 520–1.

3 Barkley DO, Hohermuth HF, Howard A, et al. IgA deficiency in juvenile chronic arthritis. J Rheumatol 1979; 6: 219–24.

4 Bauer W: What should the patient with arthritis eat? J Am Med Assoc 1935; 104: 1.

5 Beighton P, Solomon L, Valkenburg HA: Rheumatoid arthritis in a rural South African Negro population. Ann Rheum Dis 1975; 34: 136–41.

6 Bennett JC: The infectious etiology of rheumatoid arthritis—new considerations. Arthritis Rheum 1978; 21: 531–8.

7 Bergström K, Havermark C: Enzymes in intestinal mucosa from patients with rheumatoid diseases. Scand J Rheumatol 1976; 5: 29–32.

8 Bitter T, Calin A, Hughes GRV, eds: Reiter's syndrome. Ann Rheum [Suppl 1] 1979; 38: 1–150.

9 Bourne JT, Huskisson EC, Kumar P et al: Arthritis and coeliac disease. Ann Rheum Dis 1985; 44: 592–8.

10 Brown M, Gibney M, Husband PR, Radcliffe M: Food allergy in polysymptomatic patients. Practitioner 1981; 225: 1651–4.

11 Chandra RK: Immunology of nutritional disorders. London: Edward Arnold, 1980.

12 Cook RA: Hayfever and asthma. NY Med J 1918: 107: 577–83.

13 Coombs RRA, Oldham G: Early rheumatoid joint lesions in rabbits drinking cow's milk. Int Arch Allergy Appl Immunol 1981; 64: 287–92.

14 Cooper BT, Holmes GKT, Cooke WT: Coeliac disease and immunological disorders. Br Med J 1978; i: 537–9.

15 Criep LH: Allergy of joints. J Bone Joint Surg 1946; 28: 276–9.

16 Cunningham-Rundles C, Brandeis WE, Pudifin DJ et al: Autoimmunity in selective IgA deficiency: relationship to antibovine protein antibodies, circulating immune complexes and clinical disease. Clin Exp Immunol 1981; 45: 299–304.

17 Darlington LG, Mansfield JR: Food allergy and rheumatoid disease. Ann Rheum Dis 1983; 42: 218.

17a Darlington LG, Ramsey NW, Mansfield JR: Placebo-controlled, blind study of dietary manipulation therapy in rheumatoid arthritis. Lancet 1986; i: 236–8.

18 Delamere JP, Baddeley RM, Walton KW: Jejuno-ileal by-pass arthropathy: its clinical features and associations. Ann Rheum Dis 1983; 42: 553–7.

19 Denman AM, Mitchell EB, Ansell BM: Dietary exclusion in patients with rheumatoid arthritis. Proc Second Fison Food Allergy Workshop 1983; 84–5.

20 Denman AM, Mitchell B, Ansell BM: Joint complaints and food allergic disorders. Ann Allergy 1983; 51: 260–3.

21 Dicken CH: Bowel associated dermatosis–arthritis syndrome. Bowel by-pass syndrome without bowel by-pass. Mayo Clin Proc 1984; 59: 43–6.

22 Dong CH, Banks J: New hope for the arthritic. New York: Ballantine, 1975.

23 Eastmond CJ, Calguneri M, Shinebaum R, et al: A sequential study of the relationship netween faecal *Klebsiella aerogenes* and the common clinical manifestations of ankylosing spondylitis. Ann Rheum Dis 1982; 41: 15–20.

24 Ebringer RW, Cooke D, Cawdell DR, et al: Ankylos-

ing spondylitis: *Klebsiella* and HLA B27. Rheumatol Rehabil 1977; 16: 190-6.

25 Egger J, Carter CM, Wilson J, et al: Is migraine food allergy. Lancet 1983; ii: 865.

26 Emery P, Panayi G, Symmons D, Brown G: Mechanisms of depressed delayed-type hypersensitivity in rheumatoid arthritis—the role of protein energy malnutrition. Ann Rheum 1984; 43: 430-4.

27 Epstein S: Hypersensitivity to sodium nitrate: a major causative factor in case of palindromic rheumatism. Ann Allergy 1969; 27: 343-9.

28 Gendre J-P, Luboinski J, Prier A, et al: Anomalies de la muqueuse jejunale en polyarthrite rheumatoide: 30 cas. Gastroenterol Clin Biol 1982; 6: 772-5.

29 Gerrard JW: Food intolerance. Lancet 1984; ii: 413.

30 Goldman JA, Klimek GA, Ali R: Allergy in systemic lupus erythematosus IgE levels and reagenic phenomenon. Arthritis Rheum 1976; 19: 669-76.

31 Grant M, Engelhart K, Bray C, Wojtulewski JA: A study of dietary elimination and food challenge in rheumatoid arthritis. Abstract, X European Congress of Rheumatology, 97.

32 Greenstein AJ, Janowitz HD, Sachar DB: The extraintestinal complications of Crohn's disease and ulcerative colitis: a study of 700 patients. Medicine 1976; 55: 401-11.

33 Hansen TM, Lerche A, Kassis V, et al: Treatment of rheumatoid arthritis with prostaglandin E, precursors *cis*-linoleic acid and *γ*-linolenic acid. Scand J Rheumatol 1983; 12: 85-8.

34 Helliwell M, Coombes EJ, Moody BJ, et al: Nutritional status in patients with rheumatoid arthritis. Ann Rheum Dis 1984; 43: 386-90.

35 Hench PS, Rosenberg EF: Palindromic rheumatism. Proc Staff Meet Mayo Clinic 1941; 16: 808-15.

36 Hicklin JA, McEwen LM, Morgan JE: The effect of diet in rheumatoid arthritis. Clin Allergy 1980; 10: 463.

37 Horrabin DF, Campbell A, McEwan CG: Treatment of the sicca syndrome and Sjögren's syndrome with EFA, pyridoxine and vitamin C. Essential fatty acids and prostaglandins. Prog Lipid Res 1981; 20: 253-4.

38 Hunder GG, Gleich GJ: Immunoglobulin E levels in serum and synovial fluid in rheumatoid arthritis. Arthritis Rheum 1974; 17: 955-63.

39 Kaufman HS, Hobbs JR: Immunoglobulin deficiencies in an atopic population. Lancet 1970; ii: 1061-3.

39a Kremer JM, Michaelek AV, Liniger L et al: Effects of manipulation of dietary fatty acids on clinical manifestations of rheumatoid arthritis. *Lancet* 1985; i: 184-7.

40 Kunkel SL, Ogawa H, Ward PA, Zurier RB: Suppression of chronic inflammation by evening primrose oil. Essential fatty acids and prostaglandins. Prog Lipid Res 1981; 20: 885-8.

41 Lancaster Smith MJ, Perrin J, Swarbrick ET, Wright JT: Coeliac disease and autoimmunity. Postgrad Med J 1974; 50: 45-8.

42 Landré-Beauvais AJ: Doit-on admettre une nouvelle espèce de goutte sous la dénomination de goutte asthénique primitive? Paris: 1800.

43 Lessof MH, Wraith DG, Merrett TG et al: Food allergy and intolerance in 100 patients—local and systemic effects. Q J Med 1980; 195: 259-71.

44 Lewin P, Taub SJ: Allergic synovitis due to ingestion of English walnuts. J Am Med Assoc 1936; 106: 2144.

45 Little CH, Stewart AG, Fennessy, MR: Platelet serotonin release in rheumatoid arthritis: a study in food intolerant patients. Lancet 1983; ii: 297-9.

46 Malinow MR, Bardana EJ, Pirofsky B: Systemic lupus-erythematosus-like syndrome induced by diet in monkeys. Clin Res 1981; 29: 626A.

47 Mandell M, Conte A: The role of allergy in arthritis, rheumatism and associated polysymptomatic cerebroviscero-somatic disorders: a double-blind provocation test study: Ann Allergy 1980; 44: 51.

48 Mansfield JR, Darlington LG: Dietary elimination therapy and neutralisation therapy in patients with rheumatoid disease. A prospective double-blind placebo controlled study. Food and Environmental factors in Human Disease. Torquay, 1984, abstract.

49 Mansson I, Norberg R, Olhagen B, Björkland N-E: Arthritis in pigs induced by dietary factors. Clin Exp Immunol 1971; 9: 677-93.

50 Marcolongo R, Bayeli PF, Montagnani M: Gastrointestinal involvement in rheumatoid arthritis: a biopsy study. J Rheumatol 1979; 6: 163-73.

51 Marquardt JL, Snyderman R, Oppenheim JJ: Depression of lymphocyte transformation and exacerbation of Behçet's syndrome by ingestion of English walnuts. Cell Immunol 1973; 9: 263-73.

52 Meyers OL, Daynes G, Beighton P: Rheumatoid arthritis in a tribal Xhosa populaion in the Transkei, Southern Africa. Ann Rheum Dis 1977; 36: 62-5.

53 Minford AMB, Macdonald A, Littlewood JM: Food intolerance and food allergy in children: a review of 68 cases. Arch Dis Child 1982; 742-7.

54 Moolenburgh, JD, Moore S, Valkenburg HA, Erasmus MG: Rheumatoid arthritis in Lesotho. Ann Rheum Dis 1984; 43: 40-3.

55 Morrow WJW, Levy JA: Dietary fat and autoimmune disease. Arthritis Rheum 1983; 26: 1532.

56 Muller AS: Population studies on the prevalence of rheumatic diseases in Liberia and Nigeria. Leiden: 1970, MD thesis.

57 Nesterov AI: The clinical course of Kashin-Beck disease. Arthritis Rheum 1964; 7: 30-9.

58 Olhagen B: On the aetiopathogenesis of rheumatoid arthritis. Ann Clin Res 1975; 7: 119-28.

59 Olhagen B, Mansson I: Intestinal *Clostridium perfringens* in rheumatoid arthritis and other collagen diseases. Acta Med Scand 1968; 184: 395-402.

60 O'Morain C, Segal AW, Levi AJ: Elemental diets in Crohn's disease. Br Med J 1980; 281: 1173-5.

61 Osler W: The visceral lesions of purpura and allied conditions. Br Med J 1914, 1: 517-25.

62 Panush RS, Carter RL, Katz P, et al: Diet therapy for rheumatoid arthritis. Arthritis Rheum 1983; 26:462-71.

62a Panush RS, Stroud RM, Webster EM: Food-induced (allergic) arthritis. Inflammatory arthritis exacerbated by milk. Arthritis Rheum 1986; 29: 220-6.

63 Parke AL, Hughes GRV: Rheumatoid arthritis and food: a case study. Br Med J 1981; 282: 2027-9.

64 Parke AL, Fagan EA, Chadwick VS, Hughes GRV: Gut permeability in Sjögrens syndrome, rheumatoid arthritis and coeliac disease. Ann Rheum Dis 1983; 42: 216.

65 Parke AL, Fagan EA, Chadwick VS, Hughes GRV: Coeliac disease and rheumatoid arthritis. Ann Rheum Dis 1984; 43: 378-80.

66 Peskett SA, Platts-Mills TAE, Ansell BM, Stearnes GN: The incidence of atopy in rheumatic diseases. J Rheumatol 1981; 8: 321-4.

67 Prickett JD, Wight D, Robinson R, Steinberg AD: Effect of dietary enrichment with eicosapentaenoic acid upon autoimmune nephritis in female NZB × NZW/F₁ mice. Arthritis Rheum 1983; 26: 133.

68 Randolph TG: Allergic myalgia. J Mich State Med Soc 1951; 50: 487.

69 Randolph T: Ecologically oriented rheumatoid arthritis. In: Dickey LD, ed. Clinical ecology. Springfield: CC Thomas, 1976, 201-12.

70 Robinson WD: Nutrition and rheumatic disease. In: Kelly WN, Harris E, Ruddy S, Sledge CS, eds. Textbook of rheumatology. Philadelphia: WB Saunders, 1980; 337-49.

71 Rooney PJ, Kennedy AC, Gray GH, et al: Serum immunoreactive gastrin in rheumatoid arthritis. Ann Rheum Dis 1976; 35: 246-50.

72 Ropes MW, Bennett GA, Cobb S, et al: Diagnostic criteria for rheumatoid arthritis. 1958 Revision. Bull Rheum Dis 1959; 9: 175.

73 Rowe AH: Allergic toxaemia and migraine due to food allergy. Calif West Med 1930; 33: 785.

74 Rowe AH, Rowe A Jr: Food allergy: its manifestations and control and the elimination diets. A compendium. Springfield: CC Thomas, 1972.

75 Scott BB, Losowsky MS: Coeliac disease: a cause of various associated diseases? Lancet 1975; ii: 956-7.

76 Shagrin JW, Frame B, Duncan H: Polyarthritis in obese patients with intestinal by-pass. Ann Intern Med 1971; 75: 377-80.

77 Shinebaum R, Neumann V, Hopkins R, et al: Attempt to modify *Klebsiella* carriage in ankylosing spondylitic patients by diet: correlation of *Klebsiella* carriage with disease activity. Ann Dis 1984; 43: 196-9.

78 Short CD, Klouda PT, Smith L: *Campylobacter jejuni* enteritis and reactive arthritis. Ann Rheum Dis 1982; 41: 287-8.

79 Siurala M, Julkunen H, Toivonen S, et al. Digestive tract in collagen disease. Acta Med Scand 1965; 178: 13-25.

80 Sköldstam L, Larsson L, Lindström FD: Effects of fasting and lactovegetarian diet on rheumatoid arthritis. Scand J Rheumatol 1979; 8: 249-55.

81 Solis-Cohen S: On some angioneural arthroses commonly mistaken for gout or rheumatism. Am J Med Sci 1914; 147; 228.

82 Solomon L, Robin G, Valkenburg HA: Rheumatoid arthritis in an urban South African Negro population. Ann Rheum Dis 1975; 34: 128-35.

83 Stroud RM, Kroker CE, Rea WJ, et al: Comprehensive environmental control and its effect on rheumatoid arthritis. Clin Res 1980; 28: 791A.

84 Sunqvist T, Lindström F, Magnusson K-E, et al: Influence of fasting on intestinal permeability and disease activity in patients with rheumatoid arthritis. Scand J Rheumatol 1982; 11: 33-8.

85 Tagesson C, Bengtsson A: Intestinal permeability to different sized polyethylene glycols in patients with rheumatoid arthritis. Scand J Rheumatol 1983; 12: 124-8.

86 Talbot FB: Role of food idiosyncrasies in practice. NY State J Med 1917; 17: 419-25.

87 Uden A-M, Trang L, Venizelos N, Palmblad J: Neutrophil functions and clinical performance after total fasting in patients with rheumatoid arthritis. Ann Rheum Dis 1983; 42: 45-51.

88 Vaughan WT: Palindromic rheumatism among allergic persons. J Allergy 1943; 14: 256-63.

89 Vaz GA, Tan LK-T, Gerrard JW: Oral cromoglycate in treatment of adverse reactions to foods. Lancet 1978; i: 1066.

90 Wands JR, LaMont JT, Mann E, Isselbacher KJ: Arthritis associated with intestinal by-pass procedure for morbid obesity. N Engl J Med 1976; 294: 121-4.

91 Williams B: Palindromic rheumatism: a request. Med J Aust 1972; ii: 390-1.

92 Williams R: Rheumatoid arthritis and food: a case study. Br Med J 1981; 283: 563.

93 Wojtulewski JA, Fan YS, Model DG: Gluten sensitive enteropathy presenting as polyarthritis. Abstracts VII Panamerican Congress of Rheumatology 1978; 34.

94 Wordsworth P, Pack S, Brostoff J: Food allergens in rheumatoid arthritis. British Assocation for Rheumatology and Rehabilitation Annual Meeting April 1983, abstract.

95 Wraith DG: Clinical aspects of food allergy. Abstract Proceedings Fourth Charles Blackley Symposium 1981: 44.

96 Zeller M: Rheumatoid arthritis—food allergy as a factor. Ann Allergy 1949; 7: 200-5.

97 Ziff M: Diet in the treatment of rheumatoid arthritis. Arthritis Rheum 1983; 26: 457-61.

98 Zussman BM: Food hypersensitivity simulating rheumatoid arthritis. South Med J 1966; 59: 935-9.

SECTION G
CARDIOVASCULAR

Chapter 42
Cardiovascular Disease in Response to Chemicals and Foods

William J. Rea and Ollie Dawkins Brown

Introduction

Environmental insults have long been known to influence man's health. Even Hippocrates emphasized environmental effects (*see Air, Water, and Places* in ref. [39]). Early environmental records indicate that excess heat and cold influence bodily functions with extreme exposure resulting in death. Present-day thought and technology have allowed us to substantiate and augment the view that health and disease are a function of how man deals with his environment. It has become evident that treatment and prevention of cardiovascular disease must not only encompass views on biological (pollen, bacteria, virus, fungus, parasites) but also chemical factors (organic and inorganic) and physical forces (weather, cyclic phenomena, sound and electromagnetic effects).

737

AGENTS AFFECTING THE CARDIOVASCULAR SYSTEM

Chemical agents

While chemical incitants may trigger a maladaptation response in virtually any of the smooth muscle systems, those of the cardiovascular system appear to be the most susceptible (Lichtwitz in [37]). Recent literature has verified previous findings regarding the harmful effects of a variety of chemicals on the cardiovascular system as shown in Table 42.1.

Table 42.1 Chemical agents affecting the cardiovascular system.

	Reference		Reference
Fluorocarbons	37, 86	Formaldehyde	72
Phenol	56	Chlorine	21
Petroleum alcohol	98	Cigarette smoke	24
Glycerine	26	Chlorophenothane (DDT)	72
Toluene	72	Turpentine	72
Hydralazine	84		

Physical agents

Physical agents such as heat, cold, weather changes, light and cycles have for centuries been known to influence health. The increase in modern technology has augmented our environment with noise and with electric and electromagnetic fields. The induction of disease and the maintenance of cardiovascular health can be regarded as functions of how the individual manipulates the total load of these pollutants through his immune and biochemical detoxification mechanisms.

Water

Water usually contains minerals, organic chemicals, particulate matter and radiation. Chemically contaminated water is a major component of the total environmental load. Most public water systems are loaded with organic and inorganic chemicals which may increase the body burden of some chemicals several fold. These include trihalomethanes [97], pesticides [9, 61, 76, 92], formaldehyde [55], solvents [55], oils [98], heavy metals [55], and other metals such as copper [55]. Public drinking water has been described by Laseter [46] and others [81] as containing most of the contents of an organic chemical laboratory.

Hard water. When water is ingested, all of its components must be metabolized, catabolized

or excreted. In developed nations, the prevalence of many chronic diseases, particularly cardiovascular diseases, can be associated with various water characteristics related to hardness. Those involved include coronary heart disease, hypertension and stroke. The theorized protective agents found in hard water are calcium, magnesium, vanadium, lithium, chromium and manganese [55]. Recent studies report fewer heart attacks, less coronary disease and lower mortality rates in patients with existing cardiovascular disease in areas where there is hard water [25].

Soft water. Suspected harmful agents include the metals cadmium, lead, copper and zinc which tend to be found in higher concentrations in soft water as a result of its relative corrosiveness. Nitrates in water pose immediate threats to children under 3 months of age. Excessive levels have been known to react with haemoglobin in the blood to produce methaemoglobinaemia. Though barium occurs naturally in the environment, it can enter water supplies through industrial waste discharges. Barium can bring about an increase in blood pressure and even death [19]. Patients susceptible to water contaminants may exhibit multiple sensitivities and be especially sensitive to airborne chemicals [68].

Food

There are at least three aspects of food to consider in evaluating a patient's cardiovascular health. These are: (a) food sensitivity, (b) additives (natural and manmade toxins) and (c) the nutritive quality.

Food sensitivity

Involvement of the cardiovascular system in food sensitivities has been reported by a number of researchers. It was first shown by Hare [36] in 1905. He recognized tachycardia and bradycardia in patients following ingestion of some foods. Since then a variety of cardiovascular disease states have been reported to be related to food, including increased heart rates, angina pectoris, arrhythmias, myocardial infarction, extrasystoles and atrial and ventricular fibrillation [37]. Other reports have found phlebitis and vasculitis to be triggered by foods [69, 75, 89] (see also Chapter 56).

Food additives

The widespread contamination of food supplies is witnessed by the increasing use of food additives, preservatives and dyes in the manufacturing and processing of commercially available food products. Urticarial reactions, vascular abnormalities and immunological changes as a function of exposure to a number of chemicals and food additives have been reported by a number of authors [6, 8, 35, 41, 48, 54, 71, 73, 97] and are discussed in detail in Chapters 22a and 22b.

Food constituents. Intake of high fat plus sugar in combination with additive-rich food will damage blood vessels yielding plaque deposition with resultant arteriosclerosis. Many discussions appear in the literature on this subject and it will not be further discussed here.

Air

The physical factors of the weather include not only heat and cold but humidity, barometric pressure, electromagnetic and electric fields, seasons and weather cycles as well. It has been estimated that 25–30% of the population is sensitive to weather changes [38]. Some authors have suggested that triggering of cardiovascular disease including myocardial infarction may be related to the weather [38, 17].

Outdoor air pollution

Outdoor air pollution has long been thought to enhance disease processes. Prior to the 19th century, air pollution as we know it was virtually unknown. The term 'smog' was first used in England to denote a combination of smoke and natural fog, which may produce ill-effects [32]. The term is now used in all industrialized countries but often denotes air pollution of vastly different compositions. For example, Los Angeles smog is largely composed of petrochemicals and their by-products [32], while in China it is composed mainly of coal effluent. According to Environmental Protection Agency studies [32], there has been no 'fresh' air in the United States in 20 years! Contaminants involved in air pollution include inorganic chemicals (sulphur dioxide, carbon monoxide, nitrogen oxides, lead etc.), organic chemicals (petroleum-derived hydrocarbons, etc.), particulates (pollen, moulds, dust, car and factory emissions) and electromagnetic and electric emission [17].

London smog. A combination of weather inversions occurred in London during a 4-day period in December 1952. The London-type smog of particulates, sulphur oxides and fog caused approximately 4000 deaths in the following week. Between 80% and 90% of the deaths were due to respiratory and cardiovascular disease which were mainly of a chronic nature. A majority of deaths occurred in people over the age of 65 years [93]. A similar incident occurred in Donora, Pennsylvania, a highly industrialized valley, during a 6-day period in October 1984. Out of a population of 44 000, 42% became ill and 18 deaths resulted [50]. This highlights the clinical effect of outdoor air pollution.

Indoor air pollution

Historically, contaminated indoor air began with the soot on the ceilings of prehistoric caves resulting from open fires. Home air was very bad for health during the times of the great plagues and tuberculosis outbreaks. Changes in cleanliness in the home resulted in the virtual elimination of many diseases such as tuberculosis. More recently, the use of rapidly disintegrating synthetic materials, fossil fuels and pesticides, coupled with the sealing of buildings in an attempt to conserve fuel by prevention of heat loss, lead to a new type of indoor pollution.

Electrical phenomena can also contribute to indoor air pollution. Sources of indoor electric fields include most electrical appliances ranging from electric blankets (250 V/m) to light bulbs (2 V/m)[5].

Time spent indoors. Typically, people spend more than 90% of their time indoors. Some contaminants have been found to be in higher concentrations indoors than outdoors. Indoor contaminants which have been found to be associated with health include aeroallergens, microorganisms, asbestos fibres, formaldehyde, pesticides, nitrogen dioxide, carbon monoxide, radon decay products and tobacco smoke.

Electrical phenomena

Although not strictly within the remit of this chapter, there seems little doubt that electromagnetic fields (EMF) can have clinical effects, and that EMF may contribute to the overall environmental load. This in turn may make patients more susceptible to chemicals in foods.

Electromagnetic fields

Some natural areas of the earth have higher levels of EMF than others. These are found over water veins and geological faults. There are increased areas found radiating from the poles and widening over the equator [5].

High frequency emitters in the United States consist of the whole of the EMF spectrum including AM radio band (0.535–1.604 MHz) and FM and TV band (54–806 MHz). Low-frequency electromagnetic exposures emanate from the electrical power systems (60 Hz in the US, 50 Hz in Europe and the USSR). The main sources of indoor electromagnetic fields include hair dryers (10–25 gauss), electric shavers (5–10 gauss) and televisions (1–5 gauss) [5]. However, environmental exposures are very small compared with the 10^{-1}V/m across a live cell membrane [5].

Clinical effects of electromagnetic fields

Cardiovascular effects. Animals exposed to EMF may exhibit significant changes in electrocardiograms [7], sinus arrhythmia [7] and brachycardia [22, 67] (Fig. 42.1). Alterations

in heart function such as falling arterial pressure [67] and increased heart rate [30] have been noted in humans. Both short- and long-term hypotensive effects have been reported [51] along with decreases in efficient cardiac output [23]. Autonomic nervous system dysfunction was reported in individuals who were continuously exposed to higher levels of EMF, whereas very low frequency exposures were found to cause neurovascular instability in some individuals [80].

Haematological effects. Changes in the cellular composition of blood of a variety of laboratory animals exposed to EMF have been shown. Changes in number of red and white blood cells have been noted and the changes were found to be dependent on time and the magnitude of the EMF. A variety of other changes in haematological parameters in response to EMF have been reported and are discussed elsewhere [34, 43, 45, 50, 80]. These include changes in iron metabolism, fibrinolytic activity and coagulation [45].

Charged electrical conditions

Negative ions have been shown to affect the carbon dioxide combining power of plasma and to increase blood pH [95, 96]. Stimulation of heart rate and cortical alpha-rhythm [20, 79] with decreases in alpha-frequency have been seen in humans exposed to air ions of either polarity. Increases in blood pressure and 17-ketosteroids under positive ionization have been noted accompanied by cholesterol decreases. Tchijevsky [87] and Vasiliev [91] proposed as a mechanism the penetration of charged particles through the alveolar wall into the blood vessels where the charges are transferred to blood cells and colloids.

MECHANISMS OF ENVIRONMENTALLY INDUCED VASCULAR DAMAGE

There are probably numerous ways that environmental pollutants trigger vascular responses while disturbing the immune and biological detoxification systems.

Effects on vessel walls

As the pollutants enter the body, they may create free radicals [52]. These may be O^-, OH^+, lipid peroxide or others and may dam-

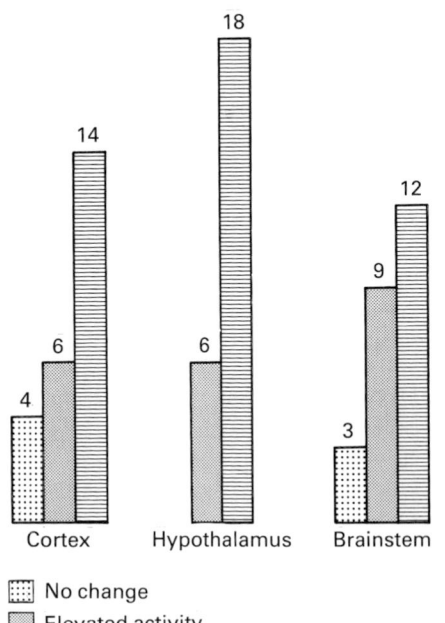

Fig. 42.1 Relation of EEG response from the cortex, hypothalamus and brainstem due to exposure at 3 GHz. The numbers indicate rabbits with a given response. From Becker and Marino [5], with permission. © State University of New York Press.

age mitochondrial and cellular membranes of the vascular tree causing vessel leakage.

According to Zeek [99], vessel wall damage may be mild with leak of fluid, but as it progresses the leaks get larger allowing red blood cells to migrate. With severe damage to the wall, clotting may occur giving distal peripheral tissue damage.

Attempts at healing may occur in various ways leading to granulomatous or fibrous scar formation. Triggering agents may be infectious (bacteria, virus, fungi, parasitic), chemical (sulphur dioxide, phenol, hydrocarbon), [65, 70] nutritional [70] or traumatic (physical environmental agents, as discussed above).

Effect on the clotting system

Countless medical and surgical procedures have been associated with chemically triggered reactions. Nickel sensitivity has been reported secondary to the use of skin clips, and in a patient with a nickel steel heart valve who developed valve thrombosis. All synthetic heart valves and artificial hearts and lungs are known to be able to trigger the clotting mechanism. Haemolysis has been associated with necrotizing dermatitis, and this can occur after exposure to the epoxy resin in needles and polyvinylchloride tubing.

Effect on cells

Some chemicals like dichlorodiphenyltrichloroethane (DDT) suppress the mast cells so thoroughly that anaphylaxis is less likely to occur [28, 29].

Cadmium can suppress the mononuclear phagocyte system [3]. Ozone can cause lipid plastic parathyroiditis with leukocytic infiltration and capillary proliferation [83]. Some substances such as phenol have an affinity for the cardiovascular system [56]. Yervick [98] demonstrated cardiovascular changes in sea animals exposed to oil spills. Chloracne perivasculitis lesions have been produced in monkeys fed a pesticide, Arochlor 1248 (polychlorinated biphenyl).

Types of mechanism in vascular damage

Immune mediated

The intrinsic mechanisms by which blood vessels are damaged can be mediated either via the immune system or via the non-immune biological detoxification system. The immune hypersensitivity responses in the vessel wall can be any of four types (see Chapters 24 and 44) and frequently can be a combination of types.

Type I hypersensitivity is mediated through the IgE mechanism on the vessel wall. The classic examples are angiodema, urticaria and anaphylaxis due to sensitivity to pollen, dust, mould or food [89].

Type II cytotoxic damage may occur with direct injury to the cell. A clinical example of this is seen with exposures to mercury [31], although this might be directly toxic rather than antibody mediated.

Type III immune complex syndromes include lupus vasculitis. Numerous chemicals including procaineamide [78] and chlorothiazide [78] are known to trigger the autoantibody reactions of lupus. Other chemicals such as vinyl chloride [47] will produce microaneurysms.

Type IV cell-mediated immunity occurs with sensitization and stimulation of T lymphocytes. Numerous chemicals such as phenol, pesticides, organohalides and some metals will also alter immune responses possibly triggering lymphokines giving a Type IV reaction [94]. Clinical examples are polyarteritis nodosa, hypersensitivity angitis, Henoch–Schönlein purpura and Wegener's granulomatosis [69].

Non-immune mechanisms: mediators

Non-immune triggering of the vessel wall may also occur. Complement may be triggered directly via the alternative pathway by moulds, foods or toxic chemicals [73]. Mediators like kinins and prostaglandins may also be directly triggered (see Chapter 44a). Interestingly, in addition to allergic responses, pollens have been shown to have toxic substances which will trigger haemolysis and other responses [27] (see also Chapter 21).

Endocrine effects in the vascular system

Oestrogen has long been known to have a mildly suppressive effect on the cardiovascular system. The late onset of arteriosclerosis in females with the onset of menopause is commonly observed. A study by Couch and Wortman [13] supports this observation in that they found a significantly greater number of occurrences of migraine in pathologically anovulatory females (polycystic ovary, galactorrhoea, amenorrhoea) compared with pregnant women or women taking the contraceptive pill. It was suggested that this might also be due to hypothalamic problems [13]. Excess oestrogen has been shown to have an adverse effect on vessel walls giving rise to venous inflammation which results in thrombophlebitis and pulmonary emboli [13].

Neurogenic vascular responses to external stimuli

When noxious stimuli are first detected there is a retrograde impulse to the dorsal nerve root ganglia through the afferent fibres of peripheral nerves (slow C or rapid delta A), or the gastrointestinal plexus. The sensory neurotransmitter, substance P, will cause immediate vasodilatation and increased permeability of the microcirculation in the area of the nerve and activate the non-IgE-mediated release of histamine via the mast cells. In addition, the release of leukotactic factors and leukotrienes is stimulated. Somatostatin is released in other cells of the dorsal root, but can also be released from the central nervous system and the pancreas. The relationship between somatostatin and substance P is complicated and both have effects on other cell interactions (see also Chapter 24).

Clinical manifestations of vascular injury

Vascular injury gives rise to a variety of clinical manifestations depending on the types of vessels involved (vein, capillary, large or small artery) and the intensity and duration of the insult.

Hypersensitivity vasculitis

The hypersensitivity vasculitides are a group of disorders characterized by small vessel inflammation. Manifestations are often mild and self-limited. Although any organ can be involved, the most common is the skin, lesions being found on the buttocks, ankles and legs. Causes for some of these have now been found. Theorell [89] showed occurrences of purpura and other signs of vasculitis after challenge with moulds, cedar and some foods. We have also observed such vascular lesions after challenge with phenol, formaldehyde and beef. Hypersensitivity vasculitis is a diverse group of disorders including serum sickness reactions, Henoch–Schönlein purpura (Fig. 42.2), essential mixed cryoglobulinaemia and

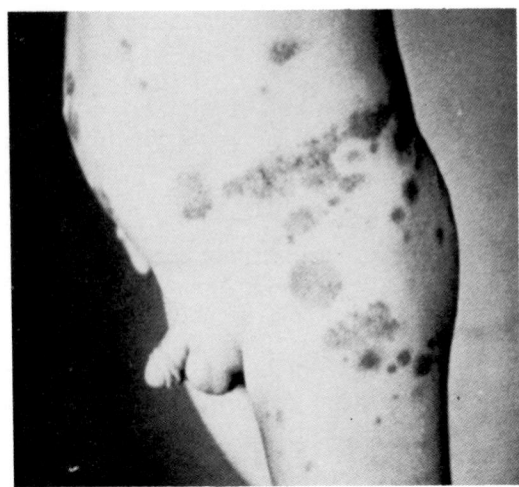

Fig. 42.2 Henoch–Schönlein purpura (anaphylactoid purpura) in a 14-year-old boy, with associated urticarial erythematous lesions with purpura, painful articular swelling and microscopic haematuria. From Olsen [57], with permission.

the connective tissue diseases particularly rheumatoid and lupus vasculitis [40].

Foreign serum proteins can cause serum sickness reactions and similar reactions may occur after use of penicillin [85], sulphonamides [77], streptomycin [11], thiouracils [11] and hydencompounds [11]. We have seen a case of Henoch–Schönlein purpura triggered by pollen, dust, moulds, foods and chemicals.

Periarteritis nodosa (PAN)

Periarteritis nodosa generally follows a prodromal fever with arthralgia and malaise; it may manifest itself as acute gastrointestinal distress, myocardial infarction, neuritis, muscle pain and/or gangrene of the extremities. It generally presents in the muscular arteries involving all three layers of the arterial wall and adjacent veins and is usually segmental.

Biopsy. Biopsy of skin, subcutaneous nodules or smooth muscle reveals acute healing vasculitis without giant cells (Fig. 42.3). The infiltrative process involves polymorphonuclear leukocytes, eosinophils and oedema followed by fibrinoid necrosis. The areas of fibrinoid necrosis are subsequently replaced by fibroblasts and scar tissue is formed.

Systemic lupus erythematosus

Apparently, many foreign substances can trigger a systemic lupus erythematosus-like syndrome. Chemical triggering of lupus has

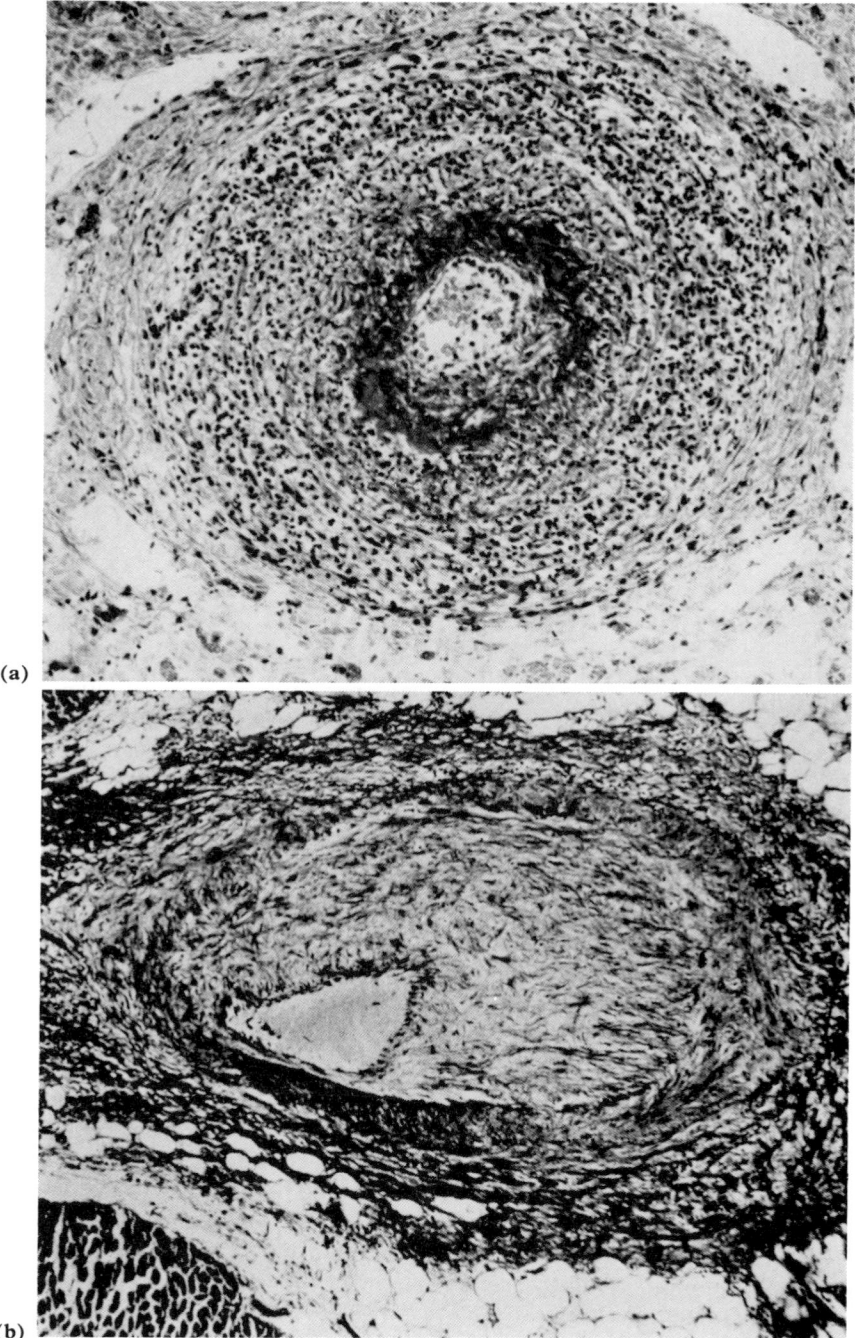

(a)

(b)

Fig. 42.3 Polyarteritis nodosa (PAN). (a) Acute inflammatory stage of PAN is characterized by panarteritic and periarteritic inflammation with polymorphonuclear leukocytes, eosinophils and round cells, destruction of vascular tissues and fibrinoid necrosis (dark, amorphous material about lumen). (b) In healing and healed stages of PAN, reparative fibrosis distorts vascular wall with loss of most of internal lamina (black wavy line) and marked narrowing of original lumen by organized thrombus and reparative fibrosis. From Titus and Kim [90], with the kind permission of the authors and C.V. Mosby Co.

been well established in the literature [88]. The following case report is an example of a patient whose symptoms were environmentally induced (Table 42.2).

Case study 1. A 36-year-old, white female had developed recurrent bouts of vomiting at the age of 5; these gave way to migraine at the age of 11 and the latter persisted. At the age of 16

Table 42.2 Case report of a patient with systemic lupus erythematosus.

		Patient	Control
Patient	36-year-old white female		
Symptoms	Vomiting, migraine, bruising, petechiae, peripheral oedema		
Laboratory	Sedimentation rate	48	10 ± 10 mm/h
	Total complement CH50	181%	$100 \pm 20\%$
	C-reactive protein	Positive	Negative
	Total eosinophil count	325	$125 \pm 75\% \, m^3$
	Antinuclear antibody	+	−
	LE test	+	−
Triggering agents	Moulds	Dust	20 foods
	Chemicals: phenol, formaldehyde, pesticides, chlorine, petroleum alcohol		
Discharge status	Improving. Clear of symptoms without medication on discharge		
Follow-up	Long term follow-up (5 years): doing well without medications. Occasional mild symptoms following acute exposures		

she developed a polyarthritis, and a diagnosis of systemic lupus erythematosus (SLE) was made. Her disease progressed over the next several years, with further involvement of the gastrointestinal, genitourinary, respiratory and vascular systems. Spontaneous bruising and petechiae occurred, together with peripheral oedema. She was eventually placed on cortisone and cytotoxic drugs. Antinuclear antibodies and LE preparations were positive on numerous occasions. She was placed in the environmental control unit, and all medications were discontinued. The stiffness and swelling of her joints gradually disappeared. Her sedimentation rate fell from 63 to 15 mm. This was the lowest it had been for many years. The circumference of her fingers diminished by 1.5–2 cm while fasting, reflecting the massive decrease of oedema. She was able to open and close her hands for the first time in many years. Challenges with 20 out of 30 different foods precipitated a return of her symptoms. The inhalation of chemicals such as perfume, phenol and natural gas also triggered symptoms. She has done well without medications on an avoidance programme for several years.

Wegener's granulomatosis

PAN is closely related to Wegener's granulomatosis, which is characterized by necrotizing granulomas in the respiratory tract and vasculitis of the medium-size arteries, veins, arterioles and venules. The onset may be acute or chronic. Though pathologically well defined, the aetiology of the disease is still obscure. Recent studies indicate that it is worthwhile looking for incitants.

Rheumatoid vasculitis

Diseases such as rheumatoid arthritis exhibit a variety of vascular manifestations and biopsy evidence of vasculitis. Although the aetiology of this disease is generally not known, evidence of immune changes in patients with rheumatoid arthritis following food and chemical challenges has been found. Two controlled series have been reported defining triggering agents in rheumatoid arthritis [44, 58] and a recent report has clearly shown the efficacy of diet in rheumatoid arthritis [15].

Eosinophilic vasculitis

Eosinophilic vasculitis has now been reported in some disease processes, i.e. eosinophilic granulomas and Goodpasture's syndrome. Lymphocytic vascular inflammation has been seen in some infectious diseases [58] and other syndromes [44].

Diagnosis of vasculitis

A variety of laboratory tests can be performed with the most relevant ones being indicated by clinical experience. Angiograms should be carried out to rule out fixed lesions as required. Frequently, spasm will be seen if the larger vessels are involved. If skin lesions are present, biopsies may show either necrotizing vasculitis with polymorphonuclear leukocyte infiltration or non-necrotizing lesions with eosinophils and/or lymphocytes around or in the vessel wall. However, only active lesions are likely to be positive when biopsy of the petechiae and bruises is done.

Challenge tests. Challenge tests should be done to define triggering agents. These may be done via oral, inhaled and/or interdermal routes. Care should be taken to do challenge tests under steady-state environmental conditions in order to reduce variability.

Environmental control unit. The use of an environmental control unit with its reduction of pollutants in air, food and water can lead to the most precise diagnosis and treatment for the environmental aspects of cardiovascular diseases, and is particularly useful for the severely compromised patient (see Chapter 55). Since these units are not commonly available, controlled areas in hospitals and offices may have to be used as a less satisfactory substitute. An improvement on reduction of the total load with deterioration on subsequent challenge is the key to diagnosing triggering agents of cardiovascular disease.

CLINICAL SYNDROMES

Vasculitis

Small vessel vasculitis

Rea et al [71] described a group of patients with multisystem involvement distinguished by a wide variety of symptoms. All evidenced frequent peripheral vasospasms, spontaneous cutaneous bruising and/or petechiae and peripheral oedema.

Following challenge, most patients produced a sequential progression of symptoms of colour change of the hands, feet, nose and skin, followed by pulse alteration, periorbital and peripheral oedema, petechiae and/or spontaneous bruising. Biopsies showed perivascular lymphocytic infiltrates.

Large vessel vasculitis

Large vessel involvement associated with sensitivities has also been reported [18, 33]. Rea detailed the case of a 65-year-old female who exhibited large-vessel involvement. She was found to be sensitive to 10 foods and three synthetic chemicals. All appeared to trigger spasm of her femoral arteries [74] (Fig. 42.4).

Large vessel vasculitis may ultimately have more devastating results than other vascular disorders since the blood supply to major organs is affected. Organ ischaemia and/or necrosis may result in severe disability or even death. The author has now seen five patients

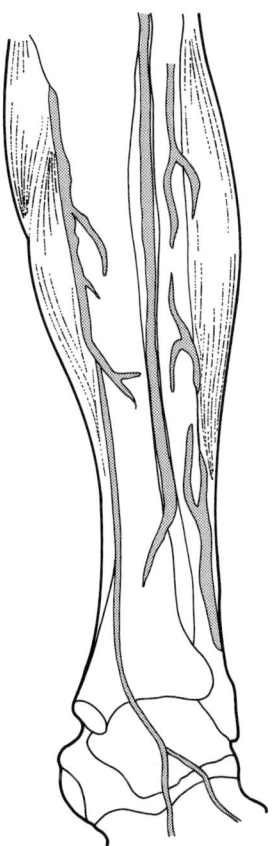

Fig. 42.4 Angiogram of femoral artery showing spasm associated with sensitivities.

with spastic carotid phenomena resulting in transient cerebrovascular accidents.

Case study 2. One patient with large-vessel involvement was a 42-year-old surgeon who developed involuntary arm movements, accompanied by asthma-like symptoms, spontaneous bruising, petechiae and acneiform lesions [33]. A carotid arteriogram revealed a decrease in left carotid and left intracerebral flow due to arterial spasm (Fig. 42.5). Double-blind challenges with foods and synthetic chemicals revealed the following sequence of events: (a) immediate right-sided peripheral cyanosis, (b) tenderness in left neck, (c) decrease of superficial temporal pulse, (d) loss of use of right arm and hand followed by (e) severe digital oedema accompanied by very foggy thinking and memory loss.

Vasculitis: Raynaud's disease?

Raynaud's disease refers to any localized peripheral digital vascular spasm or collapse of unknown aetiology. It may lead to gangrene [74].

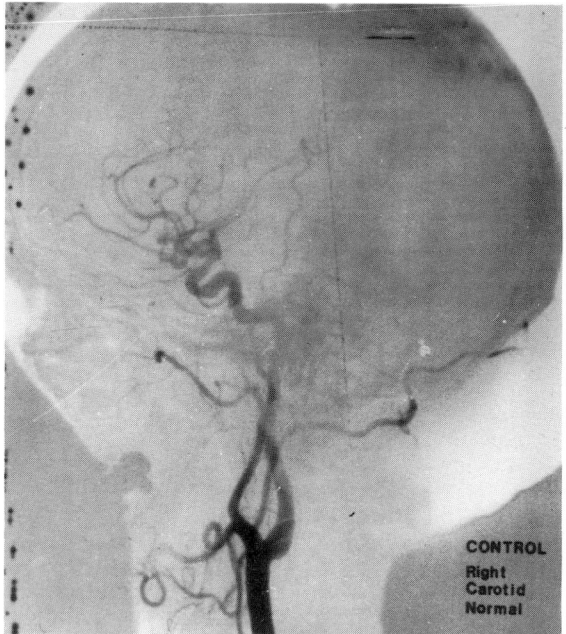
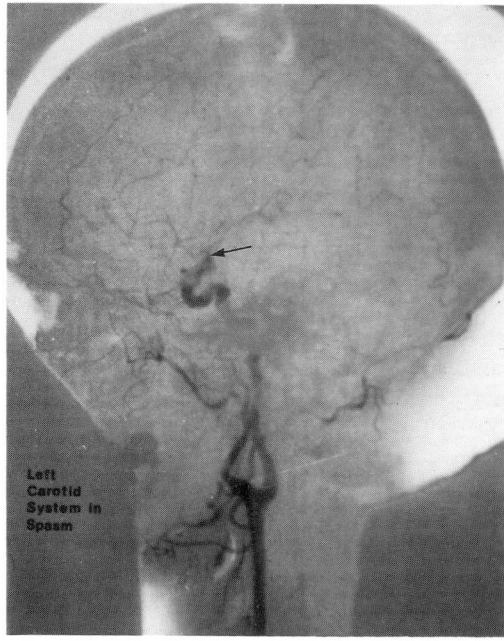

Fig. 42.5 Cerebral arteriograms revealing decreased carotid and left intracerebral flow due to arterial spasm.

Triggering agents can be identified and culprits include both foods and chemicals. One patient's symptoms could be reproduced by challenge with multiple foods and five inhaled chemicals. Follow-up over an 8-year period showed total clearing of the problem with exacerbations occurring only when massive exposures occurred.

Recurrent phlebitis

Conner (in [37]) noted two patients whose phlebitis was triggered by fish and citrus fruits. Others have identified numerous triggering agents including foods, chemicals and inhalants. It has become apparent that, in many patients, phlebitis is only part of a more generalized and severe vasculitis [74]. A study of 10 patients (see Table 42.4) treated in an environmental control unit (ECU) shows that symptoms can generally be reproduced following the relevant challenge and that treatment is effective both in the short-term and the long-term. The treated group showed a remarkable improvement in walking distance and exercise on a stationary bicycle (Tables 42.3 and 42.4). These results have both clinical and important financial implications, since all 10 of the treated patients were able to return to work whereas only 1 out of the 10 patients with triggering agents not defined was able to do so.

Cardiac arrhythmias

Food and chemical inhalation and ingestion can cause cardiac arrhythmias or coronary spasm. [82, 86]. The causal role of coffee and cigarettes in the triggering of atrial arrhythmias is well known. Pollutants can also harm the heart [73].

Details of 12 patients and their cardiovascular response to chemical exposure are shown in Appendix 42.1.

Case study 3. An undertaker had a myocardial infarct at the age of 35 and a quadruple bypass operation at the age of 37. This did not clear his recurrent chest pain and ventricular arrhythmias and he was refractory to medication. In addition, this patient had recurrent sinusitis, bronchitis and gastrointestinal upsets. After 5 days in the ECU he became symptom-free, in sinus rhythm and on no medication. Following the ambient dose bronchial challenge with formaldehyde (less than 0.2 ppm) the patient sequentially developed rhinorrhoea, sinus pain, coughing, chest pain and ventricular ectopic beats (Fig. 42.6). He continued to run his business in an office distant to the mortuary.

Case study 4. A 45-year-old, white male had a 6-month history of uncontrollable bradycardia–tachycardia syndrome with associated

Table 42.3 Thrombophlebitis: associated signs and symptoms and results of challenge studies in 10 patients in an environmental control unit.

Associated signs and symptoms reproduced	Offending agents	Phlebitis reproduced
1 Diarrhoea, pulse increase (30 beats/min), nasal congestion, bigeminy, multifocal premature ventricular contractions	Beef, chicken, cigarette smoke, shrimp, pork, gas heat, ingested chemicals	Pork, shrimp, inhaled chemicals
2 Vomiting, pulse increase	Wheat, rice, inhaled chemicals	No
3 Wheezing, rhinorrhoea, red nose, nasal stuffiness, tender muscles, cystitis	Corn, cane sugar, eggs, inhaled chemicals	Corn, eggs, inhaled chemicals
4 Peripheral pulse from 4 to 1 +, tachypnoea, shortness of breath, cyanosis, belching	Beef, potatoes, corn, ingested chemicals	Beef, corn, inhaled chemicals
5 Oedema (generalized), tender muscles, colitis, dizzy	Pork, pork fumes, ingested chemicals, inhaled chemicals	
6 Syncope, wheezing, muscle tenderness, hives, paroxysmal atrial tachycardia	Legumes, seafood, cane sugar, wheat, chicken, cigarette smoke, inhaled chemicals	Cigarette smoke, ingested chemicals, inhaled chemicals, seafood
7 GI bloat, belching, premature ventricular contractions, ventricular tachycardia	Beef, chicken, lettuce, ingested chemicals, inhaled chemicals	Wheat, potatoes
8 Decrease in pulse left arm only, left neck and arm tenderness, tender over arm veins	Turkey, chicken, peas, beef, cigarette smoke, inhaled chemicals	No
9 Dyspnoea, wheezing, eyes watering, hoarse, pulse increase (50 beats/min)	Coffee, peanut butter, cane sugar, chemicals	Apple, corn, wheat, inhaled chemicals
10 Cystitis, diarrhoea, skin rash, itching, dyspnoea, pulse increase	Corn, wheat, beef, eggs, inhaled chemicals	Chicken, beef, inhaled chemicals

Table 42.4 Results of thrombophlebitis treated in an environmental control unit.

	Phlebitis		Exercise			
			Before treatment		After treatment	
	Cleared	Reproduced	Times walking round a 10 ft × 10 ft room	Exercycle miles at 150 kpm resistance	Walking round a 10 ft × 10 ft room	Exercycle miles 150 kpm resistance
ECU	10	8	0.5	0	36.6	2.85
Control	0	10 (continued)	2.1	0	3.1	0

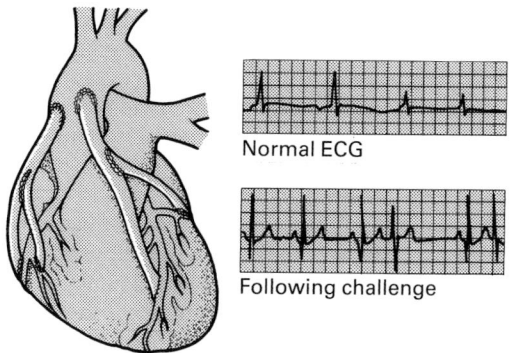

Normal ECG

Following challenge

Fig. 42.6 ECG before and after challenge with formaldehyde in a 37-year-old undertaker.

irritable bowel syndrome. Following challenge with phenol he developed bradycardia and then sinus arrest (Fig. 42.7). On another oc-casion he responded to a natural gas exposure with a tachycardia of over 200 beats/min for over an hour.

TREATMENT

Systematic avoidance treatment for inflammatory vascular disease can now be used in addition to drug therapy. The two should go hand in hand, but avoidance with removal of triggering agents should be emphasized. This has been the cornerstone of treatment of infectious disease and applies as well to other non-infectious inflammatory diseases.

The best mode of treatment and prevention of most cardiovascular disease is avoidance of incitants and replacement of nutrients.

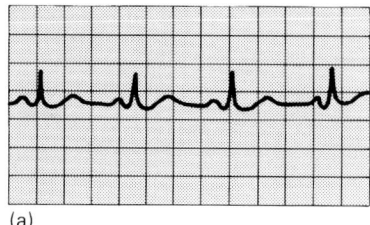
(a)

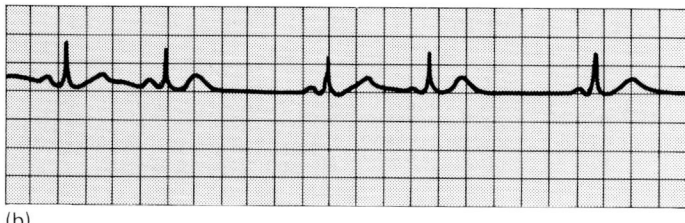
(b)

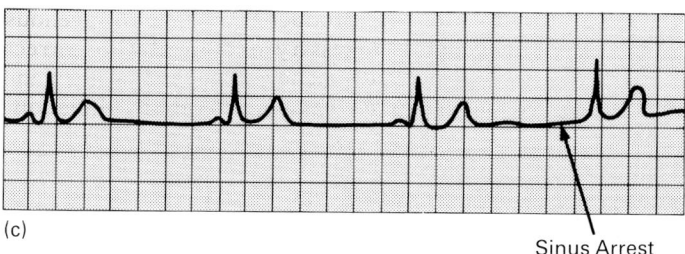
(c)

Sinus Arrest

Fig. 42.7 ECG: (a) prechallenge; (b) 30 seconds after chemical challenge with Spa spring water, showing sinus arrhythmia; and (c) sinus bradycardia and sinus arrest 5 minutes after challenge with phenol.

Avoidance

Acute reactions

Acute reactions triggered by a sudden exposure can best be treated by avoidance or removal of the offending substance(s). This can be done by placing the individual in a less polluted office, room at home or hospital. If the toxin is ingested, treatment should be given as outlined in Table 42.5. Rapid institution of these procedures within the first 1–2 hours after exposure will usually stop an acute reaction and allow the patient to return to his basal state. This regime may be effective up to 24 hours after an acute exposure.

Chronic inflammatory vascular disease

The treatment of recurrent inflammatory vascular disease (whether it be phlebitis, arthritis or vasculitis) again involves avoidance of as many triggering agents as possible. This can be done by drinking less polluted water (spring, distilled, charcoal filtered), and eating less contaminated food (less additives, preser-

Table 42.5 Treatment of acute reactions.

Laxative
Oxygen 40–100% for 2 hours
Sodium bicarbonate, 50 mEq i.v.
Vitamin C 7.5–15 g i.v. oral to GI tolerance (oral 2 tsp.)

vatives, pesticides etc.). If a patient has a food sensitivity (usually non-IgE-mediated), avoidance of those foods is necessary. Injection therapy is usually needed.

An oasis in the home

For severely affected patients an oasis should be created in the bedroom removing all possible pollutants including pesticides, fossil fuels, carpets, toxic matresses, formaldehyde-saturated plywood, particle board etc., synthetic and dry-cleaned clothes and curtains. Some severely ill patients may have to change jobs or areas of work. Complete cessation of smoking in the home is mandatory.

Nutrition

Nutritional deficiencies

Correction of nutritional deficiencies is important when trying to correct vascular damage.

Vitamin C. Vitamin C can be depleted with chemical exposures particularly to substances like benzene [1, 42], carbon monoxide [10], ethanol, smoking [2], nitrous compounds [94], vinyl chloride [94], heavy metals [94] and pesticides [46]. Amorphous ground substance of the vessel wall is somewhat dependent on vitamin C. Vitamin C supplements can be used not only to strengthen the blood vessel wall but also as a free radical scavenger and antioxidant [60]. Usually a dose of 1–10 g per day of powdered vitamin C has been used in patients with vascular dysfunction. One must be careful of the source since many individuals become intolerant of the food of origin, such as corn, sago palm, potato and carrot.

Vitamin A. β-Carotene (precursor of vitamin A) is used as a potent antioxidant and has been shown to positively affect free radical activity. Up to 5000 units daily has been used in our centre without side-effects. The patients with vascular acne-like lesions sometimes will respond to vitamin A–*cis*-retinoic acid. Care has to be taken in order to avoid multiple potential side-effects [63]. Careful monitoring of vitamin A compounds should be carried out to avoid liver damage. Vitamin A has been shown to blunt the effects of radiation, probably through its free radical scavenger effect [66]. It should not be taken for a long period of time without attempting to find the triggering agents.

Vitamin D. Vitamin D is needed to help regulate calcium metabolism. Those who live in northern climates have more difficulty generating vitamin D due to less exposure time to the sun. It has been shown that those persons living where oxidant pollutant levels are high may have a concomitant decrease in vitamin D accumulations by as much as 15% over a 25-year period. Pasteurization also eliminates vitamin D. Supplementation must be carefully monitored in order to avoid toxicity. The safest therapy is exposure to sunlight [62].

Vitamin E. Vitamin E has been used in some vascular patients. It has been shown to be an effective antipollutant. From 400 to 1400 units has been used [16].

Calcium. Calcium is clearly one mineral that is necessary for membrane stability and thus vascular wall tone. It is also a cofactor in many metabolic steps. Calcium level has been found to be inversely proportional to radiostrontium, thus it would be of use in protecting a patient against this pollutant. One to three grams of calcium has been given daily to patients with vascular disease without problems. Many forms have been used due to the patient's sensitivity. These are calcium plus magnesium, calcium chloride, calcium gluconate plus calcium carbonate. The complications of excess calcium ingestion are well known.

Magnesium. Magnesium is a membrane stabilizer. It is complexed with ATP and ADP and therefore is a mandatory cofactor for all kinases and other enzymes with nucleotides as a substrate or product cytosol. Intravenous challenge is necessary occasionally to correct a total body deficiency. Magnesium is an integral factor for vascular membrane function. Up to 500 mg may be used. A combination of calcium and magnesium in a 2 or 3 to 1 ratio may be necessary [64].

Zinc. Zinc is needed for wound healing. Zinc supplements are capable of reducing lipid peroxidation. Because of this, zinc loading has been found to stabilize cell membranes. It has reduced the damage induced by carbon tetrachloride in animals. Zinc also catalyses many other metabolic reactions in the body. Up to 45 mg of elemental zinc has been used in patients with vascular disease without problems [63].

Selenium. Selenium has immune stimulating properties. It enhances the capacity of PHA to increase blastogenic transformation of lymphocytes [53, 59]. Up to 300 μg of selenium has been given safely. It is necessary for many biochemical detoxification reactions [59]. Care should be taken to avoid overdose since severe toxic symptoms of weakness and muscle pain may occur [53].

Drugs

Prednisone (10 mg four times daily) may be given and usually will diminish reactivity in some patients by the anti-inflammatory and immunosuppressive properties. Just as often prednisone will aggravate the problem making the patient much worse. The complications of long-term use of prednisone are well known and will not be discussed here.

Cytotoxic agents have been used in some patients with leukocytoclastic vasculitis. Cyclophosphamide has been used but may not induce a significant long-term remission since the patient is well into fixed end stage disease at this point.

Immunostimulants such as transfer factor have been used by a few groups. We have a small group of patients who appeared to respond to biweekly injections of transfer factor. However, no patient was totally cleared of his vascular malady. Levamisole and thymosin have been suggested as immune stimulants. No reports, however, were found in the literature of their use in vascular disease.

Exercise

Exercise as a treatment for cardiovascular disease is like a double-edged sword. When used early in the preventive and treatment cycle, it may well blunt reactions and exclude incitants from harming the vessel wall. When it is used later in the disease process the vasculitis patient responds just as in exercise-induced asthma. We have seen many patients attempting to exercise in a late stage of vascular disease only to be incapacitated with muscular aches, dizziness and weakness. It is well known that marathon runners who ignore their cardiac signs and symptoms can die suddenly. Clearly exercise in moderation appears to help strengthen the cardiac muscle in other patients.

CONCLUSION

The prospect for the future is very bright. A concept and method has now been established for the scientific definition of chemical and food triggering agents for inflammatory cardiovascular diseases including spastic vascular phenomena such as migraines and other vascular headaches, angina due to coronary spasm, Raynaud's disease etc., many autoimmune vasculitides, i.e. lupus, rheumatoid and other early collagen vasculitis, in addition to small and large vessel vasculitis with Henoch-Schönlein purpura etc., cardiac arrhythmias and non-traumatic phlebitis. There are now many articles in the scientific literature supporting the view that cardiovascular diseases can be caused by reactions to food and environmental irritants.

APPENDIX

Reaction to double-blind exposure to fumes of chemicals (1–15-minute exposure) (ambient doses) in environmental control unit.

Patient	Saline control (3 challenges)	Petroleum alcohol (<0.5 ppm)	Phenol (<0.002 ppm)	Chlorine (<0.33 ppm)	(Mixture) pesticides (<0.134 ppm)	Pine-scented floor wash	Formaldehyde (<0.2 ppm)	Arrhythmia spectrum	
1	−	+	+	+	+	+	+	Sinus tachycardia (above 130/min)	10
2	−	+	+	+	−	+	+	Sinus bradycardia (below 45/min)	10
3	−	−	+	+	+	+	−	Sinus arrhythmia	11
4	−	−	+	+	−	+	+	Atrial fibrillation (PAT)	4
5	−	+	+	+	+	+	−	Coronary sinus rhythm	12
6	−	+	+	+	+	+	−	1° AV block	8
7	−	+	+	−	−	+	+	PVC	8
8	−	+	+	+	+	+	+	Ventricular tachycardia	2
9	−	+	+	+	+	−	−		
10	−	+	+	+	+	+	+		
11	2−,1+	−	−	−	−	−	−		
12	−	−	−	−	−	−	−		

REFERENCES

1 Askari EM, Galiks J: DDT and immunological responses. I. Altered histamine levels and anaphylactic shock in guinea pigs. Arch Environ Health 1979; 26(6):309-19.

2 Astaldi G, Karanoic D, Vettori PP, et al: Phytohemagglutinin (PHA) stimulation of peripheral-blood lymphocytes and stem cell. Biol Ist Seroten Milanesi 1974; 53:599.

3 Barnes DW, Munson AE: Cadmium-induced suppression of cellular immunity in mice. Toxicol Appl Pharmacol 1978; 45(1):350.

4 Bass HN, Hildreth BF: Paroxysmal atrial fibrillation and exposure to smoke. Lancet 1979; i:1036.

5 Becker RO, Marino AA: Electromagnetism and life. Albany: State University of New York Press, 1982.

6 Bell I, King D: Psychological and physiological research relevant to clinical ecology: an overview of the recent literature. Clin Ecology 1982; Vol. 1, No. 1.

7 Blanchi D, Cedrini L, Ceria F, et al: Exposure of mammals to strong 50-Hz electric fields. Arch Fisiol 1980; 70:33.

8 Bjorkner BH: Sensitization capacity of acrylated prepolymers in ultraviolet curing inks tested in the guinea pig. Acta Derm Venereol (Stockh) 1981; 61(1):7-10.

9 Bunter RG, Carroll JH, Randolph JC: Water in the urban environment: Real Estate Lakes. US Dept of Interior/Geological Survey, 11-19. 49. Pestic Monit J 1980; 14(3):102-7.

10 Calabrese EJ: Pollutants and high risk groups: the increased human susceptibility to environmental and occupational pollutants. New York: John Wiley and Sons, 1978.

11 Cluff LE: Serum sickness and related disorders. In: Wintrobe MM, Thorn GW, Adams RD, et al (eds.) Harrison's principles of internal medicine. New York: McGraw-Hill, 1970; 374-6.

12 Collman JD: Diseases of the peripheral vessels. In: Beeson PB, McDermott W (eds): Textbook of medicine, 14th edn. Philadelphia, Pennsylvania: WB Saunders, 1975:1076.

13 Couch JR, Wortman J: Anovulatory states as a factor in occurrence of migraine. Paper presented at The Migraine Trust, Fifth International Symposium, Sept., 1984.

14 Crapo JD, Sjostiam K, Drew RT: Tolerance and cross-tolerance using NO_2 and O_2. I. Toxicology and biochemistry. Appl Physiol 1978; 44:364.

15 Darlington LG, Ramsey NW, Mansfield JR: Placebo-controlled, blind study of dietary manipulation therapy in rheumatoid arthritis. Lancet 1986; i:236-8.

16 Davis A: Let's get well. New York: Harcourt, Brace and World, 1965; 41-2.

17 De Pasquale NP, Burch GE: The seasonal incidence of myocardial infarction in New Orleans. Am J Med Sci 242:468-78.

18 Dickey JW Jr: Drifting hematomas. Surg Gynecol Obstet 1979; 148:209.

19 Environmental Protection Agency (EPA): Is your drinking water safe?

20 Erban L: A study of biochemical and haematological changes under the application of ionized air. Int J Bioclimatol Biometeorol 1958; 3(vi).

21 Finn R: Food allergy. Lancet 1979; ii:249.

22 Fischer G, Waibel R, Richter T: Influence of line-frequency electric fields on the heart rate of rats. Zentralbl Bakteriol Mikrobiol Hyg [B] 1976; 162:374.

23 Fischer G, Waibel R, Richter T: Influence of line-frequency electric fields on the heart rate of rats. Zb1 Bakt Hyg, I. Abt Orig B 1976; 162:374.

24 Fisher SA: Dermatitis due to the presence of formaldehyde in certain sodium lauryl sulfate (SLS) solutions. Cutis 1981; 27(4):360-2, 366.

25 Fourth International Symposium on Magnesium, and American College of Nutrition 26th Annual Meeting. 1985; 4(3):303-404.

26 Fregert S: Irritant dermatitis from phenol-formaldehyde resin powder. Contact Dermatitis 1980; 6(7):493.

27 Freed DJL, Buckley CH, Tsiviori Y, et al: Non-allergic haemolysis in grass pollens and housedust mites. Allergy 1983; 38:477-86.

28 Gabliks J, Askari EM, Yolen N: DDT and immunological responses. I. Serum antibodies and anaphylactic shock in guinea pigs. Arch Environ Health 1975; 26(6):305-8.

29 Gabliks J, Al-Tubaidy T, Askari E: DDT and immunological responses. III. Reduced anaphylaxis and mast cell population in rats fed DDT. Arch Environ Health 1975; 30(2):81-4.

30 Gann D: Final report, Electric Power Research Institute Project RP 98-02. Palo Alto, California.

31 Gaworski CL, Sharma RP: The effects of heavy metals on (3H) thymidine uptake in lymphocytes. Toxicol Appl Pharmacol 1978; 46(2):305-13.

32 Gilpin A: Air pollution, 2nd edn. St. Lucia, Queensland. University of Queensland Press, 1978.

33 Grant EC: Oral contraceptives, smoking, migraine and food allergy. Lancet 1968; ii:581-9.

34 Groza P, Nicolescu E, Laz'ar D, et al: The influence of magnetic fields on some humoral parameters and on resistance to hyperthermia in rats. Physiologie 1982; 19(1):15-24.

35 Hanington E: Diet and migraine. J Hum Nutr 1978; 34:175-80.

36 Hare F: The food factor in disease. Chapter 10. London: Longmans, 1905.

37 Harkavy J: Vascular allergy and its systemic manifestations. Washington: Butterworths, 1963.

38 Heyter HE, Teng HC, Barris WB: The increased frequency of acute myocardial infarction during summer months in warm climates. Am Heart J 1953; 45:741.

39 Hippocrates: On the theory and practice of medicine. Citadel Press, 1964.

40 Katz P: Hypersensitivity vasculitis. AFP 1982; 26(1):171-5.

41 Kleibel K, Rackova M: Cutaneous allergic reactions to dithiocarbonates. Contact Dermatitis 1980; 6(5):348-9.

42 Kollwe LD: Altered immune response by environmental contaminants. International Symposium On Pathobiology of Environmental Pollutants: Animal Models and Wildlife As Monitors, CPI (59), Reg No. A7722, 1977.

43 Korobetson MA, Malenuik BU: Glucocorticoids and the blood anticoagulation system under the effect of SHF-range electromagnetic waves. Kosm Biol Aviakosm Med 1978; 1213:60-3.

44 Kroker GF, Stroud RM, Marshall R, et al: Fasting and rheumatoid arthritis: a multi-center study. Clin Ecology 1984; 2(3):137-44.

45 Kuksinsky VYe: Coagulative properties of blood and tissue of the cardiovascular system following exposure to an electromagnetic field. JPRS 1978; 71595;1.

46 Laseter JL, DeLeon IR, Rea WJ, Butler JR: Chlori-

nated hydrocarbon pesticides in environmentally sensitive patients. Arch Clin Ecol 1983; 2(1).

47 Lelbach WK, Marsteller HJ: Vinyl chloride associated disease. Ergeb Inn Med Kinderheilkd 1981; 47:1–100.

48 Lindemayer H, Schmidt J: Intolerance to acetylsalicylic acid and food additives in patients suffering from recurrent urticaria. Wien Klin Wochenschr 1979; 91(24):817–22.

49 McMillan R: Environmental thrombocytopenic purpura. J Am Med Assoc 1979; 2(22):2432–5.

50 Marino AA, Berger TJ, Mithcell JT, et al: Electric field effects in selected biologic systems. Ann NY Acad Sci 1974; 238:436.

51 Markov VV: The effects of continuous and intermittent microwave radiation on weight and atrial pressure of animals in chronic experiments. JPRS 63321:95.

52 Mustafa MG, Tierney DF: Biochemical and metabolic changes in the lung with oxygen, ozone, and nitrogen dioxide toxicity. Am Rev Respir Dis 1978; 118:1061–90.

53 Martin J, Spallholz J: Proceedings of the Symposium On Selenium-Tellurium In The Environment, Pittsburg, Pennsylvania: Industrial Health Foundation, 1976; 204–25.

54 Monroe EW, Schulz CI, Maize JC, Jordan RE: Vasculitis in chronic urticaria: an immunopathologic study. J Invest Dermatol 1981; 76(2):103–7.

55 National Research Council: Water hardness and health. In: Drinking water and health. New York National Academy of Sciences, 1977:439–47.

56 Nour-Elden R: Uptake of phenol by vascular and brain tissue. Microvasc Res 1970; 2:224.

57 Olsen T: Peripheral vascular diseases, necrotizing vasculitis and vascular-related diseases. In Moschella SL, Hurley HJ, eds. Dermatology, Vol. 1, 2nd edn. Philadelphia: WB Saunders, 1985.

58 Parish WR: Studies on vasculitis, immunoglobulins, β1C, C-reactive proteins and bacterial antigens in cutaneous vasculitis lesions. Clin Allergy 1971; 1:97–110.

59 Passwaters RA: Selenium as food and medicine. New Canaan, Connecticut: Keats Publishing, 1980;88–95.

60 Pauling L: Vitamin C, common cold and flu. San Francisco: WH Freeman, 1976; 191–3.

61 Pestic Toxic Chem News 1984; 12(32).

62 Pfeiffer CC: Mental and elemental nutrients. New Canaan, Connecticut: Keats Publishing, 1975; 199–202.

63 Pfeiffer, CC: Mental and elemental nutrients. New Canaan, Connecticut: Keats Publishing, 1975; 190–9.

64 Pfeiffer CC: Mental and elemental nutrients. New Cannan, Connecticut: Keats Publishing, 1975, 277–9.

65 Pollutants. In: Clean up your room: a compendium on indoor pollution. California: Dept of Consumer Affairs, 1982.

66 Primer on allergy and immunologic disease. J Am Med Assoc 1982; 248:20.

67 Prokhvatilo YeV: Reduction of functional capacities of the heart following exposure to an electromagnetic field of industrial frequency. JPRS 1977; 70101:76.

68 Randolph TG: Human ecology and susceptibility to the chemical environment. Springfield, Illinois: Charles C Thomas, 1962.

69 Rea WJ: Environmentally triggered small vessel vasculitis. Ann Allergy 1977; 38:245–51.

70 Rea WJ: Elimination of oral food challenge reaction by injection of food extracts: a double-blind evaluation. Arch Otolaryngol 1984; 110:248–52.

71 Rea WJ: Recurrent environmentally triggered thrombophlebitis. Ann Allergy 1981; 47:338–44.

72 Rea WJ, Mitchell MJ: Chemical sensitivity and the environment. Immunol Allergy Prac 1982; Sept/Oct:21–31.

73 Rea WJ, Suits CW: Cardiovascular disease triggered by foods and chemicals. In: Gerrard JW (ed.) Food allergy: new perspectives. Springfield, Illinois: Charles C Thomas, 1980.

74 Rea WJ, Bell IR, Smiley RE: Large vessel vasculitis. In: Johnson F, Spence JT (eds.) Allergy: immunology and medical treatment. Chicago: Symposia Specialist, 1975.

75 Rea WJ, Smiley RE, Edgar RE, et al: Recurrent environmentally triggered thrombophlebitis: a five-year followup. Ann Allergy 1981; 47:338–44.

76 Rea WJ, Butler JR, Laseter JL, DeLeon IR: Pesticides and brain-function changes in a controlled environment. Arch Clin Ecol 1984; 2(3):145–50.

77 Read H, Holt S, Housley E, et al: Raynaud's phenomenon induced by sulphasalzine. Postgrad med 1980; 56:106–7.

78 Romaquera C, Grimalt F: Sensitization to benzoyl peroxide, retinoic acid and carbon tetrachloride. Contact Dermatitis 1980; 6(6):422.

79 Silverman D, Kornblueh IH: Effect of artificial ionization of the air on the electro-encephalogram. Am J Phys Med 1957; 36:352–8.

80 Smith CW: Electromagnetic phenomena. In: Living biomedical systems, frontiers of engineering and computing. Health Care. Sept. 15–16, 1984.

81 Spalding RF, Junk GA, Richard JJ: Water: pesticides in ground water beneath irrigated farmland in Nebraska. Pestic Monit J 1980; 1(2):70–3.

82 Spizer FE, Wegerman DH, Ramires A: Palpitation rate associated with fluorocarbon exposure in a hospital setting. N Engl J Med 1975; 272:624.

83 Stokingert HE: Ozone toxicology: a review of research and industrial experience: 1954–1964. Arch Environ Health 1965; 10.

84 Suhonen R: Contact allergy to dodeayl-di-(aminoethyl) glyane (Desimex i). Contact Dermatitis 1980; 6(4):290–1.

85 Svedhem A, Alestis K, Jertborn M: Phlebitis induced by parenteral treatment with fluxoxacillin and doxacillin: a doubleblind study. Antimicrob Agents Chemother 1980; 18:349–52.

86 Taylor GS, Hern WS: Cardiac arrhythmias due to aerosol propellents. J Am Med Assoc 1970; 219:8.

87 Tchijevsky AL: Die Wege des Eindringens von Luftionen in den organismus und die physiologische wirkung von luftionen. Acta Med Scand 1934; 83: 219–72.

88 Tumulty PA: Systemic lupus erythematosus. In: Wintrobe MM, Thorn GW, Adams RD, et al (eds.) Harrison's principles of internal medicine. New York: McGraw-Hill, 1970; 1962–7.

89 Theorell H, Blombock M, Kockum C: Demonstration of reactivity to airborne and food antigen in cutaneous vasculitis by variation in fibrino peptide and others, blood coagulation, fibrinolysis, and complement parameters. Thrombo Haemo Sts (Stattz) 1976; 36:593.

90 Titus JM, Kim H-S: Blood vessels and lymphatics. In Kissane JM, ed. Anderson's pathology, Vol. 1, 8th edn. St Louis: CV Mosby, 1985; 684–729.

91 Vasiliev LL: Theory and practice of aeroionotherapy. Leningrad: University of Leningrad Press, 1951.

92 What everyone should know about the quality of drinking water. Greenville, Massachusetts: Channing L Bette 1977.

93 Whehner AP: Electro-aerosols, air ions and physical medicine. Am J Phys Med 1969; 48(3):119–49.

94 Winslow SG: The effects of environmental chemicals on the immune system; a selected bibliography with abstracts. Oak Ridge, Tennessee: Toxicology Information Response Center, Oak Ridge National Laboratory, 1981; 1-36.

95 Worden JL: The effect of unipolar ionized air on the relative weights of selected organs of the golden hamster. Sci Stud 1953; 15:71-82.

96 Worden JL: The effect of air ion concentrations and polarity on the CO_2 capacity of mammalian blood plasma. Fed Proc 1954; 13:557.

97 Wuthrich B, Fabio L: Acetylsalicylic acid and food intolerance in urticaria, bronchial asthma, and rhinoplathy. Schweiz Med Wochenschr 1981; 1(39):1445-50.

98 Yervick P: Oil pollutants in marine life. Eighth Advanced Seminar, Society of Clinical Ecology, Instatape, Tape II.

99 Zeek PM: Periateritis nodosa and other forms of necrotizing angitis. N Engl J Med 1953; 248:764.

SECTION H
OTHER ORGANS

Chapter 43a
Food Sensitivity: The Kidney and Bladder

D. Sandberg

Introduction

Of the organ systems referred to in this book, the kidney has been most subjected to investigation of immunological mechanisms of disease. A majority of these studies have focused on reactions to microorganisms, self-antigens, tumour antigens, drugs etc. There has been only slight interest in a possible role of food components as sensitizing agents. In part this reflects the lack of adequate published data suggesting such a link. Some of the renal disorders in which immune mechanisms appear to play an important role are shown in Table 43a.1 [13, 24, 25].

Perhaps the clearest published reports sug-

Table 43a.1 Renal disorders in which immune mechanisms play a role.

Glomerulonephritis
Goodpasture's syndrome
Systemic lupus erythematosus
Nephrosis
Proteinuria

gesting a relationship of food allergy to renal disease are those of Matsumura's group in Japan and our group's studies of food sensitivity in childhood nephrosis [27, 29, 43, 44]. We have also studied a small number of children with the nephrotic syndrome associated with membranous glomerulopathy and anaphylactoid purpura nephritis. Williams recently reviewed the subject of allergy and the kidney and could find no other information implicating food allergy in renal disease except in nephrosis and anaphylactoid purpura nephritis [54].

The lower urinary tract and bladder have also been investigated for a possible role of allergy, and specifically of food sensitivity as a cause of recurrent and chronic symptoms such as frequency, dysuria, enuresis etc. [2–4, 8, 11, 14, 32, 41, 45, 56]. In addition, haematuria, and interstitial and eosinophilic cystitis have characteristics suggesting a relationship to environmental sensitivities [18, 19]. There is substantial clinical evidence collected over many years suggesting that in some individuals allergy, and specifically food sensitivity, may be a significant factor in aetiology of these symptoms.

FOOD SENSITIVITY AND THE KIDNEY

There is general agreement among nephrologists that immunological mechanisms play a major role in many diseases involving the kidney. Poststreptococcal glomerulonephritis and serum sickness are prototypes of disease processes involving renal injury by humoral and/or cellular immune mechanisms. Both of these disorders have been studied in great detail both in humans and in animal models. Extension of those studies has identified a number of other diffuse disease processes in which immunological mechanisms appear to be related to renal tissue injury [13, 25].

Through study of these various diseases, it has become evident that the entire range of pathophysiological immune mechanisms may be involved, including IgE-mediated processes. A considerable part of what is known about immune mechanisms in disease has been learned through study of those renal disorders in which hypersensitivity plays a role.

Minimal change disease nephrosis

Of those kidney disorders investigated, childhood nephrosis is the disease most clearly identified as having foods as precipitating factors. This association has been reported both by Matsumura and co-workers in Japan and by our group [27, 29, 43, 44]. Triggering of nephrotic relapses by inhaled allergens had previously been reported to occur in a minority of individuals with minimal change disease (MCD) [43, 54]. More recently this has been noted by others [9, 20, 21, 38]. However, other investigators have questioned an aetiological relationship between allergy and the nephrotic syndrome, although accepting that childhood nephrosis occurs more frequently in atopic than non-atopic individuals [7, 30].

Nephrotic syndrome

The nephrotic syndrome is the most frequent presentation of persistent glomerular disease in the paediatric age group [15]. It occurs more frequently in children than in adults.

Histopathology. The predominant histopath-ological lesion in children is minimal change disease, although when the nephrotic syndrome presents in older children, the likelihood increases that it may be associated with another histological lesion. In biopsies from patients with minimal change type of childhood nephrosis, no abnormality can be recognized under light microscopy and immunofluorescence microscopy does not demonstrate immunoglobulin or complement deposition in the kidney (see Fig. 43a.1). There is also no evidence of an inflammatory response in the kidney. A report of deposition of IgE in the glomerulus has not been confirmed [43].

Response to prednisone therapy. This is so consistent in MCD that induction of remission with prednisone provides sufficient support for the clinical diagnosis. Renal biopsy is not considered necessary in most children with MCD (see Fig. 43a.2). The decrease in weight associated with diuresis and the decrease in protein excretion after approximately 1 week of therapy are indicative of a good clinical response with induction of remission. Biopsy is reserved for patients who do not respond, older children or adults who may have other disease processes and children whose course is complicated by frequent relapses and poor control with prednisone leading to consideration of immunosuppressive therapy with cyclophosphamide or other cytotoxic drugs.

Inhalant allergy and minimal change disease

Many years ago association in an adult of MCD and pollen sensitivity was described by Hardwicke and co-workers [16]. In that patient immunotherapy appeared to induce prolonged remission. Subsequently other investigators reported coexistence of nephrosis with allergy [9, 43]. More recently still, Laurent and co-workers have reported similar patients with nephrosis and relapse associated with inhaled allergens such as house dust, pollen and cat dander [20, 21]. Reeves et al have documented a seasonal pattern of nephrotic syndrome [38]. Thompson in Soothill's group demonstrated an incidence of atopic disease in children with steroid-responsive nephrotic syndrome twice that of a group of age-matched controls [47]. Meadow and colleagues have noted a similar relationship with steroid-responsive nephrosis and atopy, although they did not find a relationship between atopic status and tendency to relapse [30].

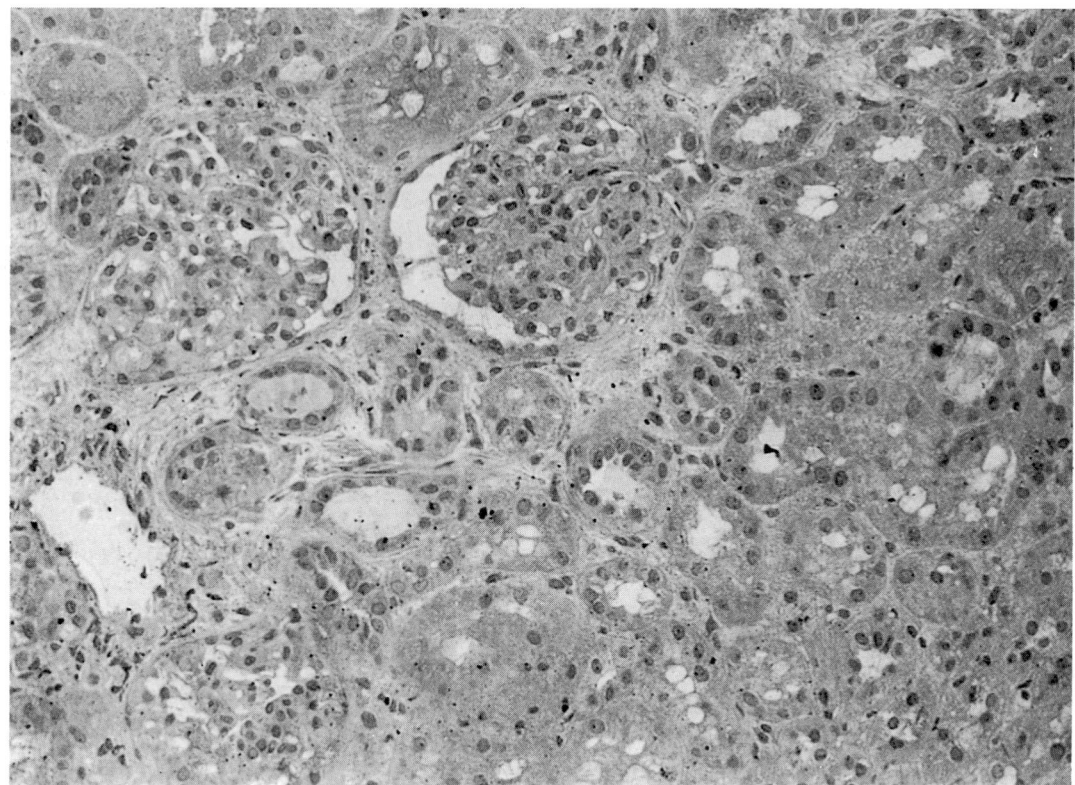

Fig. 43a.1 Haematoxylin and eosin stain of a renal biopsy from a 3-year-old, WM, with minimal change nephrotic syndrome (×100). The essentially normal appearance of the glomeruli is evident.

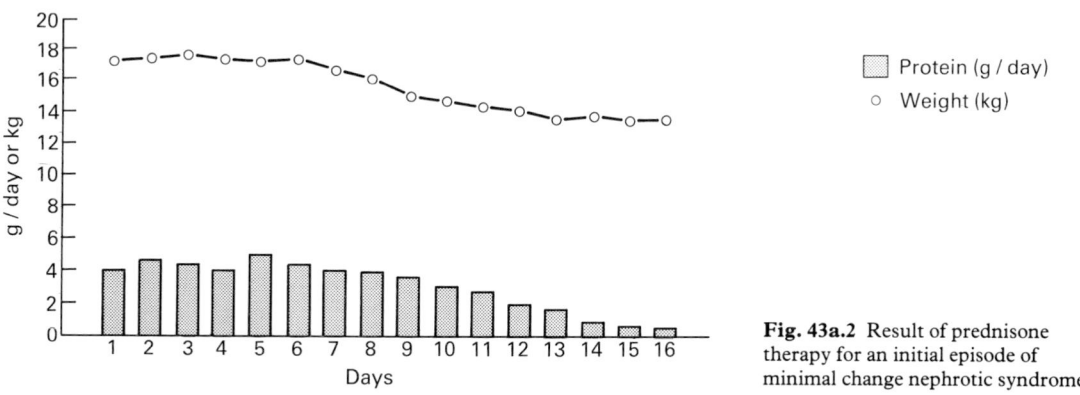

Fig. 43a.2 Result of prednisone therapy for an initial episode of minimal change nephrotic syndrome.

Further adding to the confusion, therapy with antihistamines, sodium cromoglycate or doxantrazole has been shown to be ineffective in preventing relapse [9]. Levinsky and co-workers demonstrated the presence of unusual circulating immune complex-like particles in patients with nephrosis [22]. Moorthy and colleagues [31] and Eyres and co-workers [12] have provided data suggesting involvement of the cellular immune system in MCD. Further supporting evidence for a role for allergy or hypersensitivity in MCD includes reports that a variety of environmental substances including drugs, insect stings, poison ivy etc., have triggered relapses [43]. Trompeter with Soothill's group has also reported an association of short time to relapse after cyclophosphamide treatment with an increased frequency of HLA-B12 in steroid-responsive nephrotic syndrome in children [48] (see

Table 43a.2). An association with atopy was not shown. No significant differences were observed in incidence of atopic history, elevated serum total IgE concentration, positive prick tests for grass pollen or house dust mite or elevated serum IgE antibody to those two antigens. This is consistent with the view that a non-IgE related mechanism for food sensitivity is involved in this disease process [48]. Although substantial data have accumulated linking allergy to childhood nephrosis, it has not been clear whether the relationship is a direct one or whether the relationship is between allergy and the tendency to relapse.

in a group of 19 blood donors ($P < 0.001$). Only nine showed one sensitization; eight reacted to two and three to three foods. All five foods were found to be reactive in multiple patients; this included five patients reactive to egg, six to milk and beef, and nine to wheat and pork. The HBDT was positive whether patients were in relapse or remission, whether on or off corticosteroid therapy, and whether serum immunoglobulin E was elevated or not. There was little correlation between standard skin tests, radioallergosorbent tests and HBDT.

Matsumura's group of patients with ne-

Table 43a.2 Frequency of HLA-B12 and relation with atopic features in children with steroid responsive nephrotic syndrome [33].

| | | Group A | | Group B | | Combined | | British blood donors |
		(+)	(−)	(+)	(−)	(+)	(−)	(+)
HLA-B12	(%)	54	46	44	56	50	50	24
Atopic history	(%)	37	3	15	32	29	16	
Total IgE > 150 U	(%)	48	13	17	32	34	24	

Group A consisted of 71 children who were consecutive outpatients; group B comprised 72/81 children treated with cyclophosphamide. All were in remission and off treatment. Twenty-seven of group B were included previously in group A while 45 were a new series not previously evaluated for HLA type and atopy.

Food sensitivity

Matsumura and his group reported in 1961 and again in 1971 results of clinical studies of a large number of children with nephrosis who were shown to have sensitivity to foods and in whom the use of limited diets was apparently helpful in achieving prolonged remission of their disease [27, 29]. They also reported an association of food sensitivity with postural proteinuria (see below). In 1977, our group reported studies of six children with frequently relapsing steroid-dependent MCD in whom cow's milk sensitivity was associated with relapse [44]. We subsequently described further studies in the same children and investigation of an additional group of 13 children [43]. Richards and co-workers in 1977 described a girl who had nephrosis as well as a history of asthma, eczema and urticaria who appeared to have relapsed on ingestion of chicken eggs [39]. Lagrue and his colleagues [19a] have reported results of study of the human basophil degranulation test (HBDT) to investigate food sensitivity in 34 patients with MCD nephrosis. Five food allergens were used (wheat, milk, egg, beef and pork). Sixty four per cent of the 34 patients had at least one positive test whereas it was positive only once

phrosis is of importance to our understanding since they were not selected for a pattern of frequent relapse. In contrast, the children studied in Miami had had numerous relapses requiring frequent administration of prednisone or had been treated with an immunosuppressive agent such as cyclophosphamide [43]. Matsumura reported a high degree of successful control of the nephrosis in his patients using limited diets. Evidence of food sensitivity was obtained in those patients by individual oral food challenges.

Milk allergy and relapsing minimal change disease

The six children with frequently relapsing steroid-responsive MCD studied in Miami [44] were shown to be sensitive to cow's milk by intradermal titration skin testing, and by in vivo alteration of plasma C3 complement using crossed immunoelectrophoresis. Oral challenge with cow's milk provoked relapse in five patients. Fig. 43a.3 indicates one patient's response to challenge with cow's milk. The changes in protein excretion following milk ingestion were dramatic. Transient changes in serum IgG and IgM were also demonstrated. One girl did not relapse when prednisone was

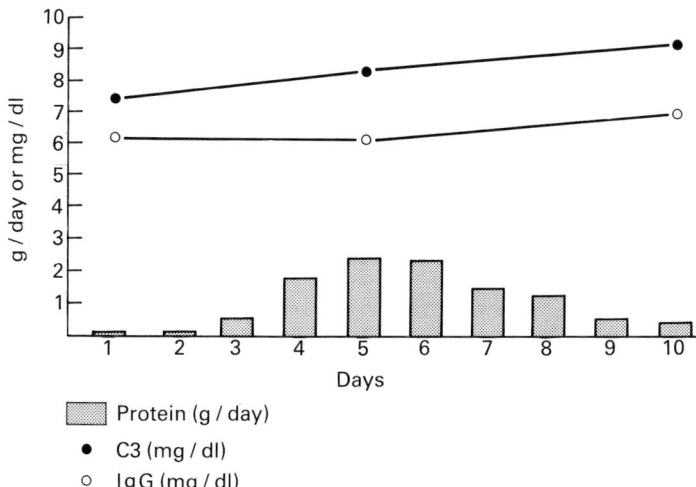

Protein (g / day)

● C3 (mg / dl)

○ IgG (mg / dl)

Fig. 43a.3 Effect of milk ingestion on protein excretion in a child with minimal change nephrotic syndrome. The solid bars depict values for 24-hour protein excretion.

discontinued, although she had requiredinter-mittent, frequent prednisone therapy for several years because of relapse whenever prednisone was discontinued previously. Subsequently 13 more children with steroid-dependent MCD were studied and reported in 1980 [43], as well as further studies of three of the original group. All 19 had had persistent disease; in nine, treatment with cytotoxic drugs was undertaken because of inadequate control with prednisone or undesirable side-effects of the latter drug. In 17 children, sensi-tivity to one or more foods was documented. Although these patients were not selected because of a history of allergic disease, seven had asthma, four eczema, one allergic rhinitis and one chronic urticaria. Thirteen of 19 children had positive intradermal skin tests to one or more foods. One child was unrespon-sive to prednisone; however, he responded well to diet restriction and food extract injec-tions with good control of his nephrosis. Although our initial report documented prov-ocation of relapse with cow's milk, all but two patients who could not be adequately evalua-ted, were found to be sensitive to multiple foods.

Study protocol. The study protocol consisted of discontinuance of prednisone while in re-mission, and admission to the Clinical Re-search Center when relapse occurred. Vivo-nex, a chemically defined formula feed, was provided as the sole diet, and, following de-crease in proteinuria, oral challenge with cow's milk was carried out. Urinary 24-hour protein excretion, weight and fluid intake and output were monitored daily. Four patients developed increased proteinuria while on Vivonex. Protein excretion decreased in those patients when another limited diet or spring water was substituted for the Vivonex [43, 44]. Eleven of the 19 patients were treated with food extracts either subcutaneously or sublingually, in addi-tion to limited diets. In some instances, patients were also tested for inhaled allergens and, when appropriate, were given immuno-therapy for those antigens for which they had positive reactions.

Long-term follow-up: case histories. Long-term follow-up of three of the original six patients has been possible (see Table 43a.3). One boy

Table 43a.3 Studies of food sensitivity in nephrosis. Long-term follow-up of three children with MCD.

Patients	Number of significant relapses	Prednisone therapy*	Other problems
EN	2	2	None
JR	1	1	None
TN	0	0	None

* Number of relapses since beginning management for food sensitivity, requiring prednisone therapy.

had no further relapses and no further need for prednisone. He was treated with a limited diet and food extract injections twice weekly for several months; after that period, other foods were gradually added to his diet after skin testing. When skin tests were positive, he was treated subcutaneously or sublingually with the appropriate food extract, and later that food was included in his diet. Treatment was discontinued after 2 years without subsequent recurrence of the nephrotic syndrome and with maintenance of normal urine and plasma laboratory values.

The two other boys had a few brief relapses lasting a few days which were either associated with acute infections or lapses in their restricted diets. The last relapse noted was at age 16 years in one and at age 19 years in the other. All three individuals are now on normal diets. Table 43a.4 shows results of the last

laboratory values in those six patients. One (THo) had early evidence of renal failure at that time, while values for the other five individuals were within normal limits. Two boys continued to have relapses, one in spite of careful diet and environmental control and food and inhalant injection therapy.

Gastrointestinal candidiasis

These patients are at risk from gastrointestinal colonization with *Candida albicans* as a result of chronic prednisone therapy as well as frequent antibiotic treatment, and are prone to hypersensitivity (see Chapter 49). It is possible that *Candida albicans* could serve as an allergen to which such patients are chronically exposed. This could explain why some children with MCD develop a pattern of frequent relapses and why evaluation and treatment of

Table 43a.4 Studies of food sensitivity in nephrosis. Laboratory values with long-term follow-up of four children with MCD.

Patients	Protein excretion (mg/24 hours)	albumin TP/albumin (mg/dl)	Cholesterol (mg/dl)	IgG (mg/dl)	BUN/creatinine (mg/dl)
EN	80	7.2/4.8	—	950	14/0.9
JR	45	6.9/4.3	—	1150	16/1.1
TN	35	7.8/5.2	190	1260	14/1.0
JM*	40	7.2/4.9	205	920	11/0.8

* This patient did not relapse when prednisone was discontinued.
BUN, blood urea nitrogen; TP = total protein.

laboratory values obtained on four of the six patients.

Long-term follow-up was also available for six other patients with MCD. Two had no subsequent relapses; one had two relapses and then none thereafter, but did develop a chronic anaemia of uncertain aetiology. Table 43a.5 shows results of the most recent

food and inhaled allergen sensitivity does not explain persistent disease in some patients. Truss has suggested that the known capacity of *Candida albicans* for altering the immune system can lead to multiple food sensitivities through interference with immunoregulation [49–51].

Table 43a.5 Studies of food sensitivity in nephrosis. Laboratory values with long-term follow-up of 6/19 patients with MCD*.

Patients	Protein excretion (mg/24 hours)	TP/albumin (mg/dl)	Cholesterol (mg/dl)	IgG (mg/dl)	BUN/creatinine (mg/dl)
VL	40	6.2/3.9	201	800	7/0.8
YB	65	7.3/4.2	165	940	9/0.8
TL	195	5.6/3.4	187	695	9/0.4
TW	60	6.2/3.8	230	580	13/0.8
THo†	1800	5.4/3.2	330	410	27/1.2
TH	35	6.8/4.5	180	1130	10/0.6

* These values were obtained from a recent follow-up visit.
† These values were representative of the status prior to dialysis and transplantation.
TP = total protein; BUN = blood urea nitrogen.

Membranous glomerulopathy

A role for food sensitivity in membranous glomerulonephropathy (MG) and the nephritis associated with anaphylactoid purpura has been reported [43]. Close study of a small number of patients suggests that such a relationship exists; however, further confirmation is needed through study of more patients with those disorders.

Histopathology

MG is an uncommon cause of the nephrotic syndrome in children; it is somewhat more frequent in older children and adults. The histopathological lesion comprises minimal mesangial proliferation and hypertrophy of glomerular epithelial cells. The glomerular capillary walls are thickened by diffuse subepithelial deposits (see Fig. 43a.4). Immuno-

Clinical features

This disorder is usually associated with a mild nephrotic syndrome, although occasionally the process will be severe and chronic and may progress to renal failure [33]. It has not been shown that therapy with corticosteroids or other immunosuppressive drugs alters the course of this disease process. Its variable clinical expression makes is difficult to evaluate response to a specific therapy.

The immune deposits have been considered to be immune complexes. The subepithelial site of deposition suggests that these complexes are small. A variety of antigens have been demonstrated to be present in a few patients with concomitant diseases such as hepatitis B or malignancy [43]. In addition, MG has been associated with other infections such as syphilis and streptococcal disease, and with sickle-cell disease and lupus erythematosus.

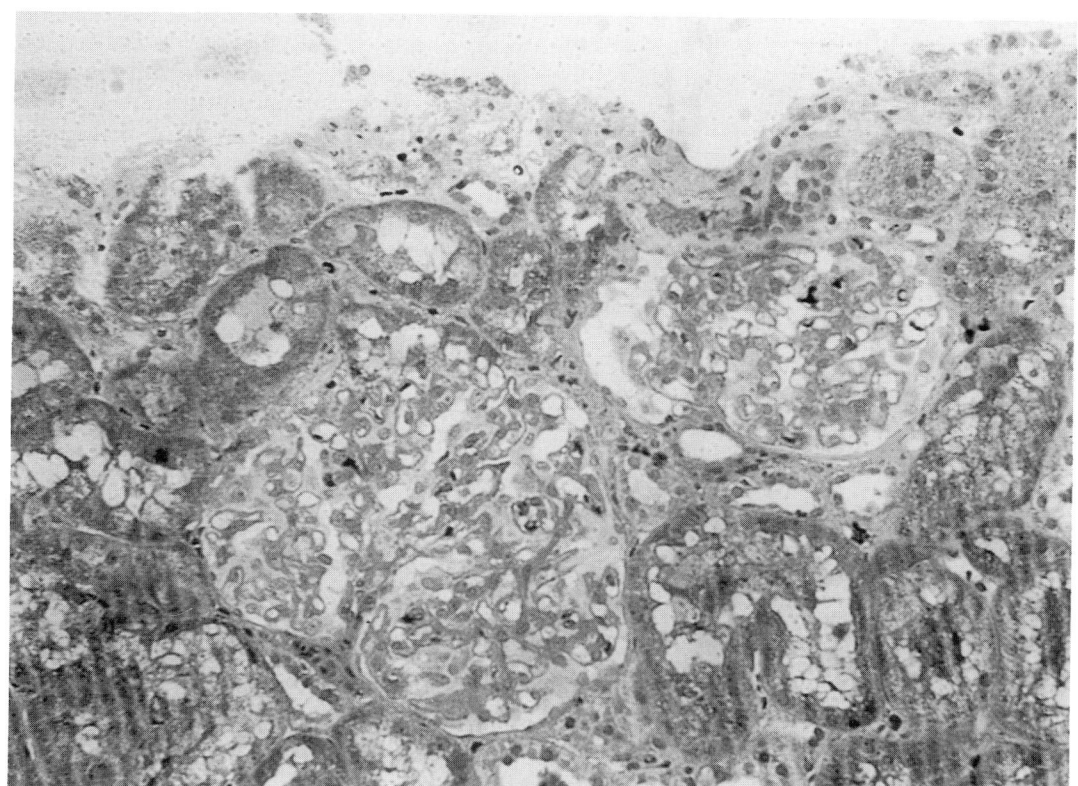

Fig. 43a.4 Haematoxylin and eosin stain of a renal biopsy from a child with membranous glomerulopathy and the nephrotic syndrome (× 100). The diffuse deposits along the glomerular capillary basement membrane are clearly visible.

fluorescence staining of these deposits usually indicates the presence of IgG and less commonly IgA and IgM; in addition, complement components are commonly present [25].

This renal lesion has also been related to reactions to some medications, i.e. troxidone (trimethadione , penicillamine, gold etc. So far food or inhaled allergens have not been detected in immune deposits or circulating immune complexes from these patients.

Food allergens

In a study of three children, age 13–15 years, with MG [43] and with asthma (one had atopic dermatitis), all were demonstrated to be sensitive to multiple foods both by oral challenge and by intradermal skin testing. They were also demonstrated to have acute in vivo alteration of plasma C3 following oral milk challenge. It was possible in all three to demonstrate increased protein excretion following ingestion of cow's milk as well as following other foods. Fig. 43a.5 depicts changes in

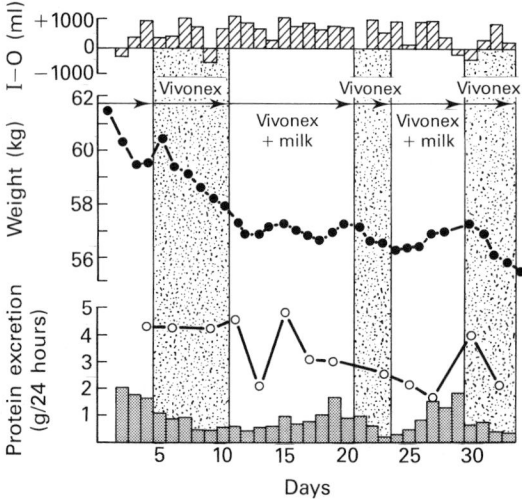

Fig. 43a.5 Changes in weight, net water balance and protein excretion during dietary changes in a patient with the nephrotic syndrome associated with membranous glomerulopathy. I−O = 24-hour fluid intake minus urine output. g/24 hours = protein excretion during a 24-hour period. From Sandberg et al [43], courtesy of Charles C. Thomas, Publisher, Springfield, Illinois.

protein excretion and body weight following successive challenges with milk in one female patient [43]. It also shows the decrease in proteinuria and oedema indicated by decrease in body weight, when she was taking only Vivonex.

Two of the children showed an excellent response to treatment using some diet limitation and food and inhalant extract injection therapy; with long-term follow-up, both are free of demonstrable renal disease at this time although neither have allowed repeated renal biopsy. One of the two is still on weekly injections for inhaled allergens and a milk product-free diet. The third patient had more severe and chronic renal disease from onset. She did not respond adequately to treatment, eventually developed renal failure and required renal transplantation. Table 43a.6 shows laboratory values obtained after long-term remission of the nephrotic syndrome in two patients and shows continued presence of the nephrotic syndrome in the third patient.

Anaphylactoid purpura nephritis

Anaphylactoid purpura involves the skin, gastrointestinal tract, joints and kidney. The incidence of renal involvement has been variously estimated at 22–70% (25% is a generally accepted figure). The nephropathy is an important component since prognosis of the disease is related to severity of the renal lesion. In fact, the severity of skin, gastrointestinal and joint involvement has no apparent relationship to severity of the kidney disease. Renal manifestations include gross or microscopic haematuria, proteinuria and occasionally renal failure. Approximately 50% of patients develop the nephrotic syndrome, but it may also be a presenting manifestation.

Family history of allergy

There is a strong history of allergy in approximately 25% of patients and recurrent bouts of acute nephrotic syndrome apparently related to food allergy have been described [43]. Other reported associated factors include medications, immunizations, tuberculosis and insect stings. There is a tendency to relapse. Successive episodes may be accompanied by further renal involvement and episodes of acute

Table 43a.6 Studies of food sensitivity in nephrosis. Follow-up of three patients with membranous glomerulopathy.

Patients	Protein excretion (mg/24 hours)	TP/albumin (mg/dl)	Cholesterol (mg/dl)	IgG (mg/dl)	BUN/creatinine (mg/dl)
SS	40	7.4/5.3	175	1150	12/0.8
SL	50	6.8/3.9	195	1250	10/0.8
JW*	2410	5.3/2.9	340	520	45/3.7

* These values were representative of this patient's status shortly before institution of dialysis.
TP = total protein.

nephrotic syndrome may occur in the absence of other manifestations of anaphylactoid purpura.

Laboratory findings

There are no characteristic laboratory abnormalities in anaphylactoid purpura. Serum C3 concentrations are usually normal, but decreased concentration of C4, C5 and C3PA have been reported suggesting activation of the alternative pathway. Cryoglobulinaemia has been reported; these cryoglobulins contained predominantly IgA. An increased incidence of demonstrable circulating antibody to bovine proteins with simultaneous presence of circulating bovine γ-globulin and casein antigen have also been noted. Immunohistological studies reveal predominantly mesangial deposits of IgA and, to a lesser extent, fibrinogen, complement, IgG and IgM. These suggest an immune complex pathogenesis. In general, this syndrome is a benign, self-limiting disorder; long-term prognosis is almost entirely related to renal involvement.

Histopathology

The predominant renal lesion observed is a focal and segmental proliferative glomerulonephritis. Other lesions described include minimal change, focal and segmental endocapillary glomerulonephritis, diffuse endocapillary proliferation and membranoproliferative glomerulonephritis. Treatment is considered to have no influence on the course of the renal disease.

Food sensitivity: case histories

Case 1. We have reported food sensitivity in two patients with nephrotic syndrome related to anaphylactoid purpura nephritis [43]. Renal biopsy was obtained from both children, and showed severe nephritis in one and moderately severe nephritis in the other. In the latter patient, renal biopsy showed crescent formation in over 50% of glomeruli in the specimen (see Fig. 43a.6). The renal lesion as indicated by this biopsy was very severe with a high probability of subsequent development of renal failure. The patient was found to have widespread sensitivity to foods as well as to

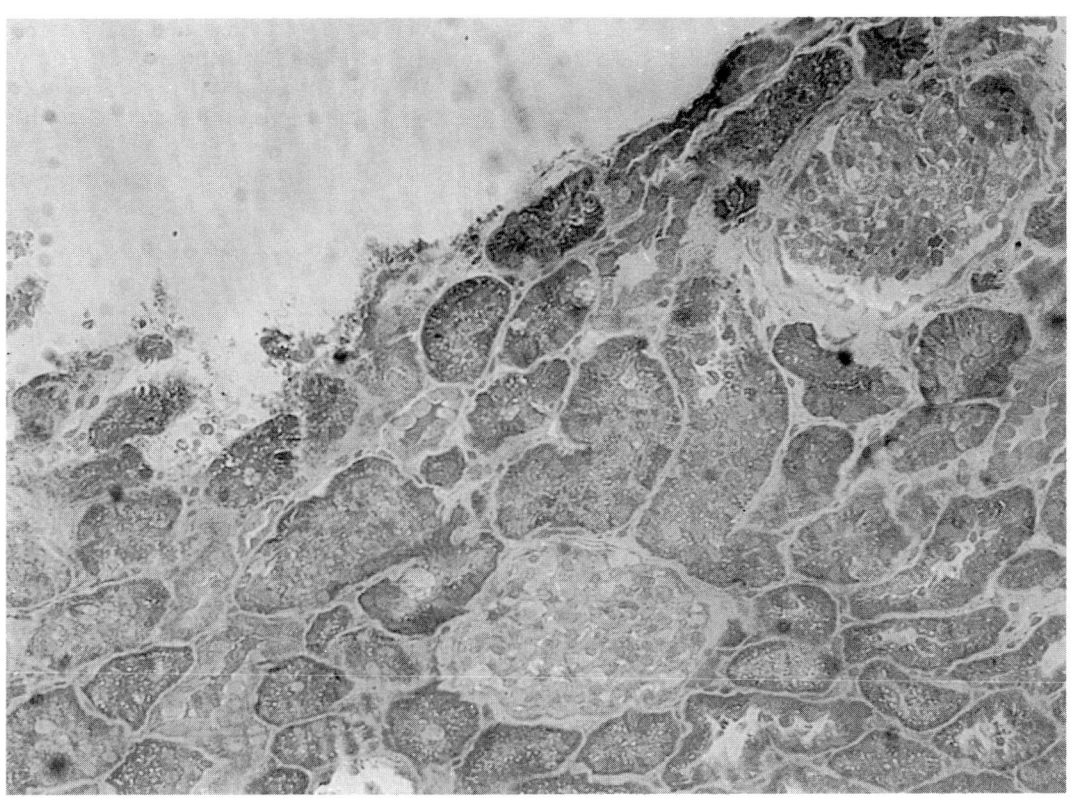

Fig. 43a.6 Haematoxylin and eosin stain of a renal biopsy from a patient with severe anaphylactoid purpura nephritis and the nephrotic syndrome (× 100). The glomeruli show severe injury with crescent formation.

inhaled allergens and various chemical agents. He was maintained on rigid environmental control in the home and a meticulous limited diet with food and inhalant extract injections for approximately 4 years. The strict regimen was gradually relaxed and he is presently living a relatively normal life except for some dietary restrictions. Renal function studies have been normal except for a slightly increased 24-hour urine protein excretion in the range of 300 mg/24 hours. He and his parents have not consented to a second biopsy.

Case 2. The other child had a milder but chronic course with continued protein excretion in the range of 1–2 g/24 hours and mild hypoproteinaemia and minimal oedema. During initial studies while taking only Vivonex, protein excretion decreased and serum IgG, C3, total protein and albumin concentrations increased towards normal. Oral challenge with cow's milk caused an increase in protein excretion to 2.4 g/24 hours which decreased following removal of milk from the diet. Urinary red blood cell excretion increased in both children following milk feeding, and decreased on Vivonex as the sole diet. Intradermal skin testing was positive to multiple food and inhaled allergens. Nephritis was undetectable after approximately 1 year and all therapy was discontinued.

Postural proteinuria

Matsumura and co-workers have reported very interesting clinical studies of food sensitivity associated with postural proteinuria [26, 28]. They evaluated both orthostatic and lordotic proteinuria in 36 patients using standard clinical methods including history, food diaries, elimination diets and challenge with individual foods.

Food challenge

The foods were tested by inclusion in the diet for 3 days in usual amounts or as a single meal with a food suspected to be the cause of postural proteinuria. They identified 72 foods as a cause of postural proteinuria in the 36 patients. Milk, egg and soya were identified 30, 20 and 17 times, respectively; pork, red beans and tuna were also found to precipitate postural proteinuria. Frequently more than one food was identified for an individual, with one food in 14 patients, two in 12, three in six, and four in four individuals.

Other symptoms. Other associated symptoms were commonly observed, including headache, abdominal pain, fatigue and diarrhoea. Fig. 43a.7 shows lordotic proteinuria produced by a single feeding of cow's milk. Fig. 43a.8 illus-

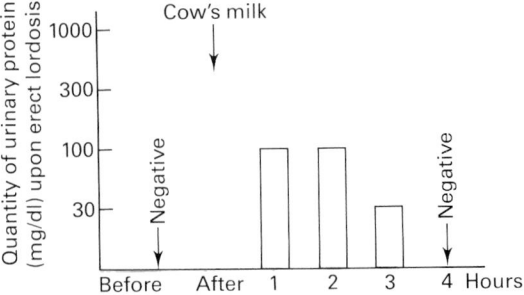

Fig. 43a.7 Lordotic proteinuria resulting from administration of a single feeding of cow's milk. From Matsumura [26], courtesy of Charles C. Thomas, Publisher, Springfield, Illinois.

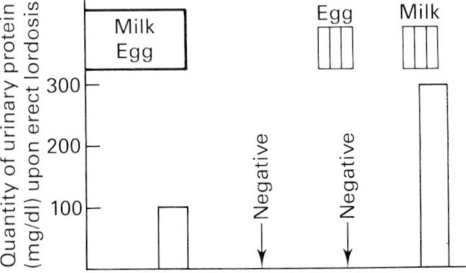

Fig. 43a.8 Lordotic proteinuria resulting from successive 3-day periods of administration of egg and milk. From Matsumura [26], courtesy of Charles C. Thomas, Publisher, Springfield, Illinois.

trates results from 3-day challenges with milk and egg and also shows disappearance of lordotic proteinuria on a diet eliminating those foods. The sensitivity of this testing procedure allowed documentation of proteinuria following ingestion of minute amounts of an offending food.

FOOD SENSITIVITY AND THE LOWER URINARY TRACT

Recurrent cystitis and/or symptoms of dysuria, frequency, suprapubic pain or bleeding are common medical problems which have been reported by physicians and their patients for over 50 years to be triggered by environmental agents [2–4, 8, 11, 14, 32, 41, 45, 52, 53, 56]. A large number of clinical observations suggest that food components may induce these problems. In many instances the urinary symptoms accompanied other system involvement; however, it has also been pointed out that the urinary tract may be the sole target of an allergic reaction.

Enuresis

Enuresis, or involuntary emptying of the bladder beyond an age when bladder control should have been established, has been studied extensively and reasonable data have been obtained supporting a role for food sensitivity. In 1954, Powell and Powell reported a study of 82 women with lower urinary tract allergy [35]. They followed this paper with reports of continuing study of allergy of the lower urinary tract [34, 36, 37]. These investigators could demonstrate that foods caused urinary tract symptoms in a majority of the women studied; the foods causing symptoms are shown in Table 43a.7. Speer commented on his experi-

Table 43a.7 Foods causing lower urinary tract symptoms in 82 women.

Food	Percentage affected
Citrus	60
Tomato	34
Condiments	20
Chocolate	15
Grape	15
Apple	9
Water melon	7

ence that milk was a common offender [46]. He also noted (as did the Powells) that black pepper was the most common triggering condiment. The authors did not provide evidence of the mechanism operating in these reactions. Specific mechanisms, in fact, have not been demonstrated in any of these studies, leaving room for doubt as to participation of immune factors in the process.

Pointers to an allergic cause

In evaluating possible allergic mechanisms of recurrent urinary tract infections, a positive history for other allergic problems in the patient and in the family may be helpful in supporting the need for further allergic study. Blood and urine eosinophilia and elevated serum total IgE concentrations may be helpful, but if not present do not rule out an allergic aetiology for the urinary tract symptoms [17]. The only valid confirming evidence is ability to provoke symptoms with specific challenges and ability to control symptoms

with avoidance of incriminated substances such as foods or treatment with specific extracts in the absence of other environmental changes.

Food sensitivity

Breneman, Pastinszky, Gerrard and Crook among others have provided studies supporting a role for food sensitivity in evocation of lower urinary tract symptoms [3, 4, 6, 11, 32]. Bray, many years before, had noted that when children with asthma avoided food allergens to which they were sensitive, their enuresis sometimes disappeared [2]. Enuresis, of course, has other possible aetiological factors, as listed in Table 43a.8. Cystoscopic findings

Table 43a.8 Aetiology of enuresis.

Allergy, including bladder spasm
Difficulty in arousal from deep sleep
Nocturnal diuresis after daytime water retention
Genetic factors
Psychological–emotional factors
Nocturnal epilepsy
Urinary tract infection
Increased urine volume secondary to diabetes mellitus or insipidus
Obstructive uropathy
Chronic renal failure with impaired concentrating ability

included mucosal pallor and oedema, occasionally accompanied by bleeding. The urine may be clear or may contain red or white blood cells and on occasion eosinophils.

Benign chronic haematuria

This condition is another disorder for which some reports have implicated food sensitivity in the aetiology [19, 40]. That immune reactions can produce haematuria is recognized. In 1930, Coca described allergic haematuria in the absence of protein and red cell casts consistent with lower urinary tract origin [5]. Ammann and Rossi also reported investigation of allergic haematuria and have noted it to be related to sensitivity to foods [1].

Eosinophilic infiltration

Eosinophilic infiltration of the bladder and lower urinary tract have been described associated with symptoms typical of cystitis. Horowitz reported a patient with chronic eosinophilic cystitis and asthma, and reviewed nine patients with the same disorder; two of those had coexistent asthma [18]. His patient progressed to renal failure in spite of treatment with corticosteroids. More recently Sanchez and co-workers [42], and Yamada and colleagues [55] described patients with food-induced interstitial and eosinophilic cystitis. Littleton and colleagues have recently reviewed the literature pertaining to eosinophilic cystitis [23]. They found 39 cases reported and noted that a variety of antigens were implicated as aetiological factors, including medications, topical agents and foods. Parasites also have been identified as possible antigenic sources. That group emphasized the necessity for including other forms of cystitis in the differential diagnosis. A recent editorial in the *Lancet* discussed chronic interstitial cystitis but did not mention allergy or food sensitivity as a possible aetiological factor [10].

The provoking agents of lower urinary tract symptoms include foods, although drugs and inhaled allergens such as moulds may play an important role in some individuals. The foods commonly implicated have been milk, wheat, corn, chicken, tomato, chocolate, cola drinks, citrus, egg, food colours, nuts and some condiments such as black pepper. Some instances of food-related bladder symptoms may be a result of non-specific irritation by spicy foods such as red pepper, etc. rather than due to an immunological mechanism.

SUMMARY

This survey of reported investigations of food sensitivity and disorders of the upper and lower urinary tract underscores the need for further study of the various types of nephrotic syndrome as well as many aspects of lower urinary tract disease. The availability of objective measures of renal function and the ability to monitor relatively easily renal and urinary tract function make this an excellent organ system for study of a potential role of environmental factors in these disorders. If the reported observations are confirmed, control of diet and other environmental factors should provide more specific and effective approaches to therapy.

REFERENCES

1 Ammann P, Rossi E: Allergic hematuria. Arch Dis Child 1966; 41:539.

2 Bray GW: Enuresis of allergic origin. Arch Dis Child 1931; 6:251.

3 Breneman JC: Allergic cystitis: the cause of nocturnal enuresis. Gen Pract 1959; 20:85.

4 Breneman JC: Nocturnal enuresis: a treatment regimen for general use. Ann Allergy 1965; 23:185–91.

5 Coca AF: Specific sensitiveness as a cause of symptoms in disease: essential hematuria and localized retinal edema as possible allergic symptoms. Bull NZ Acad Med 1930; 6:593.

6 Crook WG: Genito-urinary allergy. In: Speer F, Dockhorn RJ, eds. Allergy and immunology in childhood. Springfield: Charles C Thomas, 1974.

7 Dippell J, Wonne R: Atopie, HLA-System, und steroidsensibles nephrotisches Syndrome in Kindesalter. Monatsschr Kinderheilkd 1981; 129:684–7.

8 Duke WW: Food allergy as a cause of irritable bladder. J Urol 1923; 10:173.

9 Editorial: Atopy and steroid-responsive childhood nephrotic syndrome. Lancet 1981; i:964–5.

10 Editorial: Chronic interstitial cystitis. Lancet 1985; ii:134.

11 Esperanca M, Gerrard JW: Nocturnal enuresis. Comparison of the effect of imipramine and dietary restriction on bladder capacity. Can Med Assoc J 1969; 101:721.

12 Eyres K, Mullick NP, Taylor G: Evidence for cell mediated immunity to renal antigens in minimal-change nephrotic syndrome. Lancet 1976; i:1158.

13 Fish AJ, Michael AF, Good RA: Pathogenesis of glomerulonephritis. In: Strauss MB, Welt LG, eds. Diseases of the kidney. 2nd edn. Boston: Little, 1963.

14 Gerrard JW: Nocturnal enuresis. In: Gerrard JW, ed. Food allergy: new perspectives. Springfield: Charles C Thomas, 1980;169.

15 Grupe WE: Primary nephrotic syndrome in childhood. In: Advances in pediatrics. Chicago: Year Book Medical Publishers, 1979;163.

16 Hardwicke J, Soothill JW, Squire JR et al: Nephrotic syndrome and pollen hypersensitivity. Lancet 1959: i:500–2.

17 Horesh AJ: Allergy and recurrent urinary tract infections in childhood (Part II). Ann Allergy 1976; 36:174.

18 Horowitz J, Slavin S, Pfau A: Chronic renal failure due to eosinophilic cystitis. Ann Allergy 1972; 30:502.

19 Kittredge WE, Johnson C: Allergic hematuria due to milk. New Orleans Med Surg J 1948–9; 101:419.

19a Lagrue G, Heslan JM, Belghiti D et al: Basophil sensitization for food allergens in idiopathic nephrotic syndrome. Nephron 1986: 42:123–7.

20 Lagrue G, Laurent J: Role de l'allergie dans la néphrose lipoidique. Nouv Presse Med 1982; 11:1465–6.

21 Laurent J, Lagrue G, Belghiti D et al: Is house dust allergen a possible causal factor for relapses in lipoid nephrosis? Allergy 1984; 39:231.

22 Levinsky RJ, Malleson PN, Barratt TM et al: Circulating immune complexes in steroid-responsive nephrotic syndrome. N Engl J Med 1978; 298:126.

23 Littleton RH, Rarah RN, Cerny JC: Eosinophilic cystitis: an uncommon form of cystitis. J Urol 1982; 127:132–3.

24 McIntosh RM, Ozawa T: Immunologically mediated cell injury. In: Strauss J, ed. Pediatric nephrology: epidemiology, evaluation and therapy, Vol. 2. Miami: Symposia Specialists, 1976;161.

25 McIntosh RM, Griswold WR, Chernack W et al:

The glomerulonephropathies—etiopathogenesis. In: Strauss J, ed. Pediatric nephrology: current concepts in diagnosis and management, Vol. 1. Miami: Symposia Specialists, 1974;89.

26 Matsumura T: Postural proteinuria. In: Dickey L, ed. Clinical ecology. Springfield: Charles C Thomas, 1976;233.

27 Matsumura T, Kuroume T: The role of allergy in the pathogenesis of the nephrotic syndrome. Jpn J Pediatr 1961; 14:921.

28 Matsumura T, Kuroume T, Fukushima I: Significance of food allergy in the etiology of orthostatic albuminuria. J Asthma Res 1966; 3:325.

29 Matsumura T, Kurome T, Matsui A et al: Therapy of the nephrotic syndrome by eradication of foci and elimination diets. Proc 13th Int Cong Pediatr 1971;41.

30 Meadow SR, Sarsfield JK: Steroid-responsive nephrotic syndrome and allergy: clinical studies. Arch Dis Child 1981; 56:509–16.

31 Moorthy AV, Zimmerman SW, Burkholder PM: Inhibition of lymphocyte blastogenesis by plasma of patients with minimal change nephrotic syndrome. Lancet 1976; i:1160.

32 Pastinszky I: The allergic diseases of the male genitourinary tract with special reference to allergic urethritis. Urol Int 1959; 9:258–305.

33 Pollak VE, Pirani CL, Clyne DH: The natural history of membranous glomerulo-nephropathy. In: Kincaid Smith P, Mathew TH, Becker EL, eds. Glomerulonephritis, Part 1. New York: Wiley, 1973;429.

34 Powell NB: Allergies of the genitourinary tract. Ann Allergy 1961; 19:1019–20.

35 Powell NB, Powell BB: Vesical allergy in females. South Med J 1954; 47:841.

36 Powell NB, Boggs PB, McGovern JP: Allergy of the lower urinary tract. Ann Allergy 1970; 28:252–5.

37 Powell NB, Powell BB, Thomas OC et al: Allergy of the lower urinary tract. J Urol 1972; 107:631–4.

38 Reeves WG, Cameron JS, Johansson SGO et al: Seasonal nephrotic syndrome. Clin Allergy 1975; 5:121–37.

39 Richards W, Olson D, Church JA: Improvement of idiopathic nephrotic syndrome following allergy therapy. Ann Allergy 1977; 39:332–3.

40 Rowe AH, Rowe AH Jr: Diagnosis and control of the causes of hematological allergy. In: Food allergy: its manifestations and control and the elimination diets. Springfield: Charles C Thomas, 1972; 430.

41 Rowe AH, Rowe AH Jr: Urogenital allergy-bladder allergy. In: Food allergy: its manifestations and the elimination diets. Springfield: Charles C Thomas, 1972;409.

42 Sanchez-Palacios A, Quintero-de-Juana A, Martinez-Sagarra J et al: Eosinophilic food-induced cystitis. Allergol Immunopathol 1984; 12:463–9.

43 Sandberg DH, McLeod TF, Strauss J: Renal disease related to hypersensitivity to foods. In: Gerrard JW, ed. Food allergy: new perspectives. Springfield: Charles C Thomas, 1980;144.

44 Sandberg DH, McIntosh RM, Bernstein CW et al: Severe steroid-responsive nephrosis associated with hypersensitivity. Lancet 1977; i:388.

45 Siegel S, Rawitt L, Sokoloff B et al: Relationship of allergy, enuresis and urinary tract infections in children 4 to 7 years of age. Pediatrics 1976; 57:526.

46 Speer F: Food allergy. 2nd edn. Boston: J Wright, 1983;34.

47 Thompson PD, Stokes CR, Barratt TM et al: HLA antigens and atopic features in steroid-responsive nephrotic syndrome of childhood. Lancet 1976; ii:765–8.

48 Trompeter RS, Barratt TM, Kay R et al: HLA, atopy, and cyclophosphamide in steroid-responsive childhood nephrotic syndrome. Kidney Int 1980; 17:113–7.

49 Truss CO: Tissue injury induced by *Candida albicans*: mental and neurologic manifestations. J Orthomol Psychiatry 1978; 7:17–37.

50 Truss CO: Restoration of immunologic competence to *Candida albicans*. J Orthomol Psychiatry 1980; 9:287–301.

51 Truss CO: The role of *Candida albicans* in human illness. J Orthomol Psychiatry 1981; 10:225–38.

52 Unger DL, Kubik F, Unger L: Urinary tract allergy. J Am Med Assoc 1959; 70:1380.

53 Walter CK: Allergy as the cause of genitourinary symptoms: clinical considerations. Ann Allergy 1958; 16:158.

54 Williams DG: Allergy and the kidney. In: Lessof MH, ed. Allergy: immunological and clinical aspects. New York: Wiley, 1984;373.

55 Yamada T, Taguchi H, Nisimura H et al: Allergic study of interstitial cystitis. I. A case of interstitial cystitis caused by squid and shrimp hypersensitivity. Arerugi 1984; 33:264–8.

56 Zaleski A, Shokeir MHK, Gerrard JW: Enuresis: familial incidence and relationship to allergic disorders. Can Med Assoc J 1972; 106:30.

Chapter 43b
Food Sensitivity: The Eye

D. Sandberg

Introduction

Many ophthalmological disorders have an immunological component in their aetiology. Although, at present, most patients with such disease are considered to have unknown factors operating, there is some evidence suggesting allergy or hypersensitivity may be involved in pathogenesis [7, 10–13, 15]. Some disorders in which hypersensitivity is or may be involved are listed in Table 43b.1. Ocular symptoms may also accompany other illnesses with an allergic component; e.g. the visual changes accompanying migraine.

Because this group includes such a wide range of disorders, this review will concentrate on those medical problems in which there is a proven or possible link to food sensitivity.

Table 43b.1 Hypersensitivity disorders of the eye.

External eye
  Angioedema
  Eczema of the eyelids
  Allergic blepharitis
  Meibomitis
  Allergic conjunctivitis
  Vernal conjunctivitis
  Phlyctenular keratitis
  Corneal ulcer
  Keratoconus
  Hordeolum
  Interstitial keratitis

Intraocular processes
  Glaucoma
  Allergic cataract
  Uveitis
  Ciliary spasm
  Retinal detachment?

ALLERGY OF THE EXTERNAL EYE

Clinical characteristics

Allergic conjunctivitis. This is one of the most common allergic disorders involving the eye. In most instances it appears to be most directly related to inhaled allergens, especially to pollens and moulds. It may, however, be caused by a variety of other inhalants, by topical medications and by foods [1, 5, 14]. The major symptoms produced are itching, often severe, and watery secretion from the eye. One often observes marked subconjunctival oedema and excessive stringy mucoid secretions which usually contain many eosinophils. Conjunctival scrapings frequently reveal eosinophilia. It is commonly associated with typical allergic rhinitis. A severe form, termed vernal conjunctivitis, occurs more or less seasonally, particularly during spring and summer. It is more likely to be seen in children than adults. It usually involves both eyes; no specific allergens have been demonstrated to play a major aetiological role. In particular, foods have never been identified as aetiological agents. Concentrations of IgE in tears have been reported to be high by some investigators. Recurrent bouts of atopic conjunctivitis may lead to chronic conjunctival changes which predispose to keratitis. Corneal vascularization, ulceration and opacification may occur.

Phlyctenular keratoconjunctivitis. This is described as small nodules on the conjunctivae, cornea or limbus. They evolve as microabscesses with ulceration but do not produce scarring. They are associated with irritation and itching, eye pain, tearing and photophobia. The lesions eventually resolve spontaneously. Sensitivity to microorganisms is suspected; i.e. to staphylococci, *Mycobacterium tuberculosis*. Bothman and Lehrfeld have reported a possible relationship to sensitivity to food [4, 8].

Eczema and blepharitis. Eczema involving the eyelids is common and may be the only manifestation of atopic dermatitis [1]. However, usually other skin involvement is evident. Blepharitis, an inflammatory reaction of the eyelid margins, may be due to infection, allergy or a combination of the two [1]. Allergic blepharitis is considered to be due primarily to reactions to microorganisms or their products. The differential diagnosis for blepharitis should include seborrhoea and pediculosis. Foods have not been demonstrated to be a causative factor. Angioedema and urticaria may involve the eyes and periorbital tissues. These occur as part of a more generalized process as a rule, and may be associated with reaction to a specific food.

Stye. Hordeolum, or stye, is another common lesion which may have an allergic component in aetiology [14]. Reactions to foods may exert a permissive effect on their appearance.

Recurrent chalazion. This is a chronic inflammation of a meibomian gland due to obstruction of the gland duct, and may be associated with sensitivity to food, although the only information supporting this concept is from clinical reports [4].

Lemoine has described a patient with a corneal ulcer possibly related to allergy to food and pollen [9]. Balyeat and Rinkel have reported episcleritis associated with food sensitivity in a patient with concomitant hay fever and urticaria [3], and Bothman reported study of a patient with episcleritis related to eating pork [4].

Interstitial keratitis has been reported to be related to allergy. Dean and co-workers published a report of six patients in whom food sensitivity appeared to be an important factor in this chronic disorder [6].

INTRAOCULAR PROCESSES

Cataract

Allergic cataract may at times accompany severe eczema. The pathophysiology is not known. Bilateral anterior or posterior subcapsular cataracts have been reported in 1–16% of patients with atopic dermatitis. However, adrenocorticosteroid therapy can also induce posterior subcapsular cataracts in susceptible individuals. Typically an allergic cataract begins in early adulthood. It is localized to either the anterior or posterior pole of the lens and involves the superficial lens cortex. Most patients with allergic cataract have a long-standing history of severe atopic dermatitis. The lesions tend to worsen during acute exacerbations of the eczema. No specific association with food allergy has been demonstrated.

Keratoconus

There is also an increased frequency of keratoconus in patients with atopic dermatitis. This conical protrusion of the cornea occurs bilaterally in young adults and of those affected, about one-half also have cataracts.

Uveitis

Inflammation of the uveal tract has been associated with a number of chronic diseases of unknown aetiology which have immune phenomena as an important component of their disease process [12]. These include rheumatoid arthritis, inflammatory bowel disease etc. Uveitis has also been related to a variety of infections; here it appears likely that the uveitis is due to an immune response to the organism rather than active infection at the site. However, an immune reaction may also activate a quiescent infection. Increased vascular permeability as a result of reactions to antigens may be an important element of recurrent disease [2]. No report of chronic uveitis secondary to reactions to foods has been published.

Another entity which may have a component of food sensitivity is Coat's disease associated with residual *Toxocara* larvae in the eye. These lesions can be dormant and asymptomatic for years; flare-up of symptoms related to inflammation in the lesion may occur as a result of a variety of insults including infection. However, such exacerbations may occur as a secondary effect of a reaction to a food or other allergen.

Other conditions

Some unusual chronic eye diseases for which evaluation of a role for food sensitivity might be worthwhile are Thygeson's superficial punctate keratitis and marginal ulcers. The former is characterized by multiple epithelial corneal opacities. The conjunctivae are not affected. Symptoms are caused by microerosions overlying the elevated opacities. Attempts to isolate microorganisms have been unsuccessful. The disease has a chronic course, usually lasting 6 months to 4 years, with fluctuating symptoms. No evidence of a role for food sensitivity has been published. The marginal ulcers are thought to be related to hypersensitivity to staphylococcal antigens,

although this hypothesis has not been confirmed. Both disorders usually respond to topical corticosteroid therapy.

CONCLUSIONS

There is little evidence at present for any role of food allergens in the pathogenesis of eye diseases. However, the eye has special attributes which make it an excellent organ for study. The cornea allows direct access to intraocular tissues for observation using the ophthalmoscope and slit lamp. In addition, alteration of visual function by even subtle inflammatory processes allows qualitative and quantitative observations not easily possible with other organ systems during reactions. This accessibility and ability to use objective measures of function should encourage further study of food sensitivity as it relates to disorders of the eye.

REFERENCES

1 Allansmith MR: Allergy of the lids. In: Golden B, ed. Ocular inflammatory disease. Springfield: Charles C. Thomas, 1974.

2 Aronson SB, Goodner EK, Yamamoto E et al: Mechanisms of the host reponse in the eye. I. Changes in the anterior eye following immunization of a heterologous antigen. Arch Ophthalmol 1965; 73:402.

3 Balyeat RM, Rinkel HJ: Episcleritis due to allergy. J Am Med Assoc 1932; 98:2054.

4 Bothman L: Clinical manifestations of allergy in ophthalmology. In: Year book of the eye, ear, nose and throat. Chicago: Year Book Publishers, 1941.

5 Conlon FA: Conjunctivitis due to food anaphylaxis. Am J Ophthalmol 1919; 2:486.

6 Dean AM, Dean FW, McCutchan GR: Interstitial keratitis caused by specific sensitivity to ingested foods. Arch Ophthalmol 1940; 23:48.

7 Easty DL: Allergy of external eye. In: Lessof MH, ed. Allergy: immunological and clinical aspects. New York: Wiley, 1984;339.

8 Lehrfeld L: Visual allergy to light and intolerance to light. Arch Ophthalmol 1975; 70:992.

9 Lemoine AN: Ocular anaphylaxis. Arch Ophthalmol 1929; 1:706.

10 Liebman SD: Ocular allergy in children. In: Berman BA, MacDonnell KF, eds. Differential diagnosis and treatment of pediatric allergy. 1981;391.

11 Maumenee AE: The contributions of immunology to clinical ophthalmology. Am J Ophthalmol 1964; 58:230.

12 Maumenee AE, Silverstein AM, eds. Immunopathology of uveitis. Baltimore: Williams and Wilkins, 1964.

13 Nussenblatt RB, Palestine AG, Rook AH et al: Treatment of intraocular inflammatory disease with cyclosporin A. Lancet 1983; ii:235–8.

14 Ruedemann AD: Ocular manifestations of allergy. In: Thomas JW, ed. Allergy in clinical practice. Philadelphia: Lippincott, 1941.

15 Theodore FH: Allergy of the eye. American Academy of Ophthalmology and Otolaryngology, 1971.

Chapter 44a
Mediators in Food Allergy

Colin H. Little

Introduction

If we accept that food allergy includes the full spectrum of immune responses, then the mediators released during an allergy reaction will depend on the particular type of reaction involved.

At least three forms of food allergy have been identified:

1 IgE-based hypersensitivity;
2 immune complex reactions;
3 cell-mediated immunity.

In some instances more than one process may be involved.

Mediators will be released in each type of reaction, some specific to that type, others present in more than one type. The mediators may be derived from a number of cellular sources including lymphocytes (lymphokines), macrophages (monokines) and effector cells—platelets, basophils, mast cells, eosinophils or neutrophils.

Some of these mediators are only *locally* active, such as certain lymphokines. Demonstration of their release during an allergic reaction may perhaps only be possible using in vitro methods. The detection of leukocyte inhibitory factor (LIF) in food-allergic subjects [26] is an example of this.

Other mediators may be released into the general circulation in significant amounts and are detectable in blood samples. The timing of blood collection may be critically important. The half-life of the mediator may be brief, or its release may be phasic. Studies on histamine [7, 34] and serotonin [25, 29] release illustrate these points well.

Although blood sampling is the most usual form of collection, other fluids are available in particular instance, such as faecal fluid [2] nasal secretions [30] and sputum.

The establishment of a suitable baseline is critically important in demonstrating a meaningful pattern of in vivo mediator release. Initially a large number of samples may need to be taken to define the optimal time of sampling. Because allergies are often multiple, unless other allergies are controlled, 'background' release of mediator can obscure any pattern of change in response to an antigenic challenge. Observing patients in an environmental control unit, where exposure to other allergens can be prevented, gives a unique opportunity to overcome this problem.

As has been mentioned, mediators released during a food allergy reaction will depend on the type of reaction involved. Listed in Table 44a.1 are some of the important mediators in each case.

The variety of mediators produced

The measurement of lymphokines at sites of tissue damage has begun in disorders such as rheumatoid arthritis where, for example, interferon can be assayed in samples of joint fluid [19]. In food allergy, direct [5, 6, 26] and possibly indirect measurement [22] of lymphokines has been performed in only a few instances.

Recent research [12, 13, 35–37] has indicated that hormones and other peptides can be released by activated lymphocytes. These include adrenocorticotrophic hormone (ACTH), thyroid-stimulating hormone (TSH), human chorionic gonadotrophin (HCG) and opioid peptides.

It is possible that one or several of these molecules can signal the central nervous system, particularly the hypothalamus [10, 11] during immune reactions. Such a process could account for some of the cerebral symptoms and other constitutional effects reported in food allergy. Preliminary work has indicated that the particular hormone-like substances released will depend on how the immune system is activated [12]. Different types of allergy reactions may perhaps be associated with different 'hormones'.

MEDIATORS IN IgE-BASED HYPERSENSITIVITY

To date, because of the wider acceptance of IgE-based reactions as clinical entities, most work has been done in this area.

Histamine

This has probably been the most studied mediator. In a laboratory context the basophil histamine release test has been used as a diagnostic assay. However, in vivo studies of histamine release after food challenge are relatively few. Atkins et al [7] studied a group of patients in whom reactions were immediate and relatively mild in most instances. No significant rise in plasma histamine after food challenge was observed except in one patient (Fig. 44a.1). Also there were no significant

Table 44a.1 Mediators produced during food allergy reactions.

1 *IgE-based hypersensitivity*
Vasoactive mediators: Histamine, SRS-A (leukotrienes C, D and E), platelet aggregating factor (PAF), serotonin, prostaglandins

Chemotactic mediators: ECF-A, ECF(S), neutrophil chemotactic factor (NCF), leukotriene B (LTB), prostaglandin D_2

Other enzymes: Arylsulphatase, β-glucuronidase, β-hexosaminidase, chymase, heparin, other lysosomal enzymes

Of these mediators, histamine, prostaglandins, NCF and leukotrienes have been measured during allergy reactions. Only histamine and NCF have been measured in food allergy reactions, as will be discussed in text

2 *Immune complex reactions*
Serotonin from platelets

Lysosomal enzymes, platelet aggregating factor, cationic proteins, all derived from neutrophils

C-reactive protein

Prostaglandins

Leukotrienes

Interleukin-1 (IL-1)

To date only serotonin and prostaglandins have been measured during allergy reactions of this type

3 *Cell-mediated immunity*
Lymphokines—interleukin-2 (IL-2), α-interferon, α-interferon, interleukin-3 (Il-3), B cell growth factor (BCGF), leukocyte inhibition factor (LIF), macrophage inhibition factor (MIF), colony stimulating factor (CSF), mast-cell activator

Monokines IL-1, interferon, prostaglandin F_2, leukotriene C, PAF

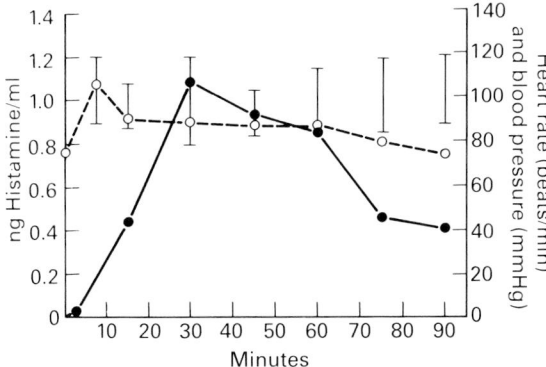

Fig. 44a.1 Plasma histamine levels (●), heart rate (○) and blood pressure (I) after oral food challenge in a patient. From Atkins et al [7], with permission.

changes in urinary histamine (Fig. 44a.2). The doses used in this study may have been insufficient to produce a significant rise in histamine post challenge, or the principal mediators of the reaction may not have included histamine. In another study [9] elevated plasma histamine levels were reported after subcutaneous administration of food antigens, but here the clinical reactions were apparently more severe than in the Atkins study. In the Atkins study most of the patients were skin test positive to the food producing a clinical reaction.

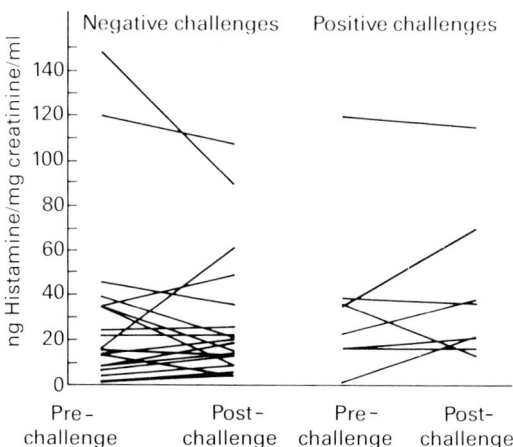

Fig. 44a.2 Urinary histamine levels obtained before and during oral food challenges. There was no significant difference between prechallenge and postchallenge urinary histamine levels obtained during challenge procedures scored as negative or positive by use of the paired sample *t*-test. From Atkins et al [7], with permission.

Atopic eczema. An interesting study [34] on histamine release was performed recently on a group of eczema patients. These patients were generally atopic and developed skin re-

actions within 90 minutes of ingestion of the test food. Positive food challenges showed a significant rise in mean plasma histamine as a group; no such rise occurred with negative challenges or challenge with placebo. Of 35 positive challenges, 28 showed a significant rise in the plasma histamine level after challenge. In all but one case, the positive clinical reactions were associated with positive prick tests to the food.

Gastric challenge. Local histamine release has been detected on intragastric provocation [33]. There was associated mast-cell degranulation and visible changes including oedema and erythema. Not only was there a reduction in tissue histamine content in positive reactions (Fig. 44a.3), but in most cases a rise in plasma histamine concentrations. The local histamine release showed a good correlation with a history of clinical reaction to the food (see also Chapter 53).

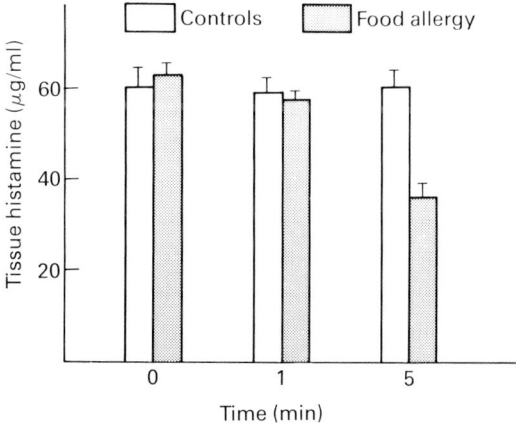

Fig. 44a.3 Tissue histamine content of corpus mucosa at different time intervals after intragastral provocation in patients with food allergy ($n = 14$) and normal controls ($n = 10$). There was a significant ($P < 0.01$) decrease in tissue histamine content 5 minutes after allergen challenge in food-allergic patients. From Reiman et al [33], with permission.

Limitations of studies of histamine release

Studies on histamine release show a number of limitations. The histamine release may occur at a site distant from the point of sample collection, e.g. from the skin in eczema patients. Histamine is also rapidly catabolized, with probably some variation between individuals in the rate of catabolism. The role of histamine is best documented for immediate hypersensitivity reactions and the basophil histamine release test is to some extent a suitable in vitro model for this. It is possible that histamine release is important in some cell-mediated reactions as the mast cell is also involved in this type of reaction [4].

Neutrophil chemotactic factor (NCF-A)

This mediator has been studied in asthmatics. It has been shown to be released during both early and late phases of asthmatic reactions [31]. Papageorgiou and co-workers studied its release in four milk-sensitive subjects. In three subjects a characteristic immediate-type asthmatic response developed which was accompanied by a rise in NCF-A (Fig. 44a.4). Skin tests, specific IgE, basophil histamine release and precipitins against milk extracts were all negative. The chemotactic activity was principally associated with a protein having a molecular weight around 600 000.

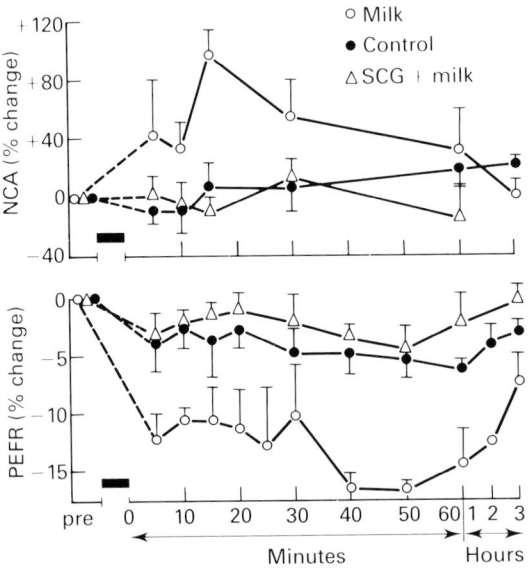

Fig. 44a.4 Mean percentage change in NCA and PEFR in three asthmatics during the control day after milk ingestion. The effect of prior administration of oral sodium cromoglycate (SCG) on the changes in PEFR and NCA has also been shown. Each point represents the mean ± SEM. The mean prechallenge NCA on the control day was 121 neutrophils/10 hpf, milk day 101.5 neutrophils/10 hpf and SCG + milk day, 126.2 neutrophils/ 10 hpf. Solid bar = period of challenge. From Papageorgiou et al [31], with permission.

Leukotrienes

There have been many studies which have measured the release of leukotrienes after antigen challenge. In one study [17] leukotrienes were present in nasal washings following the

inhalation of ragweed pollen in sensitive patients. In another study lung tissue was used [18]. As yet there has been no application of these measurements to the field of food allergy. It may be worthwhile to measure leukotrienes in intestinal secretions following food challenge.

Prostaglandins

Prostaglandin release during food reactions was demonstrated by Buisseret et al [15] who measured prostaglandins E_2 and F_2 in blood and stool samples in several patients developing acute gastrointestinal symptoms after the ingestion of specific foods. A rise in the levels of these mediators was noted following food challenge, and the use of prostaglandin-synthetase inhibitors controlled the reactions on subsequent challenge. The onset of reactions was usually within 1–2 hours and skin tests were negative (Fig. 44a.5).

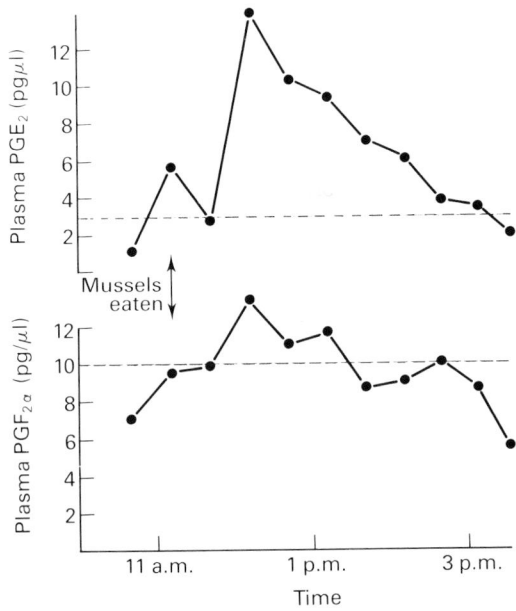

Fig. 44a.5 Peripheral venous blood plasma PGE_2 and F_2 concentrations during unprotected challenge with mussels. Dashed lines indicate upper limits of normal. From Buisseret et al [15], with permission.

Irritable bowel syndrome

An important study [2] has implicated food intolerance in the irritable bowel syndrome. PGE_2 was measured in rectal fluid after food challenge and in those patients developing diarrhoea after the challenge significant and sustained elevations of PGE_2 occurred; the prostaglandin level correlated well with faecal wet weight (see Chapter 32). However, patients who experienced pain rather than diarrhoea did not show such elevations. This would suggest that more than one mechanism was involved. Prostaglandin release is not specific for any type of immune response. In this group of patients there was no change in plasma histamine levels after challenge or evidence of histamine release from basophils after incubation with the test food.

Platelet aggregating factor (PAF)

This mediator is released in Type I and Type III immune reactions from a variety of cellular sources. It is possibly a key mediator in both 'intrinsic' asthma and IgE-mediated bronchospasm [28]. PAF can be produced locally from mast cells or alveolar macrophages [38], particularly the latter and can produce a dual response in the skin following intradermal injection [8]. As assays for PAF become available, studies on its release in food-induced asthma may shed light on underlying mechanisms. Food antigen may bind to specific IgE on alveolar macrophages, or alternatively immune complexes containing food antigen may possibly localize in alveolar macrophages [23]. In either case PAF could be released.

In animals, bronchospasm and the intravascular aggregation and activation of platelets may accompany an intravenous injection of PAF. PAF can stimulate the release of platelet factor 4 and serotonin from human platelets. In one study [24] a significant rise in platelet factor 4 was detectable following the inhalation of ragweed pollen in allergic subjects. There have been no comparable studies yet performed in food-induced asthma. In a number of patients we have observed a fall in whole blood serotonin (5-hydroxytryptamine, 5-HT) and a rise in its principal metabolite 5-hydroxyindoleacetic acid (5-HIAA), following a positive food challenge (Fig. 44a.6), to-

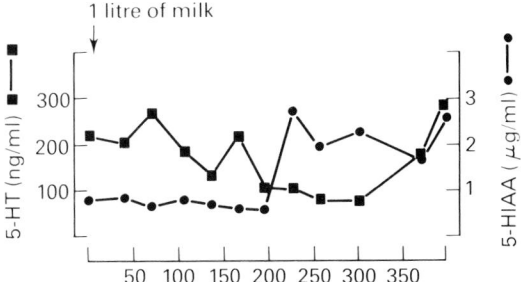

Fig. 44a.6 Fall in blood serotonin (5-HT) and rise in 5-hydroxyindoleacetic acid (5-HIAA) following positive food challenge in patient.

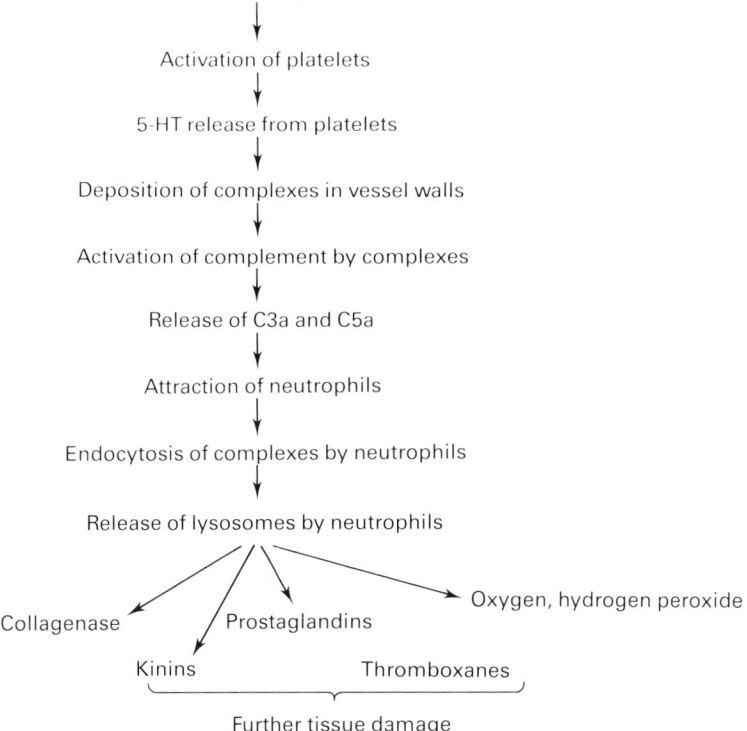

Fig. 44a.7 Immunopathological processes in Type III hypersensitivity. From Little et al [25], with permisssion.

gether with a significant degree of broncho-spasm.

MEDIATORS IN TYPE III AND TYPE IV REACTIONS

Type III reactions

The process involved in Type III hypersensitivity reactions may be summarized as shown in Fig. 44a.7. Local measurement of prostaglandins can be performed at sites of inflammation. Alternatively serotonin can be measured in whole blood samples as its release would occur primarily in the circulation.

Type III reactions have been implicated in food allergy. Examples include coeliac disease, dermatitis herpetiformis, idiopathic nephrotic syndrome and Henoch–Schönlein purpura. There is also growing evidence that food allergy may be involved in two common disorders: rheumatoid arthritis [25] and migraine [20, 27]. Immune complex formation is certainly important in the former, and may possibly play a role in the latter.

Rheumatoid arthritis

We have studied serotonin release in patients with rheumatoid arthritis whose condition was clearly exacerbated by the ingestion of certain foods [25]. There was a fall in whole blood serotonin levels and a subsequent increase in 5-HIAA following positive food challenges in these patients (Fig. 44a.8). In some patients the change in blood levels was particularly striking, as shown in Fig. 44a.9. Clearly further studies are required to confirm and extend our observations in rheumatoid arthritis.

Migraine

Several studies have demonstrated changing serotonin levels in migraine. In particular, a fall in whole blood serotonin and a subsequent rise in 5-HIAA has been repeatedly observed during the headache phase [3, 29]. This may be due to the formation of immune complexes, particularly where substantial serotonin release occurs. Measurements of whole blood serotonin and 5-HIAA in migraine patients following food challenge could be performed along with serial measurements of immune complexes. We have performed a limited number of such studies (unpublished observations).

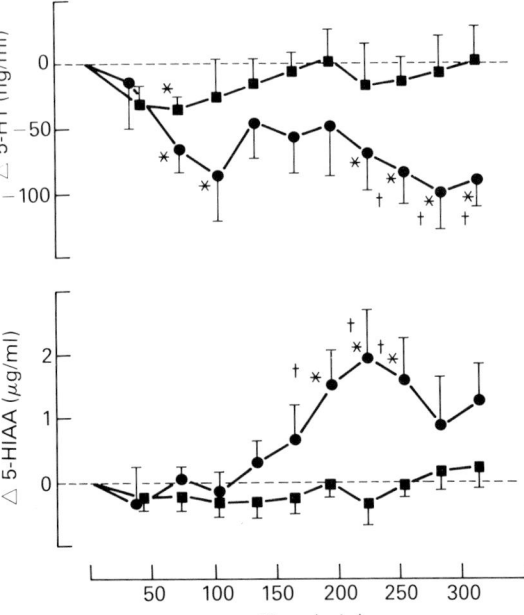

Fig. 44a.8 Changes in 5-HT and 5-HIAA in PRP after ingestion of positive foods in food-intolerant patients (●) and healthy controls (■). Results are expressed as mean of changes from control levels (average of two estimations on samples taken before food ingestion) and 1 SEM. There were seven subjects in each group. * $P < 0.05$, Student's paired t-test, compared with control concentrations. † $P < 0.05$, Student's unpaired t-test, indicates a difference in magnitude of mean changes from concentrations in controls compared with patients at certain times after food ingestion. From Little et al [25], with permission.

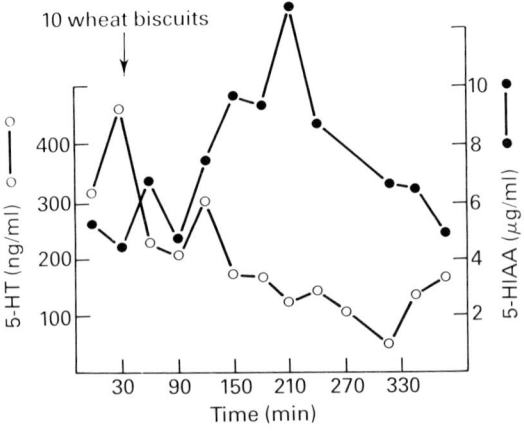

Fig. 44a.9 5-HT and 5-HIAA in PRP after ingestion of wheat at 30 minutes. Control samples were taken before ingestion of wheat followed by sampling every half hour for 330 minutes.

Case study. In one particular patient (Figs. 44a.10 and 44a.11) there was a fall in whole blood serotonin, a rise in 5-HIAA and the phasic appearance of immune complexes fol-

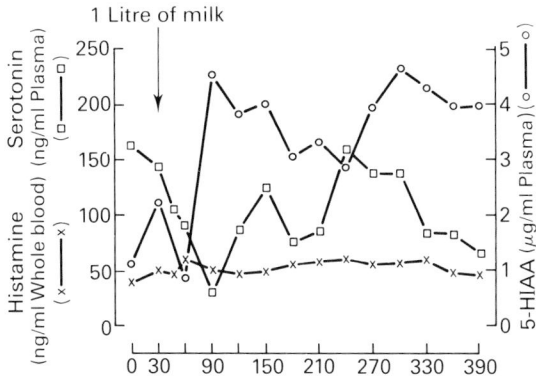

Fig. 44a.10 Fall in 5-HT and rise in 5-HIAA following ingestion of 1 litre of milk.

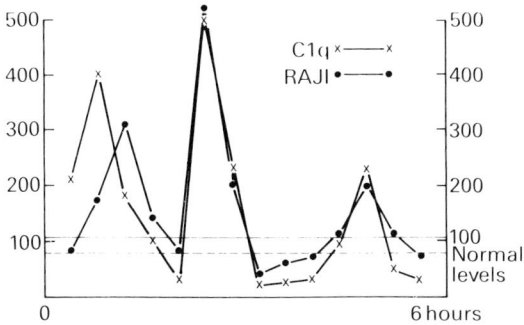

Fig. 44a.11 Circulating immune complexes following milk challenge.

lowing the ingestion of 1 litre of milk. In the course of the challenge the patient developed classic migraine with visual scotomata, parasthesiae, chills and restlessness; rhinitis and conjunctivitis were also observed. A drop in specific IgE antibody against milk was recorded (Fig. 44a.12). Perhaps both IgE- [27] and IgG-containing immune complexes were

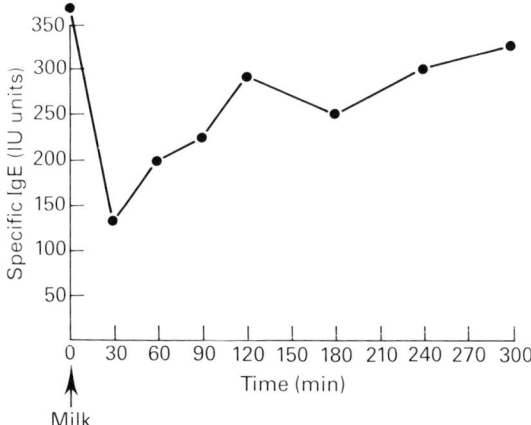

Fig. 44a.12 Drop in specific IgE antibody following milk challenge.

present in this patient during the migraine attack.

Cell-mediated immunity

Cell-mediated immunity has been documented in a number of disorders where food allergy is present. These include coeliac disease and milk-induced enteropathy. In both these conditions delayed-type hypersensitivity (DTH) is the principal cause of tissue damage and there are appropriate animal models [16]. In other disorders such as rheumatoid arthritis cell-mediated immunity plays an important role in the inflammatory process [19]. Food allergy may be implicated in at least some cases of rheumatoid arthritis, as mentioned above [16, 25]. Numerous lymphokines and monokines have been detected in the synovial fluid and synovial tissue of patients with rheumatoid arthritis [19] and give an indication of the range of mediators that can be measured (Table 44a.2).

Table 44a.2 Lymphokines and monokines detected in synovial fluid from patients with rheumatoid arthritis.

Lymphocyte products
Macrophage chemotactic factor
Macrophage inhibition factor (MIF)
Leukocyte inhibition factor (LIF)
Lymphocyte mitogenic factor
Fibroblast activating factor

Macrophage products
Interleukin 1
Plasminogen activator
Collagenase
Prostaglandins
Lysosomal enzymes
Fibroblast activating factor

Cow's milk allergy

In one study [6] of infants and children with cow's milk allergy, lymphocytes were cultured in vitro with β-lactoglobulin and the production of LIF was measured. All the patients with milk allergy showed significant LIF production in response to β-lactoglobulin compared with controls. Manifestations of cow's milk allergy were fairly severe with diarrhoea, vomiting, rashes, bloody stools and weight loss. At least some of these patients may have had milk-induced enteropathy. A similar study has been performed on patients with coeliac disease [5] with comparable results.

Table 44a.3 Peptide hormones released from lymphocytes.

Stimulus	Cell	Peptide hormone
Newcastle disease virus (NDV)	T + B	Opioids, ACTH
Tumour cells	T + B	Opioids, ACTH
Lipopolysaccharide (LPS)	B, macrophage	Opioids, ACTH
Staphylococcal enterotoxin A (SEA)	T	TSH
Corticotrophin-releasing factor (CRF)	T + B	Opioids, ACTH

LIF production

Minor et al [26] studied the production of LIF by leukocytes incubated with food antigen. Patients had a range of disorders including rhinitis, diarrhoea, vomiting, abdominal pain, asthma and eczema. The food antigens used were α-lactalbumin, β-lactoglobulin, casein and corn. Almost 60% of patients who improved with the elimination of cow's milk from the diet showed a significant LIF production when their leukocytes were cultured with whole cow's milk or its main fractions. Only 2 out of 26 controls showed significant LIF production. Similar results were obtained with corn. These results suggest a possible diagnostic usefulness of such an assay.

Peptide hormone release from lymphocytes

Over the past 5 years it has become apparent that the immune system, when signalled in certain ways, can release hormonally active substances. Blalock et al [14] have carried out a series of pioneering studies which appear to show that different subpopulations of lymphocytes can be activated to release peptide hormones, depending on the stimulus. The particular hormones released and the population of lymphocytes involved will then vary according to the nature of the stimulus [14] as is shown in Table 44a.3.

Other hormones that may be produced by lymphocytes include chorionic gonadotrophin, growth hormone, FSH, luteinizing hormone (LH), vasoactive intestinal peptide (VIP) and somatostatin [14]. There are possibly a number of different opioids that can also be produced.

Symptoms induced by peptide hormones. It is possible that certain of these hormones may account for some of the constitutional symptoms such as headache, malaise and muscle pain which occur in infectious diseases, particularly during the prodromal phase. Besedovsky et al [11] have shown that secreted immune products can affect brain function, the hypothalamus being a key target area. They found that supernatants from lymphocytes stimulated by concanavalin A (con A) substantially reduced the noradrenaline turnover in hypothalamic neurones when injected into rats.

We have wondered whether such immune products could account for certain symptoms frequently reported in food allergy. A representative list [32] is shown in Table 44a.4.

Table 44a.4 Symptoms possibly associated with release of peptide hormones.

Lethargy	Palpitations
Headache	Abdominal pain or heartburn
Abdominal swelling or discomfort	
Depression	Dizziness
Bowel disturbance	Sleep disturbance
Paraesthesiae	Breathlessness
Nausea	Mood swings
Irritability	Chest pain
Poor concentration	Peripheral oedema
Anxiety or panic attacks	Joint pains
Itch	Poor memory

These symptoms have often been dismissed as hysterical but at least in some instances may be due to mediators. Opioid peptides are a possible candidate as a cause for these symptoms which principally affect gut and brain. Indeed, a number of workers [1] have implicated opioids in the pathogenesis of migraine. A recent study by Harvath et al [22] showed that when the leukocytes of patients with coeliac disease are incubated with α-gliadin there is inhibition of leukocyte migration. This effect was blocked by naloxone and reproduced by morphine indicating that an opioid was responsible for the effect (Table 44a.5). There are a number of interpretations of the test, one being that the sensitized lymphocytes released an opioid on exposure to α-gliadin which in turn inhibited leukocyte migration. Studies are required on the possible release of opioid peptides in food allergy. The author is engaged in such a study at the present time.

Table 44a.5 Effect of gliadin, phytohaemagglutinin (PHA) and morphine on leucokyte migration in gliadin-sensitive (positive) and not-sensitive (negative) patients. From Horvath et al [22], with permission.

M	Without maloxone	With naloxone	P*
α-Gliadin			
Positive	$0.71 \pm 0.08(13)$	$0.96 \pm 0.14(13)$	0.001
Negative	$1.01 \pm 0.10(19)$	$1.03 \pm 0.09(19)$	0.5
PHA	$0.46 \pm 0.10(11)$	$0.48 \pm 0.11(11)$	0.6
Morphine			
Positive	$0.75 \pm 0.08(6)$	$0.99 \pm 0.11(6)$	0.01
Negative	$0.99 \pm 0.09(11)$	$1.07 \pm 0.14(11)$	0.01

Migration given as mean $\pm$ SEM; number of measurements in parentheses.
* Students t-test.

CONCLUSION

It is clear from this review that there have been relatively few studies on the release of mediators in food allergy. The reasons for this are the difficulties in assaying many of the mediators, and a tendency to narrow the definition of food allergy, thereby underrating its importance as a subject for serious study. It is anticipated that with technical advances assays will become more widely available, but judgment in choosing the site and time to collect samples will be important. For too long food allergy has been associated almost exclusively with Type I hypersensitivity. However, as with any other class of antigen, foods can induce several types [I–IV] of immune response, depending on the molecular form of the antigen. As a result there may be complex patterns of mediator release particular to type (or types) of immune response involved.

REFERENCES

1 Agnoli A, Denaro A, Ceci E, Falaschi P: On the etiopathogenesis of migraine: a possible link between the amines and the endorphin hypothesis. Adv Neurol 1982; 33:99–105.

2 Alun Jones V, Laughlan P, Shorthouse M et al: Food intolerance: a major factor in the pathogenesis of irritable bowel syndrome. Lancet 1982; i:115–7.

3 Anthony M, Hinterberger H, Lance J: Plasma serotonin in migraine and stress. Arch Neurol 1967; 16:544–52.

4 Ashkenase P, Van Loveren H: Delayed-type hypersensitivity: activation of mast cells by antigen-specific T cell factors initiates the cascade of cellular interactions. Immunol Today 1983; 4:259–64.

5 Ashkenazi A, Idar D, Handzel ZT et al: An in vitro immunological assay for diagnosis of coeliac disease. Lancet 1978; i:627.

6 Ashkenazi A, Levin S, Idar D et al: In vitro cell-mediated immunological assay for cow's milk allergy. Paediatrics 1980; 66:399–402.

7 Atkins F, Steinberg S, Metcalf D: Evaluation of immediate adverse reactions to foods in adult patients. J Allergy Clin Immunol 1985; 75:356–63.

8 Basran G, Page C, Paul W, Morley J: Platelet-aggregating factor: a possible mediator of the dual response to allergen? Clin Allergy 1984; 14:75–9.

9 Bellanti, J, Nerukor L, Willoughby J: Measurement of plasma histamine in patients with suspected food hypersensitivity. Ann Allergy 1981; 47:260.

10 Besedovsky H, Felix D, Haas H: Hypothalamic changes during the immune response. Eur J Immunol 1977; 7:323.

11 Besedovsky H, del Ray A, Sorkin E, et al: The immune response evokes changes in brain noradrenalin neurones. Science 1983; 221:564.

12 Blalock J: The immune system as a sensory organ. J Immunol 1984; 132:1067–70.

13 Blalock J, Smith E: Human leucocyte interferon: potent endorphin-like opioid activity. Biochem Biophys Res Commun 1981; 101:472.

14 Blalock J, Harbour-McMenamim D, Smith E: Peptide hormones shared by the neuroendocrine and immunologic systems. J Immunol 1985; 135:8585–615.

15 Buisseret P, Youlten L, Heinzelmann D, Lessof M: Prostaglandin-synethetase inhibitors in prophylaxis of food intolerance. Lancet 1978; i:906–8.

16 Coombs R, Olsham G: Early rheumatoid-like joint lesions in rabbits drinking cow's milk. Int Arch Allergy Appl Immunol 1981; 64:287–92.

17 Creticos P, Peters D, Adkinson N et al: Peptide leukotriene release after antigen challenge in patients sensitive to ragweed. N Engl J Med 1984; 310:1626–9.

18 Dahlen S, Hansson G, Hedqvist P et al: Allergen challenge of lung tissue from asthmatics elicits bronchial contraction that correlates with the release of leukotrienes C_4, D_4, and E_4. Proc Natl Acad Sci USA 1983; 80:1712–6.

19 Decker J, et al: Rheumatoid arthritis: evolving concepts of pathogenesis and treatment. Ann Intern Med 1984; 101:814.

20 Egger J, Carter C, Wilson J et al: Is migraine food allergy. Lancet 1983; ii:863–9.

21 Ferguson A, Mowat A, Strobel S, Barnetson R: Induction and expression of cell-mediated immunity in the small intestine. In: Regulation of the immune response. New York: 1982; 288–98. [Basel: Karger, 1983].

22 Horvath K, Graf L, Walcz E et al: Naloxone antagon-
   ises effect of α-gliadin on leucocyte migration in
   patients with coeliac disease. Lancet 1985; ii:185–6.

23 Kanayama Y, Amatsu K, Takeda T, Inoue T: Uptake
   of intravenously administered soluble immune complexes by Type I alveolar cells and macrophages in
   mice. Int Arch Allergy Appl Immunol 1985; 78:108–
   11.

24 Knauer KA, Lichtenstein LM, Adkinson NF, Fish J:
   Platelet activation during antigen-induced airway reactions in asthmatic subjects. N Engl J Med 1981;
   304:1404–7.

25 Little C, Stewart A, Fennessy M: Platelet serotonin
   release in rheumatoid arthritis: a study in food-intolerant patients. Lancet 1983; 297–9.

26 Minor J, Tolber S, Frick O: Leucocyte inhibition factor in delayed-onset food allergy. J Allergy Clin Immunol 1980; 66:313–21.

27 Monro J, Carini C, Brostoff J: Migraine is a food allergic disease. Lancet 1984; ii:719–21.

28 Morley J, Sanjar S, Page C: The platelet in asthma.
   Lancet 1984; ii:1142–4.

29 Muck-Seler D, Deanovic Z, Dupely M: Serotonin-re-
   leasing factors in migrainous patients. Adv Neurol
   1983; 33:257–64.

30 Naclario R, Proud D, Togias A et al: Inflammatory
   mediators in late antigen-induced rhinitis. N Engl J
   Med 1985; 313:65–70.

31 Papageorgiou N, Lee T, Nagakura T et al: Neutrophil
   chemotactic activity in milk-induced asthma. J Allergy
   Clin Immunol 1983; 72:75–82.

32 Pearson D, Rix K, Bentley S: Food allergy: how much
   in the mind. Lancet 1983; i:1259–61.

33 Reiman H, Ring J, Ultsch B, Wendt P: Intragastric
   provocation under endoscopic control in food allergy:
   mast cell and histamine changes in gastric mucosa.
   Clin Allergy 1985; 15:195–202.

34 Sampson H, Jolie P: Increased plasma histamine concentrations after food challenges in children with
   atopic dermatis. N Engl J Med 1984; 311:372–6.

35 Smith E, Blalock J: Human lymphocyte production of
   ACTH and endorphin-like substances: association
   with leucocyte interferon. Proc Natl Acad Sci USA
   1981; 78:7530.

36 Smith E, Meyer W, Blalock J: Virus-induced increases
   in corticosterone in hypophysectomised mice: a possible lymphoid-adrenal axis. Science 1982; 218:1311.

37 Smith E, Phan M, Coppenhaver D et al: Human lymphocyte production of immuno-reactive thyrotropin.
   Proc Natl Acad Sc: USA 1983; 80:6010.

38 Tonnel A, Joseph M, Gosset P et al: Stimulation of
   alveolar macrophages in asthmatic patients after local
   provocation test. Lancet 1983; i:1406–8.

Chapter 44b
Allergy and Autoimmune Endocrinopathy: APICH Syndrome

Phyllis L. Saifer and Nathan Becker

Introduction

In the complex allergy patient who presents with multiple sensitivities to foods and chemicals and with symptoms in many organ systems, it is well to consider the possibility of a complicating factor which touches on the immune, endocrine, and neurological systems. Such an entity is autoimmune endocrine disease, in particular thyroiditis and oophoritis.

Historically there is a correlation between Hashimoto's lymphocytic thyroiditis and allergic disease [4]. In our own patient population we found a substantial number of allergic patients who complained of morning fatigue and intolerance to temperature change who had thyroid antibodies. Within this group we found a subset of women who had symptoms of premenstrual syndrome with ovarian antibodies and, frequently, thyroid antibodies, but who presented with respiratory allergies and positive prick and intradermal skin tests.

APICH syndrome

The complete picture of these patients includes autoimmune polyendocrinopathy, immune dysregulation in the form of abnormal helper/suppressor 'T' cell ratios, low serum IgA, response to nystatin, and hypersensitivity states with positive allergy skin tests and improvement on elimination diets. For want of a better acronym we have assigned the label *APICH* syndrome to this constellation of findings (Fig. 44b.1). (*A*utoimmune, *P*olyendocrinopathy, *I*mmune dysregulation, *C*andidiasis, *H*ypersensitivity.)

In autoimmune endocrinopathy, an organ-specific disease, genetic predisposition is foremost in aetiology, with periods of high hormone stress such as puberty, childbirth, and menopause accounting for triggers.

Evidence for environmental chemical triggers has been accumulating in recent years. Bahn et al [3], for example, noted the increased prevalence of thyroid antibodies among workers exposed to polybrominated biphenyls.

A defect in T suppressor cells is postulated by Arulanantham et al [2] and Thielemans et al [16]. Autoimmune endocrinopathies result from multiple gene interactions: organ-specific

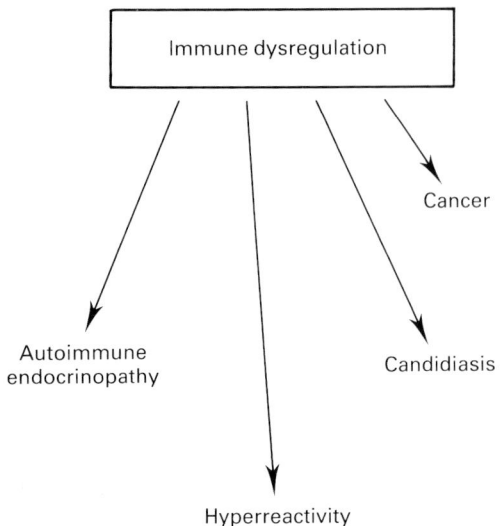

Fig. 44b.1   Clinical consequences of immune dysregulation.

and immune responsiveness control (see Volpé [17]). Antibodies may react with hormones or their receptors. Hormone antibodies react with the gland and with secreted hormone. Receptor antibodies block receptor sites. Thyrotoxicosis is an example of a hormone receptor disease (see Doniach et al [8]). Autoantibodies blocking β_2-adrenergic receptors may be a factor in some cases of asthma and allergic rhinitis.

For a full list of the organ-specific and non-organ-specific autoimmune diseases which the allergist may find in his more complex, difficult 'thick chart' patients, see Appendix 44b.1.

CLINICAL PICTURE

These patients may present to two different medical specialists: the endocrinologist and the clinical immunologist and allergist.

The endocrinologist

It is estimated [9] that approximately 4% of the population has thyroiditis. About 3% of the population has functional hypothyroidism secondary to thyroiditis. Sixteen per cent of elderly females have some degree of lymphocytic infiltration in the thyroid gland. Most spontaneous primary hypothyroidism occurs as a result of an autoimmune process that gradually destroys the thyroid gland and is reflected by lymphocytic infiltration and fibrosis

of the gland accompanied by elevated abnormal levels of thyroid antibodies in the serum.

Onset of symptoms. The onset of Hashimoto's thyroiditis is often so insidious that the classical clinical manifestations can take years to appear. The signs and symptoms are frequently interspersed with those of hypothyroidism and thyrotoxicosis. The patient is simultaneously agitated and fatigued with all symptoms reaching a crescendo at menses. Consequently, the symptoms are compounded by a premenstrual syndrome and dysfunctional menses in women, lability of mood and depression in both men and women, inappropriate fatigue despite normal thyroid indices, and concomitant allergies and other autoimmune disorders (see Table 44b.1).

Table 44b.1   Symptoms of thyroiditis.

(1) Morning fatigue.
(2) Short-term memory loss.
(3) Asthma (and other allergies).
(4) Difficulty with weight control.
(5) Depression (and other mood disturbances).
(6) Bladder disorders (frequency, urgency).
(7) Temperature change intolerance.
(8) Irregular menses.

The clinical immunologist and allergist

This very same complicated patient presents to the allergist with symptoms of rhinitis, asthma, urticaria, eczema, headache, irritable bowel syndrome, myalgia, arthralgias and multiple food, drug and chemical intolerances.

The patient may often have seen many other specialists, but with no abnormal findings. These patients may then become typical treatment failures, be labelled 'difficult' and become an example of the 'thick note' syndrome (the 'crock').

Patient symptoms. The APICH patient or polyendocrinopathy-allergy patient has so many symptoms in so many systems that the sympathetic physician is quite overwhelmed. The unsympathetic physician quickly does a mental review of all the psychiatrists he likes least. (For symptom review and treatment follow-up tabulation form, see Appendix 44b.2.)

The patient's asthma and allergic rhinitis have become perennial with associated chronic urticaria. A frequent complaint is difficulty with short-term memory, unrelenting fatigue with depression and poor concentration. The inappropriate fatigue is so outstanding that it deserves more detail. Patients frequently call themselves 'night people'. The fatigue is most prominent on arising and resolves only in the late afternoon (4–6 p.m.). Subsequently, stamina and mental clarity return late in the evening and are often followed by insomnia or easily disturbed sleep. Vascular headache adds to the picture. Typical allergic ear, nose and throat symptoms are present along with tinnitus, sore throat and difficulty in swallowing.

The patient has a poor tolerance for temperature change: she complains of easy chilling and of wilting in hot weather. She also has difficulty maintaining a stable weight.

Examination. The allergic thyroiditic presents the '3 Ps' on first glance: 'pallor, puffiness, and pastiness'.

On palpation of the thyroid gland one finds a normal-sized to modestly enlarged organ. The lobes are often asymmetrical. The gland may be firmer than normal and have an irregular, bosselated surface. Nodules may be present. The firm areas are frequently tender. Tenderness is more common in the younger thyroiditic patient. Goitre is not commonly present.

Lymphadenopathy is palpable along the course of the cartoid artery, in the postauricular and supraclavicular chain. The signs of thyroiditis are summarized in Table 44b.2.

Table 44b.2 Signs of thyroiditis.

(1) Firm, bosselated, sometimes tender thyroid gland.
(2) Cervical lymphadenopathy.
(3) Costochondral tenderness.
(4) Transverse ridging of thumb nails.
(5) Pallor, coarse complexion, generalized mild oedema.
(6) Thin, sparse hair.
(7) Hypotension and basal hypothermia.
(8) ECG: sinus bradycardia and elongated P-wave.

HOW DO YOU MAKE THE DIAGNOSIS?

Very careful history taking and detailed attention to *all* symptoms, not just the classical allergic symptoms, lead directly to the diagnosis.

Patient's history

The patient may be male or female but autoimmune diseases predominate in females. In a recent study there were ten females to one male with thyroid antibodies. A few males may have been missed because of low index of suspicion (Saifer, unpublished observation).

The patient appears in her early 20s or again in her early 40s with a story that goes back to childhood when she had recurrent otitis media, sore throats for which she received courses of antibiotics, eczema, stomach-aches, allergic rhinitis or asthma. Instead of the expected improvement of all these disorders at puberty, the allergic diseases began to be more severe and worsened throughout adolescence. A late teenage tonsillectomy may have been performed. Many patients will have been given thyroxine.

Menarche occurred at the normal time but menses were never regular and cycles tended to be extended. Oral contraceptives were not well tolerated.

The patient was said to be moody, withdrawn, negative, irritable, and disagreeable—a very difficult person, sleeping a great deal and tending to be a night person.

After delivery of any one of her several children, she may have suffered a prolonged period of depression in spite of being happy with the child and marriage. From ages 25 to 40 allergies persisted along with fatigue, but she was able to care for her family and maintain her job. A summary of the main points in the patient's history is shown in Table 44b.3.

Table 44b.3 Patient's history.

(1) Female: Male > 10:1.
(2) Allergies in childhood and worse after puberty.
(3) Irregular menses.
(4) 'Difficult' adolescence.
(5) Trial of thyroid hormone.
(6) Postpartum depression and other psychiatric problems.
(7) Poor tolerance of oral contraceptives.
(8) Frequent need for antibiotics.
(9) Recurrent *Candida* vaginitis.
(10) Mitral valve prolapse, cystic breasts, endometriosis, prematurely gray hair.
(11) Multiple system involvement (especially bladder).
(12) Uncontrolled allergies.
(13) Sore throats and late tonsillectomy, peri- or post-pubertal.
(14) Irradiation for acne, thymus, birth marks, tumours.
(15) Always short on energy.
(16) Premenstrual syndrome.
(17) Mononucleosis.
(18) Prostatitis.

The patient may also have developed cystic breasts, endometriosis, mitral valve prolapse (see Marks [13]), and prematurely gray hair. She may also have had a number of psychiatric consultations and now has premenstrual syndrome.

Now at age 40, the patient has uncontrollable allergies and is complaining that she is 'falling apart at the seams'. Her nose runs; all foods cause reactions; perfumes, cigarette smoke and car exhaust provoke symptoms. She can no longer tolerate alcohol. She itches and her asthma is no longer seasonal but perennial and is difficult to control. She has been on multiple allergy programmes throughout her life and none has been particularly successful. She has muscle aches, bowel problems, recurrent *Candida* vaginitis, and all of the above are making her life intolerable.

Family history

The family history can be enormously helpful in unravelling such a complicated patient. It is frequently necessary and very important to send the patient back to her mother, in particular, for more details about family disease patterns.

The females in the family have histories of thyroid disease, goitres, thyroidectomies and 'nervous breakdowns'. There are allergies, cancer, drug sensitivities, autoimmune diseases such as pernicious anaemia and rheumatoid arthritis, premenstrual syndrome, alopecia, and juvenile onset diabetes. There are also other endocrine disorders, prematurely gray hair, and alcoholism (see Table 44b.4).

Table 44b.4 Family history.

(1) Thyroid disease.
(2) Mental disorders.
(3) Allergy.
(4) Cancer.
(5) Alcoholism.
(6) Autoimmune disorders:
　　Diabetes mellitus (Type I), rheumatoid arthritis, pernicious anaemia, vitiligo, alopecia, prematurely gray hair.
(7) Female problems.
(8) Drug sensitivities.

Laboratory tests

Thyroid. The key laboratory tests in diagnosing autoimmune thyroiditis are the antithyroid antibodies: antithyroid microsomal antibodies and antithyroglobulin antibodies measured by radioimmunoassay (RIA). Haemagglutination is too insensitive.

In our opinion, investigation of autoimmune thyroiditis is not complete until a 24-hour radioactive iodine (^{123}I) thyroid scan is performed. The scan often demonstrates irregularity of function with the uptake being paradoxically elevated. Rarely are distinct 'cold' areas noted.

Thyroid investigation includes thyroid indices: T_3 uptake, T_4 RIA (free thyroid index). We can also measure T_3 and TSH (thyroid-stimulating hormone): frank hyperthyroidism is confirmed by an elevated T_3 RIA; primary hypothyroidism is determined by an elevated TSH.

In thyroiditis, however, these indices are not helpful. They are usually within the normal range.

There are immunological abnormalities in the thyroid and also systemically as shown by:

(a) lymphocytic infiltration in the thyroid,
(b) immunoglobulins in thyroid stroma,
(c) immune complexes in the circulation,
(d) thymic enlargement,
(e) thyroid-stimulating immunoglobulins, and
(f) evidence of cell-mediated immunity.

Other autoantibodies may also be present in these patients, e.g. against ovary, adrenal, and islet B cells (see Appendix 44b.1).

Allergy. These patients are evaluated for allergic disease in the same manner as the non-thyroiditic patients. Skin prick tests and intradermal testing are followed by an investigative elimination diet coupled with environmental control.

MANAGEMENT

Endocrinological

Thyroid hormone is the hallmark of therapy in these patients. L-Thyroxine is given in a small dose to start with, i.e. 0.025 mg daily gradually increasing to approximately 0.15–0.20 mg daily over a 4–6-week period. The patient is alerted to three possible difficulties in starting treatment with L-thyroxine. (1) Increased fatigue: the patient is instructed to increase by 0.025 mg weekly until the fatigue subsides. (2) Painful thyroid: often with the initiation of treatment the autoimmune thyroid gland will become tender and painful. The patient is advised to continue taking L-thyroxine as prescribed. The pain can be treated symptomatically with any non-steroidal anti-inflammatory compound. (3) Palpitations, nervousness, and irritability: the patient is advised to discontinue the L-thyroxine for approximately 3 days to alleviate the symptoms, then restart the L-thyroxine at the same dose. If the symptoms recur the patient is again advised to stop taking the L-thyroxine for 3 days and then return to the non-symptom-producing dose until seen at the follow-up visit.

Thyroid gland suppression

The ultimate plan is to suppress the diseased thyroid gland, establish thyroid indices in the high-normal range, suppress the often measured elevated TSH level, and monitor thyroid antibodies. A concomitant goitre often regresses in size, fatigue resolves, lability of mood and depression improve and allergic symptoms diminish. Such therapy may have long-term beneficial effects on suppressing thyroid antibodies and immune-related processes. *A rationale therefore exists for early treatment of thyroiditis prior to the development of functional deficiency of the thyroid.* We treat the patients *before* the laboratory indices document hypothyroidism, as recommended by Cooper et al [6].

Rarely L-thyroxine treatment has precipitated thyroxicosis; this can be managed with propylthiouracil in much the same way as Graves' disease is treated. The pharmacological effects of propylthiouracil are: (1) it blocks the organification of iodine and interferes with iodotyrosine coupling; (2) it interferes with peripheral conversion of thyroxine to triiodothyronine; (3) it reduces lymphocytes within the thyroid gland; (4) it is weakly immunosuppressive.

In a small group of patients in whom symptomatic thyroiditis and elevated antibodies persist, total thyroidectomy may have a place in management. In keeping with our concept described above, it is our impression that complete removal of the immunogenic thyroid tissue may account for the marked improvement observed in some patients after a total thyroidectomy (Becker and Galante, unpublished observations).

Allergological

When a maintenance dose of thyroxine has been reached (see Appendix 44b.3 for excipients in common American preparations) the patient begins immunization therapy for dusts, pollens, moulds, and danders, in addition to elimination of troublesome foods and chemicals. Polyendocrinopathy is not uncommon in this particular allergic patient population. The second most common presumed endocrinopathy (ovarian autoimmune disease) presents itself as premenstrual syndrome with the usual symptoms, from ovulation to menstruation, of mood lability, fluid retention, hunger, increased allergic reactivity, mastalgia, diarrhoea, irritability, inability to cope, and poor concentration. A proportion of these women have autoantibodies to the ovary and abnormal oestrogen/progesterone ratios.

Premenstrual syndrome

Premenstrual syndrome frequently becomes apparent in the thyroiditic patient after treatment of the thyroid disease for two reasons: (1) after thyroid treatment the patient is no longer ill all the time and so the cyclical element emerges; and (2) premenstrual syndrome worsens later in life than thyroid disease does—after age 35.

Treatment of this disorder involves a number of modalities but the most relevant in the allergic patient with thyroid disease, premenstrual syndrome and ovarian antibodies is the restoration of oestrogen/progesterone balance with supplementary progesterone. In 1947 an exhaustive, pioneering, landmark study [18] revealed the existence of allergy to oestrogen and progesterone. We have found that 20% of patients who presented with allergies and premenstrual symptoms responded to allergy testing and immunization therapy with hormones, most especially progesterone (Saifer, unpublished observations). The most commonly relieved symptom was headache.

Nystatin

After treatment of the thyroid component, the allergic components and the ovarian components, the use of nystatin in the polyendocrinopathy patient should be considered. The literature [1,5,7,10,11,14,15] is replete with polyendocrinopathy-candidiasis patient histories (see Chapter 49). Based on the literature and clinical experience, we treat the allergic polyendocrinopathy patient with nystatin for 3 weeks as a clinical trial. Kudelko [12] described a number of allergic cases with chronic monilial vaginitis where the vaginitis resolved when the allergies were controlled. Because of the histories of antibiotic use, oral contraceptives, steroids, and recurrent yeast vaginitis, and the association in the literature, the clinical trial seems justified. Because of the results in these immunologically disordered patients, we have tried it in the endocrine–allergy patients who do not give a history of antibiotics, etc., and we have been surprised and pleased with the results. We begin with 500 000 units q.i.d. and then increase as needed for 6 months or more. Stopping treatment at 3 months allows for relapses. Control of carbohydrate intake is essential (see also Chapter 49).

Case history. This patient had onset of menarche at age 10 at which time she underwent a major personality change from an outgoing, curious child to a depressed, sedentary, suicidal teenager. School work suffered because of apathy. At age 14 the goitre was noted along with a very slight elevation in antithyroglobulin antibodies (Fig. 44b.2a). She did not tolerate the synthetic T₄ preparations but did respond well to the natural thyroid extract and the dose was gradually increased over the next 3 years to a maintenance dose of 4 grains (Fig. 44b.2b).

Since age 4 she had a recognized milk hypersensitivity which produced urinary incontinence, allergic shiners, nasal congestion and insomnia. As thyroid therapy progressed she developed a greater interest in adhering to her

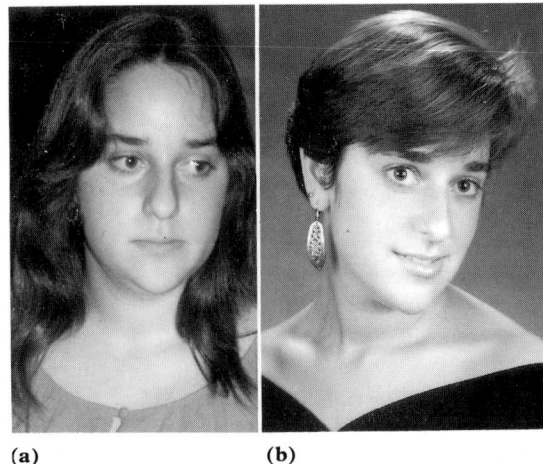

(a)   **(b)**

Fig. 44b.2 Before (a) and after (b) thyroid and allergy treatment. (a) 1982: typical thyroiditic facies. Note oedema, depressed apathetic expression, mild exophthalmos, and small goitre. (b) 1985: after 3 years of therapy with thyroid extract and elimination of milk and food colouring from diet.

milk-free diet and thus showed even greater improvement in well-being.

It has recently become apparent that she has 5–7 days of premenstrual depression and fatigue. Ovarian antibody studies are negative

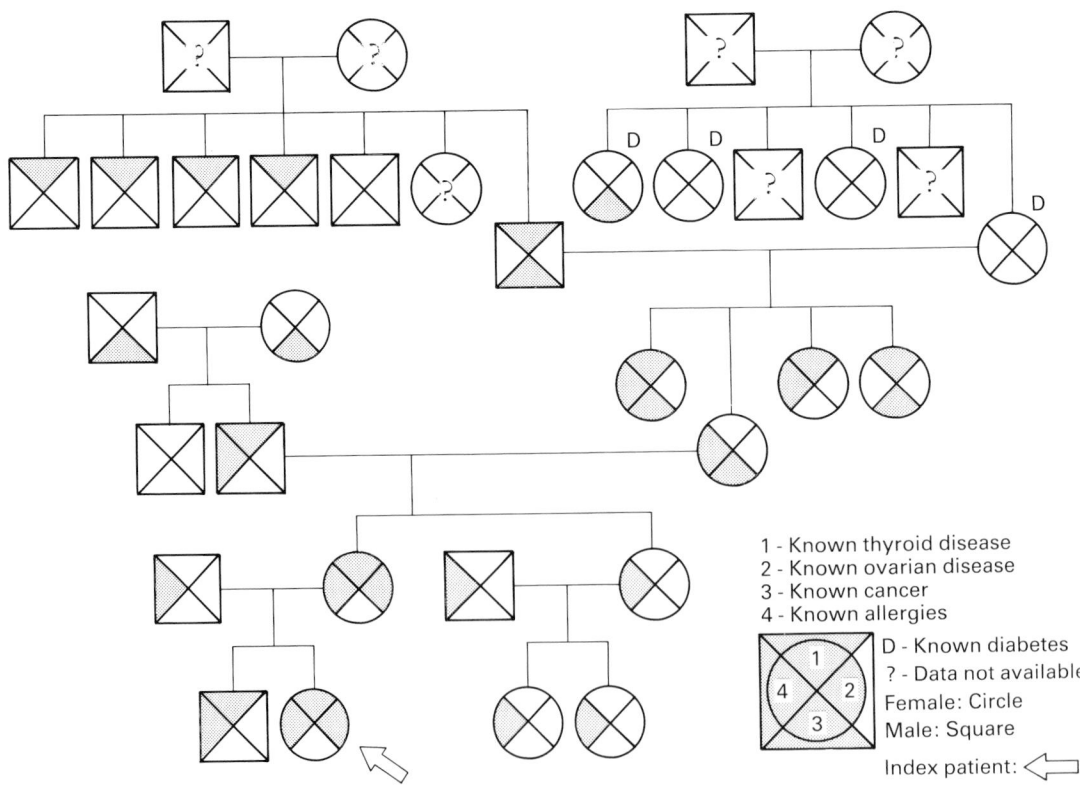

1 - Known thyroid disease
2 - Known ovarian disease
3 - Known cancer
4 - Known allergies

D - Known diabetes
? - Data not available
Female: Circle
Male: Square

Index patient: ⟵

Fig. 44b.3   Family tree of patient A.S.

at this time, but will be repeated in the future.

She reported that a 1-month trial of nystatin eliminated a chronic vaginal discharge. *Candida*-specific IgG, A, M antibodies are markedly elevated. Her family tree is presented to show the multiplicity of clinical syndromes in a single family, this emphasizing the importance of recording a meticulous family history (Fig. 44b.3).

SUMMARY

There exists a patient population presenting with signs and symptoms of allergy and endocrinopathy. Successful management of these patients requires attention to both environmental and autoallergens.

The availability of modern immune diagnostic procedures which permit the detection of antibodies to endocrine-related antigens provides a rational basis for therapy in the face of apparently normal gland function (as in the case of the euthyroid thyroiditic).

Management of environmental allergens is much more likely to be beneficial if concomitant autoallergy is effectively treated. The full spectrum of antigens to be considered must include *Candida* and other 'normal' flora. The patient response to this comprehensive approach is often remarkable.

Appendix 44b.1   Antigens of organ specific autoimmune diseases and systemic autoimmune diseases.

Antigen	Organ	Diseases
1. Microsomes Thyroglobulin TSH	Thyroid	Hashimoto's thyroiditis Graves' disease
Eye muscle	Eye muscle	Endocrine exophthalmos
2. Islet cells Insulin	Pancreas	Juvenile onset diabetes
3. Adrenal cortex	Adrenals	Addison's disease (Cushing's disease)
4. Parietal cells Gastrin Intestinal secretin Intrinsic factor	Gut	Pernicious anaemia, sprue, coeliac disease
5. Pituitary cell Prolactin Growth hormone	Pituitary	Pituitary deficiency
6. Ovaries Oocyte and stroma	Ovary	Oophoritis, premenstrual syndrome, premature menopause, ovarian failure
7. Parathyroid chief cell	Parathyroid	Idiopathic hypoparathyroidism
8. Melanocytes	Skin	Vitiligo
9. Acetylcholine receptors	Neuromuscular	Myasthenia gravis
10. Nuclei (antinuclear antibody 'diffuse') Smooth muscle Liver and kidney microsomes Mitochondria	Liver	Chronic active liver disease, 'lupoid variant', primary biliary cirrhosis, etc.
11. Hormone receptors	Hair	Alopecia
12. Squamous intercellular space	Skin	Pemphigus
13. Platelet membrane	Bone marrow	Idiopathic thrombocytopenia purpura
14. Choroid plexus	Brain	Schizophrenia, autism

Systemic autoimmune diseases
(1) Goodpasture's syndrome
(2) Rheumatoid arthritis
(3) Sjögren's syndrome
(4) Systemic lupus erythematosus

Appendix 44b.2   Symptom record and progress.

Suggested abbreviations:

Symptoms:	B = better	S = same
	W = worse	0 = cleared
Treatment (Rx):	E = endocrine treatment	
	I = immunization	
	BED = basic elimination diet	
	BOED = basic organic elimination diet	
	RD = rotary diet	
	EC = environmental control	

Name:_____

Date: _____

Check symptoms in left-hand column

		FOR DOCTOR'S USE ONLY					
√ = Current	Cause	Date & Rx	Date & Rx	Date & Rx	Date & Rx	Date & Rx	Date & Rx
NERVES & FEELINGS-(CNS) Headache—mild, moderate, severe							
Migraine							
Fainting							
Depression							
Mood swings							
Hyperactivity							
Irritability							
Hallucinations							
Forgetfulness							
Spacey feeling							
Fatigue							
Apathy							
Confusion							
Seizures							
Insomnia/nightmares							
Sleepiness							
Feelings of rage							
Poor concentration							
Learning disorders							
Numbness and tingling							
Anxiety (panic)							
Dizziness							
Other							
SKIN Itching							
Rash (hives/eczema/other)							
Flushing							
Sores, infections							
Pallor—white							
Acne							
Dryness/oiliness							
Dandruff							
Athlete's foot, fungus							
Other							

Check symptoms in left-hand column

√ = Current	Cause	Date & Rx	Date & Rx	Date & Rx	Date & Rx	Date & Rx	Date & Rx
FOR DOCTOR'S USE ONLY							
EYES Itch							
Burn							
Pain							
Tearing							
Red eyes							
Sensitive to light							
Circles under eyes							
Puffy eyes							
Other							
VISION Blurring							
Spots or floaters							
Other							
EARS Itching							
Full, blocked, pressure							
Reddening of ears							
Ringing in ears							
Earache							
Very sensitive to sound							
Other							
NASAL Sneezing fits							
Itchy nose							
Stuffy nose							
Runny nose							
Postnasal drip							
Sinus discomfort/face pain							
Nosebleeds							
Other							
THROAT-MOUTH-GUMS Itching							
Sore							
Tight							
Swollen							
Difficulty in swallowing							
Choking							
Hoarse voice							
Increased salivation							
Mucus							

Check symptoms in left-hand column

			FOR DOCTOR'S USE ONLY					
√ = Current	Cause	Date & Rx	Date & Rx	Date & Rx	Date & Rx	Date & Rx	Date & Rx
Bad metallic taste/bad breath							
Mouth ulcers							
Tongue coated							
Dry lips							
Sensitive teeth							
Other							
LYMPH SYSTEM Swollen, tender glands							
BLOOD VESSELS Sweating							
Chilly feeling							
Generalized swelling							
Puffy face							
Cold hands and feet							
Spontaneous bruising							
Low/high blood pressure							
Low body temperature							
Other							
HEART & LUNGS Coughing							
Wheezing							
Chest feels tight							
Not enough air							
Rapid breathing							
Chest pain							
Rapid or irregular pulse							
Pounding pulse							
Short of breath							
Other							
GASTROINTESTINAL Nausea							
Stomach-ache							
Belching							
Full or bloated							
Vomiting							
Pain							
Cramps							
Rumbling							
Diarrhoea							
Constipation							
Hunger/thirst							
Soiling							
Burning sensation							

Check symptoms in left-hand column

√ = Current	Cause	Date & Rx	Date & Rx	Date & Rx	Date & Rx	Date & Rx	Date & Rx
Rectal itch							
Gas							
Other							
WEIGHT PROBLEM Can't gain							
Can't lose							
Easy gain							
Easy lose							
Fluid retention							
Food cravings sugar/salt							
Arise at night to eat							
Food aversions							
Other							
GENITOURINARY Frequent urination							
Painful urination							
Urgency to urinate							
Bed wetting							
Breast swelling							
Vaginal discharge							
Yeast infections							
Menstrual irregularities							
Impotence							
Loss of libido							
Other							
MUSCLES Aching or pain Neck							
Weakness Upper back							
Shakiness Lower back							
Legs							
Other							
JOINTS Ache or pain							
Swelling							
Red and warm							
Other							

What type of work have you done?   Members of your household?

Any chemical exposures?

Home environment:

House _____   Apartment _____   Other _____
Type of heat: Gas forced air _____   Steam _____   Electric _____   Other _____

Type of range: Gas _____   Electric _____
Floors: Synthetic wall-to-wall carpets _____   Area rugs: Wool _____   Synthetic _____ Other _____

Pillows: Feather _____   Synthetic _____
Blankets: Natural fibres _____   Synthetic _____
Clothing: Natural fibres _____   Synthetic _____
Location of home: Heavy traffic _____   Light traffic _____   Agriculture _____
Animals present in home: Dogs _____   Cats _____   Other _____ None _____
Smokers present in home: Yes _____   No _____

Highest grade completed in school _____

Approximate date of last complete physical examination _____
Right-handed? _____   _____   Left-handed? _____   _____
         Yes   No   Yes   No

Appendix 44b.3   Thyroid sources.

Sodium levothyroxine (thyroxine sodium) preparations

Flint	Synthroid 0.05 mg	Levothyroxine sodium, lactose, powdered sugar, cornstarch, acacia, povidone, magnesium stearate, talc, gelatin
Armour Pharmaceutical	Levothroid 0.05 mg	Sodium levothyroxine, lactose *USP*, magnesium stearate, silica, colloidal avicel

Natural thyroid preparations

Armour Pharmaceutical	Thyroid 1 grain	Thyroid powder *USP*, calcium stearate, Cerelose, anhydrous (*not* cellulose, but a corn-derived product tradename)
Lanpar	Parloid 1 grain	Thyroid *USP* (porcine), lactose, magnesium stearate, stearic acid, and a *sugar* coating
Lanpar	Naturoid 1 grain	Thyroid *USP* (porcine), magnesium stearate, stearic acid, methylcellulose (ingredients give natural buff colour)
Western Research Labs	Westhroid 1/2 grain, 1, 2, 3, 4 & 5 grain	Avicel, thyroid *USP* (uncoated no colouring, lactose, corn starch). New Westhroid preparations do have corn and lactose.

Triiodothyronine preparations

Smith, Kline & French Laboratories	Cytomel 5 μm, 25, 50	Triiodothyronine-synthetic, sugar, cornstarch, calcium sulphate, no dyes, no inks, gelatin, stearic acid, sucrose, talc

---

REFERENCES

1 Appelboom T, Flowers F: Ketoconazole in the treatment of chronic mucocutaneous candidiasis secondary to autoimmune polyendocrinopathy–candidiasis syndrome. Cutis 1982; 30:71–2.

2 Arulanantham K, Dwyer JM, Genel M: Evidence for defective immunoregulation in the syndrome of familial candidiasis endocrinopathy. N Engl J Med 1978; 300(4):164–8.

3 Bahn AK et al: Hypothyroidism in workers exposed to polybrominated biphenyls. N Engl J Med 1980; 302:31.

4 Brostoff J: personal communication.

5 Dempsey A, DeSwiet M, Dewhurst J: Premature ovarian failure associated with candida endocrinopathy syndrome. Br J Obstet Gynaecol 1981; 88:563–5.

6 Cooper D, Halpern R et al: L-Thyroxine therapy in subclinical hypothyroidism. Ann Intern Med 1984; 101:18–24.

7 Dolen J, Varma S, South MA: Chronic mucocutaneous candidiasis endocrinopathies. Cutis 1981; 27:592.

8 Doniach D, Bottazzo G, Drexhage H: The auto-

immune endocrinopathies. In Lachman P, ed. Clinical immunology. London: Blackwell Scientific, 1982.

9 Fisher D, Beall GN: Hashimoto's thyroiditis. Pharmacol Ther 1976; C1:445-58.

10 Kaffe S, Petigrew CS et al: Variable cell-mediated immune defects in a family with *Candida* endocrinopathy syndrome. Clin Exp Immunol 1975; 20:397-408.

11 Kenny FJ, Holliday M: Hypoparathyroidism, moniliasis, Addison's and Hashimoto's diseases. N Engl J Med 1964; 27(4):708-13.

12 Kudelko NM: Allergy in chronic monilial vaginitis. Ann. Allergy 1971; 29:266-7.

13 Marks AD, Bertram J et al: Chronic thyroiditis and mitral valve prolapse. Ann Intern Med 1985; 102:479.

14 Morse WI, Cochrane WA, Landrigan PL: Familial hypothyroidism with pernicious anemia, steatorrhea and adrenocortical insufficiency. N Engl J Med 1961; 264(20):1021-6.

15 Odds F, Evans E et al: Prevalence of pathogenic yeasts and humoral antibodies to candida in diabetic patients. J Clin Pathol 1978; 31:840-4.

16 Thielemans C, Vanhaelst L et al: Autoimmune thyroiditis: a condition related to a decrease in T-suppressor cells. Endocrinology 1981; 15:259-63.

17 Volpé R: Autoimmunity in the endocrine system. Monographs in endocrinology, Vol 20. New York: Springer-Verlag, 1981.

18 Zondek B, Bromberg Y: Endocrine allergy: clinical reactions of allergy to endogenous hormones and their treatment. J Obstet Gynaecol Br Empire 1947; 54(1):1-19.

RECOMMENDED READING

Clinical Immunology I. Med Clin North Am 1985; 69(3).

Hyperthyroidism. Clin Endocrinol Metab 1985; 14(2).

Thyroid disease. Med Clin North Am 1985; 69(5).

Volpé R: Autoimmunity and endocrine disease. New York: Marcel Dekker, 1985.

PART IV

DIAGNOSIS OF FOOD ALLERGY AND INTOLERANCE

SECTION A
CLINICAL DIAGNOSIS

Chapter 45
Food Hypersensitivities: Historical Perspectives, Diagnosis and Clinical Presentations

Armond S. Goldman, Anand G. Kantak, Antony J. Ham Pong and Randall M. Goldblum

Introduction

Untoward reactions to foods were recognized in ancient times by Hippocrates (460–370 BC) [21] and some 600 years later by Galen (131–210 AD) [15]. Systematic inquiries regarding food-induced diseases were not initiated however until the 20th century when fulminating reactions attributed to foods were observed [23, 35, 43]. Because of certain similarities between those acute, alarming symptoms and systemic anaphylaxis induced in animal models [34, 37, 45], it was assumed that the clinical disorders were immunological in nature. Indeed, the putative antibodies for immediate-type hypersensitivity reactions in humans were discovered in the 1920s by in-jecting serum from a fish-sensitive subject intradermally into a non-allergic individual, reinjecting the test site with an extract of fish tissue and noting the subsequent local wheal and erythema [39]—the classical Prausnitz-Küstner reaction.

During the next three decades increasing numbers of cases of allergic reactions to foods were described and the spectrum of the clinical abnormalities in these cases was broadened to include reactions that were often slower in onset and solely involved the gastrointestinal tract, skin or respiratory system [5, 10]. In these reports, however, a cause–effect relationship between the exposure to the food and the production of the clinical abnormalities was often not established. In that regard, the diagnoses were usually based solely on the case history and improvement following elimination of the suspected allergen from the diet. The reactions were not verified by subsequent oral challenge with the food and appropriate immunological methods to investigate the problem were not available.

DESIGN OF CLINICAL INVESTIGATIONS

Because of the paucity of objective information, many leaders in academic medicine felt that very little if any credence could be given to the concept of food allergy, and they cautioned that non-allergic mechanisms would be responsible for most food-related disorders. In concert with those concerns, one of us considered at that time that certain postulates would be useful in designing investigations of food hypersensitivities (Table 45.1).

Table 45.1   Criteria for the diagnosis of food allergy.

1   The symptoms should disappear after the suspected allergen has been eliminated

2   The allergen should be isolated in a pure form for experimental use

3   The administration of the allergen by the natural route should produce reactions in experimental subjects that are similar to the original symptoms

4   The allergen should be identified in its natural or modified form to react with cells or immunological factors from the patient

5   The immunological responses generated by the allergen should be shown to be responsible for the pathogenesis of the untoward reaction

Several leaders in the academic community recommended that controlled test feedings with the suspected allergens to reproduce the symptoms would be the 'gold standard' for deciding whether the patient was allergic to a food. The lack of purified food allergens for oral challenges, however, precluded investigations until the 1960s when sufficient quantities of isolated cow's milk proteins were made available for such a study [16]. In that study a large group of children (mainly infants) who were suspected of being sensitive to cow's milk were first taken off milk to determine if their symptoms disappeared. If that occurred, then the child was challenged orally, first with a standard preparation of cow's milk, and then, if reactive, with casein, β-lactoglobulin, α-lactalbumin or bovine serum albumin. The

results demonstrated a number of important points that served as guidelines for future studies (Table 45.2).

The immunological basis of these reactions was investigated by direct skin testing [17] and serological measurements [42] with the antigens that were employed in the oral challenge experiments, but few clues to an immunological basis for the reactions were found.

Some years later a double-blind design was employed in oral challenge tests for the investigation of food hypersensitivity, to minimize the bias of the observers [32]. Although purified food proteins were not employed and the initial investigations were limited to a highly selected group of older children with severe asthma, it was demonstrated that certain individuals with food hypersensitivities could be detected by provoking the reactions by oral challenge. The coupling of dietary elimination with oral challenge has remained the cornerstone of experimental studies and practical clinical diagnosis of food hypersensitivities.

Table 45.2   Important findings from trial of food elimination and challenge.

1   Past symptoms suggestive of food allergy were provoked by the oral administration of specific protein antigens

2   The onset, duration and type of reactions were highly reproducible in individual patients

3   The reactions varied in their onset, duration, intensity and system involvement amongst the subjects in the study

4   Multiple symptoms involving one or more organ systems were common

5   There seemed to be an inverse relationship between the dose of the allergen that was necessary to provoke a reaction and the rapidity with which the reaction developed.

6   Reactions to cow's milk proteins occurred principally in non-breast-fed infants and usually did not persist in school-age children

DIAGNOSIS OF FOOD ALLERGY

Since non-immunological causes of adverse food reactions are common and may mimic food hypersensitivities [4] (Chapter 23), it is important to consider those disorders in a given case. These include: (a) food contaminants such as pathogenic microorganisms or their toxins [12], (b) food additives such as tartrazines, (c) enzymatic defects (e.g. galactosaemia [26]) which block the metabolism of a nutrient and (d) acquired insults to the intestinal tract that interfere with the digestion or absorption of food (e.g. disaccharidase deficiency [24]). In addition, common infections and other pathological processes that produce respiratory, gastrointestinal or skin abnormalities must be considered in the differential diagnosis [4].

The principal foods responsible for allergic reactions may be age-dependent and may be contingent upon ethnic-cultural practices. Food allergens in infants are usually limited to the major types of foreign proteins in the diet. These include cow's milk, cereals, eggs, fish and soya. In older children and adults, chocolate, peanuts, nuts and berries are common allergens (see Chapter 17 for further information).

Elimination of food

If the history suggests that a food is the responsible allergen, it is eliminated from the diet and the patient is observed to determine if the symptoms disappear. The test period of elimination depends upon the type of food-induced disorder. In more common types of sensitivities, the symptoms disappear within several days after the food responsible is removed from the diet, whereas in more complex types of food hypersensitivities such as cow's milk-induced pulmonary haemosiderosis the pathology resolves more slowly.

The degree of difficulty in eliminating a suspected food allergen depends upon the age of the patient, the compliance of the patient and the type of food. In general, the diet of young infants is easily controlled. If cow's milk is the suspected allergen, the diet can be restricted to a soya milk, a meat-base milk or a casein hydrolysate formulation. A casein hydrolysate preparation may be preferable because of its low antigenicity [13]. If other foods are suspected offenders, then the infant's diet can be restricted to cow's milk for the test period. The elimination of basic foods such as cow's milk is much more difficult in older children because their occurrence is widespread in food products. Elimination of such foods even for a test period therefore requires careful planning and often the aid of a dietician (see Chapters 4 and 5).

Oral challenge

Although oral challenge with the suspected food allergen is necessary for the diagnosis, there are certain pitfalls and shortcomings in the procedure (Table 45.3). Cases that present with urticaria should be particularly monitored for anaphylaxis during the challenge [16].

In order to avoid these difficulties, oral challenges should be conducted by a physician in a medical facility, and the diagnostic criteria limited to objective findings such as vomiting, diarrhoea, blood or eosinophils in stool mucus [38], inflammatory changes in intestinal tissue [44] or abnormalities in pulmonary function. The steps that should be taken are as follows. (a) The decision is made whether it is safe to conduct the challenge and what safeguards should be employed to minimize a serious reaction. This can be predicted to a degree by the history of the severity and duration of the clinical symptoms and the time of onset of the

Table 45.3 Disadvantages and pitfalls of oral challenge.

1 In the face of a history of severe reactions such as anaphylaxis, oral challenge is usually precluded

2 The oral dose of the allergen may not be large enough to provoke a reaction, although the patient is sensitive to the agent

3 The reaction may be missed because of a delayed onset

4 Positive challenges may be due to an intercurrent disease such as an infection

5 If the challenge is conducted with a food mixture, the offending agent may not be identified

6 Bias by the observer or the subject (if old enough) may be confounding

7 Even when patients with a history of anaphylaxis are excluded, anaphylaxis may nevertheless occur during oral challenges [13, 16, 18]

reaction following ingestion of the suspected allergen. (b) An interim history is obtained to document that the patient has become asymptomatic during the dietary elimination of the suspected allergen and has not been exposed to contagion or medication which would mimic or suppress a reaction. (c) This is then confirmed by a thorough physical examination. (d) If the history suggests that the reaction might be serious, an intravenous line should be established to administer fluids, electrolytes and antiallergic medications and the oral dose of the allergen should be reduced considerably. Aqueous epinephrine (adrenaline), parenteral corticosteroids, antihistamines and equipment for respiratory resuscitation should be immediately available. It is essential that the personnel who are conducting the challenge have the expertise to detect and properly treat serious allergic reactions.

Method of challenge

The oral challenge is then given using a single food (preferably a purified component) in a dose which is judged to incite a reaction. Double-blind challenges with or without the suspected allergen hidden in an elemental diet or in capsules [33] are undoubtedly preferable for research purposes, but the procedure is impractical for standard clinical use. The start of the challenge is timed. The patient is monitored intensively during the first hour following the challenge to detect and treat early signs of anaphylaxis. The time of appearance and the intensity of abnormal findings should be carefully recorded to document the outcome of the challenge. An example of such a documentation is included in Table 45.4 (see also Chapter 46).

disorders. As will be discussed in other parts of this book (see Chapter 50), some food reactions in humans appear to be mediated by IgE antibodies, but that type of hypersensitivity does not appear to be responsible for many cases. Aas has demonstrated a close correlation between the presence of IgE antibodies to cod and allergic reactions following feedings with that antigen [1] (see Chapter 19). Currently employed in vivo and in vitro techniques for detection of IgE antibodies to food allergens, however, do not appear to be generally useful in predicting clinical reactions to the foods. Skin testing and radioallergosorbent techniques have limited reliability because of the paucity of purified food allergens (Chapter 50) and poor correlation between the results of those tests and the results of oral challenge [6, 17, 42]. In fact, both types

Table 45.4 Example of one oral challenge.

Patient's name: B.P.
Patient ID number: 24001–X
Sex: Male
Age: 4 months

Date of birth: 6/2/84
Date of challenge: 10/8/84
Observer: G.P.

Suspected food allergen:	Cow's milk
Symptoms before allergen elimination:	Vomiting, diarrhoea and weight loss
Period of dietary elimination:	Two weeks
Effects of dietary elimination:	Disappearance of symptoms. Weight gain of 400 g in 2 weeks.
Prechallenge physical examination:	No abnormalities
Type and time of challenge:	100 ml of skimmed cow's milk given by mouth at 10.00 a.m.

Time	General	Pulse rate	Respiration rate	BP	Skin	Respiratory system	Gastrointestinal system	Other	Treatment
9.30 a.m.	Active	100	24	84/62	N	N	N	—	—
10.00 a.m.	Challenge	104	26	82/62	N	N	N	—	—
10.05 a.m.	N	102	24	82/60	N	N	N	—	—
10.10 a.m.	Crying	116	30	86/64	N	N	Vomiting	—	—
10.15 a.m.	Crying	112	30	88/62	N	N	Vomiting	—	—
10.30 a.m.	N	104	26	80/64	N	N	N	—	—
11.00 a.m.	N	104	26	80/64	N	N	N	—	—
1.40 p.m.	Crying	112	30	88/64	N	N	Diarrhoea	—	—
2.00 p.m.	Fussing	108	28	86/62	N	N	Diarrhoea	—	—
3.00 p.m.	N	108	26	80/60	N	N	Diarrhoea	—	—
4.00 p.m.		120	28	84/60	N	N	N	—	—

Specific remarks: Stool mucus obtained at 3.00 p.m. containing many eosinophils

B.P = arterial blood pressure, N = normal.

Laboratory tests

Because of the cumbersome nature of the oral challenge method and the potential for self-deception with that method, many efforts have been made to discern the immunological basis of food sensitivities and thereby develop appropriate laboratory methods to diagnose these

of tests tend to greatly overestimate the population of patients who will react clinically to specific foods. Although strongly positive skin tests to certain foods may be useful in diagnosis [17], such reactions are uncommon. Therefore, the predictive value of tests for IgE antibodies to foods appears to be too limited for standard clinical use.

The measurement of serum or secretory antibodies of other immunoglobulin classes produced in response to food antigens, the detection of blood lymphocytes sensitized to these allergens [29], investigations of oral tolerance [25] (see Chapter 14), complement activation [31] and other abnormalities of the immunological functions of the gastrointestinal tract (Chapters 1 and 2), are promising but as yet are not clinically applicable. It should also be stressed that the clinical usefulness of such laboratory diagnostic methods will require validation by careful oral challenge experiments in selected patients with the food allergens in question [2].

DISORDERS ASSOCIATED WITH FOOD ALLERGENS

Based upon the use of dietary elimination–oral challenge studies and the exclusion of other disorders, certain clinical manifestations have been suspected to be due to immunological reactions to food proteins.

Gastrointestinal reactions

Gastrointestinal disorders are the most common reactions to food allergy (see Chapters 29–33). The manifestations include perioral erythema, fissuring of the mouth, palatal itching, abdominal pain, colic, diarrhoea, gastrointestinal blood loss, protein-losing enteropathy, carbohydrate and/or fat malabsorption and ulcerative colitis. The most common problems are as follows.

Vomiting

Vomiting is one of the most common symptoms in food allergy and usually occurs within 10–30 minutes after ingestion of the allergen. The vomit usually consists of gastric secretions and ingested food. The emesis ranges from mild spitting to projectile vomiting.

Abdominal pain–colic

In children who are old enough to describe their symptoms, abdominal pain due to food allergy varies from dull to severe. The pain is usually located in the upper abdomen or the periumbilical region. Even in those cases where the pain is severe, abdominal tenderness is usually absent.

A great deal of controversy persists regarding the role of food allergy in the production of colic in human infants. Although there are convincing reports of colic induced by ingested foods, it is unclear whether food allergens commonly cause colic for the following reasons. In some studies objective criteria for the diagnosis of colic by history or oral challenge were not stated. In fact, the degree of irritability or crying that constitutes pathological colic is difficult to define [9]. In addition, it was not clarified in some investigations whether the subjects in studies were selected at random from cases of colic in the community or whether the cases were chosen because of a strong suspicion of food allergy. Furthermore, certain studies suggest that crying is a natural behaviour in most infants during the first 2–3 months of life [9].

Diarrhoea

Diarrhoea is probably the most common clinical manifestation of food allergy. The degree of diarrhoea ranges from loose to explosive watery stools. In cow's milk and soya protein-induced enterocolitis [18, 38], stool mucus obtained after oral challenge often contains eosinophils and proctoscopy reveals an erythematous, friable, ulcerated mucosa.

Gastrointestinal bleeding

Gastrointestinal blood loss often occurs in infants who are allergic to cow's milk [18, 49]. The blood loss may occur in the presence or absence of diarrhoea and the bleeding may be gross or more often occult. Those infants who experience blood loss in the absence of diarrhoea are usually iron deficient and the degree of loss in those infants appears to be directly proportional to the amount of ingested cow's milk [50]. The bleeding ceases within a few days after the elimination of cow's milk, and the disorder disappears in most infants by age two years.

Allergic gastroenteropathy

A few cases of protein-losing enteropathy due to cow's milk have been reported [47]. Affected infants present with oedema due to hypoproteinaemia. Fat malabsorption, gastrointestinal blood loss, iron-deficiency anaemia or eosinophilia are found in some cases.

Fat malabsorption

Directly following the Second World War, Dicke and his colleagues in The Netherlands recognized a large number of infants and preschool-age children who displayed steatorrhoea and growth failure due to wheat and related cereals [11]. The responsible component in the cereal proved to be gluten (see Chapter 30). Although the number of reported cases decreased as the amount of gluten in the diet of infants declined, gluten intolerance continues to be one of the principal causes of fat malabsorption [11]. In this condition the villi of small intestines are flattened and an increased number of inflammatory cells are often found in the lamina propria [36]. The steatorrhoea and intestinal pathology usually resolve a few weeks after eliminating gluten from the diet. A very similar, if not identical, syndrome may be provoked by cow's milk [28].

Ulcerative colitis

A few decades ago there was considerable enthusiasm for the role of food allergens in the pathogenesis of ulcerative colitis [46]. Comparatively few cases, however, appear to be due to ingested foods. The role of foods in the production of the irritable bowel syndrome is discussed in Chapter 3.

Respiratory diseases

A wide variety of respiratory symptoms including rhinitis, cough and asthma [8, 16] have been documented to be triggered by food allergens (see Chapters 26–28). It is not clear how frequently food allergens are responsible for many of these cases. For example, the majority of asthma attacks in young infants are associated with viral respiratory infections, especially respiratory syncytial virus and rhinovirus [48]. Nevertheless, food allergens should be considered in the pathogenesis of allergic respiratory disease, particularly in infants who present with dermal and/or gastrointestinal symptoms in addition.

There is considerable controversy regarding the possible association of otitis media with food allergy. Some reports suggest that such an association is likely [6], but other studies have not confirmed that impression [14] and investigations of unselected cases of acute otitis media indicate that infections are the most common cause [22] (see Chapter 26).

Cow's milk-induced pulmonary haemosiderosis

In the early 1960s Douglas Heiner and his colleagues discovered a novel type of cow's milk hypersensitivity in young infants [19, 20]. The disorder is characterized by pulmonary haemosiderosis, gastrointestinal blood loss, iron-deficiency anaemia, failure to thrive, eosinophila and high serum titres of precipitating antibodies to cow's milk proteins. The manifestations of the sensitivity disappeared within several weeks after elimination of cow's milk from the diet and the abnormalities reappeared when cow's milk was reintroduced into the diet. Although this syndrome is less common than the gastrointestinal reactions to cow's milk, it is perhaps the best documented type of cow's milk sensitization because of the close relationship between the exposure to cow's milk, the elevation of serum antibodies to the allergens and the clinical abnormalities.

Skin diseases

Two types of dermal reactions, urticaria and atopic dermatitis, have been found to be provoked by food allergens, but the number of cases that can be attributed to food allergens is controversial. In surveys of chronic recurrent urticaria [30], a cause is found in only 10–15% of cases. In the absence of other symptoms, a search for food allergens may be fruitless unless there is a temporal relationship between the food ingestion and the onset of urticaria or if the reactions occur in young infants (see Chapters 34–36).

The role of food allergens in the pathogenesis of atopic dermatitis is puzzling. Some investigators have presented reasonable evidence that certain cases of this chronic dermatitis are provoked by food allergens, but it is unclear whether those patients are representative of most cases of atopic dermatitis, or whether they were selected for study because of a strong suspicion of food allergy. For example, in one study the median age of affected cases supposedly due to food allergy was 11 years [41], whereas atopic dermatitis usually begins in the first year of life and remits by age five years [40]. It is therefore difficult to decide whether food allergens are aetiological agents in a subpopulation of patients with atopic dermatitis or whether the dermatological manifestations of those cases are only similar to atopic dermatitis (see Chapter 34).

Systemic anaphylaxis

The manifestations of anaphylaxis due to food allergens are identical to those reported in anaphylaxis due to other agents. Those include urticaria, angioedema, laryngeal oedema, bronchospasm, diarrhoea, convulsions and shock. Anaphylactic reactions are not as common as other disorders induced by food allergens. In most cases the diagnosis is evident because of the rapid onset of the reaction following food ingestion (see Chapter 25). It is difficult, however, to identify the responsible allergen in some patients because of the complexity of the mixture of food ingested or because of food additives (see Chapter 22b).

Recently, a few adults have presented with anaphylaxis which appears to have been caused by an interaction between physical exercise and the ingestion of a particular food allergen [27]. The nature of this interaction in the pathogenesis of the reaction is unknown.

Central nervous system abnormalities

Seizures, anxiety, lethargy, headaches and other central nervous symptoms have been reported to be due to food allergens. There is little objective evidence for the occurrence of only central nervous abnormalities in food allergies. In particular, there is little evidence for a role of food allergens in the production of the tension–fatigue syndrome, in learning disorders or in chronic behavioural disturbances (see Chapters 37–40).

The role of food allergens in the production of headaches is also controversial, since the finding is subjective and few double-blind trials with suspected food antigens have been performed in affected subjects (see Chapter 37). The problem is further compounded by the occurrence of vasoactive amines in many foods (tyramine in cheese, phenylethylamine in chocolate) (see Chapter 23) which may trigger vascular headaches. Thus, such reactions associated with foods may not be due to specific immunological events.

Miscellaneous symptoms

Although many other symptoms or disorders such as sudden infant death syndrome, thrombocytopenia, enuresis, vasculitis syndromes, cardiac arrhythmias and disorders of the musculoskeletal system such as rheumatoid arthritis have been attributed to food allergens, there is little scientific evidence as yet to support these claims [3] (see Chapters 41–43).

SUMMARY

Food sensitivities are most likely to occur in young infants who are not breast fed. The principal food allergens are cow's milk, cereals, eggs, soya protein, fish, nuts and berries. The most frequent symptoms that are produced by food allergens are gastrointestinal reactions. In addition, respiratory symptoms, dermatoses, anaphylaxis and certain specific disorders such as fat malabsorption and pulmonary haemosiderosis are attributable in some cases to food allergens. The diagnosis of food hypersensitivity is dependent upon the amelioration of symptoms following elimination of the suspected food antigen and the development of similar clinical reactions following oral challenge with the food antigen. The oral challenge method should be conducted under careful medical supervision to recognize and quickly abort serious reactions and to obtain objective information about the presence or absence of reactions. Other diagnostic procedures though of considerable research interest have not been proved to be reliable in the diagnosis of food sensitivities.

Because of the paucity of absolute laboratory criteria in the diagnosis, it is important to understand that it is often uncertain whether reactions to foods are based upon immunological mechanisms. Despite an explosion of information concerning macromolecular absorption (see Chapter 11), oral tolerance (see Chapter 14) and the genesis of secretory immune responses (see Chapter 15), our understanding of the complex way that the gastrointestinal tract deals immunologically with food antigens remains incomplete. It is anticipated that a more rational understanding of the role of the hypersensitivities in reactions to foods will be forthcoming in the near future. If that proves to be the case, then it is likely that the categorization of these reactions may be subject to re-examination and possibly to revision.

REFERENCES

1 Aas K: The diagnosis of hypersensitivity to ingested foods: reliability of skin prick testing and the radioallergosorbent test with different materials. Clin Allergy 1978; 8:39–50.

2 American Academy of Allergy: Position statements— controversial techniques. J Allergy Clin Immunol 1981; 67:333–8.

3 American Academy of Allergy and Immunology Committee on Adverse Reactions to Foods and National Institute of Allergy and Infectious Diseases. DHEW publication no. (NIH) 4-2442, 1984; 43–102.

4 American Academy of Allergy and Immunology Committee on Adverse Reactions to Foods and National Institute of Allergy and Infectious Diseases. DHEW publication no. (NIH) 4-2442, 1984; 103–24.

5 Bachman KD, Dees SC: Milk allergy. II. Observations on incidence and symptoms of allergy in allergic children. Pediatrics 1957; 20:400–7.

6 Bahna SL: RAST or skin test versus oral challenge in food sensitivity. Presented at the 5th International Food Allergy Symposium. Atlanta: American College of Allergists, 1984.

7 Bluestone CD: Eustachian tube function and allergy in otitis media. Pediatrics 1978; 61:753–60.

8 Bock SA, Lee W-Y, Remigio LK, May CD: Studies of hypersensitivity reactions to foods in infants and children. J Allergy Clin Immunol 1978: 62:327–34.

9 Brazelton TB: Crying in infancy. Pediatrics 1974; 29:579–88.

10 Clein NW: Cow's milk allergy in infants and children. Int Arch Allergy Appl Immunol 1958; 13:245–56.

11 Dicke WK, Wiejers HA, van de Kamer JH: Coeliac disease. II. The presence in wheat of a factor having a deleterious effect in cases of coeliac disease. Acta Paediatr 1953; 42:34–42.

12 Finberg L: Toxic substances in the food supply in infants and children. Pediatr Ann 1979; 8:706–9.

13 Fontaine JL, Navarro J: Small intestinal biopsy in cow's milk protein allergy in infancy. Arch Dis Child 1975; 50:357–62.

14 Friedman RA, Doyle WJ, Casselbrent MC et al: Immunologic-mediated eustachian tube obstruction: a double-blind crossover study. J Allergy Clin Immunol 1983; 71:442–7.

15 Galen: De sanitate tuenda (Hygiene). Translated by RM Green. Springfield: Charles C Thomas, 1951; 210.

16 Goldman AS, Anderson DW Jr, Sellers WA et al: Milk allergy. I. Oral challenge with milk and isolated milk proteins in allergic children. Pediatrics 1963; 32:425–43.

17 Goldman AS, Sellers WA, Halpern SR et al: Milk allergy. II. Skin testing of allergic and normal children with purified milk proteins. Pediatrics 1963; 32:572–9.

18 Gryboski JD: Gastrointestinal milk allergy in infants. Pediatrics 1967; 40:354–62.

19 Heiner DC, Sears JW: Chronic respiratory disease associated with multiple circulating precipitins to cow's milk. Am J Dis Child 1960; 100:500–2.

20 Heiner DC, Sears JW, Kniker WT: Multiple precipitins to cow's milk in chronic respiratory disease. A syndrome including poor growth, gastrointestinal symptoms, evidence of allergy, iron deficiency anemia and pulmonary hemosiderosis. Am J Dis Child 1962; 103:634.

21 Hippocrates: The Hippocratic Collection. Encyclopedia Britannica. Chicago: Encyclopedia Britannica, 1983; 8:942–3.

22 Howie V, Pollard RB, Kpeyn K et al: Presence of interferon during bacterial otitis media. J Infect Dis 1982; 145:811–14.

23 Hutinel V: Intolérance pour le lait et anaphylaxie chez les nourrissons. Clinique (Paris) 1908; 3:227–31.

24 Johnson JD, Kretchmer N, Simoons FJ: Lactose malabsorption: its biology and history. Adv Pediatr 1974; 21:197–237.

25 Kagnoff MF: Induction and paralysis: a conceptual framework from which to examine the intestinal immune system. Gastroenterology 1974; 66:1240–56.

26 Kalckav HM, Kinoshita JH, Donnell GN: Galactosemia, biochemistry, genetics, pathophysiology, and developmental aspects. In: Gaull GE, ed. Biology of brain dysfunction, vol 2, New York: Plenum Press, 1973; 31.

27 Kidd JM III, Cohan SH, Sosman AJ, Fink JN: Food dependent exercise induced anaphylaxis. J Allergy Clin Immunol 1983; 71: 407–11.

28 Kuitunen P, Visakorpi JK, Savilahti E, Pelkonen P: Malabsorption syndrome with cow's milk intolerance. Arch Dis Child 1975; 50:351–6.

29 McDonald PJ, Goldblum RM, Van Sickle GJ, Powell GK: Food protein-induced enterocolitis: altered antibody response to ingested antigen. Pediatr Res 1984; 18:751–5.

30 Mathews KP: Management of urticaria and angioedema. J Allergy Clin Immunol 1980; 66:347–57.

31 Mathews TS, Soothill JF: Complement activation after milk feeding in children with cow's milk allergy. Lancet 1970; ii: 893–5.

32 May CD: Objective clinical and laboratory studies of immediate-hypersensitivity reactions to food in asthmatic children. J Allergy Clin Immunol 1976; 58:500–15.

33 May CD, Bock SD: A modern clinical approach to food hypersensitivity. Allergy 1978; 33:166–88.

34 Otto R: Zur Frage der Serum-Ueberemfindlichkeit. München Med Wochenschr 1907; 54:1665–70.

35 Park EA: A case of hypersensitivity to cow's milk. Am J Dis Child 1920; 19:46–54.

36 Paulley JW: Observations on aetiology of idiopathic steatorrhoea: jejunal and lymph-node biopsies. Br Med J 1954; 2:1318–21.

37 Portier P, Richet C: De l'action anaphylactique des certaines venins. C R Soc Biol (Paris) 1902; 54:170–2.

38 Powell GK: Milk and soy induced enterocolitis of infancy. Clinical features and standardization of challenge. J Pediatr 1978; 93: 553–60.

39 Prausnitz C, Küstner H: Studien über die Ueberemfindlichkeit. Zentralbl Bakteriol Orig 1921; 86:160–9.

40 Rasmussen J E, Provost TT: Atopic dermatitis. In: Middleton E Jr, Reed CE, Ellis EF, eds. Allergy, principles and practice. St Louis: Mosby 1983; 2:1297–312.

41 Sampson HA: Role of immediate food hypersensitivity in the pathogenesis of atopic dermatitis. J Allergy Clin Immunol 1983; 71:473–80.

42 Saperstein S, Anderson DW, Goldman AS, Kniker WT: Milk allergy. III. Immunological studies with sera from allergic and normal children. Pediatrics 1963; 32:580–7.

43 Schlossman A: Ueber die Giftwirkung des artfremden Eiweisses in der Milch auf den Organismus des Sauglings. Arch Kinderheilkd 1905; 41:99–103.

44 Shiner M, Ballard J, Brook CGD et al: Intestinal biopsy in the diagnosis of cow's milk protein intoler-

ance without acute symptoms. Lancet 1975; ii:1060-3.

45 Talbot FB: Idiosyncrasy to cow's milk: its relationship to anaphylaxis. Boston Med Surg J 1916; 175:409-10.

46 Truelove SC: Ulcerative colitis provoked by milk. Br Med J 1961; 1:154-65.

47 Waldman TA, Wochner RD, Laster L et al: Allergic gastroenteropathy. A cause of excessive gastrointestinal protein loss. N Engl J Med 1967; 276:762-9.

48 Welliver RC: Viral infections and obstructive airway disease in early life. Pediatr Clin North Am 1983; 30:819-28.

49 Wilson JF, Heiner DC, Lahey ME: Studies on iron gastrointestinal dysfunction in infants with iron deficiency anemia: a preliminary report. J Pediatr 1962; 60:787-800.

50 Wilson JF, Lahey ME, Heiner DC: Studies on iron metabolism. V. Further observations on cow's milk-induced gastrointestinal bleeding in infants with iron-deficiency anemia. J Pediatr 1974; 84:335-44.

Chapter 46
Diagnostic Use of Dietary Regimes

M. J. Radcliffe

Introduction

Whatever laboratory or clinical techniques may be deployed to assist in the diagnosis of food allergy or intolerance, at some stage it is necessary to attempt to demonstrate a cause and effect relationship between food ingestion and the precipitation of symptoms. Indeed, whilst for the food-intolerant patient exclusion offers the most effective form of management, the establishment of an appropriate avoidance regime is also an essential stage in education.

A clinically significant maladaptive response to a specific food substance cannot be diagnosed by the presence of a positive serological or skin prick test alone, neither can the diagnosis be invalidated by their absence. Even when the food allergy is of the immediate type, skin prick test and measurement of allergen-specific IgE may be negative [8].

Clearly, serological and skin test results will be of even less value in delayed response types of allergy, where immune mechanisms are less well substantiated, or in which pharmacologi-cal, toxic or enzyme-mediated effects are of more importance than immune effects.

Therefore, the ability of the clinician to make an accurate, reproducible assessment of a dietary cause and effect relationship is an essential prerequisite for the diagnosis of food allergy or intolerance.

THE IMPORTANCE OF AN ACCURATE, REPRODUCIBLE DIAGNOSTIC DIETARY TEST

Whilst the many possible mechanisms of food intolerance remain ill understood, it is clearly impossible to devise diagnostic dietary regimes which will satisfactorily discriminate between all these pathological processes. Conversely, tests of food intolerance which depend on a specific pathological mechanism will remain inefficient in producing a clinically useful re-sult. This lack of pathological specificity im-parts to the dietary test a fundamental unique-ness and means that accurate and reproducible challenge studies are likely to remain the diagnostic yardstick.

Sadly, dietary challenge studies, even when performed with the utmost care on the part of patient and investigator, are inefficient in many respects when compared to the characteristics of an ideal test. Because of the shortcomings of dietary challenge studies, it can be argued that accurate diagnosis of food-allergic disease is virtually impossible for some of our patients.

Inherent weaknesses of food challenge studies

Firstly, food challenge studies are laborious and time consuming both for patient and clinician. An essential prerequisite for this approach is an intelligent and well-motivated patient.

Secondly, there is considerable risk of underachievement with respect to four important functions of any test:

1 Reproducibility—this can be affected by multiple variables in the process of presentation, ingestion and absorption of food.
2 Specificity—coincidental factors are highly likely to affect the outcome.
3 Sensitivity—false negatives commonly occur.
4 Discrimination—false positives commonly occur.

Thirdly, so wide is the range of possible clinical responses (Fig. 46.1) and the possible

frustrating. However, it is abundantly clear that numerous patients with both classical and more bizarre symptom complexes have been cured by the use of diagnostic and therapeutic food elimination regimes.

Thus, whilst a circumspect approach is necessary when using antigen avoidance regimes, this should not detract from the need to advocate their use in the wide range of common, readily confirmable though not yet commonly accepted, food-allergic diseases.

Immediate and delayed versus fixed and cyclic food allergy

A knowledge of the empirical nature and mechanism of food allergy and of specific features producing modification of the clinical response is essential for the establishment of a specific diagnosis.

Whilst there has been a tendency in recent texts to refer to food reactions as immediate or late in type, it is helpful when considering phenomena which both complicate and facilitate the diagnostic process to refer also to the concept of cyclic as opposed to fixed food allergy [20].

Fixed food allergy

In the typical case of fixed food allergy, a food which has not been eaten for a period of several years will, upon first reingestion, produce definite and often severe symptoms. Such

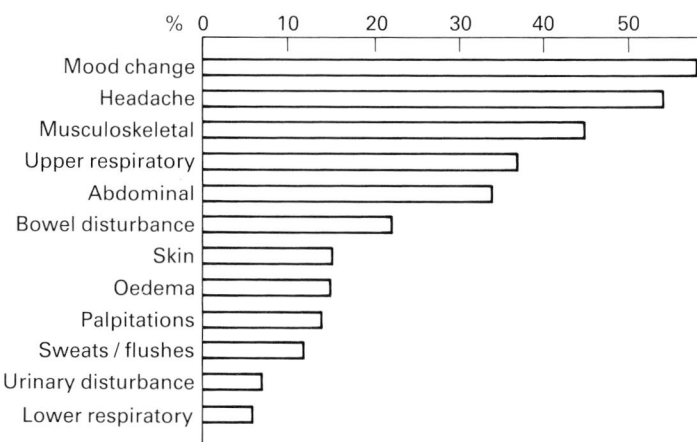

Fig. 46.1 Percentage of patients with specific symptom relief in 100 polysymptomatic responders to dietary exclusion. From Radcliffe MJ: Clinical methods for diagnosis. Clin Immunol Allergy 1982; 2: 205–20, with permission.

range of implicated substances (Fig. 46.2) that a standardized form of testing is difficult to conceive. Certainly nothing remotely resembling a standard test exists at the present time.

All of these shortcomings make the scientific study of food intolerance cumbersome and

fixed food reactions, usually immediate in type, with a positive RAST (radioallergosorbent test) and skin prick test, are usually clearly apparent to the patient and do not, therefore, require diagnostic tests for their identification.

Cyclic food allergy

Cyclic food allergy, although a relative term, refers to food intolerance in which the implicated food can be tolerated when eaten infrequently following prolonged avoidance. The likelihood of sensitization is proportional to the frequency of occurrence of the food in the diet. Increased intake increases the risk of sensitization. Common examples are, therefore, to be found among the staple foods (Fig. 46.2).

Initial allergic symptoms. Symptoms occurring on first encounter may well be forgotten. Vomiting, diarrhoea, colic or temporary failure to thrive with bottle or breast feeding or on weaning may give evidence of initial sensitization. Tolerance seems to be associated with subsequent regular use of the offending food, though this appears to be a genuinely symptom-free state, avoidance and challenge at this stage producing no evidence of a masked state.

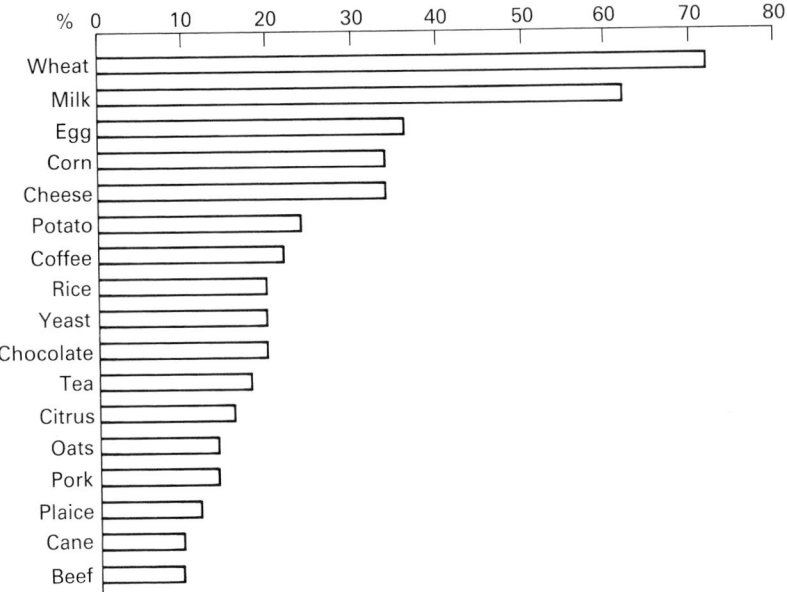

Fig. 46.2 Percentages of individual food 'allergies' in 50 exclusion diet responders identified by sequential food ingestion challenge. From Radcliffe MJ: Clinical methods for diagnosis. Clin Immunol Allergy 1982; 2: 205–20, with permission.

Sufferers are usually skin prick test and RAST negative, though it is claimed that the RAST would yield more positives in this group with a more sensitive and patient-specific scoring system [14]. Whilst there has been a tendency to use the term 'food intolerance' rather than 'food allergy' when speaking of such reactions [8], it seems appropriate to include all reproducible food challenge-related reactions in an examination of phenomena and methodology.

An examination of the effects of first encounter, of regular ingestion with the successive development of tolerance and masked sensitivity and of the effects of temporary or prolonged omission and rechallenge at this masked stage, forms the basis of the 'cyclic concept' (Fig. 46.3). First described in 1944 [19], it remains a valid account of the clinical phenomena encountered in the investigation of 'non-fixed' food allergy.

Whilst it can be argued that in many cases this stage of tolerance can last indefinitely, in other cases a stage of masked sensitivity supersedes after months or years of regular use. The degree and rate of this progression seems to depend, in part at least, upon the frequency of exposure to the food in question.

The phenomena of masking and addiction

The patient who presents himself for possible food allergy diagnosis is most likely to present in this masked state. In contrast, the presence of a fixed, unmasked allergy to an infrequently ingested food such as prawn or peanut is seldom a diagnostic problem. Most commonly, when the patient is able to detect the food which precipitates a particular symptom, it is a food which is eaten less commonly than one

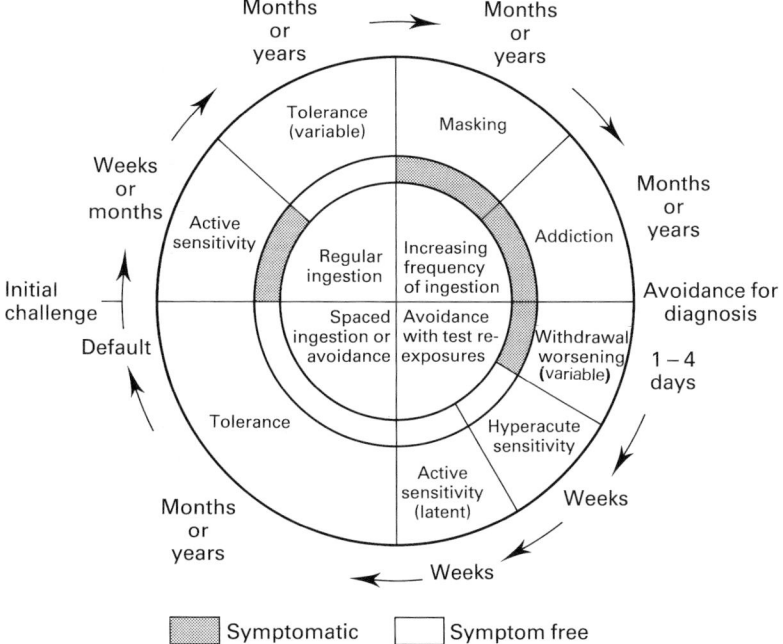

Fig. 46.3 The cyclic concept of food allergy. The upper part represents the natural history prior to diagnosis, the lower part the sequence which follows specific diagnosis.

day in five. Conversely, when the patient is totally unaware which food is causing symptoms, or doubts the presence of a food allergy at all, it is likely that the most important implicated food(s) will be eaten more than once in five days and most likely more than once a day.

Masking

The phenomenon of masking, therefore, involves an inversion of the expected response. Avoidance, accidental or otherwise, results in a transient worsening of symptoms, whereas the eating of the food produces initial improvement. It seems unlikely to the sufferer that a chronically occurring symptom could be associated with the ingestion of a food which tends to make him feel 'better'.

Case history 1. Paul, aged 10, had been referred for child guidance by his headmaster. Disruptive behaviour had rendered him unteachable, due to increasingly frequent episodes of unprovoked aggression and regressive behaviour amounting at times to animal-like crawling around the classroom floor. Following such episodes he would return to a withdrawn and sulky state, usually with pallor and stomach pain. His two sisters had eczema and urticaria, respectively, an aunt had asthma and a cousin coeliac disease. Paul had previously

suffered from migraine and had had little uninterrupted good health for four years.

A dietary history revealed an addictive pattern of wheat ingestion with wheat cereal being regularly consumed at breakfast and on return home from school. He took frequent snacks of biscuits or bread, and would frequently wake for biscuit snacks during the night. Favourite meal-time foods were spaghetti and beans on toast.

A wheat-free diet produced a marked improvement. Formerly lethargic and pale-faced, he became robust and healthy in appearance. His school reported a marked improvement in his performance, with complete cessation of the 'attacks'. Overt challenge with wheat produced reactions within two hours, lasting up to 36 hours. Subsequent single-blind challenges were organized, with wholewheat flour masked in mashed potato. Similar reactions followed on each of three separate oral challenges. These reactions were characterized by marked behaviour and mood disturbance, stomach pain and bloating, head pains and pallor. The disturbance of mood would follow a distinct pattern, the overactive behaviour receding and giving way to a withdrawn and depressed state usually ending quite abruptly at some time on the second or third day.

Three subsequent reactions, unexpected at the time, occurred over a period of two years. These were traced to 'liquorice allsorts', an

'Oxo' cube and 'Robertson's Mincemeat', all of which contain wheat. These reactions apart, he has remained well for five years.

Milder addictive patterns of food intolerance are more usual and have been well described by Randolph [15], who has made similar observations with sugars [17] and alcoholic beverages [18]. Hypothesizing a common mechanism, he has identified the addictant in each case as the botanical source of the specific sugar or alcohol.

Use of the diet diary

An examination of the pattern of food ingestion and also the pattern of symptom response provides a valuable initial dietary assessment and can help the physician decide what form of exclusion regime it would be most helpful to employ.

To this end, a frequently used device is the diet diary (Fig. 46.4). The patient records the

likely to have already been spotted by the patient, they should nevertheless be looked for at this stage. Diets high in chemical additives or nutritionally unsound should be earmarked for correction prior to the commencement of an exclusion regime. Not uncommonly, marked improvement occurs with simple dietary advice about wholefood nutritional principles, making the complex process of food allergy diagnosis unnecessary. Specific reaction to food additive or additives should be borne in mind at this stage (Chapter 22b).

Pattern of symptoms

As exemplified in the above case history, an addictive food ingestion pattern may be apparent from the food diary. More subtle single food responses can come to light provided that it is remembered that symptoms from a single ingestion may occur later the same day or during the night or following day. In some cases, symptoms from a single inges-

DIET DIARY

Name _____   Date _____

	DAY 1		DAY 2		DAY 3	
a.m. 8.00	Food	Symptoms	Food	Symptoms	Food	Symptoms
9.00						
10.00						
11.00						
12.00						
p.m. 1.00						
2.00						
3.00						
4.00						
5.00						
6.00						
7.00						
8.00						
9.00						
10.00						

Fig. 46.4 The diet diary. Immediate food reactions and food addictions may be revealed. Delayed food reactions are not as easily seen.

nature and time of consumption of all foods, beverages and snacks, together with a timed record of activity and symptoms. It may be necessary to instruct the patient in the evaluation of symptoms, as often the patient tends to disregard lower levels of symptoms as a symptom-free state. Those with complex allergic problems should in addition record such activities as exposure to dust, moulds, feathers, animals and chemical odours. Women should note also the possible correlation of symptoms with the menstrual cycle.

Although immediate cause and effect relationships between food and symptoms are

tion may occur on two or three consecutive nights with relative freedom from symptoms during the intervening day-time hours.

Certain diurnal patterns of symptom occurrence can suggest a masked food allergy without necessarily implicating a specific food [20]. Such diurnal patterns, made up of exacerbations and quiescent periods, are the characteristic response to the staple foods, e.g. wheat, milk, corn, egg, potato, etc.

With a low-grade response, the only clear exacerbation of symptoms may be during the first 1–2 hours following sleep.

With a high degree of sensitivity to a food

allergen, increase in both the frequency and intensity of exacerbations has been noted. Typically, such episodes occur 1–2 hours after rising, at 11.00 a.m., at 4.00–5.00 in the afternoon, at 9.00–10.00 in the evening and sometimes early in the morning (2.00–4.00 a.m.). However, the exacerbation occurring 1–2 hours after rising remains the most troublesome.

'Catalytic' effect of alcohol

One other factor in symptom provocation is worth noting as it is quite helpful in diagnosis. This is the apparent ability of alcohol to 'catalyse' the food-allergic response. For example a rhinitis sufferer might notice that a particular alcoholic beverage produces sneezing and rhinorrhoea. Closer study might reveal such a sufferer to be sensitive to corn, for example, and suffer no such reaction on consuming a non-grain-derived alcoholic beverage (e.g. Jamaica rum). Similarly, a masked sensitivity to potato can show up as an immediate exacerbation after a meal containing potato and alcohol.

Hidden allergies: incomplete avoidance

Finally, the diet diary may show up that a specific food is being half-heartedly avoided. Such is the ubiquity in the modern diet of many of our staple foods, that the individual's own attempts to avoid that which is known to cause symptoms is usually ineffective. Thus the child who avoids 'milk' but eats yoghurt, and the adult who avoids 'fish' but eats ice-cream (which usually contains fish oils), may well become completely symptom free with a complete avoidance of the already suspected food allergen.

METHODS OF DIETARY ELIMINATION

Whether the elimination planned is a selective elimination of one to three foods, a basic elimination diet, a trial fast or an elemental diet, the method of implementation of the dietary procedure is the same in each case. The patient (or the parents in the case of a child) will be responsible for the recording of symptoms, so it is desirable that a baseline period of self-observation precedes the test diet. This should be conducted on the patient's 'normal' diet. All non-essential drugs should be

stopped. (In the case of drugs that produce withdrawal effects, this should be done well in advance.) In certain circumstances, essential drugs (e.g. thyroxine, insulin) will have to be continued. In other circumstances, disease-modifying drugs (e.g. corticosteroids in Crohn's disease or asthma) can be continued and possibly later tailed off if a good response to dietary control is established.

Doctor and patient then decide what symptoms should be the subject of daily scores. Any self-measurable parameter of disease activity (e.g. peak flow rate, grip strength) can be added to the score sheet (Fig. 46.5).

'Simple' elimination diets

Some fortunate patients can be quite easily helped as their symptoms are provoked by only one or two foods. If the food to be eliminated is not widely used as an ingredient by the food industry (e.g. coffee) its elimination is fairly straightforward.

Unfortunately, an increasing number of foods are now used in this way and their elimination is no simple matter. The help of a dietician experienced in this work would be invaluable.

Milk. Casein, caseinate, lactose and whey are all milk derivatives. Most 'non-dairy' milk and cream substitutes contain one of these derivatives. Powdered artificial sweeteners contain lactose, as do many medications. For the following foods it should be assumed that milk is present unless one has specific evidence to the contrary: bread, margarine, ice-cream (even labelled 'non-milk fat'), sausages, hamburgers, *plain* chocolate, sherbet and other sweets.

Egg. Vitellin, ovovitellin, livetin, ovomucin, ovomucoid and albumin are all egg derivatives. They are found both labelled *and unlabelled* in baking powder, cakes, cake mixes, croissants, glazed bread and rolls, pastry, meringue, sauces, salad dressings, icing, sweets, sausages and luncheon meats. Egg is used in the production of wines, coffee and root beer.

Wheat. This category includes wheat grain, germ, starch and 'food' starch, flour, bran and farina. Wheat starch may be classified as gluten-free if its purity is within the codex alimentarius definition. However, this may be a quite unsuitable standard for the wheat-allergic patient. Major wheat-containing foods

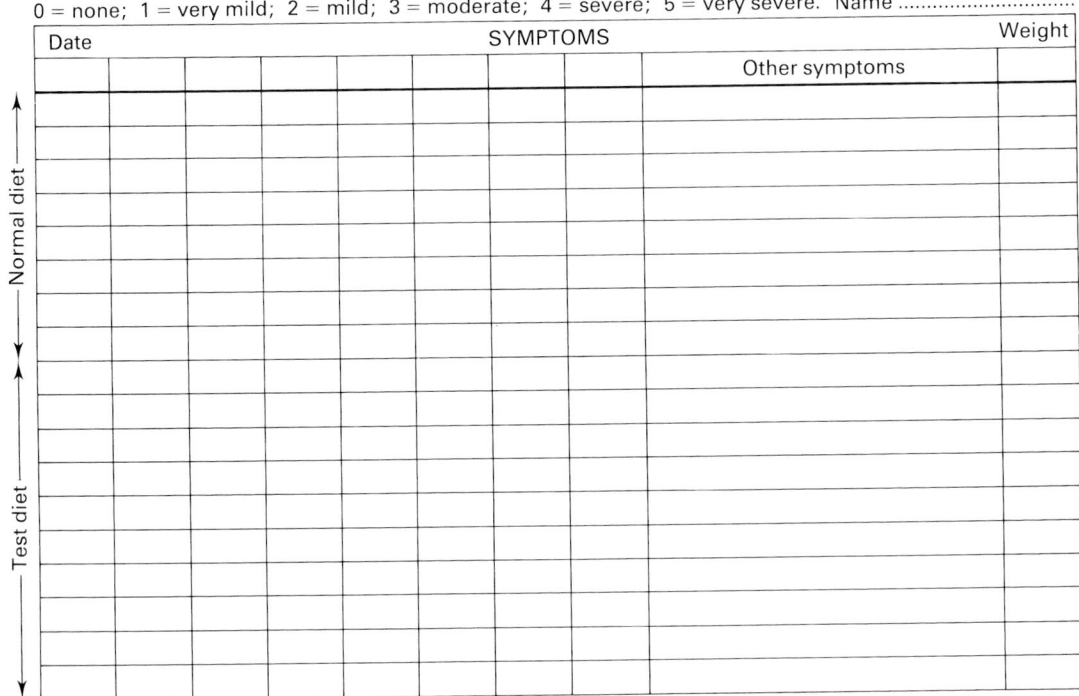

Fig. 46.5 Symptom chart.

are fairly easily identifiable. Hidden sources include baking powder, sausages, vinegars and alcoholic beverages. Rye and barley frequently cross-react with wheat and for practical purposes should be classified together. (Even '100%' rye contains up to 10% wheat as the seed is commonly so contaminated.) Malt is derived from barley, sometimes from wheat or corn as well, and is present in many non-wheat breakfast cereals.

From the above it can be seen that a number of foods commonly contain all three of these frequently encountered food allergens. For this reason the author frequently uses a diet eliminating all three, giving the patient a list of foods to be avoided together with recipes for biscuits, cakes and crackers made from rice, soya, sago, chick-pea and potato flours. Books containing recipes for such patients are now readily available [6, 25].

Hidden ingredients

Other foods commonly found as allergens and widespread as hidden ingredients include corn, soya, yeast, fish, pork and beef. Of all food allergens, corn is the most difficult to avoid. As oil, starch, syrup or sugar (e.g. glucose, fructose, dextrose), it is present in virtually all factory-processed foods. It is also very widely distributed in alcoholic beverages. A fuller account of hidden 'natural' ingredients has been prepared by Miller [13].

Quite clearly, 'simple' elimination diets are far from simple. It follows that if the patient is to avoid more than one or two foods, a simpler approach is needed.

'Basic' elimination diets

Basic elimination diets are based on the inescapable fact that giving the patient one list of foods to be avoided (containing, for example, milk) is difficult enough, but adding together numerous lists for various avoidances (for example, food additives, milk, egg, wheat, corn and soya) would make adherence complex and compliance virtually impossible to achieve. Diets which tell the patient what to eat rather than what not to eat are simpler to apply.

Numerous basic regimes have been used. Those employed most frequently by the author are shown in Table 46.1. Another widely used regime gives one meat, perhaps an unusual one such as rabbit, one vegetable and one fruit (containing no pips).

With all these 'basic' regimes the two biggest difficulties for the average patient are a

Table 46.1 Elimination diets: (1) exclusion of major offenders (after Mackarness [10]); (2) use of rarely implicated foods.

Elimination diet 1	
Fresh meat	Any kind including offal
Fresh fish	Any kind
Fresh vegetables	Any kind except potato and tomato
Fresh fruit	Any kind except citrus
Drinks	Spring water
	Additive-free juices of allowed fruits
	Herb and fruit teas e.g. mint, linden flower, rosehip, Rooibosch, Ruby Red
Seasoning	Fresh black pepper, herbs, sea salt
Cooking and salad oils	Olive, sunflower, safflower
Elimination diet 2	
Meat	Venison, rabbit
Fish	Cod, haddock, herring, mackerel
Poultry	Turkey
Game	Pheasant
Parsley family	Carrot, parsnip, celery, parsley
Mustard family	Cabbage, cauliflower, Brussels sprout, turnip, watercress, radish, mustard, horseradish
Plum family	Plum, prune, peach, apricot
Melon family	Watermelon, cucumber, cantaloup, pumpkin, melon
Pineapple family	Pineapple
Drinks	Spring water, additive-free juices of above fruits
	Herb and fruit teas
Seasoning	Sea salt, herbs
	Olive oil

Data from Radcliffe MJ: Clinical methods for diagnosis. Clin Immunol Allergy 1982; 2: 205–20, with permission.

substitute for tea or coffee and a substitute for bread. There are no truly satisfactory grain-free bread substitutes, although reasonable tea and coffee substitutes are available (e.g. Rooibosch tea and dandelion coffee).

None of these basic diets can be regarded as nutritionally 100% sound, and it must be stressed that they are for short term diagnostic use only, especially in young children.

The trial fast and elemental diets

Two other avoidance regimes have been used in food allergy investigation. Both are an attempt to approximate to 'total' removal of the gastrointestinal antigen load.

Fasting regimes

Trial fast was first advocated by Randolph [15] who has subsequently hospitalized, fasted and challenge tested over 10 000 individual patients using this method [16]. The technique has been extended to incorporate the inhaled component through the development of a comprehensive environmental control programme. Several such environmental units now exist in the USA. By their use, contaminants of both industrial and biological derivation in air, food and water are reduced to a minimum by the use of carefully chosen materials of construction and cleansing, specialized techniques of barrier nursing and air filtration and the use of chemically less contaminated water sources (see Chapter 55).

Patients fasted and later challenge tested with chemically less contaminated (organically grown) foods in such units have been relieved of a wide range of clinical conditions. In particular, patients with both large and small vessel vasculitis of unknown aetiology have been noted to have evidence of compromised immune function prior to treatment (e.g. marked reduction of absolute T lymphocyte count) with evidence of a return to normal during 'environmental control' and the restoration of a symptom-free state (see Chapter 42).

Elemental diets

Alternative techniques include the use of proprietary 'elemental' diets (e.g. Vivonex, Eaton Laboratories). These have been employed where it has been thought that the number of involved allergens may be large, and in particular when prolonged avoidance is thought necessary to secure a remission. They have been used in the investigation of eczema in children [24], rheumatoid arthritis [4], in the investigation of children with complex food allergies [5] and following 7–10-day intravenous nutrition in the investigation of inflammatory bowel disease [7].

However, neither of these forms of alternative nutrition can be claimed to be free of antigenic activity. Both contain sugar derivatives of corn which have been shown to perpetuate chronic effects attributable to corn when administered both orally and intravenously [17].

Such extreme measures can be advocated only for the most complex of problems. In most cases the simple elimination diets described above and administered with careful preparation and attention to detail will produce good results.

Prerequisites for successful fast or elimination diet

For either a fast or an elimination diet the following prerequisites are necessary for a successful result.

Aperient. The patient should take a large dose of epsom salts or milk of magnesia on the first morning to obtain a satisfactory bowel evacuation.

Fluid intake. A large quantity of fluid should be drunk. Bottled spring water is to be preferred, especially in the fasting patient who is likely to find his taste heightened after the initial withdrawal phase. This also allows for the testing of tap water as a challenge test.

Absolute adherence. There must be absolutely no break in the diet. For example, spurious reactions have been traced to the licking of a food-soiled finger in the preparation of food for others.

Fresh foods. Foods used in exclusion diets should be fresh if possible, but frozen or dried if not. However, the latter two heighten the risk of hidden ingredients of both natural and synthetic origin. Ideally chemically less contaminated food of 'organic' origin should be used to eliminate the possibility of reactions occurring to pesticide or herbicide residues (see Chapters 22a and b).

Pharmaceutical preparations. Toothpaste, drugs and medicines (including the contraceptive pill) contain food substances and should be discontinued to avoid false-negative challenge tests due to incomplete unmasking. Cigarettes carry the same risk as they contain sugars. Also, tobacco is botanically related to potato and tomato (Solanaceae) and may cross-react and therefore cross-mask.

Knowledge of hidden food and synthetic ingredients is essential for the accurate diagnosis and management of food allergy. Such information is inadequate in the UK. A review of this problem by Miller [13] gives a useful guide to the unexpected pitfalls.

Daily diary. A daily diary of symptoms should be kept by the patient, who should be warned about the possibility of exacerbation of symptoms on withdrawal (even though this can be criticized on the grounds of suggestion). So marked are withdrawal effects in some cases that, despite such forewarning, craving at the height of withdrawal becomes so extreme that the patient, failing to understand what is happening, breaks the diet. Careful note should be made of the craved-for food or foods in this situation as it is likely that they may be those responsible for the original symptoms.

Withdrawal effects

The precipitation of a withdrawal response and its nature can be extremely variable. In some cases the effect can be a worsening of the presenting problem, in other cases the symptoms may be apparently unrelated.

Early symptoms

An early occurrence towards the end of the first day, whatever the presenting complaint, is headache, frequently migrainous in type. It should not be assumed that withdrawal effects will be entirely physical, as agitation or depression are common. There is, quite clearly, a direct comparison to be made between the withdrawal effects of foods, alcohol, drugs and tobacco.

Late symptoms

Later manifestations of withdrawal include extreme muscle aching, and the worst affected individuals may need to spend the second and third days of the test in bed. On the second, third and fourth days fatigue, physical weakness and tachycardia with minimal exertion commonly occur, leading the sufferer and others to ascribe the symptom state to hunger and a break in the dietary regime may follow. Patients may describe the experience as resembling the manifestations of a viral illness. Such symptoms are temporary and perseverance results in their rapid amelioration.

Length of elimination period

The elimination regime or trial fast should be continued until there is convincing evidence of a positive or negative response. No hard and fast rule can be laid down as to the necessary duration, but in general 5–10 days are needed. Young patients seem to clear in a shorter time and some conditions such as asthma may require longer to clear [9].

The features of the withdrawal response as described above are sufficiently characteristic to act as an aid in the diagnosis of the positive response. Whilst such withdrawal effects do not invariably occur, their occurrence may lead the physician to proceed to challenge testing after the first symptom-free day, rather than waiting for a more prolonged remission to indicate a positive response.

INDIVIDUAL SEQUENTIAL FOOD INGESTION CHALLENGE AFTER EXCLUSION

The method of dietary exclusion and challenge in the diagnosis of food allergy was first described by Rowe [21] and later expanded [22]. Reference has already been made to the cyclic concept of food allergy, described first by Rinkel [19]. Deliberate unmasking and the subsequent utilization of the 'hyperacute' stage of reactivity for challenge testing was first described by him. If a food is avoided for at least four days or at least long enough for withdrawal phenomena to subside (though not long enough for tolerance to develop) and is then taken in normal amounts, the original symptoms will return often in a markedly exaggerated form. Moreover, this reaction normally occurs within a short time, from a few minutes to a few hours, when compared to symptom provocation by the same food in the unmasked state.

Failure to establish the hyperacute state

Failure to establish this hyperacute state, so useful in diagnosis, can result from the incomplete unmasking of the specific food allergy. Causes of incomplete unmasking include incomplete elimination (the food being still consumed inadvertently or in a 'hidden' form), incomplete withdrawal, or overprolonged elimination (the hyperacute state though variable in its timing appears to recede in three to six

weeks). Clearly a more complete state of tolerance can eventually occur, although how soon after elimination is far from clear.

Prolonged challenges

It is not universally accepted that such a hyperacute state of immediate postchallenge reactivity can be induced and it has been suggested that 'delayed' food allergy must be tested by prolonged challenges of up to one week per food. The author believes that this approach is both time consuming and unnecessary, and that ingestion challenge of a single food need take no more than one day. An exception to this is the cereal grains which tend to produce delayed responses even in the 'unmasked' state and for which a two-day test is wise.

A satisfactory response. Although a satisfactory response to an elimination diet cannot on its own be considered diagnostic of food allergy, certain characteristics of the response as indicated above lead to the suspicion that food allergy is present. However, a satisfactory response to an elimination regime is a necessary prerequisite for individual food testing. There is little point proceeding with challenge tests in the absence of a relatively symptom-free state. Where withdrawal worsening has occurred it is important that symptoms should have completely subsided prior to testing.

The pulse test

The most useful addition to subjective symptom assessment is measurement of the pulse rate. This can be satisfactorily carried out by the patient when conducting the test at home, and it forms the basis of the pulse test originally described by Coca [3] (see also Chapter 56). The authors have recently completed a study which demonstrates the validity of the pulse test under conditions of double-blind challenge (unpublished, Table 46.2). Pulse acceleration (or deceleration) in excess of ten beats per minute when compared with the preprandial level is usually taken as a positive response.

The original description

As originally described, the test relied on a diet structured in respect of single-food meals. Without preliminary elimination, challenge tests did not utilize the hyperacute state de-

Table 46.2 Significant (>10 beats per minute) pulse changes ($+$) in response to double-blind allergen challenge, with double-blind sodium cromoglycate (SCG) pretreatment.

Challenge Pretreatment	A Allergen Placebo	B Allergen SCG	C Placebo Placebo	D Placebo SCG
Patient				
1	+	−	−	−
2	−	−	−	−
3	+	+	−	−
4	+	+	+	−
5	+	+	−	+
6	+	+	−	−
7	+	+	−	+
8	+	+	−	−
9	+	−	−	−
10	−	−	−	−
11	+	−	−	−

A significant difference was observed between allergen and placebo challenge (A vs. C, $P=0.01$). A significant effect of SCG pretreatment on this response was not noted (B vs. D, n.s.; A vs. B, n.s.; C vs. D, n.s.).

scribed. The pulse test was, therefore, critical to the prediction of the delayed symptom response. Fourteen pulse counts were taken on each day, one on rising, one on retiring and pulse counts preprandially, 0.5 hour, 1 hour and 1.5 hours postprandially, three single food meals being consumed on each day of the test. An attempt was made to minimize pulse-accelerating factors, both non-specific (e.g. exertion) and specific (e.g. infection and inhaled allergens such as house dust).

Used in conjunction with elimination and challenge, symptom and pulse responses are recorded. Whilst symptom provocation is, quite clearly, the most reliable indicator of a positive response, in practice the pulse provides a useful cross-check and in many instances helps avoid false negatives. It must be stressed, however, that a significant pulse change is neither pathognomonic of food allergy, nor a universal accompaniment of a significant symptom response.

Practical aspects

As usually practised now, the resting pulse is taken before taking a normal-sized, unadulterated portion of the food to be tested. If normally eaten when cooked, it should be tested in the cooked state and vice versa. Postprandial pulse rates are taken after 20, 40, 60 and 80 minutes (longer in some cases, e.g. cereal grains). Symptom responses are monitored for a minimum of four hours, though responses delayed as long as 48 hours can occur, particularly with the cereal foods. No more than two foods should be tested on each day. One

food can be tested at breakfast and, provided that no response is apparent, another at lunch. The evening meal can consist of test-negative foods together with the foods tested earlier in the day. Only if no symptom response is suspected up to and including the early morning should another two foods be tested the following day.

Variations in the testing regime

Whether because of a waning of the 'hyperacute' stage which follows elimination, or because of the development of tolerance or because of the risk of specific nutritional deficit, there is general agreement that neither the elimination regime nor the period of challenge testing should continue for too long. If by the end of six weeks the individual food challenges are incomplete, consideration should be given to introducing as a block challenge over a three- or four-day period those foods still untested. This assumes that the most likely suspects have already been tested and that one or more have been identified as possible provocants. As well as giving the patient a break, this manoeuvre acts as a possible short cut if no new symptoms arise. If the introduction does trigger a fresh reaction, it can be argued that the risk of tolerance development producing false negative test results is thereby minimized. A general scheme of diet elimination and challenge is shown in Fig. 46.6.

Another system which reduces the duration of challenge tests has been suggested by some authors (Eaton 1984, personal communica-

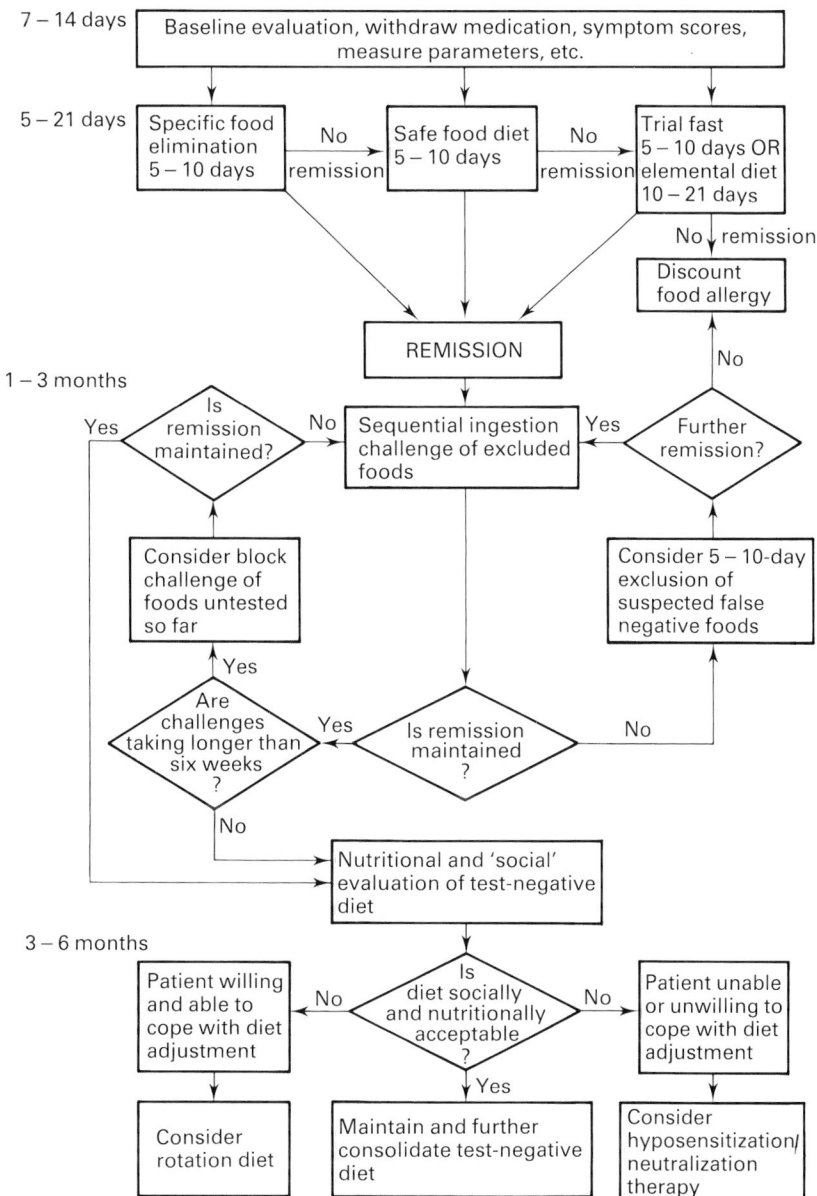

Fig. 46.6 A general scheme of diet elimination and challenge.

tion). Foods to be tested are arranged in groups to be introduced together and tested over a one-week period. As cross-reaction occurs not infrequently between foods of the same botanical or zoological family, this suggests a logical basis for the grouping of foods (see Chapter 17).

Case history 2. Patricia, a 40-year-old housewife, presented in August, 1979, with a 30-year history of multiple health problems. In the preceding five years she had been a frequent hospital inpatient and outpatient, a very frequent attender at the doctor's surgery and

had consumed appreciable quantities of medication. Her worst year was 1977, when she spent 30 days in hospital, made 20 outpatient attendances and 28 general practitioner visits, and was taking as many as 11 different medications concurrently.

She had suffered severe migraine since the age of 12, urinary difficulties since her teens with subsequent 'sterile' dysuria and episodes of severe renal pain. Assuming a microangiopathy, she had been treated with warfarin since 1977. She had a history of depression, with suicide attempts in 1972 and 1975, and electroconvulsive therapy in 1972 and 1973.

As a child she had tonsillitis and since childhood had had perennial rhinitis. She was known to be sensitive to the house dust mite.

She was initially started on a simple egg- and milk-free diet and suffered severe withdrawal effects resulting in the worst migraine she had ever known. This provided the opportunity to fast her for the next few days and she became symptom free and felt better than she had for a long time. The results of her challenge tests are given in Table 46.3. Since

studies are subjective. However, it has also been suggested from animal experiments that an immunological response resulting in histamine release can be produced by a classical conditioning procedure [23].

Reasons for false negative results

Other studies, which claim to demonstrate the need for double-blind placebo control in every case of food allergy diagnosis, reach this con-

Table 46.3 Individual sequential food ingestion challenge.

| | Preingestion | Pulse rate | | | | | | Symptoms in next four hours |
| | | Minutes after ingestion | | | | | | |
		20	40	60	80	100	120	
Turkey	92	92	92	92	92			None
Potato	92	92	92	92	92			None
Cow's milk	90	90	98	**104**	**120**			Sneezing, chest tight, runny nose, pain in temples
Plaice	92	92	92	92	90			None
Soya	88	88	88	88	88			None
Pork	88	96	**100**	96	88			None
Tomato	80	80	88	88	88			Slight headache
Rice	92	92	92	94	94			None
Butter	84	84	**104**	**96**	**96**			Headache, agitated
Onion	82	82	82	82	82			None
Wheat 1	94	94	96	94	94	90	82	None
Wheat 2	82	84	**96**	84	80	80	80	None
Wheat 3	80	80	80	80	84	—	—	16 hours very depressed, 22 hours severe migraine
Banana	78	78	78	76	78			None
Egg	88	88	**100**	**116**	**120**			Frontal headache, nausea, renal pain
Mushroom	92	92	88	92	92			None
Corn 1	86	88	96	**100**	88	90	84	Nausea and fatigue, 12 hours
Corn 2	—	—	—	—	—	—	—	—
Corn 3	—	—	—	—	—	—	—	—

Bold type indicates a significant rise in pulse rate.

the establishment of a compatible diet, she has led a happy healthy family life. Her medical requirements in the last five years have been met by four visits to the surgery, and she has required no medication. Details of her medical needs over the past 10 years are summarized in Fig. 46.7.

OTHER DIETS AND CHALLENGE TESTS

Double-blind challenge tests

Placebo-controlled double-blind ingestion challenge studies of patients whose food allergies have been diagnosed by open challenge have demonstrated an heterogeneity of response [2]. The responses measured in these

clusion merely on the failure of active challenge to reproduce symptoms [1, 11]. In the absence of accurate quantification of placebo response it is difficult to substantiate such a claim because of many possible reasons for false-negative responses. Some of these reasons have been discussed above. Other possible reasons for false negative responses may be inherent in the particular method of ingestion challenge chosen. For example, ingestion challenge with powdered foods in capsules revealed as many as 80% non-responders amongst subjects demonstrated to be prick-test positive to the relevant foods [12]. It is possible that two mechanisms of failure of reaction result from the use of capsules. Firstly, the relatively small amount of food used in the challenge, and secondly the bypassing of the oral mucosa. Nasogastric tube introduction of

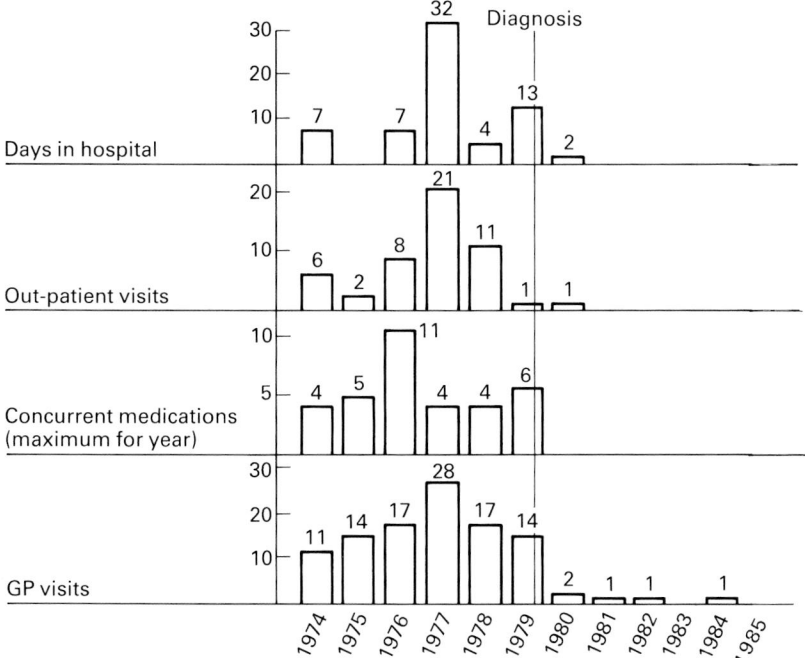

Fig. 46.7 Medical requirements of food allergy sufferer before and after the diagnosis of food allergy in 1979.

foods avoids the first of these drawbacks but not the second. Probably the most satisfactory methods of 'blind' administration of foods involves the use of homogenates of strongly textured and flavoured compatible foods to provide a base with which to mask the food under test [2]. The integrity of such techniques of masking should, of course, be tested.

Placebo-controlled ingestion challenge

As long as the ingestion challenge test remains the yardstick of food allergy diagnosis, and whilst it provides information about the patient's sensitivities which cannot be obtained in any other way, then the double-blind placebo-controlled administration of the test will remain an essential part of the research in this field. However, to argue that such techniques are required in every case is to place a major and unjustifiable obstacle in the way of food allergy diagnosis.

The rotary diversified diet

An extension of the concept of masking is the idea that foods eaten less often than once in four days will fail to mask, and will therefore produce self-evident cause and effect responses. A practical application of this principle, which serves as both a diagnostic and a management regime for the patient with

multiple intolerances, has been termed the rotary diversified diet (Table 46.4) [20].

The reasons for rotation of foods

Eating foods in rotation serves three purposes. Firstly, it helps in the identification of specific food allergies. As individual foods are eaten no more often than one day in four, each ingestion becomes an 'unmasked' challenge and identification of intolerances is facilitated. Secondly, it reduces the frequency of exposure of foods to which the individual is already sensitive. For the patient with numerous intolerances, this produces a compatible diet which is neither restricted, hence the description 'diversified', nor nutritionally inadequate. Thirdly, it avoids the risk of further sensitization to foods well tolerated. Not infrequently, a patient who substitutes one staple food for another eventually develops a sensitivity to the new staple food. This is particularly likely when the foods belong to the same botanical family, for example rice in place of wheat.

Four-day rotation. In a four-day rotation of foods, if beef is eaten for dinner on Monday, it should not be eaten again in any form (for example in a soup or as dripping) until dinner on Friday. Rice, if eaten on Wednesday, should not be eaten again until Sunday. This

Table 46.4 Four-day rotary diversified diet.

Day	Meat Poultry Fish	Vegetables	Fruits	Beverages	Grains Flours	Nuts	Oils Fats	Sweetener
1	Beef Lamb Cheese	*Parsley family* Carrot, celery, parsnip, parsley *Fungi* Mushroom, yeast	*Rose family* Strawberry, raspberry *Apple family* Apple, pear	Milk Tea Apple juice	Oats	Brazil Cashew	Beef dripping Butter	Beet sugar
2	Fish Shellfish	*Sunflower family* Lettuce, chicory, endive, artichoke (Jer.) *Potato family* Tomato, peppers, potato	*Citrus family* Orange, lemon, grapefruit, lime Avocado Rhubarb (buckwheat family)	Orange juice Grapefruit juice Chamomile tea (sunflower family)	Buckwheat Sunflower seeds Tapioca	Filbert Hazel	Olive Sunflower oil Safflower oil	Maple Maple sugar
3	Poultry Eggs	*Mustard family* Cabbage, broccoli, cauliflower, turnip *Gourd family* Marrow, cucumber, courgette	Banana Melon (gourd family) Pineapple *Gooseberry family* Gooseberry, currant	Pineapple juice Mint tea	Wheat Corn (maize) Rice Sago	Walnut	Corn oil	Cane sugar Molasses
4	Pork Rabbit	*Legume family* Peas, beans, lentil, chick-pea, soya Sweet potato *Lily family* Onion, garlic, chive, asparagus, leek	*Grape family* Grape, raisin *Plum family* Cherry, peach, apricot *Palm family* Coconut, date	Grape juice Rosehip tea	Lentil Chick-pea Soya	Peanut (legume) family Almond (plum family)	Peanut oil Soya oil Pork lard	Date sugar Honey

Use unprocessed foods, fresh, frozen or dried; avoid tins.
Data from Radcliffe MJ: Clinical methods for diagnosis. Clin Immunol Allergy 1982; 2: 205–20, with permission.

obviously requires a fair degree of commitment on the part of the patient as it requires careful forward planning. The diet plan is continually modified according to the patient's sensitivities and preferences.

Whilst such a dietary prescription is unnecessarily complicated for the vast majority of food allergy sufferers, it provides a means of treatment for the occasional patient with very numerous intolerances. For such patients, particularly young children, dietary rotation provides a method of symptom control which avoids the risk of nutritional deficiency inherent in the grossly restricted diet. Whilst rotation diets can be criticized on the grounds that they are in some circumstances unnecessarily complicated and socially isolating, they should not be criticized on nutritional grounds. Indeed the basic advice, to eat from a wide range of fresh, unprocessed foods, must surely be sound wisdom.

Apart from its long-term use, the short-term adoption of a rotation diet provides the food allergy sufferer with an alternative method of identification of dietary intolerances.

SUMMARY

Despite the failure of food avoidance and challenge techniques to meet the criteria of an ideal diagnostic test, they remain the yardstick for the diagnosis of dietary allergy and intolerance. Properly performed, they provide information about the patient's intolerances which cannot be obtained in any other way. Undue emphasis on the cellular and biochemical mechanisms of disease has resulted in a failure of some of the medical profession to consider seriously the reproducible techniques of avoidance and challenge, essential to the diagnosis of food allergy, which were well described over 30 years ago.

For such studies to be valid, it is necessary for the clinician to take into account the empirical phenomena of masking addiction and tolerance and to take into account the ubiquitous nature of many of our staple foods. Considering the importance of the psychological factor, a circumspect approach is needed, and double-blind ingestion challenge techniques must be used and perfected. However, the routine use of such techniques would place an unacceptable barrier in the way of food allergy diagnosis. At the same time it must be remembered that the elimination diet, carrying as it does the risk of nutritional inadequacy, is a potentially dangerous tool.

All these techniques are subject to certain limitations, particularly to human error. At its most extreme this means that, for some of our patients, the diagnosis of food allergy with currently available techniques remains impossible. This human factor must not be overlooked. The techniques requires time and patience on the part of the diagnostician, and dedication and care, together with appropriate objectivity, on the part of the patient. Accurate diagnosis is only possible when the patient's cooperation is enlisted from the outset, and when careful training of the patient in the method of diagnosis is a planned part of the diagnostic regimen.

REFERENCES

1 Bock SA, Lee W-Y, Remigio LK, May CD: Studies of hypersensitivity reactions to foods in infants and children. J Allergy Clin Immunol 1978; 62:327.
2 Brown M, Gibney MJ, Husband PR, Radcliffe MJ: Food allergy in polysymptomatic patients. Practitioner 1981; 225:1651-4.
3 Coca AF: Familial non-reaginic food allergy. Springfield: Charles C Thomas, 1942.
4 Denman AM, Mitchell EB, Ansell BM: Dietary exclusion in patients with rheumatoid arthritis. In: The second Fisons food allergy workshop. Oxford: Medicine Publishing Foundation, 1983; 84-5.
5 Goldsborough J, Francis DEM: Dietary management. In: The second Fisons food allergy workshop. Oxford: Medicine Publishing Foundation, 1983; 89-94.
6 Golos N, Golbitz FG, Leighton FS: Coping with your allergies. New York: Simon and Schuster, 1979.
7 Hunter JO, Alun Jones V, Freeman AH et al: Food intolerance in gastrointestinal disorders. In: The second Fisons food allergy workshop. Oxford: Medicine Publishing Foundation, 1983; 69-72.
8 Lessof MH, Wraith DG, Merrett TG et al: Food allergy and intolerance in 100 patients—local and systemic effects. Q J Med 1980; 49:259.
9 McEwen LM, Constantinopolous P: The use of a dietary and antibacterial regimen in the management of intrinsic asthma. Ann Allergy 1970; 28:256-66.
10 Mackarness R: Stone age diet for functional disorders. Med World (Lond) 1959; 9:114.
11 May CD: Objective clinical and laboratory studies of immediate hypersensitivity reactions to foods in asthmatic children. J Allergy 1977; 58:500-15.
12 May CD, Bock SA: A modern clinical approach to food hypersensitivity. Allergy 1978; 33:166-88.
13 Miller JB: Hidden food ingredients, chemical food additives and incomplete food labels. Ann Allergy 1978; 41:93-8.

14 Monro JA, Brostoff J, Carini C, Zilkha K: Food allergy in migraine. Lancet 1980; ii:1-4.

15 Randolph TG: Descriptive features of food addictions, addictive eating and drinking. Q J Stud Alcohol 1956; 17:198.

16 Randolph TG: An ecological orientation in medicine—comprehensive environmental control in diagnosis and therapy. Ann Allergy 1965; 23:7.

17 Randolph TG: The role of specific sugars. In: Dickey LD, ed. Clinical ecology. Springfield: Charles C Thomas, 1976; 310-20.

18 Randolph TG: The role of specific alcoholic beverages. In: Dickey LD, ed. Clinical ecology. Springfield: Charles C Thomas, 1976; 321-33.

19 Rinkel HJ: Food allergy. I. The role of food allergy in internal medicine. II. The technique and clinical application of individual food tests. Ann Allergy 1944; 2:504.

20 Rinkel HJ, Randolph TG, Zeller M: Food allergy. Springfield: Charles C Thomas, 1951. (Reprinted 1971 by the New England Foundation for Allergic and Environmental Diseases.)

21 Rowe AH: Food allergy, its manifestations, diagnosis and treatment. J Am Med Assoc 1928; 91:1623.

22 Rowe AH, Rowe MD: Food allergy, its manifestations and control and the elimination diets. Springfield: Charles C Thomas, 1972.

23 Russell M, Dark KA, Cummins RW et al: Learned histamine release. Science 1984; 225:733-4.

24 Warner JO, Hathaway MJ: Dietary treatment of eczema due to food intolerance. In: The second Fisons food allergy workshop. Oxford: Medicine Publishing Foundation, 1983; 105-8.

25 Workman E, Hunter JO, Alun Jones V: The allergy diet—how to overcome your food intolerance. Martin Dunitz, 1984.

Chapter 47
Diagnosis of Gastrointestinal Food-allergic Diseases in Childhood

R. P. K. Ford, A. D. Phillips and J. A. Walker-Smith

Introduction

Various approaches have been taken to the problem of diagnosis of gastrointestinal food-allergic disease. As described in Chapter 33, the types of adverse reaction can be broadly divided into quick and slow onset reactions. The quick onset reactions are relatively easy to recognize whereas the slow onset reactions are difficult to diagnose, hence the search for reliable and practical objective diagnostic tests. So far the gastrointestinal tests which have been employed in the diagnosis of the slow onset reactions have been based either on proximal small intestinal biopsy or on tests of gut function (Table 47.1). This chapter primarily concentrates on the diagnosis of gastrointestinal milk hypersensitivity since the majority of studies have dealt with this food. Other foods will be mentioned as appropriate.

Table 47.1 Gastrointestinal tests so far employed in the diagnosis of gastrointestinal food-allergic disease.

Small intestinal biopsy
  Light microscopy
  Morphometry
  Electron microscopy
  Mucosal immunoglobulins
  Disaccharidase estimation
One-hour blood-xylose test
Breath hydrogen test
Colonoscopy
Colonic biopsy

SMALL INTESTINAL BIOPSY

Light microscopy

The diagnostic role of small intestinal biopsy for gastrointestinal milk hypersensitivity has evolved with time. The first observation made with this technique was that cow's milk protein could produce severe small intestinal mucosal damage in young infants who were failing to thrive. This relationship between cow's milk protein and mucosal damage was recognized by means of serial biopsies taken before and after milk provocation [32,73]. It has been suggested that evidence of small intestinal mucosal damage should be included in the criteria for the routine diagnosis of gastrointestinal milk hypersensitivity in infancy [26], but this is not generally practicable. This approach has however led to the recognition of cow's milk sensitivity enteropathy as a definite diagnostic entity [74] but it has also established that histological damage following cow's milk ingestion does not always lead to the development of clinical symptoms [67,69]. However, it is also clear that not all children with gastrointestinal symptoms that are clearly produced by cow's milk ingestion have recognizable small intestinal mucosal damage [15,21].

Milk-induced small intestinal mucosal damage

There are widely conflicting reports on the incidence and degree of small intestinal mucosal damage following cow's milk challenge, as seen by light microscopy, ranging from 0 to 100% of patients studied (Table 47.2). There

reaction to milk. The degree of damage observed will depend upon the amount of time elapsed between milk ingestion and small intestinal biopsy. Mucosal changes have been observed to occur within the first 24 hours [68,69], and after several weeks [67] of continuing milk ingestion. More often they occur within 24–28 hours [74]. With quick onset reactions usually only small amounts of milk can be taken because either it is rapidly vomited, or serious reactions may preclude further drinking. This would give little opportunity for mucosal damage to occur. However, from experimental studies in animals it would appear likely in any event that minimal histological changes would be seen [10]. Thus normal mucosa may be present with quick onset reactions. However, both Type I and IV reactions may coincide.

2 The degree of mucosal damage is to some extent related to the amount of milk ingested. In the first reports of mucosal damage due to cow's milk [34], infants had had prolonged exposure to milk and correspondingly severe damage to the gastrointestinal mucosa. Later studies [21], with biopsies performed at the onset of symptoms when relatively little milk had been given, reported both a lower incidence and decreased severity of mucosal damage.

Table 47.2 Light microscopy mucosal changes in gastrointestinal milk hypersensitivity.

Authors	Symptomatic patients		Biopsy timing*	Number (%) of abnormal biopsies
	Number	Age range		
Kuitunen et al [31]	6	2–4 months	varied	6 (100%)
Walker-Smith et al [74]	5	0–3 months	24 hours	5 (100%)
Iyngkaran et al [26]	7‡	0–3 months	24 hours	7 (100%)
Kuitunen et al [34]	48	0–9 months	when symptomatic	47 (98%)
Fontaine and Navarro [11]	31	3–7 months	varied	30 (97%)
Morin et al [57]	7	3–24 months	when symptomatic	5 (71%)
Silver and Douglas [70]	3	2–4 months	NS†	2 (66%)
Shiner et al [68,69]	6	5–8 months	6–23 hours	4¶ (66%)
Freier et al [15]	6	0–3 months	NS	2 (33%)
Hill et al [21]	9	7–17 months	at onset of symptoms	3 (33%)
Lubos [41]	18	3 months–8 years	NS	0 (0%)

* Time elapsed from cow's milk ingestion to small bowel biopsy.
† NS = not stated.
‡ Four other children had moderate changes but no symptoms.
¶ Two of these children were asymptomatic.

are many important variables to take into account when interpreting small intestinal mucosal changes which may explain most of these differences.

1 Time and the type of allergic reaction induced in the gut are important. Time is needed for histological damage to occur after cow's milk ingestion in those with slow onset

3 Age and nutritional status are likely to influence the degree of small bowel mucosal damage. With increasing age, an increased tolerance to milk is seen and mucosal damage may be more limited. This may explain the lack of mucosal damage in the older group of patients studied by Lubos [41]. In children with a poor nutritional status, as in some of the earlier studies, mucosal damage may be modified by the associated depression of the immune and inflammatory response.

4 Coincidental gastrointestinal infection and parasitic infestation (mostly giardiasis) must be carefully excluded.

5 Technical details of the biopsy, the numbers of biopsies taken, the orientation and interpretation of the section and application of quantitative techniques must be also taken into consideration when evaluating the literature on this subject.

6 The selection of the patients in the above studies was varied. In some studies only those patients who had less severe small intestinal mucosal damage were studied.

Small intestinal biopsy on its own is not the specific test for gastrointestinal food allergy but it plays a useful diagnostic role in detecting gastrointestinal food allergy, especially in infants less than a year of age. Its main value has been to establish by means of a serial biopsy that a number of foods namely soya [1], chicken meat, ground rice, fish [72] and eggs [23] may all temporarily damage the small intestinal mucosa, thus introducing the concept of food-sensitive enteropathy. However, it is clear that a normal small intestinal mucosa may be found in some children with gastrointestinal food allergy.

Morphometry

In addition to histological evaluation of the small intestinal mucosa by light microscopy, accurate measurements of tissue dimensions and cell numbers can be made, providing a quantitative, objective assessment of small bowel appearance. This technique of quantitative morphometry has been applied to the mucosa of children with cow's milk-sensitive enteropathy [30, 62, 71]. When on a milk-containing diet the mucosa is thinner than in normal controls, with crypt depth lengthening, shortening of the villi and reduction of epithelial cell height (Table 47.3) [47]. The numbers of intraepithelial lymphocytes are increased in the untreated disease. When treated with a cow's milk-free diet, their numbers diminish

Table 47.3 Morphometric changes in the intestinal mucosa in milk-sensitive enteropathy.

Thin mucosa
Crypt lengthening
Villus shortening
Epithelial cell height reduced
Intraepithelial lymphocytes increased

to below normal levels, and on challenge rise to within the normal range [62].

This mucosal lesion is quite different to that seen in coeliac disease. In food-sensitive enteropathy there is less crypt lengthening, a thinner mucosa, typically a patchy enteropathy [48] and usually smaller numbers of intraepithelial lymphocytes, whereas in coeliac disease the crypts are long, the mucosal is of normal thickness, of uniform severity and with very high levels of intraepithelial lymphocytes.

Electron microscopy

This technique gives greatly improved resolution allowing study of cellular detail. There are however only a few studies of electron microscopic changes in small bowel mucosa in children with gastrointestinal food hypersensitivity. The problems encountered with electron microscopy are similar to those of small bowel biopsy but also include the following.

1 Ultrastructural changes may be apparent before histological changes.

2 Only small areas of mucosa can be examined and so the possibility that observed changes may not be representative must always be borne in mind.

3 Helps to exclude viral or bacterial infection—both in tissue and by negative staining electron microscopy of stools.

4 Orientation, as in light microscopy, is important. Full mucosal thickness must be studied and not just part of the mucosa.

Ultrastructure following food challenge

Kuitunen et al [33] first described electron microscopic changes in three infants aged 3–7 months. One child developed vomiting, diarrhoea and a shock-like state within two hours of drinking 5 ml of fresh milk. A duodenal biopsy at 20 hours showed shortening of microvilli, abnormality of nuclear shape, loss of perpendicular orientation of nuclei, increased numbers of lysosomes in the apical part of cell and infiltration of lymphocytes into the surface epithelium. The other two children had very late onset reactions with the development of anorexia, tiredness and failure to thrive after 20 and 38 days, respectively, of continued milk ingestion. The electron microscopic changes were similar, but more marked than those of the first child, and in addition there were continuous accumulations of undulating and whirled collagen fibres at the thickened basal lamina. These abnormalities disappeared after four weeks of a strict milk-free diet. All three children had light microscopic abnormalities of bowel mucosa prechallenge which makes interpretation of the electron microscopic changes after challenge very difficult.

Rossipal [66] described electron microscopic changes after milk ingestion in three children, but their ages, the types of adverse reaction and the timing of biopsies were not stated. As well as enterocyte changes, he reported swelling and vacuolation of capillary endothelial cells, perivascular membrane thickening and infiltration by active plasma cells and numerous lymphocytes. Also Shiner et al [68, 69] described six infants from 5 to 11 months old, again with similar electron microscopic changes after milk ingestion. Two children out of three had electron microscopic changes but no clinical symptoms. Finally, two infants with soya-sensitive enteropathy had been shown to have mucosal changes demonstrated by scanning electron microscopy [63].

Evaluation with the electron microscope adds a further important dimension to the assessment of small intestinal mucosal biopsy. Its particular role is to exclude acute viral infection which can be misinterpreted as an acute reaction to milk. Rapid electron microscopy of stools is of more practical value. This may preclude the necessity for a small intestinal biopsy in the situation where a child develops acute vomiting and diarrhoea after a cow's milk challenge.

Mucosal immunoglobulins

Immunoglobulins can be demonstrated in the gastrointestinal mucosa by immunofluorescence and immunoperoxidase-staining techniques (see Chapter 7), but there is conflicting evidence over the classes of antibodies that are involved in the immune response in children with gastrointestinal milk hypersensitivity (Table 47.4).

Shiner et al [68, 69] have presented evidence that an IgE-mediated reaction occurs within the first 24 hours, followed by mast-cell degranulation. They studied six infants aged 3–8 months who had a history of diarrhoea and vomiting after drinking milk, but postchallenge only two had adverse reactions. Small bowel biopsies were performed on all children before milk challenge and again within the following 24 hours. Four children, including the two with positive milk challenge, had immunoglobulin changes in the small bowel mucosa, particularly with increases in IgM- and IgE-containing plasma cells. No changes were found in the numbers of IgA-containing plasma cells.

An increase in IgE-producing plasma cells was also demonstrated in children with colic related to cow's milk ingestion [18]. Seven children with a history of colic related to drinking milk had duodenal biopsies repeated after seven days of milk challenge. A significant rise of IgE-producing plasma cells was seen in the lamina propria. These children were not troubled with diarrhoea or any other symptom except colic.

Increases of IgA-producing plasma cells have been found by others [28, 67, 71], as well as some elevation of IgM-producing plasma cells. Small bowel biopsies in these studies were performed after a longer exposure to milk and the increased mucosal IgA levels were reflected by increased IgA levels in serum and faeces. This increase in IgA-producing plasma cells is likely to be a morphological response

Table 47.4 Immunoglobulin mucosal changes in gastrointestinal milk hypersensitivity.

Authors	Number	Patient age	Biopsy timing*	Immunoglobulin-producing plasma cells†			
				IgG	IgA	IgM	IgE
Shiner et al [68, 69]	4	5–8 months	6–23 hours	+	−	+ +	+ +
Kilby et al [29]	2	2–4 months	4–6 days	ND‡	ND	ND	+ +
Harris et al [18]	7	2–6 months	NS¶	−	−	−	+ +
Savilahti [67]	8	2–8 months	2–24 days	−	+ + +	+	−
Jos [28]	7	NS	NS	−	+ +	±	ND
Maffei et al [46]	10	2–20 months	NS	ND	+ +	−	ND
Stern et al [71]	10	9 months, mean	NS	+ +	+ +	+ +	+ +

* Time elapsed from cow's milk challenge to small bowel biopsy.
† Increase in numbers of immunoglobulin-producing plasma cells: − = no change, + = variable, + = slight, + + = moderate, + + + = marked.
‡ ND = not done.
¶ NS = not stated.

of the small intestine to damage and not a primary abnormality [46]. Proliferation of IgA-producing plasma cells seems to take several days to appear.

Disaccharidase estimation

Disaccharidases are the enzymes, situated on the brush border of the small intestine, which hydrolyse disaccharides into their component monosaccharides. The disaccharidase activity of the mucosa is usually depressed when there is mucosal damage. Lactase activity appears to be the most vulnerable of the disaccharidase activities. Disaccharidase measurements share many of the problems of small intestinal biopsy (see above).

Adverse gastrointestinal reactions to cow's milk protein may result in damage to the small bowel mucosa, which in turn may cause secondary lactase depression. The reported degree of lactase depression in children with milk-sensitive enteropathy varies from 0 to 100% and this appears to be closely related to the extent of mucosal damage caused by the cow's milk protein (Table 47.5). Poley et al

lenge. McNeish [43] has suggested that biochemical lactose malabsorption may be common in milk hypersensitivity, but that frank clinical lactose intolerance was probably uncommon.

In vitro challenge tests

The technology is available to keep small intestinal biopsy tissue growing in tissue culture medium for several days or weeks [2]. It is therefore theoretically possible to challenge the small bowel mucosa in vitro with suspected foods and observe any subsequent tissue damage. This type of procedure has been applied in coeliac disease [28]. However, there are many problems that arise from this approach of studying an isolated piece of tissue which severely complicate the interpretation of any tissue damage.

1 Digestion of food protein commences as soon as it has been ingested and this may change both the quantity and nature of the food antigen to which the mucosa is exposed.

2 The concentration of the ingested antigen will be reduced as it becomes diluted with in-

Table 47.5 Lactase levels in gastrointestinal milk hypersensitivity.

Authors	Number	Patients' ages	Abnormal biopsies	Reduced lactase	Reduced sucrase
Lubos et al [41]	18	3 months to 8 years	0 (0%)	0 (0%)	NS*
Hill et al [21]	8	8–16 months	3 (30%)	2 (25%)	NS
Iyngkaran et al [25]	18	1–13 months	18 (100%)	17 (94%)	17 (94%)
Poley et al [64]	7	1–11 months	7 (100%)	7 (100%)	7 (100%)

*NS = not stated.

[64] found mucosal abnormalities and lactase depression in all their patients, while Lubos et al [41] found none.

Although generally the degree of lactase depression seems to correspond to the amount of intestinal mucosal damage, Harrison and Walker-Smith [20] found that in individual patients the levels of lactase did not necessarily closely correlate with mucosal morphology.

Lactose intolerance may play an important part in the symptoms of children with cow's milk protein intolerance. It has been clearly demonstrated that, although cow's milk protein alone can cause adverse gastrointestinal symptoms in milk-hypersensitive infants, these symptoms of diarrhoea, abdominal pain and irritability can also be potentiated by the addition of lactose [39]. Harrison et al [19] found both lactase depression and a degree of lactose malabsorption in the majority of their milk-hypersensitive children after milk chal-

testinal secretion and its contact with the mucosa will be limited by intestinal transit.

3 Absorption of the antigens and their subsequent entry into the systemic circulation may occur. This may be associated with stimulation of hormones and chemical mediators, all of which may play a part in, or even be the major cause of, symptoms which in turn may not necessarily be related to any pathological changes at the site of antigen entry.

4 The immune response is intimately related to the circulation, and thus in an isolated piece of tissue the immunological response will be severely curtailed. Some of these responses are protective, such as the limiting action of antigen entry, whereas other responses may be required to allow the full expression of the pathological changes.

Thus the response of an isolated piece of small intestinal mucosa in the tissue culture to food antigens may be quite unrelated to events in vivo. At present this technique can only be viewed as a research tool and great caution is needed when extrapolating the results to the clinical situation.

GUT FUNCTION TESTS

Other methods have been used to try and measure the effects of food upon the function of the small intestinal mucosa. In principle, the integrity of the small bowel can be assessed by its ability to absorb various substances and the tests used to determine changes in permeability will be discussed.

Intestinal permeability

Principles

The intestinal mucosa is a major interface between the body and the external environment. It acts as a selective barrier, actively taking up some molecules whilst excluding others. This barrier is by no means absolute and there is a degree of leakiness which allows molecules which are not actively taken up to permeate passively through the intestinal wall. The rate of this permeation depends upon many factors which include the size of the molecule, its lipid solubility, the osmolality of the intestinal fluid and the health of the intestinal mucosa. Therefore the measurement of intestinal permeability should be an indication of the state of mucosal integrity so long as these other variables are taken into account.

The clinical assessment of intestinal permeability in vivo to relatively small sugar molecules is now practicable. Three techniques are currently available which are all based on the measurement of the fraction of an orally administered molecular probe that is subsequently recovered in the urine. This can be considered as a measure of intestinal permeability provided that it is established both that the chosen probe permeates the intestinal wall by immediate diffusion and that the absorbed fraction is completely excreted in the urine [52].

The differential absorption of two or more inert sugars appears to be the most promising test. A major advantage of this technique is that by expressing the urinary excretion of the sugars as a ratio, the effects of the many variables influencing the individual sugar probes can be overcome. These variables include the adequacy of ingesting the oral load, gastric emptying time, intestinal transit time, the dilution of the marker by intestinal secretions, renal clearance and the completeness of the urine collection. The disadvantages are the difficulty in collecting any urine in small children with diarrhoea and the complexity of the assay. The relation of diarrhoea to protein permeability is unknown.

This test has been reported to be a simple, accurate and non-invasive method of measuring changes in intestinal permeability in coeliac disease [8, 54] and in gastroenteritis [59]. There is also a close correlation between this measurement of intestinal permeability and proximal intestinal mucosal morphology [13, 54] (Fig. 47.1).

This test of differential sugar absorption therefore appears to have great potential in the investigation and diagnosis of gastrointestinal food-allergic disease. It is a non-invasive test and should give an objective measurement of significant changes in the integrity of the intestinal mucosa following provocation with

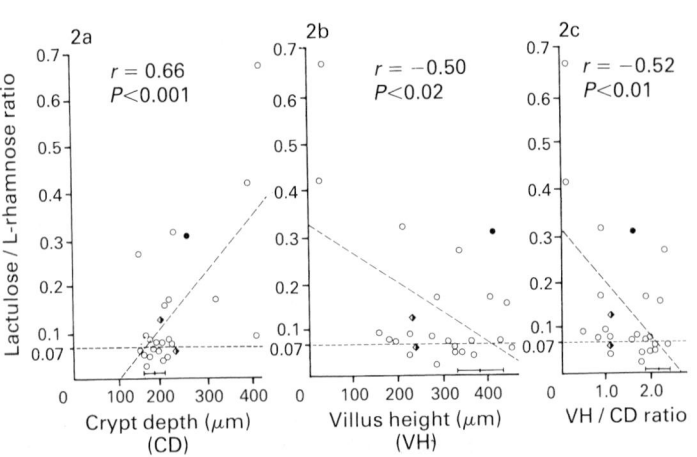

Fig. 47.1 Relationship between intestinal permeability and proximal small bowel morphology.

food. So far we have made sequential permeability measurements on three children with milk hypersensitivity using this technique (Table 47.6 and Fig. 47.2).

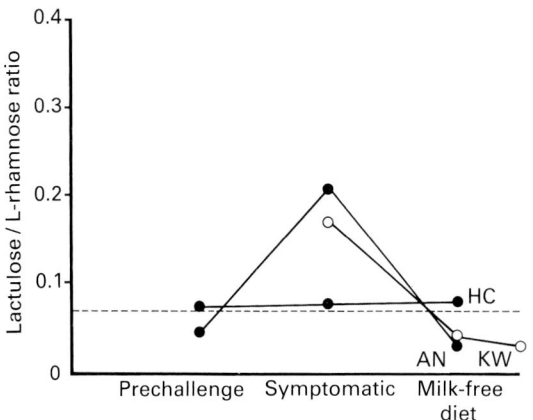

Fig. 47.2 Sequential permeability measurements in three children with milk hypersensitivity reactions.

tested, which may have a bearing on her overall tolerance to milk. The persistence of the milk permeability abnormality could indicate either some underlying gastrointestinal abnormality that might predispose to food hypersensitivity, or perhaps the existence of subclinical reactions to other foods.

This pilot study demonstrated that there were significant permeability disturbances in some children with milk allergic disease, and that sequential permeability measurements might help to objectively document clinical adverse reactions. The potential of this test of intestinal permeability apears great for the diagnosis and investigation of children with food hypersensitivity and obviously requires further development.

The other techniques available to measure intestinal permeability have serious drawbacks. The ^{51}Cr-labelled EDTA method [3] uses only one probe molecule and this loses the advantage of the differential absorption

Table 47.6 Intestinal permeability study in three patients with milk hypersensitivity.

Patient	Sex	Age (months)	Atopy					Milk reaction	
			Skin prick tests			Total IgE	Clinical	Timing	Symptoms
			Milk	Egg	Inhalants				
KW	F	2	+ +	+	0	783	Eczema	Quick	Diarrhoea, vomiting, urticaria, angioedema
AN	M	15	0	0	0	4	Nil	Slow	Diarrhoea, irritability
HC	F	35	0	+	0	72	Eczema	Slow	Diarrhoea, pallor, anorexia, irritability

Clinical findings

Child KW was atopic with a marked positive skin prick test response to milk. She had a quick onset reaction to milk and her dominant symptoms were urticaria, angioedema and vomiting. She also had diarrhoea. When on milk her intestinal permeability was quite abnormal, returning to normal when milk was again excluded from her diet.

The other two children had slow onset reactions with diarrhoea and irritability as their major symptoms. Both had negative skin prick tests to milk. Whereas child AN developed abnormal permeability with milk provocation, child HC had no such change. However, her intestinal permeability was marginally abnormal at all times. She was also mildly atopic and had exacerbation of her eczema when on milk. The possible reasons for the lack of any permeability change in this child can only be speculative. She was the eldest of the children

technique. It is dependent upon a radioisotope and thus not suitable for regular or repeated use in children. It also requires an accurate 24-hour urine collection which is not practicable for routine use with children. The other method is based on the differential absorption of polyethyleneglycol fractions [5], which also requires a 24-hour urine collection. In addition, the smaller fractions of polyethylene glycol are lipid soluble and thus its absorption is not only a function of its permeability [53].

One-hour blood-xylose test

The one-hour blood-xylose test has been widely used as a test of the function of small intestinal mucosa. It was developed as a screening test for the diagnosis of coeliac disease [65] but its accuracy and value have been severely questioned [7, 35, 36]. This test has been reported [57] as a simple and useful test in the diagnosis of milk hypersensitivity, but again this has been disputed [14, 23, 42].

Xylose is a pentose sugar which is partially absorbed by normal small intestinal mucosa. The one-hour blood-xylose test is performed by giving an oral load after a fast and then collecting a blood sample one hour later for blood-xylose measurement. About 60% of absorbed xylose is metabolised in the liver, and 40% is excreted unchanged in the urine [75]. If there is extensive damage to the small bowel mucosa then there is reduced absorption of xylose and the blood-xylose level at one hour would be expected to be low.

There are many factors that influence the absorption and the subsequent blood levels of xylose, and this test might be made more reliable if it was incorporated into a differential absorption test as in the assessment of permeability. The one-hour blood-xylose test does not appear to have any advantages over clinical observation.

Breath hydrogen test

The breath hydrogen test is a clinical method by which sugar malabsorption can be measured. The breath hydrogen test is performed by giving an oral sugar load, after a fast, and measuring exhaled breath hydrogen concentration at regular intervals for several hours. A rise in breath hydrogen concentration of more than 10–20 parts per million is evidence that the sugar has been malabsorbed. This test was first described as a method for detecting disaccharide malabsorption by Levitt and Donaldson [38]. Subsequently it has been validated and refined [4, 56, 58] and has been successfully applied to children [45, 61]. A major advantage of this test is that it is non-invasive.

The basis of the test is as follows. Unabsorbed sugar is fermented in the colon by the commensal bacterial flora; this process produces gases, including hydrogen. Hydrogen is rapidly absorbed through the mucosal wall and circulated to the lungs where gas exchange takes place, and then exhaled in the expired breath. Thus a rise in breath hydrogen concentration can be used as an indication of sugar malabsorption. Hydrogen is almost exclusively produced in the large bowel [37] although bacterial overgrowth in the small bowel has been reported to be a source [55]. The amount exhaled is proportional to the amount of intestinal hydrogen produced which in turn is related to the amount of malabsorbed sugar available for fermentation and the number and type of bacteria in the colon.

This test, using lactose as the test sugar, has been used to try and measure lactose depression caused by milk-sensitive enteropathy [13]. This test did not prove to be specific enough to use as a definitive test, but like the one-hour blood-xylose test it can be used to give objective evidence of small intestinal damage in some patients.

MUCOSAL APPEARANCE

Colonoscopy

Those infants and children who have chronic bloody diarrhoea require colonoscopy with multiple colonic biopsies. The colonoscopic features of cow's milk-sensitive colitis are erythema, friability of the mucosa and sometimes ulceration. This appearance is not specific and it needs to be distinguished from inflammatory bowel disease [6].

Colonic biopsy

Multiple mucosal biopsies taken at the time of colonoscopy characteristically show an eosinophilic infiltration of the mucosa [27], although Gryboski [17] describes changes not unlike ulcerative colitis. Cow's milk, soya protein and probably other foods can produce such a colitis.

DIAGNOSTIC APPROACH TO FOOD HYPERSENSITIVITY

We have discussed the techniques that are presently available to assess the gastro-intestinal status of a patient in relation to gastrointestinal food-allergic disease. Many of these tests may be impracticable for routine use, may not be reliable or may not yet have been sufficiently validated to be worthwhile. We therefore present our approach to the child presenting with possible gastrointestinal food-allergic disease.

Quick onset reactions

Children with quick onset reactions to foods are usually not a diagnostic problem as the symptoms are usually florid and closely associated with the ingestion of a particular food.

The children are usually atopic and investigations show an elevated total IgE. Also the response to skin prick test and RAST are positive. The approach to these children is discussed in detail in Chapter 33.

Slow onset reactions

Food-sensitive enteropathy

This diagnosis should be suspected in a child with chronic diarrhoea and poor weight gain. Food-allergic disease is only one of a number of causes for such a clinical picture, many of which can be identified by small intestinal biopsy (see Table 47.7). A scheme for approaching this problem is given in Fig. 47.3.

Small intestinal biopsy is most helpful when performed at the presentation of the illness

Table 47.7 Conditions causing chronic diarrhoea and poor growth which may be distinguished from food-sensitive enteropathy by small intestinal biopsy.

Coeliac disease
Giardiasis
Sucrase–isomaltase deficiency
Lactase deficiency
A β-lipoproteinaemia
Lymphangiectasia
Hypogammaglobulinaemia
Cystic fibrosis

when the child is still on the original diet. If the child has an enteropathy, i.e. a light microscopic abnormality, then the major diagnostic decision is between coeliac disease and food-sensitive enteropathy, although other conditions must be considered (Table 47.8). It is therefore of paramount importance to determine whether or not the child has been taking gluten in the diet.

Table 47.8 Conditions in which an enteropathy is found.

Coeliac disease
Food-sensitive enteropathies
Giardiasis
Gastroenteritis
Tropical sprue
Acquired hypogammaglobulinaemia
Congenital microvillus atrophy

Flat mucosa, on gluten. If gluten has been taken and the biopsy appears uniformly damaged, and there is a high intrapithelial lymphocyte count then coeliac disease is the most likely diagnosis and a gluten-free diet should be implemented. However, if there is no response to this diet, then the elimination of other foods should be considered as a small number of children with coeliac disease may subsequently develop sensitivities to other food proteins [11]. Where there is a positive clinical

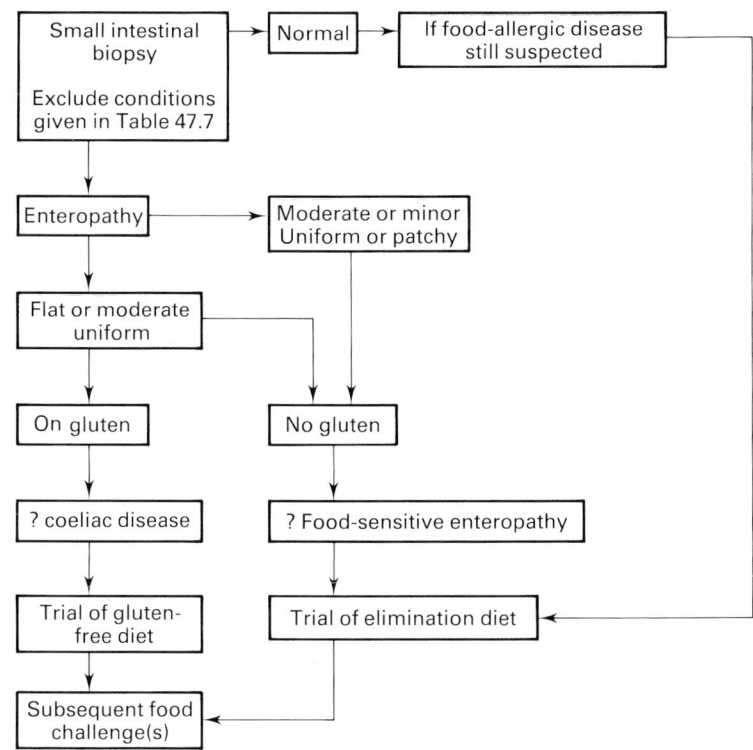

Fig. 47.3 Diagnostic approach to the investigation of possible food-sensitive enteropathy.

response to a gluten-free diet it is necessary to perform serial biopsies while off and on gluten to confirm the diagnosis [51].

Transient gluten intolerance. There are now clear criteria for the scientific diagnosis of 'transient gluten intolerance'. These are, first, the need to provide evidence that gluten toxicity was in fact present and that the apparent response to gluten restriction was not fortuitous [44]. In practice this is very difficult to do. Second is the need to show the presence of a normal small intestinal mucosa two years or more after the return to a normal gluten-containing diet. A retrospective diagnosis of transient gluten intolerance can be made when a child with features of an abnormal mucosa previously has responded to a gluten-free diet but after two years on a normal diet has a normal mucosa. However, reports of the delayed relapse of coeliac disease after more than two years on a gluten-containing diet makes the definitive diagnosis of transient gluten intolerance very difficult.

Mucosal damage, no gluten. If there is an enteropathy that is not uniformly flat then this is more likely to be caused by food sensitivity. This type of mucosal damage is characteristically patchy [48]. Most children presenting in this way are in their first six months of life and not taking gluten. A trial elimination diet, usually avoiding cow's milk, is then indicated. If there is a positive clinical response then subsequent food challenge is necessary to confirm the diagnosis.

Normal mucosa. If there is no enteropathy this does not necessarily exclude the possibility of food-allergic disease. If other conditions have been excluded and food is still suspected as causing the symptoms, then the only practical approach is a trial elimination diet. Again, milk is the most commonly implicated food but other foods may be incriminated by a carefully taken dietary history. If there is a clinical response to such an elimination diet then food provocation is needed to confirm the diagnosis.

Food-sensitive colitis

As outlined earlier, children with chronic bloody diarrhoea require colonoscopy with multiple colonic mucosal biopsies.

Food challenge

There are many problems encountered when attempting to provoke symptoms and small intestinal mucosal changes with foods. These problems need to be carefully appraised in order to achieve a balanced and practical approach to food challenges. Again milk hypersensitivity reactions have been the ones most commonly investigated and to which this discussion will be primarily related.

An objective approach to the diagnosis of milk hypersensitivity by milk provocation was first made by Goldman et al [16] whose diagnostic rules have become known as Goldman's criteria. They are as follows:

(a) Symptoms should subside following milk elimination.
(b) Symptoms should occur within 48 hours following a trial feeding of milk.
(c) Three such challenges should be positive and similar with respect to onset, duration and clinical features.
(d) Symptoms should subside following each challenge reaction.

These criteria have subsequently been adopted for the diagnosis of hypersensitivity to other foods. This approach to the diagnosis of cow's milk hypersensitivity was an important milestone in the history of the study of food intolerance. Although these criteria led to the collection of more objective evidence, and seemed to eliminate both coincidental illness with milk challenge and fortuitous recovery with milk elimination, these criteria had many serious drawbacks (see Chapter 45).

1 Some children are so sensitive to some food proteins that it may be considered unsafe to give repeated food challenges which would impose unnecessary morbidity to the child, and distress to the parents.

2 The time of onset of symptoms may be greater than 48 hours [34].

3 Symptoms may change with successive challenges depending upon circumstances such as the rate of food administration and the age of the child [15].

4 The child may have out-grown the hypersensitivity to milk by the time of the second or third challenge, and thus the diagnosis of food hypersensitivity may be incorrectly excluded.

5 Conditioned reflexes to the challenge food might have been developed, and thus adverse reactions may be predominantly psychological manifestations [40]. Double-blind studies showing this effect have been on older children and adults [49, 50] and not on infants.

6 The adverse reaction may be due to other factors and not related to the food protein at all; e.g. lactose or sucrose intolerance.

7 Subclinical reaction may be missed if the assessment is purely clinical [34].

Although Goldman himself recognized many of these faults, much use has nevertheless been made of these criteria over the past two decades, but they are no longer used in routine clinical practice. Improved criteria for the diagnosis of food hypersensitivity must therefore take these problems into consideration and may need to incorporate variations to suit the circumstances of individual adverse clinical reactions.

Generally we favour the use of open challenges. In our experience we have found that the rate of positive double-blind challenge has been the same as the rate of positive open challenges in children under five years of age. This suggests that psychological conditioning is not an important factor in the persistence of symptoms in the early years of life and most children that we see can tolerate milk by three or four years of age. In addition, children with food-sensitive enteropathies often require large amounts of milk over several days to provoke symptoms and it becomes logistically very difficult to give these volumes under double-blind conditions.

We would advocate double-blind studies in older children with persisting symptoms especially in those who report unusual symptoms. Adults who report bizarre symptoms have been found to be uniformly unresponsive to food provocation under double-blind conditions [60].

Age at challenge

The age at which the initial food provocation challenge should be done is debatable. By performing challenges in the first six months of life there is more likelihood of observing a positive reaction as the child has had little time to develop tolerance to the food. But such a reaction is likely to be more severe in this age group than in older children, with the risk of life-threatening reaction occurring [9]. It is our practice in children with a convincing history of a food hypersensitivity who have clinically responded to an elimination diet, to wait until they are 12 months old before formally challenging them. The drawback of this approach is that the diagnosis cannot be confirmed in children who have outgrown their hypersensitivity by the time of their food provocation and one then merely establishes the safety of reintroducing milk. One then has to revert to the less satisfactory diagnosis of milk elimination responsive enteropathy [22].

We recommend that the initial food challenges should be commenced under careful supervision because of both the occasional occurrence of severe reactions and the need for careful observation. There may be a considerable time delay until the development of symptoms and so it is often impossible to definitely state whether or not the food provoked the symptoms. Hence the need for some reliable objective test that indicates if an adverse response has occurred.

SUMMARY

The diagnosis of gastrointestinal food-allergic disease remains a predominantly clinical one, i.e. the response to food elimination and subsequent challenge, and so the various laboratory and clinical tests put forward for its diagnosis must still be evaluated and compared with the clinical response. It is important to ensure that symptoms associated with food provocation are not due to coincidental illness or psychological conditioning.

Small intestinal biopsy seems to be the most useful investigation test, but it is not pathognomonic. It helps exclude other gastrointestinal conditions. Mucosal damage due to food hypersensitivity might be detected with more sensitivity by tests of gut function but such tests as the one-hour blood-xylose and breath hydrogen tests have not been found to be particularly helpful. Tests of gut function require further study. The measurement of intestinal permeability appears promising at present—but likewise it is also not pathognomonic or 100% predictive.

REFERENCES

1 Ament ME, Rubin CE: Soy protein—another cause of the flat intestinal lesion. Gastroenterology 1972; 62:227–34.

2 Ashkenazi A, Idor D, Mairron M et al: Alkaline phos-phatase activity in fresh intestinal mucosa and cultured mucosal explants. J Pediatr Gastroenterol Nutr 1984; 3:210–14.

3 Bjarnason I, Peters TJ, Veall N: A persistent defect in

intestinal permeability in coeliac disease demonstrated by a ^{51}Cr-labelled EDTA absorption test. Lancet 1983; i:323–5.

4 Bond JH, Levitt MD: Quantitative measurement of lactose malabsorption. Gastroenterology 1976; 70:1058–62.

5 Chadwick VS, Phillips SF, Hofmann AF: Measurements of intestinal permeability using low molecular weight polyethylene glycols (PEG 400). Gastroenterology 1977; 73:247–51.

6 Chong SKF, Bartram C, Campbell CA et al: Chronic inflammatory bowel disease in childhood. Br Med J 1982; 284:101–4.

7 Christie DL: Use of the one-hour blood-xylose test as an indicator of small bowel mucosal disease. J Pediatr 1978; 92:725–8.

8 Cobden I, Rothwell J, Axon ATR: Intestinal permeability and screening test for coeliac disease. Gut 1980; 21:512–8.

9 De Peyer E, Walker-Smith JA: Cow's milk intolerance presenting as necrotizing enterotozing enterocolitis. Helv Paediatr Act 1977; 32:509.

10 Ferguson A: Pathogenesis and mechanisms in the gastrointestinal tract. In: Proceedings of the first Fisons food allergy workshop. Oxford: Medicine Publishing Foundation, 1980; 28–38.

11 Fontaine JL, Navarro J: Small intestinal biopsy in cow's milk protein allergy in infancy. Arch Dis Child 1975; 50:357–63.

12 Ford RPK, Barnes GL, Hill DL: Gastrointestinal milk hypersensitivity: the diagnostic value of gut function tests. Aust J Paediat 1986 (in press).

13 Ford RPK, Menzies IS, Phillips AD et al: Intestinal sugar permeability: relationship to diarrhoeal disease and small bowel morphology. J Pediatr Gastroenterol Nutr 1985; 4:568–75.

14 Ford RPK, Saxon S, Barnes GL: One-hour blood-xylose in cow's milk intolerance (Letter). Lancet 1981; ii:312.

15 Freier S, Kletter N, Gery I et al: Intolerance to milk protein. J Pediatr 1969; 75:623–631.

16 Goldman AS, Anderson DW, Sellers WA et al: Milk allergy. I. Oral challenge with milk and isolated milk protein in allergic children. Paediatrics 1963; 31:425–43.

17 Gryboski JD: Gastrointestinal milk allergy in infants. Pediatrics 1967; 40:354–62.

18 Harris M, Petts V, Renny P: Cow's milk allergy as a cause of infantile colic: immunofluorescent studies on jejunal mucosa. Aust Paediatr J 1977; 13:276–81.

19 Harrison M, Kibly A, Walker-Smith JA et al: Cow's milk protein intolerance: a possible association with gastroenteritis, lactose intolerance, and IgA deficiency. Br Med J 1976; i:1501–4.

20 Harrison M, Walker-Smith JA: Re-investigation of lactose intolerant children: lack of correlation beween continuing lactose intolerance and small intestinal morphology, disaccharidase activity and lactose tolerance tests. Gut 1977; 18:48–52.

21 Hill DJ, Davidson GP, Cameron DJS, Barnes GL: The spectrum of cow's milk allergy in childhood: clinical, gastroenterological and immunological studies. Acta Paediatr Scand 1979; 68:847–52.

22 Hutchins P, Walker-Smith JA: End-organ effects. The gastrointestinal system. Clin Immunol Allergy 1982; 2:34–77.

23 Iyngkaran N, Abidain Z: One-hour blood xylose in the diagnosis of cow's milk protein-sensitive enteropathy. Arch Dis Child 1982; 57:40–43.

24 Iyngkaran N, Abidain Z, Meng LL, Yadav M: Egg-protein-induced villous atrophy. J Pediatr Gastroenterol Nutr 1982; 1:29–35.

25 Iyngkaran N, Davis K, Robinson MJ et al: Cow's milk protein-sensitive enteropathy: an important contributing cause of secondary sugar intolerance in young infants with acute infective enteritis. Arch Dis Child 1979; 54:39–43.

26 Iyngkaran N, Robinson MJ, Prathap K et al: Cow's milk protein sensitive enteropathy: combined clinical and histological criteria for diagnosis. Arch Dis Child 1978; 53:20.

27 Jenkins HR, Milla PJ, Pincott TR et al: Food allergy: the major cause of infantile colitis. Pediatr Arch Dis Child 1984; 59:326–9.

28 Jos J: Immunohistochemical study of the intestinal mucosa in children (Abstract). Acta Paediatr Scand 1970; 59:447.

29 Kilby A, Walker-Smith JA, Wood CBS: Small intestinal mucosa in cow's milk intolerance. Lancet 1975; i:351.

30 Kuitunen P, Kosnai I, Savilahti E: Morphometric study of the jejunal mucosa in various childhood enteropathies and special references to intraepithelial lymphocytes. J Pediatr Gastroenterol Nutr 1982; 1:525–31.

31 Kuitunen P, Visakorpi JK, Hallman N: Histopathology of duodenal mucosa in malabsorption syndrome induced by cow's milk. Ann Paediatr 1965; 205:54–63.

32 Kuitunen P, Rapola J, Savilahti E, Visakorpi JK: Light and electron microscopic changes in the small intestinal mucosa in patients with cow's milk induced malabsorption syndrome. Acta Paediatr Scand 1972; 61:237.

33 Kuitunen P, Rapola J, Savilahti E, Visakorpi JK: Responses of jejunal mucosa to cow's milk in the malabsorption symptoms with cow's milk intolerance. A light- and electron-microscopic study. Acta Paediatr Scand 1973; 62:585–95.

34 Kuitunen P, Visakorpi JK, Savilahti E, Pelkunen P: Malabsorption syndrome with cow's milk intolerance, clinical findings and course in 54 cases. Arch Dis Child 1975; 50:351–6.

35 Lamabadusuriya SP, Packer S, Harries JT: Limitations of xylose tolerance test as a screening procedure in childhood coeliac disease. Arch Dis Child 1975; 50:34–9.

36 Leibman WM: Xylose test in malabsorption (Letter). J Pediatr 1979; 94:508–9.

37 Levitt MD: Production and excretion of hydrogen gas in man. N Engl J Med 1969; 281:122–7.

38 Levitt MD, Donaldson RM: Use of breath hydrogen in study of carbohydrate malabsorption. Clin Res 1968; 16:287.

39 Liu HY, Tsao MU, Moore B, Giday Z: Bovine milk protein induced intestinal malabsorption of lactose and fat in infants. Gastroenterology 1968; 54:27–34.

40 Loveless MH: Milk allergy: a survey of its incidence: experiments with masked ingestion test. J Allergy 1950; 21:489–99.

41 Lubos MC, Gerrard JW, Buchan DJ: Disaccharidase activities in milk-sensitive and celiac patients. J Pediatr 1967; 70:325–31.

42 McDonald PJ, Powell K, Goldblum RM: Serum D-xylose absorption tests: reproducibility and diagnostic usefulness in food-induced enterocolitis. J Pediatr Gastroenterol Nutr 1982; 1:533–6.

43 McNeish AS: The role of lactose in cow's milk intolerance (Abstract). Acta Paediatr Scand 1974; 63:651.

44 McNeish AS, Rolles CJ, Arthur LJH: Criteria for diagnosing temporary gluten intolerance. Arch Dis Child 1976; 51:275–8.

45 Maffei HV, Metz GL, Jenkins DJA: Hydrogen breath test: adaption of a simple technique to infants and children. Lancet 1976; 1:1110.

46 Maffei HV, Kingston D, Hill ID, Shiner B: Histopathologic changes and the immune response within the jejunal mucosa in infants and children. Paediatr Res 1979; 13:733–6.

47 Maluenda C, Phillips AD, Briddon A, Walker-Smith JA: Quantitative analysis of small intestinal mucosa in cow's milk sensitive enteropathy. J Pediatr Gastroenterol Nutr 1984; 3:349–56.

48 Manuel PD, Walker-Smith JA, France NE: Patchy enteropathy in childhood. Gut 1979; 20:211–5.

49 Maslansky L, Wein G: Chocolate allergy: a double blind study. Conn Med 1971; 35:5–9.

50 May CD: Objective clinical and laboratory study of immediate hypersensitivity reaction to foods in asthmatic children. J Allergy Clin Immunol 1976; 58:500–15.

51 Meeuwisse G: Diagnostic criteria in coeliac disease. Acta Paediatr Scand 1970; 59:461–3.

52 Menzies IS: Absorption of intact oligosaccharides in health and disease. Biochem Soc Trans 1974; 2: 1042–7.

53 Menzies IS: Transmucosal passage of inert molecules in health and disease. Falk Symposium 1984.

54 Menzies IS, Laker MF, Pounder R et al: Abnormal intestinal permeability to sugars in villous atrophy. Lancet 1979; ii:1107–9.

55 Metz G, Draser BS, Gassull MA et al: Breath-hydrogen test for small intestinal bacterial colonisation. Lancet 1976; 1:668–9.

56 Metz G, Jenkins DJA, Peters TJ et al: Breath hydrogen as a diagnostic method for hypolactasia. Lancet 1975; i:1155–7.

57 Morin CL, Buts JP, Weber A et al: One-hour blood-xylose test in diagnosis of cow's milk protein intolerance. Lancet 1979; 1:1102–4.

58 Newcomer AD, McGill DB, Thomas PJ, Hofmann AF: Prospective comparison of indirect methods for detecting lactase deficiency. N Engl J Med 1975; 293:1232–6.

59 Noone C, Menzies IS: Intestinal permeability in acute gastroenteritis of infants and adults (Abstract). Br Soc Gastroenterol 1983.

60 Pearson DJ, Rix KJB, Bently SJ: Food allergy: how much in the mind. Lancet 1983; 1:1259–61.

61 Perman JA, Barr RG, Watkins JB: Sucrose malabsorption in children. Non invasive diagnosis by interval breath hydrogen determination. J Pediatr 1978; 93:17–22.

62 Phillips AD, Rice SJ, France NE, Walker-Smith JA: Small intestinal lymphocyte levels in cow's milk protein intolerance. Gut 1979; 20:509–12.

63 Poley JR, Klein AW: Scanning electron microscopy of soy protein-induced damage of small bowel mucosa in infants. J Pediatr Gastroenterol Nutr 1983; 2:271–278.

64 Poley JR, Bhatia M, Welsh JD: Disaccharidase deficiency in infants with cow's milk protein intolerance: response to treatment. Digestion 1978; 17:97–107.

65 Rolles CJ, Kendall MJ, Nutter S, Anderson CM: One-hour blood-xylose screening-test for coeliac disease in infants and young children. Lancet 1973; ii:1043–5.

66 Rossipal E, Aubock L: Electron microscope studies on the morphological changes of the small intestinal mucosa in three infants with cow's milk intolerance (Abstract). Acta Paediatr Scand 1974; 63:654.

67 Savilahti E: Immunochemical study of the malabsorption syndrome with cow's milk intolerance. Gut 1973; 14:491–501.

68 Shiner M, Ballard J, Smith ME: The small-intestinal mucosa in cow's milk allergy. Lancet 1975; i:136–140.

69 Shiner M, Ballard J, Brook CGD, Herman S: Intestinal biopsy in the diagnosis of cow's milk protein intolerance without acute symptoms. Lancet 1975; ii:1060–3.

70 Silver H, Douglas DM: Milk intolerance in infancy. Arch Dis Child 1968; 43:17–22.

71 Stern M, Dietrich R, Muller J: Small intestinal mucosal in coeliac disease and cow's milk protein intolerance. Morphometric and immunofluorescent studies. Eur J Pediatr 1982; 139:101–5.

72 Vitoria JC, Camarero C, Sojo A et al: Enteropathy related to fish, rice and chicken. Arch Dis Child 1982; 57:44–8.

73 Walker-Smith JA: Cow's milk protein intolerance. Transient food intolerance of infancy. Arch Dis Child 1975; 50:347–50.

74 Walker-Smith JA, Harrison M, Kilby A et al: Cow's milk sensitive enteropathy. Arch Dis Child 1978; 53:375–80.

75 Wyndgaarden JB, Segal S, Foley JB: Physiological disposition and metabolic fate of infused pentoses in man. J Clin Invest 1957; 36:1395–407.

Chapter 48
Food Intolerance Masquerading as Food Allergy: False Food Allergy

D. A. Moneret-Vautrin

Introduction

Food pathology comprises different components, depending on whether the nutritional anomaly is quantitative (food illnesses from deficiencies or excesses) or qualitative. Qualitative nutritional anomalies include food toxicity, intolerances arising from enzyme deficiencies and a large group of ailments that are either immunological (food allergy) or non-immunological (false food allergies or pseudoallergic reactions).

Toxicity

Acute or chronic food toxicity, which is rarely due to foodstuff, is usually the result of a mishap. An example is death following consumption of a goulash made with tulip bulbs that had been confused with onions [42] and another is the demise of the mother of President Lincoln, following ingestion of milk from cows that had eaten the toxic plants *Eupato-rium rugosum* and *Applopappus heterophyllus* [76]. Death due to accidental consumption of *Tetraodon* fishes is another example. However, toxicity may be the result of a secondary product that appears following fermentation (polyamines of bad meat) or contamination by bacteria (botulism) or fungi (ergotism due to *Claviceps purpurea* that parasitizes cereals). It may even be due to a substance that has been fraudulently introduced, such as methyl alcohol or ethylene glycol in alcoholic drinks [54].

Enzyme deficiency

Food intolerances due to enzyme deficiency may be well defined by similar aetiological mechanisms, but the clinical symptoms may be quite different. Thus there is no clinical link among haemolytic anaemia due to deficiency of glucose-6-phosphodehydrogenase; brain and liver disease due to galactosaemia from deficiency of galactose-1-phosphate-uridyltransferase; renal intolerance to fructose caused by deficiency, predominantly of 1-phosphofructoaldolase; diarrhoea due to lactose because of deficiency of lactase; and the neuropathy of Refsum's disease from impaired oxidation of phytanic acid derived from food phytols. Toxicity and intolerance can be differentiated, since in the case of toxicity the food is entirely responsible, whilst the accident of intolerance is due to conjunction of the patient anomaly (enzyme deficiency) and a particular type of food.

Food allergy or sensitivity

The third group of qualitative food pathologies is composed of adverse reactions that are often divided, according to the mechanism, into food allergy (or food hypersensitivity) and non-immunological reactions that are variously called food sensitivity, food idiosyncrasy, pharmacological food reactions, false food allergies and pseudoallergic reactions to foods [3, 11, 46].

It has become possible to diagnose food allergy by two series of tests: firstly, by skin tests, radioallergosorbent tests and basophil degranulation tests that show evidence of specific IgE; secondly, single or double-blind provocation tests, that support the involvement of these antibodies in the pathology that is under investigation [4, 7, 47].

Having defined immediate-type food allergy and whilst retaining reservations such as where a food allergy evolves by a different mechanism, it becomes possible to diagnose the non-immunological adverse reactions. Amongst these, the false food allergies due to the histamine mechanism were the first to be recognized [45].

'False' food allergy

Three major mechanisms are recognizable in the production of symptoms by a 'false' food allergy: excessive consumption of biogenic amines, non-specific liberation of chemical mediators by mucosal mast cells and interference with the autonomic nervous system. After discussion of the clinical symptomatology, this chapter will consider these, before indicating the ways in which these reactions influence intestinal inflammatory disease, as opposed to psychological reactions to foods. Finally, the diagnostic approach to these reactions, necessarily complex because of the multiplicity of mechanisms, will be indicated.

CLINICAL SYMPTOMS OF PSEUDOALLERGIC FOOD REACTIONS

The frequency of non-immunological reactions is much greater than that of food allergy.

May [44] considers food allergy to be present in only a third of the subjects who show an intolerance and Bock only in 20% of the children [8]. In chronic urticaria, food allergy is found in less than 3% of cases [31]. Generally, false food allergy is found three times more often than food allergy when the two types of illness are investigated at the same time [47].

Clinical syndromes include anaphylactoid shock, chronic urticaria, defects of intestinal function, vasomotor headaches, rhinitis and asthma.

Anaphylactoid shock

Anaphylactoid shock is rare (1.7% of 230 cases of false food allergy) and is often due to histamine, appearing later than anaphylactic shock. Two hours after the meal the subject suffers generalized erythema with nausea, vomiting, diarrhoea and a moderate and transitory fall in blood pressure. However, serious anaphylaxis has been ascribed to metabisulphites [59].

Chronic urticaria

Chronic urticaria is very frequent and in more than 40% of cases there is a food factor, which is often due to additives. In confirming the work of Juhlin [31], Ortolani has shown the involvement of benzoic acid (20%), tartrazine (13%), metabisulphites (10%), butylhydroxytoluene and butylhydroxyanisole (10%) in the provocation of episodes [56].

Defects of intestinal function

The defects of intestinal function include slowing of digestion, epigastric acceleration, abdominal pains and intermittent diarrhoea and afflicts more than 40% of patients with chronic urticaria. When these symptoms are found, they may be diagnosed as irritable bowel syndrome. Systematic investigation for false food allergy may be helpful in this kind of patient [37].

Vasomotor headaches

Vasomotor headaches, as well as some forms of rhinitis, indicate an intolerance to amines. The presentation is most often with pain in the temporal areas, only rarely as a one-sided migraine.

Asthmatics may show symptoms on exposure to metabisulphites in legally accepted amounts. Asthma in response to exposure to benzoates, butylated hydroxytoluene (BHT) or sodium glutamate is exceptional [2, 8, 31, 37, 44, 45, 47, 56, 59]. Of patients with rhinitis 11% show intolerance to benzoic acid, tartrazine or metabisulphites [56].

Psychological symptoms

A variety of psychological symptoms which together constitute the 'hyperactive child' syndrome may be due to food intolerance or to additives. In spite of great controversy, a recent study accepts that there is a relationship, which may be indirect, between food intake and psychological symptoms [12] (see Chapters 38b and 39).

Other symptoms

Symptoms due to other causes may be aggravated secondarily by the pharmacological action of some categories of foods. For example, atopic dermatitis is aggravated by the histamine-liberating effect of tomatoes, strawberries, egg white and chocolate.

MECHANISMS OF FALSE FOOD ALLERGIES

Mechanisms of false food allergies include excessive intake of biogenic amines, liberation of mast cell mediators by non-specific stimuli; and interference by foods with the autonomic nervous system.

EXCESSIVE INTAKE OF BIOGENIC AMINES

Biogenic amines arise from decarboxylation of amino acids. In small amounts, they exert a physiological influence, in particular vasoactivity. They are present in different foods or are synthesized locally in the intestine by microorganisms (Table 48.1) [75].

Table 48.1 Amounts of biogenic amines in different foods, in mg/100 g or mg/100 ml according to Hanington [24], Moneret-Vautrin [47].

Aliments	Histidine	Histamine	Tyramine	Phenylethylamine
Fermented cheese		Up to 133		
Camembert	600		2–8.6	
Brie			18	
Gruyère			51	
Cheddar	600		146	1.2–3.5
Roquefort			Raised, variable	
Parmesan	1050			
Brewer's yeast				
Baker's yeast		Up to 283	150	
Soused herrings		350	303	
Wine		2		
Chianti			2.5	
Cream cheese	93			1.2–6
Chocolate				2–12 ppm
Sauerkraut		16		
Dry pork and sausage	1400	22		
Tinned anchovy, tuna		2–3		
Tinned smoked herring's eggs		35		
Tuna		0.5		
Sardine		1.5		
Salmon		0.7		
Anchovy fillets		4.5		
Meats		1		
Roast venison	1290			
Milk	12			
Peanuts, avocado	680		2.3	
Tomato		2	0.4	
Spinach		3.7		

Table 48.2 Duodenal instillation of histamine (1.75 mg/kg) or placebo in 13 healthy volunteers (double-blind study).

Substance	n	Pulse		Systolic BP		Diastolic BP	
		Before	After	Before	After	Before	After
Placebo	6	81	73	128	113*	69	64
Histamine	7	78	105*	132	116*	72	58*

After = 3 mins after.
BP = blood pressure.
*$P < 0.05$.

Accidents from excessive ingestion of food rich in histamine

Clinical symptoms. The symptoms vary and include histamine shock, urticaria, headaches or migraines and anomalies of intestinal function [45]. Duodenal intake of histamine in normal subjects does not provoke symptoms up to 2.75 mg/kg. At 1.75 mg/kg the only clinical signs were a tachycardia and a transient diastolic hypotension which lasted less than 5 minutes (Table 48.2). In 77 patients who presented with this pathology, an abnormal response was observed in 58%. As well as the symptoms already quoted, headaches occurred in 64%, tachycardia in 40%, urticaria in 28%, abdominal disturbance in 9%, hypotension in 6.5% and bronchospasm in 2%. Overall, the signs are long-lasting, observed in the 10th minute and often persisting for half an hour. Similar anomalies of response following intestinal provocation with histamine have been reported by other authors [29].

Histamine can be synthesized in excess by the normal flora of the colon and this may assume a significant secondary role following abuse of starchy foods that are rich in cellulose and starch. Histamine of bacterial origin passes through the intestinal mucosa that has been already irritated by organic acids generated by fermentation. This may explain some of the urticarias in those who eat large amounts of starchy foods.

Excessive consumption of foods that are rich in histidine may favour endogenous synthesis of histamine and this, at doses much less than that of exogenous histamine, seems to be much more reactive [22].

Intolerance to tyramine

This was characterized following accidents seen in subjects undergoing antidepressive treatment with inhibitors of monoamine oxidase. Foods rich in tyramine cause flushing followed by a pulsating headache and sudden hypertension.

Several deaths have been described following tyramine ingestion whilst the patients were taking monoamine oxidase inhibitors. Very small doses, (± 6 mg) can start the symptoms.

Tyramine is present in some foods (Table 48.1) or is formed from tyrosine by intestinal microorganisms. It is catabolized by a monoamine oxidase, intestinal and renal, or eliminated by the intestine and kidney in either the free form or as a conjugate (Fig. 48.1). A potent vasoconstricting amine, it also liberates noradrenaline from the adrenergic neurones as

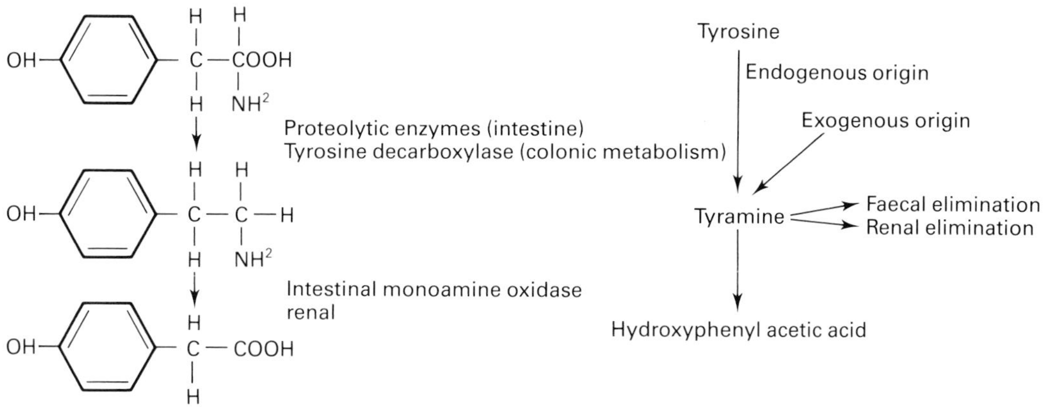

Fig. 48.1 Metabolism of tyramine.

well as histamine and prostaglandins from mast cells [24]. This intolerance is expressed as headaches or true migraines or as urticaria. A dose of 100 mg, normally well tolerated, triggers headaches in 15% of patients who suffer from migraine [24]. Urticaria to tyramine is provoked in 11% of cases of chronic urticaria by a dose of 100 mg and 5% of subjects react at a dose of 40 mg.

Phenylethylamine

Phenylethylamine has been detected in chocolate and fermented cheeses and arises from decarboxylation of phenylalanine. The titre increases with the degree of maturity of the cheese and the roasting of the cocoa seeds [66]. This vasoactive amine can cause migraines at a dose of 3 mg (found in 50 to 100 g of chocolate) [24, 65, 66].

Failure of protective mechanisms

Excessive intake of whatever biogenic amine does not seem to be enough to explain all the accidents seen clinically. Failure of normal protective mechanisms can be postulated at two levels (Fig. 48.2).

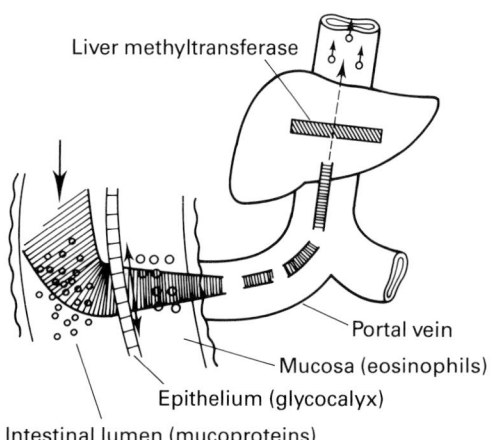

Fig. 48.2 The route of exogenous histamine in the digestive tract.

At the intestinal level

Parrot and Mordelet-Dambrine have shown in the guinea pig the importance of the mucoproteins that are secreted locally by the intestinal epithelium [53]. The mucoproteins pass into the intestinal juice and cover the brush border of the enterocytes. They fix and inactivate some histamine. That part of histamine which

is unfixed at this level passes into the mucosa and is subject to enzymic destruction (monoamine oxidase and acetylase) or undergoes phagocytosis by the eosinophils [33, 40, 43].

At the hepatic level

Histamine that is transmitted through the portal vein may be degraded by hepatic histaminase : methyltransferase [40]. The synthesis of this enzyme is decreased by 50% in viral hepatitis [73].

A study on volunteers who have had a cholecystectomy has shown that portal histamine remains stable if 72 mg of histamine is instilled into the duodenum. If more than 108 mg is instilled, the digestive mucosa allows histamine to pass into the portal vein. Up to a dose of 180 mg there is a corresponding raised portal histamine level, but the liver maintains a normal posthepatic level [52].

It can be seen, therefore, that healthy subjects tolerate high levels of histamine in food. The causes of intolerance may be due to abnormal permeability of the intestinal mucosa, enzymic insufficiency (inhibition of histaminase by isoniazid) or to portocaval shunts in cirrhosis.

Sodium nitrite. Sodium nitrite, currently used, sometimes in large amounts, as a preservative in preserved meats [47] may provoke intolerance to amines by its multiple actions. Experimentally, it damages the digestive epithelium, provokes vasodilation that enhances permeability and inhibits monoamine oxidases. It may also denature the mucoproteins of the intestinal juice and alters their capacity to handle histamine [63].

Monoamine oxidases

A common requirement for vasoactive amines (histamine, tyramine, phenylethylamine) is monoamine oxidases of types A and B which are present in the intestinal mucosa, the liver, the kidneys, etc. Platelet monoamine oxidase of type B metabolizes tyramine and phenylethylamine. A deficiency of platelet monoamine oxidase has been described in patients with migraine and also as a functional abnormality of platelet aggregation [64]. Vasoconstriction initiated by the amines enhances platelet aggregation and is itself followed by release of 5-hydroxytryptamine, thereby augmenting the amount of vasoactive amines, which are insufficiently degraded because of the deficiency in monoamine oxidase. These processes explain migraines caused by amines [24].

LIBERATION OF CHEMICAL MEDIATORS FROM MAST CELLS BY NON-SPECIFIC STIMULI

Foods implicated

The best documented examples of damage are those due to the release of histamine. Some foods have the properties of histamine liberators, such as ovomucoid from egg white, crustaceans (prawns especially), strawberries, tomatoes, fish, pork, chocolate [67] and also pineapple and papaya that contain proteolytic enzymes (bromelain, papain), as well as alcohol from acetaldehyde. The roles of leguminous plants and peanuts are probably connected with their contents of histidine and lectins [26].

Clinical syndrome in childhood

Histamine-release illnesses follow a different course in children and adults. In the young child between 3 and 8 years old, this type of disorder is often observed where there is an atopic background (atopic dermatitis, asthma due to dust mites, or hay fever) with a particular tendency to release histamine. The child, often not weighing a great deal, is greedy and the ingestion of histamine-releasing foods, which it likes (strawberry, chocolate), is excessive.

Apart from the common histamine-dependent symptoms (urticaria, angioedema), there may be exacerbation of aphthous stomatitis or of atopic dermatitis. In 300 infants with eczema, the foods most often incriminated in the attacks are histamine liberators: fish (43% of cases), eggs (24%) and chocolate (20%) [61]. The growing child becomes less sensitive to histamine release as it gets older. After 8 years of age, the previously incriminated foodstuffs can be ingested without causing a reaction. However, the patient faithfully retains the notion of the 'allergy to strawberries' that never was. More than 100 of these subjects were studied by skin tests and basophil degranulation: not one case was positive.

Clinical syndrome in adults

In the adult, non-specific histamine release effects result from the excessive consumption of 'fast' or readymade foods (chocolate, egg, fish, pork chops, tomatoes, etc.). An example is provided by the individual who develops localized urticaria and erythema on the forehead (or more florid symptoms of histamine shock), in the quarter hour following the ingestion of an aperitif on an empty stomach, together with peanuts, almonds, etc.

The site of non-specific histamine release

In the case of constitutional eczema, excess consumption of the above-mentioned foods often provokes a pruritus that is localized around the lesions. There is a secondary extension of the eczema following scratching. The eczematous skin is very rich in mast cells [30] and local degranulation is therefore very likely.

However, it seems possible that degranulation may be more pronounced in the particularly numerous ($20\,000/mm^3$) [6] mast cells of the digestive mucosa than in the skin which has only $7000/mm^3$. Several authors have shown degranulation in the course of food allergy [69]. The experimental models, however, seem to indicate that they are refractory to non-specific histamine liberation by Compound 48/80, peptide 401 of bee venom or phosphatidylserine [58]. In man, mast cells are refractory to formyl-methionine peptide, though they react with anti-IgE serum [16]. In subjects who present a false food allergy, duodenal mucosal biopsies show massively degranulated mast cells in sharp contrast to those seen in controls [51]. This supports the hypothesis that the digestive mucosal mast cells may be abnormally sensitive to histamine liberation in some subjects, children in particular.

Triggering mechanisms for non-specific histamine release

Lectins. Some substances act directly on the cell membrane, such as basic oligopeptides or proteolytic enzymes [70]. The lectins of vegetables and peanuts are glycoproteins, reinforced in activity by different sugars. Lectins bind to carbohydrate residues on enterocytes and in experimental situations lead to epithelial changes and hyperpermeability of the mucosa [41]. This may facilitate their access to mucosal mast cells. Lectins may also act by bridging the membrane IgE, by linking either the carbohydrates of the Fc fragments, like concanavalin A, or the Fab fragments like staphylococcal protein A [11]. We have seen human mucosal mast-cell degranulation in five cases of false food allergy after in vitro incubation of a mucosal biopsy with concanavalin A [51] (see Chapter 21).

Endotoxin. It has also been suggested that bacterial endotoxin or substances from fungi that have contaminated foods may activate the alternative complement pathway and lead to the formation of anaphylatoxins C3a and C5a, which are histamine liberators [11].

Mineral or enzyme deficiency. There are other factors that favour the appearance of food histamine accidents. For example, a deficiency of cellular magnesium has been observed in about half of those who present with false food allergy. This deficiency can alter histamine release and increase the sensitivity of histamine in the same way as has been shown in rats [9, 19, 25]. A deficiency of the enzyme acetaldehyde dehydrogenase, which is frequent amongst Japanese, is accompanied by signs of histamine liberation on ingestion of alcohol. These symptoms are due to the badly metabolized acetaldehyde, large quantities of which are present in the plasma [25].

Chemical mediators other than histamine

Aspirin and benzoate intolerance

Metabolism of membrane phospholipids is modified by certain additives. Around 10% of patients who are intolerant to aspirin show rhinitis, asthma or urticaria to tartrazine, other azo dyes, benzoic acid, butylhydroxytoluene or butylhydroxyanisole [68].

The mechanism of intolerance to aspirin and to other non-steroid anti-inflammatory drugs is linked to their capacity to inhibit cyclooxygenase. Sodium salicylate, which is close to aspirin, but which does not have this property, is better tolerated by these patients. For this reason there is no need for a diet that is low in salicylates. In contrast, for subjects who are very sensitive to benzoates, a temporary diet is indicated that is low in fruits such as grapes and in vegetables, which are naturally rich in benzoic acid. These subjects risk serious reactions with injectable drugs that contain this preservative [50].

The mechanism of action of these additives is obscure, as they do not inhibit cyclooxygen-

ase. Larsen believes that they may act as competitive substrates to arachidonic acid [36].

Prevention of clinical reactions. The possibility of prevention of clinical reactions to benzoic acid by pretreatment with free radical scavengers presupposes that these free radicals are the cause of the clinical problem [48]. Some reactions of intolerance to metabisulphites may be the result of free radicals produced by the oxidizing effect of the sulphites on the unsaturated membrane fatty acids. Sulphurous anhydride can also combine with the epoxide of HPETES, forming a conjugate that may have the properties of slow reacting substance A (SRSA) [60].

Release of inflammatory mediators. A possible disequilibrium of the catabolism of arachidonic acid, with excessive production of prostaglandins, has been postulated by Lessof [39] to be present in some subjects intolerant of milk. Abnormal production of other mediators of cytoplasmic origin, such as neutrophil chemotactic factor, has been noted in some cases of asthma due to milk, where immunological mechanisms have not been found [39].

Whatever chemical mediators are liberated in some reactions to foods, the possibility that the mucosal mast cells are involved is of great importance. The local consequences of mast-cell degranulation are hyperpermeability of the epithelium and small vessels and the absorption of a battery of food substances. This may lead to further sensitization so that false food allergy may be complicated by true food hypersensitivity.

INTERFERENCE BY FOODS WITH THE AUTONOMIC NERVOUS SYSTEM

Interference by foods, or most often, food additives, occur with the receptors of the autonomic nervous system, sometimes peripheral (adrenergic and cholinergic receptors) and sometimes in the central nervous system (medullary transmission and the hypothalamus).

Methylxanthines

Intolerance to the methylxanthines, caffeine, theobromine, theine, that are contained in coffee, Coca-Cola, chocolate and tea, has been well described. Some subjects when given a normally well-tolerated dose of 100 mg of caffeine, develop headaches, tachycardia, anxiety, abdominal pains and even cardiac arrhythmia or hypertension [13]. It is known that caffeine produces endogenous secretion of catecholamines [18]. These subjects show particular sensitivity to adrenergic stimuli, which can be demonstrated by perfusion with isoprenaline [23]. The same patients experience reactions to dental local anaesthetics, because of intolerance of the sympathomimetic vasoconstrictor associated with the anaesthetic (see Chapter 23).

Metabisulphites

Intolerance to metabisulphites, which is a frequent preservative in carbonated drinks, wines and raw vegetable salads, has been frequently described [17, 28, 71]. It seems to be most frequent in those patients who have nasal polyps, intrinsic asthma and intolerance to aspirin. In these subjects skin manifestations or anaphylactoid shock are sometimes seen. Most often the symptoms consist of rhinitis or asthma, which may occur within 2 minutes following the ingestion. Symptoms seem to appear in response to a vagal reflex, triggered by irritation of the tracheobronchial receptors by sulphurous anhydride inhaled during the ingestion [17, 71]. Stimulation of production of free radicals may explain some slower reactions [60].

Monosodium glutamate

Intolerance to sodium glutamate provokes the 'Chinese restaurant' syndrome [34]. Ingestion of a usual amount, at least 0.5 g, triggers flushing, sweating, loss of coordination, headache and hypotension. The clinical picture is that of an acute intoxication with acetylcholine. Glutamic acid and sodium are precursors in the synthesis of acetylcholine and ingestion of sodium glutamate provokes a sudden synthesis of acetylcholine [20]; a diminution of pseudocholinesterases can also be seen. This is especially noted in subjects who have a high plasma level of sodium glutamate because of reduced metabolism, probably due to a deficiency of vitamin B_6.

Metabisulphites. Triggering of an asthma attack has only been observed in those who present with the Chinese restaurant syndrome, or in asthmatics with intolerance to metabi-

sulphites. Allen, using much higher doses (2.5–5 g) than the usual European consumption, obtained asthmatic reactions in 12 of 32 patients tested [1]. In our studies a dose of 2.5 g did not lead to reduced forced expiratory volume in seven allergic asthmatic subjects, 17 patients with intrinsic asthma and nasal polyps (of whom 10 had intolerance to aspirin) or 4 of 5 patients who presented with the triad and in addition intolerance to metabisulphite or benzoates. Only one responded with moderate bronchospasm, several hours afterwards (Fig. 48.3).

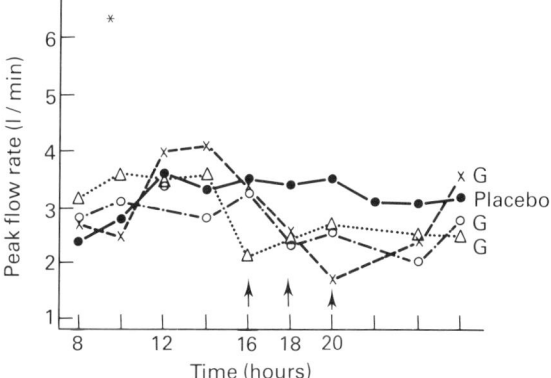

Fig. 48.3 Results of challenges with sodium glutamate (2.5 g) in a 36-year-old male. Challenges, on separate days, with placebo (once) or sodium glutamate (three times), in a patient with triad: nasal polyposis, intrinsic asthma, intolerance to metabisulphites. ⋆ = normal value of peak flow rate, according to age and height.

It is probable that only those asthmatics who are extremely sensitive to cholinergic stimuli produce asthma with doses of sodium glutamate that are higher than those usually used. However, the frequency of reactions detected by Allen invites consideration that the sodium glutamate used in Australia, without doubt from sugar cane, may be different from that which is available in Europe from sugar beet. It could be postulated that contaminants, products of the metabolism of moulds of sugar cane, may be responsible for the reactions that are observed with glutamate of Asian origin.

Effect of additives on hypothalamic neurones

A new concept concerning the action of certain additives such as glutamate and aspartate, concerns their action on immature hypothalamic neurones. Work on newborn rats has led Olney to make a hypothesis under the name of 'excitotoxins' and to launch an alarm cry against the great usage of these additives for infants [55]. Other experimental studies in vitro have shown possible interference by dyes (xanthines and erythrosine) in cholinergic and dopaminergic neurotransmission [5, 35].

In newborn mice, exposure to butylated hydroxytoluene and butylated hydroxyanisole in utero induces a fall in cerebral serotonin and noradrenaline as well as cholinesterase activity. The animals also show behavioural problems, such as aggressiveness, sleepiness and disorientation [72].

Although these data do not establish an actual link with clinical symptoms in man, this work does suggest the hypothesis that behavioural problems in children (the hyperactive child with no organic cerebral alteration) may be linked with abuse of consumption of additives such as dyes and benzoic acid. This hypothesis, which has been passionately contested, has rarely been given serious consideration [12, 74]. Some disturbing observations, in a sea of non-scientific publications, suggest that this possibility should not be rejected absolutely (see Chapter 38b).

DIAGNOSIS OF FALSE FOOD ALLERGY

Alcoholic intolerance

Diagnosis of false food allergy is difficult because of the multiplicity of mechanisms which cause multiple possibilities of action of a single food. Intolerance to alcohol is particularly instructive, since it may, exceptionally, provoke an anaphylactic shock to the alcohol, to cereal antigens (whisky, bourbon), potato (vodka), aniseed (pastis), papain (beers), quinine (aperitifs), etc. Many delayed-onset headaches from white wine are due to an intolerance to tyramine, whilst flush and erythema suggests a histamine reaction that is more often found with red and fortified wines. Almost immediate rhinitis and asthma show an intolerance to metabisulphites. If the reaction is delayed, it is necessary to look for an intolerance to benzoic acid or dyes of aperitifs and digestifs (tartrazine, patent blue V, erythrosine, etc.). The vasodilator effect of alcohol may also potentiate the rapid absorption of foods that are ingested at the same time and mask a weak food allergy. The cocktail syndrome is itself potentiated by physical effort [49].

Diagnosis of non-immunological reactions

Skin tests

Diagnosis of non-immunological reactions to foods should never be made without a previous search for food allergy. Negative prick tests to 12 common foods should be followed with intradermal tests on the extensor surface of the arm to milk, egg, fish, flour, pork, tomato, peas, hazelnuts, celery, peanuts, soya and prawns. If these are also negative and the patient is not able to incriminate the foods in any other way, then the hypothesis of food allergy is unlikely.

If the prick test is positive then food allergy is almost certain. The intradermal reaction is positive when the diameter of the oedema, after injection of 0.05 ml of a 1 : 10 (w/v) solution of the food, is greater than 10 mm. If it is positive, laboratory tests to seek specific IgE should be made and if these are detected, provocation tests with either lyophilized extracts or the original food, to confirm clinical food allergy must follow (Fig. 48.4).

The methods of diagnosis must centre around digestive equilibrium, the functional state of the mucous membrane, the characteristics of the organ that may produce an abnormal liberation of chemical mediators, possible insufficient degradation of these substances or perhaps an abnormal organ sensitivity to the mediators.

Diet diary

In the search for an alimentary cause involving the food categories which have been described above, it is essential to analyse the dietary intake of amines and nitrites, as well as starch and dairy foods, coffee and alcoholic beverages (Fig. 48.4).

The assessment begins with the study of the patient's diet over a period of a week, in which the objective is to analyse all ingested substances in categories that include foods that are rich in tyramine or histamine, those which release histamine, starchy foods, milk and dairy products, alcohol or coffee. The subject notes down all the food and liquid that is taken, together with the quantity. This list is then analysed, both in quantity and category, assigning one point to a 'usual' quantity of each particular food. The same food may appear simultaneously in two or three different categories and the total of weekly points

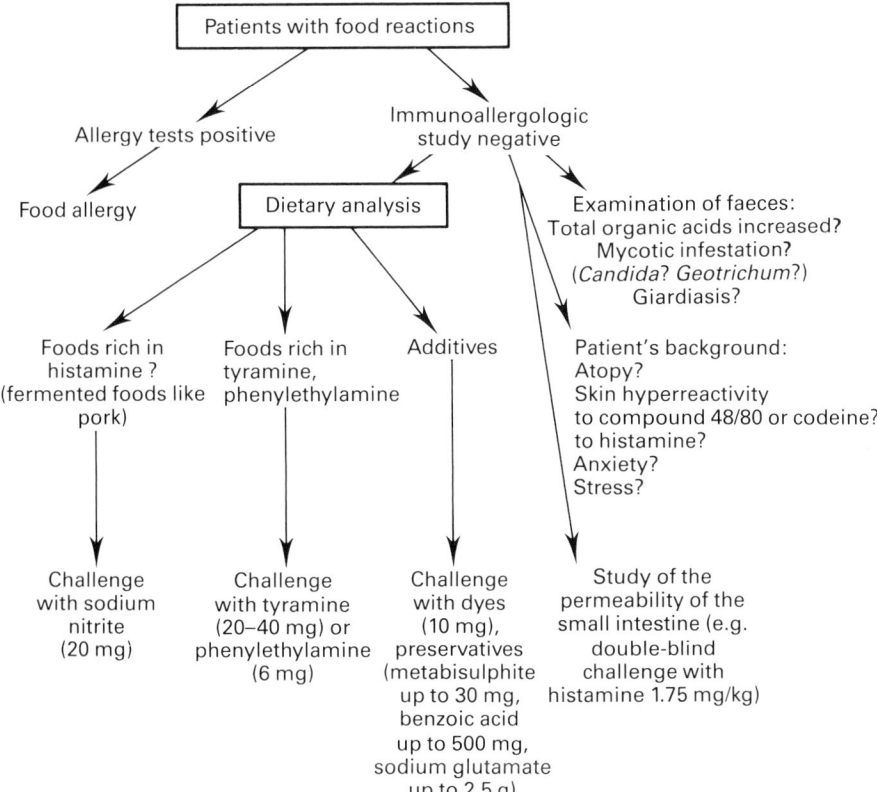

Fig. 48.4 The diagnosis of false food allergy.

for each category is reduced to an average daily index, to be compared with a normal range obtained from a group of randomly chosen healthy subjects.

Initially, this type of enquiry allowed us to establish the frequency of ingestion of food additives and to identify the provocation tests that were indicated in the individual cases. We have since continued to use it clinically and have found it to be valuable as a diagnostic tool.

Oral provocation tests

Oral provocation tests are not practicable with foods as in food allergy but they permit the testing of amines or additives when the symptoms are in the skin.

Daily challenge tests. Daily challenge tests may be done at home, after a morning fast. The patient is previously informed of the inclusion of one or several placebos amongst the substances tested. Explanation of the methodology used and the inclusion of a placebo lead to a great reduction in the subjective effects (placebo effect), making interpretation easier. Re-

ports of symptoms by the patient then requires checks under medical supervision, both single- and double-blind, where the dose is suitably adjusted. When the symptoms are of shock or bronchospasm, the tests should be done in a hospital, where adequate supervision can be given.

Additives. Approximately 16% of subjects with the triad of nasal polyps–asthma–intolerance to aspirin also have an intolerance to additives (Table 48.3) whereas only 3% of

Table 48.3 Oral provocation tests to food additives in 34 patients presenting with the Fernand–Widal syndrome (triad).

Additives	n	Negative	Positive
Tartrazine	21	19	2
Sodium benzoate	17	15	2
Sodium metabisulphite	5	2	3
Total	43	36	7 (16%)

patients who have isolated nasal polyposis are similarly sensitive. In 245 patients who presented with clinical symptoms linked to food, after exclusion of a food allergy, 189 consumed additives or were suspected of amine intolerance. Provocation tests were positive in 15.8% of all cases (Table 48.4). In patients with chronic urticaria systematic multiple challenges with food additives reveal intolerance in 60% of cases [56].

Table 48.4 Oral provocation tests in 245 subjects presenting with a false food allergy.

Additives	n	Positive
Sodium nitrite	59	5
Sodium benzoate	9	1
Butylhydroxytoluene-butylhydroxyanisole	6	1
Lecithin	2	5
Diphenyl	1	0
Tartrazine	33	3
Yellow–orange S	6	0
Brilliant black	1	0
Tyramine	64	16
Phenylethylamine	6	0
Total	189	36 (15.8%)

Integrity of the intestinal mucosa

The study of the digestive mucosa is important. Questioning reveals that, in 60% of cases of false food allergy, drugs that irritate the mucous membrane were being taken. Aspirin and the non-steroidal anti-inflammatory compounds are responsible for mucosal erosion, breaking of inter-enterocyte 'tight junctions' and inhibition of the synthesis of mucoproteins [27, 32]. A low dose of aspirin greatly increases the intestinal permeability, similar to that shown by dextrans [14]. General use of irritant laxatives, such as those based on derivatives of phenolphthalein, has now fortunately fallen into disuse. It is still useful to seek chronic candidiasis or a mycosis from *Geotrichum candidum* as factors that alter gut integrity. Studies of mucosal permeability that use non-metabolizable molecules are directed to the cellobiose–mannitol association, or to polyethylene glycol. It has been shown in this way that spiced food seems capable of increasing intestinal permeability [38].

Digestive challenge with histamine, at a dose of 1.75 mg/kg, can be done by duodenal instillation, or by ingestion of capsules [29]. The anomalies of the responses make the interpretation very complex since they may be due to intestinal hyperpermeability, or to an anomaly of catabolism of histamine.

Factors favouring histamine reactions

Susceptibility of the organ to histamine liberation, as well as hyperreactivity to histamine, may be seen in intradermal reactions with normally non-reactive doses of Compound 48/80, codeine and histamine (0.01 and 0.1 μg/ml). Low cellular magnesium is sought by measuring the magnesium of erythrocytes. The adrenergic reactivity is investigated by isoprenaline perfusion by the method of Grilliat [23].

MANAGEMENT OF FALSE FOOD ALLERGY

Bad dietary habits

Correction of dietary errors is of the utmost importance. Since the beginning of the century, patterns of food consumption in France have undergone great changes, with increases of sugars, fruits and vegetables, as well as of cooked pork meats, which doubled between 1950 and 1968. Similar developments have been noted in other countries. Since 1965 the consumption of vegetables has diminished, whilst there has been an increase of 18% in the consumption of eggs since 1974. There are some local differences in eastern France, where consumption of meat, green vegetables and fruit is at its lowest and we may suppose that these have been replaced by starchy and sugary foods in this part of the country. Storage provides an added problem and the length of time spent on the commercial circuit makes fish a potent cause of histamine-induced illness, as histidine changes to histamine during storage. So, histamine-provoked symptoms can be seen that are dependent on changes of consumption and regional eating habits. In children, the present excess of sugary foods conceals a regular consumption of additives, preservatives and dyes, that the allergist must systematically take into account. Finally, some reducing diets, which are based on the intake of a single food during a week, seem to us to encourage the development of histamine-mediated symptoms.

Dietary re-education

At present we do not have much evidence about eating habits with regard to the above-mentioned foods. In the absence of this, the rule in clinical treatment is to re-establish a balanced and varied everyday diet which is free from alimentary or pharmacological irritants. The question is never one of totally eradicating a category of food, but should be one of restricting its excessive intake. However, a diet that eliminates food additives, as was proposed by Freedman [17], seems to be reasonable and is worth considering in certain children.

General rules

Some general rules may be of value:

1 Regular meal times, which presupposes regular times of work and sleep.
2 Protection of the epithelium by bland agents (colloidal aluminium phosphate), enzymatic preparations such as cellulases and sulphurated drugs in children.
3 Protective measures that are directed at the mucous membrane, including the possible complementary role of anti-H_2 drugs (e.g. cimetidine), must be added to the classic antihistamines which block the H_1 receptors, but drugs with a coloured coating should be avoided.

In contrast to this, sodium cromoglygate does not seem to be very effective in adults, in contrast to its actions in food allergy. However, it appears to be very effective in some histamine-releasing illnesses in children.

CONCLUSIONS

Approach and understanding of a mysterious foreign country often starts with a survey of the frontier zones.

So, in the complex area of false food allergies, the frontier zones can be established around two subjects that are radically different. Firstly, the psychological reactions to foods and, secondly, the chronic inflammatory diseases of the intestines, where the role of certain foods is often suggested by the patients themselves.

The population of mast cells of the digestive mucosa is embedded in a lattice of exquisitely sensitive amyelinic fibres of type C and Aδ. These fibres are capable of liberating neuropeptides in the mucosa, such as substance P and somatostatin, by axon reflex in response to harmful stimuli or a local inflammatory reaction [57]. Substance P provokes histamine liberation from the mucosal mast cells as well as activating macrophages and polymorphonuclear leukocytes and causing vasodilation [21].

This neuromodulation of mast-cell degranulation, of which the starting point may be a harmful stimulus, gives logical support to the explanation of intolerance to some foods in the case of an inflammatory condition of the intestine, for example by the expedient of the epithelial irritative effect of lectins. It also allows the concept of a psychological dislike for a food with a conditioned reflex, to lead to release of chemical mediators, giving rise to urticaria and abdominal pains [62].

Currently one of the most important advances in the diagnosis of food allergy is surely the contribution of better characterization of the non-immunological reactions to foods rather than the screening of adverse reactions to food through sophisticated immunological tests.

Acknowledgement

I am grateful for the English translation provided by Dr Brighton.

REFERENCES

1 Allen DH: Monosodium glutamate induced asthma. New Trends Allergy 1985; 11:306.
2 Allen DH, Baker GJ: Chinese-restaurant asthma. N Engl J Med 1981; 305:1154-5.
3 Atkins FM, Metcalf DD: The diagnosis and treatment of food allergy. Annu Rev Nutr 1984;4:233-55.
4 Atkins FM, Steinberg SS, Metcalf DD: Evaluation of immediate adverse reactions to foods in adult patients. II. A detailed analysis of reaction patterns during oral food challenge. J Allergy Clin Immunol 1985; 75: 356-63.
5 Augustine JG, Levitan H: Neuro-transmitter release from a vertebrate neuro-muscular synapse affected by a food dye. Science 1980; 207:1489-90.
6 Barrett DE, Metcalf DD: The mucosal mast cell and its role in gastrointestinal allergic diseases. Clin Rev Allergy 1984; 2:39-53.
7 Bock SA, Lee WY: Studies of hypersensitivity reactions to foods in infants and children. J Allergy Clin Immunol 1978; 62:327-34.
8 Bock SA, Martin M: The incidence of adverse reactions to foods. A continuing study. J Allergy Clin Immunol 1983; 74:98.
9 Bois P: Effect of magnesium deficiency on mast cells and urinary histamine in rats. Br J Exp Pathol 1963; 44:151-5.
10 Desse G, Drouet J et al: Intoxications par consommation de filets congelés tétraodons. Bull Acad Natl Med (Paris) 1978; 162:469-74.
11 De Weck AL: Pathophysiologic mechanisms of allergic

and pseudo-allergic reactions to foods, food additives and drugs. Ann Allergy 1984; 53:583–6.

12 Egger J, Carter CM, Graham PJ et al: Controlled trial of oligoantigenic treatment in the hyperkinetic syndrome. Lancet 1985; i:540–5.

13 Finn R, Cohen MN: Food allergy: fact or fiction. Lancet 1978; i:426–8.

14 Flemstrom G, Marsden VB et al: Passsive anaphylaxis in guinea pigs elicited by gastric absorption of dextran induced by acetylsalicylic acid. Int Arch Allergy Appl Immunol 1976; 51:627–36.

15 Folkers K, Willis R, Takemura K et al: Biochemical correlations of a deficiency of vitamin B_6, the carpal tunnel syndrome and the Chinese restaurant syndrome. IRCS Med Sci 1981; 9:444.

16 Fox CC, Dvorak AM, Peters SP et al: Isolation and characterization of human intestinal mucosal mast cells. J Immunol 1985; 135:483–91.

17 Freedman BJ: Asthma induced by sulfur dioxide, benzoate and tartrazine contained in orange drinks. Clin Allergy 1977; 7:407–15.

18 Froeberg J, Carlson LA, Karlsson CG et al: Effects of coffee on catecholamine excretion and plasma lipids. In: Heim F, Ammon HP, eds. Caffein und andere Methylxanthine. Stuttgart: Schattauerverlag, 1969;65–73.

19 Geelen MJ, Van Cogten MJ: Effet d'un régime pauvre en magnésium sur la toxicité de l'histamine chez le rat. Rev Fr Allergol 1975; 15:155–7.

20 Ghadimi H, Kumar S et al: Studies on monosodium glutamate ingestion: biochemical explanations of Chinese restaurant syndrome. Biochem Med 1971; 5:447–56.

21 Goetzl EJ, Chernou T, Renold F, Payan D: Neuropeptide regulation of the expression of immediate hypersensitivity. J Immunol 1985; 135:802–5.

22 Granerus G: Effects of oral histamine, histidine and diet on urinary excretion of histamine, methylhistamine and 1-methyl-4-imidazole acetic acid in man. Scand J Clin Lab Invest [Suppl 104] 1968; 22:49–58.

23 Grilliat JP, Le Van D, Mayeux D, Kohler C: Spasmophilie, rhinite, urticaire, et activité béta-adrénergique. Rev Fr Allergol 1982; 22:211–6.

24 Hanington E: Migraine. In: Lessof MH, ed. Clinical reactions to food. Chichester: John Wiley, 1983;155–80.

25 Harada S, Misawa S, Agarwal DP, Goedde HW: Liver alcohol dehydrogenase and aldehyde dehydrogenase in the Japanese; isozyme variation and its possible role in alcohol intoxication. Am J Genet 1980; 32:8–15.

26 Helm RM, Froese A: Binding of the receptors for IgE by various lectins. Int Arch Allergy Appl Immunol 1981; 65:81–4.

27 Ivey KJ, Baskin WN et al: Effect of aspirin and acid on human jejunal mucosa. An ultrastructural study. Gastroenterology 1979; 76:50–6.

28 Jamieson DM, Guill MF, Wray BB, May JR: Metabisulfite sensitivity: case report and literature review. Ann Allergy 1985; 54:115–21.

29 Joelt SV, Sondergaard I, Svendsen UG, Weeke B: Intestinal provocation with histamine. Proceedings from XV Nordic Congress of Allergology Turkin Finland June 5-8, 1984. Allergy 1984; 39:2.

30 Juhlin L: Localization and content of histamine in normal and diseased skin. Acta Dermatol 1967; 47:383–91.

31 Juhlin L: Recurrent urticaria: findings in 330 cases seen from 1974 to 1978. Br J Dermatol 1981; 104:369–81.

32 Konturek SJ, Obtulowicz W et al: Distribution of prostaglandins in gastric and duodenal mucosa of healthy subjects and duodenal ulcer patients: effects of aspirin and paracetamol. Gut 1981; 22:283–9.

33 Kusche J, Lorenz W et al: Oxidative deamination of biogenic amines by intestinal amine oxidases: histamine is specifically inactivated by diamine oxidase. Hoppe Seylers Z Physiol Chem 1975:1485–96.

34 Kwok RHM: Chinese restaurant syndrome. N Engl J Med 1968; 278:796.

35 Lafferman JA, Silbergerd EK: Erythrosin B inhibits dopamine transport in rat caudate synaptosomes. Science 1979; 205:410–12.

36 Larsen JC: Absorption and biotransformation: intolerance to certain foreign chemicals. In: Allergy and hypersensitivity to chemicals, Interim Document, WHO Regional Office for Europe, Copenhagen, 1983; 162–214.

37 Lessof MH, Anderson JB: Prostaglandins and other mediators in food intolerance. Clin Rev Allergy 1984; 2:70–93.

38 Lessof MH, Baker RWR et al: Intestinal permeability in food intolerance. Allergol Immunopathol (Madr) 1980; 8:463.

39 Lessof MH, Buisseret PD et al: Mechanisms involving prostaglandins in food intolerance. In: Pepys J, Edwards AM, eds. The mast cell: its role in health and disease. Tunbridge Wells: Pitman Medical, 1979;407–40.

40 Lindhall KM: The histamine methylating enzyme system in liver. Acta Physiol Scand 1960; 22:964–70.

41 Lorenzsonn V, Olsen W: In vivo responses of rat intestinal epithelium to intraluminal dietary lectins. Gastroenterology 1982; 82:838–48.

42 Maretic Z, Russell FE: Tulip bulb poisoning. Period Biol 1978; 80:141–3.

43 Marley E, Thomas DV: Histamine and its metabolites in cat portal venous blood and intestine after duodenal instillation of histamine (Proceedings). J Physiol 1976; 263: 273P-4P.

44 May CD, Bock SA: Adverse reactions to food due to hypersensitivity. In: Elliot Middleton ED, Reed CE, Ellis EF, eds. Allergy: principles and practice. St Louis: CV Mosby, 1978; 1159–71.

45 Moneret-Vautrin DA: False food allergies. In: Pepys J, Edwards AM eds. The mast cell: its role in health and disease. Tunbridge Wells: Pitman Medical, 1979; 431–7.

46 Moneret-Vautrin DA: False food allergies: nonspecific reactions to foodstuffs. In: Lessof MH, ed. Clinical reactions to food. Chichester: John Wiley, 1983; 135–53.

47 Moneret-Vautrin DA, André C: Immunopathologie de l'allergie alimentaire et fausses allergies alimentaires. Paris: Masson, 1983.

48 Moneret-Vautrin DA, Martin R: Intolerance to aspirin: a role for free radicals? Lancet 1985; i:929.

49 Moneret-Vautrin DA, Wayoff M: Allergie et intolérance aux alcools. Med Hyg 1985; 43:1125–30.

50 Moneret-Vautrin DA, Moeller R, Malingrey L, Laxenaire MC: Anaphylactoid reaction to general anaesthesia: a case of intolerance to sodium benzoate in patient suffering of following triad: nasal polyposis, asthma, idiosyncrasy to aspirin. Anaesth Intensive Care 1982; 10:156–7.

51 Moneret-Vautrin DA, De Korwin JD, Tisserant J et al: Ultrastructural study of the mast cells of the human duodenal mucosa. Clin Allergy 1984; 14:471–9.

52 Moneret-Vautrin DA, Viniaker J et al: Effets de

l'instillation d'histamine dans l'intestin grêle chez l'homme. I. Variation de l'histaminémie portale et périphérique. Ann Gastro-Entérol Hépatol 1981; 17: 395-400.

53 Mordelet-Dambrine M, Parrot JL: Action de l'histamine introduite par voie buccale ou formée dans le tube digestif. Med Nutr 1970; 6:59-73.

54 Morgan JP, Penovich P: Jamaica ginger paralysis. Forty seven year follow-up. Arch Neurol 1978; 35:530-2.

55 Olney JW, Labruyer J: Brain damage in mice from voluntary ingestion of glutamate and aspartate. Neurobehav Toxicol 1980; 2:125-9.

56 Ortolani C, Pastorello E, Luraghi MR et al: Diagnosis of intolerance to food additives. Ann Allergy 1984; 53:587-91.

57 Payan DG, Levine JD, Goeltz EJ: Modulation of immunity and hypersensitivity by sensory neuropeptides. J Immunol 1984; 132:1601-4.

58 Pearce FL, Befus AD, Gauldie J, Bienenstock J: Mucosal mast cells. II. Effects of anti-allergic compounds on histamine secretion by isolated intestinal mast cells. J Immunol 1982; 128:2481-6.

59 Prenner BM, Stevens JJ: Anaphylaxis after ingestion of sodium bisulfite. Ann Allergy 1976; 37:180.

60 Pryor WA: Free radical biology: xenobiotics, cancers, and aging. Ann NY Acad Sci 1982; 393:1-22.

61 Queille C, Saurat JG: Dermatite atopique (eczéma constitutionnel). Etude informatisée de 300 observations. Journ Parisiennes Pédiatr Paris: Ed Flammarion, 1981; 293-301.

62 Russel M, Dark KA, Cummins RW: Learned histamine release. Science 1984; 225:733-4.

63 Saint-Blanquat G: Aspects toxicologiques et nutritionnels des nitrates et des nitrites. Ann Nutr Aliment 1980; 34:827-64.

64 Sandler M, Youdim MBH et al: A clinical and biochemical correlation between tyramine and migraine. Headache 1970; 10-12:43-51.

65 Sandler M, Youdim MBH et al: A phenylethylamine oxidising defect in migraine. Nature 1974; 250:335-7.

66 Saxby MJ, Chaytor JP, Reid RG: Changes in the levels of 2-phenylethylamine in cheese and chocolate during processing and storage. Food Chem 1980-81; 6:281-8.

67 Schachter M, Talesnik J: The release of histamine by egg-white in non-sensitized animal. J Physiol 1952; 118:258-63.

68 Schlumberger HD: Drug-induced pseudo-allergic syndrome as exemplified by acetylsalicylic acid intolerance. In: Pseudo-anaphylactoid reactions. Basel: Karger, 1980; 125-203.

69 Selbekk BH: Mast cell reaction in human jejunal mucosa in vitro. In: Pepys J, Edwards Am, eds. The mast cell: its role in health and disease. Pitman Medical, 1979; 710-15.

70 Stanworth DR: Oligopeptide-induced released of histamine. In: Pseudo-anaphylactoid reactions. Basel: Karger, 1980; 56-107.

71 Stevenson DD, Simon RA: Sensitivity to ingested metabisulfites in asthmatic subjects. J Allergy Clin Immunol 1981; 68:26-32.

72 Stokes JD, Scudder CL: The effect of butylated hydroxyanisole and butylated hydroxytoluene on behavior development of mice. Dev Psychobiol 1974; 7:343-50.

73 Stopik D, Beger HG et al: Uber den Einfuss der Leber auf die prä-und posthepatischen Konzentrationen des Plasma-histamins beim Menschen. Klin Wochenschr 1974; 52:696-8.

74 Swanson JM, Kinsbourne M: Food dyes impair performance of hyper-reactive children on a laboratory learning test. Science 1980; 207:1485-6.

75 Tarjan V, Janossy G: The role of biogenic amines in foods. Nahrung 1978; 3:281-5.

76 Wilson BJ: Naturally occurring toxicants of foods. Nutr Rev 1979; 37:305-12.

Chapter 49
Chronic Candidiasis and Allergy

George F. Kroker

Historical introduction

Clinical descriptions of chronic fungal disease date back to antiquity, when Hippocrates described the manifestations of oral thrush [29].

Historically, earlier studies made clear the infectious potential of the *Candida* organism to invade a wide variety of human tissues and to cause human disease [15, 22, 35, 66, 75, 97]. Unfortunately, however, many physicians considered the role of *Candida* in chronic disease processes to be strictly limited to the clearly definable instances of direct tissue invasion previously described (Table 49.1). The emphasis in this chapter, however, will be towards outlining the broader role for *Candida* species in causing chronic illness from tissue *sensitivity* to the organism and/or its by-products rather than from direct tissue *invasion* by the organism itself.

Table 49.1 *Candida albicans*—infectious disease.

Cutaneous involvement
  Intertriginous candidiasis
  Onychia/paronychia
  Candida granuloma

Mucocutaneous involvement
  Oral—thrush, glossitis, cheilitis, stomatitis, perleche
  Genital—vaginitis, balanitis
  Bronchial—bronchitis, laryngeal candidiasis
  Alimentary—oesophagitis, enteric and perianal candidiasis
  Chronic mucocutaneous candidiasis

Systemic involvement
  Urinary—renal candidiasis, cystitis, urethritis
  Cardiovascular—myocarditis, endocarditis
  Musculoskeletal—arthritis, osteomyelitis
  Central nervous system—meningitis
  Eye/ear/nose—endophthalmitis, conjunctivitis, sinusitis

  Septicaemia

  Iatrogenic candidiasis

GENERAL ASPECTS OF *CANDIDA ALBICANS*

Clinical microbiology of *Candida*

Candida is a heterogeneous genus presently grouped with the Fungi Imperfecti. There are over 80 species of *Candida*, which are seen microscopically as gram-positive thin-walled ovoid budding yeasts which are 4 to 6 µm in diameter (Fig. 49.1). The principal group

Candida albicans is found only in human and animal reservoirs, so acquisition from the environment is unlikely.

Isolation rates of *Candida albicans* from the mouth, vagina and faeces was higher for hospitalized patients than for normal subjects [61], although both groups did have significant colonization rates (Table 49.2) for *Candida albicans* and other yeast organisms [61]. However, *Candida albicans* is only rarely recovered from human skin [10].

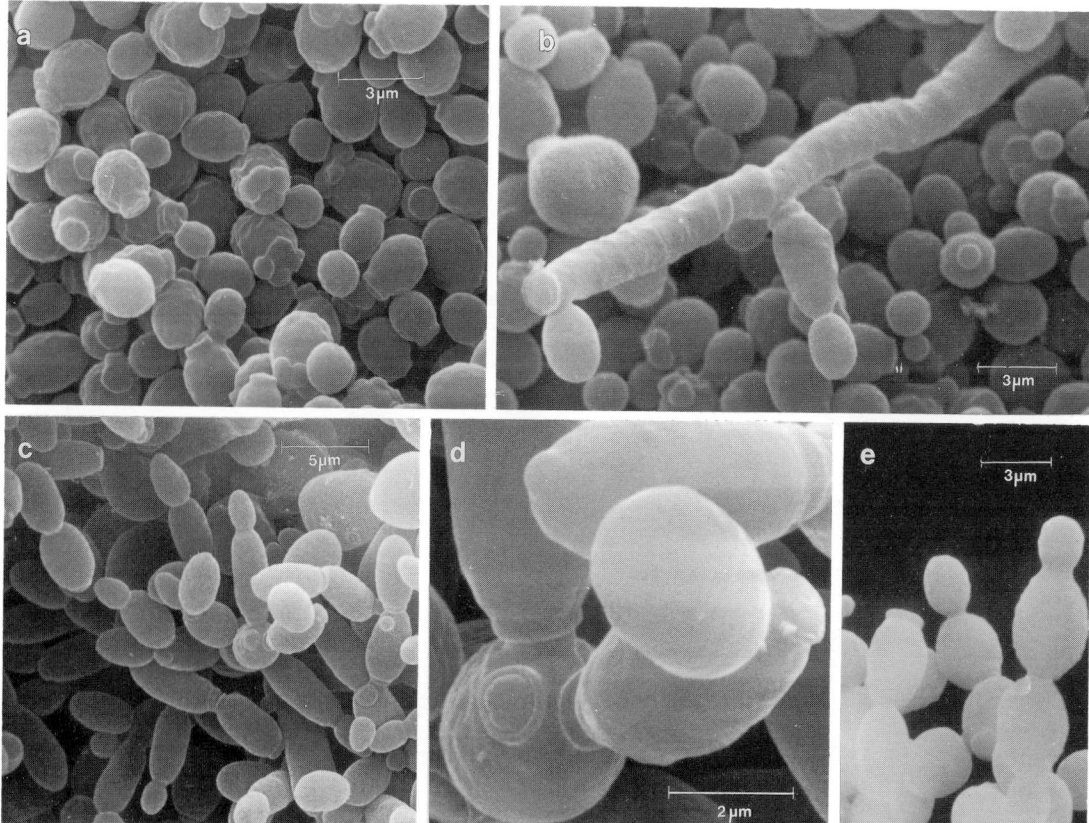

Fig. 49.1 Scanning electron micrographs of various pathogenic *Candida* species. (a) *C. albicans* blastospores. (b) *C. albicans* hypha in foreground, with multiple blastospores in background. (c) *C. pseudotropicalis* blastospores. (d) Higher magnification of (c). (e) *C. quilliermondii* blastospores. Reproduced from Odds [61], with permission.

characteristic of all *Candida* species is their ability to produce pseudohyphae (elongated chains of yeast cells) from budding unicellular yeast forms when cultured on certain media (Fig. 49.2). At least six *Candida* species have been implicated as human pathogens [61], but the majority of *Candida* infections are caused by *Candida albicans* and *Candida tropicalis*. *Candida* grow readily at 37°C on Sabouraud's glucose agar and on blood agar, forming soft creamy-coloured colonies with a characteristic yeasty odour (Fig. 49.3).

Table 49.2 Mean isolation rates of *Candida albicans* carriage.

Location	Normal subjects (%)	Hospital patients (%)
Mouth	10.3	42.9
Faeces	14.6	22.0
Vagina	7.8	14.9

Adapted from Odds [61], with permission.

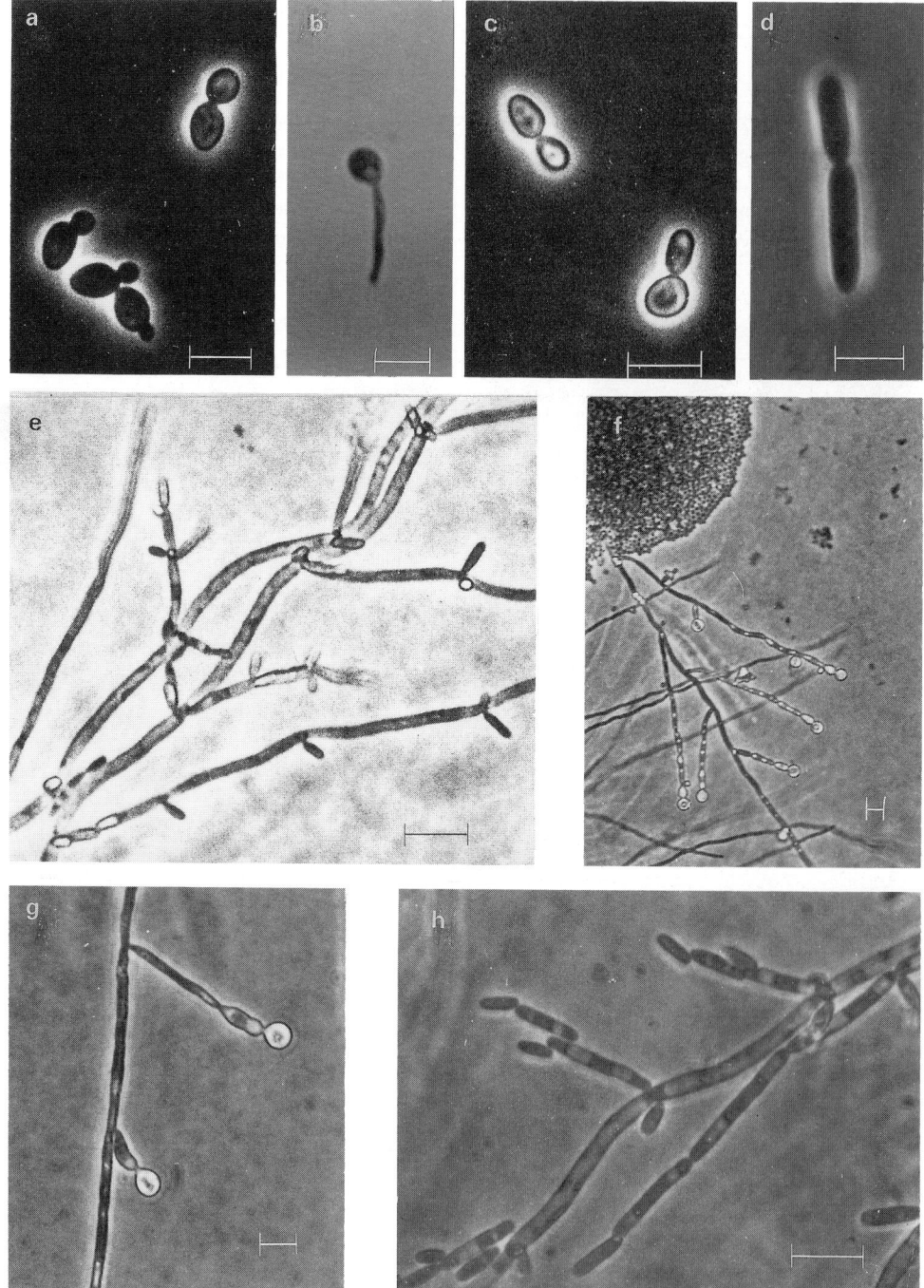

Fig. 49.2 Light microscopic appearance of several morphological forms of *Candida* species. (a) *C albicans* blastospores by phase contrast microscopy. (b) *C. albicans* germ tube produced in serum; phase contrast microscopy. (c) *C. parapsilosis* blastospores by phase contrast microscopy. (d) *C. krussei* blastospores by phase contrast microscopy. (e) *C. pseudotropicalis* pseudomycelium grown in corn meal agar; stained with lactophenol cotton blue. (f) *C. albicans* mycelium, pseudomycelium, and chlamydospores grown in corn meal agar; phase contrast microscopy. (g) *C. albicans* chlamydospores under high magnification with phase contrast microscopy. (h) *C. krusei* pseudohyphae; phase contrast microscopy. Reproduced from Odds [61], with permission.

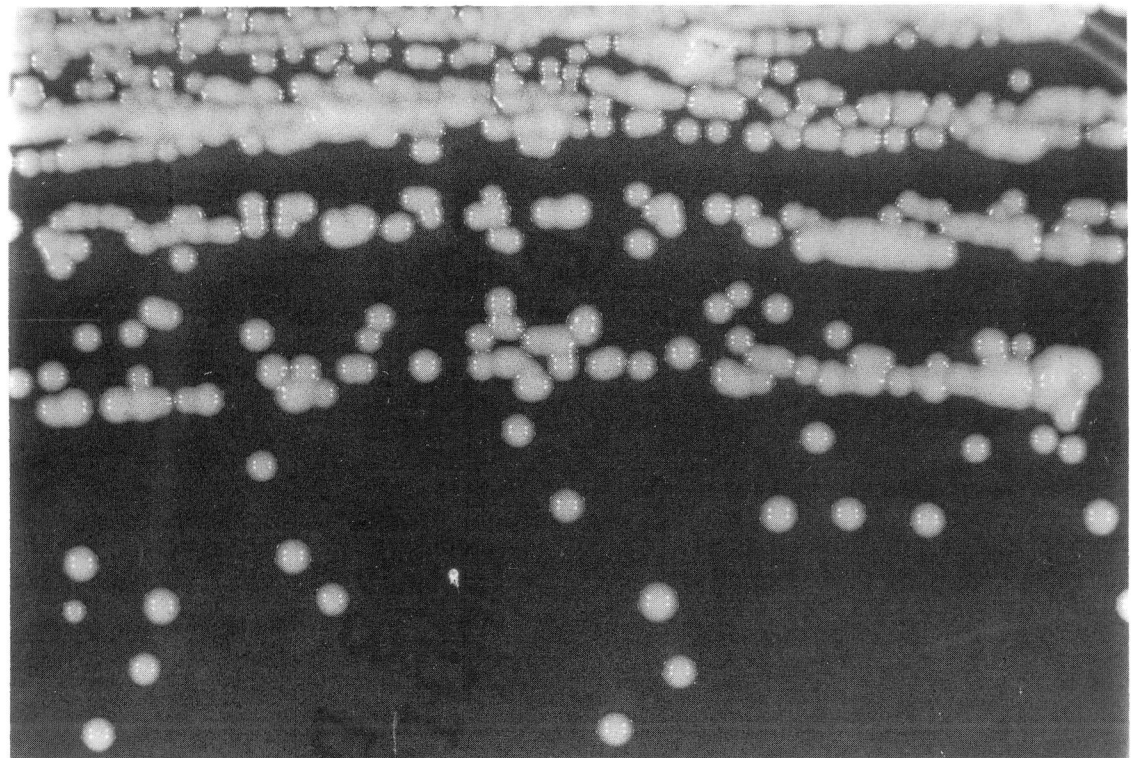

Fig. 49.3 Macroscopic appearance of *Candida albicans* colonies, as grown on blood agar culture.

If this organism has *sensitization* potential as well as *infectious* potential, then the frequency with which it is found points to the enormous potential epidemiological impact such sensitization might have on the population at large.

Clinical immunology of *Candida albicans*

Candida albicans is a polyantigenic organism; 79 immunologically distinct antigenic determinants have been described for *Candida albicans*—principal cell-wall antigen (mannan and glucan), 77 cytoplasmic antigens and a mycelial antigen [5]. The cell-surface polysaccharide components which include glucans and mannans appear to be the important antigens of *Candida* [61]. Each strain of *Candida albicans* is thought to contain 30–35 of these antigens, and each individual may harbour more than one strain of organism.

Antibody response

By virtue of widespread mucosal contact with this organism, antibody formation against the organism is common and begins early in life. *Candida* antibodies have been shown to belong to the IgA, IgG, IgM and IgE immunoglobulin classes [17]. The predominant antibody in patients with systemic infectious candidiasis is anti-*Candida* IgG [46], whereas in patients with recurrent vaginal candidiasis, the antibody response has been reported to be primarily local and consists mainly of secretory immunoglobulin IgA [51]. The potential diagnostic value of antibody profiles to *Candida* antigens in patients with *Candida* sensitivity diseases will be discussed further below.

***Candida* sensitization and clinical syndromes**

There is theoretical and clinical support for the sensitization potential of *Candida albicans* [31, 39, 65, 77] since *Candida* glycoproteins have been shown to stimulate histamine release from isolated rat mast cells in vitro [58] and *Candida* antigen-induced histamine release from human leukocytes has been noted in selected cases as well [59]. *Candida albicans* has been reported to be a pathogenic factor in selected cases of urticaria, asthma, irritable bowel disease and psoriasis (Table 49.3).

Table 49.3 *Candida albicans*—sensitivity disease.

Localized sensitivity
  Cutaneous—urticaria, psoriasis
  Pulmonary—asthma
  Gastrointestinal—irritable bowel syndrome
Generalized sensitivity
  Chronic candidiasis sensitivity syndrome (CCSS)

Urticaria

Early studies suggested that fungi may have a pathogenic role in certain cases of urticaria [78,95,100]. Later studies by Holti [30] as well as James and Warin [36] examined the potential role of *Candida albicans* in contributing to selected cases of chronic urticaria (Table 49.4).

nystatin medication coupled with a yeast-free diet in certain cases of resistant urticaria [103].

Asthma

Candida albicans is a potent experimental bronchial antigen. Several investigators have reported immediate and late-phase responses on skin testing and provocation inhalation challenge with *Candida albicans* extracts [26,64]. Itkin and Dennis showed that bronchial hypersensitivity to *Candida albicans* aerosols correlated with immediate (but not delayed) cutaneous hypersensitivity to the fungus [33]. A few cases of immediate hypersensitivity *Candida*-induced asthma have been reported in the literature [38,41,48]. However, based on these reports alone it is not easy

Table 49.4 Chronic urticaria and *Candida albicans*.

Study	Number of patients with positive skin test	Number of patients cured: nystatin treatment	Number of patients cured: diet + nystatin	Total cured
Holti [30]	49*	9	18	27
James and Warin [36]	36†	3	23	26

* Intradermal test.
† Prick test.

Treatment with nystatin. Holti reported on a *Candida albicans* sensitivity in a population of 255 patients who had chronic urticaria. Forty-nine (19%) of these patients had immediate intradermal whealing reactions to *Candida albicans* extract, and 27 (11%) also had immediate whealing responses to baker's and/or brewer's yeast. Treatment for 3 weeks with nystatin tablets resulted in a clinical cure for 27 out of these 49 patients. Eighteen of these patients lost their urticaria only when they also adhered to a yeast-free diet, and two of these patients also required long-term desensitization to *Candida albicans* to bring adequate relief of their urticaria.

James and Warin in 1970 studied *Candida albicans* sensitivity in 100 patients with chronic urticaria. Thirty-six patients (36%) had a positive prick test to *Candida albicans* extract. When these 36 patients were treated, three patients responded to antifungal therapy alone, and 23 required a yeast-free diet and nystatin for satisfactory resolution of their symptoms (Table 49.4).

Zamm also stressed the causative role of *Candida albicans* in certain cases of chronic urticaria, and advocated a therapeutic trial of

to accept *Candida albicans* as a definitive causative agent of bronchial asthma. Recently, allergic bronchopulmonary candidiasis has been described in the literature and has been documented with selected antigen-specific serological studies [1].

Irritable colon

Candida albicans has also been implicated as being a causative factor in certain cases of irritable colon syndrome. Holti reported on the treatment of 57 patients with irritable bowel syndrome who had positive stool cultures for yeast [30]. Nystatin therapy resulted in permanent cures in 17 patients (30%) and partial relief in 31 patients (54%). In the 31 patients experiencing only partial relief with nystatin, institution of a yeast-free diet resulted in 23 additional patients experiencing further significant improvement. Five of the patients who experienced relief of their symptoms with the therapy mentioned above were subsequently challenged orally in a double-blind manner with 5 ml of a commercially available *Candida albicans* antigenic extract; they subsequently experienced various levels of gastrointestinal distress after the challenge. Five control patients similarly challenged experienced no symptoms when tested.

Unfortunately, further studies in this area have not been forthcoming. However at least one other author has felt that *Candida albicans* might be involved allergenically in the pathogenesis of certain cases of irritable bowel syndrome, and that patients with chronic diarrhoea and positive *Candida* cultures may respond excellently to antifungal therapy [2].

Psoriasis

Candida species may have a pathogenic role in selected cases of psoriasis. Early investigators reported higher than normal occurrences of intestinal carriage of *Candida* in patients with psoriasis [92]. More recent reports have suggested that administration of oral nystatin may result in improvement of psoriasis in selected patients [6], even though nystatin is an agent with antifungal properties largely limited to the gut lumen. Rosenberg noted improvement in scalp psoriasis with ketoconazole usage; more interestingly he observed some patients had improvement in psoriasis in distant skin sites as well, where the surface microflora harboured few yeast organisms, suggesting a systemic effect [72]. Subsequently, it has been suggested that *Candida* may contribute to psoriasis in certain patients susceptible to alternative complement pathway activation through stimulation by *Candida* cell-wall products [73].

CHRONIC CANDIDIASIS SENSITIVITY SYNDROME

The literature presented above provides evidence that under selected conditions *Candida albicans* can produce localized manifestations of sensitivity in selected tissues (skin, respiratory tract, colon). Truss in 1978 theorized that multiple other organ systems, remote from the actual site of *Candida* carriage in the body, could also be sensitized to this organism [85], and outlined the characteristic clinical presentations of such patients and selected therapeutic regimens for them [86,87]. These clinical findings were confirmed by other physicians [7,15] and subsequently extended and presented in detail as the 'chronic candidiasis sensitivity syndrome' (CCSS) [101,102].

Clinical presentation

Age and sex

Patients presenting with CCSS have variable presentations, depending on such factors as age, sex, host resistance and environmental exposure to various factors promoting *Candida* carriage. Generally, young women are affected with this disease process to a greater extent than men (Table 49.5).

Table 49.5 Chronic candidiaisis sensitivity—clinical manifestations.

Sex: Adult female
Age: Young/middle age
Presenting symptoms
  Central nervous system (multiple symptoms)
  Endocrine (multiple symptoms)
  Multiple other organ system complaints
  Localized symptoms yeast overgrowth (mouth, vagina, intestine)
  Cravings for carbohydrates/yeast foods
Past history
  Chronic yeast infections
  Chronic antibiotics for acne, infections
  Oral birth control pill usage
  Oral steroid usage
Associated conditions
  Endocrinopathies
  Mitral valve prolapse
  Premenstrual syndrome
  Inhalant, food, chemical sensitivities
Physical examination:
  Signs of yeast infection (oral, vaginal)
  Signs of fatty acid deficiencies
  Signs of respiratory allergy

Polysymptomatology

Polysymptomatic illness with multiple complaints referable to various organ systems is the rule. Symptoms especially common to see and extremely distressing to patients include those referable to the central nervous system and endocrine system. Fatigue, mood lability, depression, inability to concentrate, headaches and loss of energy are especially common [14].

Women often are aware of menstrual irregularities, loss of libido and premenstrual accentuation of their symptoms [12]. Many women with this illness have been previously diagnosed as having 'premenstrual syndrome' (PMS). However, even though symptoms are similar to PMS, there is no characteristic symptom-free period following menstruation and typically symptoms are present throughout the menstrual cycle.

Other organ systems may be involved, including: musculoskeletal (aching, myalgia), cardiac (palpitations), respiratory (wheezing, sinusitis), gastrointestinal (bloating, gas, constipation or diarrhoea), cutaneous (pruritus, urticaria) and genitourinary (persistent vaginal discharge, cystitis).

Food cravings

Dietarily, patients with CCSS often have intense food cravings for foods rich in carbohydrates or yeast, and many patients have been previously diagnosed as having 'hypoglycaemia'. Carbohydrate and/or yeast cravings is such a characteristic finding in this disorder that one should seriously doubt the diagnosis of this illness if it is not present. Often, patients will also experience gastrointestinal upset after ingestion of rich carbohydrate foods, noting uncomfortable bloating, flatulence or bowel irregularity after ingestion.

Mould sensitivity

In addition to food intolerance, many patients exhibit strong intolerance to mould antigens. Not only may patients develop classical respiratory symptomatology from mould exposure, but they may also develop such non-IgE-mediated delayed-onset symptomatology as fatigue, depression and headache from mould exposure as well. An environmental history with relevance toward daily mould exposure is especially important.

Multiple food and chemical intolerance

As CCSS progresses, patients may also start developing multiple food and chemical intolerances, making it increasingly difficult for them to work and maintain a normal life style. Many of these patients suffer from environmental chemical sensitivity syndrome, as described by Randolph [67]. In this syndrome, patients react adversely to small, non-toxic amounts of commonly encountered environmental chemical stimuli, such as perfumes, tobacco smoke, pesticides, automobile exhaust etc. It is especially important, therefore, to take a pertinent food and chemical history on any patient suspected of having CCSS.

Mucosal involvement

Symptoms of recurrent localized yeast overgrowth in the mouth, vagina and intestine are particularly common, and often there is a history of chronic prior mucocutaneous fungal

infections (thrush, vaginitis, oesophagitis, intestinal candidiasis) or prior dermatophytosis. There may be a dramatic increase in chronic low-grade symptoms following broad-spectrum antibiotic administration, or use of oral contraceptives or steroids.

Presentation in children

There are variations to this typical clinical presentation in both young children and adult males (Table 49.6). The characteristic constellation of findings in children with CCSS include: recurrent infections with multiple antibiotic therapy, chronic bowel disturbances, central nervous system dysfunction (including irritability, hyperactivity and learning disabilities) and localized manifestations of past or present yeast overgrowth (thrush, nappy rash). Coexisting allergies to foods or inhalants may be present.

Table 49.6 Chronic candidiasis sensitivity—clinical manifestations.

History	Symptoms	Examination
Infant child		
Chronic infection and multiple antibiotics	Carbohydrate cravings	Oral thrush
	Hyperactivity and irritability	Nappy rash
		Usual signs of allergy
Yeast infection as infant	Chronic bowel disturbances	
Prior diagnoses: 'failure to thrive' 'hyperactivity'		
Adult male		
Chronic infection and multiple antibiotics	Fatigue, depressed bowel disturbances	Dermatophyte infections
		Usual signs of allergy
Chronic fungal infection of skin	Carbohydrate and yeast cravings	
Chronic steroid use for allergies etc		
Sexual partner with yeast infections		

Presentation in adult males

In adult males, polysymptomatic illness is the rule, with fatigue and low-grade irritability and depression being particularly common complaints. There may be a history of chronic dermatophytosis and/or prostatitis. Often there are characteristic carbohydrate and/or yeast food cravings (Table 49.6).

In most patients with this disease, the onset of localized yeast symptoms usually precedes the systemic response, although occasionally remote tissue reactions to *Candida* may antedate symptoms of mucosal involvement by several years.

DIAGNOSIS

There is no single diagnostically specific test for CCSS. This lack of diagnostic specificity coupled with the variable polysymptomatic clinical picture explains why this condition may be easily missed by the physician in daily clinical practice. There are, however, several diagnostic factors which when taken as a whole allow the clinician to confidently arrive at a diagnosis of this condition. The most important criteria are: (a) a suggestive history, (b) a positive provocative challenge to *Candida albicans* and yeast antigenic extracts and (c) a favourable response to a 1–2 month trial of therapy (Table 49.7).

Table 49.7 Chronic candidiasis sensitivity—diagnosis.

Most helpful diagnostic factors
  History
  Provocative challenge to *Candida* and yeast antigens
  Response to 1–2 month trial of therapy

Partially helpful diagnostic factors
  Antibody levels to selected *Candida* antigens
  Microbiological cultures of selected tissues

Unhelpful diagnostic factors
  Routine skin test to *Candida albicans*

History

The history is most important and if as described above under 'Clinical presentation' is highly suggestive of this illness. However, histories may be misleading and falsely negative if the patient is a poor historian, or has been partially treated (with diet or medications) prior to consultation. Certain authors have devised point-scored questionnaires which are helpful in diagnosis [13] but these cannot replace a careful assessment by the physician with attention directed towards certain essential key points in the history (Table 49.8).

Provocative challenge

A helpful diagnostic manoeuvre in assessing CCSS is a provocative challenge to *Candida*

Table 49.8 Essential points to consider in history-taking for CCSS.

1 What factors in the patient's history might predispose to excessive *Candida albicans* carriage?

2 Is there historical evidence of previous *Candida albicans* infections?

3 Does there appear to be a correlation between increasing *Candida* antigenic load and increasing systemic symptoms?

4 Is there a positive environmental history of food, mould, or chemical sensitivity?

5 In taking the general medical history, are there any co-existing medical conditions which are usually associated with *Candida albicans* carriage?

albicans and food yeast extracts as outlined in Chapter 54. All patients challenged to *Candida albicans* should also be provocatively challenged to yeast antigen extract, due to the likelihood of overlapping sensitivities in these two areas.

Negative tests. The testing may be negative for several reasons, including (a) difficulty with inherent variability in extract potencies and/or patient anergy on intradermal testing, (b) delayed-onset symptomatology missed in the patient during testing or (c) 'allergenic overload' from multiple other sources, with such a high pretest baseline that correct interpretation of the test is difficult. Although the technique of provocative neutralization is generally extremely safe when used in trained and competent hands, it is not without some hazard, particularly in the brittle, allergically 'overloaded' patient who has evidence of gross *Candida* antigenic overload coupled with multiple severe food, mould and chemical sensitivities. In such a patient it is advisable to defer provocative testing until the patient's total environmental overload can be reduced.

Therapeutic trial

A useful test is the patient's response to a 1–2 month course of diet and antifungal therapy. This trial is obviously only useful diagnostically if the patient responds. However, this test may be falsely negative due to technically inadequate antifungal therapy, or it may be falsely positive due to a 'placebo' effect or due to simultaneous avoidance/treatment of another sensitivity (food, chemical, mould) which may be the patient's real problem—and not *Candida albicans*.

Antibody measurements

Candida antibodies can be measured by a variety of techniques, including agglutination, complement fixation, precipitin (Fig. 49.4) fluorescent antibody and radioimmunoassay tests [83].

Opinions on the diagnostic value of yeast antibody detection differ, largely due to three factors: (a) lack of standardization of testing techniques and antigen preparation, (b) the common occurrence of antibodies to *Candida albicans* in normal human hosts without disease and (c) lack of established blood levels of *Candida* antibodies in disorders characterized by excessive *Candida* colonization.

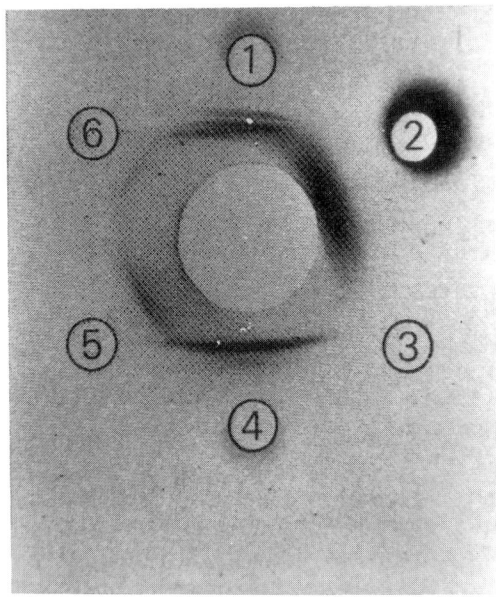

Fig. 49.4 Ouchterlony double diffusion test for precipitating antibodies to *Candida* antigens in a patient with systemic candidiasis. The patient's serum was placed in the centre large well; the surrounding small wells were filled with various soluble *Candida* extracts: (1) *C. albicans* culture filtrate, 2 mg/ml. (2) *C. albicans* 'cytoplasmic' antigen, 10 mg/ml. (3) Saline solution (negative control). (4) *C. albicans* culture filtrate, 20 mg/ml. (5) *C. albicans* 'cytoplasmic' antigen, 1 mg/ml. (6) Purified *C. albicans* mannan, 5 mg/ml. Note presence of lines of identity and non-identity between the different antigens. Reproduced from Odds [61], with permission.

IgE radioallergosorbent test (RAST) to *Candida albicans* may be helpful to document Type I hypersensitivity but is usually negative in advanced stages of CCSS.

Some authors have suggested a correlation between *Candida*-specific antibody levels and colonization level [45,76]. Others have reported that enzyme-linked immunosorbent assay (ELISA) against purified cytoplasmic protein antigens of *Candida* have good sensitivity (92%) and high specificity (89%) in diagnosing CCSS [25], and show correlation between certain antibody profiles and the clinical likelihood of CCSS [24]. Changes in antibody titre with appropriate antifungal therapy may be a useful clinical indicator of response.

However, immune-suppressed or immune-deficient patients may not mount an appropriate antibody response to *Candida albicans*. Also, if the patient's predominant yeast organism is not *Candida albicans*, a negative antibody result might occur when measuring *Candida albicans*-specific antibodies.

Thus, the role of serodiagnosis of CCSS through anti-*Candida* antibody measurements is promising but is yet unproven in clinical application.

Culture of Candida albicans

There are inherent limitations to the use of *Candida* cultures in the diagnosis of CCSS: culture tells us nothing about the host response and sensitization. In addition, cultures may be alternately positive and negative in the same individual, depending on culturing techniques. Thus, although culturing *Candida albicans* verifies yeast colonization, it is a useful aid but not a diagnostic test of CCSS.

Routine intradermal testing

Occasionally, routine intradermal skin testing to *Candida albicans* may reveal strong immediate whealing and may correlate with Type I hypersensitivity manifestations of *Candida albicans* mentioned above (urticaria, asthma). However, it is not helpful in distinguishing patients with CCSS from normal controls [86].

PATHOGENESIS OF CHRONIC CANDIDIASIS SENSITIVITY

CCSS is largely a disease of the host—not the organism. Even the most virulent *Candida* species (*Candida albicans*) occurs as a human commensal and is able to invade and damage tissues only when host defences are locally and systemically impaired. Figure 49.5 shows a proposed model for the pathogenesis of this illness. Three factors are proposed as key elements in the evolution of this illness: (a)

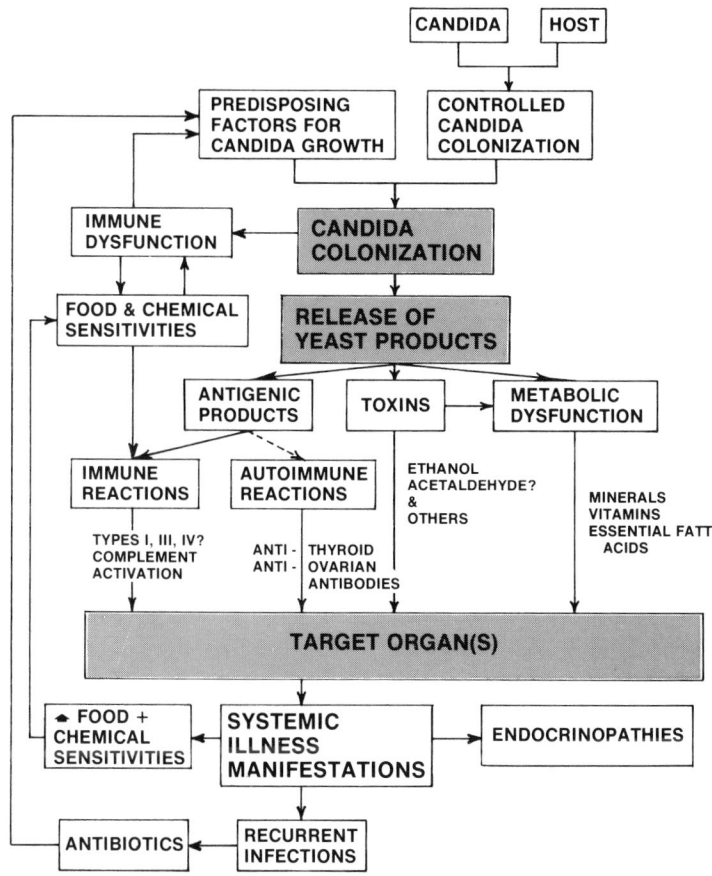

Fig. 49.5 Proposed model for the pathogenesis of chronic candidiasis sensitivity.

altered host/pathogen balance with increased *Candida* colonization, (b) release of yeast products (both antigenic and non-antigenic) into the system and (c) distant end-organ effects of these products (both immunological and non-immunological).

Increased colonization

Intrinsic host resistance

Many factors have been implicated as increasing *Candida* carriage in the human host (Table 49.9). Immunological, nutritional and mechanical host defences are important intrinsic predeterminants in a person's susceptibility towards *Candida* carriage. Disorders associated with increased chronic *Candida* carriage include: disorders of cell-mediated immunity and phagocytic dysfunction [79], nutritional deficiencies [11, 20, 27, 28, 53], skin burns/abrasions/wounds [44, 81], suppression of gastric acid [9, 84], altered glucose metabolism [80, 96] and pregnancy [61].

Iatrogenic factors

Although intrinsic host defences are important predeterminants in a person's susceptibility towards chronic *Candida albicans* carriage, iatrogenic medical factors are equally important.

Antibiotics. Prolonged antibiotic usage is clinically the most important external factor associated with enhanced *Candida* carriage in the host and the development of CCSS. Broad-spectrum antibiotics, through suppressing intestinal bacteria, remove natural restraints in the control of gastrointestinal *Candida* carriage [8]. Very often a 'vicious cycle' is created, whereby a patient with lowered immunological resistance is more susceptible to chronic infections, resulting in increased usage of antibiotics. This in turn increases *Candida* carriage; increased *Candida* carriage may further suppress the patient's ability to resist further infections.

Corticosteroids. In addition to antibiotics, chronic corticosteroid usage has been asso-

Table 49.9 Factors predisposing to chronic candidiasis carriage.

Impaired immunity
  Phagocytic cells (neutrophils and macrophages)
  Decreased numbers—leukaemias, radiation treatment, chemotherapy
  Intrinsic dysfunction—myeloperoxidase deficiency chronic granulomatous disease
Cell-mediated immunity
  Intrinsic defects—thymoma, DiGeorge's syndrome, chronic mucocutaneous candidiasis
  Acquired defects—chemotherapy, steroids, radiation, environmental chemical sensitivity

Nutritional and dietary factors
  Hypovitaminosis A
  Low serum iron
  High carbohydrate diet
  Low serum folate

Mechanical factors
  Skin barrier—burns, maceration, wounds, catheters
  Mucosal barrier—dentures, increased gastric pH, mucosal tumours, increased glucose in secretions (diabetes)

Hormonal factors
  Pregnancy
  Oral contraceptives
  Menses

Medications
  Antibiotics
  Oral steroids
  Oral contraceptives
  Metronidazole
  Cimetidine

Underlying disease states
  Diabetes mellitus
  Polyendocrinopathies—thyroid, parathyroid, adrenal
  Malignancies

ciated with increased carriage of *Candida* in the host [61]. Corticosteroids have the capability to depress cell-mediated immunity, including lymphocyte migration inhibition and lymphocyte transformation in response to *Candida albicans* [21]. Patients predisposed towards CCSS may symptomatically worsen following usage of high-dose steroids.

Oral contraceptives. Oral contraceptives are often poorly tolerated by women who have a history suggestive of CCSS; their use is often associated with central nervous system dysfunction, including depression, emotional lability, fatigue and other symptoms. Chronic yeast vaginal carriage is heightened when progesterone levels are high, as in pregnancy and the luteal phase of the menstrual cycle. Although five studies have reported significantly higher rates of yeast carriage in users of combined-formulation oestrogenic contraceptives than in users of sequential-formulation progestagenic contraceptives [3, 16, 43, 82, 94] it is better to discontinue oral contraceptive use if possible, and their 'avoidance is mandatory if chronic *Candida* is to be successfully controlled' [86].

Release of *Candida* antigens/toxins

Candida colonization is clinically relevant, since invasion and disease due to *Candida* has been related to the magnitude of host colonization with this organism [79].

Candida albicans interference with proper immune function may occur at several levels, including (a) generation of increased populations of T suppressor cells, with alterations in the T4/T8 lymphocyte ratio, (b) interference with correct *Candida* antigen presentation by macrophages to autologous T lymphocytes and (c) secretion of hyphal substances impairing immune function [79]. This generalized impairment in cellular immunity may augment the development of further *Candida* colonization and mycelial phase transformation, with the eventual release of yeast by-products—both antigenic and non-antigenic—into the circulation.

Antigenic/allergic effects

Antigen quantity or presentation may be responsible for a variety of clinical disease states in patients with chronic candidiasis carriage:

1 Type I hypersensitivity reactions—urticaria, asthma;
2 Type III sensitivity reactions—allergic bronchopulmonary candidiasis;
3 Alternative complement pathway activation;
4 Type IV reaction—altered cellular immune response to *Candida* antigens.

Activation of these mechanisms may lead to release of multiple primary and secondary mediators of inflammation (prostaglandins, kinins, histamine) which in turn may be responsible for some of the distant end-organ effects seen in clinical illness.

Metabolic/toxic effects

The pathogenic potential of *Candida albicans* may be partly related to its ability to aggravate subclinical metabolic dysfunction and nutrient deficiencies in genetically susceptible individuals. The following metabolic factors may be responsible for some of the symptomatology in patients with CCSS.

Toxins. Various strains of *Candida albicans* have the capacity to produce multiple toxins. Toxins from several *Candida* strains have a variety of effects on the host as can be seen in Table 49.10.

Table 49.10 Effect of *Candida* toxins.

Suppression of T cell number and function
Enhanced vascular permeability
Augmentation of histamine release with induction of anaphylaxis [15]
Behavioural changes (in animals) [18]

Sugar metabolism. The metabolism of sugars by yeast organisms may have pathological consequences for the host as well. Yeasts are able to convert sugars to pyruvate; this in turn is anaerobically converted to acetaldehyde and carbon dioxide. (Chronic carbon dioxide production may account for the persistent bloating and gas noted clinically by many patients with CCSS.) Some strains of *Candida albicans* are able to reduce acetaldehyde to ethanol. In certain individuals harbouring an ethanol-producing strain of *Candida*, central nervous system effects similar to a state of chronic alcohol intoxication can ensue. This syndrome, called *Meitei-sho* ('drunk disease') in Japanese has been described in the foreign medical literature since the 1950s [34] and reported in the popular press recently in the United States [15].

Acetaldehyde production. It may be that chronic acetaldehyde production—rather than chronic ethanol production—is responsible for a large number of signs and symptoms in CCSS. Truss [88] proposes that chronic acetaldehyde production may be responsible for multiple central nervous system symptoms through (a) acetaldehyde-induced loss of red blood cell flexibility with resultant diminished oxygen tissue delivery, (b) acetaldehyde binding to amine groups of neurotransmitters and (c) acetaldehyde oxidation leading to a chronically elevated NADH/NAD ratio with multiple potential neuronal metabolic problems.

Urinary amino acid profile. Truss found abnormal patterns of urinary amino acid profiles in patients with CCSS. Certain amino acids (especially glutamine, glutamate and asparagine) were found to be particularly low (Table 49.11). These amino acids are derived from intermediates in the citric acid cycle, and may be low secondary to acetaldehyde-induced depression of acetyl-coenzyme-A production, with consequent depression of the citric acid cycle.

Vitamin B_2 and B_6. In a recent paper on nutrition and candidiasis, Galland reported on metabolic abnormalities found in patients with CCSS [23]. Deficiencies in certain vitamins and minerals were frequently found in patients with CCSS (Table 49.12). Lowered vitamin B_6 activity was found in a large percentage [67%] of a series of 39 patients with CCSS. This lowered B_6 activity was found to correlate with lowered B_2 activity also. Although lowered vitamin B_6 activity is probably a result of other metabolic abnormalities rather than a primary problem, its deficiency could present symptomatic difficulties for patients with CCSS and conceivably contribute to multiple symptoms, including fatigue, depression, neuropathic problems, heightened oedema formation and additional metabolic dysfunction.

Fatty acid metabolism. Clinical expression of fatty acid deficiency is often seen in patients with CCSS. Galland reported nearly 66% of CCSS patients he studied had two or more clinical signs of fatty acid deficiency [23]. Such non-specific signs as dry stiff hair, dry scaly skin, brittle nails and follicular dermatitis may be associated with essential fatty acid deficiency. In no patient was a normal fatty acid profile found [23].

Table 49.11 24-Hour urinary amino acid levels in 24 patients with CCSS. The results for each amino acid are expressed as the percentage of these 24 patients with values that were normal, low or elevated.

Amino acids	Normal	Below normal	Above normal
Taurine	87.5	12.5	0
Phosphoethanolamine	29.2	70.8	0
Aspartic	95.8	0	4.2
Threonine	25.0	75.0	0
Serine	50.0	45.8	4.2
Asparagine	0	100.0	0
Glutamic	4.2	95.8	0
δ-Amino adipic	8.3	91.7	0
Glycine	95.8	0	4.2
Glutamine	37.5	62.5	0
Alanine	91.7	4.2	4.2
α-Amino n-butyric	62.5	37.5	0
Valine	50.0	50.0	0
Cystine	83.3	0	16.7
Methionine	29.2	70.8	0
Cystathionine	8.3	91.7	0
Isoleucine	20.8	79.2	0
Tyrosine	50.0	50.0	0
Phenylalanine	54.2	33.3	12.5
Ethanolamine	54.2	4.2	41.7
Lysine	62.5	33.3	4.2
1-Methylhistidine	20.8	75.0	4.2
Histidine	83.3	16.7	0
3-Methylhistidine	83.3	0	16.7
Leucine	45.8	54.2	0

Reproduced from Truss [88], with permission.

Table 49.12 Nutrient deficiencies in CCSS.

Nutrient	Number of patients	Percentage low
Pyridoxal-5-phosphate	39	67
Riboflavin	17	28
Zinc	83	17.3
Folate	101	15
Vitamin A (< 25 mg/dl)	101	13
Ferritin	101	10
Vitamin C	101	5

Adapted from Galland [23].

Table 49.13 Essential fatty acid metabolism abnormalities in CCSS.

EFA lesion	Number of patients	Percentage
Deficient ω-3 versus ω-6	27	73
ω-6 desaturase block	24	65
Abnormal ω-6 metabolism	25	68
Elevated arachidonic acid	25	68
Decreased DGLA	15	40
Low DGLA/arachidonic ratio	21	57

DGLA = dihomogammalinolenic acid.
EFA = essential fatty acid.
Adapted from Galland [23].

Multiple abnormalities were noted in both the ω-3 and ω-6 series, but the ω-6 series appeared to be more severely affected. Essential fatty acid lesions found are listed in Table 49.13.

Magnesium metabolism. In addition to deficiencies in vitamin B₆ and certain essential fatty acids, red blood cell levels of magnesium have also been reported to be low in as many as 50% of patients with CCSS [23]; this may be accompanied by excessive urinary magnesium excretion. Lowered magnesium levels may in turn further interfere with formation of essential fatty acids and stimulate prostaglandin formation.

End-organ effects: *Candida* and endocrinopathy

The triad of candidiasis, autoantibody production and endocrinopathy may account for a large part of the symptom complex seen in patients with CCSS. Symptoms of menstrual dysfunction are common complaints of women with CCSS.

Autoantibodies

Mathur and his colleagues found antibodies reacting against *Candida* antigen, T helper cells and ovarian stroma; in addition these antibodies appeared to cross-react with each other [50]. The level of *Candida* colonization required to stimulate these antibodies is purportedly found in chronic vaginal candidiasis. Thus, a *Candida*-stimulated autoimmune oophoritis may contribute to the symptoms of ovarian gland dysfunction so common in patients with CCSS, and treatment with antifungal drugs and suppressive doses of progesterone usually results in dramatic improvement in symptoms [74].

Autoimmune thyroiditis

Thyroiditis is encountered in CCSS patients at a frequency greater than expected in the general population [74] and could account for multiple symptoms seen in CCSS including menstrual irregularity, fatigue, temperature intolerance, weight gain and depression. Treatment with thyroid supplements combined with anti-*Candida* therapy usually results in dramatic improvement. Some patients with chronic *Candida* infections reportedly do not respond until thyroid disease is treated [55] (see Chapter 44b).

Mitral valve prolapse

It is interesting to note that there appears to be a relationship between CCSS, mitral valve prolapse and thyroiditis. A greater than expected incidence of mitral valve prolapse is seen in patients with CCSS [23,88], and a very close association between mitral valve prolapse and chronic thyroiditis [52] has been reported.

Hormones

Hormonal influences on *Candida albicans* growth may be an important additional factor to consider in the *Candida*-endocrine connection. *Candida albicans* has a corticosteroid-binding protein which binds corticosteroids and progestins, and brewer's yeast has an oestrogen-binding protein and oestrogenic endogenous ligand [19]. The hormone–receptor interaction provides a mechanism by which the host hormonal environment could theoretically alter the infectivity of the *Candida* organism. Is this one reason why CCSS appears to have a female sexual preference, and why other fungal infections (such as *Paracoccidioides brasiliensis*) have male sexual preference [19]? Rifkind has shown that gonadal hormones influence the extent of delayed hypersensitivity in mice [69]; and changes in anti-*Candida* antibody levels are specifically associated with progesterone and oestradiol [49].

Conclusion

The *Candida*-endocrine interaction is complex, most likely involving fungal-hormonal interactions at several levels, and potentially contributing to many of the more serious symptoms of CCSS. Fortunately, with appropriate antifungal treatment and hormonal supplementation (when necessary) dramatic improvement in clinical symptoms usually ensues.

Candida and allergy

Disturbances in fungal sensitivity and load can exacerbate previously quiescent chemical sensitivities. Conversely, disturbances in the allergy reactions to foods, inhalants and chemicals can make patients more susceptible to small perturbations in their total *Candida* load. This stresses the concept of the patient's 'total load' [68].

Onset of symptoms

The onset of overt food and chemical intolerances may be traceable to a specific increase in *Candida* antigenic load (recurrent antibiotic therapy, high carbohydrate diet, steroids or oral contraceptives). Conversely, patients may begin to experience *Candida* sensitivity symptoms shortly after experiencing a heavy chemical exposure, such as to formaldehyde-containing products (mobile homes, foam insulation) or agricultural pesticides [88].

Treatment

Clinically, antifungal treatment of patients with CCSS may result in dramatic improvement in otherwise untreated mould, food and chemical intolerances, possibly through these or other mechanisms. Patients treated for *Candida* sensitivity may report improvement in seasonal mould-induced respiratory symptoms, lesser cravings for carbohydrate and improved food tolerance, and improvement in tolerance for indoor and outdoor air pollution. However, it is important to note that over-aggressive antifungal treatment early in the management of a severely chemically sensitive patient can sometimes result in *worsening* of chemical sensitivities—particularly if appropriate environmental control measures are not instituted prior to initiation of antifungal medication and immunotherapy to reduce the patient's total load.

TREATMENT OF CHRONIC CANDIDIASIS SENSITIVITY SYNDROME

The treatment of CCSS is multifactorial, involving three major areas of management: pharmacological, dietary and immunological (Table 49.14). The rapidity of recovery from

Table 49.14 Treatment of chronic candidiasis sensitivity syndrome.

Dietary and nutritional measures:
  Dietary measures to retard *Candida* growth:
  Low carbohydrate, yeast-free diet
  Adequate nutrients for optimal immune response
  e.g. vitamins: yeast-free B complex, vitamins A, E, C
      etc.
      Minerals: zinc, iron, magnesium calcium
      Fatty acids: evening primrose oil

  Supplementation to ensure favourable gut flora ecology
      e.g. *Lactobacillus*

Pharmacological measures:
  Avoidance of drugs promoting chronic *Candida* growth
  Antibiotics, steroids, oral contraceptives etc.
  Treatment of *Candida* with antifungal medication
      e.g. nystatin, ketoconazole, caprylic acid etc.

Immunological measures:
  Active immunization with *Candida albicans* extracts

Other measures:
  Treat all inhalant, food and chemical allergies
      e.g. environmental control, active immunotherapy
      hypoallergenic diets
  Rule out associated endocrinopathic conditions
      e.g. thyroid, ovarian, adrenal etc.

CCSS is influenced by several factors, including (a) the ability of the patient to avoid those factors promoting yeast growth, (b) the sensitivity of the yeast organism to the antifungal medication administered and (c) the degree and speed of immune response to *Candida* immunotherapy.

Diet and nutrition

Diet: low-carbohydrate and yeast-free diet

Diet is the single most important management step likely to help the patient. It is extremely unlikely that a seriously ill patient with CCSS will recover from his or her disease unless adequate dietary measures are instituted.

Carbohydrate restriction. Carbohydrate is the chief nutrient of *Candida albicans*. There is general agreement that a low-carbohydrate diet is mandatory in the treatment of CCSS, but there are no hard data to support this opinion. Most patients do well on a diet simply avoiding refined sugars and large amounts of honey, maple syrup and fruit juice. Milk should also be restricted due to its high lactose content. Some patients will not feel optimal unless a rigid carbohydrate restriction diet is prescribed (60–80 g carbohydrate per day). Strict carbohydrate restriction is generally not recommended for youngsters with CCSS. A representative diet which appears helpful to the majority of patients is shown in the Appendix, and others are available [15, 70].

Difficulty in compliance

Patients may have considerable difficulty in coping with these dietary changes, due to (a) withdrawal effects from removal of coexisting food allergens from the diet and (b) intense continued carbohydrate cravings. Patients should be reassured that these symptoms are usually temporary in nature and improve with time.

Yeast restriction. Elimination of yeast-containing foods is also recommended, due to the high degree of apparent cross-sensitization between *Candida albicans* and brewer's/baker's yeast. Major foodstuffs containing yeast include: fermented (alcoholic) beverages, cheeses, mushrooms, vinegar and vinegar-containing foods, dried fruits and breads. A hidden source of yeast commonly overlooked is found in nutritional supplements—especially yeast-derived B-complex. Hence, all supplements taken by the patient should be carefully examined for yeast content. However, (a) not all patients sensitive to *Candida albicans* will be sensitive to yeast-containing foods and (b) ingestion of a yeast-containing food does not in itself augment *Candida albicans* growth.

Thus, there are occasional patients who do not need to avoid yeast-containing foods when being treated long-term for CCSS, although they are definitely in the minority.

Finally, it should be noted that the safest and best diet for the patient with CCSS and a history of multiple food allergy/intolerance is a *rotary diversified diet* limiting carbohydrate and yeast-containing foods (see Chapter 17).

Nutritional supplementation

Specific nutritional supplementation must be tailored to the unique needs of each individual patient. Certain principles should be followed: (a) yeast-free hypoallergenic supplements are best tolerated; (b) nutrient supplements are often better tolerated (and perhaps more effective) after the total load of *Candida albicans* has been reduced by dietary and drug measures; and (c) patients with CCSS may have greater than expected deficiencies in the following: vitamin B_6/B_2, vitamin A, iron, magnesium, zinc, certain amino acids and essential fatty acids. Specific blood and/or urine nutrient assays may be helpful to detect nutritional deficiencies, but for most patients with CCSS such assays are not necessary provided appropriately designed dietary and nutrient supplementation measures are instituted.

Lactobacillus supplementation

The literature on the effect of *Lactobacillus* on *Candida albicans* growth is conflicting; *Lactobacillus* has been claimed both to enhance and to inhibit the growth of *Candida albicans* [61]. Clinically, it is difficult to re-establish *Lactobacillus* in the bowel, and commercial *Lactobacillus acidophilus* supplements vary greatly in potency—with some commercial brands apparently not containing appreciable numbers of *Lactobacillus* [91]. 'High-potency' *Lactobacillus acidophilus* preparations are now available, and may be derived from a variety of sources—including cow's milk, goat's milk, soya, carrot and synthetic processes [60].

The source is of practical importance, since some patients sensitive to milk products may also react adversely to the standard milk-derived *Lactobacillus acidophilus* products. Addition of a high-potency *Lactobacillus acidophilus* preparation to the diet may be helpful.

Other supplements

Garlic extracts have known antifungal prop-

erties; the active component of garlic extracts, allicin (allyl-allylthiosulphonate), has broad antifungal activity in vitro [4]. Commercial garlic preparations have gained popularity among patients with CCSS due to their relative cheapness and non-prescription status. Similarly, other treatments (such as 'Taheebo tea') are popular for similar reasons. Their use remains questionable and without proven merit in the treatment of CCSS.

Pharmacological treatment

Antifungal therapy for *Candida albicans* is an exceedingly important part of treatment of CCSS. Although dietary measures may passively reduce *Candida* colonization, active pharmacological eradication of existing *Candida albicans* reservoirs is nearly always necessary in any patient with serious CCSS.

There are certain general principles which apply to the institution of any antifungal regimen in patients with CCSS.

'Die-off' reactions

Early in treatment, patients may exhibit a transient worsening of symptoms, sometimes lasting 1-2 weeks in duration. This phenomenon is only rarely an allergic reaction to the medication; it is possibly a systemic 'Herxheimer' reaction due to the rapid killing of *Candida albicans* organisms and consequent transient absorption of large quantities of fragmented yeast products into the circulation [15]. 'Die-off' reactions can be minimized through:

1 attempts at passively controlling *Candida* load by diet for 1-2 weeks prior to institution of antifungal medications;
2 starting medication in low doses and slowly increasing the dose over time;
3 lowering chemical and food 'overload' situations *before* institution of antifungal therapy.

Long-term treatment

Most seriously ill patients with CCSS need antifungal medication (nystatin) for at least a 4-6-month initial period, in a dose of 8-10 million units daily while following their diet and receiving immunotherapy, although the exact duration of antifungal therapy needed varies with each patient. There is no diagnostically reliable test to indicate with certainty when patients are able to reduce or discontinue antifungal therapy. An attempt should be made to slowly taper patients off antifungal medication if they are doing well and after several months of comprehensive treatment. If symptoms recur, treatment should be started again. Diet and immunotherapy constitute the preferred long-term management for patients with CCSS, especially for those who suffer from food and chemical sensitivities and who run a heightened risk of developing drug intolerance to any antifungal agent.

Treatment of sexual partners. Candida infections may be spread by sexual activity [71]. However, sexual transmission is probably responsible for a minority of reinfections and most women with CCSS do not need simultaneous treatment of their sexual partner.

Nystatin

Nystatin, a polyene-class antimycotic derived from *Streptomyces noursei*, is both fungistatic and fungicidal, damaging yeast cell walls through binding to membrane sterols (primarily ergosterol) and is the principal treatment for CCSS. There is negligible absorption from the gastrointestinal tract, and it is excreted in the stool. Although it is generally non-sensitizing and extremely well tolerated by most patients, it can occasionally cause nausea when administered, as well as the 'die-off' effects mentioned earlier.

Formulation. Nystatin is available in several forms, including tablets (500 000 units nystatin/tablet), pure powder (500 000 units nystatin per 1/8 teaspoon), vaginal suppositories and topical creams and powders.

Nystatin powder is preferred when patients with CCSS have mouth or oesophageal evidence of *Candida* as well as lower gastrointestinal tract symptoms; otherwise nystatin tablets may be used. A suggested regimen for treatment of CCSS in an adult patient is given below:

500 000 U nystatin p.o. q.i.d. × 1 week
1 000 000 U nystatin p.o. q.i.d. × 1 week
1 500 000 U nystatin p.o. q.i.d. × 1 week
2 000 000 U nystatin p.o. q.i.d. therafter

Children 6–12 years old will usually tolerate one-third to one-half of the dosage regimen listed above.

Minimal toxicity of nystatin at similar high dosages (6–24 million units/day) is seen in trials utilizing nystatin to treat immunosup-

pressed leukaemic patients [93]. Occasionally, patients will need dosages even higher than the induction regimen given above in order to relieve symptoms. This may be partially due to drug-resistant organisms.

Response to treatment. Response to therapy is generally prompt, usually occurring within 2–4 weeks of therapy. Earliest symptoms to improve are bowel function disturbances, followed later by improvement in distant end-organ systems, including central nervous system functioning and proper endocrine regulation.

Uncommon symptoms such as urticaria, angioedema, depression, muscle weakness and uncontrolled diarrhoea have been reported to occur in exquisitely environmentally sensitive individuals with CCSS upon taking nystatin [89]. Some of these patients respond favourably to low-dose nystatin. Others simply cannot tolerate nystatin at all and need other treatment.

Ketoconazole

Ketaconazole, a piperazine derivative of imidazole, is a potent inhibitor of ergosterol synthesis in *Candida albicans* and is completely absorbed from the gastrointestinal tract. It is metabolized in the liver and excreted in the bile. Due to its broader antifungal properties it may be the drug of choice in CCSS patients who have coexisting severe dermatophyte infections or who do not tolerate and/or respond to nystatin therapy.

The normal dose is one 200 mg tablet once or twice a day. However, ketoconazole requires intact stomach acidity to become soluble. In CCSS patients taking concomitant antacids, anticholinergics and H_2-receptor blockers, ketoconazole should be given at least 2 hours beforehand.

Side-effects include nausea and vomiting as well as a reported incidence of 1% liver enzyme abnormalities and 0.01% symptomatic hepatitis. Liver function tests should be monitored at least monthly for patients on ketoconazole. Other reported adverse reactions include gynecomastia, anaphylaxis and altered testosterone synthesis [90].

Reports of *Candida* organisms with clinical and in vitro resistance to ketoconazole have emerged [47], and patients who fail to respond completely to ketoconazole may have an improved response to nystatin or other antifungal medications.

Other antifungal preparations

In addition to nystatin and ketoconazole, other antifungal medications are available [48]. For the treatment of CCSS, the use of drugs other than nystatin and ketoconazole has been limited, largely due to toxicity and route of administration. Two potentially promising agents which may overcome these difficulties are caprylic acid and orally administered amphotericin.

Caprylic acid. Caprylic acid has been reported in the early medical literature as being effective in treating patients with mucocutaneous candidiasis [40] as well as patients with severe symptomatic enteric candidiasis [57]. It is available commercially as an enteric-coated tablet containing coconut-derived caprylic acid adsorbed to a non-resinous ion exchange moiety for gradual release through the intestine. Caprylic acid exhibits fungistatic and fungicidal properties in vitro and in vivo. Its major side-effects are gastrointestinal (nausea, abdominal pain) but the incidence is low, particularly with the enteric-coated formulations. To date, no long-term studies utilizing caprylic acid in the long-term management of CCSS have been reported.

Amphotericin. Amphotericin is a polyene antifungal medication similar to nystatin. Although its inevitable toxicity when given intravenously makes it unsuitable for long-term treatment of CCSS by that route, it has been reported to be effective against chronic mucocutaneous candidiasis and surprisingly non-toxic as well when given orally [54]. Although potentially a promising agent, no long-term studies have been reported with this agent in the treatment of CCSS.

Immunotherapy

Immunotherapy with *Candida* vaccines has been reported to be helpful for a variety of problems associated with *Candida albicans*. Several authors have reported favourably on *Candida* hyposensitization treatment with vaccine extracts for recurrent vaginal candidiasis [32, 42, 62, 63].

In addition, other authors have reported that hyposensitization injections of *Candida albicans* may relieve other symptoms in end organs distant from vaginal colonization [48, 86].

Clinically, immunotherapy with *Candida* antigenic extracts appears to be useful for many patients with CCSS. Often, *Candida* immunotherapy has been able to provide additional clinical improvement in CCSS patients who have 'plateaued' in their response to diet and antifungal therapy. Many patients can be successfully managed long-term on immunotherapy and diet alone, without recourse to chronic antifungal medication.

Mechanism of action. It is known that repeated intracutaneous administration of *C. albicans* glycoprotein in rabbits stimulates both cellular and humoral responses [37], and it is possible that *Candida albicans* injection therapy in man is non-specifically stimulating the immune system and acting as an adjuvant. Nevertheless, the exact mechanism of action of *Candida* immunotherapy is unclear and the reason for its effectiveness in CCSS is purely speculative.

Side-effects. Clinically, in attempting to immunize with *Candida albicans*, it is important to note that patients can have their symptoms made worse if immunotherapy is begun too early in treatment, especially if such patients have coexisting food and chemical sensitivities and/or florid *Candida* overgrowth.

Techniques. Various immunotherapy techniques are advocated by different practitioners for the treatment of CCSS; these can generally be grouped into four basic techniques—low-dose injection therapy, high-dose provocation/neutralization therapy, serial dilution titration therapy and repeated intradermal injections for stimulation of cellular immunity.

1 Low-dose injection immunotherapy as described by Truss involves administration of subcutaneous dosages of 0.10 ml of 10^{-7} to 10^{-15} dilution of serial 1 : 10 dilutions of commercial *Candida albicans* extracts. The usual starting dose is 0.1 ml of 10^{-14} or 10^{-15} dilution biweekly. Further details of this technique are published elsewhere [86].
2 Provocative intradermal neutralizing dose immunotherapy for *Candida albicans* has been described elsewhere [98] and is based on intradermal or sublingual administration of *Candida albicans* antigenic extracts, with initial provocation of the patient's symptoms followed by subsequent relief of symptoms when an appropriate neutralization dose is found.
3 In serial dilution titration immunotherapy, described elsewhere [99], the treatment dose

is determined through observing for a progressive '5-7-9' mm immediate whealing response to intradermal administration of *Candida* vaccine; no attempt is made to provoke or neutralize symptoms with this technique. Treatment is given either by subcutaneous injection or sublingual administration of *Candida* vaccine.

4 Intradermal administration of *Candida* extracts is an important index of delayed hypersensitivity in CCSS; if there is no delay seen on *Candida* intradermal testing with 2000 PNU (protein nitrogen units), then repeated intradermal injections of this dilution will encourage the development of an appropriate delayed hypersensitivity response [56].

Comparison of Candida immunotherapy techniques

Unfortunately, the immunotherapy techniques outlined above have not been compared for efficacy in the treatment of CCSS. Clinically, the response to immunotherapy in CCSS is mixed, and is dependent on many variables, including the immunotherapy technique utilized, the mechanism of CCSS (immunological versus metabolic/toxic), variations in extract strengths and antigenic potency, host variations in immunopathology, other treatments concurrently being employed etc. For patients with true fungal hypersensitivity and a strong immediate whealing response to *Candida* antigenic extracts, serial dilution titration with appropriate suppressive doses of antigen administered may be helpful. In contrast, for patients with an absence of an immediate and delayed 24 hour-whealing response to *Candida*

antigen, repeated intradermal stimulatory injections of *Candida* extract 2000 PNU may encourage the development of an appropriate delayed response.

In conclusion, *Candida* immunotherapy may be valuable in the treatment of CCSS, but remains an empirical tool at best, with techniques and results that vary among practitioners.

CONCLUSIONS

1 *Candida albicans* has sensitization potential as well as infective potential in certain susceptible individuals.

2 *Candida albicans* may exert its sensitization response on the human host through immunological-allergic, or toxic-metabolic processes; these processes may occur individually or together in the same host.

3 *Candida albicans* sensitization may result in a polysymptomatic condition involving multiple symptoms in distant end organs remote from actual localized *Candida* colonization. This condition, termed chronic candidiasis sensitivity syndrome, may involve not only polysystemic illness involving multiple organ systems, but also may be associated with other specific illnesses, including environmental food and chemical sensitivities, polyendocrinopathies and mitral valve prolapse.

4 Therapy of chronic candidiasis sensitivity syndrome involves utilization of diet, drug and immunotherapy to aid the body in controlling *Candida albicans* carriage, and is generally safe and effective in nature.

REFERENCES

1 Akiyama K, Mathison DA, Riker JB et al: Allergic bronchopulmonary candidiasis. Chest 1984; 85:699–701.

2 Alexander JG: Allergy in the gastrointestinal tract. Lancet 1975; ii:1264.

3 Anyon CP, Desmond FB, Eastcott DF: A study of *Candida* in one thousand and seven women. NZ Med J 1971; 73:9–13.

4 Appleton JA, Tansey MR: Inhibition of growth of zoopathogenic fungi by garlic extract. Mycologia 1975; 67:882–5.

5 Axelson NH: Analysis of human *Candida* precipitins by quantitative immunoelectrophoresis: a model for analysis of complex microbiol antigen–antibody systems. Scand J Immunol 1976; 5:177–90.

6 Baker SM: Nystatin in the treatment of psoriasis.

Presented at the *Candida albicans* conference, Dallas Texas, 10 July, 1982.

7 Baker SM: The yeast problem. Gesell Institute of Human Development Update 1982;2(5):3–6.

8 Bolivar R, Bodey GP: Candidiasis of the gastrointestinal tract. In: Bodey GP, Fainstein V, eds. Candidiasis. New York: Raven Press, 1985:184.

9 Brooks JR, Smith HE, Pease FB: Bacteriology of the stomach immediately following vagotomy: the growth of *Candida albicans*. Ann Surg 1974;179:859–62.

10 Clayton YM, Noble WC: Observations on the epidemiology of *Candida albicans*. J Clin Pathol 1966;19:76–8.

11 Cohen BE, Elin RJ: Enhanced resistance to certain infections in vitamin A-treated mice. Plast Reconstr Surg 1974;54:192–4.

12 Crook WG: PMS and yeasts: an etiological connection? Hosp Pract 1983;18:21-4.

13 Crook WG: *Candida* questionnaire and score sheet. In: The yeast connection. 2nd edn. Jackson, Tennessee: Professional Books, 1984;29-33.

14 Crook WG: Depression associated with *Candida albicans* infections. J Am Med Assoc 1984;25:2928-9.

15 Crook WG: The yeast connection. 2nd edn. Jackson, Tennessee: Professional Books, 1984.

16 Davis BA: Vaginal moniliasis in private practice. Obstet Gynecol 1969;34:40-5.

17 Edge G, Pepys J: Antibodies in different immunoglobulin classes to *Candida albicans* in allergic respiratory disease. Clin Allergy 1980;10:47-58.

18 Edwards DA: Depression and candida. J Am Med Assoc 1985;253:3400.

19 Feldman D: Steroids produced by yeasts and steroid receptor sites in yeasts. Presented at the Yeast-Human Interaction Symposium, San Francisco, California, 29-31 March, 1985.

20 Fletcher J, Mather J, Lewis MJ, Whiting G: Mouth lesions in iron-deficient anemia: relationship to *Candida albicans* in saliva and to impairment of lymphocyte transformation. J Infect Dis 1975;131:44-50.

21 Folb PI, Trounce JR: Immunological aspects of *Candida* infection complicating steroid and immunosuppressive drug therapy. Lancet 1970;ii:1112-14.

22 Forbes JG: A case of mycosis of the tongue and nails in a female child aged 3½ years. Br J Dermatol 1909;21:221-3.

23 Galland L: Nutrition and candidiasis. J Orthomol Psychiatry 1985;15:50-60.

24 Guilford FT, Der-Balian GP: Human isotype levels to *Candida albicans* in patients with candidiasis. Presented at the Yeast-Human Interaction Symposium, San Francisco California, 29-31 March, 1985.

25 Haggland H, Bauman DS: Antibody studies in patients with candidiasis. Presented at the Yeast-Human Interaction Symposium, San Francisco, California, 29-31 March, 1985.

26 Herxheimer H: The late bronchial reaction in induced asthma. Int Arch Allergy Appl Immunol 1952;3:328.

27 Higgs JM: Chronic mucocutaneous candidiasis: iron deficiency and the effects of iron therapy. Proc R Soc Med 1973;66:802-4.

28 Higgs JM, Wells RS: Chronic mucocutaneous candidiasis: associated abnormalities of iron metabolism. Br J Dermatol 1972;86:88-102.

29 Hippocrates, Circa 460-377 BC: Epidemics. Book 3. Translated by F. Adams. Baltimore: Williams and Wilkins, 1939.

30 Holti G: *Candida* allergy. In: Winner HI, Hurley R, eds. Symposium on *Candida* infections. Edinburgh and London: E & S Livingstone, 1966;74-81.

31 Holti G: Some skin hazards and allergy problems in dentistry. Newcastle Med J 1969;30:245-4.

32 Hosen H: Focal fungal infections treated by immunological therapy with emphasis on vaginal moniliasis. Tex Med 1971;67:56-8.

33 Itkin IH, Dennis M: Bronchial hypersensitivity to extract of *Candida albicans*. J Allergy 1966;37:187-94.

34 Iwata K: A review of the literature on drunken symptoms due to yeasts in the gastrointestinal tract. In: Iwata K, ed. Yeasts and yeast-like microorganisms in medical science. International specialized symposium on yeasts. Tokyo: University of Tokyo Press, 1976;184-90.

35 Jacobi E: Ein besondere Form der Trichophytie als Folgeerscheinung des permanenten Bades. Arch Dermatol Syphilogr 1907;84:289-300.

36 James J, Warin RP: An assessment of the role of *Candida albicans* and food yeasts in chronic urticaria. Br J Dermatol 1971;84:227-37.

37 Jenssen HL, Kohler H, Kaben Y, Westphal HJ: Cell electrophoretic studies on the cellular immune response to *Candida albicans* in rabbits. Sabouraudia 1975;13:123-31.

38 Kabe J, Aoki Y, Ishizaki T et al: Relationship of dermal and pulmonary sensitivity to extracts of *Candida albicans*. Am Rev Respir Dis 1971;104:348-57.

39 Kashkin PN, Krassilnikov NA, Nekachalov VY: *Candida* complications after antibiotic therapy. Mycopathol Mycol Appl 1961;14:173-88.

40 Keeney EL: Sodium caprylate: a new and effective treatment of moniliasis of the skin and mucous membrane. Bull Johns Hopkins Hosp 1946;78:333-9.

41 Keeney EL: *Candida* asthma. Ann Intern Med 1951;34:223-6.

42 Kudelko NM: Allergy in chronic monilial vaginitis. Ann Allergy 1971;29:266-7.

43 Lapan B: Is the 'pill' a cause of vaginal candidiasis? Culture study. NY State J Med 1970;70:949-51.

44 Law EJ, Kim OJ, Steritz DD, McMillan BG: Experience with systemic candidiasis in the burn patients. J Trauma 1972;12:543-52.

45 Lehmann P, Reiss E: Comparison by ELISA of serum anti-*Candida albicans* mannan IgG levels of normal population and in diseased patients. Mycopathologia 1980;70:89-93.

46 Lehner T: Serum fluorescent antibody and immunoglobulin estimations in candidosis. J Med Microbiol 1970;3:475-81.

47 Levine HB: Resistance to ketoconazole. Lancet 1982;i:211.

48 Liebeskind A: *Candida albicans* as an allergic factor. Ann Allergy 1962;20:394-6.

49 Mathur S, Mathur RS, Dowda H et al: Sex steroid hormones and antibodies to *Candida albicans*. Clin Exp Immunol 1978;33:79.

50 Mathur S, Melchers JT, Ades EW et al: Antiovarian and anti-lymphocyte antibodies in patients with chronic vaginal candidiasis. J Reprod Immunol 1980;2:247-62.

51 Mathur S, Virella G, Koistinen J et al: Humoral immunity in vaginal candidiasis. Infect Immun 1977;15:287-94.

52 Marks AD, Channick BJ, Adlin EV et al: Chronic thyroiditis and mitral valve prolapse. Ann Intern Med 1985;102:479-83.

53 Montes LF, Krumdieck C, Cornwell PE: Hypovitaminosis A in patients with mucocutaneous candidiasis. J Infect Dis 1973;128:227-30.

54 Montes LF, Bradford LG, Lauderdale RO, Taylor CD: Prolonged oral treatment of chronic mucocutaneous candidiasis with amphotericin B. Arch Dermatol 1971;104:45-56.

55 Montes LF, Pittman CS, Moore WJ et al: Chronic mucocutaneous candidiasis: influence of thyroid status. J Am Med Assoc 1972;221:156-9.

56 Morris DL: Value of delayed hypersensitivity index in patients with malignancy. Ann Allergy 1977;38:182-4.

57 Neuhauser I, Gustus EL: Successful treatment of intestinal moniliasis with fatty acid resin complex. Arch Intern Med 1954;93:53-60.

58 Nosal R: Histamine release from isolated rat mast

cells due to glycoprotein from *Candida albicans* in vitro. J Hyg Epidemiol Microbiol Immunol 1974;18:377-8.

59 Numata T, Yamamoto S, Yamura T: The role of mite, house dust and *Candida* allergens in chronic urticaria. J Dermatol (Tokyo) 1980;7:197-202.

60 Nutrition Department, Environmental Health Center Dallas Texas: *Lactobacillus acidophilus.* In: Cummings RA, ed. Twentieth century living. Dallas: Environmental Health Association, July/Aug 1984;5.

61 Odds FC: *Candida* and candidosis. Leicester: Leicester University Press, 1979.

62 Palacios HJ: Hypersensitivity as a cause of dermatologic and vaginal moniliasis resistant to local therapy. Ann Allergy 1976;37:110-13.

63 Palacios HJ: Desensitization for monilial hypersensitivity. Virginia Med J 1977;393-9.

64 Pepys J, Faux JA, Longbottom JL et al: *Candida albicans* precipitins in respiratory disease in man. J Allergy 1968;41:35.

65 Planes M, Brunet D, Dalayeun H et al: Allergie à *Candida albicans* chez l'enfant. Rev Fr Allerg 1972;12:115-23.

66 Rafin M: Muguet et calcul de la vessie. J Urol 1927;23:32.

67 Randolph TG: Human ecology and susceptibility to the chemical environment. Springfield, Illinois: Charles C Thomas, 1962.

68 Rea WJ: Diagnosing food and chemical susceptibility. Continuing Education for the Family Physician 1979;16:47-59.

69 Rifkind D, Frey JA, Davis JR: Influence of gonadal factors on skin test reactivity of CFW mice to *Candida albicans.* Infect Immun 1973;7:322-8.

70 Rockwell, SJ: Coping with *Candida* cookbook. Seattle, Washington: Diet Design, 1984.

71 Rosen T: Cutaneous candidiasis. In: Bodey GP, Fainstein V, eds. Candidiasis. New York: Raven Press, 1985;230.

72 Rosenberg EW, Belew PW: Improvement of psoriasis of the scalp with ketoconazole. Arch Dermatol 1982;118:370-1.

73 Rosenberg EW, Belew PW, Skinner RB, Crutcher N: Crohn's disease and psoriasis. N Engl J Med 1983;308:101.

74 Saifer P: Endocrinopathies in patients with chronic candidiasis. Presented at the Yeast-Human Interaction Symposium, San Francisco California, 29-31 March, 1985.

75 Schmorl G: Ein Fall von Soormetastase in der Nier. Zentralbl Bakteriol 1890;7:329-35.

76 Schonheyder H, Johansen JA, Moller-Hansen C, Senderup A: IgA and IgG serum antibodies to *Candida albicans* in women of child-bearing age. Sabouraudia 1983;21:223-31.

77 Sclafer J: l'Allergie à *Candida albicans*; clinique, diagnostique et traitment. Sem Hop Paris 1957;33:1330-9.

78 Shelley WB, Florence R: Chronic urticaria due to mold hypersensitivity. Arch Dermatol 1961;83:549.

79 Smith CB: Candidiasis: pathogenesis, host resistance, and predisposing factors. In: Bodey GP, Fainstein V, eds. Candidiasis. New York: Raven Press, 1985;62-5.

80 Sonck CE, Somersalo O: The yeast flora of the anogenital region in diabetic girls. Arch Dermatol 1963;88:846-52.

81 Spebar MJ, Pruitt BA: Candidiasis in the burned patient. J Trauma 1981;21:237-9.

82 Spellacy WN, Zaias N, Buhi WC, Birk SA: Vaginal yeast growth and contraceptive practices. Obstet Gynecol 1971;38:343-9.

83 Tomsikova A, Tomaierova V, Kotal L, Novackova D: An immunologic study of vaginal candidiasis. Int J Gynaecol Obstet 1980;18:398-403.

84 Triger DR, Slater DN, Goepel JR, Underwood JCE: Systemic candidiasis complicating acute hepatic failure in patients treated with cimetidine. Lancet 1981;ii:837-8.

85 Truss CO: Tissue injury induced by *Candida albicans*: mental and neurologic manifestations. J Orthomol Psychiatry 1978;7:17-37.

86 Truss CO: Restoration of immunologic competence to *Candida albicans.* J Orthomol Psychiatry 1980;9:287-301.

87 Truss CO: The role of *Candida albicans* in human illness. J Orthomol Psychiatry 1981;10:228-38.

88 Truss CO: Metabolic abnormalities in patients with chronic candidiasis: the acetaldehyde hypothesis. J Orthomol Psychiatry 1984; 13:66-93.

89 Truss CO, O'Shea JA: Truss, O'Shea discuss candidiasis. SCE Scene 1982;3-5.

90 Utz JP, Drouhet E: Treatment of *Candida* infections. In: Bodey GP, Fainstein V, eds. Candidiasis. New York: Raven Press, 1985;253-69.

91 Von Hilsheimer G: *L. acidophilus* and the ecology of the human gut. J Orthomol Psychiatry 1982;11:204-7.

92 Wachowiak W, Stryker GV, Marr J, et al: The occurrence of *Monilia* in relation to psoriasis. Arch Dermatol 1929;19:713-31.

93 Wade JC, Schimpff SC, Hargadon MT et al: A comparison of trimethoprim-sulfamethoxazole plus nystatin with gentamicin plus nystatin in the prevention of infections in acute leukemia. N Engl J Med 1981;304:1057-62.

94 Walsh H, Hildebrandt RJ, Prystowsky H: Oral progestational agents as a cause of *Candida* vaginitis. Am J Obstet Gynecol 1968;101:991-3.

95 Weary PE, Guerrant JL: Chronic urticaria in association with dermatophytosis. Response to the administration of griseofulvin. Arch Dermatol 1967;95:400.

96 Weinstein IW, Duke LB, Peters RS, Bahn AN: *Candida albicans* in the saliva of diabetics. J Dent Res 1959;38:656.

97 Wilkinson JS: Some remarks upon the development of epiphytes with the description of new vegetable formation found in connexion with the human uterus. Lancet 1849;ii:448.

98 Williams ML, Slack S: Technical protocols. Environmental Health Center, Dallas Texas. 1983; Section 3:4.

99 Willoughby JW: Diagnosis of allergy by serial dilution skin end point titration. Continuing Education for the Family Physician 1979;11:21-44.

100 Winkelmann RK: Chronic urticaria. Proc Staff Meet Mayo Clin 1957;32:329-34.

101 The Yeast-Human Interaction Symposium, Birmingham Alabama, 9-11 Dec, 1983.

102 The Yeast-Human Interaction Symposium, San Francisco California, 29-31 March, 1985.

103 Zamm AV: Chronic urticaria: a practical approach. Cutis 1972;9:27-37.

APPENDIX

Representative *Candida* control diet.

Note: dietary suggestions listed below are intended only as general guidelines; they should be modified as necessary for the unique needs of individual patients.

The diet consists of:

1 *Avoiding foodstuffs high in carbohydrate content* that may lead to an increase in yeast growth in the body. These include: refined sugars (sucrose, fructose, dextrose), fruit juices, excessive honey and maple syrup.

2 *Avoiding yeast-containing foodstuffs.* These include: alcoholic beverages, cheeses, mushrooms, vinegars, breads, dried fruits, certain vitamins. Although these foods do not contribute to intestinal yeast growth, they often cross-react allergenically with *Candida* species.

Vegetables

All vegetables acceptable; see examples below.
★ Limit intake of high carbohydrate vegetables.

Artichokes	Cabbage	Eggplant	Kohlrabi	Potato★
Asparagus	Carrots	Endive	Leeks	Pumpkin
Bean sprouts	Cauliflower	Escarole	Lentils★	Radishes
String beans	Celery	Garlic	Lettuce	Rutabaga
Lima beans★	Chard	Greens	Okra	Soya beans
Beets	Cucumbers	beet	Onions	Peas★
Broccoli	Corn★	collard	Parsley	Squash
Brussel sprouts		kale	Parsnip★	Tomato
		mustard	Peppers	Turnips
		spinach	Pimento	Yams★

Proteins

All meat, poultry, fish acceptable; examples below.
Eggs and non-sweetened yoghurt acceptable.

Red meat		Poultry		Fish	
Beef	Veal	Chicken	Goose	Tuna	Haddock
Pork	Rabbit	Turkey	Quail	Salmon	
Lamb		Duck	Pheasant	Halibut	

Nuts and seeds

All nuts acceptable; examples below.
★ Limit peanuts (mould content).
★ Limit cashews (carbohydrate content).

Almonds	Hazel nuts	Pine nuts	Walnuts
Brazil nuts	Macadamia nuts	Pistachios	
Cashews★	Peanuts★	Pumpkin seeds	
Filberts	Pecans	Sunflower seeds	

Grains

All whole grains may be eaten.
★ Avoid yeast-containing cereal-grain products.

Barley	Millet	Oatmeal
Brown rice	Rye	Wheat
Corn	Barley	

Beverages

All non-sugar, non-fermented beverages acceptable.
★ Avoid milk due to high lactose content.
★ Limit coffee and diet soda due to poor nutritional content.
Plain and sparkling water
Sugar-free diet sodas
Herbal teas★
Coffee (non-sweetened)

Fruits

2–3 servings of the following fruits can be eaten per day. Fruit should be fresh or frozen; avoid overripe items. Each serving below contains approx 15–20 g of carbohydrate.
★ Limit melons (mould content).
Note: For severe candidiasis, a fruit-free diet may initially be necessary for a period of time. Consult with your physician for your particular case.

1 medium apple	1 cup cherries	1 cup grapes
1 cup blueberries	1 cup shredded coconut	3 lemons

APPENDIX-*cont.*

Representative *Candida* control diet.

1 cup blackberries	1/2 large grapefruit	1 orange
1 cup papaya cubes	1 cup fresh pineapple	1 medium pear
1 banana	1 cup raspberries	3 medium plums
1 wedge melon★	20 large strawberries	3 peaches

Sweeteners
★ Limit honey and maple syrup to 1–2 tsp/day maximum.
★ Limit aspartame–sweeteners if have dextrose or lactose additives.
Honey★
Maple syrup★
Aspartame★

Fats
Butter and oils acceptable.

Chapter 50
Laboratory Diagnosis of Food Intolerance

D. L. J. Freed

BASIC PRINCIPLES

The need for laboratory tests

If all food intolerance syndromes were typical and occurred within a few minutes of ingestion every time the food were taken there would be no need for laboratory tests and little need for allergists. Unfortunately, the onset of some food intolerance syndromes is delayed for several hours or days (perhaps longer) after taking the food. This statement can be made with confidence because of the efforts of numerous physicians (and patients) who over the years have taken the time and trouble to embark upon challenge programmes, sometimes double-blind [93, 157].

It can also confidently be stated that even when true food intolerance exists, food challenges will not necessarily cause symptoms every time. Some food reactions require the simultaneous presence of another stress factor, such as exertion [130, 155], histamine [109, 247] or aspirin [52]. One needs to be exceptionally lucky to uncover such synergistic factors, so we do not know how often they are important. It follows from this that food challenges must give an unknown number of false-negative results. False-negatives also occur when the dose is not large enough or not repeated often enough [94] or when the challenge is delivered direct to the stomach via tube or capsules in an individual whose main route of antigen uptake is buccal [153, 175]. After a period of avoidance, a patient may not respond again to a damaging food for several doses [110, 148], or indeed ever again [177] and it must also be remembered that reactivity can fluctuate with season, with menstrual cycle or with intercurrent infections [100]. It follows therefore that it is never completely possible to disprove food intolerance, even in those rare cases when the patient is convinced that her symptoms (or her children's symptoms) are caused by foods and the doctor is convinced that they are not [187, 242]. Failure to respond to 'oligoallergic diets' or fasting does not formally disprove food intolerance either since we cannot be certain that the illness will remit before either starvation supervenes or the patient loses patience. In published series, the proportion of apparently food-sensitive patients who are confirmed by double-blind challenge tends to be rather low [33, 42, 100, 177, 187], which suggests either that patients and clinicians are easily fooled or that the false-negative rate of this procedure is uncomfortably high.

Double-blind challenges (Table 50.1)

It is sometimes forgotten that the opposite proviso also applies, namely, that double-blind challenges cannot formally *prove* the existence of food intolerance [188]. At best they can make the null hypothesis implausible as in the cases reported by Finn and Cohen [93] who correctly distinguished active challenge from water each time in a series of 10 double-blind challenges. The probability of correctly guessing the answer in any single double-blind challenge is 50%, i.e. $p = 0.5$. The probability of correctly guessing two in a row is $p = 0.5 \times 0.5 = 0.25$ and so on. To get below the conventional 5% probability level therefore requires five consecutive correct identifications, in a randomized series, as $p = (0.5)^5 = 0.031$, and clinicians who frequently subject their patients to the rigours of such challenge series should be aware that one in every 32 patients who 'pass' that test will have done so by chance. If the clinician recognizes that false-positive and false-negative challenges can occur, and permits one mistake in a series of six challenges [187], the probability of passing that test by chance is $p = 0.11$ (binomial theorem), i.e. one in every nine patients [188].

Added to these fundamental weaknesses of

the double-blind challenge approach are the practical difficulties of expense, laboriousness, patient compliance, the choice of a placebo that is truly inert and the danger that simply initiating a challenge programme will switch on a hypochondriacal response in patients predisposed to neuroticism [242]. In the case of children who must be challenged without understanding or giving consent the question of real suffering cannot be evaded. It is not therefore surprising that so few clinicians routinely subject their patients to double-blind challenges, presumably taking the view that the risks of unnecessary elimination diets are lower than the risks of prolonged drug treatment. The only absolute indication for double-blind challenges is in order to convince sceptical doctors.

Some emphasis has been given to the question of double-blind challenge procedures as these are the best clinical diagnostic tool available. Even the most skilfully elicited case history is unreliable [189] and skin tests are only a general guide to systemic sensitivity, and even then only in Type I (IgE-associated) allergies. A reliable laboratory test for food intolerance would be immensely valuable.

The validation of laboratory tests

The requirement is simply stated: laboratory tests should be positive in all patients who have a food sensitivity and negative in all people who do not. But if we cannot be certain of making the correct clinical diagnosis we have no yardstick against which to measure the reliability of our tests. We can only try to get as close as possible to accuracy.

Definitive clinical diagnosis can be approached most closely and relatively easily in Type I allergies in which response to challenge is usually swift and convincing and occurs every time. As the control group we need, *not* apparently food-sensitive patients with negative challenges (since the challenge results may have been false) but rather a group of healthy or sick volunteers, matched for age, sex, social class, smoking and dietary habits, who have no history or family history of allergies or food reactions, who are also challenged and emerge without reactions. Of course it is very difficult to assemble two comparable groups of this kind but at least it is theoretically feasible and examples will be alluded to below. A comparison of true-positive, true-negative, false-positive and false-negative rates allows a computation of the accuracy, most

Table 50.1 Difficulties with double-blind challenges.

Theoretical
  Positive challenges do not prove intolerance
  Negative challenges do not disprove intolerance

Practical
  Expense of time, effort, money
  Organization
  Patient compliance
  Choice of truly inert placebo
  Danger of hypochondria

Table 50.2 Example of the χ^2 approach to validation of a test, applied to RAST diagnosis of allergic rhinitis.

	Test result positive	Test result negative	Totals
Clinically sensitive	19 (true-positives)	14 (false-negatives)	33
Clinically not sensitive	2 (false-positives)	48 (true-negatives)	50
Totals	21	62	83

$\chi^2 = 27.4$; $P < 0.00025$.

This statistic tells us how probable it is that the test results and the clinical diagnoses are non-correlated. The lower the P value, the better the test's accuracy. Only P values below 0.05 (preferably below 0.01) need be of interest. Data taken from Freed et al [97a].

conveniently using the χ^2 or similar test (Table 50.2).

Statistically acceptable studies

Statistically acceptable double-blind challenge studies in delayed-onset non-IgE-associated food intolerances are rather rare; a flavour of the daunting difficulties involved can be obtained by a close perusal of the methods sections of the papers by Egger et al [80] on childhood migraine and Alun Jones et al [123] on irritable bowel syndrome. In a disease that may not be provoked unless challenges last for a week or more one cannot reasonably expect a series of five challenges to be administered to each patient. The reader who calculates the probabilities as outlined above on these two papers will conclude that food intolerance is virtually proven in a substantial proportion of these patients—but one cannot say *which* patients. As we do not know which patients to allot to which block in our contingency table, it would be impossible to work out the accuracy of laboratory tests by the χ^2 method; as it happens however the 'true-positive' rate for the radioallergosorbent test (RAST) in these diseases is so low that we do not need to seek control data. Since it is so immensely difficult to establish the necessary clinical yardstick in diseases of this type, it is not yet possible to assess the reliability in such cases of most of the tests alluded to in this chapter. It is of course quite illogical to argue that since a particular test is reasonably accurate in Type I allergies its positivity in a non-IgE condition proves the condition to be allergic—or (more insidiously) that its negativity disproves food intolerance [126].

A more popular approach to the validation of tests is to prescribe a diet based on the test results and see whether the patient feels better. If a good proportion of patients improve, at least in the short term, the test is considered valid. This kind of evidence—the evidence of success—was correctly termed 'treacherous' as far back as 1827 by the *Edinburgh Medical and Surgical Journal* [11] for at least three good reasons:

1 Those patients who do badly tend either not to return to the doctor to report or else give a falsely favourable report in order to please him, while

2 placebo-sensitive patients will improve, at least for a while, after any dietary change—exclusion diets are stressful and expensive and cause radical realignments in family tensions and

3 there is always coincidence; a proportion of patients who improve on elimination dieting would have improved anyway.

It should also be acknowledged that exclusion diets of the kind that forbid additives and convenience foods usually force the patient to eat a more healthful diet, so that a marginal unsuspected vitamin or mineral deficiency that might have been causing immunological imbalance [95, 104] is inadvertently corrected. The evidence of success is therefore not to be trusted—a point that should be borne in mind by users of the so-called cytotoxic test (see below).

Reproducibility and specificity

Before we can consider the accuracy of a test we need to consider its reproducibility when replicates of the same specimen are tested on the same, and on separate, occasions by the same and by different laboratories and staff, and when different specimens from the same patient are tested. The ideal test has a reproducibility of 100% but it may come as a distressing surprise to some clinicians to realize that most clinical laboratories consider an error rate of around 10% rather good. The ideal laboratory test is also specific, measuring only the substance being sought and being unaffected by other substances in the specimen. Lastly, tests should be cheap and not rely over much on high technology and should be useful if done only once on a small blood sample to minimize expense and suffering. This chapter considers how closely current tests approach these desiderata.

THE VALUE OF A LABORATORY TEST IN THE DIAGNOSIS OF FOOD ALLERGY

I do not intend to cover the use of laboratory tests in initially deciding that an allergic diagnosis is appropriate since that is properly done by taking a careful history. To base the initial diagnosis of allergy on a high total IgE level, for example, will yield many false results. The use of initial screening tests for this purpose is also an invitation to the doctor to stop thinking. Hamburger notes [108] that 'no serum IgE level, no matter how low, precludes a diagnosis of atopic allergy', and the same certainly goes for non-atopic allergy. The only established value for screening for total IgE is in infancy, since a high cord-blood IgE level predicts the development of later atopy and should make exclusive breast-milk feeding mandatory [50]. The IUIS/WHO working group report on laboratory tests [119] states that a total IgE estimation is never essential except for the diagnosis of the hyperimmunoglobulinaemia E—recurrent infection syndrome (Buckley's syndrome)—in which the information does not determine treatment.

I shall make the assumption that the doctor has already formed the view that an allergy or intolerance may be the cause of the patient's illness and is now seeking guidance on the identification of the damaging ingestant. This is the rational way to use laboratory tests. Although history, skin tests, challenge studies and laboratory tests are each individually unreliable to some degree, if most or all of them point in the same direction the physician is justified in feeling some confidence in that identification.

General unsolved problems: which allergen preparation?

Before considering each laboratory test in detail it will be profitable to contemplate the un-

Table 50.3 General unsolved problems in laboratory food allergy diagnosis.

Raw or cooked allergens?
Whole foodstuffs or digests?
Complex mixtures of antigens in each foodstuff
Antigenic cross-reactivity
Labelling and chemical handling problems
Lectins
Stability of allergens
Limitations of the antibody titre
Non-immunological food intolerance
Interpretation of 'false-positive' results

certain foundations upon which our edifice is built, that is, the unsolved problems that apply to all tests (Table 50.3).

To cook or not to cook? Prausnitz and Küstner [193] noted that whereas Küstner was exquisitely sensitive to cooked fish he could consume large doses of raw fish without problem. The reverse of this situation is rather more common [150, 172]. In spite of these observations, extracts of uncooked foods are usually used in tests. The question breeds subquestions. How hot and how long? Dry heat, hot water or steam? With or without salt or spices? This subject is obviously in need of investigation but has not been properly approached because of the awesome size of the task.

Should digests be used? Peptic/tryptic digestion of proteins leads to the destruction of some antigens [225] and creation of new ones [107]. The former process is probably more common than the latter [210] although failure to detect allergenic activity in digests is fraught with dangers of artefact. Foods change their antigenic clothing continuously in the journey from plate to portal vein but undigested foods are almost universally used in tests. This problem likewise has not been properly approached except for the case of gliadin in coeliac disease, in which digests retain toxicity [72] and lectin activity [135].

Which part of the foodstuff should be looked at? All foods are complex mixtures and any or all of the components might be clinically relevant. The mixture may vary from batch to batch and from season to season. If saline extracts are used the test ignores all materials in the insoluble residue, which are usually the majority.

Cow's milk, for example, contains over 20 separate antigenic proteins [19]. The principal whey antigens are α-lactalbumin, β-lactoglobulin, casein and bovine serum albumin (BSA); different patients have antibodies to one, several or all of these proteins. The fat globule membrane has its own separate antigens [69] besides adsorbing casein and other proteins from the milk plasma (Shakib, personal communication). To save effort many investigators use whole pasteurized milk as test reagent, yet this approach is also risky since the various antigens may mask each other in the test [106, 121]. The extent of this might vary from one run to the next so that it is conceivable that the antibodies detected on a Monday are different from those detected on a Wednesday. With the exception of cow's milk and wheat, most foods used in tests are not chemically fractionated, although the use of highly purified individual proteins in RAST greatly increases the test's accuracy, at least for fish allergy [3, 67] (see Chapter 19). This approach is only possible for foods that contain just one major allergen and these are unusual [53]. Turner et al [228] wryly observe that 'the choice of allergen for screening purposes is never clear-cut and some compromise is necessary'.

In view of the complex mixtures of allergens in most foods there is some relevance in finding out which are significant in each individual patient. The crossed radioimmunoelectrophoretic technique (CRIE) separates food antigens by cross-electrophoresis into a rabbit antiserum, after which the various peaks are developed with patient's serum and radiolabelled anti-IgE [140]. The technique is expensive in terms of animal antiserum and can only detect those antigens that this serum sees [22]. There is little clinical experience of this technique as yet and even less with its more recent variant of 'immunoblotting'. Developments are awaited.

Antigenic cross-reactivity. Now that highly sensitive methods for antibody detection are used (radioisotope and enzyme techniques), antigenic cross-reactions are frequently found. It is no surprise to find that wheat and rye share several antigenic determinants [38, 87] since these grasses are closely related botanically, and with more sensitive methods some cross-reactivity is also demonstrated with (in decreasing order) barley, oats [85, 225] and even to some extent rice and maize [41] (see Chapter 17). Similarly, there is considerable cross-reactivity between goat and cow milks [19, 150] and, indeed, between different species of mite [88]. Unexpected cross-reactions between totally different botanical families also occur. In Scandinavia where a short but vicious birch pollen season causes considerable allergy, high degrees of sensitization to birch pollen (assessed by RAST and skin prick testing) are strongly correlated with food intolerance, particularly to apple [76, 83, 84]; this clinical cross-sensitivity is reflected in the RAST [37] (see below). Even more startling is the in vitro discovery by Aalberse et al [1] of a carbohydrate antigen (not starch) that is shared by a very wide range of foods, inhalants and venoms across many species, both plant and animal. This antigen appears not to be a lectin (see below). All of these instances of cross-reactivity—and the many others no doubt yet undiscovered—have the potential to cause a lot of false-positive test results. Curiously, the one instance in which cross-reactivity is predictable—grass pollen and wheat flour—does not cause a problem in practice [225].

Solid-phase support and labelling problems. Most radioimmunoassays for food antibody require the food extract either to be chemically coupled on to a solid particle (paper, cellulose, Sepharose, etc.) or radiolabelled. These procedures affect antigenicity to a variable degree and are responsible for an unknown number of false-negatives. Some proteins in the mixture always bind better than others to the solid phase or interfere with their expression once bound.

Lectins. These are carbohydrate-binding proteins of variable chemical nature, prominent in edible seeds such as grains and beans, and to a lesser extent in other plant, and some animal, tissues [143]. Their binding affinities are in the same range as those of antibodies and often higher. The known and potential in vivo effects of ingested lectins are reviewed in Chapter 21.

Human immunoglobulin molecules have carbohydrate side-chains as well as antigen-binding sites, and when an antibody binds to a foodstuff this could be because of antigen-antibody binding, lectin–carbohydrate binding or both [218]. Extracts of pea, for example, bind all IgE molecules so that any individual with a detectable serum IgE will also have an apparent positive RAST for pea [1]. The same is probably true for other legumes and, to a lesser extent, grains, and this will inevitably reduce the 'signal-to-noise' ratio. Peanut lectin, exceptionally, is a poor allergen in RAST and does not bind IgE non-specifically [25]. Lectins could be removed from most foodstuffs, albeit laboriously, but the lectin molecules might already be attached to relevant allergens. A better scheme would be to neutralize the lectin activity with simple sugar inhibitors (if they were known) leaving the antigenicity of the lectin unaltered. The complexities of this situation are enormous and have hardly begun to be explored.

Confusingly, there is a suggestion that allergen-bound IgE of food-allergic patients may be more susceptible to lectin competition than the IgE of patients allergic only to pollens [147]. If true, this confuses the interpretation of the RAST further but might also become a useful marker of food allergy. Food lectins are particularly confusing in tests of lymphocyte activation, since many lectins are polyclonal mitogens.

Stability and reliability of allergen extracts. Most water-based extracts deteriorate on storage, some (e.g. apple) within minutes [76], unless preservatives are used, and sometimes even then [9, 252]. The extent of this deterioration is usually unspecified and unknown [173]. Although solid phase allergens are generally very stable some can apparently fall off the matrix on storage [127].

The limitations of a titre. The titre of an antibody is a function both of its concentration and its average binding avidity. Since the latter can vary by up to two orders of magnitude for IgE [238] and by more than that for other immunoglobin classes, the concentration and function of antibodies can vary widely between different sera having the same titre. This has important biological consequences which we are only just beginning to explore. The term 'antibody level' is a convenient shorthand whose limitations should be understood.

Non-immunological food toxicity. Foods contain an impressive array of potential poisons, including alkaloids, lectins, anti-enzymes, antivitamins, hormone mimics, toxic amino acids, mycotoxins, saponins, goitrogens and many other classes [59, 195], some of which are resistant to cooking and digestion. May [157] notes that 'the prevalence of toxic reactions ... is unknown and while the possibilities are legion, cases proven by blind challenge are uncommon'. This is not surprising as food toxins whose effects are rapid are well known in folklore, which is why acorns, sweet pea seeds and deadly nightshade berries—full of nourishment though they are—are not generally eaten. The toxins that exist in foodstuffs are by definition those whose effects are gradual and insidious. If their effects become apparent within a week or two they might be detected by the kind of long-term challenges discussed in relation to migraine [80], though some toxins take months or years to build up and are undetectable except by epidemiology, e.g. chickpea lathyrism [216] and carcinogens [222]. Some people are inevitably more sensi-

tive to these poisons than others. No laboratory tests currently available can detect this kind of intolerance and immunological tests are negative unless present by coincidence.

The significance of false-positive results. When a test result is positive for a food but the patient can consume the food without obvious harm, we usually conclude that the test result is wrong. But it could also mean (a) that a previous allergy has waned while the immune function remains still abnormal [58], (b) that the patient has a subclinical degree of sensitization which could become clinical in the near future [156] or (c) that there is a silent pathological mechanism in progress which might manifest itself in years ahead in an apparently non-allergic guise, like heart attacks [69] or rheumatoid arthritis [60].

TESTS FOR FOOD INTOLERANCE

Antibodies against foodstuffs

Precipitating antibodies against cow's milk proteins were observed at the turn of the century by Moro [171] in the blood of a baby suffering from cow's milk-induced marasmus. Food antibodies have been sought in serum since the 1920s for the diagnosis of food intolerance but it is now abundantly clear that the presence of these antibodies is normal. The subject has been well reviewed [58, 227]. Antibodies to cow's milk and/or its constituents are occasionally found in cord blood and are usual by the age of 1–3 months, although initial feeding at the breast (or on protein hydrolysates) reduces the titres and delays their appearance [78, 106, 133, 206]. Though food antibodies are normal, titres and prevalence are raised in selective IgA deficiency [26, 48, 207] (even though most of these patients can tolerate cow's milk), and in coeliac disease, inflammatory bowel disease and acute infectious gastroenteritis as well as in proven symptomatic food intolerance [227]. Most workers agree that *very* high titres are significant of current intolerance (though my own high anticow's milk titre is not). Overt food intolerance in infancy commonly remits spontaneously after which the antibody titre may gradually fall; the same is observed after successful treatment of coeliac disease and inflamatory bowel disease [58, 128, 205, 206]. Raised cow's milk antibody titres are associated with challenge-proven food intolerance (not necessarily milk intolerance [162]), chronic recurrent pulmonary diseases, iron deficiency anaemia in children, Wiskott–Aldrich syndrome, systemic lupus erythematosus (SLE) and conditions predisposing to aspiration, such as familial dysautonomia and Down's syndrome [26, 139].

Coeliac disease

This condition is a paradigm for food intolerances that are associated with immunological sensitization but apparently not caused by it. Of all food intolerances it has the firmest clinical diagnostic criteria, which makes it the ideal condition against which to judge laboratory tests. Coeliac patients have high titres of antibodies (though not usually IgE) against not only gliadin but also most of the various wheat proteins as well as the proteins of rye, barley and oats [57, 131]. This could be related to increased permeability of the gut in coeliac disease [34, 186], although the existence of hyperpermeability is controversial [178, 192]. The ability to become orally sensitized to wheat proteins is a species characteristic; normal rabbits have as much antibody as coeliac humans, whereas guinea pigs can only be immunized parenterally to produce such antibodies [61]. This supports an alternative explanation which is that the coeliac intestinal mucosa is more heavily bound by gluten lectins [136], which then become the target for secondary immunological attack (see also Chapters 30 and 36).

This explanation is further supported by the curious 'antireticulin' antibodies (Fig. 50.1) of many coeliac sera which bind to the intercellular matrix of mammalian tissues. Wheat lectin binds directly to connective tissue fibres in mammalian tissues, and when the 'reticulin' antibody test is done using sections of tissue that have been pretreated with wheat protein, the test becomes highly specific, excluding the diagnosis of coeliac disease when negative [231]. When antibodies of different classes are examined, antigliadin antibodies of the IgA class are found to be highly specific, falling on a gluten-free diet and rising after challenge [208, 230]. A combination of these two tests would offer a very firm diagnosis. It is ironic that coeliac disease, which seems not to be caused by an immunological mechanism, is so well diagnosed by means of immunological tests, and doubly ironic because in a disease that can be firmly diagnosed clinically, reliable laboratory tests are not needed.

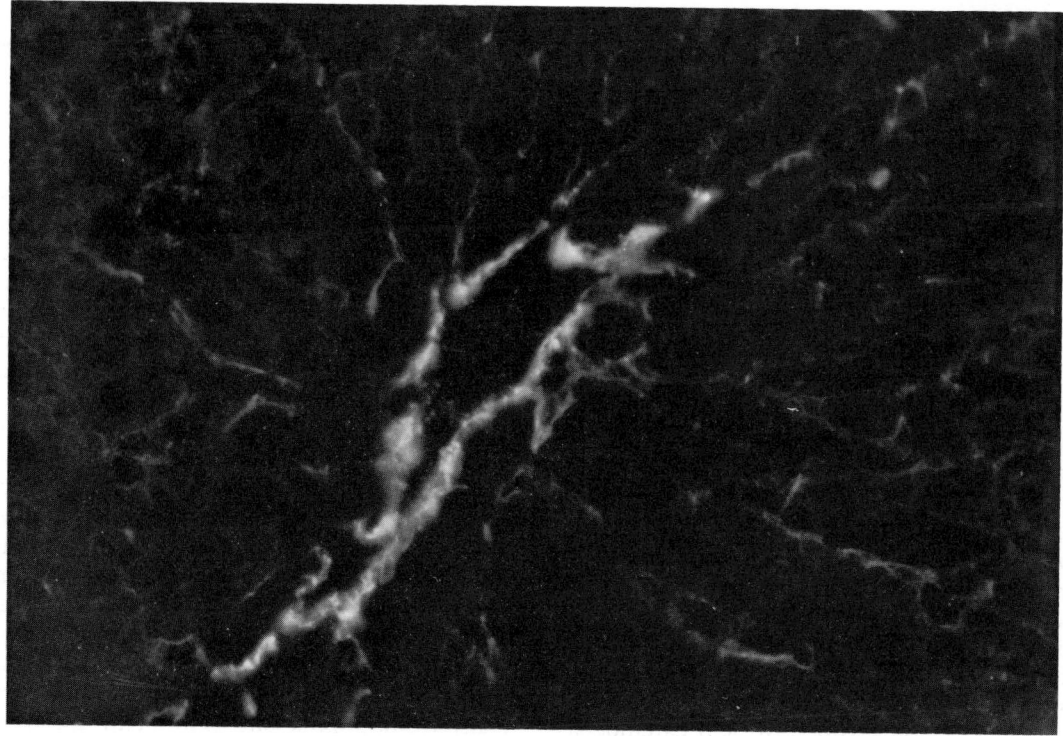

Fig. 50.1 Immunofluorescent demonstration of antireticulin antibodies.

Assay methods

The classical immunological techniques (pre-cipitation, passive haemagglutination, comple-ment fixation, passive cutaneous anaphylaxis (PCA) in guinea pigs) have all been employed with no one technique showing consistent su-periority over the others, although Saperstein et al [94] reported that the PCA technique dis-criminated far better than the others between milk-intolerant and tolerant children. Since this technique requires the killing of several animals each time, it has never been popular (Fig. 50.2).

By contrast, May et al [160] reported an im-pressive discriminating power of the Farr radioimmunoassay as applied to 11 double-blind-challenge proven milk-intolerant child-ren versus 30 challenge-disproven children (who returned to drinking milk without symp-toms). In this test radiolabelled milk proteins that are bound by antibodies are precipitated by ammonium sulphate; the radioactivity of the precipitate is a direct function of the anti-body titre. A group of children with 'non-allergic' diarrhoea also had raised anti-cow's

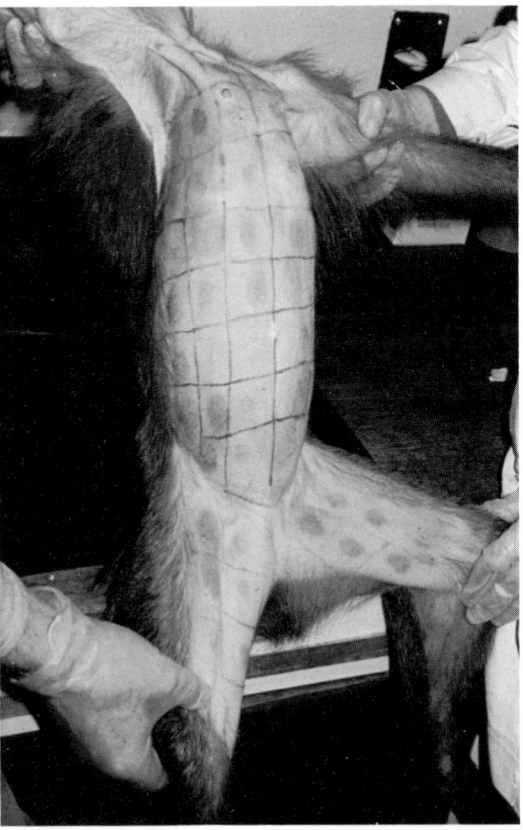

Fig. 50.2 Demonstration of passive cutaneous anaphy-laxis in monkey.

milk antibody titres and the test did not help in the diagnosis of challenge-proven soya in-tolerance, perhaps because that condition is partly lectin-mediated [75].

Direct binding tests

Direct binding tests of this kind also include the enzyme-linked immunosorbent assay (ELISA) in its various forms, the fluorescent immunosorbent test [49] and the indirect fluorescent antibody test [85]. This last tech-nique has the advantage that the whole food stuff—a thin cross-section of a grain or bean, for example—is used as substrate, so worries about incomplete extraction are eliminated (Fig. 50.3a-d). The section can also be cooked if desired. This is incubated with the patient's serum and, after washing, bound antibodies are 'developed' with fluorescein-labelled anti-human immunoglobulin serum (Fig. 50.4). With this method one may see which portion of the foodstuff is binding the antibody; for wheat, antibodies to gluten are easily distin-guished from antibodies to other components of the grain. It is more sensitive to small changes in antibody titre than solid-phase techniques [124]. Of course, the test cannot be applied to such foodstuffs as milk and egg nor (like the other tests listed) does a positive re-sult reliably indicate clinically important in-tolerance.

Radioactive and other direct binding tech-niques can be used to distintuish antibodies of different immunoglobulin classes but apart from the case of coeliac disease there seems as yet to be no diagnostic advantage in separately measuring the non-IgE classes of antibody (except for one isolated report of clinically relevant IgD antibodies) [101]. These tech-niques are far more sensitive than the classical methods but because of this very sensitivity false-positive rates are high and antigenic cross-reactivity is a serious problem (see above).

Antibodies in faeces and other secretions

Coproantibody studies have not been followed with enthusiasm, not only because of the nature of the specimens but because of the enormous difficulties involved. Unlike blood, whose composition is kept steady by many homeostatic mechanisms, faeces and other secretions vary greatly in concentration and composition, so that it is difficult to assign meaningful units to antibodies found therein

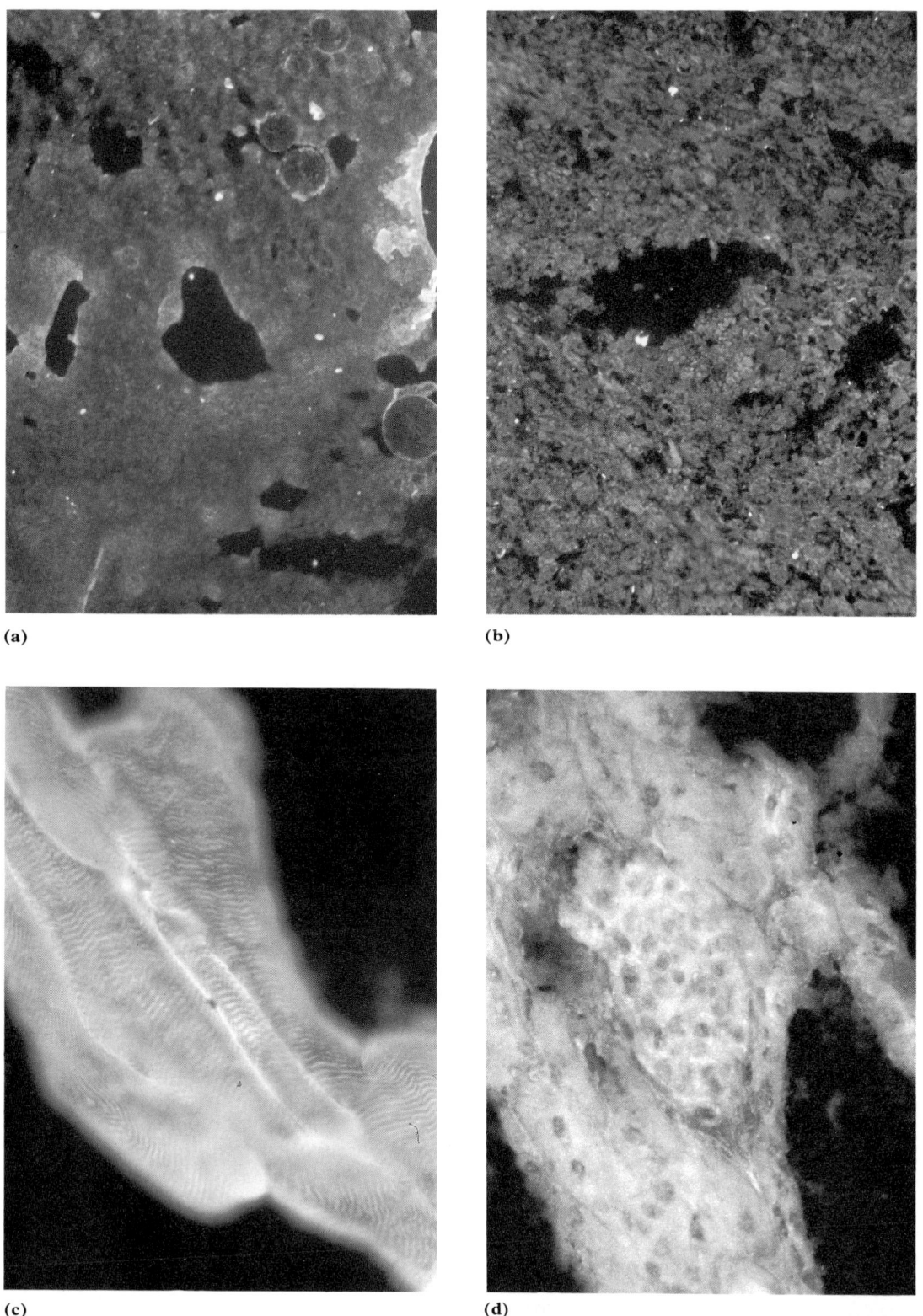

Fig. 50.3 Immunofluorescent demonstration of human antibodies against (a) yeast, (b) peanut, (c) lamb's kidney, (d) chicken.

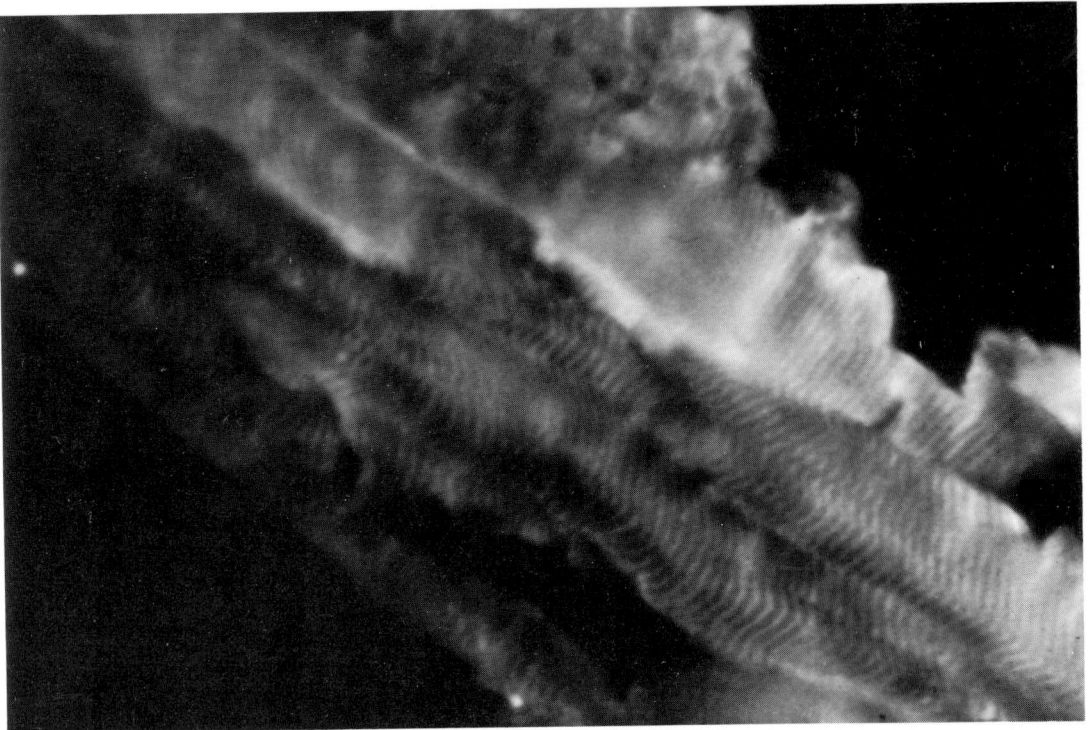

Fig. 50.4 Section of beef muscle showing fluorescent staining of anti-beef antibody. This is not auto-antibody to striated muscle, although the appearances are identical (× 400 approx.). Reproduced from Freed [96a], with permission.

[97, 154]. When measuring nasal IgA levels in this laboratory we estimated our error as ±400% [97] and regarded that as acceptable. In addition, most secretions contain antiprotease enzymes, so protease inhibitors must be incorporated into the assay to prevent the destruction or desorption of the antigen. The choice of antiprotease is difficult as it must be effective and, at the same time, must not itself interfere with either antigen or antibody; phenylmethylsulphonyl fluoride is the best reported so far [112, 239].

IgA and IgG antibodies against cow's milk, wheat and pollen appear in faeces, tears and colostrum and appear to be a normal physiological phenomenon, while corresponding serum antibodies are frequently absent [23, 70, 125, 132]. IgE antibodies are found in jejunal aspirate and faeces (albeit in semi-digested form) but appear to have no diagnostic value [24, 134]. The levels of IgE and IgD antibodies to cow's milk and soya protein in duodenal fluid appear to be under the control of pancreozymin and secretin, raising the possibility that these antibodies play a role in normal digestion [98].

IgE antibodies against foodstuffs—RAST (Fig. 50.5)

The radioallergosorbent test (RAST) was first described by Wide et al [246] in 1967, 3 months after the initial description of the IgE myeloma that had made possible the production of anti-IgE sera. In this test, solid-phase-immobolized allergen is incubated with the patient's serum and, after washing, the solid phase (nowadays usually a paper disc) is 'developed' with radiolabelled anti-IgE. The radioactivity bound by the disc is a function of the antibody titre [4–6, 73, 119, 167]. The isotope label can be replaced by an enzyme label with little difference in results [179].

Of all the tests reviewed in this chapter, RAST and its enzyme counterpart are currently the most popular because they are readily available at reasonable cost, cause no risk or discomfort to the patient, give a quantitative result that remains relatively constant over long periods of time, have a certain air of immunological glamour and are well advertised in the trade press (Phadebas[R] and Phadezym[R], Pharmacia).

Nevertheless, Adkinson [6] warns that 'indiscriminate wholesale replacement of skin testing with RAST ... is fraught with numerous difficulties.' It is also partly responsible for the regrettable view among some physicians and immunologists [79, 152] that only a RAST-positive disease is a true allergy.

Difficulties with RAST

1 The solid phase has a non-specific trapping effect so that sera having a high level of total IgE may give spurious positive RAST results [122]. This can be avoided by diluting sera that have total IgE levels greater than 1000 units/ml. Total IgE levels (and the RAST antibodies that constitute them) are artifactually raised by extraneous influences, such as cigarette smoking [21, 243, 253], this being in contrast to the immunosuppressive effect of smoking on other immunoglobulin classes [10]. Malnutrition [197], acute infections [117] and particularly infectious mononucleosis [20], and recent ingestion of the relevant food [105] can also elevate IgE levels which may also vary seasonally [220].

2 RAST results are artifactually low in the presence of IgG or IgD antibodies against the same antigen [6, 44, 55, 176, 191]. This may pose a special problem when patients are being desensitized. This can be overcome to some extent by further diluting the specimen [55, 176] by using extra allergen [191] or by pretreating the specimen with staphylococcal protein A (though this may present further

problems as some IgE is also removed by this procedure) [191].

3 Because the labelled second antibody is expensive it is often used at suboptimal doses, leading to underestimation at high levels of IgE antibody [151]; the opposite, too high a dose, would run the risk of falsely high results when the true RAST level is low. This can be overcome by repeating the estimation on further diluted sera, or by eluting the bound IgE antibodies from the solid-phase allergen and measuring them immunochemically. It must be added that there is little to be gained from accurately quantifying very high RAST levels.

4 There is a suggestion that IgE molecules are not all equally efficient at binding to basophils and inducing histamine release [15]. IgE antibodies that are free in the serum, and not tissue bound, may be considered as blocking antibodies while in that state. These are precisely the antibodies which RAST measures. It could therefore be argued that a histamine-release assay (see below) is more relevant as it also assesses the bound antibody and the 're-leasability' of the cells.

5 Because of chemical limitations, RAST can only be used to study allergens containing amino acids, although polysaccharide antigens can sometimes be immobilized by adsorption on to plastic instead [122].

6 Because of variable IgE avidities and the inherent problems of standardizing multicomponent allergens, RAST can never be more than semiquantitative [164]. Results obtained by the Phadebas RAST system cannot be meaningfully compared with those of other RAST or equivalent systems [119], nor can RAST grades with regard to one allergen be compared with those for other allergens [119].

7 The problem of cross-reaction artefacts has been alluded to above and is particularly troublesome in RAST [1, 28, 37, 138].

8 Problems with the anti-IgE specificity have arisen in the past [32] and still cause some controversy [122] but these are less of a problem with more recent anti-IgE antibodies [74, 190]. 'Home-made' anti-IgE sera are dangerous unless raised by experts.

9 Many atopic sera contain autoantibodies against IgE (a type of rheumatoid factor though not linked with rheumatoid disease) [118], which can interfere with the binding of the second antibody.

10 RAST gives no indication of the avidity of the IgE antibodies (see above), although it could theoretically be adapted to do so [238].

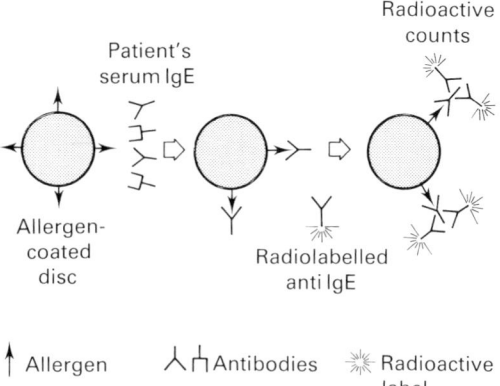

Fig. 50.5 Radioallergosorbent test (RAST). The allergen is made insoluble on a paper disc and the patient's serum containing IgE is then placed on the disc, allowing the IgE to bind to the allergen. Radiolabelled anti-IgE is added; the radioactive counts obtained reflect the amount of allergen specific IgE in the serum.

11 RAST is far more expensive than skin testing when a wide range of allergens is to be investigated. It is also susceptible to commercial abuse, as for instance kits that at one time purported to detect IgE antibodies against X-ray contrast media or drugs [4].

12 There are notable inter- and intralaboratory errors [86, 114].

Conclusions. With these provisos in mind the IUIS/WHO working group on laboratory tests concludes [119] that RAST is 'not essential in any clinical situation' and 'no alternative to careful history taking and skin tests'. The working group disputes the contention [184] that RAST can be used as a screening test for allergy. But these difficulties are not the only side of the coin and some advantages of RAST are listed in Table 50.4.

Table 50.4 Advantages of RAST over skin testing [119].

1 When dermographism or antihistamine use make skin testing impossible

2 When very severe sensitization makes skin testing too hazardous

3 When the allergens are too toxic for in vivo use

4 For hysterics, patients with needle phobia and children, a single venepuncture is sometimes more merciful than a series of prick or intradermal tests

Clinical accuracy of RAST

Early enthusiasm for the usefulness of RAST [249] has given way to a more realistic assessment (Table 50.5). In 'immediate', Type I syndromes, most workers now agree on an overall accuracy of about 75%, which means that a patient having a positive RAST to a food has a 3 : 1 chance of being clinically allergic to it. This is usually enough to allow a clinical suspicion of a food intolerance to be confirmed. This overall figure conceals the fact that some foods perform considerably better than others. RAST is most reliable in egg white and codfish allergies for which single major allergens are responsible. Cow's milk and cereal RAST are less accurate while at the other end of the scale the RAST results for white beans and soya beans are virtually random [2, 3, 67, 102], presumably because of the lectin problem noted above.

Since IgE antibody levels are usually well

Table 50.5 Reported accuracy, false-positive and false-negative rates of food RAST in selected papers.

Reference and year of publication	Accurate (%)	False-positives (%)	False-negatives (%)
249 (1979)	92	6	2
36 (1983) (if delayed reactions are classed as positive)	66	9	26
36 (1983) (if delayed reactions are classed as negative)	74	9	17
2 (1978)	78	20	2
144 (1983) egg	19	—	28
144 (1983) wheat	6	38	21
144 (1983) cow's milk	10	—	47

correlated with antibodies of other classes [160, 226] there is likely to be some clinical profit to be derived from measuring RAST and antibodies of other classes simultaneously.

In 'slow' reactions as exemplified by the migraine and irritable bowel studies cited above, early enthusiasm for RAST [249] has largely evaporated [80, 123, 167]. A novel use for RAST in migraine was reported by Monro et al in 1980 [170]. Although results were generally low (approaching perilously close to background error), when they were arranged relative to each other in a RAST profile those foods that stood out above the others were well correlated with clinical migraine triggers and enabled clinically efficacious diets to be prescribed in 23 of 26 patients. Other workers failed to confirm this claim [163] but seem to have missed the point that conventional cutoff points are useless in this kind of study. The initial results therefore still stand unrefuted, in stark contradiction of the consensus view. At the time of writing this controversy is unresolved.

Non-RAST IgE tests

Red cells and enzyme labels can be substituted for radioisotope with little overall change in sensitivity or discriminating power [17, 89] and the allergens can be adsorbed on to polyvinyl chloride (PVC) plates (which allow carbohydrate allergens better scope) instead of the more usual cyanogen bromide-activated paper or Sepharose [196].

Predictably, RAST and ELISA results were not in perfect agreement even when the same bank of sera was examined, with neither test being more clinically accurate [89]. A fluorescent label was found to be inferior to the isotopic label [63]. Further variations [62, 73, 165, 224, 251] are limited only by the ingenuity of laboratory scientists though none so far has progressed beyond the laboratories of isolated enthusiasts. The conventional RAST continues to set the standard.

RAST in patients recovered from food allergy

After recovery from a food allergy the RAST levels may remain high for many years [56], like antibodies of other classes [58]. IgE and IgG antibody levels are in general well correlated [226] and tend to wane gradually in parallel fashion, although an early high IgG : IgE ratio is said to be a good prognostic sign [66].

Cellular studies

Lymphocyte activation

Committed lymphocytes are involved in various capacities in all immunological responses and should be detectable by blastoid transformation in the presence of the relevant antigen (Fig. 50.6). Food antigens are problematic though because of their lectin content (see above). Frew et al [99] reported that a proportion of healthy people show lymphocyte transformation in response to wheat gliadin, or its chemical subunits. There were some day-to-day fluctuations. Also the lymphocytes of atopic people are likely to be somewhat different in their intrinsic responsiveness from those of normals [18, 90, 223]. Any work involving living cells is technically more demanding than antibody work and therefore expensive and slow by comparison. Experience is in general rather limited for this reason.

The results of different groups have been in conflict. On the credit side, Baudon et al [27] found positive lymphocyte transformation in response to β-lactoglobulin, although not α-lactalbumin or casein, in a majority of milk-sensitive children, and Shibasaki et al [213] found the same with rice protein in sensitive

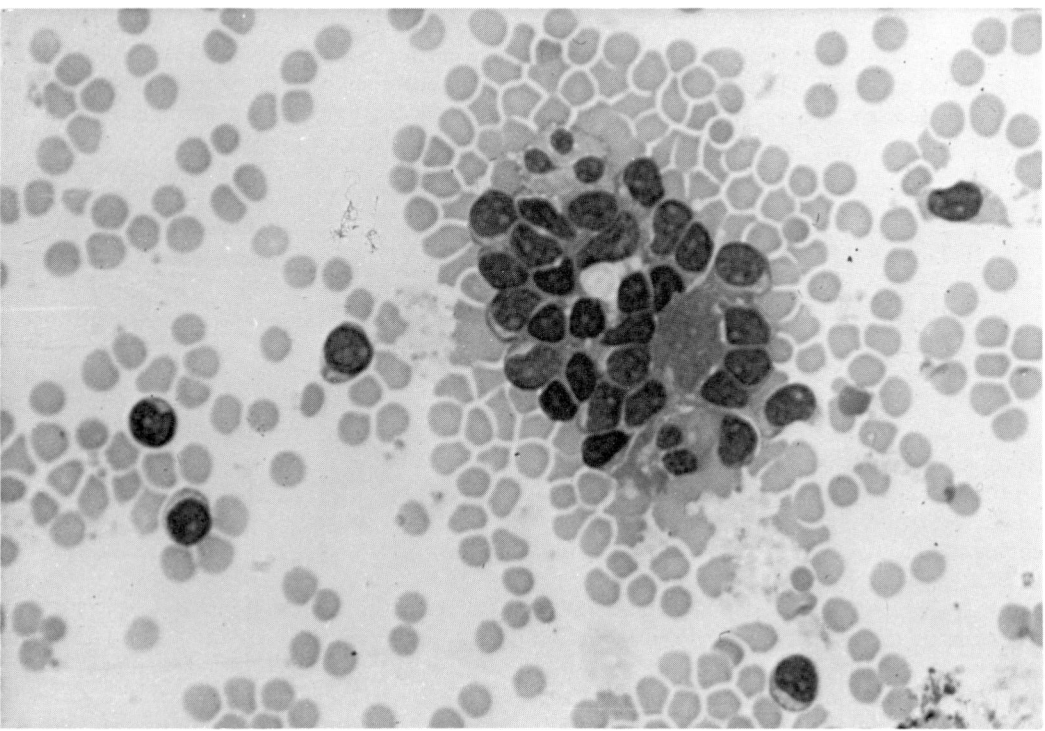

Fig. 50.6 Blastoid transformation of lymphocytes; small lymphocytes and many lymphoblasts can be seen.

patients; the IgE-binding determinants of rice protein were quite distinct from the lymphocyte-stimulating moiety. Endre and Osvath [82] found lymphocyte transformation to β-lactoglobulin or bovine serum albumin in 15 of 17 milk-allergic patients and in only one of eight control people.

In contrast, May and Alberto [158] were unable to distinguish patients from normals when testing milk- and egg-sensitive cells against the relevant antigens. These workers recorded false-positive rates of 87% and 64% for the two foods. Scheinmann et al [209] on the other hand, reported a false-negative rate of 62% and a false-positive rate of only 10% in cow's milk intolerance. To some extent these differences are reflections of the very many variables between laboratories in performing this test. In a remarkable pair of papers from Spain, Valverde et al [233, 234] reported positive transformation rates in response to foods and/or food additives of 238 out of 258 (92%) patients with chronic urticaria, and 42 out of 44 (95%) children suffering from a syndrome of hyperactivity, tiredness, tension and other indefinable symptoms. There were no positives among 20 healthy people. Prescription of the appropriate diets led to complete remission of symptoms in 61 and 86% of cases of the two syndromes respectively. These workers ascribe their excellent discrimination to the use of a higher cut-off point (200% of control) than that of May and Alberto [158]. These studies deserve to be repeated by others to establish their credibility.

Gliadin adheres to the B lymphocytes of coeliac patients more than to normal lymphocytes [237], presumably because of differences in lectin receptors (see Chapter 21). It is therefore not surprising that coeliac lymphocytes transform in response to gliadin and, provided a precise gluten subfraction is used, their stimulation is far greater than that of normal lymphocytes, with very little overlap [215].

Lymphokine production

Of the various lymphokines produced by activated lymphocytes, only the leukocyte migration inhibition factor (LIF) has been extensively investigated for diagnosis of food intolerance. Peripheral blood leucocytes from atopic patients are somewhat different from those of normals in their intrinsic responsiveness to adrenaline and methacholine [194, 198] so their responsiveness to lymphokines might also be different; the LIF test in such patients is therefore susceptible to at least two separate variables.

Ashkenazi et al [13] applied a variation of the LIF test to cow's milk allergy using β-lactoglobulin as stimulant (Fig. 50.7), reporting virtually no overlap between challenge-proven milk-intolerant patients and controls (including patients with acute gastroenteritis, whose milk *antibody* levels were presumably raised or rising). Five out of 18 children who had become tolerant of milk after previously being sensitive were also positive. Three of these children in whom a previous LIF test

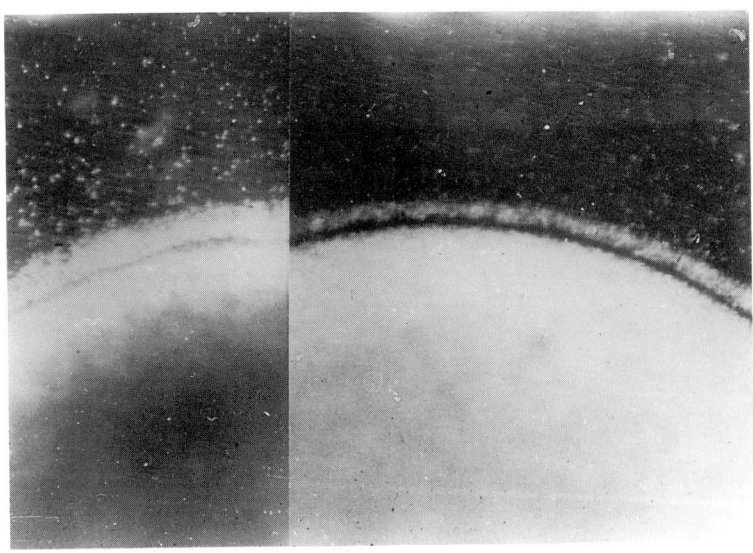

Fig. 50.7 Demonstration of positive LIF test. Left: control. Right: 40% inhibition by 10 μg/ml β-lactoglobulin. Reproduced by courtesy of Dr A. Ashkenazi.

had been done during the active illness now had lower results than when they were ill.

A similar good discrimination was observed when using gliadin for coeliac disease, provided a defined subfraction of gliadin was used [12]. Once again, after healing of the disease on a gluten-free diet, 50% of the hitherto positive LIFs became negative after (in some cases) a transient rise [14]. Reversion to normal of the test thus appears to follow within months, on resolution of the illness—unlike antibody levels.

Considerable manual skill and experience is required of the technician who performs these tests (in common with most technologies involving living cells) but results are reproducible once this level is attained. Gettinby et al [103] criticized Ashkenazi's technique on methodological grounds and Minor et al [168] obtained poor discrimination when using the test in milk allergy and corn allergy. Thus, the test requires wider evaluation to establish its reliability although the expense makes it unpopular.

Mediator release from basophils

Histamine release from peripheral blood leukocytes or basophils in response to antigen is a function of the final common pathway of Type I and Type III allergy. Although there is some correlation between serum and cell-bound IgE, the relationship is far from linear [7]; the two types of IgE may not be quite the same with respect to histamine-releasing efficiency [15]. The 'releasability' of atopic mast cells and basophils is also probably different from that of normal cells [92] and thus a functional measurement of cell-bound IgE is theoretically more likely to be clinically accurate than a RAST. Histamine release can either be measured chemically or indirectly by observing degranulation of basophils. Both methods can be automated and give results consistent with each other [71, 161, 236].

However, there are theoretical grounds for concern. The basophils of food-allergic children have high spontaneous histamine release which can appear after positive food challenge and last for months [159]. If the test is done in the presence of plasma, normal and atopic plasma will have different effects [159, 166]. Histamine release is elevated in the presence of factors from activated platelets [137] and non-steroidal anti-inflammatory drugs [248], and the binding of IgE to basophils is also influenced by interferon [214]. All of these

effects are likely to modulate the response of the cells to antigen.

Nevertheless, Soifer and Hirsch [217] applied the test to 17 'selected patients with distinct and reliable clinical [food intolerant] syndromes' and 31 normal controls, reporting an accuracy of 69%. These authors did not find any fundamental difference in releasability between the two groups. Benveniste [31] has popularized a semiautomated version of the test in France (TDBH: test de degranulation des basophiles humaines) and reports that true-positive results may be obtained in cases of drug reactions that do not usually show up with other methods. The test is reliable for pollen allergy and is marketed for a wide range of foods as well, although other workers [169] reported nine normal volunteers without histories of food intolerance and with negative food challenges, whose basophils produced positive response in the test. The TDBH is in need of further evaluation. McLaughlan and Coombs [149] reported histamine release in reponse to cow's milk proteins in 25% of normal infants and to a marked degree in 10%; they interpreted this not as a false-positive rate, but as evidence of silent and potentially harmful allergy.

Another consequence of mast-cell and basophil degranulation is attraction of neutrophils. Although atopic neutrophils are somewhat deficient in this regard [194], Papageorgiou et al observed the activation of neutrophil chemotaxis after clinically positive milk challenge in four patients whose skin tests, RAST and IgG4 antibody levels, precipitins and histamine-release results were all negative [185]. This is an intriguing result which deserves further investigation.

Cytotoxic test

Of all the tests reviewed in this chapter, this is the test that most frequently distinguishes doctors of the 'clinical ecology' persuasion from conventional allergists who consider it to be 'controversial' [8], 'untested' [145], 'not proven' [146] and (to be honest, if unkind) totally unbelievable.

The test is based on the original observation of Squier and Lee [219] that after incubation of the whole blood of ragweed-sensitive hay fever patients with ragweed in vitro, there was a pronounced fall in its white cell count, whereas this did not occur with the blood of successfully treated patients. Two years later a paper appeared that purported to refute this observation [96] but it has been independently rediscovered since then [116, 202], and there seems to be no doubt that the phenomenon exists. In the 1950s and 1960s Black [39] and later the Bryans [47] popularized the test for the diagnosis of both inhalant and ingestant allergies, claiming success rates of up to 95% for patients who adopted the diets indicated by the test results. This test has been taken up by a number of commercial laboratories in various countries (one such laboratory in Honolulu, apparently possessed of particular 'chutzpah', marks its reports 'Immunology') and a 1981 paper from Finland reported that the test had been in routine use at the Ear, Nose and Throat hospital of Helsinki since 1975 [203]. The criteria of test positivity are slowing and rounding of polymorphs, with (in very strong reactions) apparent disintegration of polymorphs and degenerative changes in platelets and erythrocytes. Results are usually graded from 0 to 3.

Theoretical considerations. The test is performed in autologous plasma, this being essential for some but not all reactions [113]. It is often forgotten (by all but first-year physiology students) that the pH of blood is largely maintained by the buffering action of carbonic acid and bicarbonate ions; when whole citrated blood or serum is left to stand, the pH rises due to outgassing of carbon dioxide (Fig. 50.8), thus providing a culture medium in

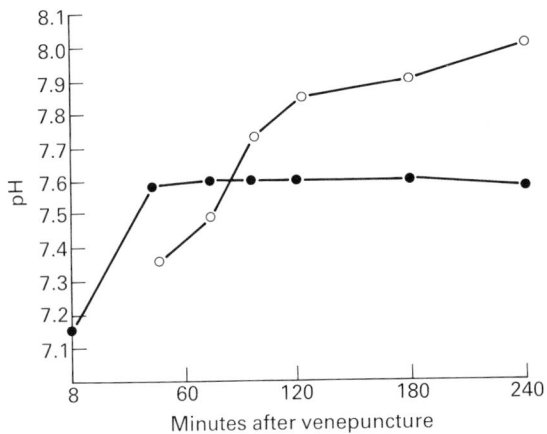

Fig. 50.8 Changes in pH of whole citrated blood (●) and serum (○) with time. The specimens were allowed to stand at room temperature in sealed screw-top tubes. Demonstration performed by Ms K. Collison.

which the cells are already considerably stressed, to a variable and unknown degree. Although plasma is of fairly uniform composition, variations in its lipoprotein and mineral levels occur, and have a strong influence on lymphocyte function [95, 104, 221]. To the buffy-coat cell suspension in autologous plasma is added an unspecified concentration of food extract or chemical, usually with some distilled water to counteract its 'dryness'. The resulting medium has an unknown pH, osmolarity and microbial content, and its composition must vary between laboratories and within laboratories, and between different foods and chemicals. This is clearly a test devised and performed by enthusiastic amateurs, which may partly explain the prejudice against it.

Clinical reliability: reproducibility. In common with the RAST, it is reasonable to bear in mind that a difference between adjacent grades could be discounted as the distinction is hard to make for borderline results. Several workers have noted that about 20–30% of results vary from day to day over two or more grades [30, 54, 141, 203] which agrees with the variability reported to me in a joint ongoing study by the York Medical and Nutritional Laboratory, UK. In our study, about 2% of specimen replicates, whether taken from the same blood sample or from the same patient on different days, varied across three grades at least once (i.e. were said to be both grade 0 ['not allergic'] and grade 3 ['severely allergic']). Although this error rate may horrify the clinician reader, it is not much worse than that of some conventional laboratory tests of cellular immunology [103].

Clinical reliability: accuracy. Although the initial observations [39, 219] implied that the test might be valuable for inhalant allergy, the Bryans [47] and most other users now consider that these are better diagnosed by RAST, and that the cytotoxic test should be reserved for use in 'masked food allergy', i.e. that kind of food intolerance that is associated with craving or addiction to the food in question and only becomes apparent after prolonged avoidance. A cynic might observe that thus limiting the claims restricts the test to those very cases in which its validation is most difficult, if not impossible. That this circumspection is wise is clear from a small collaborative study with the

York Medical and Nutritional Laboratory on grass pollen and house dust mite allergy (unpublished) which yielded the results in Table 50.6.

Table 50.6 Cytotoxic test result in patients with grass pollen or house dust mite allergy.

	Positive	Negative	Totals
Clinically sensitive	20	19	39
Clinically not sensitive	19	36	55
Totals	39	55	94

The χ^2 of this analysis was 1.99, which means that although these results do indeed point in the right direction (60% accurate) this could easily have been due to chance. Of course, this result does not predict the outcome of a trial of the test in 'slow' food intolerance, which is currently in progress.

Being controversial, the test has provoked some workers into making unfair criticisms without having become adept in its use [54, 141]. Nevertheless, some well-conducted trials have been done [30, 140] and report false-positive rates of up to 70%, noting that in several patients a strict adherence to the indicated diet would inevitably lead to malnutrition [30]. Clearly, the results need to be interpreted with great caution, preferably by an experienced physician [250]. In its 'Position Statement on Controversial Techniques' of 1981, the American Academy of Allergy asserted that (a) there is no proof that the test is effective, (b) there is evidence that it is ineffective and (c) it should be reserved for experimental work [8]. This restrained statement is still entirely correct.

Further comments. In spite of the above discussion it would be unfair and incautious to deny that many patients do become better, or well, when they embark on the diets indicated by the cytotoxic test [43, 229, 232], even though the uncharitable might attribute this to coincidence [229] or a placebo effect. It is entirely possible that were the test done in a defined, stable and sterile culture medium, with and without added serum, using food extracts of defined composition and concentration and using replicate estimations, a clinically accurate test might emerge. Under these conditions it is demonstrable that the neutrophils of

different people show wide variations to the cytotoxic effects of cigarette smoke [116]. These variations are stable in the individual person and unrelated to age, sex or smoking habit. Patients with smoking-related emphysema or chronic bronchitis have cells that are killed at lower doses of smoke extract, and the converse is true of healthy individuals over the age of 70 [115]. The mechanism of this cytotoxicity is presumably toxic and not immunological, so that one would expect such a test to be more reliable in 'slow, non-allergic' food intolerances than in immunological reactions.

Intestinal permeability and the detection of dietary antigens in the blood

The human intestine appears to undergo 'closure' in utero at around 34 weeks of gestation [29, 200, 245] so that except for premature infants (especially during an episode of bloody stools [244]) only trace amounts of protein survive intact the translation from intestine to systemic blood [181]. Nevertheless, such small doses are often capable of evoking antibody formation and ingestion of food is normally followed by the appearance of circulating immune complexes, which presumably constitute a physiological pathway for clearance of these antigens [46, 181]. Food-allergic patients appear to form more of these complexes [181], which are larger [46], often contain IgE and/or Clq [45, 181] and are more slowly cleared [204] than normal complexes. Abnormal postprandial immune complexes are also associated with selective IgA deficiency [64, 65] and some cases of glomerulonephritis [51, 235]. Although these statements have been challenged [81] this is largely because of the bewildering array of available immune-complex assays, most of which give results somewhat at variance with each other [201], so that the assay to be used has to be selected intelligently.

Postprandial immune complexes. The abnormal postprandial immune complexes of food allergy seem to be a reflection of an increased gut permeability [120] although this is controversial [77]. Food-allergy patients whose symptoms are limited to the gastrointestinal tract have been reported to have *lower* intestinal permeability than normals [91], presumably because the antigens are trapped within local gut immune complexes [142, 199] and do not proceed further. Gut permeability is non-specifically enhanced by alcohol [35, 241], trauma [129, 174] and inflammation, whether induced by carrageenan [174] or intestinal anaphylaxis [40]. Thus, the causal antigen may be prevented by local immune complexes from passing into the circulation at the same time as the uptake of 'bystander' antigens is encouraged. The presence of free dietary antigens in the circulation is not therefore diagnostic of allergy to that food [180] and if antibodies are also present these will mask the antigen [68, 180].

Several workers have attempted to split postprandial immune complexes in order to find out which antigens are involved. There are several methods for doing this [16, 65, 111, 182] and clinically relevant antigens have been detected [65, 182, 183]. It is too early to say if such complex splitting will prove to have diagnostic value.

CONCLUSIONS

1 Immunological reactivity against foods is a normal and possibly physiological phenomenon.

2 No laboratory test can prove food intolerance; at best it can add meaningful weight to a clinical suspicion.

3 RAST and histamine release are fairly (75%) reliable in 'immediate' Type I allergies but unhelpful in slow (possibly non-IgE) types of intolerance.

4 RAST accuracy varies from food to food, being good for codfish and egg white, intermediate for milk and cereals and poor for soya and white beans.

5 Food antibody measurements are more helpful when antibodies of several or all immunoglobulin classes are measured on the same specimen.

6 Certain food antibody measurements (see text) have become quite accurate in coeliac disease.

7 Promising techniques for the diagnosis of food allergy include neutrophil chemotaxis, LIF and immune-complex splitting.

8 The 'cytotoxic test' as currently performed is unreliable, though with modification it might be made more accurate.

9 The case history, skin tests, challenges and laboratory tests are all individually unreliable to some extent, but can serve to strengthen diagnosis when they agree. There will always be cases in which food intolerance can be neither proved nor disproved.

REFERENCES

1 Aalberse RC, Koshte V, Clemens JGJ: Immuno-globulin E antibodies that crossreact with vegetable foods, pollen and Hymenoptera venom. J Allergy Clin Immunol 1981;68:356–64.

2 Aas K: The diagnosis of hypersensitivity to ingested foods. Reliability of skin prick testing and the radio-allergosorbent technique with different materials. Clin Allergy 1978;8:39–50.

3 Aas K, Lundkvist V: The radioallergosorbent test with a purified allergen from codfish. Clin Allergy 1973;3:255–63.

4 Adkinson NF: The radioallergosorbent technique: uses and abuses. J Allergy Clin Immunol 1980;65: 1–4.

5 Adkinson NF: The radioallergosorbent test. J Allergy Clin Immunol 1980; 66:174–5.

6 Adkinson NF: The radioallergosorbent test in 1981—limitations and refinements. J Allergy Clin Immunol 1981;67:87–9.

7 Allen KR, Osmond S, Alston WC: A method for the simultaneous determination of serum and cell bound IgE. Clin Allergy 1977;7:273–7.

8 American Academy of Allergy: Position statements—controversial techniques. J Allergy Clin Immunol 1981;67:333–8.

9 Anderson MC, Baer H: Antigenic and allergenic changes during storage of a pollen extract. J Allergy Clin Immunol 1982;69:3–10.

10 Andersen P, Pedersen OF, Bach B, Bonde GJ: Serum antibodies and immunoglobulins in smokers and non-smokers. Clin Exp Immunol 1982;47:467–73.

11 Anonymous: On acupuncture. Edinburgh Med Surg J 1827;27:190–200.

12 Ashkenazi A, Levin S, Idar D et al: Immunological assay for the diagnosis of coeliac disease: interaction between purified gluten fractions. Pediatr Res 1980;14:776–8.

13 Ashkenazi A, Levin S, Idar D et al: In vitro cell-mediated immunologic assay for cow's milk allergy. Pediatrics 1980;66:399–402.

14 Ashkenazi A, Levin S, Idar D et al: Effect of gluten-free diet on an immunological assay for coeliac disease. Lancet 1981;i:914–16.

15 Assem ESK, Attallah NA: Increased release of his-tamine by anti IgE from leucocytes of asthmatic patients and possible heterogeneity of IgE. Clin Allergy 1981;11:367–74.

16 Baatrup G, Petersen I, Svehag S-E, Brandslund I: A standardized method for quantitating the complement-mediated immune complex solubilizing capacity of human serum. J Immunol Methods 1983;59:369–80.

17 Bamdad S, Goodwin BFJ, Hill JE: IgE antibodies to food allergens detected by ELISA, RAST and mon-key PCA. Clin Allergy 1983;13:89–97.

18 Badger A, Young J, Poste G: Inhibition of PHA induced proliferation of human peripheral blood lym-phocytes by histamine and histamine H1 and H2 agonists. Clin Exp Immunol 1983;70:205–6.

19 Bahna SL, Heiner DC: Cow's milk allergy: patho-genesis, manifestations, diagnosis and management. Adv Pediatr 1978;25:1–37.

20 Bahna SL, Heiner DC, Horwitz CA: Sequential changes of the five immunoglobulin classes and other responses in infectious mononucleosis. Int Arch Allergy Appl Immunol 1984;74:1–8.

21 Bahna SL, Heiner DC, Myhre BA: Immunoglobulin E pattern in cigarette smokers. Allergy 1983;38:57–64.

22 Baldo BA: Standardization of allergens: examination of existing procedures and the likely impact of new techniques on the quality control of extracts. Allergy 1983;38:535–46.

23 Ballow M, Mendelson L, Donshik P et al: Pollen-specific IgG antibodies in the tears of patients with allergic-like conjunctivitis. J Allergy Clin Immunol 1984;73:376–80.

24 Barnetson R St C, Merrett TG, Ferguson A: Studies on hyperimmunoglobulinaemia E in atopic diseases with particular reference to food allergens. Clin Exp Immunol 1981;46:54–60.

25 Barnett D, Baldo BA, Howden MEH: Multiplicity of allergens in peanuts. J Allergy Clin Immunol 1983; 72:61–8.

26 Barnett DJ, Bertani L, Wara DW, Amman AJ: Milk precipitins in selective IgA deficiency. Ann Allergy 1979;42:73–6.

27 Baudon JJ, Fontaine J-L, Mougenot JF et al: L'intolerance digestive aux proteins du lait de vache chez le nourisson et l'enfant. Arch Fr Pediatr 1975;32:787–802.

28 Baur X: Studies on the specificity of human IgE-antibodies to the plant proteases papain and bro-melain. Clin Allergy 1979;9:451–7.

29 Beach RC, Menzies IS, Clayden GS, Scopes JW: Gastrointestinal permeability changes in the preterm neonate. Arch Dis Child 1982;57:141–5.

30 Benson TE, Arkins JA: Cytotoxic testing for food allergy: evaluation of reproducibility and correlation. J Allergy Clin Immunol 1976;58:471–6.

31 Benveniste J: The human basophil degranulation test as an in vitro method for the diagnosis of allergies. Clin Allergy 1981;11:1–11.

32 Bernier GM, McIntyre OR: Contaminating anti-bodies in anti IgE antisera. J Immunol Methods 1976;13:81–5.

33 Bernstein M, Day JH, Welsh A: Double-blind food challenge in the diagnosis of food sensitivity in the adult. J Allergy Clin Immunol 1982;70:205–10.

34 Bjarnason I, Peters TJ, Veall N: A persistent defect in intestinal permeability in coeliac disease demon-strated by a ^{51}Cr-labelled EDTA absorption test. Lancet 1983;i:323–5.

35 Bjarnason I, Ward K, Peters TJ: The leaky gut of alcoholism: possible route of entry for toxic com-pounds. Lancet 1984;i:179–82.

36 Björksten B, Ahlstedt S, Björksten F et al: Immuno-globulin E and immunoglobulin G^4 antibodies to cow's milk in children with cow's milk allergy. Allergy 1983;38:119–24.

37 Björksten F, Halmepuro L, Hannuksela M, Lahti A: Extraction and properties of apple allergens. Allergy 1980;35:671–7.

38 Björksten F, Backman A, Järvinen KAJ et al: Immuno-globulin E specific to wheat and rye flour proteins. Clin Allergy 1977;7:473–83.

39 Black AP: A new diagnostic method in allergic dis-ease. Pediatrics 1956;17:715–23.

40 Bloch KJ, Walker WA: Effect of locally induced in-testinal anaphylaxis on the uptake of a bystander anti-gen. J Allergy Clin Immunol 1981;67:312–16.

41 Block G, Tse KS, Kijek K et al: Baker's asthma: studies of the cross-antigenicity between different cereal grains. Clin Allergy 1984;14:177–85.

42 Bock SA, Lee W-Y, Remigio LK, May CD: Studies of hypersensitivity reactions to foods in infants and children. J Allergy Clin Immunol 1978;62:327–34.

43 Boyles JH: The validity of using the cytotoxic food test in clinical allergy. Ear Nose Throat J 1977; 56:168–73.

44 Bringel H, Vela C, Ureha V et al: IgD antibodies in vitro blocking activity of IgE mediated reactions. Clin Allergy 1982;12:37–46.

45 Brostoff J, Johns P, Stanworth DR: Complexed IgE in atopy. Lancet 1977;ii:741–2.

46 Brostoff J, Carini C, Wraith DG et al: Immune complexes in atopy. In: Pepys J Edwards AM, eds. The mast cell. London: Pitman, 1979;380–93.

47 Bryan WTK, Bryan MP: Cytotoxic reactions in the diagnosis of food allergy. Laryngoscope 1969;79:1453–72.

48 Buckley RH, Dees SC: Correlation of milk precipitins with IgA deficiency. N Engl J Med 1969;281:465–9.

49 Bürgin-Wolff A, Signer E, Friess HM et al: The diagnostic significance of antibodies to various cow's milk proteins (fluorescent immunosorbent test). Eur J Pediatr 1980;133:17–24.

50 Businco L, Marchetti F, Pellegrini G, Perlini R: Predictive value of cord blood IgE levels in 'at-risk' newborn babies and influence of type of feeding. Clin Allergy 1983;13:502–8.

51 Cairns SA, London A, Mallick NP: Circulating immune complexes following food delayed clearance in idiopathic glomerulonephritis. J Clin Lab Immunol 1981;6:121–6.

52 Cant AJ, Gibson P, Dancy M: Food hypersensitivity made life-threatening by ingestion of aspirin. Br Med J 1984;288:755–6.

53 Catsimpoolas N, ed: Immunological aspects of foods. Westport, Connecticut: Avi Publishing, 1977.

54 Chambers VV, Hudson BH, Glaser J: A study of the reactions of human polymorphonuclear leukocytes to various antigens. J Allergy 1958;29:93–102.

55 Cheung N-KV, Blessing-Moore J, Reid MJ et al: Reduction of interference by specific IgG with a modified microtiter solid-phase radioimmunoassay to measure honeybee venom IgE. J Allergy Clin Immunol 1983;71:283–93.

56 Chua YY, Bremner K, Llobet JL: Diagnosis of food allergy by the radio-allergosorbent technique. J Allergy Clin Immunol 1976;58:477–82.

57 Ciclitira PJ, Ellis HJ, Evans DJ: A solid-phase radioimmunoassay for measurement of circulating antibody titres to wheat gliadin and its subfractions in patients with adult coeliac disease. J Immunol Methods 1983;62:231–9.

58 Collins-Williams C, Salama Y: A laboratory study on the diagnosis of milk allergy. Int Arch Allergy 1965;27:110–28.

59 Conning DM, Lansdown ABG, eds: Toxic hazards in food. London: Croom Helm, 1983.

60 Coombs RRA, Oldham G: Early rheumatoid-like joint lesions in rabbits drinking cow's milk. Int Arch Allergy Appl Immunol 1981;64:287–92.

61 Coombs RRA, Kieffer M, Fraser DR, Frazier PJ: Naturally occurring antibodies to wheat gliadin fractions and to other cereal antigens in rabbits, rats, guineapigs on normal laboratory diets. Int Arch Allergy Appl Immunol 1983;70:200–4.

62 Cuevas M, Moneo I, Urena V et al: Reverse enzyme immunoassay for the determination of *Lolium perenne* IgE antibodies. Int Arch Allergy Appl Immunol 1983;72:184–7.

63 Cukor P, Woehler ME, Persiani C, Fermin A: Iodinated versus fluorescent labelling in the RAST for the determination of serum IgE levels. J Immunol Methods 1976;12:183–92.

64 Cunningham-Rundles C, Brandeis WE, Good RA: Bovine antigens and the formation of circulating immune complexes in selective IgA deficiency. J Clin Invest 1979;64:272–9.

65 Cunningham-Rundles C, Brandeis WE, Safai B et al: Selective IgA deficiency and circulating immune complexes containing bovine proteins in a child with chronic graft vs. host disease. Am J Med 1979;67:883–9.

66 Dannaeus A, Inganäs M: A follow-up study of children with food allergy. Clinical course in relation to serum IgE and IgG antibody levels to milk, egg and fish. Clin Allergy 1981;11:533–9.

67 Dannaeus A, Johansson SGO, Foucard T, Ohman S: Clinical and immunological aspects of food allergy in childhood. I. Estimation of IgG, IgA and IgE antibodies to food antigens in children—food allergy and atopic dermatitis. Acta Paediatr Scand 1977;66:31–7.

68 Dannaeus A, Inganäs M, Johansson SGO, Foucard T: Intestinal uptake of ovalbumin in malabsorption and food allergy in relation to serum IgG antibody and orally administered sodium cromoglycate. Clin Allergy 1979;9:263–70.

69 Davies DF: Immunology of human atheroma. In: Freed DLJ, eds. Health hazards of milk. Eastbourne: Baillière Tindall, 1984;202–13.

70 Davis SD, Bierman CW, Pierson WE, et al: Clinical non-specificity of milk copro-antibodies in diarrhoeal stools. N Engl J Med 1970;282:612–13.

71 Diamant B, Patkar S: Histamine release from washed whole blood. A method suitable for routine diagnosis of Type I allergy. Int Arch Allergy Appl Immunol 1982;67:13–17.

72 Dissanayake AS; Coeliac disease. In: Truelove SC, Jewell DP, eds. Topics in gastroenterology. Vol. 1. Oxford: Blackwell, 1973;167–83.

73 Dockhorn RJ: Using the RAST and PRIST with an overview of clinical significance. Ann Allergy 1982;49:1–8.

74 D'Onofrio I: Clinical accuracy of updated versions of Phadebas RAST. In: Kemeny DM, Lessof MF, eds. Recent developments in RAST and other solid-phase immunoassay systems. Amsterdam: Excerpta Medica, 1983;86–92.

75 Donovan K, Torres-Pinedo R: Effects of D-galactose on the fluid loss in soy bean protein intolerance (abstract). Pediatr Res 1978;12:433.

76 Dreborg S, Foucard T: Allergy to apple, carrot and potato in children with birch pollen allergy. Allergy 1983;38:167–72.

77 DuMont GCL, Beach RC, Menzies IS: Gastrointestinal permeability in food-allergic eczematous children. Clin Allergy 1984;14:55–9.

78 Eastham EJ, Lichauco T, Grady MI, Walker WA: Antigenicity of infant formulas: role of immature intestine on protein permeability. J Pediatr 1978;93:561–4.

79 Editorial: Food allergy and intolerance. Lancet 1980;ii:1344–5.

80 Egger J, Carter CM, Wilson J et al: Is migraine food allergy? Lancet 1983;ii:865–8.

81 Elkon KB, Lanham JG, Dash AC, Hughes GRV: The effect of a protein meal on a three fluid-phase assays for circulating immune complexes. Clin Exp Immunol 1981;45:279–82.

82 Endre L, Osvath P: Antigen-induced lymphoblast

transformations in the diagnosis of cow's milk allergic diseases in infancy and early childhood. Acta Allergologica 1975;30:34-42.

83 Eriksson NE, Formgren H, Svenonius E: Food hypersensitivity in patients with pollen allergy. Allergy 1982;37:437-43.

84 Eriksson NE, Wihl J-A, Arrendal H: Birch pollen-related food hypersensitivity: influence of total and specific IgE levels. Allergy 1983;38:353-7.

85 Eterman KP, Hekkens WThJM, Pena AS et al: Wheat grains: a substrate for the determination of gluten antibodies in serum of gluten-sensitive patients. J Immunol Methods 1977;14:85-92.

86 Evans R (Committee on in vitro tests, American Acad Allergy): Variability in the measurement of specific immunoglobulin E antibody by the RAST technique. J Allergy Clin Immunol 1982;69:245-52.

87 Ewart JAD: Immunochemistry of wheat proteins. In: Immunological Aspects of foods. Westport, Connecticut: Avi Publishing, 1977;87-116.

88 Falk ES, Dale S, Bolle R, Haneberg B: Antigens common to scabies and housedust mites. Allergy 1981;36:233-8.

89 Fällstrom SP, Ahlstedt S, Hanson LA: Specific antibodies in infants with gastrointestinal intolerance to cow's milk protein. Int Arch Allergy Appl Immunol 1978;56:97-105.

90 Fällström S-P, Lindholm L, Ahlstedt S: Cow's milk protein intolerance in children is connected with impaired lymphoblastic responses to mitogens. Int Arch Allergy Appl Immunol 1983;70:205-6.

91 Fälth-Magnusson K, Kjellman N-IM, Magnusson K-E, Sundqvist T: Intestinal permeability in healthy and allergic children before and after sodium cromoglycate treatment assessed with different sized polyethylene glycols (PEG 400 and PEG 1000). Clin Allergy 1984;14:277-86.

92 Findlay SR, Lichtenstein LM: Basophil 'releasability' in patients with asthma. Annu Rev Respir Dis 1980;122:53-9.

93 Finn R, Cohen HN: Food allergy: fact or fiction? Lancet 1978;i:426-8.

94 Ford RPK, Hill DJ, Hosking CS: Cow's milk hypersensitivity: Immediate and delayed onset clinical patterns. Arch Dis Child 1983;58:856-62.

95 Fraker PJ: Zinc deficiency: a common immunodeficiency state. Surv Immunol Res 1983;2:155-63.

96 Franklin W, Lowell FC: Failure of ragweed pollen extract to destroy white cells from ragweed-sensitive patients. J Allergy 1949;20:375-7.

96a Freed DLJ: Laboratory diagnosis of food intolerance. Clin Immunol Allergy 1982;2:181-203.

97 Freed DLJ, Sinclair T, Topper R et al: IgA levels in rhinitic nasal secretions during short-term therapy with sodium cromoglycate, beclomethasone and antihistamine. In: Pepys J, Edwards AM, eds. The mast cell. London: Pitman, 1979;795-804.

97a Freed DLJ, Wilson P, Downing NPD, Musgrove D: The cytotoxic test in immediate-type respiratory allergies. Int J Biosoc Res (in press).

98 Freier S, Lebenthal E, Freier M et al: IgE and IgD antibodies to cow's milk and soy protein in duodenal fluid: effects of pancreozymin and secretin. Immunology 1983;49:69-75.

99 Frew AJ, Bright S, Shewry PR, Minro A: Proliferative response of lymphocytes of normal individuals to wheat protein (gliadins). Int Arch Allergy Appl Immunol 1980;62:162-7.

100 Fries JF: Food allergy: current concerns (editorial). Ann Allergy 1981;46:260-3.

101 Galant S, Nussbaum E, Wittner R et al: Increased IgD milk antibody responses in a patient with Down's syndrome, pulmonary hemosiderosis and cor pulmonale. Ann Allergy 1983;51:446-9.

102 Gavani UD, Hyde JS, Moore BS: Hypersensitivity to milk and egg white, skin tests, RAST results and clinical intolerance. Ann Allergy 1978;40:314-18.

103 Gettinby G, Connolly PJ, Anderson JM: Immunological assays for coeliac disease. Lancet 1981;i:1156.

104 Good RA: Nutrition and immunity. J Clin Immunol 1981;1:3-11.

105 Goodwin BJF: IgE antibody levels to ingested soya protein determined in a normal adult population. Clin Allergy 1982;12:55-62.

106 Gunthur M, Aschaffenburg R, Matthews RH et al: The level of antibodies to the proteins of cow's milk in the serum of normal human infants. Immunology 1960;3:296-306.

107 Haddad ZH, Kalra V, Verma S: IgE Antibodies to peptic and peptic tryptic digests of β lactoglobulin: significance in food hypersensitivity. Ann Allergy 1979;42:368-71.

108 Hamburger RN: The immunogenetics of IgE provides predictive value for the development of allergy. Ann Allergy 1982;49:9-11.

109 Haraparsad D, Wilson N, Dixon C, Silverman M: Oral tartrazine challenge in childhood asthma: effect on bronchial reactivity. Clin Allergy 1984;14:81-5.

110 Hill DJ, Davidson GP, Barnes GL: The spectrum of cow's milk allergy in childhood. Clinical, gastroenterological and immunological studies. Acta Paediatr Scand 1979;68:847-52.

111 Höffken K, Bosse F, Steih V, Schmidt CG: Dissociation and isolation of antigen and antibody from immune complexes. J Immunol Methods 1982;53:51-9.

112 Hohmann A, LaBrooy J, Davidson GP, Shearman DJC: Measurement of specific antibodies in human intestinal aspirate: effect of the protease inhibitor phenylmethylsulphonyl fluoride. J Immunol Methods 1983;64:199-204.

113 Holopainen E, Palva T, Stenberg P, et al: Cytotoxic leukocyte reaction. Acta Otolaryngeal 1980;89:222-6.

114 Homburger HA, Jacob GL: Analytic accuracy of specific immunoglobulin E antibody results determined by a blind proficiency survey. J Allergy Clin Immunol 1982;70:474-80.

115 Hopkins JM, Gorecka D: Tough cells and old age. Lancet 1983;ii:1170-3.

116 Hopkins JM, Tomlinson VS, Jenkins RM: Variation in response to cytotoxicity of cigarette smoke. Br Med J 1981;283:1209-11.

117 Hsieh KH: Interferon-induced suppression of in vitro IgE biosynthesis in asthmatic children. Ann Allergy 1982;48:302-4.

118 Inganäs M, Johansson SGO, Bennich H: Anti-IgE antibodies in human serum: occurrence and specificity. Int Arch Allergy Appl Immunol 1981;65:51-61.

119 IUIS/WHO working group report: Use and abuse of laboratory tests in clinical immunology: critical considerations of eight widely used diagnostic procedures. Clin Exp Immunol 1981;46:662-74.

120 Jackson PG, Lessof MH, Baker RWR et al: Intestinal permeability in patients with eczema and food allergy. Lancet 1981;i:1285-6.

121 Johansson SGO, Bennich HH: The clinical impact of the discovery of IgE. Ann Allergy 1982;48:325-30.

122 Johansson SG, Björksten F: Standardization of in vitro methods of atopic allergy. Allergy 1980;35:177-80.

123 Jones VA, McLaughlan P, Shorthouse M et al: Food intolerance: a major factor in the pathogenesis of irritable bowel syndrome. Lancet 1982; ii:115-17.

124 Jonsson J, Schilling W: Some characteristics of immunofluorescence tests for antibodies against gluten using wheat grain sections or gliadin coated sepharose beads. Acta Pathol Microbiol Immunol Scand [C] 1981;89:253-62.

125 Jonsson J, Schilling W, Forsberg M: Colostral IgA binding to wheat gluten and gliadin. Clin Exp Immunol 1982;50:203-8.

126 Kaplan GW, Wallace WW, Orgel HA, Miller JR: Serum IgE and incidence of allergy in group of enuretic children. Urology 1977;10:428-30.

127 Kemeny DM, Mackenzie-Mills M Lessof MH: Allergen-cellulose interactions in RAST: specificity and stability with purified bee venom proteins. In: Kemeny DM, Lessof MH, eds. Recent developments in RAST and other solid-phase immunoassay systems. Amsterdam: Excerpta Medica, 1983;3-13.

128 Kenrick KG, Walker-Smith JA: Immunoglobulins and dietary protein antibodies in childhood coeliac disease. Gut 1970;11:635-40.

129 Kessel D, Cuthbert AW: Sidedness of the reaction to β lactoglobulin in sensitized colonic epithelia. Int Arch Allergy Appl Immunol 1984;74:113-19.

130 Kidd JM, Cohen SH, Sosman AJ, Fink JN: Food-dependent exercise-induced anaphylaxis. J Allergy Clin Immunol 1983;71:407-11.

131 Kieffer M, Frazier PJ, Daniels NWR, Coombs RRA: Wheat gliadin fractions and other cereal antigens reactive with antibodies in the sera of coeliac patients. Clin Exp Immunol 1982;50:651-60.

132 Kletter B, Freier S, Davies AM, Gery I: The significance of copro-antibodies in cow's milk proteins. Acta Paediatr Scand 1971;60:173-80.

133 Kletter B, Gery I, Freier S, Davies AM: Immune responses of normal infants to cow's milk. II. Decreased immune reactions in initially breast-fed infants. Int Arch Allergy Appl Immunol 1971;40:667-74.

134 Kolmannskog S, Haneberg B, Marhang G, Bolle R: Immunoglobulin E in extracts of feces from children. Int Arch Allergy Appl Immunol 1984;74:50-4.

135 Köttgen E, Kluge F, Volk B, Gerok W: The lectin properties of gluten as the basis of the pathomechanism of gluten sensitive enteropathy. Klin Wochenschr 1983;61:111-12.

136 Köttgen E, Volk B, Kluge F, Gerok W: Gluten, a lectin with oligomannosyl specificity and the causative agent of gluten sensitive enteropathy. Biochem Biophys Res Commun 1982;109:168-73.

137 Krauer KA, Kagey-Sobotka A, Adkinson NF Jr, Lichtenstein LM: Platelet augmentation of IgE-dependent histamine release from human basophils and mast cells. Int Arch Allergy Appl Immunol 1984; 74:29-35.

138 Lahti A, Björksten F, Hannuksela M: Allergy to birch pollen and apple and cross reactivity of the allergens studied with the RAST. Allergy 1980;35:297-300.

139 Lee SK, Kniker WT, Cook CD, Heiner DC: Cow's milk-induced pulmonary disease in children. Adv Pediatr 1978;25:39-57.

140 Lehman CW: The leukocyte food allergy test: a study of its reliability and reproducibility. Effect of diet and sublingual food drops on this test. Ann Allergy 1980;45:150-8.

141 Lieberman P, Crawford L, Bjelland J et al: Controlled study of the cytotoxic test. J Am Med Assoc 1975;231:728-30.

142 Lim PL, Rowley D: The effect of antibody on the intestinal absorption of macromolecules and on intestinal permeability in adult mice. Int Arch Allergy Appl Immunol 1982;68:41-6.

143 Lis H, Sharon N: The biochemistry of plant lectins (phytohemagglutinins). Annu Rev Biochem 1973;42:541-74.

144 Littlewood JM: RAST measurements in childhood. In: The Second Fisons Food Allergy Workshop. Oxford: Medicine Publishing Foundation 1983;49-51.

145 Lowell FC: Some untested diagnostic and therapeutic procedures in clinical allergy. J Allergy Clin Immunol 1975;56:168-9.

146 Lowell FC, Heiner DC: Food allergy: cytotoxic diagnosis technique not proven. J Am Med Assoc 1972;220:1624.

147 Lowenstein H, Eriksson NE: Hypersensitivity to foods among birch pollen-allergic patients. Immunochemical inhibition studies for evaluation of possible mechanisms. Allergy 1983;38:577-87.

148 McGovern JJ: Re: sublingual provocative food testing (letter). Ann Allergy 1981;46:44-6.

149 McLaughlan P, Coombs RRA: Latent anaphylactic sensitivity of infants to cow's milk proteins: histamine release from blood basophils. Clin Allergy 1983;13:1-9.

150 McLaughlan P, Anderson KJ, Widdowson EM, Coombs RRA: Effect of heat on the anaphylactic-sensitising capacity of cow's milk, goat's milk and various infant formulae fed to guineapigs. Arch Dis Child 1981;56:165-71.

151 Magnusson CGM, Masson PL: Particle-counting immunoassay after immunoglobulin E antibodies after their elution from allergosorbents by pepsin: an alternative to the radioallergosorbent test. J Allergy Clin Immunol 1982;70:326-36.

152 Malm L, Wihl JA, Lamm CJ, Lindqvist N: Reduction of metacholine-induced nasal secretion by treatment with a new topical steroid in perennial non-allergic rhinitis. Allergy 1981;36:209-14.

153 Mathews JB, Fivaz BH, Sewell HF: Serum and salivary antibody responses and the development of oral tolerance after oral and intragastric antigen administration. Int Arch Allergy Appl Immunol 1981;65:107-13.

154 Matthews KP: Calculation of secretory antibodies and immunoglobulins. J Allergy Clin Immunol 1981;68:46-50.

155 Maulitz RM, Pratt DS, Schocket AL: Exercise-induced anaphylactic reaction to shellfish. J Allergy Clin Immunol 1979;63:433-4.

156 May CD: Food allergy: lessons from the past. J Allergy Clin Immunol 1982;69:255-9.

157 May CD: Food sensitivity. Proc N Engl Soc Allergy 2:198-203.

158 May CD, Alberto R: In vitro responses of leukocytes to food proteins in allergic and normal children: lymphocyte stimulation and histamine release. Clin Allergy 1972;2:335-44.

159 May CD, Remigio L: Observations on high spontaneous release of histamine from leucocytes in vitro. Clin Allergy 1982;12:229-41.

160 May CD, Remigio L, Bock SA: Usefulness of measurement of antibodies in serum in diagnosis of sensitivity to cow's milk and soy proteins in early childhood. Allergy 1980;35:301-10.

161 May CD, Lyman M, Alberto R, Cheng J: Procedures for immunochemical study of histamine release from leucocytes with small volume of blood. J Allergy 1970;46:12-20.

162 May CD, Remigio L, Feldman J et al: A study of serum antibodies to isolated milk proteins and oval-bumin in infants and children. Clin Allergy 1977;7:583–95.

163 Merrett J, Peatfield RC, Rose FC, Merrett TG: Food related antibodies in headache patients. J Neurol Neurosurg Psychiatry 1983;46:738–42.

164 Merrett TG, Merrett J: The RAST principle and the use of mixed-allergen RAST as a screening test of IgE-mediated allergies. Methods Enzymol 1980;70(A):376–87.

165 Metzger WJ, Butler JE, Swanson P et al: Amplification of the enzyme-linked immunosorbent assay for measuring allergen-specific IgE and IgG antibody. Clin Allergy 1981;11:523–31.

166 Miadonna A, Tedeschi A, Zanussi C: Plasma of normal, but not atopic, persons reducing basophil degranulation induced by anti-IgE. Clin Allergy 1984;14:29–35.

167 Minford AMB, Macdonald A, Littlewood JM: Food intolerance and food allergy in children: a review of 68 cases. Arch Dis Child 1982;57:742–7.

168 Minor JD, Tolber SG, Frick OL: Leukocyte inhibition factor in delayed-onset food allergy. J Allergy Clin Immunol 1980;66:314–21.

169 Moneret-Vautrin DA, Gerard H, Grilliat JP: Allergie alimentaire de type immediat: évaluation critique du RAST et du teste degranulation des basophiles. Nouv Press Med 1979;8:3176.

170 Monro J, Brostoff J, Carini C, Zilkha K: Food allergy in migraine. Study of dietary exclusion and RAST. Lancet 1980;ii:1–4.

171 Moro E: Kühmilchpräzipitin im Blute eines 4½ Monate alten Atrophikers. Munch Med Wochenschr 1906;53:214.

172 Morrow Brown H: Milk allergy and intolerance: clinical aspects. In: Freed DLJ, ed. Health hazards of milk. Eastbourne: Baillière Tindall, 1984;92–113.

173 Nelson HS: Effect of preservatives and conditions of storage on the potency of allergy extracts. J Allergy Clin Immunol 1981;67:64–9.

174 Nicklin S, Miller K: Local and systemic immune responses to intestinally presented antigen. Int Arch Allergy Appl Immunol 1983;72:87–90.

175 Niinimäki A, Hannuksela M: Immediate skin test reactions to spices. Allergy 1981;36:487–93.

176 Oggell JD, Dockhorn RJ: Staphylococcal protein A and enhancement of disc RAST sensitivity. Ann Allergy 1983;50:178–81.

177 Ogle KA, Bullock JD: Children with allergic rhinitis and/or bronchial asthma treated with elimination diet: a five year follow-up. Ann Allergy 1980;44:273–8.

178 O'Mahony CP, Stevens FM, Bourke M et al: ⁵¹Cr-EDTA test for coeliac disease. Lancet 1984;i:1355.

179 Ormonroyd P, Robertshaw D: A comparison of the Phadebas^R and Phadezym^R IgE paper immunosorbent test kits. Clin Allergy 1983;13:51–5.

180 Paganelli R, Levinsky RJ: Solid phase radioimmunoassay for detection of circulating food protein antigens in human serum. J Immunol Methods 1980;37:333–41.

181 Paganelli R, Atherton DJ, Levinsky RJ: Differences between normal and milk allergic subjects in their immune responses after milk ingestion. Arch Dis Child 1983;58:201–6.

182 Paganelli R, Levinsky RJ, Atherton DJ: Detection of specific antigen within circulating immune complexes. Validation of the assay and its application to food antigen/antibody complexes found in healthy and food-allergic subjects. Clin Exp Immunol 1981;46:44–53.

183 Paganelli R, Levinsky RJ, Brostoff J, Wraith DG: Immune complexes containing food proteins in normal and atopic subjects after oral challenge and effect of sodium cromoglycate on antigen absorption. Lancet 1979;i:1270–1.

184 Pantin CFA, Merrett TG: The microcomputer as an aid to allergy investigation. Ann Allergy 1982;49:12–15.

185 Papageorgiou N, Lee TH, Nagakura T et al: Neutrophil chemotactic activity in milk-induced asthma. J Allergy Clin Immunol 1983;72:75–82.

186 Pearson ADJ, Eastham ET, Laker MF et al: Intestinal permeability in children with Crohn's disease and coeliac disease. Br Med J 1982;285:20–1.

187 Pearson DJ, Rix KJB, Bentley SJ: Food allergy: how much in the mind? Lancet 1983;i:1259–61.

188 Pearson DJ, Bentley SJ, Rix KJB, Roberts C: Food hypersensitivity and irritable bowel syndrome. Lancet 1983;ii:746–7.

189 Pecoud A, Bonstein HS, Frei PC: Value of the case history in the diagnosis of allergic state and the detection of allergens. Clin Allergy 1983;13:141–7.

190 Pecoud A, Ochsner M, Arrendal H, Frei PC: Improvement of the radioallergosorbent test (RAST) sensitivity by using an antibody specific for the determinant D2. Clin Allergy 1982;12:75–81.

191 Perelmutter L, Bergeron M, Mandy F: Assessment of the effect of IgG antibodies to ragweed and rye grass on the IgE antibody disc RAST. Ann Allergy 1983;50:393–7.

192 Pitcher-Wilmott RW, Booth I, Harries J, Levinsky PJ: Intestinal absorption of food antigens in coeliac disease. Arch Dis Child 1982;57:462–6.

193 Prausnitz C, Küstner H: Studies on supersensitivity. Centralbl f Bakteriol 1 Abt Orig 1921;86:160–9.

194 Radermecker M, Maldague M-P: Depression of neutrophil chemotaxis in atopic individuals: an H2 histamine receptor response. Int Arch Allergy Appl Immunol 1981;65:144–52.

195 Rechcigl M, ed: CRC handbook of naturally occurring food toxicants. Boca Raton, Florida: CRC Press, 1983.

196 Reid MJ, Cheung N-KV, Lewiston NJ: Microtiter solid-phase radioimmunoassay for specific immunoglobulin E. J Allergy Clin Immunol 1981;67:263–71.

197 Reyes MA, Saravia NG, Watson RR, McMurray DN: Effect of moderate malnutrition on immediate hypersensitivity and immunoglobulin E levels in asthmatic children. J Allergy Clin Immunol 1982;70:94–100.

198 Ring J, Mathison DA, O'Connor R: In vitro cyclic nucleotide responsiveness in leukocytes and platelets in patients suffering from atopic dermatitis. Int Arch Allergy Appl Immunol 1981;65:1–7.

199 Roberts SA, Reinhardt MC, Paganelli R, Levinsky J: Specific antigen exclusion and non-specific facilitation of antigen entry across the gut in rats allergic to food proteins. Clin Exp Immunol 1981;45:131–6.

200 Robertson DM, Paganelli R, Dinwiddie R, Levinsky RJ: Milk antigen absorption in the preterm and term neonate. Arch Dis Child 1982;57:369–72.

201 Rote NS, Caudle MR: Detection of circulating immune complexes with a Raji cell enzyme immunoassay. J Immunol Methods 1983;56:33–42.

202 Rubin JL, Griffiths RW, Hill HR: Allergen-induced depression of neutrophil chemotaxis in allergic individuals. J Allergy Clin Immunol 1978;62:301–8.

203 Ruokonen J, Holopainen E, Palva T, Backman A:

Secretory otitis media and allergy with special reference to the cytotoxic leucocyte test. Allergy 1981;36:59–68.

204 Sancho J, Egido J, Rivera F, Hernando L: Immune complexes in IgA nephropathy: presence of antibodies against diet antigens and delayed clearance of specific polymeric IgA immune complexes. Clin Exp Immunol 1983;54:194–202.

205 Saperstein S, Anderson DW Jr, Goldman AS, Kniker WT: Milk allergy. III. Immunological studies with sera from allergic and normal children. Pediatrics 1963;32:580–7.

206 Savilahti E: Cow's milk allergy. Allergy 1981;36:73–88.

207 Savilahti E, Pelkonen P, Visakorpi JK: IgA deficiency in children. A clinical study with special reference to intestinal findings. Arch Dis Child 1971;46:665–70.

208 Savilahti E, Viander M, Perkkiö M et al: IgA antigliadin antibodies: a marker of mucosal damage in childhood coeliac disease. Lancet 1983; i:320–2.

209 Scheinmann P, Gendrel D, Charles J, Paupe J: Value of lymphoblast transformation test on cow's milk protein intestinal intolerance. Clin Allergy 1976;6:515–21.

210 Schwartz HR, Nerurkar LS, Spies JR et al: Milk hypersensitivity: RAST studies using new antigengenerated by pepsin hydrolysis of beta-lactoglobulin. Ann Allergy 1980;45:242–5.

211 Scott ML, Thornley MJ, Coombs RRA: Comparison of red-cell linked anti IgE and ^{125}I-labelled anti IgE in a solid-phase system for the measurement of IgE specific for castor bean allergen. Int Arch Allergy Appl Immunol 1981;64:230–5.

212 Sepulveda R, Longbottom JL, Pepys J: Enzymelinked immunosorbent assay (ELISA) for IgG and IgE antibodies to protein and polysaccharide antigens of *Aspergillus fumigatus*. Clin Allergy 1979;9:359–71.

213 Shibasaki M, Suzuki S, Nemoto H, Kuroume T: Allergenicity and lympho-stimulating property of rice protein. J Allergy Clin Immunol 1979;64:259–65.

214 Shurkovich S, Shurkovich B, Bellanti JA, Banergee DK: Interferon increases IgE binding to basophils. Ann Allergy 1983;50:505–8.

215 Sikora K, Anand BS, Truelove SC, Ciclitira PJ: Stimulation of lymphocytes from patients with coeliac disease by a subfraction of gluten. Lancet 1976;ii:389–91.

216 Silverstone GA: Possible sources of food toxicants: plants, some foods of animal origin, microorganisms, food additives. In: Seely S, Freed DLJ, Silverstone GA, Rippere V, eds. Diet-related diseases: The modern epidemic. London: Croom Helm (in press).

217 Soifer MM, Hirsch SR: The direct basophil degranulation test and the intracutaneous test: a comparison using food extracts. J Allergy Clin Immunol 1975;56:127–32.

218 Spengler GA, Weber R-M: Interactions of PHA and human normal serum proteins. Lectins. Biol Biochem Clin Biochem Vol. I. 1981;231–40.

219 Squier TL, Lee HJ: Lysis in vitro of sensitized leukocytes by ragweed antigen. J Allergy 1947;18:156–63.

220 Stempel DA, Davis VL, Morissey LJ, Helms RW: Seasonal variations of serum IgE levels in normal children. Ann Allergy 1981;47:14–16.

221 Stenback EI: The influence of human plasma lipoproteins and fatty acids in immunological reactions. Allergy 1984;39:1–11.

222 Stoddart RW: The generation of cancer: initiation, promotion, progression and the multiple influences of the environment. Nutr Health 1983;2:153–62.

223 Strannegard O, Strannegard IL: In vitro differences between the lymphocytes of normal subjects and atopics. Clin Allergy 1979;9:637–43.

224 Subba Rao PV, NcCartney-Francis NL, Metcalfe DD: An avidin-biotin micro ELISA for rapid measurement of total and allergen-specific human IgE. J Immunol Methods 1983;57:71–85.

225 Sutton R, Hill DJ, Baldo BA, Wrigley CW: Immunoglobulin E antibodies to ingested cereal flour components: studies with sera from subjects with asthma and eczema. Clin Allergy 1982;12:63–74.

226 Taylor B, Fergusson DM, Mahoney GN et al: Specific IgA and IgE in childhood asthma, eczema and food allergy. Clin Allergy 1982;12:499–505.

227 Truelove SC, Jewell DP: The intestine in allergic diseases. In: Gell PGH, Coombs RRA, Lachman PJ, eds. Clinical aspects of immunology. Oxford: Blackwell, 1975;1441–65.

228 Turner MW, Paganelli R, Levinsky RJ, Williams A: Antigen-binding radioimmunoassays for human IgG antibodies to bovine β-lactoglobulin. J Immunol Methods 1983;56:175–83.

229 Ulett GA, Perry SG: Cytotoxic testing and leucocyte increase as an index to food sensitivity. Ann Allergy 1974;33:23–32.

230 Unsworth DJ, Kieffer M, Holborow EK et al: IgA anti-gliadin antibodies in coeliac disease. Clin Exp Immunol 1981;46:286–93.

231 Unsworth DJ, Manuel PD, Walker-Smith JA et al: A new immunofluorescent blood test for gluten sensitivity. Arch Dis Child 1981;56:864–8.

232 Updegraff TR: Food allergy and cytotoxic tests. Ear Nose Throat J 1977;56:450–9.

233 Valverde E, Vich JM, Garcia-Calderon JV, Garcia-Calderon PA: In vitro response of lymphocytes in patients with allergic tension-fatigue syndrome. Ann Allergy 1980;45:185–8.

234 Valverde E, Vich JM, Garcia-Calderon JV, Garcia-Calderon PA: In vitro stimulation of lyphocytes in patients with chronic urticaria induced by additives and food. Clin Allergy 1980;10:691–8.

235 Van der Woude FJ, Hoedemaeker PhJ, Van der Giessen M et al: Do food antigens play a role in the pathogenesis of some cases of human glomerulonephritis? Clin Exp Immunol 1983;51:587–94.

236 van Toorenenbergen AW, Kramps JA, van der Burgh JF, Dijkman JH: Use of automatic counting of basophil leukocytes: correlation of basophil degranulation with histamine release. J Immunol Methods 1982;49:209–13.

237 Verkasalo MA: Adherence of gliadin fractions to lymphocytes in coeliac disease. Lancet 1982;i:389–91.

238 Vervloet D, Bongrand P, Charpin J: Absolute determination of IgE antibodies to grass pollen allergens. Allergy 1978;33:203–10.

239 Viscidi R, Laughton BE, Hanvanich M et al: Improved enzyme immunoassays for the detection of antigens in fecal specimens. Investigation and correction of interfering factors. J Immunol Methods 1984;67:129–43.

240 Wahn U, Herold U, Danielsen K, Lowenstein H: Allergoprints in horse allergic children. Allergy 1982;37:335–43.

241 Walzer M: Allergy of the abdominal organs. J Lab Clin Med 1941;26:1867.

242 Warner JO, Hathaway MJ: Allergic form of Meadow's syndrome (Munchausen by proxy). Arch Dis Child 1984;59:151–6.

243 Warren CPW, Holford-Strevens V, Wong C, Manfreda J: The relationship between smoking and total immunoglobulin E levels. J Allergy Clin Immunol 1982;69:370–5.

244 Weaver LT, Laker MF, Nelson R: Enhanced intestinal permeability in preterm babies with bloody stools. Arch Dis Child 1984;59:280–1.

245 Weaver LT, Laker MF, Nelson R: Intestinal permeability in the newborn. Arch Dis Child 1984;59:236–41.

246 Wide L, Bennich H, Johansson SGO: Diagnosis of allergy by an in vitro test for allergen antibodies. Lancet 1967;ii:1105–7.

247 Wilson N, Vickers H, Taylor G, Silverman M: Objective test for food sensitivity in asthmatic children: increased bronchial reactivity after cola drinks. Br Med J 1982;284:1226–8.

248 Wojnar RJ, Hearn T, Starkweather MS: Augmentation of allergic histamine release from human leucocytes by NSAI—analgesic agent. J Allergy Clin Immunol 1980;66:37–45.

249 Wraith DG, Merrett J, Roth A et al: Recognition of food-allergic patients and their allergens by the RAST technique and clinical investigation. Clin Allergy 1979;9:25–36.

250 York Alternative Medical Practice: Physician's cytotoxic handbook: explanatory literature.

251 Zeiss CR, Grammer LC, Levitz D: Comparison of the RAST and a quantitative solid-phase RIA for the detection of ragweed-specific immunoglobulin E antibody in patients undergoing immunotherapy. J Allergy Clin Immunol 1981;67:105–10.

252 Zetterström O, Öhman S, Nilson G, Dreborg S: Stability of freeze-dried and reconstituted Timothy pollen allergen extract and hymenoptera venoms reconstituted in saline with and without albumin. Allergy 1982;37:25.

253 Zetterström O, Osterman K, Machado L, Johansson SGO: Another smoking hazard: raised serum IgE concentration and increased risk of occupational allergy. Br Med J 1981;283:1215–17.

Chapter 51
The Role of IgG4 in Food Allergy

Farouk Shakib

BIOLOGICAL PROPERTIES OF IgG4

IgG4 represents a very small proportion of total IgG in normal sera [38]. It has an average biological half-life of 21 days [28] and, in contrast to IgE, it can cross the placenta into the fetus [25, 30]. It differs from other IgG subclasses in its inability to activate complement by the classical pathway [2]. However, recent observations suggest that the IgG4 subclass also possesses a C1q binding site within its $C\gamma 2$ domain, but that this is shielded by the molecules Fab regions [46]. IgG4 exists in two genetic forms, termed IgG4a and IgG4b [20]. The 4a antigenic determinant is shared by IgG1 and IgG3, whilst the 4b determinant is shared by the IgG2 subclass only. In normal sera these two variants of IgG4 are found either alone or in mixture, but it appears that the IgG4a form is the predominant one. However, the available methods of measuring total and specific IgG4 do not generally distinguish between these two variants (Table 51.1).

Interest in the role of IgG4 in allergic disease stems from the capacity of this subclass to bind to basophils and presumably to mast cells. Thus the initial demonstration of the selective inhibition of IgE-mediated passive cutaneous anaphylactic reactions in subhuman primates by a myeloma IgG4 protein [47] was later confirmed by other investigators [52]. Since then more direct evidence for the presence of receptors for IgG4 molecules on human basophils has been reported. Several studies have shown that IgG4 can bind to basophils in such a way that subsequent challenge with an anti-IgG4 antibody causes cell degranulation [31] and histamine release

Table 51.1 Comparison of biological activity of IgE and IgG4.

	IgE	IgG4
Serum concentration	100 ng/ml	300 μg/ml
Biological half-life (days)	2.5	21
Cross placenta	−	+
Complement fixation	−	−
Binding of C1q	−	+
Monocyte binding (Fc)	±	+
Reactivity with protein A	−	+
Mast cell binding—primate	+	+
—guinea-pig	+	−
Genetic variants	+	+

Table 51.2 Reactivity of the IgG subclasses and IgE with basophils and mast cells.

Property	IgG1	IgG2	IgG3	IgG4	IgE
Basophil/mast cell binding	−	−	−	+	+
Basophil mediator release with					
allergen	−	−	−	−	+
antiserum	−	−	−	+	+
oligomers	−	−	−	−	+

[11, 53]. Challenge with specific allergen, however, does not result in a similar effect [50]. Recently the ability of covalently cross-linked oligomers of purified myeloma IgG subclass proteins to release histamine from human leukocytes has been examined [56]. It was found that oligomers of IgG4, and those of other subclasses, failed to release histamine from leukocytes of donors whose basophils released histamine when challenged with IgE dimers (Table 51.2).

Perhaps the most striking conclusion drawn from these studies is that IgG4 can bind to basophils, but mediator release can only be initiated upon cross-linking with a specific anti-IgG4 antibody. Interestingly, such anti-IgG4 antibody can also trigger off mediator release from basophils of non-atopic individuals passively sensitized with IgG4 [53].

METHODS OF IgG4 DETECTION

In the early days of IgG subclass work one of the major difficulties in quantitating IgG subclasses was the production of satisfactory anti-IgG subclass antisera [14, 37]. The necessity for exhaustive absorption with the undesired specificities often made these antisera either weak or highly restricted in their reactivity. However, recent advances in immunology have made possible the production of mouse monoclonal antibodies to IgG subclasses [24]. These reagents are of such specificity [24, 51] that their use in IgG4 assays will have an important impact on current efforts aimed at delineating the role of IgG4 in allergic disorders.

The IgG4 subclass can be measured as total and as food specific.

Total IgG4

Total IgG4 levels have been measured with polyclonal anti-IgG4 antiserum using radial immunodiffusion [42, 49, 55], radioprecipitation [22] and radioimmunoassay [26, 29, 34]. More recently monoclonal reagents have been employed to measure total IgG4 by a radial immunodiffusion system [13]. We have also employed monoclonal antibodies in a highly economical and sensitive enzyme-linked immunosorbent assay (ELISA) inhibition system to measure IgG4 concentrations in serum [44]. In this assay IgG4 standards and sera are allowed to compete with the immobilized IgG4 phase for binding to an IgG4 specific monoclonal antibody. The extent to which the binding of the monoclonal antibody to the solid phase is reduced by the unknown serum is used to determine total IgG4 concentration by comparison to a set of standards.

Food-specific IgG4

Methodology. The principle of the radioallergosorbent test (RAST) has also been applied to measure IgG4 antibodies to cow's milk [5, 26], hen's egg white, codfish, wheat flour, peanut and almond nut [26].

In our own laboratory we have developed a very sensitive ELISA for the measurement of IgG4 to three cow's milk proteins and two hen's egg proteins [39]. In this ELISA system the allergen is coated onto the solid phase (microtitre plate) and allowed to react with the specific IgG4 in the added serum. Any bound IgG4 is then detected with a mouse monoclonal antibody to IgG4 which is in turn detected with a peroxidase-conjugated rabbit anti-mouse IgG (Fig. 51.1). The use of a con-

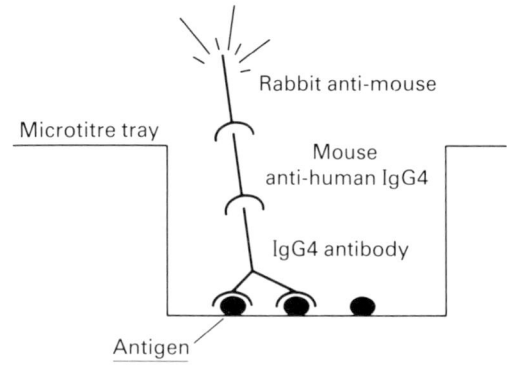

Fig. 51.1 ELISA method for IgG4 antibody.

jugated anti-mouse IgG rather than conjugated mouse monoclonal anti-IgG4 (i.e. the introduction of an extra layer), would serve to amplify the sensitivity of the assay and allow the detection (when desired) of food-specific antibodies of all immunoglobulin classes and subclasses with the same conjugated antiserum. Contrary to some reports [6, 45] the so-called 'microtitre plate edge effect' was not encountered in our ELISA system [39] or in that of others [21]. The use of human serum albumin as a blocking protein was found to be essential in our system in that it reduced background readings.

Assays based on measuring the amount of allergen binding to the patient's immobilized IgG4 (i.e. labelled antigen-binding assay) are obviously influenced by the valency of the antibody under measurement. In the light of a recent report [1] showing that IgG4 might act as a monovalent antibody, such assays are bound to underestimate the amount of specific IgG4 in the sample tested.

Calculation of results. Results of food-specific IgG4 assays are for the time being expressed in arbitrary units by comparison to a normal serum pool or a positive serum pool. A recent report [21] warned against the use of normal serum pools as negative reference because such an approach presupposes that food-specific IgG4 antibodies either (a) are not present, and that any activity observed is due to non-specific binding, or (b) represent normal levels and only higher values are significant. Either of these suppositions could lead to the false interpretation of data. Pooling sera positive for food-specific IgG4 is also to be avoided because, as will be indicated later, some allergic sera might contain precipitating anti-IgG4 antiglobulins. For these reasons, it is far better to express results as a percentage of a highly active (positive) sample than as a percentage increase from a non-active (negative) sample or pool.

There is now a method available for quantitating circulating levels of food-specific IgG4 [21]. The demand for such quantitative procedures would obviously become greater when the diagnostic value of current IgG4 tests are firmly established.

LEVELS OF IgG4 IN NORMAL INDIVIDUALS

Although all reports [13, 26, 30, 40, 42, 49] agree that IgG4 is the least abundant of all IgG subclasses, its percentage contribution to total IgG in the sera tested varies from one series to another (Table 51.3). These differences could possibly be attributed, at least in part, to the adoption of different assay procedures in different laboratories and to the variation in the frequency of certain genetic markers in the human populations studied [35, 36, 40]. Thus G2m(n) homozygotes are known [35] to have the highest levels of IgG4, individuals negative for G2m(n) have the lowest levels and heterozygotes have levels of IgG4 between the two. Such a gene–dosage effect on the concentration of serum IgG4 may well be connected with the relative abundance of the two allotypic variants of IgG4, 4a and 4b, in the sera tested [20].

Extremely high levels of IgG4 were reported in a study of a group of normal sera obtained from an isolated community in Iceland [54]. We have also found higher levels of IgG4 in one Middle Eastern population [40] compared with a British population [42]. Obviously, further work is needed, particularly with regard to the distribution of genetic markers, in order to compare IgG4 values from different populations.

Ontogeny of IgG subclasses

In the newborn baby, levels of IgG4 (and IgG2) develop much more slowly than those

Table 51.3 Variation in reported IgG4 levels.

Series reference	Number of sera studied	Method employed	IgG4	
			Mean (g/l)	Percentage of total IgG
[30]	108	Radioassay	0.46	4.3
[42]	111	Mancini	0.08	0.7
[49]	107	Mancini	0.60	4.9
[40]	91	Mancini	0.25	3.0
[26]	156	Radioassay	0.38	?
[13]	172	Mancini	0.24	2.5

of IgG1 and IgG3. Thus, whilst IgG1 synthesis starts before 3 months of age and concentrations are close to adult values at 8 months, IgG4 synthesis is still far from maturity at the age of 2 years [29]. These findings were later confirmed by other authors [49] who showed that the amount of IgG4 (and IgG2) rises slowly with age, not having yet reached the adult level at the age of 12 years. Levels of IgG4 also tend to drop more quickly than those of IgG1 and IgG3 in the very old age group, i.e. individuals above 95 years of age [34].

Serum levels of IgG4, like those of other subclasses, show no significant weekly or monthly variations in the absence of a sudden antigenic exposure [42] (Fig. 51.2).

Incidence of food-specific IgG4 in the general population

A community survey of 156 adults from a small town in South Wales demonstrated that high serum levels of IgG4 antibodies specific to foods, especially egg and milk, were frequently present in the population studied [26]. In a more recent study [39] we found raised IgG4 specific to one or more egg proteins in 12 (46.2%) out of 26 non-atopic individuals (two adults and 24 children); 11 had raised IgG4 specific to ovalbumin and one to both ovalbumin and ovomucoid (Fig. 51.3). Raised IgG4 specific to one or more milk proteins, on the other hand, were found in only three (11.5%) out of these 26 individuals; one had raised IgG4 specific to β-lactoglobulin, one to α-casein and one to both β-lactoglobulin and α-casein. In a quantitative study of 40 non-allergic individuals, 80% of the sera tested possessed IgG4 antibodies to ovalbumin, 60% to β-lactoglobulin but only 42% to gluten [21]. These sera showed considerable variation in food-specific IgG4 levels, the Mean $\pm$ SD (μg/ml) being 1.9 $\pm$ 4.9 for ovalbumin, 1.9 $\pm$ 5.1 for β-lactoglobulin and 1.7 $\pm$ 4.5 for gluten.

Although food-specific IgG4 is frequently detectable in sera of apparently healthy individuals, its presence should not be regarded as physiological. Thus, for instance, milk- and egg-specific IgG4 antibodies are not demon-

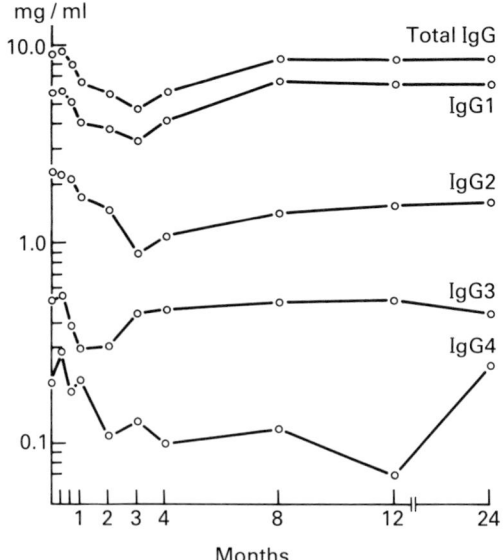

Fig. 51.2 Concentrations of total immunoglobulins and immunoglobulin subclasses throughout the first 2 years of life. Reproduced from [29] with permission.

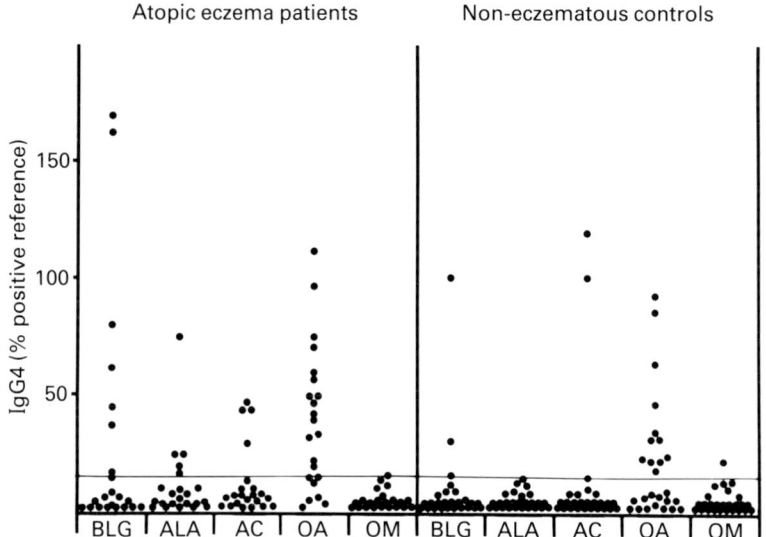

Fig. 51.3 Results of the ELISA for IgG4 specific to three cow's milk proteins and two hen's egg proteins in 22 eczema patients and 26 non-eczematous controls. The horizontal line represents the 15% cut-off point above which values were considered raised. BLG = β-lactoglobulin, ALA = α-lactalbumin, AC = α-casein, OA = ovalbumin, OM = ovomucoid. Reproduced from [39] with permission.

strable in a considerable proportion of people who constantly consume these foods. In five such individuals deliberate challenge with either half a pint of cow's milk or one boiled hen's egg failed to result in any detectable specific IgG4 when monitored over a 4-week period (author's unpublished observation). In fact, in a very recent study [44] we have demonstrated that the capacity to mount milk- and egg-specific IgG4 might be genetically predisposed.

IgG4 ANTIBODIES IN FOOD ALLERGY

Circulating IgG antibodies to foods are detectable in a proportion of patients with food sensitivity [4, 8, 12]. It is not certain, however, if such food-specific IgG is pathological. Thus, for instance, high titres of egg-specific IgG were frequently found in sera of children with eczema and other allergies, while showing increasing tolerance to egg [9]. Whether this indicates a possible 'blocking' capacity of IgG antibodies or is just the result of an increased allergenic load, is not known. IgG antibodies to the codfish muscle allergen, DS22, were, on the other hand, found only in children allergic to fish [9]. In contrast, clinical improvement following immunotherapy with fish extract in one case was accompanied by a great increase in the concentration of IgG antibodies to DS22 allergen [7] (see Chapter 19).

Cord blood. Serum IgG antibodies to milk and egg have been detected in newborns and levels reflected the corresponding maternal concentrations [8]. High levels in cord sera seemed to protect against the onset of atopic symptoms during the first 2 years of life [7]. In food-sensitive children, an early high IgG/IgE food antibody ratio was thought to be a good prognostic sign, indicating a possible protective capacity of IgG antibodies [7]. This is in line with previous work from the same group [8] showing that symptom-free children had higher titres of IgG antibodies to β-lactoglobulin and ovomucoid than those who developed allergic symptoms. A recent study showed that a delay in the introduction of cow's milk in the baby's diet reduces the development of specific IgG antibodies [12]. Trace quantities of maternal dietary protein in breast milk are also thought to be immunologically significant for the suckling infant [19].

A case of egg-white allergy and a case of fish allergy, where complement fixation by thermostable IgG-class antibody was positive at extremely high antigen dilution, have been described [4]. The antibody in egg-white allergy was of the precipitating variety and the complement fixation phenomenon was not related to the presence or absence of IgE antibody. The IgG antibody involved may be related to the complement-dependent IgG class 'short-term anaphylactic' antibody described by Parish [33], which had already been implicated in a case of allergy to shellfish [17].

IgG4 antibodies to cow's milk protein

It was because of such discrepant findings that we felt that an IgG subclass assay may provide insight into the role of IgG antibodies in food allergy. In view of our first report [43] and those that had followed [3, 15, 16], showing a remarkable increase in total IgG4 in some atopic eczema patients, it seemed important to investigate the clinical relevance of food-specific IgG4 in this condition. An ELISA was developed to measure IgG4 specific to three cow's milk proteins (β-lactoglobulin, α-lactalbumin and α-casein) and two hen's egg proteins (ovalbumin and ovomucoid) in the sera of milk- and/or egg-allergic eczema patients and non-eczematous controls [39].

Atopic eczema. The study has shown that IgG4 antibodies to milk were mainly directed against β-lactoglobulin, but also against α-lactalbumin and α-casein. IgG4 antibodies to egg were almost entirely directed against ovalbumin. Although milk- and egg-specific IgG4 antibodies were detectable in a large proportion of the eczema patients, their presence did not correlate with clinical sensitivity to these foods (Fig. 51.3). Thus, 11 out of 22 eczema patients had raised serum IgG4 specific to one or more milk proteins: three had raised IgG4 specific to β-lactoglobulin, two to α-casein, two to α-lactalbumin, two to both β-lactoglobulin and α-lactalbumin, one to both β-lactoglobulin and α-casein and one to β-lactoglobulin, α-casein and α-lactoglobulin. Only seven out of these 11 patients had milk allergy, the other four did not. There were a further 10 eczema patients who, although they were milk allergic, had no demonstrably raised level of specific IgG4. Only one out of the 11 eczema patients with raised IgG4 specific to milk proteins also had positive IgE RAST for milk.

It has, therefore, become obvious that IgG4 antibodies to the main three milk proteins are not detectable in a proportion of atopic eczema patients who are undoubtedly milk allergic. The possibility that such discrepant findings were caused by failure to measure IgG4 antibodies to another probably more relevant milk antigen was also considered. Thus, for instance, antigens present on bovine milk fat globule membrane, which separates out with the cream fraction of milk, have been implicated in eliciting pathologically important IgG responses in patients with coronary heart disease [10]. It seemed, therefore, of particular importance to investigate the occurrence of IgG4 antibodies to the fat globule membrane in atopic eczema patients and to determine whether their presence would account for milk allergy in cases where antibodies to the milk proteins are not detectable.

IgG4 antibodies to milk fat globule membrane

Although IgG4 antibodies to the fat globule membrane were detectable in some eczema patients (Fig. 51.4), their occurrence was of no additional diagnostic value as these antibodies were only present in those patients who also were previously shown to have IgG4 antibodies specific to α-casein. Thus, when levels of IgG4 antibody to the fat globule membrane in eczematous patients and controls were compared with α-casein-specific IgG4 levels, a correlation coefficient (r) of 0.93 was obtained. These findings seemed to suggest that we may have been measuring antibodies to α-casein which is either part of the fat globule membrane structure or tightly adsorbed to it. Cross-absorption experiments with four milk proteins proved beyond any doubt that the fat globule membrane antigen detectable in our assay system was in fact α-casein [41].

IgG4 antibodies to egg proteins

We have also demonstrated that 15 out of 22 eczema patients had raised IgG4 specific to the egg protein ovalbumin and none to ovomucoid. Only nine out of these 15 patients had egg allergy, the other six did not. There were a further three eczema patients who although they were egg allergic had no demonstrably raised level of specific IgG4. Only five out of the 15 eczema patients with raised IgG4 specific to ovalbumin had a positive IgE RAST for egg. Low or undetectable specific IgE found in a considerable number of eczematous patients' sera was apparently not due to interference by coexisting specific IgG4 antibodies. Thus, removal of IgG antibodies by staphylococcal protein A absorption

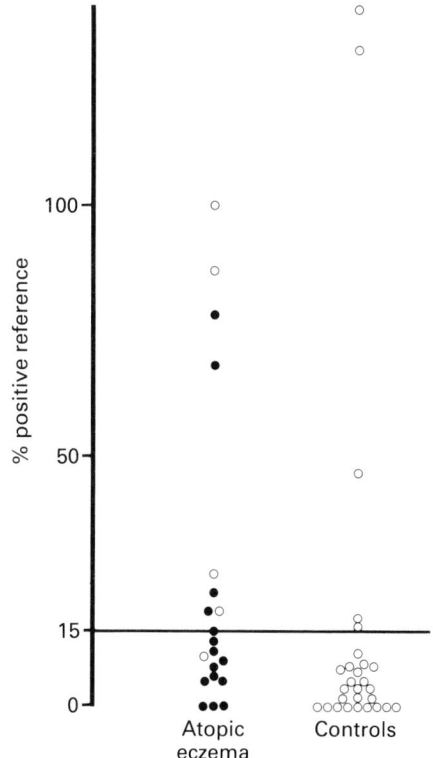

Fig. 51.4 Results of the ELISA for IgG4 specific to bovine milk fat globule membrane in 20 eczema patients and 28 non-eczematous controls. The horizontal line represents the 15% cut-off point above which values were considered raised. (○) milk allergy not present, (●) milk allergy present.

showed that only one out of six such sera scored a higher RAST result [39].

Gm marker and IgG4 antibody levels

In a recent study, many atopic eczema patients were shown to have IgG4 antibodies to grass, mites, cats, fish, wheat and nuts. However, the highest levels of IgG4 antibodies were to the foods most difficult to avoid—eggs and milk [27]. Studies conducted in our own laboratory [44] have established a relationship between serum levels of milk- and egg-specific IgG4 and the expression of the G2m(n) marker in atopic eczema patients (Fig. 51.5). Thus, grossly elevated milk- and egg-specific IgG4 (i.e. > 50% positive reference) occurred more frequently in G2m(n)-positive patients (7/12) than in G2m(n)-negative patients (2/9). This is an interesting situation where the capacity to mount food-specific IgG4 response appears to be linked to the expression of a genetic marker belonging to the IgG2 subclass. Enhanced production of IgG4 in atopic eczema patients

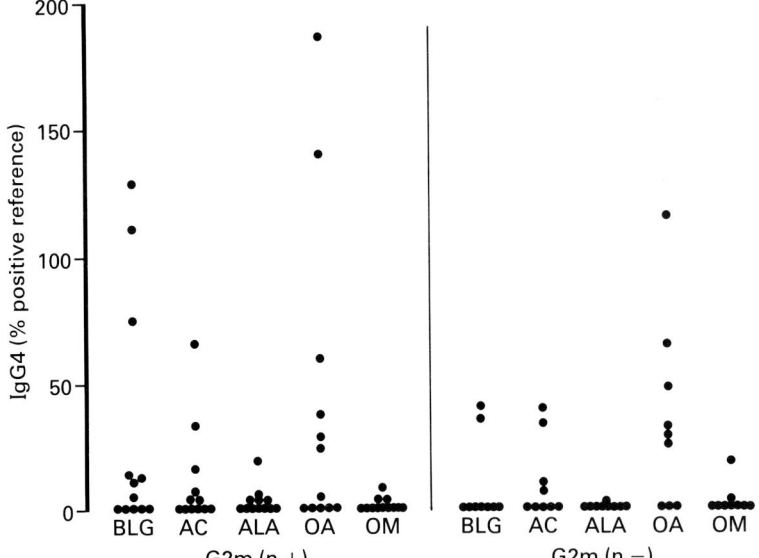

Fig. 51.5 Results of the ELISA for IgG4 specific to three cow's milk proteins and two hen's egg proteins in 12 G2m(n)-positive and nine G2m(n)-negative eczema patients. BLG = β-lactoglobulin, AC = α-casein, ALA = α-lactalbumin, OA = ovalbumin, OM = ovomucoid. Reproduced from [44] with permission.

may also be the result of failure of immunological suppression, which has already been suggested as an explanation of the high concentrations of IgE found in this condition [23, 48].

The frequent finding of IgG4 specific to milk and egg in the general population [21, 26, 39] does, however, suggest that food-specific IgG4 antibodies are part of a general immune response to dietary antigens gaining access to the immune system. In atopic excema patients this process may become amplified because of the associated increase in gut permeability [18] and decrease in clearance rate of ingested proteins [32]. As a result, these patients may experience chronic antigenic stimulation, a situation which as pointed out recently [1] would favour an IgG4 response (Fig. 51.6).

IMPORTANCE OF ANTIGLOBULINS IN FOOD ALLERGY

There is no doubt that patients with food allergies, particularly those manifesting as eczema, have large amounts of circulating food-specific IgG4 [27, 39]. Ingestion of the offending aliment by such patients will, therefore, result in excessive formation of immune complexes. The process may be preceded by an IgE-mediated hypersensitivity reaction in the gut. Such immune complexes are not likely to cause tissue damage via activation of the classical complement pathway because native IgG4 cannot fix C1q [2]. Evidence is also available to suggest that interaction of basophil- (or mast cell)-bound IgG4 with allergen does not culminate in mediator release from these cells [50].

The demonstration in vitro that IgG4-mediated release of histamine from basophils can be initiated upon interaction of IgG4 with an anti-IgG4 antibody [11, 31, 53] makes one wonder if a similar mechanism could become

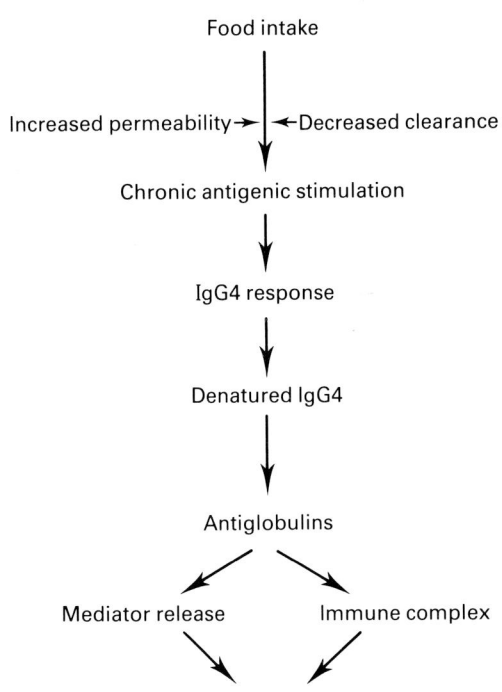

Fig. 51.6 A schematic representation of the hypothetical mechanism of IgG4 involvement in food allergy.

operative in eczema patients in the presence of an autoantibody directed against IgG4 (i.e. antiglobulin). It is interesting, therefore, that when sera from atopic eczema patients with raised food-specific IgG4 are mixed together, as in preparing a reference pool, the specific IgG4 activity in the mixture becomes undetectable (author's unpublished observation). This is a situation which could arise if these sera were to contain antiglobulins reactive with IgG4. It was for these reasons that we looked for IgG4-specific antiglobulins in sera of patients with atopic eczema; a condition known for its association with raised levels of total [3, 15, 16, 43] and food-specific IgG4 [27, 39].

Using a sensitive ELISA system, a significant proportion of eczema patients were shown to have IgM antiglobulin directed against IgG4 (author's unpublished observations). Although nothing is known, at this stage, about the clinical relevance of this antiglobulin, it is possible that its production is initiated by an abnormal load of altered IgG4 generated by excessive formation of food–IgG4 complexes (Fig. 51.5).

We are currently investigating the in vitro capacity of this antiglobulin to cross-link IgG4 bound to basophils (and mast cells) to cause mediator release in the manner demonstrable with a heterologous antiserum [11, 31, 53]. Furthermore, although IgG4 itself is incapable of activating the classical complement pathway [2], its involvement in immune complex formation with the complement fixing IgM antiglobulin may indirectly initiate complement-mediated tissue injury.

CONCLUSION

IgG4 is often raised in sera of food-allergic patients, but the detection of food-specific IgG4 in these patients is of no diagnostic value because of its frequent occurrence also in individuals who can tolerate these foods. Thus food-specific IgG4 antibodies are probably part of a general immune response to dietary antigens gaining access to the immune system. In atopic individuals this process may become amplified because of the chronic antigenic stimulation associated with abnormal handling of dietary proteins. However, the presence of an IgM anti-IgG4 in the sera of some eczema patients may be important in the the light of in vitro evidence showing that heterologous anti-IgG4 antisera can release mediators from basophils sensitized with IgG4.

REFERENCES

1 Aalberse RC, Van Der Gaag R, Van Leeuwen J: Serologic aspects of IgG4 antibodies. I. Prolonged immunisation results in an IgG4-restricted response. J Immunol 1983; 130:722–6.

2 Augener W, Grey HM, Cooper NR, Muller-Eberhard HJ: The reaction of monomeric and aggregated immunoglobulins with C1. Immunochemistry 1971; 8:1011–20.

3 Barnetson R St C, Merrett TG: Food allergy and atopic eczema. Proc Nutr Soc 1983; 42:247–56.

4 Berrens L, Van Dijk AG, Weemaes CMR: Complement consumption in egg white and fish sensitivity. Clin Allergy 1981; 11:101–9.

5 Bjorksten B, Ahlstedt S, Bjorksten F et al: Immunoglobulin E and immunoglobulin G4 antibodies to cow's milk in children with cow's milk allergy. Allergy 1983; 38:119–24.

6 Burt SM, Carter TIN, Kricka JL: Thermal characteristics of microtitre plates used in immunological assays. J Immunol Methods 1979; 31:231–6.

7 Dannaeus A, Inganas M: A follow-up study of children with food allergy. Clinical course in relation to serum IgE- and IgG-antibody levels to milk, egg and fish. Clin Allergy 1981; 11:533–9.

8 Dannaeus A, Johansson SGO, Foucard T: Clinical and immunological aspects of allergic symptoms and humoral immune response to foods in infants of atopic mothers during the first 24 months of life. Acta Paediat Scand 1978; 67:497–504.

9 Dannaeus A, Johansson SGO, Foucard T, Ohman S: Clinical and immunological aspects of food allergy in childhood. I. Estimation of IgG, IgA and IgE antibodies to food antigens in children with food allergy and atopic dermatitis. Acta Paediatr Scand 1977; 66:31–7.

10 Davies DF: Immunology of human atheroma. In: Freed DLJ, ed. Health hazards of milk. London: Baillière Tindall, 1984; 201–12.

11 Fagan DL, Slaughter CA, Captra D, Sullivan TJ: Monoclonal antibodies to immunoglobulin G4 induce histamine release from human basophils in vitro. J Allergy Clin Immunol 1982; 70:399–404.

12 Fallstrom SP, Ahlstedt S, Carlsson B et al: Influence of breast feeding on the development of cow's milk protein antibodies and the IgE level. Int Arch Allergy Appl Immunol 1984; 75:87–91.

13 French MAH, Harrison G: Serum IgG subclass concentrations in healthy adults: a study using monoclonal antisera. Clin Exp Immunol 1984; 56:473–5.

14 Goosen PCM, Van Beekhuizen S, Droogh C, De Lange G: Preparation of antibodies against subclasses of human IgG. J Immunol Methods 1981; 40:339–44.

15 Gwynn CM, Morrison Smith J, Leon Leon G, Stanworth DR: Role of IgG4 subclass in childhood allergy. Lancet 1978; i:910–11.

16 Gwynn CM, Morrison Smith J, Leon Leon G, Stanworth DR: IgE and IgG4 in atopic families. Clin Allergy 1979; 9:119–23.

17 Halpern GM: Sensitisation to shellfish. Nouv Presse Med 1977; 6:3111.

18 Jackson PG, Lessof MH, Baker RWR et al: Intestinal permeability in patients with eczema and food allergy. Lancet 1981; i: 1285-6.

19 Kilshaw PJ, Cant AJ: The passage of maternal dietary proteins into human breast milk. Int Arch Allergy Appl Immunol 1984; 75:8-15.

20 Kunkel HG, Joslin FC, Penn GM, Natvig JB: Genetic variants of γG4 globulin. A unique relationship to other classes of γG globulin. J Exp Med 1970; 132:508-20.

21 Layton GT, Stanworth DR: The quantitation of IgG4 antibodies to three common food allergens by ELISA with monoclonal anti-IgG4. J Immunol Methods 1984; 73:347-56.

22 Leddy JP, Deitchman J, Bakemeier RF: IgG subclasses measurement by radioimmunoassay in normal and hypogammaglobulinaemic sera. Arthritis Rheum 1970; 13:331-2.

23 Leung DYM, Rhodes AR, Geha RS: Enumeration of T cell subsets in atopic dermatitis using monoclonal antibodies. J Allergy Clin Immunol 1981; 67:450-5.

24 Lowe J, Bird P, Hardie D et al: Monoclonal antibodies (McAbs) to determinants on human gamma chains: properties of antibodies showing subclass restriction or subclass specificity. Immunology 1982; 47:329-36.

25 Mellbye OJ, Natvig JB: Presence and origin of human IgG subclass proteins in newborns. Vox Sang 1973; 24:206-15.

26 Merrett J, Burr ML, Merrett TG: A community survey of IgG4 antibody levels. Clin Allergy 1983; 13:397-407.

27 Merrett J, Barnetson R St C, Burr ML, Merrett TG: Total and specific IgG4 antibody levels in atopic eczema. Clin Exp Immunol 1984; 56:645-52.

28 Morell A, Terry WD, Waldmann TA: Metabolic properties of IgG subclasses in man. J Clin Invest 1970; 49:673-80.

29 Morell A, Skvaril F, Hitzig WH, Barandum S: IgG subclasses: development of the serum concentration in normal infants and children. J Pediatr 1972; 80:960-4.

30 Morell A, Skvaril F, Van Loghem E, Kleemola H: Human IgG subclasses in natural and fetal serum. Vox Sang 1971; 21:481-92.

31 Nakagawa T, Stadler BM, Heiner DC et al: Flow cytometric analysis of human basophil degranulation. II. Degranulation induced by anti-IgE, anti-IgG4 and the calcium ionophore A23187. Clin Allergy 1981; 11:21-30.

32 Paganelli R, Levinsky RJ, Brostoff J, Wraith DG: Immune complexes containing food proteins in normal and atopic subjects after oral challenge and effect of sodium cromoglycate on antigen absorption. Lancet 1979; i:1270-1.

33 Parish WE: Short-term anaphylactic IgG antibodies in human sera. Lancet 1970; ii:591-2.

34 Radl J, Sepers JM, Skvaril F et al: Immunoglobulin patterns in humans over 95 years of age. Clin Exp Immunol 1975; 22:84-90.

35 Schanfield MS: Immunoglobulins: genetic markers. In: Fudenberg HH, Stites DP, Caldwell JL, Wells JV, eds. Basic and clinical immunology. Los Altos: Lange Medical Publications, 1980; 79-83.

36 Shakib F, Barr D: The incidence of Gm allotypes in a group of Iraqi Arabs. J Immunogenet 1980; 7:369-73.

37 Shakib F, Stanworth DR: Human IgG subclasses in health and disease. Ric Clin Lab 1980; 10:463-79.

38 Shakib F, Stanworth DR: Human IgG subclasses in health and disease. Ric Clin Lab 1980; 10:561-80.

39 Shakib F, Brown HM, Stanworth DR: Relevance of milk- and egg-specific IgG4 in atopic eczema. Int Arch Allergy Appl Immunol 1984; 75:107-12.

40 Shakib F, James K, Barr D: Gm allotypes and IgG subclass levels in Iraqi Arabs. J Immunogenet 1982; 9:149-53.

41 Shakib F, Morrow Brown H, Redhead R, Phelps A: IgE and IgG4 antibodies to bovine milk fat globule membrane in atopic eczema patients: study of their occurrence, relevance and antigenic specificity. Clin Allergy 1985; 15:265-71.

42 Shakib F, Stanworth DR, Drew R, Catty D: A quantitative study of the distribution of IgG subclasses in a group of normal human sera. J Immunol Methods 1975; 8:17-28.

43 Shakib F, McLaughlan P, Stanworth DR et al: Elevated serum IgE and IgG4 in patients with atopic dermatitis. Br J Dermatol 1977; 97:59-63.

44 Shakib F, Morrow Brown H, Phelps A et al: Relationship between serum levels of total and milk- and egg-specific IgG4 and the expression of G2m(n) in atopic eczema patients. Exp Clin Immunogenet 1984; 1:185-8.

45 Sainte-Laudy J: Enzyme-linked immunosorbent assays (ELISA) for total serum IgG4 and specific IgG4 antibodies. Clin Rev Allergy 1983; 1:225-9.

46 Stanworth DR: Immunochemical aspects of human IgG4. Clin Rev Allergy 1983; 1:183-95.

47 Stanworth DR, Smith AK: Inhibition of reaginmediated PCA reactions in baboons by the human IgG4 subclass. Clin Allergy 1973; 3:37-41.

48 Strannegard IL: Lymphocyte stimulation with phorbol myristate acetate in atopic and non-atopic individuals. Int Arch Allergy Appl Immunol 1979; 58:175-81.

49 Van Der Giessen M, Rossouw E, Algra Van Veen T et al: Quantification of IgG subclasses in sera of normal adults and healthy children between 4 and 12 years of age. Clin Exp Immunol 1975; 21:501-9.

50 Van Toorenenbergen AW, Aalberse RC: IgG4 and release of histamine from human peripheral blood leukocytes. Int Arch Allergy Appl Immunol 1982; 67:117-22.

51 Vartdal F, Bird P: Imprint immunofixation of IgG subclasses using monoclonal subclass-specific antibodies. Scand J Immunol 1983; 18:367-70.

52 Vijay HM, Perelmutter L: Inhibition of reaginmediated PCA reactions in monkeys and histamine release from human leukocytes by human IgG4 subclass. Int Arch Allergy Appl Immunol 1977; 53:78-87.

53 Vijay HM, Perelmutter L, Bernstein IL: Possible role of IgG4 in discordant correlations between intracutaneous skin tests and RAST. Int Arch Allergy Appl Immunol 1978; 56:517-22.

54 Williamson N, Edwards JH, Monk K et al: Anti-tissue antibodies and immunoglobulin levels in relation to HLA and other markers in Icelandic families. J Immunogenet 1979; 6:223-44.

55 Yount WJ, Hong R, Seligmann M et al: Imbalances of gammaglobulin subgroups and gene detector in patients with primary hypogammaglobulinaemia. J Clin Invest 1970; 49:1957-66.

56 Zhou T, Conroy MC, Splengler H, De Weck AL: Failure of covalently cross-linked human IgG myeloma subclass protein to release histamine from human leukocytes. Int Arch Allergy Appl Immunol 1984; 74:108-12.

Chapter 52
What Tests Should a Clinician Ask For?

Oscar L. Frick

Introduction

For the accurate diagnosis of an allergic reaction to a particular food or additive in food, the physician must establish whether or not the particular symptoms and signs are, in fact, associated with ingestion of the suspected food. Therefore, the history of the types of symptoms, of the association of these with meals or snacks and of the association with ingestion of a particular food or group becomes of cardinal importance. Are all the patient's symptoms related to ingestion of a particular food or do different foods cause different kinds of symptoms? Have the symptoms changed in type, severity or frequency in recent weeks or months? Can the symptoms be classified according to organ system involvement, for example nausea, vomiting, diarrhoea and abdominal pain to the gastrointestinal system, or sneezing, rhinorrhoea, coughing or wheezing to the respiratory tract?

HISTORY AND EXAMINATION

History

A family history of allergic manifestations, or

of other gastrointestinal complaints such as chronic constipation, peptic ulcer, ulcerative colitis, coeliac or Crohn's disease or autoimmune states may be significant. A past personal history of allergic symptoms or gastrointestinal problems especially related to ingestion of a particular food group may be particularly significant. For example, a history of abdominal 'colic', vomiting or diarrhoea in infancy with improvement upon switching to a non-dairy formula may be particularly significant. Although, as the child matures, he might become tolerant to cow's milk or 'outgrow' his milk intolerance, there may persist a low-grade subclinical milk intolerance that can later cause symptoms if triggered by bodily insults such as a viral infection or emotional tension. In schoolchildren, we frequently observe a recurrence of vague abdominal complaints during various school adjustment crises, in children who have 'outgrown' an infantile cow's milk allergy and who respond favourably by restoration of a cow's milk-free diet. Therefore, the patient's personal or family history of food intolerances remains the most important diagnostic tool for the physician.

Physical examination

The physical examination may present clues that one is dealing with a food allergy. Prominent in many such individuals, especially in children, are 'allergic shiners' or infraorbital soft-tissue swelling and bluish discoloration that accompany a chronically obstructed nasal mucosa. A pallid complexion and flat malar facies with accompanying mouth-breathing supports this impression of allergy, especially to foods in young or school-age children. Pale congestion of the ear drums may also be sign of chronic nasal and eustachian tube oedema. Minimal ronchi on chest auscultation, and minimal scaling or thickened skin in body creases, especially of extremities, are signs of chronic allergy.

EVALUATION OF THE FOOD-ALLERGIC PATIENT

Skin prick tests

In our clinic, we use the protocol illustrated in Fig. 52.1 to evaluate a patient with suspected food allergy [29]. An initial screening by skin prick tests may include several common inhalants such as house dust mite (*Dermatophagoides pteronyssimus* or *farini*), crude house

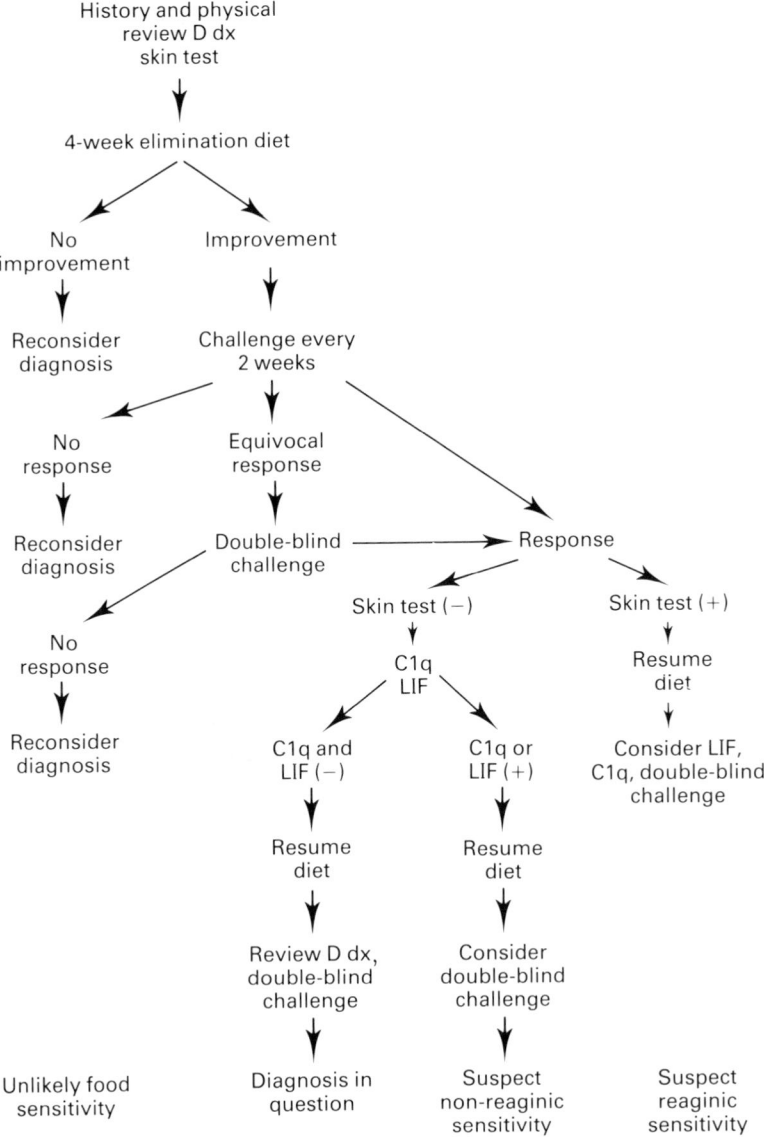

Fig. 52.1 Protocol for evaluating suspected food sensitivity. Reproduced from [29] with permission.

dust, dog and cat dander, mixed grasses and *Alternaria* and *Cladosporium* moulds, as well as food allergens, such as cow's milk, egg, wheat, corn, peanut, codfish and walnut. Such a screening series in children will detect about 80% of the IgE-mediated allergens in our experience. If anaphylaxis has occurred previously following ingestion of a particular food, skin prick tests should be replaced by an in vitro test such as the radioallergosorbent test (RAST).

Differential diagnosis

Blood count. Before proceeding with the further laboratory diagnostic work-up to identify specific food allergens in the patient, other conditions that enter the differential diagnosis should be ruled out, if possible. A complete blood count with differential white cell count may help rule out an infection with elevated leukocyte count and preponderance of neutrophils. Eosinophilia above 5% or greater than 500 per mm³ absolute suggests allergy [37]. A total leukocyte count of less than 5000 with neutropenia (< 30%) is commonly observed in food-sensitive individuals. A low haematocrit or haemoglobin may indicate anaemia which may occur in cow's milk-induced hypersensitivity and in low-grade intestinal bleeding. This reaction is probably of an Arthus type (Type III) hypersensitivity reaction, and may occasionally occur with secondary haemosiderosis [46]. Increased numbers of reticulocytes on the blood smear may also indicate correction of such an anaemia.

Sedimentation rate. This might be useful as a screening test to detect the presence of a low-grade persistent or unsuspected infection, or activity of an autoimmune process which might simulate food hypersensitivity. There is reported evidence that rheumatoid arthritis-like symptoms may be caused by foods.

Chest X-ray. A chest X-ray should be performed on every patient with wheezing to identify hyperinflation and areas of mucous plugging that cause secondary atelectasis. Food-sensitive asthma is similar to inhalant-induced asthma. Furthermore, such a chest X-ray should rule out other chest conditions, such as foreign body aspiration or neoplasia, and granulomata such as tuberculosis and sarcoidosis. X-ray of the paranasal sinuses, especially the Waters' view, should be performed

in everyone with a chronic cough which may simulate a food-induced asthma or be secondary to infected sinuses from a primary allergic rhinitis.

Tympanic membrane mobility. In children, one should measure tympanic membrane mobility simply by moving it with alternating positive and negative pressure with the pneumatic attachment to an otoscope [5]. More elaborately, one might confirm the presence of serous otitis with tympanometry using a printed pattern or with an acoustic otoscope which simply measures sound reflected off the tympanic membrane.

Sweat test. Chloride levels should be determined in children with chronic coughs or wheezing to rule out cystic fibrosis. Children with cystic fibrosis have sodium and chloride levels above 60 mEq/litre; normal children under age 14 generally have levels below 40 mEq/litre. These levels tend to rise gradually with age; some normal older adolescents and adults have sodium and chloride levels of 60–80 mEq/litre which fall with advancing age. A value of 100 mEq/litre of sodium or chloride is diagnostic of cystic fibrosis, even in adults [28]. The intestinal symptoms of cystic fibrosis, for example bulky and frequent stools and poor weight gain, may also mimic a food allergy.

Faecal fat. Mushy, foul-smelling and bulky stools with failure to gain weight are also signs of gluten-induced coeliac disease. Therefore, a stool examination for fat (Sudan III stain) and starch crystals (iodine stain) or a 1 to 3 day faeces collection should be carried out to measure total fat excretion; greater than 2 g/day would indicate a coeliac state. Symptomatic improvement should occur promptly on a gluten-free diet [14].

Hydrogen breath analysis. This test may be indicated to rule out a disaccharidase deficiency, especially of lactase, which is quite common, affecting about 14% of Caucasians, 60% of American Blacks and 70–90% of American Indians, Hispanics and orientals. Lactose intolerance is often misdiagnosed as milk allergy since the diarrhoea improves on a cow's milk-free diet. The stool pH should be neutral (pH 7), and an acid stool (pH < 5.5) and reducing substances in stool (positive Clinitest) further indicate a disaccharidase deficiency. Starch, sucrose and maltose may be similarly maldigested with appropriate primary or secondary enzyme deficiencies. Ultimately, an intraluminal small intestinal biopsy may be indicated to confirm either coeliac disease or disaccharidase deficiency [14].

Secondary disaccharidase deficiency may occur following administration of broad spectrum antibiotics or infestation with *Giardia lamblia* or other parasites.

LABORATORY TESTS

Immunoglobulins

Serum quantitative immunoglobulins IgA, IgM and IgG might show an isolated or pan-immunoglobulin deficiency. Absent or low serum IgA (< 10 mg/dl) would reflect a compromised intestinal secretory IgA barrier. Incompletely digested foods, especially proteins and proteoses, are antigenic and react to form large complexes with secretory IgA on the mucosal surface or intestinal cell vesicles. This secretory IgA complexing with food antigens inhibits or limits the absorption of the antigen into the lymphatic system and thus the systemic system (see Chapter 9). In the absence of secretory IgA (which appears to be compatible with normal asymptomatic health), food antigens are absorbed via the lymphatics to the mesenteric lymph nodes, and eventually to systemic lymph nodes. IgM and IgG circulating antibodies are induced and these can be detected by classic precipitin methods, as shown by Buckley and Dees [7]. Recently, Cunningham-Rundles et al [13] (see Chapter 12) suggested that such circulating food immune complexes cause some autoimmune diseases. In the absence of secretory IgA, sometimes secretory IgM can act as a substitute. Therefore, concomitant quantitation of serum IgM and IgG are indicated, though IgG and IgM hypogammaglobulinaemia is rare in food allergy. A caveat is that serum immunoglobulin levels change with age, especially in children and it is therefore of cardinal importance to compare the values in a patient with age-matched standards of normals for that laboratory.

Secretory IgA

A more direct determination of the presence of secretory IgA (SIgA) in the gastrointestinal tract is by quantitation of such in purged stool specimens or, alternatively, measurement of secretory IgA in saliva collected from the par-otid duct by a special cup method [1]. Monoclonal antisera to human SIgA are now available, though total SIgA trends can be measured adequately with polyclonal antisera. With the recent availability of monoclonal antisera to human IgG subclasses, more studies should be forthcoming of the role of such IgG and IgA subclasses in patients with food allergies.

IgE—total and specific

Serum IgE

Total serum IgE quantitation by radioimmunoassay (PRIST—paper radioimmunosorbent test, Pharmacia, Uppsala, Sweden) or a similar assay with enzyme or fluorescent markers may be useful in assessing the overall allergic status of the patient [9]. Serum IgE occurs in concentrations of less than 1 U/ml in the cord serum, gradually rising to a maximum of about 120 U/ml in early adolescence and regressing somewhat to a normal adult level of about 100 U/ml by age 20. Higher cord IgE levels of 0.67–1.3 U/ml have been shown to be predictors of atopy during childhood, especially in infants from atopic families [11,33]. Furthermore, Orgel et al [36] showed that an IgE level of > 20 U/ml by age 12 months was a near 100% predictor of atopy by the age of 2. A serum IgE level of over 300 U/ml generally correlates with atopy, parasitic infection or a cellular immune defect. The corollary, however, is that many atopic patients have total serum IgE levels within the range of normal, but the specific antibody IgE may be almost totally devoted to one allergen, as occurs commonly with Hymenoptera venom sensitivity or in birch pollen-sensitive patients.

Measurement of specific IgE

More important is IgE antibody to a particular allergen, which is usually measured by the radioallergosorbent test (RAST) [45]. Fluorescent or enzyme labels are commonly substituted for the radioisotope ^{125}I in an adapted assay which has a similar degree of sensitivity and specificity.

In both PRIST and RAST, an insoluble medium such as a filter paper disc [9] or microcellulose beads is activated with cyanogen bromide to provide free carboxyl groups (Fig. 52.2). Upon exposure of such activated particles to protein antigens, the free carboxyl groups of the particle bind to the free amino

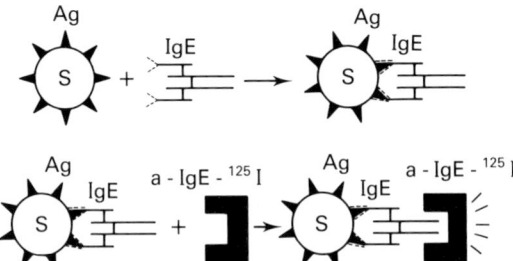

Fig. 52.2 Schematic diagram of the radioallergosorbent test (RAST). S is the sorbent, with antigenic determinants (Ag). Human IgE attaches to the antigen and is detected with radiolabelled anti-IgE. Reproduced with permission from Frick OL: Immediate hypersensitivity. In: Stites D et al, eds. Basic and clinical immunology, 5th edn. 1984.

groups of the protein forming a firm covalent attachment. These antigen-coated particles are allowed to react for 30 minutes at room temperature with the patient's serum sample. All classes of antibodies to that antigen in the patient's serum will react with the antigen-coated particles, depending upon the number of free antigen sites. In order to measure specific IgE antibodies, radiolabelled rabbit or goat polyclonal (or mouse monoclonal) antibodies to human IgE (epsilon heavy chain specific) are incubated with the antigen particle complex. The particle complexes are resuspended in buffer and washed several times by centrifugation and are counted in a gamma spectrometer. The counts per minute are directly proportional to the IgE antibodies to that antigen in the patient's serum.

IgE RAST was first used by Hoffman and Haddad [22] for the diagnosis of immediate allergic reactions to many specific foods. Wraith et al [47] employed IgE RAST in the diagnosis of both immediate and delayed onset allergic reactions to foods (see Chapter 24).

Modified RAST

In an attempt to increase the sensitivity of the RAST, Nalebuff and Fadal [35] introduced a modified RAST with longer incubation times, time controls and a finer tuning of the scoring system. In a critique of the modified RAST, Santrach et al [41] found that the threshold of positivity was set so low that there were 33% false-positive results among non-IgE-containing controls. Background binding produced by negative control sera varied considerably among different allergen discs indicating that the cut-off between positivity and negativity may vary from allergen to allergen. The modified RAST has been proposed to calculate the initial starting dose of inhalant immunotherapy [35], but such doses produced large reactions in 30% of the patients [41]. They concluded that the modified RAST does not afford any significant diagnostic advantage over the conventional RAST.

Measurement of total IgE

For PRIST, the particles are coated with anti-IgE myeloma serum, reacted with IgE-containing patient's serum and subsequently reacted with antibody to a second IgE myeloma protein [9]. Antisera to two myelomas are used to circumvent the possible problem of IgE idiotypic antibodies. The rest of the procedure is like the RAST and can be done simultaneously in semiautomated systems along with RASTs.

Instead of radioisotope labelling, several fluorescent and enzyme labels have been adapted to RAST-like techniques to circumvent the problem of exposure to and disposal of radioactivity. Enzymes such as horseradish peroxidase, alkaline phosphatase [15] and biotin–avidin have been used with sensitivities and specificities similar to RAST. Quality control and adequate numbers of standards and fresh reagents are essential for these assays. Assessment of reproducibility of a series of samples in 12 different laboratories produced over a 100-fold variability in results [16]. Therefore, one cannot overemphasize quality control.

Other tests for IgE-mediated food allergy

Other tests of IgE-mediated food allergy that have been used in investigations include (a) passive transfer of atopic serum containing IgE antibodies to the skin of a non-atopic individual (Prausnitz–Küstner reaction) [40] but this has the danger of transferring serum hepatitis or acquired immune deficiency syndrome, (b) skin-window eosinophilia (in the presence of antigen, a three-fold or greater influx of eosinophils in 6–12 hours constitutes a positive reaction [8]; (c) rat peritoneal mast cells can be passively sensitized with human IgE antibodies and added antigen causes histamine release, as with human basophils (18). These tests are generally not used clinically.

IgG antibodies

IgG antibodies to allergens can be measured by the same method outlined for IgE, except

that labelled anti-IgG serum or staphylococcus A protein which binds to IgG Fc can be
used for quantitation [17]. Again the amount
of binding is directly proportional to the
quantity of IgG antibodies to that allergen in
the serum sample. These methods have recently been applied to the measurement of
IgG subclass antibodies by using specific
mouse monoclonal antibodies to human IgG
1, 2, 3 and 4 subclasses. IgG4 antibodies have
been implicated in insect sting immunotherapy [21] and in food allergies [39].

Competitive binding of IgG antibodies to
the allergen must be considered in all assessments of IgE-specific immunoassays in atopics
who have undergone specific immunotherapy
[48]. Attempts have been made to circumvent
the problem by using diluted sera or ion exchange removal of IgG before the IgE antibody assay is performed.

IgG4 antibody

Other non-IgE-mediated immunological reactions to foods have been studied. IgG4 subclass has characteristics similar to those of IgE
[38] and has been suggested as an alternative
reaginic antibody. RAST and fluorescence al-
lergosobent tests for IgG4 antibodies are currently under study for both inhalant and food
allergies. Heiner [20] has found good clinical
correlation between IgG4 antibodies and food
antigens in patients with suspected food allergy. IgG4 may therefore become important
in food allergy diagnosis in the near future.

Basophil histamine release

Antigen-induced histamine release from sensitized human leukocytes (basophils) is a procedure that has provided much information
about the mediators of allergy and the mechanisms of their release. With automation of
much of the procedure, it is being adapted for
routine clinical use in some centres. This is a
miniature in vitro allergic reaction model
(Fig. 52.3).

Buffy coat leukocytes from a 10–20 ml sample of heparinized blood from an atopic patient
are isolated in suspension after settlement separation of erythrocytes is induced by added
dextran [32]. To aliquots of 2×10^5 washed
leukocytes are added three 10-fold dilutions of
the antigen in duplicate. Following 35 minutes
incubation at 37°C and centrifugation, the supernatant is decanted. This supernatant contains histamine released as a consequence of

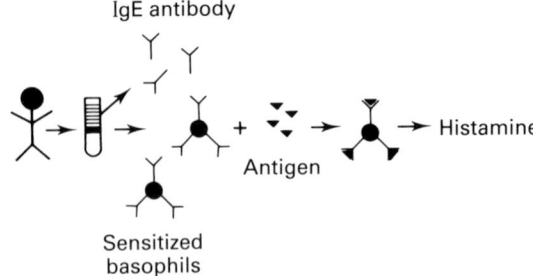

Fig. 52.3 Schematic diagram of the leukocyte (basophil)
histamine release test. Buffy coat leukocytes from an
atopic patient have attached IgE antibodies. Upon addition of antigen, histamine is released from the sensitized
basophils. Supernatant histamine is measured either spec-
trofluorometrically or isotopically. (Adapted from Stanworth DR: Immediate hypersensitivity. Amsterdam:
North-Holland, 1973).

the antigen reacting with IgE antibodies
attached to the sensitized basophils. (Basophils
are the only circulating leukocytes that contain
histamine in man.) The histamine in the supernatant is extracted and rendered fluorescent with *o*-phthalaldehyde and the quantity
of histamine is assayed on a fluorospectrome-
ter.

Automated assay

In the automated method of Siraganian et al
[43], the analysis is done on heparinized whole
blood thus skipping the leukocyte isolation
step. Alternatively, the extracted histamine
in the supernatant is radiolabelled with
[^{14}C]methyl groups from *S*-adenosylmethion-
ine by histamine-*N*-methyltransferase and
counted on a liquid scintillation counter [25].
Duplicate aliquots of leukocytes are lysed with
perchlorate in order to determine the total histamine content of the leukocytes. The results
of antigen-induced histamine release are reported as a percentage of the total histamine
present. Appropriate control cell aliquots,
with no antigen added, release up to 5–10%
histamine as a baseline. With antigen present,
histamine released may be 5–90% above baseline, but commonly is in the range of 20–60%.

Some patients with food allergies have an
elevated baseline histamine release of 20–40%
that may be due to low-grade reactions from
circulating immune complexes with ingested
food antigens causing complement activation
and release of anaphylatoxins, C3a and C5a, to
cause 'spontaneous' histamine release [30].
Specific food antigens induce histamine release
from such leukocytes above this high spontaneous release baseline in such patients.

Leukocyte histamine release—summary

The leukocyte histamine release is a valuable, if somewhat cumbersome, test in that it represents a miniature allergic reaction in the test tube with representative cells from the patient. All components of the allergic mechanism must be present, for example the appropriate antigen and specific IgE antibody to that antigen fixed to the target leukocytes (basophils) which contain the representative mediator, histamine. Experimentally, other allergic mediators, such as leukotrienes, ECF-A and NCF-A have also been measured; these are also released in amounts proportional to the severity of the allergic reaction. The leukocyte histamine release test correlates closely with the degree of clinical hypersensitivity [26] and can be used as a basis of comparison of such sensitivity in a group of patients [27] (Fig. 52.4). This test in many ways is preferred

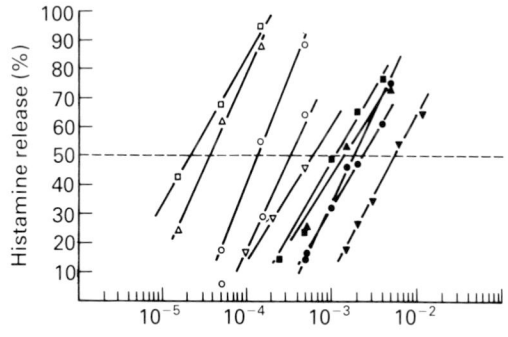

Fig. 52.4 Dose–response relationships for histamine release as a function of antigen concentration (cells from 10 ragweed-sensitive donors). (Reproduced from [27] with permission.)

to the RAST because it tests the allergic reactivity of the patient's cells, whereas RAST measures only specific IgE antibodies in the circulation, in effect a by-product, because most allergic reactions take place on sensitized basophils or mast cells in shock organ tissues.

Limitations of the leukocyte histamine release test in food allergy may be (a) the high baseline histamine release which may mask a small amount of antigen-induced histamine released, (b) digested altered food which may be the antigen (this may not be present in the raw food extracts used in testing [19]), (c) drugs in vivo and in vitro which alter the degree of histamine release.

Immune complexes

Circulating immune complexes of IgG, IgM, IgA and IgE have been demonstrated in patients with inhalant and food allergies. A huge literature has developed on tests for measuring circulating immune complexes in rheumatoid and autoimmune diseases. Lambert et al [24] evaluated 18 such tests on the same serum samples and found that the Raji cell tests and the C1q-binding tests showed the best correlation with clinically active disease.

Raji cell assay

The Raji cell is a human B cell lymphoma line that is rich in receptors for the Fc component of IgG and in complement receptors for C1q, C3b and C3d. Therefore it can bind at multiple sites to the IgG antibody component of circulating immune complexes. It is a widely used standard clinical test for measuring circulating immune complexes in patients with autoimmune diseases. Raji cells in cultures are reacted with serum containing circulating IgG and antigen-containing immune complexes. Enzyme or radiolabelled rabbit anti-human IgG is then reacted with the Raji cell-IgG-antigen complex. Binding of more than 40 μg equivalents of anti-human IgG is considered a positive result [44]; patients with systemic lupus erythematosis and rheumatoid arthritis commonly bind 100–200 μg equivalents of anti-human IgG. In our study of 25 children with delayed onset food allergies [10], 20 children had positive Raji cell tests binding between 50 and 2000 μg/ml, with a mean of 187 $\pm$ 71 μg/ml. Therefore the Raji cell technique may be useful in assessing immune complex Type III food allergy.

C1q binding assay

C1q binding by circulating immune complexes in sera of patients with autoimmune diseases is a useful routine clinical assay available in many centres for the assessment of autoimmune disease activity. There are many versions of these assays. In our study of 25 children with delayed onset food allergy [10], we used a microtitre plate assay [23]. Purified C1q in 100 μl aliquots containing 137 CH$_{50}$ units was adsorbed to the plastic in wells of a polyvinyl chloride microtitre plate for 72 hours at 4°C (Dynatech Laboratories, Inc, Alexandria, Virginia, USA). After washing, any remaining free binding sites in the plastic were covered with 1% gelatin in phosphate-buffered saline (PBS) for 2 hours at 25°C and washed. The patient's serum at a 1:10 dilution was incubated at 37°C for 1 hour and then at 4°C for 4 hours, then washed; ^{125}I-labelled staphylococcus A protein was added to each well and incubated at 37°C for 1 hour and then at 4°C for 4 hours. After washing, radioactivity in individual wells was measured in a gamma spectrometer. In this C1q assay, sera from non-allergic individuals had less than 11% binding (mean was 9.7% ± 0.8 in 13 subjects). Sera from 25 children with delayed onset food allergy had C1q binding of 5–22%, with a mean of 13.7 ± 3.2; 20 out of 25 children had greater than 11% binding which was significant at $P < 0.001$. Currently we are developing a modified C1q assay to demonstrate and measure antigen binding in such immune complexes.

Complexes in selective IgA deficiency and atopics

In patients with selective IgA deficiency, Cunningham-Rundles et al [12] have demonstrated Raji cell binding by circulating immune complexes in their sera. Bovine casein binding by these sera was also demonstrated. All these tests became more positive within 1–2 hours after ingestion of a glass of cow's milk, and returned to pre-ingestion levels in 3–4 hours. She suggested that vascular deposition of such circulating immune complexes containing cow's milk protein antigens in patients with selective IgA deficiency may cause symptoms of autoimmunity, for example, rashes, joint effusions and pain, and fever. Brostoff et al [6] have demonstrated mixed IgE- and IgG-containing immune complexes in circulation in two patients with egg allergy after ingestion of eggs. These complexes were not present before the egg challenge, rose within hours and fell again post challenge. These studies all suggest that circulating immune complexes may cause allergic-type symptoms, perhaps through the activation of complement and release of anaphylatoxins C3a and C5a which cause the release of histamine from mast cells.

Cell-mediated immunity

Finally, cellular immunity has been implicated in patients with food allergy, especially with the delayed onset type, and in coeliac disease. Initially there was enthusiasm for the lymphoproliferation assay with [³H]thymidine uptake by food antigen stimulated lymphocytes [42]. However, May et al [31] demonstrated comparable lymphoproliferation with food antigens in allergic and non-allergic individuals. A positive lymphoproliferation with a food antigen indicates an immune response to that food even though it does not apparently discriminate between allergic and non-allergic reactivity to that food.

Lymphokine production

The leukocyte migration inhibition factor (LIF) test has been used to differentiate cellular immune reactivity to foods in allergic and non-allergic subjects. The LIF test correlates highly (>95%) with positive delayed hypersensitivity skin tests to *Candida albicans*, streptokinase–streptodornase and tuberculin in man [4]. This LIF is an inflammatory mediator or factor released by non-proliferating sensitized T lymphocytes upon contact with antigen. LIF has a molecular weight of 69 000, and is a heat-stable (at 56°C for 30 minutes) protease that inhibits the migration of granulocytes.

Practical details of the LIF assay. Buffy coat leukocytes from dextran-sedimented heparinized venous blood are washed three times and suspended in TC199 suspension medium in concentrations of 2.2×10^8 cells/ml. To 50 μl aliquots of this leukocyte suspension are added 5 μl of food extract in six successive five-fold dilutions; these tubes are incubated at 37°C in a waterbath for 30 minutes. The food antigen extract used is the highest glycerinated concentration available commercially, for example 5% cow's milk or corn. As controls, several tubes have saline substituted for antigen. To 0.5 g agarose (Indubiose A-37, Industrie Biologique Française SA, Grenvilliers, France) are added 38.75 ml distilled water and this is then autoclaved for 15 minutes. Then in a 37°C waterbath, 5 ml of TC199 10× with 5 ml of horse serum, 0.25 ml of sodium bicarbonate and 1 ml of penicillin–streptomycin solution are added to the agarose after it has cooled to 47°C. The agarose–TC199 is pipetted into 60 × 15 mm Falcon petri dishes (Falcon Plastics, Oxnard, California, USA) and allowed to gel. Wells (12–16 per dish) are cut with a 7 μl well cutter and filled with cell–antigen or cell–saline suspension and then incubated for 18 hours at 37°C in 5% carbon dioxide. Cells migrate between the agarose and the plastic dish in a ring. Two ring diameters, one with and one without antigen, are multiplied. If the product of these diameters with antigen is 80% or less than that without antigen, the test is considered positive.

LIF in milk and corn allergy

In 40 patients with delayed onset food allergy to cow's milk or corn, we found 24 out of 40 with positive LIFs and only 4 out of 40 positive in non-food-allergic subjects; the difference was significant at $P < 0.001$ [34] (Fig. 52.5). In a similar study of cow's milk in allergic children, Ashkenazi et al [2] found that

LIF with bovine lactoglobulin was positive in a group of 24 children with cow's milk-induced respiratory and gastrointestinal symptoms (vomiting, diarrhoea, bloody stools and weight loss) only after two or more cow's milk challenges (mean 23.5% $\pm$ 1.3). In a similar group of cow's milk-allergic children who had recovered and were drinking cow's milk, the mean LIF was 8.5% $\pm$ 1.1%; this indicated that LIF was positive in active disease and became negative upon spontaneous recovery. In normal infants and children, the mean LIF was 3.1% $\pm$ 0.8. The difference between LIF in active cow's milk-allergic children and normals was at $P < 0.0005$. Ashkenazi et al [3] have observed a similar usefulness for LIF to gluten in children with coeliac disease.

CONCLUSIONS

In conclusion, we have reviewed a number of laboratory tests that may be useful in assessing patients with suspected adverse reactions to foods. The history and food diary are the most useful diagnostic tools along with the diagnostic elimination diet and challenge two or more times with the suspected food allergen. A careful scoring and documentation of symptoms and signs are very important in the successful application of these procedures. The double-blind encapsulated food challenge is the 'gold standard' for the diagnosis of a food allergy and should be conducted in hospital to control for accidental suspect food ingestion.

The most useful laboratory tests of IgE-mediated food allergy are the skin prick test, IgE-RAST and leukocyte histamine release test which correlate highly ($>80\%$) with double-blind food challenges. In vitro tests for circulating immune complexes, Raji cell and C1q binding, and for cellular immunity, LIF, are currently under evaluation for diagnosis and for following the progress of patients with non-IgE-mediated food allergies.

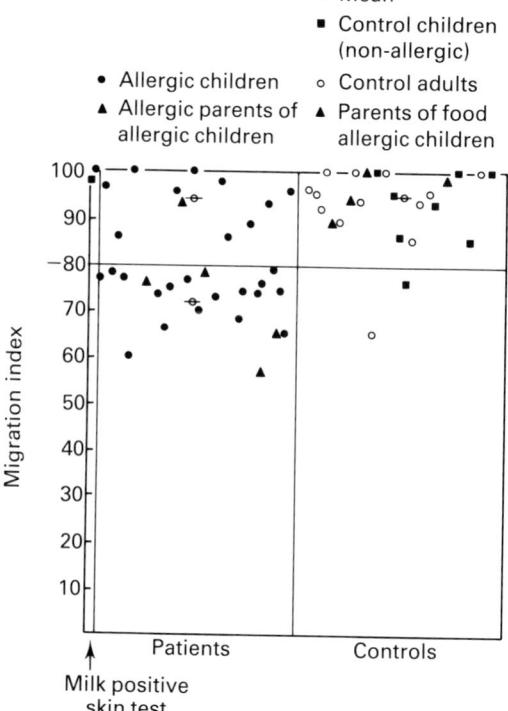

Fig. 52.5 LIF results with whole cow's milk and its fractions in children with delayed onset milk allergy and various control groups. (Reproduced from [34] with permission.)

REFERENCES

1 Ammann AJ, Hong R: Selective IgA deficiency: report of 30 cases and a review of the literature. Medicine (Baltimore) 1971; 50:223–36.

2 Ashkenazi A, Levin S, Idar D et al: In vitro cell-mediated immunologic assay for cow's milk allergy. Pediatrics 1980; 66:399–402.

3 Ashkenazi A, Levin S, Idar D et al: Effect of gluten-free diet on an immunologic assay for coeliac disease. Lancet 1981;i:914–9.

4 Astor SH, Spitler LE, Frick OL, Fudenberg HH: Human leukocyte migration inhibition in agarose using 4 antigens: correlation with skin reactivity. J Immunol 1973; 110:1174–9.

5 Bluestone CD, Douglas GS, Bernstein JM: Otitis media. In: Middleton E Jr, Reed CE, Ellis EF eds. Allergy, principles and practice, 2nd edn. St Louis: C V Mosby, 1983; 1275–96.

6 Brostoff J, Carini C, Wraith DG, Johns P: Production

of IgE complexes by allergen challenge in atopic patients and the effect of sodium cromoglycate. Lancet 1979; i:1268–70.

7 Buckley RH, Dees SC: Correlation of milk precipitins with IgA deficiency. N Engl J Med 1969; 281:465–9.

8 Bullock JD, Frick OL: Mite sensitivity in house dust-allergic children. Am J Dis Child 1972; 123:222–6.

9 Ceska M, Lundqvist U: A new and simple radioimmunoassay method for the determination of IgE. Immunochemistry 1972; 9:1021–30.

10 Chang TT, Char DH, Frick OL: Immune complexes in delayed onset food allergy. J Allergy Clin Immunol 1981; 49:4.

11 Croner S, Kjellman NIM, Eriksson B, Roth A: IgE screening in 1701 newborn infants and the development of atopic diseases during infancy. Arch Dis Child 1982; 57:364–8.

12 Cunningham-Rundles C, Brandeis WE, Good RA et al: Bovine antigens and the formation of circulating immune complexes in selective IgA deficiency. J Clin Invest 1979; 64:272–9.

13 Cunningham-Rundles C, Brandeis WE, Pudifin DJ et al: Autoimmunity in selective IgA deficiency: relationship to anti-bovine protein antigens, circulating immune complexes and clinical disease. Clin Exp Immunol 1981; 45:299–304.

14 Davidson M: Diarrhea. In: Rudolph AM, Hoffman JIE, eds. Pediatrics, 17th edn. Norwalk: Appleton-Century-Crofts, 1982; 924–37.

15 Engvall E, Perlmann R: Enzyme-linked immunosorbent assay (ELISA). Quantitative assay of immunoglobulin G. Immunochemistry 1971; 8:871–9.

16 Evans R III: A US reference for human immunoglobulin E. J Allergy Clin Immunol 1981; 68:79–82.

17 Forsgren A, Sjoquist J: Protein A from *Staphylococcus aureus*. I. Pseudoimmune reaction with human γ-globulin. J Immunol 1966; 97:822–7.

18 Gillman SA, Haddad ZH: The role of human IgE antibodies in the in vitro sensitization of rat mast cells (RMC) as determined by histamine release. J Allergy Clin Immunol 1972; 49:91.

19 Haddad ZH, Vin Kalra MS, Verma S: IgE antibodies to peptic and peptic-tryptic digests of beta lactoglobulin. Significance in food hypersensitivity. Ann Allergy 1979; 42:368–71.

20 Heiner DC: Food allergy and respiratory disease. Ann Allergy 1984; 53:657–64.

21 Heiner DC, deWeck AL, Svaril F et al; IgG4 antibody responses to 5 bee venom antigens. J Allergy Clin Immunol 1980; 65:20.

22 Hoffman DR, Haddad ZH: Diagnosis of IgE-mediated reactions to food antigens by radioimmunoassay. J Allergy Clin Immunol 1974; 54:165–73.

23 Hunt JS, Kennedy MP, Barber KE, McGiven AR: A microplate adaptation of the solid-phase C1q immune complex assay. J Immunol Methods 1980; 33:267–75.

24 Lambert PH, Dixon FJ, Zubler RH et al: A WHO collaborative study for the evaluation of eighteen methods for detecting immune complexes in serum. J Clin Lab Immunol 1978; 1:1–20.

25 Levy DA, Widra M: A microassay for studying allergic histamine release from human leukocytes using an enzyme-isotopic assay for histamine. J Lab Clin Med 1973; 81:291–7.

26 Lichtenstein LM, Norman PS: Human allergic reactions. Am J Med 1969; 46:169–73.

27 Lichtenstein LM, Osler AG: Studies on the mechanism of hypersensitivity phenomenon. Histamine release from human leukocytes by ragweed pollen antigen. J Exp Med 1964; 120:507–30.

28 Lipow HW, McQuitty JC: Cystic fibrosis. In: Rudolph AM, Hoffman JIE, eds. Pediatrics, 17th edn. Norwalk: Appleton-Century-Crofts, 1982; 1433–40.

29 McCarty EP, Frick OL: Food sensitivity: keys to diagnosis. J Pediatr 1983; 102:645–52.

30 May CD: Spontaneous release of histamine in vitro from leukocytes of persons hypersensitive to food. J Allergy Clin Immunol 1976; 55:432–7.

31 May CD, Alberto R: In vitro response of leukocytes to food proteins in allergic and normal children: lymphocyte stimulation and histamine release. Clin Allergy 1972; 2:335–44.

32 May CD, Lyman M, Alberto R, Cheng J: Procedures for immunochemical study of histamine release from leukocytes with small volume of blood. J Allergy 1970; 46:12–20.

33 Michel FB, Bousquet J, Greillier P et al: Comparison of cord blood IgE concentration and maternal allergy for the prediction of atopic disease in infancy. J Allergy Clin Immunol 1980; 65:422–30.

34 Minor JD, Tolber SG, Frick OL: Leukocyte inhibition factor (LIF) production in delayed onset food allergy. J Allergy Clin Immunol 1980; 66:314–21.

35 Nalebuff DJ, Fadal RG: The modified RAST assay: an aid in the diagnosis and management of allergic disorders. Cont Educ Fam Physician 1979; 10:64.

36 Orgel HA, Hamburger RN, Bazaral M et al: Development of IgE and allergy in infancy. J Allergy Clin Immunol 1975; 56:296–307.

37 Ottesen EA, Cohen SG: The eosinophil, eosinophilia, and eosinophil-related disorders. In: Middleton E Jr, Reed CE, Ellis EF, eds. Allergy, principles and practice, 2nd edn. St. Louis: C V Mosby 1983; 701–69.

38 Parish WE, Barrett AM, Coombs RRA et al: Hypersensitivity to milk and sudden death in infancy. Lancet 1960; ii:106–80.

39 Perelmutter L: IgG4: non-IgE mediated atopic disease. Ann Allergy 1984; 52:64–7.

40 Prausnitz C, Küstner H: Studien uber Uberempfindlichkeit. Centralbl Bakteriol [1 Abt, Orig] 1921; 86: 160–9.

41 Santrach PJ, Parker JL, Jones RT, Yunginger JW: Diagnostic and therapeutic application of a modified RAST and comparison with the conventional RAST. J Allergy Clin Immunol 1981; 67:97–104.

42 Scheinmann P, Gendrel D, Charles J et al: Value of lymphoblast transformation test in cow's milk protein intestinal intolerance. Clin Allergy 1976; 6:515–21.

43 Siraganian RP, Brodsky MJ: Automated histamine analysis for in vitro allergy testing. I. A method utilizing allergen-induced histamine release from whole blood. J Allergy Clin Immunol 1976; 57:525–40.

44 Theofilopoulos AN, Wilson CB, Dixon FJ: The Raji cell radio-immune assay for detecting immune complexes in human sera. J Clin Invest 1976; 57:169–82.

45 Wide L, Bennich H, Johansson SGO: Diagnosis of allergy by an in vitro test for allergenic antibodies. Lancet 1967; ii:1105–8.

46 Wilson JF, Lahey ME, Heiner DC: Studies on iron metabolism. V. Further observations on cow's milk induced gastrointestinal bleeding in infants with iron deficiency anemia. J Pediatr 1974; 84:335–44.

47 Wraith DG, Merrett J, Roth A et al: Recognition of food allergic patients and their allergens by the RAST technique and clinical investigation. Clin Allergy 1979; 9:25–36.

48 Zimmerman EM, Yunginger JW, Gleich GJ: Interference in ragweed pollen and honeybee venom radioallergosorbent tests. J Allergy Clin Immunol 1980; 66:386–93.

SECTION C
ALTERNATIVE DIAGNOSTIC TECHNIQUES

Chapter 53
The Pathology of Food Allergy Studied by Gastric Allergen Challenge

Bogdan Romanski

Introduction

In 1949 Ingelfinger et al [12] stated that 'Gastrointestinal allergy is a diagnosis frequently entertained, occasionally evaluated and rarely established.' Today, when diagnostic procedures for food allergy are more numerous, 'there is no doubt that laboratory investigations are only just beginning to sort out and explain some food allergy problems.' [10]

A correct diagnosis of an adverse reaction to a food may sometimes be established by a detailed history. In addition, skin tests, conjunctival, nasal and duodenal provocation (the latter with X-ray confirmation), as well as elimination diets, have been used to obtain objective proof of hypersensitivity to different foods [16]. Some immunological methods, especially the radioallergosorbent test (RAST), are occasionally useful in the diagnosis of food allergy in atopic patients [1] (see Chapter 50). The production of IgE complexes in food allergy subjects has been studied by Brostoff and Carini [7] and may be relevant to food allergy-induced multisystem disease.

Even with modern investigative methods, a definitive diagnosis of food allergy is not always easy. There is considerable controversy as to the value of skin tests with food extracts, and of the objective value of elimination diets or ingestion provocation tests with fresh non-processed foods. May and Bock [17] have pointed out that, 'throughout the discussion of food hypersensitivity the point will be repeatedly emphasized, that the presence of specific antibodies or sensitized cells is evidence of immunological sensitization, but their mere presence does not mean that clinical symptoms necessarily will occur after ingestion of the food antigen which produced the sensitization.' Even a positive RAST is not always indicative of a cause and effect relationship [31]. Thus, it is still true that there is no single diagnostic test that is completely accurate.

The major difficulties in correctly diagnosing food allergy are caused by lack of techniques for investigating both the development and the effects of allergic reactions in different tissues. Some progress in understanding the mechanisms of food allergy may be obtained, however, by the use of techniques for direct visualization of the immediate response of the gastric mucosa following an allergic challenge.

PROVOCATION OF THE GASTRIC MUCOSA WITH ALLERGENIC FOODS

Food allergy disorders occurring in atopic patients may be defined as 'those in which the adverse response to an ingested food is shown to involve an allergic or less specifically an immune response' [11]. These disorders may affect several tissues rich in mast cells and clinically may take many forms, including skin manifestations such as urticaria and eczema, respiratory manifestations such as wheezing and asthma, and conjunctival, neurocerebral and gastrointestinal symptoms.

Evidence that the stomach may be an important 'target organ' in food-sensitive individuals was first provided by Chevallier [9] and Paviot and Chevallier [19]. Using gastroscopy, they observed and subsequently described several characteristic signs in the gastric wall of their allergic patients of an adverse reaction caused by the ingestion of sensitizing foods. The signs included transitory antropyloric oedema, which could be compared to

Quincke's oedema, and more persistent haemorrhage and erosion. In some patients, ulcers were seen in sensitized areas of the gastric mucosa after food allergen ingestion. Similar experimental results from controlled observations of the mucosa were subsequently obtained by Pollard and Stuart [20].

Since the stomach is the first point of contact with ingested foods apart from the mouth and oesophagus, we have tried to develop in our Department a new technique for food allergy diagnosis based on allergen challenge made under fibrescopic observation. This technique, first elaborated by Swiatkowski and Kurek [32, 33], and subsequently refined by Kurek et al [15], makes possible direct and prolonged observations of pathological reactions in the stomach provoked by introduced foods.

Gastric challenge tests

Challenge tests with allergenic foods are performed as follows. The gastrofibrescope (GIF-type K Olympus) is introduced into the stomach after local anaesthesia of the pharynx with lignocaine. The surface mucosa, secretory activity and upper gastrointestinal tract motility are carefully evaluated beforehand. The apparatus is then introduced into the descending duodenum and, during its slow progressive removal, a few drops of a water-soluble suspension of the food under examination are placed directly on the surface of macroscopically normal gastric mucosa (Fig. 53.1). Subsequently, after placing the end of the gastrofibrescope on the border between the cardia and fundus of the stomach, close observation of the appearance of the gastric mucosa is maintained for 30 minutes. In all cases colour photographs are taken before and after food introduction and mucosal biopsies are made twice—before and after allergen challenge.

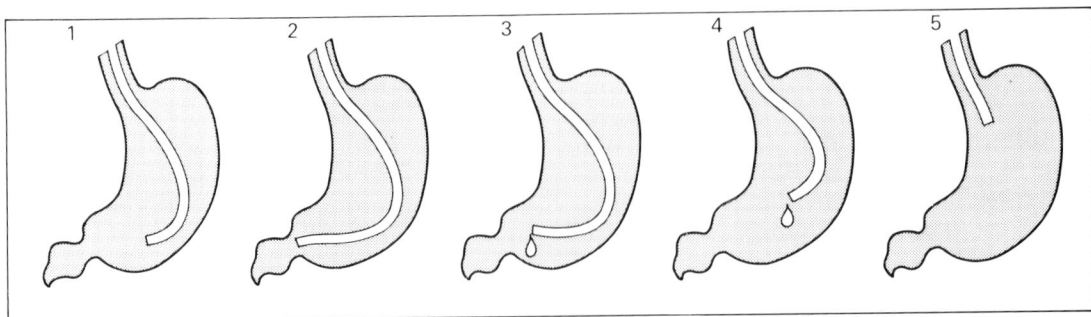

Fig. 53.1 Scheme of gastric fibrescopic investigation.

Advantages of gastric challenge tests

This method of investigation has many advantages and has been employed in our clinical practice for a number of purposes:

1 to reveal adverse reactions of the stomach to ingested foods,
2 to confirm the allergic origin of some pathological manifestations of other organs suspected to be related to food ingestion,
3 to study the efficacy of antianaphylactic drugs in food allergy patients and
4 to examine the presumed role of exogenous allergens in the development of organic lesions of the stomach and duodenum.

Adverse reactions of the stomach to food allergen challenge

In an important number of atopic patients some manifestations of gastrointestinal tract pathology, especially vomiting and abdominal pain, may be periodically observed. In others, nausea, heartburn and loose mucous stools occur after ingestion of different foods of animal or plant origin. Such symptoms, however, are not characteristic of food allergy only and are common in many gastrointestinal diseases not related to hypersensitivity mechanisms.

Macroscopic appearance

Using the method of allergen challenge on the gastric mucosa it is possible to see, in sensitive individuals, the macroscopic appearance of the gastric mucosa suddenly change within 5–20 minutes of contact with the introduced food. The normal colour of the mucosa changes, partly due to hyperaemia and partly to pallor. Afterwards, local oedema, punctate haemorrhages, hyperperistalsis of the stomach and hypersecretion of mucus may be observed. All patients deemed positive by the allergen challenge method showed the simultaneous appearance of at least four of the six above reactions [27].

Symptomatology

The characteristic clinical symptomatology of food allergy, as well as the local reaction of gastric mucosa to allergen challenge, may be illustrated by our group of 10 atopic patients,

Table 53.1 Gastrointestinal disorders occurring after ingestion of different foods, familial and personal history of atopy, suspected food allergen, skin tests results and total IgE level.

Patient number	Sex and age	Family history of atopy	Gastrointestinal symptoms	Other allergic manifestations	Suspected allergen	Skin test results	Serum IgE (PRIST) (U/ml)
1	M 41	Positive	Abdominal pains Loose mucous stools	Rhinitis and urticaria	Egg	House dust (+ + +) Feathers (+ + + +) Egg white (+ + + +)	1000
2	M 29	Positive	Pyrosis	Rhinitis	Flour	House dust (+ + + +) Wheat flour (+ + +) Rye flour (+ + +)	230
3	F 21	Positive	Abdominal pains Loose mucous stools	Bronchial asthma and rhinitis	Milk	House dust (+ + +) Moulds (+ + + +) Milk (+ + +)	1000
4	M 16	Negative	Abdominal pains Nausea Loose mucous stools	Bronchial asthma and rhinitis	Fish	House dust (+ + + +) Horse dander (+ + + +) Fish (+ +)	1000
5	F 18	Negative	Abdominal pains Nausea, vomiting Loose stools	Pollinosis and urticaria	Chicken	Feathers (+ + + +) Grass pollen (+ + + +) Chicken (+ + +)	1000
6	F 47	Negative	Abdominal pains	Angioedema	Celery	Parsley (+ + +) Celery (+ +)	440
7	M 27	Negative	Abdominal pains Heartburn Gas	Rhinitis and urticaria	Cocoa	Cocoa (+ + +) Yeast (+ + +) Pea (+ + +)	270
8	M 18	Positive	Abdominal pains Heartburn Nausea	Bronchial asthma and urticaria	Tomato	House dust (+ + +) Feathers (+ + + +) Tomato (+ + +)	1000
9	F 33	Positive	Abdominal pains Gas	Bronchial asthma and urticaria	Beer	House dust (+ + + +) Feathers (+ + +) Yeast (+ + +)	625
10	M 26	Negative	Abdominal pains Gas	Bronchial asthma and pruritus	Mustard	Mustard (+ + +) Vinegar (+ + +)	115

all suffering from respiratory and/or skin allergy, who also had a variety of gastrointestinal disorders which they thought were due to food allergy. Table 53.1 shows that the most frequent gastrointestinal symptoms in these patients were rather common and banal. The total serum IgE level was markedly increased in nine patients. All patients suffering from rhinitis and asthma had strongly positive skin tests with common inhalant allergens, and with some food extracts. It is interesting to note that a personal history suggesting intolerance to specific foods was, in all cases, subsequently confirmed by positive skin tests. The macroscopic appearance of the gastric mucosa before challenge was normal in four patients and slightly erythematous in six patients. The histology of the mucosa was normal in six cases, while in four the typical features of gastritis were found. After allergen challenge, the mucosa showed an immediate positive reaction in all patients, in addition to the characteristic microscopic changes on biopsy (Table 53.2).

The collected data suggest that different food allergens of both animal and plant actually provoke an immediate hypersensitivity reaction in the gastric mucosa following contact with allergen. This reaction is certainly specific in atopics because it was observed in our patients only after contact with the sensitizing food. For example, patients allergic to milk did not react to wheat provocation and, vice versa, patients hypersensitive to wheat showed no reaction to milk challenge. As a control, a group of 20 non-atopic subjects, aged from 14 to 52, suffering from gastritis and duodenitis, were provoked with five different natural foods, with negative results in all cases [32].

Comparison of provocation by ingestion and direct challenge

We have compared the practical value of provocation tests by ingestion and direct allergen challenge in 26 asthmatic patients aged between 17 and 59 where attacks of dyspnoea seemed to be related to ingestion of specific foods. In this group the total IgE serum level was raised in 20 patients, while the skin tests were positive in all cases. Spirographic examination after oral ingestion of about 5 g of the suspected foods enabled a diagnosis of food allergy to be established in only 11 of the 26 patients, in whom the fall of forced expiratory volume in 1 second (FEV_1) values of 13.2% to 50% was observed 5–60 minutes following allergen ingestion. The direct provocation test of gastric mucosa was positive in all 26 cases, both in macroscopic and microscopic studies [14].

It seems, therefore, that the direct provocation test may be used to obtain a correct diagnosis of food allergy in those cases in which other diagnostic methods are insufficient. Also, correct interpretation of some abdominal complaints in atopic people may be made using the direct allergen challenge method. It appears that a number of the above

Table 53.2 Macroscopic and microscopic changes of the gastric mucosa before and after direct provocation by foods.

Patient number	Sex	Before Macroscopy: Pale	Oedema	Punctate haemorrhage	Hyperperistalsis	Hypersecretion	Erythema	Before Microscopy: Oedema	Hyperaemia	Capillary haemorrhage	Eosinophilic infiltration	Inflammation	Food allergen introduced into the stomach	After Macroscopy: Pale	Oedema	Punctate haemorrhage	Hyperperistalsis	Hypersecretion	Erythema	After Microscopy: Oedema	Hyperaemia	Capillary haemorrhage	Eosinophilic infiltration	Inflammation
1	M						+					+	Egg		+ +			+ + + +	+ +					+
2	M						+					+	Wheat flour		+ +			+ + +	+		+			+
3	F												Milk		+			+ + + +			+			+
4	M												Fish		+			+ + +			+		+	
5	F						+					+	Chicken		+ +			+ + +	+ +	+				
6	F						+					+	Celery		+			+ + + +	+		+			+
7	M												Cocoa		+ +			+ + +	+		+		+ +	
8	M												Tomato		+			+ + +	+		+			
9	F						+						Beer		+			+ + + +	+ +		+			
10	M						+						Vinegar					+ + + +	+ +		+			

complaints may be caused by an allergic reaction of the gastric mucosa to ingested foods, often having the character of an acute allergic gastritis [32].

Allergic gastrointestinal disorders

Gastrointestinal disorders of allergic origin are probably more frequent in adult atopics than is generally admitted. The aetiology of these disorders, however, is not always recognized due to the atypical character of the manifestations and the frequently negative results of X-ray examinations. Such manifestations may also, in some cases, be inappropriately attributed to coadministered drugs.

Our experience with direct food allergen challenge permits us to confirm the high diagnostic value of the old method of skin testing with food allergen extracts. We were surprised to see a good correlation between history, strongly positive skin reactions and positive results from provocation of the gastric mucosa. It seems that skin reactivity in food-allergic patients reflects the actual state of sensitivity to ingested aliments.

SYSTEMIC MANIFESTATIONS OF FOOD ALLERGY

Adult atopics are often hypersensitive to both ingested and inhaled allergens and may therefore suffer simultaneously from allergic disorders of several organs, including skin, respiratory tract and gastrointestinal tract. In effect, it is not always easy in patients sensitized to numerous allergens to recognize the respective roles of each in the pathological manifestations.

The importance of food allergens in the aetiology of systemic manifestations in atopics may be confirmed by direct allergen challenge. This is convincingly demonstrated by the results of investigations made in our Department on a group of 20 patients suffering from such manifestations, and having a history of gastrointestinal complaints after ingestion of different foods. In all cases skin reactions to extracts of incriminated foods were strongly positive; it was therefore possible to suspect their causative action in patients' pathology.

Reactions in other organs after gastric challenge

In all patients the direct provocation test was performed using a water suspension of food allergens and a local positive reaction in the gastric mucosa was observed both macroscopically and on biopsy. All patients reacted within minutes with pathological manifestations in other organs. In some, excessive sialorrhoea appeared; in others, the development of an acute conjunctivitis, skin erythema and oedema of the face and fingers was observed.

Table 53.3 Multiorgan manifestations in atopic patients after direct allergen challenge in the gastric mucosa.

Patient number	Sex	Age	Food allergen used for provocation	Nasal	Conjunctival	Bronchial	Cutaneous	Intestinal	Cerebral	Oral
1	M	28	Flour	+						
2	M	47	Egg white	+	+		+	+		
3	F	41	Celery	+	+		+			
4	M	25	Flour		+	+				+
5	M	20	Orange	+	+		+	+		+
6	F	22	Milk	+		+		+		+
7	F	28	Beer	+		+				
8	M	26	Mustard			+				+
9	M	47	Flour	+		+	+			
10	F	28	Tomato	+	+		+		+	
11	M	19	Tomato	+		+				
12	M	59	Flour	+	+					
13	M	18	Milk	+						
14	F	21	Chicken	+		+	+		+	
15	M	20	Fish	+	+		+			
16	M	21	Fish	+	+					
17	F	35	Flour	+						
18	M	17	Fish	+	+		+			
19	M	43	Flour	+	+	+				
20	M	32	Flour	+	+	+				

Some patients reacted with rapid dyspnoea, acute nasal congestion with abundant aqueous secretion, or abdominal pain with diarrhoea.

In 17 of the 20 patients pathological reactions of more than one organ were seen simultaneously. The types of offending allergen, together with their associated observed symptoms, are presented in Table 53.3.

Possible target organs. The data in Table 53.3 indicate the main 'target organs' in food-allergic individuals. Besides the gastric mucosa which appears to react the most often to offending allergens, nasal and conjunctival mucosa seemed to be especially sensitive to food allergen challenge. A similar reaction, at a distance from the site of allergen penetration, may be observed in the bronchial tree, and in the skin, as well as in the mouth, bowel and cerebral nervous system. The incidence of acute headache after provocation may support the theory of an allergic origin for some cases of migraine [26].

The same multiorgan manifestations were observed during provocation with foods of both animal (egg, milk and fish proteins) and plant (vegetables, fruits and flour) origin. Among the latter allergens, flour merits special attention because it may enter the organism by both the respiratory tract and the gastrointestinal tract; in consequence, flour allergy may also have the character of an occupational disease.

Flour allergy

The multiorgan symptomatology of flour allergy has been demonstrated by our investigation undertaken on a group of 10 patients with a negative history of atopy, in whom a variety of pathological manifestations appeared during prolonged exposure to flour at their places of work. All patients suffered from chronic gastrointestinal disorders, while the symptoms of chronic perennial rhinitis, bronchial asthma, conjunctivitis and urticaria appeared in nine, eight, six and two, respectively. The total serum IgE level was raised in six patients; intradermal tests were weakly positive with house dust extracts and strongly positive with flour extract in all cases.

In this group the causative role of the flour in all the pathological disorders was confirmed by provocation tests. The nasal test was positive in six out of nine patients with rhinitis and the conjunctival test was positive in all six patients with conjunctivitis. The bronchial test with inhaled flour extract was positive in six out of eight patients with asthma, in whom a significant fall of FEV_1 was observed.

On fibroscopy, symptoms of chronic gastritis were found in six patients. The direct provocation test of the gastric mucosa with a water suspension of flour was positive in all 10 patients, where the typical oedematous and haemorrhagic changes were seen after allergen challenge. It was therefore possible to confirm the causative role of flour not only in skin, respiratory and conjunctival manifestations but also in the aetiology of gastrointestinal complaints [32]. It should be emphasized that the commonly used definition of 'baker's asthma' is inadequate because flour allergy so often involves other organs. In patients having prolonged occupational contact with flour, not only the conjunctival, nasal and bronchial mucosa, but also the gastrointestinal tract, become sensitive to flour allergens. In the light of data obtained by provocation of the gastric mucosa, it is possible to explain why people allergic to flour may also suffer from persistent gastrointestinal disorders.

Summary

In summary, objective evidence for systemic manifestations of food allergy in adult atopics can frequently be obtained by direct provocation of the gastric mucosa. The typical 'target organs' of food allergy are schematically represented in Fig. 53.2.

Studies on the systemic manifestations of food allergy subsequently undertaken by Kurek [13] in a large number of cases indicate that a causative role for ingested aliments in the aetiology of several skin, conjunctival, respiratory and gastrointestinal disorders is sometimes overlooked in adult atopics. A correct diagnosis of food allergy in such patients may frequently be difficult to obtain because its existence can often be masked by simultaneous manifestations of sensitivity to inhalant allergens. It appears that a role for food allergens should be suspected in patients whose systemic manifestations include gastric or intestinal disorders of unknown origin. The latter are highly indicative of the existence of food allergy and must therefore be carefully researched by history.

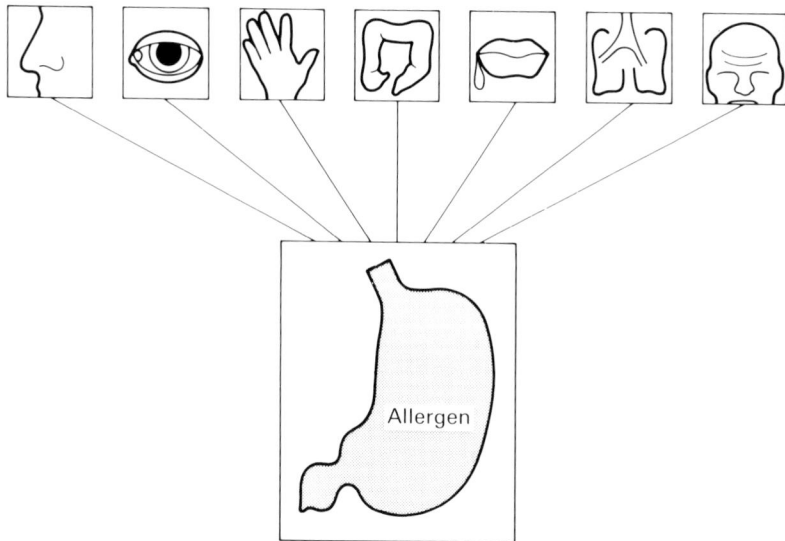

Fig. 53.2 Scheme of food allergy 'target organs'.

DIRECT GASTRIC PROVOCATION

The protective action of disodium cromoglycate and ketotifen in patients with food allergy

In the last few years we have investigated the protective action of ketotifen (Zaditen) and disodium cromoglycate (DSCG) in 50 unselected patients with the atopic form of asthma by a double-blind controlled method. We have observed that ketotifen is highly effective in 56% of patients and DSCG highly effective in 76%; the difference between the two administered products was not statistically significant. Both drugs were less effective in patients with recurrent infections of the respiratory tract [28].

It is to be emphasized, however, that clinical evaluation of the effectiveness of anti-anaphylactic drugs in man is, of necessity, indirect and based mainly on the appraisal of improvement in the state of health of treated persons. Such appraisal is certainly not very scientific and may be easily criticized. We have tried therefore to confirm the protective value of DSCG and ketotifen by a more objective method of direct provocation of the gastric mucosa.

Ketotifen

We first studied the protective anti-anaphylactic action of ketotifen in 12 atopic patients aged between 18 and 58 in whom gastrointestinal and other pathological manifesta-tions occurred after the ingestion of definite different foods of animal or plant origin. In all of them the intradermal tests with food extracts were strongly positive and the total IgE serum level was elevated. The direct provocation test with food allergens introduced into the stomach was positive in all examined cases.

Subsequently 1 mg of ketotifen was given orally twice—in syrup form in six patients and in tablet form in the other six—over 14 days and after this time the results were carefully evaluated by clinical examination, and verified by repetition of the direct provocation test with the same food extracts. It was found that all gastrointestinal, respiratory, cutaneous and conjunctival disorders disappeared in 11 patients. In the twelfth patient, suffering from both gastrointestinal and respiratory manifestations, no clinical improvement was noticed.

Repeated gastric provocation tests

The repeated direct provocation test of the gastric mucosa with the same food allergens was negative in the 11 patients with clinical improvement, but positive in the patients without amelioration after ketotifen therapy. In the former the only response was a slight change in colour of the mucosa in five cases; other pathological reactions in the stomach were not found. In the twelfth patient the pathological changes provoked by food allergens were similar to those observed after the first provocation. The macroscopic changes in the stomach are summarized in Table 53.4.

Table 53.4 Macroscopic changes of the gastric mucosa after direct provocation by foods before and after treatment with ketotifen.

	No pretreatment	After pretreatment with ketotifen
Hyperperistalsis	in 12 patients	in 1 patient
Hypersecretion	in 12 patients	in 1 patient
Mucosa: pale	in 8 patients	in 1 patient
Mucosa: hyperaemic	in 11 patients	in 4 patients
Mucosa: oedematous	in 12 patients	in 1 patient
Punctate haemorrhage	in 12 patients	in 1 patient

The above macroscopic data were confirmed by microscopy in which the picture of tissue oedema, capillary haemorrhage and eosinophilic infiltrations found after the first provocation was absent after the second. It was noticed, however, that inflammatory mononuclear infiltrations found on biopsy at the first examination were detected in the same patients on the second biopsy made after the treatment.

Summary

The results of our study with ketotifen—in patients in which the gastric mucosa constituted one out of several 'target organs' of food allergy—are highly suggestive, because the protective action of the drug on sensitized tissues was observed directly, and it was possible to confirm objectively the inhibition of immediate reactions with food allergens in the wall of the stomach. It appears that the employed drug really exerted a highly protective action in the gastric mucosa, acting probably by inhibition of allergen-induced mediator release [26].

Disodium cromoglycate (DSCG)

Subsequent to the interesting results with ketotifen therapy, we tried to determine if it were possible to inhibit the anaphylactic reaction in the gastric wall with DSCG applied locally. We therefore administered this compound in eight patients, aged from 20 to 65, in whom systemic manifestations occurred after the ingestion of foods, especially milk, eggs, wheat and fish. The intradermal tests with those allergens were positive in all patients, and their total serum IgE level was raised. The direct provocation test of the gastric mucosa was strongly positive in all cases, both in macroscopic and microscopic examinations.

Challenge. After the first allergen challenge, 80 mg of DSCG dissolved in hot water were given orally to all eight atopic patients in four daily doses over 14 days. After this period their states of health were clinically evaluated. A very great improvement was observed in five patients in whom allergic disorders of the gastrointestinal tract and other organs disappeared after treatment. In the sixth patient the gastrointestinal complaints and the rhinitis disappeared although he suffered as before from asthma. In the seventh patient all systemic allergic manifestations, excluding rhinitis, were relieved while in the eighth patient the symptoms of rhinitis cleared after therapy but he still suffered from conjunctivitis, urticaria and asthma.

In repeated provocation tests, it was found that the gastric mucosa did not react on the second allergen challenge in four patients, while these reactions were very weak in three patients and very strong (similar to the first provocation) in one patient, who showed no clinical improvement on the treatment.

Table 53.5 summarizes the pathological changes seen macroscopically in the stomach.

Table 53.5 Macroscopic changes of the gastric mucosa after direct provocation by foods, before and after the treatment with disodium cromoglycate (DSCG).

	No pretreatment	After pretreatment with DSCG
Hyperperistalsis	in 7 patients	in 1 patient
Hypersecretion	in 7 patients	in 1 patient
Mucosa: pale	in 4 patients	in 1 patient
Mucosa: hyperaemic	in 8 patients	in 2 patients
Mucosa: oedematous	in 6 patients	in 2 patients
Punctate haemorrhage	in 6 patients	in 1 patient

Conclusions

It appears, therefore, that oral doses of DSCG of as little as 80 mg per day may inhibit mediator release in the stomach and effectively protect the gastric mucosa against food allergen challenge.

This local action of the drug is fully comprehensible in the light of the data on the mechanism of its action, and our observations also support the view that DSCG taken orally may prevent allergic manifestations in organs which are distant from the point of absorption [22] (see Chapter 58).

THE ALLERGIC PATHOGENESIS OF SOME PEPTIC ULCERS

Passive mucosal sensitization

The first convincing evidence for allergic phenomena affecting the gastrointestinal tract was provided by Gray and Waltzer in 1937. They passively sensitized the rectal mucous membrane with a human reagin-bearing serum for peanut by local injection. Between 24 and 48 hours later the patient ingested the peanut antigen on a fasting stomach. Within a few minutes an inflammatory reaction developed at the sensitized rectal site as shown by oedema, hyperaemia and increased secretion of mucus [30].

Conceivably, the gastroduodenal mucosa could react similarly to ingested allergens and exposure to acid peptic activity might result in ulceration. This possibility has recently been confirmed in animals. Intramucosal injection of ovalbumin into the gastric fundus of the African rodent *Mastomys natalensis* provokes a local allergic reaction in sensitized animals, resulting three days later in the appearance of a gastric ulcer [4, 5]. It was also found that treatment with DSCG may be effective in varioliform gastritis in man [3] and could prevent the development of experimental ulcers [6].

Peptic ulcer and exogenous allergens

In our preliminary studies of a group of 50 patients with peptic ulcers, in Gdansk in 1970, strongly positive skin reactions to house dust and to mould extracts were observed in 50% and 40% of the patients, respectively. High titres of serum haemagglutinating antibodies against food and inhalant allergens were also found which were similar to those determined in a group of patients with allergic bronchial

asthma. We have therefore advanced the working hypothesis of a relationship between hypersensitivity to inhaled or ingested allergens and the development or progression of peptic ulcer disease [25].

In 1983 we examined, in Bydgoszcz, a group of 257 patients with a gastric or duodenal ulcer but without any manifestation of skin or respiratory allergy. Skin tests with both inhalant and food allergens were positive in 136 (52.9%) [23]. In 51 cases with positive skin reactions further detailed investigations have been made up to the present.

Summary of Bydgoszcz study. The examined group was composed of 29 men and 22 women aged from 17 to 55 suffering from gastric (24 cases) or duodenal (27 cases) ulcers. In all patients the disease was chronic with seasonal aggravations over several years. None of the patients had a positive personal or familial history of atopy.

In an endoscopic examination, both the characteristic gastric or duodenal ulceration and inflammatory changes of the mucosa were seen. Evidence of a chronic inflammatory process in tissues surrounding the ulceration was subsequently obtained in microscopic studies, in which the diagnosis of chronic gastritis or duodenitis was made in all cases. The typical appearance of some observed ulcers is presented in Fig. 53.3.

All patients had strongly positive immediate-type skin reactions to extracts of different allergens. The results of skin tests with 13 common foods and inhalants are presented in Table 53.6. These data show that the patients were sensitive to a number of exogenous allergens.

Table 53.6 Skin test results in 32 patients with gastric or duodenal ulcers.

Strongly positive reactions	Number positive	Percentage positive
House dust extract	26	81
Tomatoes	26	81
Chicken	21	66
Potatoes	17	53
Dermatophagoides pteronyssinus	15	47
Feathers	14	44
Moulds	10	31
Honey	7	22
Egg white	6	19
Milk	5	16
Pork	3	9
Wheat	3	9
Fish	2	6

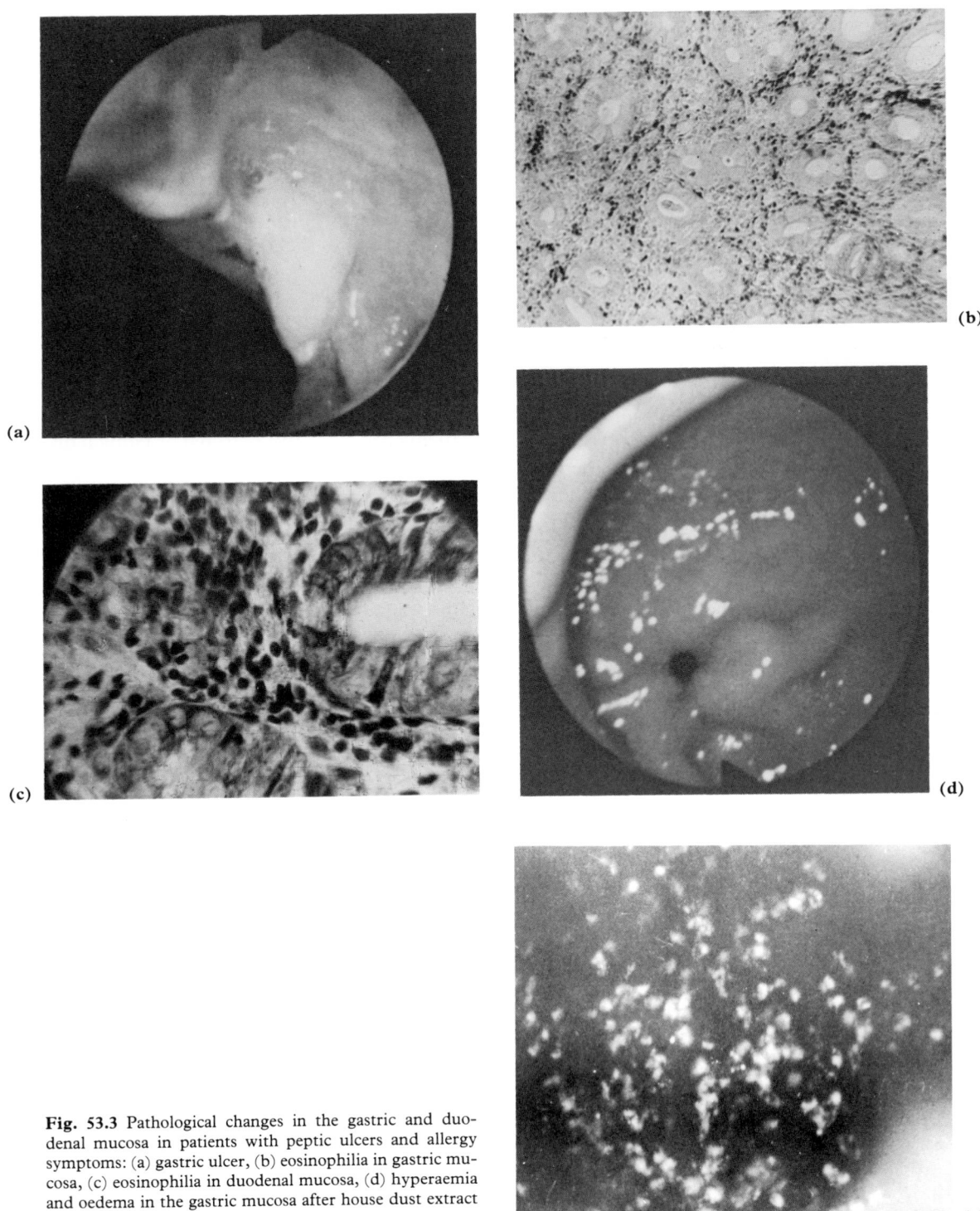

Fig. 53.3 Pathological changes in the gastric and duodenal mucosa in patients with peptic ulcers and allergy
symptoms: (a) gastric ulcer, (b) eosinophilia in gastric mucosa, (c) eosinophilia in duodenal mucosa, (d) hyperaemia
and oedema in the gastric mucosa after house dust extract
challenge, (e) IgE-bearing cells in gastric mucosa.

The total IgE level measured by Phadezym PRIST (Pharmacia) was raised in patients with positive skin tests and markedly higher than in control subjects. The mean values of total serum IgE levels were 61.78 kU/l in the 82 healthy subjects, 32.42 kU/l in the 16 patients with gastric or duodenal ulcers and negative skin tests and 143.2 kU/l in the 32 patients with gastric or duodenal ulcers and positive skin tests to exogenous allergens.

In the 48 patients with ulcers serum IgE antibodies against 15 common allergens were measured by Phadezym RAST. The results of the test are presented in Table 53.7.

From Table 53.7 it may be seen that the suspicion of sensitivity to different food and inhalant allergens, obtained initially by the skin test method in several patients with peptic ulcers, was subsequently confirmed by RAST. It is not surprising that the close correlation between skin tests and RAST results was not found in patients sensitive to exogenous allergens because it is known that, unlike the skin test, RAST cannot detect cell-bound IgE antibodies [2]. It seems, however, highly significant that serum IgE antibodies against such commonly consumed foods as wheat, tomatoes and potatoes were found in several patients with ulcers. The causative role of these and perhaps other food allergens in the development of peptic ulcers in sensitive individuals appear possible in the light of our observations on the reactivity of the gastric mucosa on food allergen challenge.

Antibodies to inhalant allergens in patients with peptic ulcers

The presence of IgE antibodies against inhalants in patients with peptic ulcers but without any detectable skin or respiratory allergic manifestation was surprising. The importance of *Dermatophagoides pteronyssinus* antigens in the aetiology of respiratory allergy is very well known. The sensitivity to cockroach allergens in some asthmatic patients, all of whom were allergic to house dust, was observed previously. It is therefore possible that cockroach allergy is in fact closely related to house dust allergy [29]. Mould allergy is also very common in patients hypersensitive to dust which normally contains several spores of Fungi Imperfecti, especially of *Aspergillus* species [21]. It seems, therefore, that patients with ulcers may be sensitized to a number of house dust antigens.

Gastric challenge with house dust allergens

The possibility of the gastric mucosa reacting to these antigens was subsequently verified by the provocation method. Allergen challenge with 1 ml of house dust or *Dermatophagoides pteronyssinus* water extract in 1:5000 concentration was made under fibrescopic control in 10 patients with ulcers and house dust allergy, and in 10 patients with ulcers but without symptoms of hypersensitivity to house dust antigens. In eight of the ulcer patients with allergy the immediate hyperaemic, oedematous and haemorrhagic reaction was seen

Table 53.7 Serum IgE antibodies measured by Phadezym RAST (Pharmacia) in patients with gastric or duodenal ulcers.

Allergen	Percentage positive RAST in patients with positive skin tests ($n = 32$)	Percentage positive RAST in patients with negative skin tests ($n = 16$)
Blatella germanica	63	12
Dactylis glomerata	53	0
Aspergillus fumigatus	50	3
Dermatophagoides pteronyssinus	25	6
Penicillium notatum	9	0
Cladosporium herbarum	6	0
House dust	6	0
Goose feathers	3	0
Wheat	41	0
Tomato	22	0
Potato	19	0
Milk	6	0
Fish	6	0
Egg white	3	0
Chicken meat	3	0

Table 53.8 The results of direct provocation of the gastric mucosa with inhalant allergens in patients with gastric and duodenal ulcers.

Patient number	Sex	Age	Ulcers	Allergen	Results of provocation		
					Hyper-aemia	Oedema	Haemorr-hage
1	M	25	Duodenal	House dust	+	+	+
2	M	40	Gastric	*Dermatophagoides pteronyssinus*	+	+	−
3	M	35	Duodenal	House dust	+	+	−
4	M	32	Duodenal	House dust	+	+	+
5	F	33	Gastric	House dust	+	+	+
6	F	32	Duodenal	*Dermatophagoides pteronyssinus*	+	+	−
7	F	41	Gastric	*Dermatophagoides pteronyssinus*	+	+	+
8	M	55	Duodenal	House dust	−	−	−
9	M	35	Several gastric	House dust	−	−	−
10	M	32	Several duodenal	House dust	+	+	−

(Table 53.8, Fig. 53.3d), while no pathological changes were observed in the latter patients.

It appears, therefore, that house dust antigenic components may really provoke some inflammatory and haemorrhagic reaction in the stomach of predisposed individuals after direct contact with the gastric mucosa.

Eosinophils and IgE B cells

In all examined cases the presence of chronic inflammatory process of the gastric duodenal mucosa was found on biopsy. We have tried to explore more fully the nature of this process and to ascertain its presumed allergic origin. We therefore searched for the presence of eosinophils and IgE-producing cells in challenged sites. Studies were made on seven healthy subjects and on 18 patients with ulcers and allergy symptoms by observing the colour of the biopsy material and by direct immunofluorescence using an anti-epsilon chain antiserum produced by the Behring Institute.

In the seven healthy control subjects with a normal gastric mucosa only single eosinophils and single IgE-bearing fluorescent cells were seen per microscopic field. Such results were considered negative. On the other hand, in patients with ulcers, the number of both eosinophils and IgE cells was much greater. The detailed results of this study are shown in Table 53.9.

The data indicate that in all 18 patients an increased number of IgE-producing cells and eosinophils were seen in the greater and lesser curvature and in the antrum of the stomach. In 12 of 13 patients in whom the duodenal

mucosa was simultaneously investigated, eosinophils and IgE cells were present in large numbers. These findings firmly suggest that an immediate-type allergic reaction takes place in gastric and duodenal tissues in patients with ulcers and hypersensitivity to exogenous allergens. Such a reaction probably often involves the whole gastric and duodenal mucosa.

Our latter observations are similar to those studies of other authors in which large numbers of IgE cells have been demonstrated in the gastric mucosa of patients with varioliform gastritis [3] and in the tissue surrounding the ulcers [8]. Recently it has also been found that the edges of peptic ulcers are characterized by a marked increase in IgE cells [6].

The typical appearances of marked gastric and duodenal eosinophilia and of an increased number of IgE cells in the gastric mucosa are presented in Fig. 53.7c, d, f.

Treatment of peptic ulcer with DSCG

The immediate-type reactions may be effectively prevented by local treatment with DSCG. We have tried, therefore, to verify its action in our patients. In 51 patients with peptic ulcers and allergy symptoms, oral DSCG was given in a small dose of 160 mg daily. The other group of 46 patients without allergy symptoms was treated simultaneously with 1.0 g of cimetidine. All patients were treated in ambulatory conditions and did not receive any other drugs. In all 97 cases the healing of ulcers was assessed every 12 days from the beginning of therapy under fibrescopic control (Fig. 53.4).

Table 53.9 Total serum IgE levels, RAST, local eosinophilia and IgE in gastric and duodenal mucosa in patients with gastric or duodenal ulcers and allergy symptoms.

Patient number	Sex	Age	Ulcers	IgE PRIST (kU/ml)	RAST		Gastric mucosa		Duodenal mucosa	
							Local eosinophilia	Local IgE	Local eosinophilia	Local IgE
1	M	35	Gastric	500.0	+	Greater curvature	+ + +	+ +		
						Lesser curvature	+ + +	+ +		
						Antrum	+ +	−		
2	M	51	Gastric	43.45	+	Greater curvature	+	+		
						Lesser curvature	+	+ +		
						Antrum	+	+ + +		
3	F	44	Duodenal gastric	8.195	+	Greater curvature	−	+		
						Lesser curvature	−	−	+ +	+
						Antrum	+ +	+		
4	M	40	Duodenal	118.25	+	Greater curvature	+ +	+ +		
						Lesser curvature	+ +	+ +		
						Antrum	+ +	+		
5	M	32	Duodenal	627.0	+	Greater curvature	+	+		
						Lesser curvature	+ +	+ +		
						Antrum	+ + +	+ + +		
6	M	33	Duodenal	>660	+	Greater curvature	−	+		
						Lesser curvature	−	−		+ + +
						Antrum	+ +	+ + +		
7	F	32	Duodenal	190.85	+	Greater curvature	−	+		
						Lesser curvature	−	+	+ + +	+ + +
						Antrum	−	+		
8	M	55	Duodenal	412.5	+	Greater curvature	−	−		
						Lesser curvature	−	−		+ + +
						Antrum	+	+		
9	M	44	Duodenal	31.075	+	Greater curvature	−	−		
						Lesser curvature	−	−	+ + +	+ + +
						Antrum	+	+		
10	F	33	Gastric	>660	+	Greater curvature	+ + +	+ + +		
						Lesser curvature	+ + +	+ + +	+ +	+ + +
						Antrum	−	+		
11	M	35	Gastric	420.75	+	Greater curvature	+	−		
						Lesser curvature	+	+	+ +	+
						Antrum	+ + +	+ + +		
12	M	42	Duodenal	213.95	+	Greater curvature	−	−		
						Lesser curvature	+	+	+ +	+ +
						Antrum	+ +	−		
13	F	48	Duodenal	44.55	+	Greater curvature	+	+ +		
						Lesser curvature	+ + +	+ + +	+ + +	+ + +
						Antrum	+	+		
14	M	47	Gastric	145.75	+	Greater curvature	−	−		
						Lesser curvature	−	−	+ +	+ +
						Antrum	+	+		
15	M	37	Gastric	41.25	+	Greater curvature	−	−		
						Lesser curvature	−	−	+	−
						Antrum	+ +	+ +		
16	M	35	Duodenal	146.3	−	Greater curvature	−	+		
						Lesser curvature	−	+	−	+
						Antrum	+	+		
17	M	28	Duodenal	89.10	+	Greater curvature	−	−		
						Lesser curvature	+	−	−	−
						Antrum	+ +	+		
18	M	47	Gastric	113.3	−	Greater curvature	+	+		
						Lesser curvature	+	+		
						Antrum	+ + +	+ + +		

After 12 days, the percentage of healed ulcers was higher in those treated by DSCG, while full healing of ulcers after 24 and 36 days of treatment was found in 73% and 82% of patients treated by DSCG, and in 65% and 78% of cases treated by cimetidine. Thus, the action of both compounds seems to be similar. It is highly surprising that DSCG, which is a

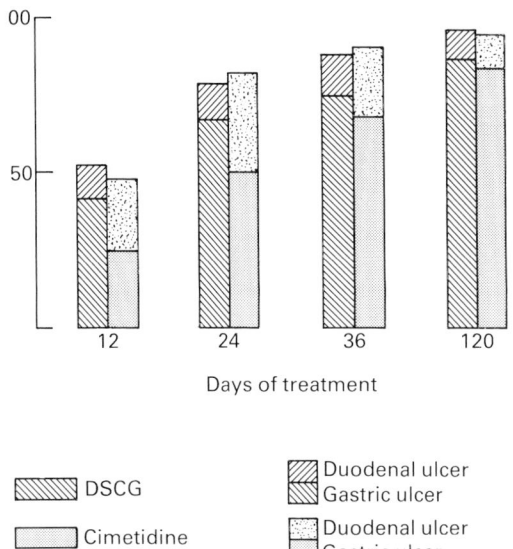

Days of treatment

DSCG

Cimetidine

Duodenal ulcer
Gastric ulcer

Duodenal ulcer
Gastric ulcer

Fig. 53.4 Percentage of healed ulcers following treatment with disodium cromoglycate (DSCG) and cimetidine.

drug without antacid properties and without anti-H2 receptor activity, appeared to be as effective as cimetidine, considered recently as the best agent employed in peptic ulcer therapy. It is also to be emphasized that the good results obtained by 'treatment' with placebo do not in general exceed the limits of 50% of treated cases [24].

Disodium cromoglycate has been shown to be of great value in the prevention of adverse reactions to food in a number of trials [34] (see Chapter 58). It appears to be both effective and well tolerated in the treatment of food allergy, particularly when used in conjunction with a maintenance elimination diet [18].

Summary. All the symptoms of allergy observed in our patients—positive immediate-type skin reactions, raised total serum IgE level, occurrence of specific IgE antibodies, reactivity of gastric mucosa to house dust and to *D. pteronyssinus* extracts, local eosinophilia in gastric and/or duodenal mucosa, presence of a significant number of IgE-bearing cells in gastric and duodenal tissues, as well as the excellent results of therapy with DSCG—when considered together, firmly support the hypothesis of an allergic origin for some peptic ulcers. An exciting path for future research on the pathology, prevention and treatment of ulcer disease seems to be open.

REFERENCES

1 Aas K: The diagnosis of hypersensitivity to ingested foods. Reliability of skin prick testing and the radioallergosorbent test with different materials. Clin Allergy 1978; 8:39.

2 Adkinson NF: The radioallergosorbent test in 1981—limitations and refinements. J Allergy Clin Immunol 1981; 67:87–9.

3 André C, Moulinier B, Lambert R, Bugnon B: Gastritis varioliformis, allergy and disodium cromoglycate. Lancet 1976; i:964–5.

4 André F, André C: Animal model of human disease: gastric ulcer disease. Gastric ulcer induced by mucosal anaphylaxis in ovalbumin-sensitized *Praomys (Mastomys) natalensis*. Am J Pathol 1981; 102:133–5.

5 André F, André C, Vialard JF: Role of homocytotropic antibodies in pathogenesis of gastric ulcer. Digestion 1979; 19:175–9.

6 André C, Moulinier B, André F, Daniere S: Evidence for anaphylactic reactions in peptic ulcer and varioliform gastritis. Ann Allergy 1983; 51:325–8.

7 Brostoff J, Carini C: Regulation of IgE complex formation in food allergy subjects. In: Proceedings of XII Congress of the European Academy of Allergology and Clinical Immunology, Rome, 1983; 33–42.

8 Brown WR, Borhistle BK, Chen ST: Immunoglobulin E (IgE) and IgE-containing cells in human gastrointestinal fluids and tissues. Clin Exp Immunol 1975; 20:227–37.

9 Chevallier R: Les gastropathies allergiques sous le contrôle du gastroscope (à propos de quatre nouvelles observations d'oedème antral fugace). Rapports du 1er Congrès International de Gastro-Entérologie, Bruxelles, 1935; 654.

10 Frankland AW: The problems of diagnosis and treatment in food allergy. In: Food Allergy. Utrecht: hal Allergy Service, 1980; 113–8.

11 Hutchins P, Walker-Smith JA: The gastrointestinal system. Clin Immunol Allergy 1982; 2:43–76.

12 Ingelfinger FJ, Lowell FC, Franklin W: Gastrointestinal allergy. N Engl J Med 1949; 241:303.

13 Kurek H: Rozpoznawanie wielonarzadowych objawów alergii na pokarmy przy pomocy prób prowokacyjnych. Bydgoszcz: Akademia Medyczna, 1982. Dissertation.

14 Kurek M, Swiatkowski M, Dziedziczko A, Romański B: Practical value of spirographic and endoscopic examinations in food allergy occurring in asthmatic patients. Xe Congrès d'Interasma (Abstracts) Paris. Respiration [Suppl 1] 1981; 42:26.

15 Kurek M, Swiatkowski M, Kazimierczak H et al: Znaczenie prób prowokacyjnych w rozpoznawaniu alergii na pokarmy u atopików. Wiad Lek 1980; 23: 1995–8.

16 Martens BPM: Some other diagnostic procedures and therapeutic possibilities in food allergy. In: Food Allergy. Utrecht: hal Allergy Service, 1980; 41–5.

17 May ChD, Bock SA: A modern clinical approach to food hypersensitivity. Allergy 1978; 33:166–88.

18 Ortolani C, Pastorello E, Zanussi C: Prophylaxis of adverse reactions to foods. A double-blind study of oral sodium cromoglycate for the prophylaxis of adverse reactions to food and additives. Ann Allergy 1985; 50:105–9.

19 Paviot J, Chavallier R: Les gastropathies allergiques. J Méd Lyon 1936; 17:31–65.

20 Pollard HM, Stuart GJ: Experimental reproduction of gastric allergy in human beings with controlled observations on the mucosa. J Allergy 1942; 13:467–73.

21 Romański B: Mold allergy. State of art. Allergol Immunopathol (Madr) [Suppl] 1980; 8:13–21.

22 Romański B: Researches on the antianaphylactic properties of disodium cromoglycate and Ketotifen. Zentralbl Pharm Pharmakother Laboratoriumsdiagnostik 1983; 122(7):775–80.

23 Romański B, Bokowski W: Alergia typu natychmiastowego u osób z choroba wrzodowa zoladka lub dwunastnicy. Pol Tyg Lek 1983; 38(10):301–4.

24 Romanski B, Bokowski W: Pol Tyg Lek 1986; 6: 181–4.

25 Romański B, Chyliński J, Swiderska A: Odczynowość alergiozna w chorobie wrzodowej zoladka i dwunastnicy. Pol Tyg Lek 1971; 26(15):550–3.

26 Romański B, Kurek M, Swiatkowski M: Study on the protective action of Zaditen in cases of allergic disorders provoked by food allergens. In: Fuchs E, Palm D, eds. Asthma bronchiale, bronchiale Übereregbarkeit, Asthmaprophylaxe. Stuttgart: T K Schattauer, 1982; 111–20.

27 Románski B, Kurek M, Swiatkowski M: Alergia na pokarmy. Bydgoszcz: Akademia Medyczna w Gdańsku, 1983.

28 Romański B, Pawlik-Miśkiewicz K, Wilewska-Kłubo T: Clinical studies on the protective effects of Ketotifen and Intal in atopic asthmatic patients. Allergol Immunopathol (Madr) 1983; 11(1):34–9.

29 Romański B, Dziedziczko A, Pawlik-Miśkiewicz K, et al: Allergy to cockroach antigens in asthmatic patients. Allergol Immunopathol (Madr) 1981; 9(5):427–32.

30 Shay H, Bun DCH: Etiology and pathology of gastric and duodenal ulcer. In: Bockus HL, ed. Gastroenterology, Vol. 1. Philadelphia: WB Saunders, 1963; 420–65.

31 Siegal SC: Food allergy controversies. In: Food allergy. Utrecht: hal Allergy Service, 1980; 25–32.

32 Swiatkowski M: Przydatnoźé endoskopowej próby prowokacji górnego odcinka przewodu pokarmowego w rozpoznawaniu alergii na pokarmy. Bydgoszcz: Akademia Medyczna, 1982. Dissertation.

33 Swiatkowski M, Kurek M, Kakol J, Romański B: Study on the multiorganal manifestations of an acquired form of flour allergy. Xe Congrès d'Interasma (Abstracts) Paris. Respiration [Suppl 1] 1981; 42:23.

34 Wraith DG: The use of sodium cromoglycate in patients with adverse reactions to food. In: Food allergy. Utrecht: hal Allergy Service, 1980; 107–11.

Chapter 54
Intradermal Provocative-Neutralizing Food Testing and Subcutaneous Food Extract Injection Therapy

Joseph B. Miller

Introduction

Since 1911 allergy immunotherapy has been utilized with emphasis on allergenic extracts of inhalants, with little or no attempt to employ immunotherapy for foods. There is obviously no essential difference in the atomic elements or molecular configurations which comprise inhalant versus food allergens, and indeed immunotherapy with food extracts can be effective [1–4, 6–9, 11–15]. However, a different testing procedure, the intradermal method, is required to achieve this effectiveness.

In food testing, the full maintenance treatment dose of each food allergen must be precisely determined during initial intradermal skin testing. Either stronger or weaker dosages than this tend to be ineffective or even symptom-inducing.

This is in contrast to the commonly employed procedure of inhalant testing and immunotherapy, in which a therapeutic extract or multiallergen mix is administered subcutaneously in gradually increasing dosages. Build-up therapy continues over months or years until the maximal tolerated subcutaneous dose, the maintenance treatment dose, of the entire mix or of the most active allergen in the mix is reached.

RESPONSES TO INDIVIDUALIZED TREATMENT DOSES

Utilizing the full optimal maintenance treatment dose of each individual food allergen in the solution from the beginning of therapy has produced some unexpected responses. The first is that relief occurs very rapidly. Most patients can begin to tolerate the majority of their allergenic foods within a few weeks; others, often after the first two or three treatment injections; and some while testing is still in progress.

A second surprising response is that the subcutaneously administered food extract injection may be therapeutic as well as prophylactic. Relief can often be obtained even after a food has been taken and produced ill-effects.

Thirdly, self-administration of the treatment dose is safe, as the end-points for each allergen have been specifically measured, thus liberating the patient from the need to visit the doctor for injections.

The rapid-relief phenomenon

During build-up inhalant immunotherapy some patients have reported rapid relief lasting several days or a week following a certain dose of the inhalant mix. However, it did not occur or went unnoticed in the majority of patients.

Until recently there was no technique for deliberately reproducing this rapid-relief effect in the patient. The purpose of this chapter is to describe clinical procedures utilized in food-sensitive patients that have achieved the rapid-relief phenomenon with a high degree of effectiveness, reliability and safety.

Definition of provocation–neutralization

Initially the test procedure required to determine precise therapeutic doses was called the intradermal 'provocative' method [5]. This was because it was felt that the aetiological role of an allergenic food could only be shown by 'provoking' symptoms with an intradermal injection of an extract of the suspect food. Provoked symptoms could then be relieved ('neutralized'), usually in minutes, by the intradermal injection of a different strength of the same food extract. It soon became evident that symptom provocation was not necessary, and indeed did not always occur during testing even in the presence of known sensitivity to the food.

It became clear that the optimal therapeutic dose could usually be found by carefully observing wheal patterns even in the absence of symptom production. This led to the description of the procedure known as the 'relieving dose method', the 'neutralizing dose method', the 'definitive dose method' and the 'individualized treatment dose method'.

The term 'neutralizing method' seems to have become the more generally accepted. It will be used in this chapter with the clear acknowledgement that the term is only descriptive of symptom relief and does not indicate a known specific molecular or cellular mechanism.

Neutralization procedure

The neutralization procedure includes both diagnostic and therapeutic facets. The diagnostic facet consists in determining the neutralizing or optimal therapeutic concentration of each allergen through intradermal testing with various concentrations of an extract of the allergen being tested.

The treatment facet consists in combining in a vial the neutralizing dose of each of the allergenic foods, and in administering the combined treatment solution subcutaneously.

Testing materials. The food extracts (Tables 54.1 and 54.2) are available on a weight vol-

Table 54.1 Extracts on the 'A' tray.

Beef	Pork
Chicken	Potato
Chocolate	Soya bean
Corn	Beet sugar
Egg	Cane sugar
Cow's milk	Wheat
Orange	Baker's yeast
Peanut	Brewer's yeast

ume basis, usually a 1:10 concentration containing 50% glycerin. The presence of 50% glycerin in the extracts provides stability over a long period of time even when not refrigerated and even when serially diluted. Aqueous (non-glycerinated) extracts tend to be less stable.

Table 54.2 Extracts on the 'B' tray.

Apple	Lettuce
Celery	Malt
Cinnamon	Oats
Coconut	Onion
Coffee	Green peas
Garlic	Rice
Grape	Stringbean
Lemon	Tomato

Dilutions. The stock extract or 'concentrate' is serially diluted in a 1:5 ratio. Thus if the concentrate is 1:10, the No. 1 vial is 1:50, the No. 2 vial is 1:250 and so on.

To simplify labelling, each vial is labelled only with the name of the food and the number of the dilution, e.g. Beef No. 1, Beef No. 2. A total of nine such vials are prepared for each food extract (Fig. 54.1). Weaker dilutions are prepared when needed. The concentrates are stored elsewhere, not on the testing tray.

Additional materials. Additional materials consist of 10 ml vials, the vial trays and sterile physiological saline diluent containing 0.4% phenol. One useful type of tray holds 16 rows, nine holes deep, for nine serially diluted vials of 16 foods (Fig. 54.2). Sterile plastic disposable 0.5-ml syringes are used for intradermal testing. A syringe once used is discarded. The vial caps and skin are cleansed with alcohol sponges or with double-strength Zephiran sponges made fresh each day. Also available

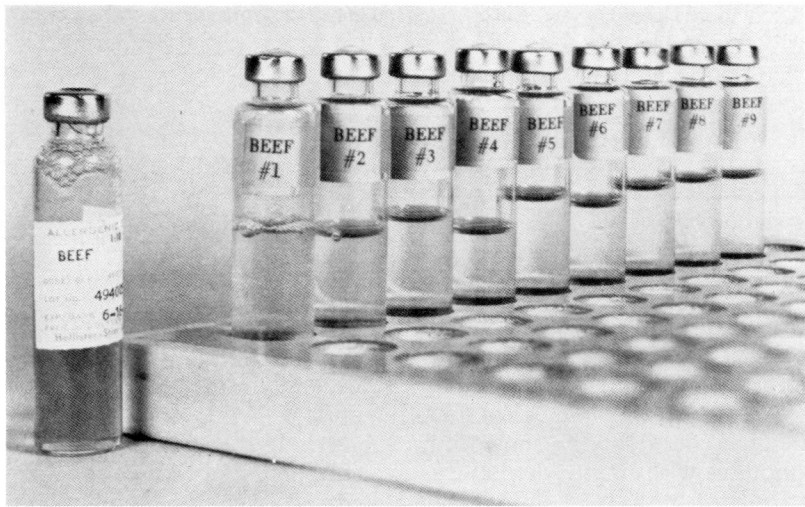

Fig. 54.1 Nine dilutions are prepared for each food concentrate in a 1:5 serial dilution ratio, the No. 1 dilution being the strongest and the No. 9 being the weakest in the series. Reproduced from Miller [7], courtesy of Charles C. Thomas, Publisher, Springfield, Illinois.

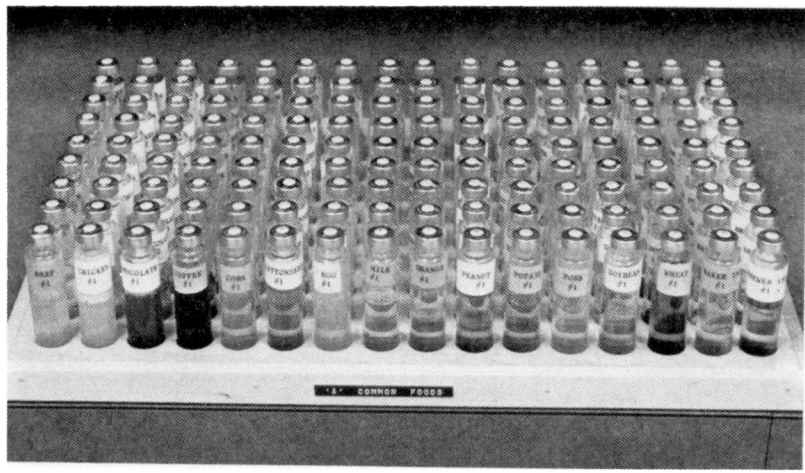

Fig. 54.2 The 'A' tray contains nine dilutions of each of the 16 most common and/or hidden foods. Reproduced from Miller [7], courtesy of Charles C. Thomas, Publisher, Springfield, Illinois.

should be disposable syringes of 3 ml and 12 ml sizes for preparing serial dilutions and treatment sets.

The wheal growth must be measured at each 10-minute interval during testing so a suitable ruler is required.

Patient materials

Pretest procedures

A detailed history is taken, and physical examination, laboratory tests (including immunoglobulin levels) and environmental and dietary instructions are given initially as indicated. Medications may be prescribed.

Non-allergic problems may need higher priority care. Testing may be postponed until an intercurrent infection, dyspnoea or other health problem has been controlled to the satisfaction of the physician. Informed consent is obtained, with the patient able to understand and participate in the test and treatment procedures.

Each patient records his or her symptoms during the testing procedure (Fig. 54.3).

Skin tests

Skin prick tests are always performed first including a negative saline control and a positive histamine control.

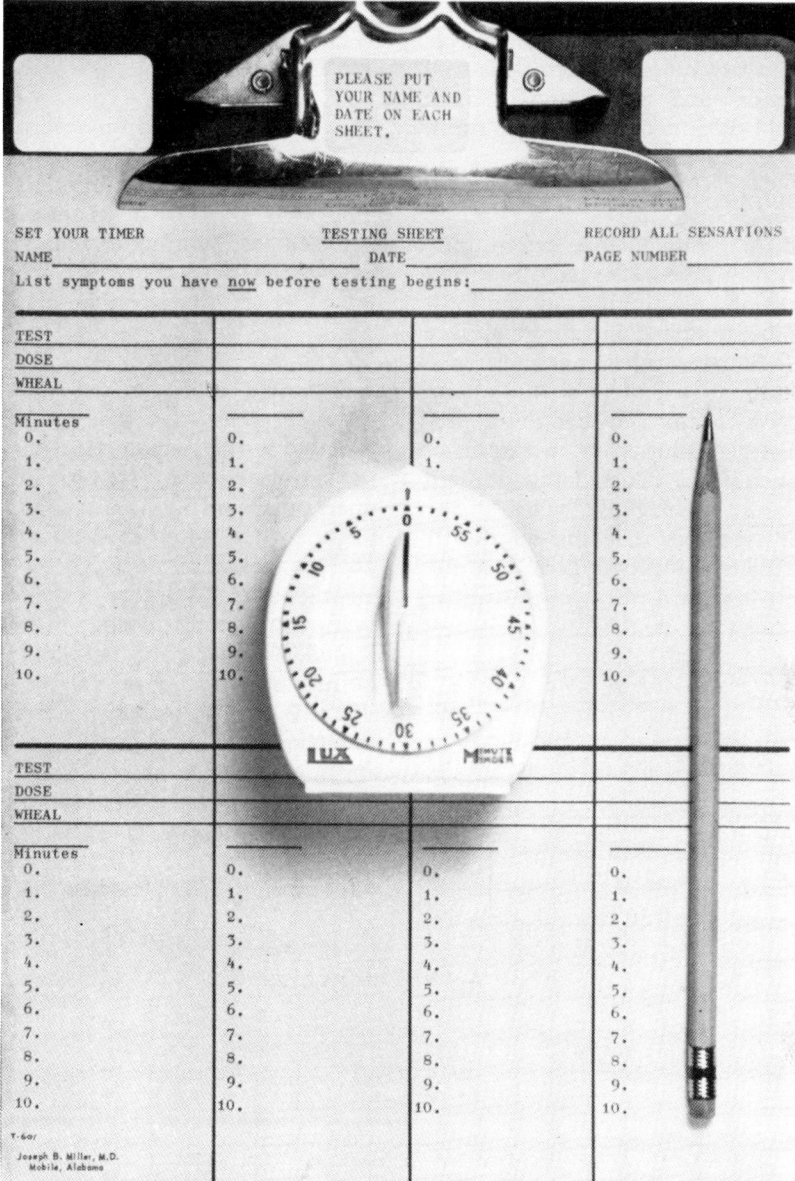

Fig. 54.3 Clipboard, timer, pencil and test sheet on which the patient records his symptoms during testing. Reproduced from Miller [7], courtesy of Charles C. Thomas, Publisher, Springfield, Illinois.

A food which has at any time produced a severe reaction such as anaphylaxis, severe laryngeal oedema or acute asthma is rarely skin tested even by the prick method. On the other hand, there are mild and intermediate degrees of reactivity and there may be some instances where a serial dilution prick test may be employed. Radioallergosorbent tests (RAST) or enzyme-linked immunosorbent assay (ELISA) may be carried out first for some foods in some patients before even considering prick testing for those foods.

Control intradermal injections

The first test injection (control No. 1) consists of a 'dry needle control', using a new empty syringe which has never contained anything, not even saline. The purpose of this injection is to select out psychological factors.

Control No. 2, administered 10 minutes later, consists of non-phenolated saline, control No. 3, saline containing 0.4% phenol and control No. 4, 2% glycerin. This is the same strength glycerin included in dilution No. 2

(1:250), which is usually the strongest dilution used in testing and treatment. These controls further highlight psychological factors as well as irritant reactions and sensitivities to some of the individual diluent materials employed.

Determining neutralizing doses

The two most important factors determining which dilution of a given allergenic food extract is the neutralizing dilution for the individual patient being tested intradermally are symptom relief and whealing. On the neutralizing dilution the patient should obtain relief from any symptoms evoked by a previously administered dilution of an extract of the same antigen. The neutralizing dilution must also produce a 'negative wheal'. The neutralizing or symptom-relieving dilution is usually the strongest dilution which does not produce a positive wheal.

WHEAL CHARACTERISTICS AND TEST VOLUMES

The following description pertains to characteristics of wheals produced by intradermal injection of 0.05 ml of solution. This is the volume which provides optimal correlation between test symptoms and wheal characteristics.

Screening and verifying

A screening test volume of 0.01 ml is also used for preliminary test doses of a given extract. Since this small volume is difficult to read on the syringe marking, the 0.01 ml volume is defined operationally as the volume required to form a wheal 4 mm in diameter. The 0.01 ml volume is accurate enough to be used in injecting various dilutions of an extract until the preliminary neutralizing dilution is determined by either symptom relief or whealing or both. Then the 0.05 ml volume is used to verify the 0.01 ml wheal characteristics and symptom changes, and to complete the test.

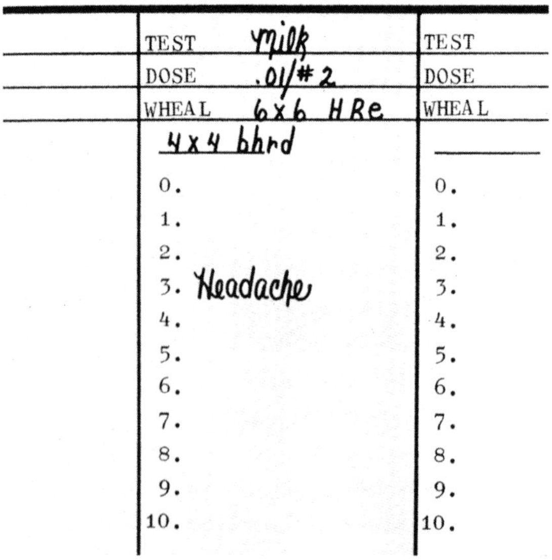

TEST	*milk*	TEST
DOSE	.01/# 2	DOSE
WHEAL	6x6 H Re	WHEAL
	4x4 bhrd	
0.		0.
1.		1.
2.		2.
3.	Headache	3.
4.		4.
5.		5.
6.		6.
7.		7.
8.		8.
9.		9.
10.		10.

Fig. 54.4 Close-up of the test sheet of a patient being tested with 0.01 ml of dilution No. 2 of the milk extract in which his wheal was initially 4 × 4 mm, blanched (b), hard (h), raised (r) and discoid (d), and at the end of 10 minutes was 6 × 6 mm, Hard (H), Raised (R) and erythematous (e). Note that at 3 minutes the patient recorded the onset of headache. Reproduced from Miller [7], courtesy of Charles C. Thomas, Publisher, Springfield, Illinois.

All tests end with a 0.05 ml volume. Thus, the whealing characteristics and symptom changes produced by the 0.05 ml volume are definitive.

Characteristics of wheal positivity

It is not the absolute size of the wheal but rather its growth in average diameter over 10 minutes which is most critical. A positive wheal characteristically grows at least 2 mm in average diameter and is also blanched paperwhite, indurated ('hard' on palpation), markedly elevated ('raised') and with a sharply demarcated peripheral edge which rises abruptly from the surface of the surrounding skin as though a disc had been cemented to the skin ('discoid'). In summary, a typical positive wheal has grown at least 2 mm and is blanched, hard, raised and discoid (Fig. 54.4).

Positive wheals. Any major sign of positivity is significant only by comparison with control wheals and wheals produced by other dilutions of the same extract in the individual patient being tested.

To determine the average diameter of wheal growth the wheal should be measured first across its shorter diameter and then across its longer diameter with an accurate ruler to reach an average (Fig. 54.5). A growth of 2 mm is exemplified by a wheal of 7×7 mm at injection which grows to 9×9 mm in ten minutes. A negative wheal is thus defined as one which grows less than 2 mm in average diameter in 10 minutes and is not blanched, hard, raised or discoid. It is usually neutral coloured and soft and its edges decline gradually into the surrounding skin.

Interestingly, the fluid flow from the underlying capillaries to the wheal is fairly quantitative. A 2 mm growth in average wheal diameter represents the addition by the body of approximately 0.05 ml of fluid into the wheal. A 4 mm growth in wheal diameter represents the addition by the body of 0.10 ml of fluid and so on. This can be verified by injecting saline intradermally in 0.05 ml, 0.10 ml and 0.15 ml volumes. This will usually result in wheals of approximately 7 mm, 9 mm and 11 mm diameters. Consequently, with a ruler, one can fairly accurately quantify the intensity of the local allergic response to a given concentration of allergen (Fig. 54.6).

Some problems in reading wheal sizes. Not all wheals are sharply positive or negative and not all clearly provoke or relieve symptoms. One wheal may grow 2 mm in diameter but not be blanched, hard, raised or discoid. In this instance, consecutively stronger dilutions should be injected until an unequivocal positive wheal is produced; then the next weaker dilution will probably be the neutralizing dilution.

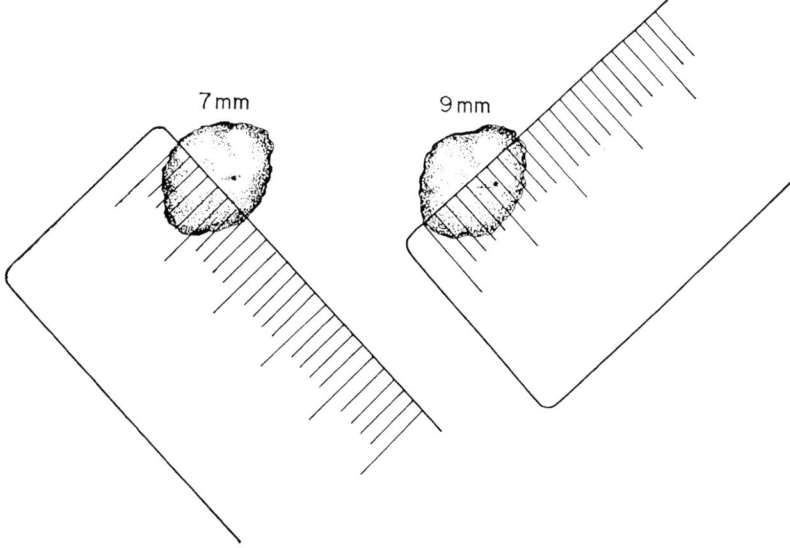

Fig. 54.5 The wheal is measured across its shortest diameter and its longest diameter with an accurate ruler to strike an average. A 7 mm × 9 mm wheal is considered an 8 mm average diameter wheal. Reproduced from Miller [7], courtesy of Charles C. Thomas, Publisher, Springfield, Illinois.

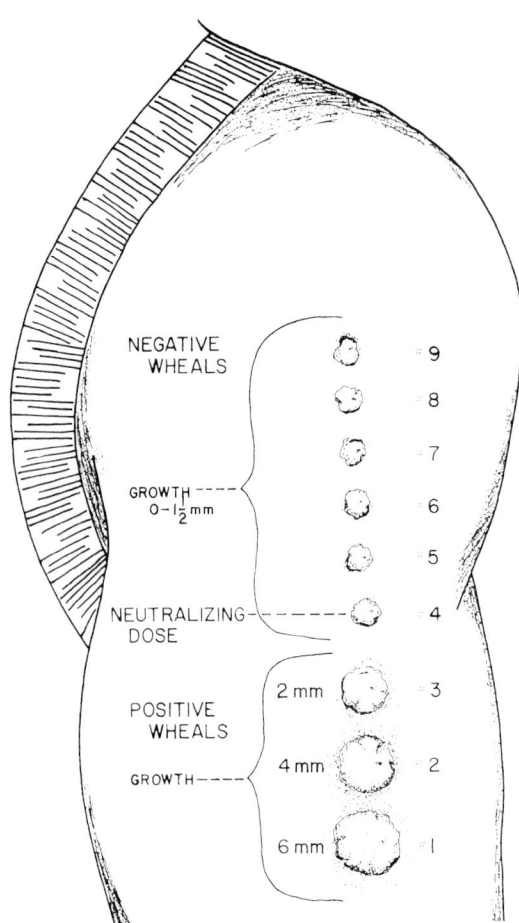

Fig. 54.6 To illustrate the whealing principle in a hypothetical patient, one can imagine that 0.05 ml of each dilution from dilution No. 9 to dilution No. 1 are all injected simultaneously in a vertical column on the arm. In this hypothetical instance, all will produce wheals of about the same size and characteristics at the moment of injection, namely approximately 7 mm average wheal diameter, blanched, hard, raised and discoid. If the neutralizing dilution for this particular antigen is dilution No. 4, then the No. 4 dilution will change to a negative wheal by 10 minutes.

However, the No. 3 will have grown 2 mm to approximately 9 mm, the No. 2 will have grown 4 mm to approximately 11 mm and the No. 1 will have grown 6 mm to approximately 13 mm. Numbers 4–9 may have grown as much as, but usually not more than, 1.5 mm to approximately 8.5 mm.

This is a generalization. The measurements must be made precisely with a ruler in each individual case to determine the growth, and each wheal must be inspected and palpated at the moment of injection and again in 10 minutes to determine the changes in wheal characteristics which accompany negativity and positivity as revealed by the 10-minute evaluation.

Reproduced from Miller [7], courtesy of Charles C. Thomas, Publisher, Springfield, Illinois.

The same procedure is used in patients whose negative wheals tend to be elevated. Proceeding to use consecutively stronger dilutions to produce an unequivocally positive wheal, then dropping back one dilution weaker, will usually produce a wheal which may be elevated but is otherwise totally negative; this is generally the neutralizing dilution.

Symptoms and syndromes often caused by food sensitivity

The syndromes most responsive to food extract injection therapy are migraine (both classical and common types) (see Chapter 37); gastrointestinal syndromes (aphthous stomatitis, irritable bowel, diarrhoea, chronic ulcerative colitis and Crohn's disease) (see Chapter 32); dermatological syndromes (atopic dermatitis, chronic urticaria, angioedema and adult acne) (see Chapters 34–36); and cerebral syndromes (attention deficit disorder, hyperkinesis, learning disability and behaviour problems) (see Chapter 38b). Respiratory and otolaryngological syndromes which have not responded optimally to inhalant immunotherapy and supportive care are also sometimes improved by food extract injection therapy.

The symptoms produced on testing are usually related to the syndrome presented. For example, the headache patient may develop a headache on one test dilution of a given food extract and gain relief of the headache on another. However, there are instances where the symptom induced by testing is not the same as the one induced by natural exposure. This is immaterial to the determination of the neutralizing dilution.

Asymptomatic test patients

Some patients are definitely sensitive to certain foods according to history, repeated oral challenge or both, yet have no symptoms when tested intradermally for these foods. The neutralizing dose can still be determined for each such food by intradermal skin testing.

The usual test method

We use the 0.01 ml volume, the screening volume, for all dilutions, until the strongest negative wheal dilution is determined (Fig. 54.7). This can be termed the presumptive neutralizing dilution.

Then 0.05 ml of this dilution is administered for verification. If this produces a negative wheal it verifies the negativity of the 0.01 ml

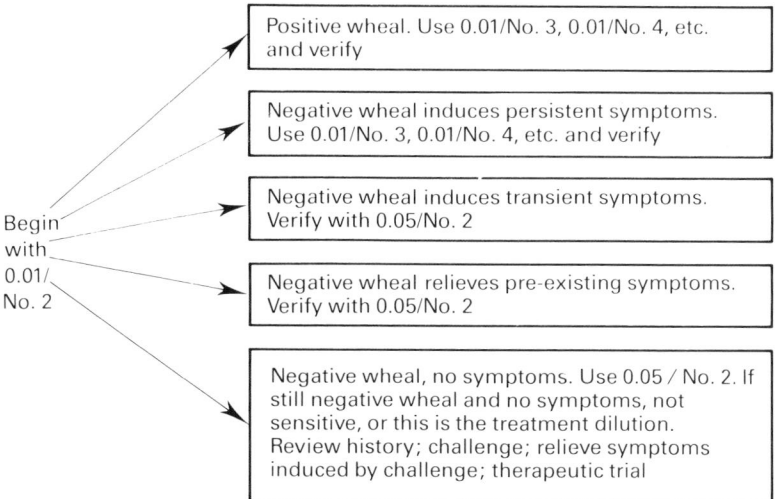

Fig. 54.7 The usual test method. After appropriate and comprehensive evaluation, including history, physical, laboratory tests and a listing of suspected food sensitivities, testing is begun with 0.01 ml of the No. 2 dilution of one of the most frequently eaten and least likely allergenic foods in order to establish the patient's test patterns. The initial dose is followed by one of the five possibilities exemplified by the arrows in this illustration. The more hyperallergenic foods in the general population, and the foods considered likely to be more allergenic in this specific patient, may be tested in the sequence illustrated in Fig. 54.8 (method for testing potentially brittle patients); or not tested at all if the history of reactivity is of a major degree or in a vital organ.

wheal. If no symptoms occur on 0.05 ml of the negative wheal dilution it is the neutralizing dilution.

On the other hand, if symptoms occur and persist or worsen with the 0.05 ml verifying dose, testing must proceed with consecutively weaker dilutions to find the strongest symptom-relieving negative wheal dilution. It is usually just one or two dilutions weaker.

In this situation, while proceeding with weaker dilutions than the strongest negative wheal dilution, one can revert to the use of 0.01-ml test volumes to minimize symptoms if indicated. However, once the strongest symptom-improving negative wheal dilution is determined with the 0.01 ml volume, the test is always concluded with a 0.05 ml volume of that dilution to provide adequate and prolonged symptom clearing.

If symptoms worsen on a given negative wheal dilution while proceeding consecutively weaker, these symptoms can be neutralized by administering consecutively *stronger* dilutions. The neutralizing dilution is usually just one dilution stronger.

The test method for potentially brittle patients

A brittle patient is one who is considered to have a greater than average potential for experiencing serious symptoms on testing. This may be because of a history of anaphylaxis, laryngeal oedema or acute asthma.

It may also be because of a history of prolonged usage of steroids, the concomitant usage of β-blockers, poor or adverse response to adrenaline (epinephrine) injections in the past, the need for multiple medications, or extreme sensitivity to a wide variety of drugs, chemicals and other substances. Included also are debilitated, very elderly, psychotic or convulsive patients; patients with lung, liver, kidney or heart disease; patients with dysrhythmia, repeated cerebral ischaemia, strokes or other cardiovascular problems; and patients who are pregnant, particularly in the first trimester. Since there are many possibilities, the prudence of the physician is critical.

Many of these patients should not be tested at all. Some can be helped by rotary diets, elimination diets with very cautious reintroduction of certain individual foods, avoidance of food mixtures and avoidance of factory-made foods with unknown or multiple ingredients [10].

If the risk/benefit ratio is such that a decision is made to test a potentially brittle patient, the first foods tested should be foods which are eaten regularly with no known symptoms and which the patient considers his 'safest' foods. The starting test dose for the first food may be 0.01 ml of dilution No. 4, No. 8 or weaker (Fig. 54.8).

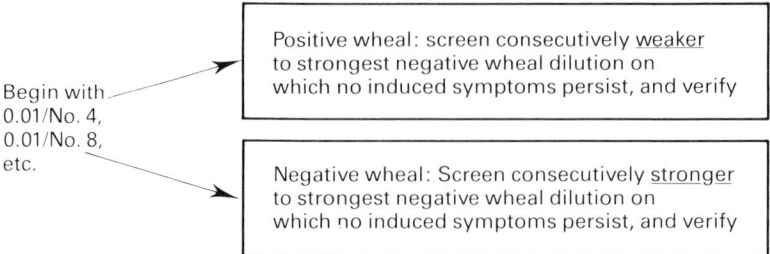

Fig. 54.8 Method for testing potentially brittle patients. Potentially brittle patients are tested with 0.01 ml of a weaker dilution than in non-brittle patients. The weakness of the first injection depends on the physician's judgment as to the severity of the patient's known or suspected reactions; whether or not the reactions were in a vital organ such as the larynx, bronchi or heart; or whether they were simply severe degrees of itching, headache, abdominal bloating or other such symptoms in non-vital organs.

As one screens with consecutively stronger dilutions, the wheals are likely to be negative in this range and only minor symptoms are likely to occur. When one finally reaches the first positive wheal dilution, e.g. dilution No. 3, the next step is to verify with 0.05 ml of the next weaker dilution, e.g. 0.05 ml of dilution No. 4 in this instance, and complete the test as already described. The second food tested in a brittle patient usually can be started with 0.01 ml of one dilution stronger than the neutralizing dilution of the first food, except that dilution No. 1 is not used.

Food test reactions can be severe in a small minority of patients. These patients should be selected out in advance and special precautions taken if indicated.

Supportive measures for potentially brittle patients

An emergency tray with adrenaline, injectable antihistamines and steroids, intravenous fluids, oxygen and other medications and equipment must be at hand in case of need.

In some patients such as asthmatics, testing should be postponed until their symptoms have been adequately controlled with medications and they are no longer wheezing, dyspnoeic, tired, infected or obstructed by impacted bronchial mucus.

Drugs that can affect whealing

Theophylline products rarely if ever affect whealing. Sus-Phrine (sustained action adrenaline) can be administered subcutaneously in small dosage (0.01–0.05 ml) before, during or after testing to prevent or lessen the degree of test symptoms, or prevent nocturnal symptoms. In such an instance a 5 cm diameter circle is drawn around the site of the Sus-

Phrine injection. Subsequent intradermal test doses are unaffected by the Sus-Phrine so long as they are not injected within this circle.

Steroids. Protective steroids do not affect whealing and should not be discontinued just prior to testing in patients who require them. Steroid dosage should be resumed, continued or increased if deemed necessary until testing has been completed and immunotherapy has progressed to the point that gradual steroid reduction can be considered.

Some patients on long-term steroid therapy now or in the past often have poor physiological and immunological reserves and possibly should not be tested at all.

Antihistamines. The effect of antihistamines is varied. Chlorpheniramine is less apt to affect whealing than hydroxyzine. Some antidepressants and tranquillizers have antihistaminic or anticholinergic effects and can diminish whealing. These as well as β-blockers, which interfere with adrenaline activity, should be discontinued if possible for a week before testing. If the prick test with histamine (the positive prick control) is negative, testing should be postponed until medications with antihistaminic properties have been eliminated long enough to allow the histamine prick test to become positive.

It is not the intention to convey the impression that the use of any or all of these medications and other protective measures makes it safe to test all patients to all foods. There are some patients who are so sensitive, or so steroid dependent, or so ill, or so potentially complicated, that they should not be tested at all.

Daily post-test injections

At the end of the first test day, a subcutaneous injection containing all the neutralizing doses clearly determined that day is administered midway on the lateral aspect of the upper arm. The patient is then observed for at least 30 minutes. The usual result of this injection is that the patient actually feels better, or at least no worse, verifying the correctness of the neutralizing doses determined thus far.

At the end of the second day, a similar subcutaneous injection is administered containing all the neutralizing doses clearly determined on both days. Each day, a cumulative post-test injection is repeated, and many patients note steady improvement while still being tested.

On the other hand, if a post-test injection induces symptoms, the patient can be given Sus-Phrine and other protective medications, and should be instructed to return the next day for retesting to determine which allergen caused the symptoms. Usually, the culprit allergen can be determined by a study of the test sheets, and it may be necessary to retest only the one allergen rather than all, or simply delete it from future treatment sets and avoid it in the diet.

Retesting

Occasionally the neutralizing dose may change, for example, following a period of therapy, a virus infection, a change of season or for no discernible reason. When this occurs the formerly effective injection may cause a local reaction at the injection site, or may no longer protect from symptoms when some foods are eaten or may even cause some symptoms.

Retesting and preparing a fresh therapeutic extract containing the currently needed doses usually eliminates local and systemic side-effects and restores effectiveness immediately. Retesting is also performed for any patient who has omitted to use his injections for 2 months, since there may have been some dosage changes during that interval.

Retesting is usually begun with 0.01 ml of the dilution one stronger than the old treatment dilution to establish the positive wheal landmark. In some patients, 0.01 ml of the old treatment dilution is used as the initial retest dose.

In patients with minor syndromes such as mild diarrhoea who have been under treatment for a long period of time and have been retested before with few, mild or no test symptoms, the beginning dose volume might be 0.05 ml after the first few allergens have been retested. However, hyperallergenic foods and foods suspected or known to have caused major symptoms in the past are usually screened with 0.01 ml, even on retesting. After the initial dose of a given allergen has been chosen, the pathways for retesting are the same as described for testing.

Emergency kits

All allergy patients are supplied with an emergency kit at the first office visit. Meticulous instructions for its use are provided verbally and then issued to the patient in printed form. The kit usually contains adrenaline 1:1000, and tablets of an antihistamine and a steroid. For those who cannot swallow tablets, prescriptions for liquid preparations are substituted. In some instances, prescriptions for a vial of Sus-Phrine 1:200 and vials of an injectable antihistamine and steroid are added. Syringes and alcohol sponges in aluminium foil are also included.

Selection and order of testing foods

All patients fill out a food history form (Fig. 54.9) before or during the first appointment, listing which foods are eaten at least daily, about twice a week or less than twice a week. They also list all foods not eaten at all because they may now or in the past have caused symptoms, or are not eaten at all even though they have never caused symptoms. Repeated food histories are then taken, a diet diary is begun (Fig. 54.10) and a four-column food ledger (Fig. 54.11) is prepared listing (a) foods eaten regularly with no known symptoms, (b) foods which definitely cause mild symptoms, (c) foods which the patient suspects of causing mild symptoms but is unsure and (d) foods either suspected or known to have caused severe symptoms now or in the past.

Testing is begun with the foods in the first column, i.e. those which form the staples of the patient's diet and are not known to cause symptoms. Although these are the best-tolerated foods so far as the patient knows, it is surprising how often on testing some of these foods do reproduce the patient's syndromes to some extent.

By the time the first column of foods has been tested and the patient has had one or more post-test treatment injections, his

FOOD HISTORY

Name _____ Date _____

Please list these foods in the appropriate columns below, as to frequency in your diet:

Beef	Salmon	Brewers yeast	Soybean
Potato	Tuna	Onion	Carrots
Apple	Green peas	Tea	Cinnamon
Chicken	Tomato	Lemon	Coconut
Rice	Lettuce	Snapper	Garlic
Stringbeans	Peach	Codfish	Malt
Pork	Turkey	Asparagus	Mustard
Banana	Sweet potato	Cabbage	Oats
Coffee	Celery	Cucumber	Grape
Milk	Orange	Pear	Spinach
Egg	Corn	Pineapple	Turnip greens
Cane sugar	Wheat	Cottonseed	Kidney beans
Beet sugar	Bakers yeast	Peanut	Lima beans

A	B	C	D	E	F	G	H
Eat more than once each day	Eat about once each day	Eat about 2-3 times a week	Eat about once each 1-2 weeks	Eat less than two weeks apart	Never eat it, as do not care for it	Eat but it may bother me	Never eat it, as it bothers me

List additional foods and beverages taken at least once a week: _____
_____

List all foods and beverages which have ever caused <u>allergic reaction</u> and the type of reaction
caused: _____
_____
_____

List all additional foods which have ever <u>disagreed</u> in any way and how: _____
_____
_____

List all foods you have ever <u>limited or avoided</u> and why: _____

List favorite, particularly enjoyed, or <u>craved</u> foods: _____
_____

SPECIAL FOODS: Circle any which have <u>ever</u> caused symptoms:

Almond	Peanut	Walnut	Crab	Lobster	Shrimp	Buckwheat	Flaxseed	Soybean
Cashew	Pecan	Clam	Fish	Cyster	Egg	Cottonseed	Mustard	Mushroom

Please use back of page for additional information.

Fig 54.9 The preliminary food history. This history is filled out by the patient before or during the first office visit, with additional notations made by the nurse and physician before testing is begun. The procedure enables the physician to choose which tests to begin with in order to establish the test pattern; which to test later once the test pattern is established; and which to omit from testing. The 'special foods list' at the bottom of the page contains many of the most hyperallergenic foods which are often deleted in testing and also avoided from the diet.

		14 DAY DIET DIARY			DATE	

NAME_____

1st DAY	2nd DAY	3rd DAY	4th DAY	5th DAY	6th DAY	7th DAY
SYMPTOMS						
MEDICATION						
BREAKFAST						
SYMPTOMS						
MEDICATION						
LUNCHEON						
SYMPTOMS						
MEDICATION						
DINNER						
SYMPTOMS						
MEDICATIONS						

RECORD FOODS AND MEDICATIONS IN BLUE AND SYMPTOMS IN RED. (over)

8th DAY	9th DAY	10th DAY	11th DAY	12th DAY	13th DAY	14th DAY
SYMPTOMS						
MEDICATION						
BREAKFAST						
SYMPTOMS						
MEDICATION						
LUNCHEON						
SYMPTOMS						
MEDICATION						
DINNER						
SYMPTOMS						
MEDICATION						

RECORD FOODS AND MEDICATIONS IN BLUE AND SYMPTOMS IN RED.

Fig. 54.10 The diet diary. This is an example of a 14-day diet diary containing space for entries concerning foods ingested and symptoms experienced, with 7 days' notations on each side of a single sheet.

NAME				DATE	
FOOD LEDGER					
TOLERATED	**POSSIBLE MILD SYMPTOMS**		**DEFINITE MILD SYMPTOMS**		**POSSIBLE OR DEFINITE SEVERE SYMPTOMS**
FOOD	FOOD	SYMPTOM	FOOD	SYMPTOM	FOOD	SYMPTOM

Fig 54.11 The food ledger. The patient begins filling out this ledger during the first office visit. It may be enlarged upon and continued indefinitely as the patient learns more about his sensitivities. It is improved upon by repeated discussions with the nurse and physician. The patient is instructed to bring both the diet diary and the food ledger to the office for re-evaluation at several subsequent visits to 'fine tune' his diet.

allergic burden has been somewhat decreased and he is often feeling better already. This is particularly true if he is careful to eat on each test day chiefly or only the foods to which he is receiving cumulative post-testing injections. However, some patients do not have the discipline to restrict their diets in this manner, and some may develop withdrawal symptoms from some foods omitted, so this dietary system cannot be applied rigidly to all patients.

Next the foods in the second and third columns are tested and cumulative post-testing injections administered subcutaneously at the end of each test day. The foods in the fourth column, i.e. those suspected or known to have caused severe symptoms, must be considered individually. If they are placed in the fourth column because of inducing severe headaches, diarrhoea, itching or other non-life-threatening symptoms, they may be considered for testing. This is particularly true if they are foods which are virtually impossible to avoid because of their presence as a hidden ingredient in many other foods.

However, foods in the fourth column which may have caused life-threatening symptoms such as anaphylaxis, laryngeal oedema or acute asthma are generally not tested at all. If there is an overriding need to test some of these because they cannot be avoided, the foods to be tested may have to be chosen carefully, the patient may have to be premedicated optimally, the test method for potentially brittle patients should be employed and preparations should be made to manage severe reactions should they occur during testing. It is our custom to completely avoid testing such foods.

Hyperallergenic foods

Some foods tend to be more 'hyperallergenic' than others. They are, therefore, approached with greater caution. These include fish, shellfish, egg, nuts, legumes such as peanuts and soya, mustard, buckwheat and mushroom. Some of these may not be tested in some patients. Flaxseed is not tested at all, and cottonseed is tested only under exceptional circumstances.

Treatment instructions

When testing is completed, one injection of the total solution is administered in the office, usually by the patient himself. The patient generally notes improvement, or at least no symptoms, from this injection, particularly since he has usually had several post-test cumulative treatment injections on previous test days to begin building his protection.

Testing may require 3 to 5 days. It is our practice to start teaching self-administration of subcutaneous food extract injections at the end of the first test day, and to continue instructing and supervising self-administration daily if necessary. All treatment injections prepared for home use are made with additional diluent so that the dose is always the same (0.5 ml), regardless of the number of foods included in the solution.

Site of injection. The fleshy portion of the lateral aspect of the arm about midway between the elbow and shoulder is the preferred injection site, although some patients use the lateral aspect of the thigh or the upper outer quadrant of the buttock. It has been our experience that thigh injections occasionally produce residual tenderness, whereas the same injections administered in the arm usually do not.

The patient is instructed to inject the treatment solution subcutaneously three times a week for the first 2 weeks for rapid response, then generally twice a week thereafter. Additional injections can be self-administered at any time for rapid relief whenever symptoms occur from ingestion of a food included in the treatment solution.

It is perfectly safe to use them daily if necessary. In fact this is sometimes prescribed for the first few days for patients who need them. As the protective effect builds up, the injections can soon be spaced to every other day and finally to twice a week.

The use of these procedures in patients with food sensitivities can clarify the issue as to whether or not food extract injection therapy can be clinically effective.

REFERENCES

1 Boris M, Shiff J, Weindorf S et al: Broncho-provocation blocked by neutralization therapy. J Allergy Clin Immunol 1983; 7:92.

2 Forman RA: Critique of evaluation studies of sublingual and intracutaneous provocative tests for food allergy. Med Hypotheses 1981; 7:1019-27.

3 Forman RA: Medical resistance to innovation. Med Hypotheses 1981; 7:1009-17.

4 King D: Can allergic exposures provoke psychological symptoms? A double-blind test. Biol Psychiatry 1981; 16:317.

5 Lee C: A new test for diagnosis and treatment of food allergies. Buchanan County Med Bull 1961; 25:9.

6 Mandell M, Conte A: The role of allergy in arthritis, rheumatism and polysymptomatic cerebral, visceral and somatic disorders: a double-blind study. J Int Acad Prev Med 1982; July: 5-6.

7 Miller JB: Food allergy: provocative testing and injection therapy. Springfield, Ill: Charles C Thomas, 1972.

8 Miller JB: Technique of intradermal testing and sub-cutaneous injection therapy. Trans Am Soc Ophthalmol Otolaryngol Allergy 1976; 16(1): 154-68.

9 Miller JB: A double-blind study of food extract injection therapy. Ann Allergy 1977; 38(3):185-91.

10 Miller JB: Hidden food ingredients, chemical food additives and incomplete food labels. Ann Allergy 1978; 41 (2):93-8.

11 Miller JB: Neutralization therapy update. In: Spencer JT, ed. Allergy—immunologic and management considerations. Miami, Florida: MEDED Publishers, 1982; 43-54.

12 O'Shea J, Porter A: Double-blind study of children with hyperkinetic syndrome treated with multi-allergen extract sublingually. J Learning Disabil 1981; 14: 189-91.

13 Rapp D: Weeping eyes in wheat allergy. Trans Am Soc Opthalmol Otolaryngol Allergy 1978; 1:149-50.

14 Rapp D: Double-blind confirmation and treatment with milk sensitivity. Med J Aust. 1978; 1:571-2.

15 Rapp D: Food allergy treatment for hyperkinesis. J Learning Disabil 1979; 12: 42-50.

Chapter 55
Concept of an Environmental Unit

Donald E. Sprague and Melody J. Milam

Introduction

For some patients, an outpatient approach to diagnosing food allergies fails to produce the desired results. Pollutants encountered in the home and in transit to the testing facility can either cloud symptoms provoked by intradermal challenge or interfere with attempts to clear symptoms through intradermal neutralization. Food and chemical overload may be so severe that any increase in stress, such as antigen testing, elicits acute and, sometimes, life-threatening symptoms. In such cases, admitting the patient to an environmental control unit (ECU) has several benefits.

OBJECTIVES FOR AN ENVIRONMENTAL CONTROL UNIT (ECU)

Pollution-free environment

First, the ECU provides a relatively pollution-free environment with respect to food, air and water. This ensures reduction of the total load of contaminants. Patients in an overload state often show sensitivity to sub-toxic levels of commonly occurring chemicals (e.g. formaldehyde) as well as foods. Physical allergens such as pollens, dust, moulds, water and food contaminants, as well as inhaled ambient doses of chemicals (e.g. car exhaust), may provoke hypersensitive reactions [5, 13, 16, 17, 24, 27]. Such agents may then interact with one another, producing multiple cellular insults in an additive or synergistic manner to produce either generalized inflammatory disease or a change in one end organ. Most food-sensitive patients have been observed to show pollutant or chemical sensitivities which either facilitate the development of food allergies and/or trigger specific food reactions [20]. Once the load is reduced, reactions occurring with allergen challenge become more clearly defined and allow more precise, reproducible relationships between allergens and reactions.

Patient education

The second major purpose of an ECU is comprehensive patient education. The ECU programme, lasting on average 2 weeks, provides an opportunity for the most intensive learning course of cause and effect relationships in environmental illness. Not only do patients experience and observe their own reactions to foods, chemicals and inhalants, but they also begin to recognize those reactions in others. Thus confidence that symptoms are not psychosomatic develops quickly and is reinforced consistently where appropriate by staff and fellow patients.

Homeostatic stability

Third, placement in a clean environment allows the patient's homeostatic mechanisms to achieve stability. Masking of symptoms has occurred as an adaptive response to repeated exposures to harmful substances, both food and chemical. Metabolic pathways adjust to those recurring events so that body functioning is altered and abnormal [26]. Randolph [16,17] observed that some patients tend to seek out exposures to the very substances that were harming them. They may even exhibit dependence (addiction) on the presence of the stressor (apparently to keep the metabolism in an altered state of homeostasis to which it had become adjusted). Sudden removal of the substance then creates a withdrawal phenomenon [15].

Caffeine. Caffeine is an excellent example of a substance to which people may become addicted, although alcohol or heroin would serve as well. Initial intake provides a pleasant stimulating experience which is followed by a return to normal (Fig. 55.1a–e). The intake is

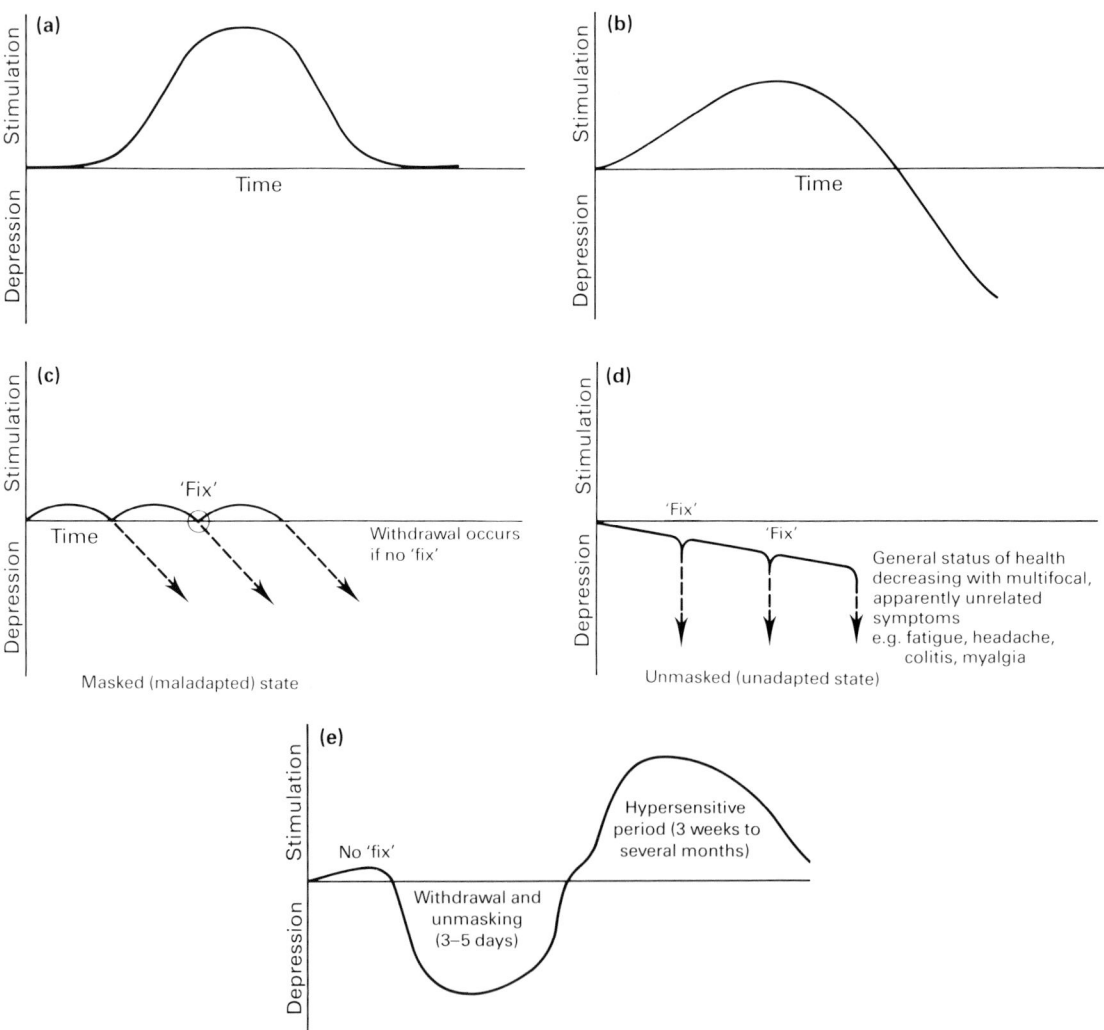

Fig. 55.1 Time course of caffeine addiction: (a) caffeine stimulation; (b) bipolarity; (c) 'fix' to mask withdrawal symptoms; (d) unmasking; (e) withdrawal.

then repeated on a regular basis. However, with repeated exposure (over months or years), the 'high' is not so high, and as the caffeine level drops, the individual doesn't feel quite up to par (Fig. 55.1b). Eventually there is no 'high', but without frequent intake of caffeine the individual begins to 'crash'. At this point, he takes a 'fix'. Thus the caffeine is taken not for its stimulatory effect but to prevent withdrawal symptoms (Fig. 55.1c). The patient enters a masked (adapted) state which may continue for years or even a life time depending on the individual's biological reserves (enzyme stores, etc.). However, once this reserve is depleted the patient will begin to unmask (unadapt), and symptoms begin to surface, often apparently unrelated to the offending substance (e.g. frequent headaches, colitis, hypertension) (Fig. 55.1d). Withdrawal symptoms can also occur if the substance to which the patient is addicted is suddenly withdrawn. These symptoms can vary from mild to life threatening. Various components of this sequence of events—stimulation (bipolarity), masking (adaptation), addiction (maladaptation), withdrawal (unmasking)—can occur with practically any substance whether food or chemical. Withdrawal symptoms following removal of sugar from the diet have certainly been frequently observed, but the same process can occur with wheat, beef, yeast or indeed any food [21].

Fasting. Extensive medically supervised fasting (1–5 days), coupled with environmental controls, allows the patient to unmask in relation to food and chemical substances. Following withdrawal, the patient enters a period of reactivity where exposure to the offending substance can provoke severe reactions (Fig. 55.1e). It is precisely this reactive state, following unmasking, that the physician strives to achieve in the ECU. In this condition, food and chemical testing is more precise and reproducible.

The severity of reaction can be well controlled in the hospital environment. Although food challenge following unmasking performed on an outpatient basis usually works well, it can be dangerous if severe reactions occur.

THE ENVIRONMENTAL CONTROL UNIT

Construction

The environmental control unit studied was constructed specially for the purpose of providing a relatively chemical-free environment and to minimize patient exposure to airborne contaminants (see Fig. 55.2). The walls and ceiling are made of porcelain-covered stainless steel and the floors are ceramic tile. Two sets of doors act as an air lock between the ECU and the rest of the hospital. Lighting consists of incandescent ceiling fixtures; fluorescent lights are avoided because of electromagnetic radiation and fumes.

Filters. The electrical heating and air-conditioning system contains both particulate matter filters (preferably steel mesh) and chemical filters composed of activated charcoal and/or aluminium oxide impregnated with potassium permanganate. In addition, specially treated charcoal filters are utilized to remove not only complex organic molecules, but also simple gas molecules such as formaldehyde. No carpet, particle board, plywood or fibreboard were used as building materials, in order to reduce formaldehyde pollution [18, 19]. Special kitchen facilities are located just adjacent to the ECU to avoid any contamination during food preparation and transport.

Furniture. Patient rooms are devoid of volatile petrochemicals and dust. To ensure this condition, beds and furniture are of metal and formica construction. Sheets, blankets and curtains are made of less chemically contaminated 100% cotton, linen or silk previously laundered in pure non-detergent vegetable or animal soap or just with water. Mattresses are composed of similar cotton with all plastic removed [18]. Rooms are cleaned regularly with borax, non-chlorinated cleaner and water. Bathrooms are equipped with ultraviolet lighting, shielded at eye level, to inhibit mould growth (mould has been a problem for some patients).

Clothing. Patients are required to remain in the ECU unless special tests are required that necessitate a brief transit to another department of the hospital. Less chemically contaminated 100% cotton clothing is provided and all hair sprays, perfumed products, cosmetics and polyester clothing must be avoided during the course of the programme. Visitors to the ECU must utilize cotton gowns over street clothing and may not enter while wearing any odorous materials or chemicals. No smoking is allowed in the ECU at any time. Patient's medications are discontinued upon admission

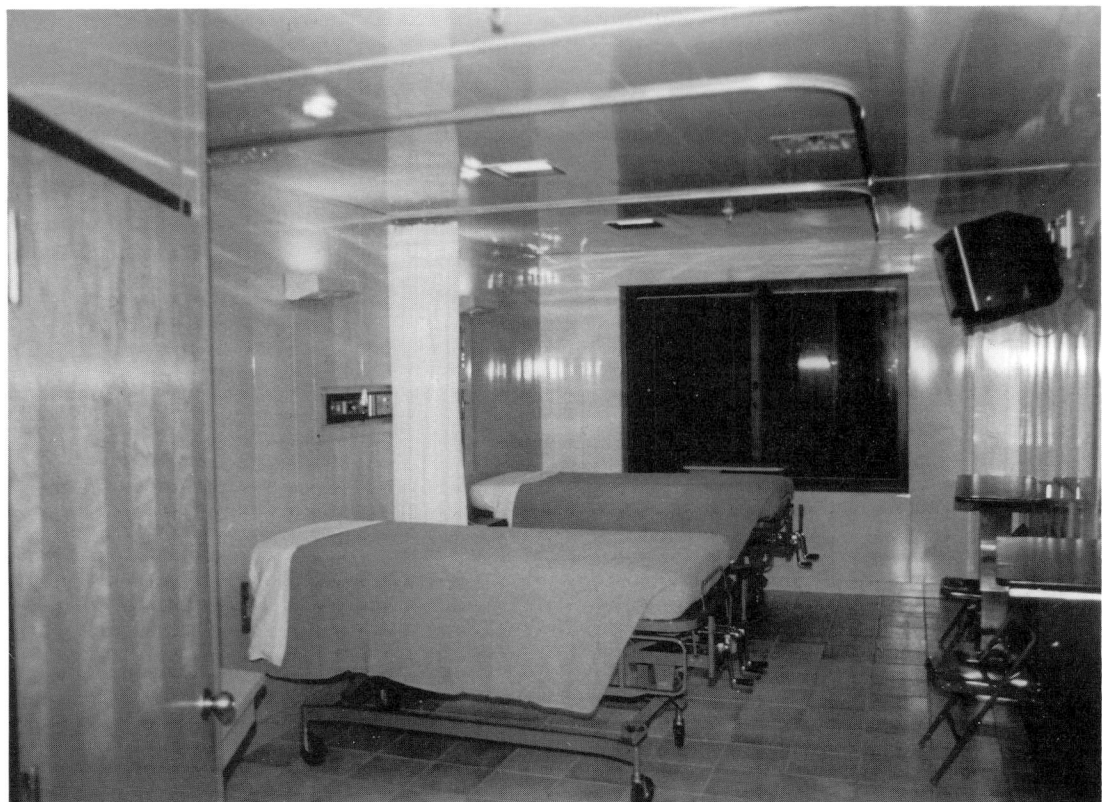

Fig. 55.2 ECU patient room.

with only rare exceptions made (e.g. cortico-steroids are gradually reduced to avoid placing the patients in a crisis).

Air analysis

Trace air analysis is performed at the ECU to determine organic, inorganic and particulate pollutants inside the Unit in comparison with non-environmentally controlled areas of the hospital and the area outside the hospital. As a result of the air-filtering system, and rigorous controls in the operation of the ECU, contaminant levels are generally significantly lower [2, 6].

Organic air pollutants. In general, the major organic air pollutants were observed in smaller concentrations inside the ECU, except for a few substances such as tetrachloroethylene (dry-cleaning fluid) where ECU concentrations exceeded corridor values. These values were probably transient, being caused by outgassing from individuals wearing dry-cleaned clothing. No polyhalogenated aromatic hydrocarbons such as pesticides or herbicides were found in the ECU.

Some contaminants such as formaldehyde originate inside the building, particularly in the conventional facilities of the hospital. An exchange of contaminants between the Unit and the rest of the hospital probably occurs as a result of the unavoidable traffic between the two.

THE ECU PROGRAMME

Patients

Individuals admitted to the ECU come from around the world with diagnoses that are rarely well established beforehand. Food and chemical hypersensitivities are frequently the underlying causes of symptoms but patients in the ECU are screened carefully to rule out other disorders.

Diagnosis

The provisional diagnoses on admission to the ECU are usually multiple since true end-organ disease of many systems is often well established, and patients may present with almost any disorder including asthma, multiple sclerosis, ventricular arrhythmia and arthritis or a full-blown psychosis. The environmental triggering phenomena are usually multifactorial and polysymptomatic.

Protocol

The present ECU protocol has evolved over the last 12 years since the Dallas programme began:

1 Preadmission evaluation provides a provisional diagnosis.
  (a) History and physical examination and study of medical records.
  (b) Psychological assessment to evaluate the patient in relation to the unit's capability to deal with any cerebral symptoms, and to evaluate the probability of environmental components.
  (c) Nutritional assessment to assess nutritional status, to order necessary diagnostic laboratory studies, to institute initial therapy and to outline an individual food testing programme.
2 Chemical cleaning.
3 Water challenge.
4 Identification of allergens:
Food challenge—oral and intradermal.
Natural inhalant challenge—intradermal.
Chemical challenge—inhalation and intradermal.
5 Laboratory analysis—summary of tests and results.
6 Patient education.
7 Stress management.

Psychobehavioural assessment

Almost all patients have symptoms associated with psychological overlay (with the possible exception of asthmatics and arthritics who tend towards a single target organ) and an extensive neuropsychological study is useful.

Psychologists administer a complete test battery consisting of the Wechsler Adult Intelligence Scale, Clinical Analysis Questionnaire, Bender Gestalt Test of Motor Ability, Psychological Rating Scale for DSM III (partial) and a brief neuroscreen. Patients are tested both pre- and post-treatment for three reasons:

1 To rule out or differentially diagnose psychological disorders.
2 To assess the neuropsychological effect of ecological disorder and to objectively demonstrate cerebral changes occurring as a result of treatment in the ECU.
3 To determine interactional effects of ecological illness with other factors (emotional stress, interpersonal relationships, etc.).

Patients may appear to fit the clinical picture of psychotic disorder, or of the neurotic triad of hypochondriasis, depression and hysteria with phobic response to disease. However, support for a somatopsychic rather than psychosomatic diagnosis can be gained from provocation and subsequent remission of symptoms during food-chemical challenge and neutralization (Butler 1981, unpublished observations).

Nutritional assessment, diagnosis and treatment

Gastrointestinal dysfunction ranging from vomiting and diarrhoea to irritable bowel syndrome has repeatedly been attributed to food allergy and intolerance (see Chapter 32). The associated malabsorption results in vitamin/mineral deficiencies that can cause further acquired immune dysfunction [1, 4, 7].

A clearcut pattern of vitamin deficiencies has emerged. In 1982, serum vitamin assays (B_{1-6}, B_{12}, folic acid, vitamins A, E and C) were performed on 120 environmental patients prior to initiation of a rotary diet. Recent functional vitamin assays on 150 patients concur (Fig. 55.3).

Why do deficiencies occur? It is not clearly understood why these deficiencies occur but several theories are proposed:

1 A diet of highly refined/processed foods, or of high sugar content may increase utilization of B and C vitamins.
2 Alteration of nutrient metabolism (reduced serum and tissue storage, impairment of transport mechanisms or destruction of enzyme systems).
3 Genetic predisposition.
4 Increased need for nutrients due to handling of environmental factors such as carcinogens, chemical by-products, pesticides/herbicides, gaseous irritants, heavy metals or drugs.
5 Stress—emotional, physical (due to disease processes) and environmental.

Range of nutritional problems. The range of nutritional problems varies from acute and life-threatening malnutrition to chronic, low-grade (apparent) digestive enzyme deficiencies resulting in true food intolerance (Fig. 55.4).

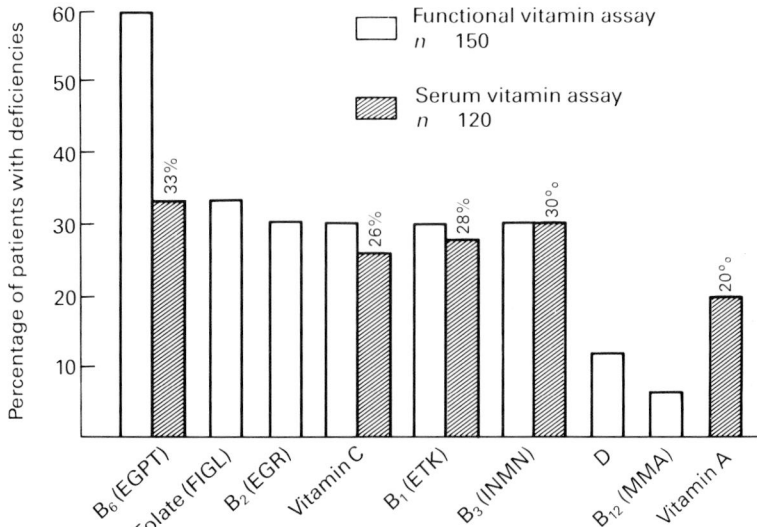

Fig. 55.3 Functional versus serum vitamin deficiencies in ecology patients. □ Functional vitamin assay, N = 150; ■ serum vitamin assay N = 120

Correction of acute deficiencies must occur before meaningful oral and intradermal food challenge can be accomplished.

In patients suffering from malnutrition (severe muscle and/or fat wasting) the therapy of choice is total parenteral nutrition [10]. Nutrients included are crystalline amino acids, dextrose, intralipid and/or vitamin infusions (Table 55.1).

Digestive aids. Some patients benefit from various digestive aids such as hydrochloric acid, betaine or glutamic acid and pancreatic enzymes (amylase, lipase and protease). These may be effective in reducing gastrointestinal distress from protein foods such as meat, fish and/or poultry.

Nutritional supplements. The food origin of most nutritional supplements is extremely important. For example, vitamin B complex produced from brewer's yeast can provoke severe reactions in yeast/mould-sensitive patients. Most of the supposedly natural supplements contain traces or are derived from food particulates (e.g. vitamin C from corn). For this reason, hypoallergenic sources (e.g. free from yeast, corn, mould and sugar) are recommended and often must be rotated.

A patient who is extremely environmentally ill with severe nutritional deficiencies, presents a unique challenge to the physician and is best managed in an environmental unit. Such an individual may react consistently to even the purest available supplements, thus presenting

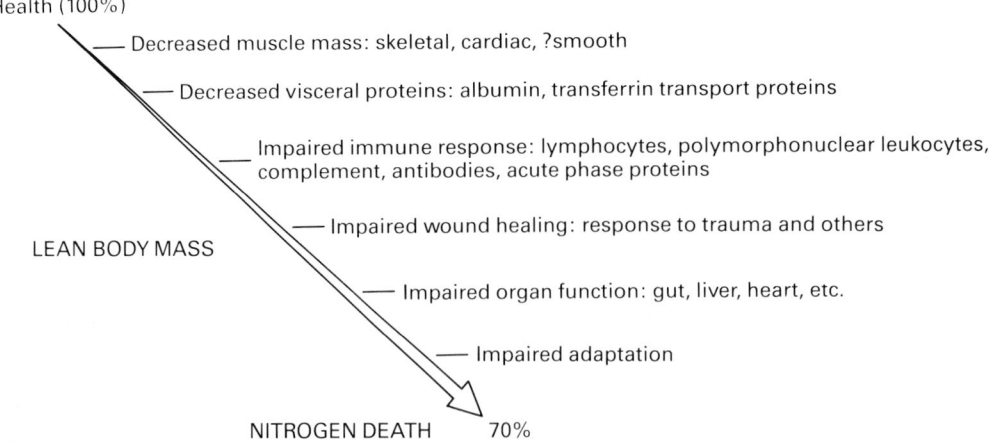

Fig. 55.4 Sequence of clinical and laboratory events in the natural history of starvation. From Heymsfield et al: Ann Intern Med 1979; 90:63–71.

Table 55.1 Nutritional support therapy.

Intravenous alimentation (IVA)
1 Crystalline amino acid solution with or without electrolytes, and multivitamins
2 Lipid solution—intravenous fat emulsion (Liposyn)
3 Regimens: 2-3 litres amino acids solutions
plus
500-1000 ml of Liposyn 10%
(if tolerated)

Enteral hyperalimentation
Vivonex HN = elemental diet of crystalline amino acids with no lactose

Caloric density	1 kcal/ml (full strength)
Protein content	42 g/litre
Protein source	Crystalline amino acids
Fat content	0.9 g/litre
Fat source	Safflower oil
CHO content	210 g/litre
CHO source	Glucose oligosaccharides
mOsm/kg	810

Other therapy
Rotary diet as tolerated—liberalize 2-4 foods/meal
Oral supplements: calcium, minerals, multivitamins, etc.

---

almost insurmountable obstacles to treatment on an outpatient basis. However, this approach is usually successful and no deaths from malnutrition have occurred.

Chemical clearing

During the first 3-5 days in the ECU the patient, unless malnourished, fasts to empty the alimentary canal of food and its associated herbicide/pesticide contamination. Fat-bound pesticides are leached into the blood stream and eliminated.

Symptoms associated with fasting

The fasting patient experiences a myriad of symptoms secondary to unmasking or the withdrawal phenomenon [5, 11]. Exacerbation of presenting symptoms is most common, including headaches, fatigue and muscle aches. Cerebral confusion often increases in the initial stages of the fast.

Hypoglycaemia. Some of the most striking and frequent symptoms are those traditionally associated with hypoglycaemia, possibly due to triggering of prostaglandins and kinins. These symptoms may vary from extreme fatigue, weakness and food craving to a strong sensation of impending loss of consciousness, and mental confusion. Repeated ingestion of the offending food or chemical agent has successfully masked those symptoms previously. An abnormal glucose tolerance test, utilizing dex-

trose (corn-derived) challenge, is an excellent indicator of corn food allergy. True hypoglycaemia, utilizing serum insulin levels, is found in only 2-3 patients per year.

Control of symptoms during fasting. Control of the symptoms produced during early fasting is accomplished by the use of various treatments as outlined in Table 55.2. Once the patient is clear of symptoms, testing and challenge begins.

Table 55.2 Control of symptoms during withdrawal phase.

Tri salts—calcium, sodium, potassium, bicarbonate

Laxatives—promote rapid elimination of incitant

Intravenous ascorbic acid—clears chemically related symptoms

Intravenous sodium bicarbonate—clears food reactions

Nasal oxygen—abates cerebral confusion

Water challenge

During the chemical clearing process, the patient endeavours to find a safe water. Double-blind studies using samples from numerous water sources reveal that approximately 90% of the chemically sensitive patients are intolerant of tap water. Recent reports show that most of our larger cities have severely contaminated water supplies [18].

When testing water, at least 3 hours must pass before a different sample can be tested.

Table 55.3 Volatile organic screening test (VOST) results* for selected EHC: Dallas water samples.

VOST component	Crystal Fresh Water in glass	Mt. Valley Water in glass	Spring House in glass	Spring House in plastic bottles
Benzene	0.01	0.03	—	0.04
Toluene	0.03	0.09	—	0.12
Ethylbenzene	—	—	—	—
Trimethylbenzene	—	0.03	—	—
Xylene	—	—	—	—
Styrene	—	—	—	—
Dichloromethane	0.33	0.05	—	0.92
Chloroform	—	—	—	0.19
Carbon tetrachloride	0.01	0.01	0.01	0.01
Bromoform	—	—	0.02	0.02
Bromodichloromethane	—	0.01	—	0.15
Dibromochloromethane	—	—	—	0.11
Trichloroethane	—	—	—	0.03
Tetrachloroethane	—	—	—	—
Trichloroethylene	—	0.17	—	0.14
Tetrachloroethylene	—	0.11	—	0.07
Chlorobenzene	—	—	—	0.05
Dichlorobenzene	—	—	—	—
Benzaldehyde	—	—	—	—
Methylmercaptan	—	—	—	—

* Reported in $\mu g/l$ = parts per billion. Results are based on gas chromatography–mass spectroscopy data.

Some patients react to distilled water and some to spring waters. Spring water, however, appears to be the most likely tolerated of the available alternatives. Occasionally, patients are unable to tolerate any of the usual sources and must resort to triple distilled, fractionally distilled or reversed-osmosis purified waters. This intolerance may be due to the presence of minerals or low-grade chemical pollution inherent in the bottling process, as contaminants may leach out of plastic containers (Table 55.3).

Identification of incitants

The purpose of food, inhalant and chemical challenge is to document the existence of the disease process and to prepare the patient for coping with the environment after discharge from the unit. The following techniques are utilized:

1 Food challenge—oral and intradermal.
2 Inhalant challenge—intradermal only (pollens, dust, mites, moulds, trees, weeds, grasses, smuts and terpenes).
3 Chemical challenge—by inhalation and intradermally (where indicated).

Food challenge (oral)

Oral food challenge is the basis of diagnosis of food allergy or intolerance, forming the standard to which other testing methods are com-

pared [8]. In an ECU setting, the patient and physician are able to identify clearly the various target organs affected by a particular food and evaluate the severity of these reactions. Thus the patient can recognize the early onset, the probable incitant, and take steps to abort or ameliorate a food reaction after returning home. For details of food challenge and rotation diets see Chapters 17, 46 and 57.

Initially, only less chemically contaminated foods are challenged as outlined in Chapter 22.

Food testing begins once symptoms provoked during fasting are cleared. The patient records symptoms such as pulse rate (see Chapter 56); at the same time, any other signs and symptoms are noted along with duration and intensity. These signs may include changes in blood pressure, ECG, pulmonary function, joint size, etc. Severe reactions are treated with alkali salts, intravenous or rectal ascorbic acid, laxatives and/or enemas made up using the patient's 'safe' water. Persistence of residual symptoms requires that fasting begin once more until the patient is clear. For an outline of the food challenge see Appendix 55.1.

Nutritional programme

Nutritional counsellors design an individual nutrition programme consisting of three phases.

Phase one is initiated upon admission to the

ECU. The diet plan chosen depends upon diagnosis, availability of foods in the patient's home area and personal preferences.

Phase two begins on completion of food testing and yields a programme for home use.

Phase three is effective upon a follow-up visit to the clinic. The diet is re-evaluated at that time and a maintenance programme is established.

Treatment of food allergy

Treatment of food allergy consists of:

1 Identifying the specific allergen by oral food challenge or intradermal testing and taking the relevant treatment (see Chapters 59, 61).
2 A rotary diversified food diet (see Chapter 17). The direct benefits of rotation are to reduce the total load and reduce the likelihood of new food sensitivities developing.

Foods producing strong reactions are eliminated from the diet for several months. After that the offending food can be rechallenged on an outpatient basis until no symptoms are noted. The majority of patients can become tolerant of most of their foods over a 1–2-year period. However, there are some foods that some patients cannot tolerate no matter how long they are avoided.

Initial work with food allergy relied strongly on elimination diets [25]. It has also been repeatedly observed that elimination combined with subsequent oral food challenge is an excellent diagnostic tool [11]. However, elimination diets have limited long-term therapeutic value. Patients treated by elimination alone frequently develop a whole new set of food allergies.

Food challenge (intradermal)

Intradermal food testing in the ECU is used primarily for symptom neutralization and thus treatment. Used on conjunction with oral food challenge, the Lee–Miller provocative neutralization technique provides a means for relieving and aborting symptoms through injections of mini-doses of specific incitant foods (see Chapter 54). Double-blind studies conducted in the ECU show that injection of food extracts protects subjects from reactions induced by food challenge [22]. The patient may utilize this technique to reduce reactivity during the re-adaptation period following discharge from the ECU.

During hospitalization, patients may devote a substantial amount of time to intradermal testing. Approximately half of this testing consists of neutralization of symptoms provoked by oral food challenge.

Natural inhalant challenge (intradermal)

In order to further reduce total load, natural inhalants (e.g. dust, moulds, weeds, grasses and trees) are tested intradermally. Intradermal testing by serial dilution titration (SDT) [23] is utilized if the patient's natural inhalant sensitivity is IgE mediated, i.e. radioallergosorbent test (RAST) positive, and his health status permits.

Frequently, however, the patient is in a state of complete overload and the amounts of antigen required for SDT are simply too much to tolerate. Also this technique is often ineffective if IgE levels are low or the patient's natural inhalant sensitivities are not IgE mediated. In this situation, provocative neutralization [13] is used (see Chapter 54).

Chemical challenge (inhalation and intradermal)

Reduction of total load requires that all sources of stress be investigated and treated. As food sensitivity diagnosis is completed and nutritional status stabilized, chemical and inhalant challenge becomes the next step in an orderly sequence of diagnostic exercises. Chemical testing serves to acquaint the patient with reactions to commonly encountered household chemicals and to document those sensitivities.

Chemical testing. Inhalation testing of common chemicals is done in a booth constructed of stainless steel and glass. The patient is challenged, in a double-blind fashion, to standardized concentrations of formaldehyde, chlorine, phenol, pesticides, ethanol and natural gas. In addition, the patients may test samples of a suspect chemical they have brought with them (e.g. petrochemically contaminated fibreglass used as housing insulation). Patients record both subjective and objective reactions (ECG by telemetry, Coca Pulse Test). The serum is analysed for changes in eosinophils, total complement and IgG. In addition several chemicals may be neutralized by the Lee–Miller technique (e.g. petrochemical alcohol), especially if the patient must return home to a contaminated environment over which he has no control.

Chemical screening tests

VOST (volatile organic screening test) screens for the presence of organic vapours and solvents in serum and reflects the patient's recent exposure history (Fig. 55.5). The organic compounds selected for analysis originate from household products, chlorination of water, paint, degreasers, natural gas, plastics, petroleum products, etc. (see Table 55.4).

CPST (chlorinated pesticide screening test) screens the blood for presence and amount of several chlorinated hydrocarbon pesticides, using gas chromatography–mass spectrographic analysis with levels to 0.01 ppb (Fig. 55.6). Pesticides are often consumed in foods or absorbed via the skin or lungs during environmental exposure. In a study of 108 environmental patients, pesticides could be detected in the blood of all but one. The mean number of pesticides detected in blood samples was 3.4 and the most frequently occurring were heptachlor epoxide, hexachlorobenzene, DDT, β-BHC and dieldrin.

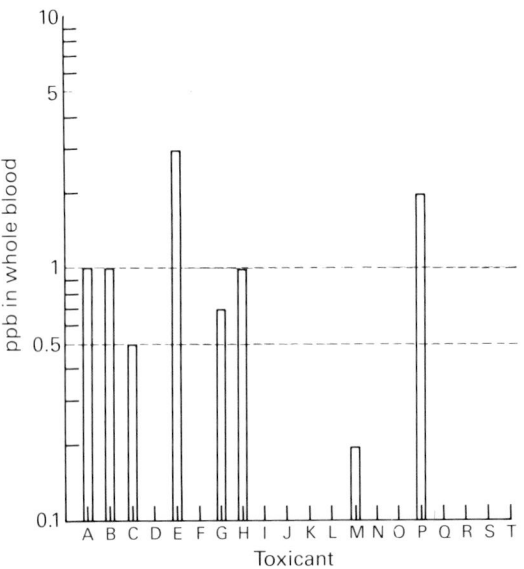

Fig. 55.5 VOST—Volatile Organics Screening Test. Examples of the levels of organic volatile compounds in the serum of a patient. A, benzene; B toluene; C, ethylbenzene; D, trimethylbenzene; E, xylene; F, styrene; G, dichlorometheine; H, chloroform; I, carbontetrachloride; J, bromoform; K, bromodichloromethane; L, dibromochloromethane; M, trichloroethane; N, tetrachloroethane; O, trichloroethylene; P, tetrachloroethylene; Q, chlorobenzene; R, dichlorobenzene; S, benzaldehyde; T, methylmercapton.

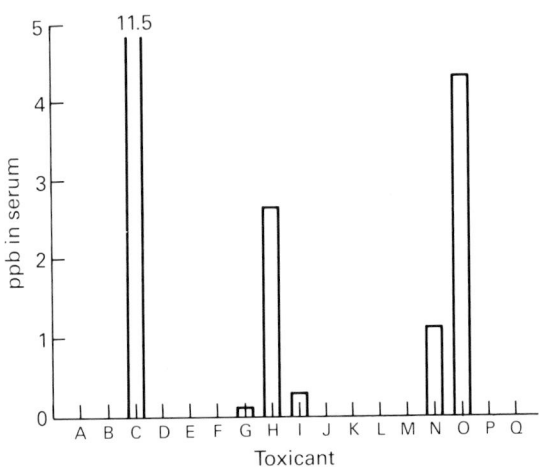

Fig. 55.6 CPST—Chlorinated Pesticide Screening Test. Levels of chlorinated pesticides in the serum of a patient. A, Aldrin; B, α-BHC; C, β-BHC; D, α-BHC (lindame); E, δ-BHC; F, α-chlordane; G, DDT; H, DDE; I, dieldrin; J, endosulfan I; K, endosulphan II; L, erdrin; M, heptachlor; N, heptachlor epoxide; O, hexachlorobenzene; P, polychlorinated biphenyls; Q, mirex.

Table 55.4 Common sources of certain volatile organics.

Volatile organic	Food additive/ flavouring agent	Product of disinfection of drinking water	Soil, grain, building fumigants	Nematocides	Industrial degreaser and solvent	Refrigerant and refrigerant impurity	Laundry dry cleaning	Fossil fuels and exhaust
Methyl bromide			X	X	X			
Chloroform		X	X		X	X		
Dichloromethane	X	X	X		X	X		
Carbon tetrachloride		X	X		X	X	X	
1, 2-Dibromoethane		X		X				
1, 2-Dichloroethane			X		X			
Trichloroethylene	X	X			X		X	
Tetrachloroethylene			X		X		X	
Dibromochloropropane			X	X				
1, 3-Dichloropropene			X	X				
Dichlorobenzenes		X	X	X				
Dichlorodifluoremethane					X	X		
Tetralin					X			X

Reduction of chlorinated pesticides

Data for 34 subjects analysed pre- and post-treatment by CPST revealed highly significant reductions in the concentration of pesticides [9].

Wagstaff and Street [28] first recognized that pesticide toxicity may be modulated by ascorbic acid. Pesticides are detoxified in part by the activity of hepatic microsomal hydroxylative enzymes whose activity is reduced in the presence of inadequate ascorbic acid levels.

Several pesticides (γ-chlordane, endosulfan and heptachlor) disappear quickly from the blood. New pesticides may appear in the blood during treatment apparently due to the mobilization of adipose tissue in the fasting process and subsequent 'dumping effect' (see Chapter 22a).

Pesticides and personality profile. A study of 200 patients [21] revealed a relationship between the most often occurring pesticides (heptachlor, β-BHC, DDT, endosulfan 1) and profiles on a personality evaluation (MMPI) that would traditionally lead a clinician to diagnose either neurosis or psychosis. Presence of any pesticide in the blood is abnormal and to date no effort has been made to assess levels in the general population for comparison.

PATIENT EDUCATION

Patients in the ECU must play an active role in their own recovery. The major goal of the education programme is to prepare patients for successful evaluation and management of their own illness. This process begins prior to admission with a mailed information package and continues after discharge from the ECU.

Later consultations of the patient with the referring physician are helpful during the transition period from a 'sterile' environment to the real world situation. The key to a successful programme lies in providing patients with as much information about their disease process as possible. This facilitates motivation and compliance with the rigorous regimen which must be followed in the ECU and at home.

Educational material

Patients are carefully orientated to the ECU upon admission. A medical education specialist and various staff members instruct new patients in the details of the programme and regulations of the ECU. Educational videotapes via closed circuit television are available in each room. These tapes cover such vital information as scheduling of unit procedures and activities, self-injection instruction, record keeping, measuring symptom severity and utilization of the ECU patient manuals.

The patient's programme manuals contain most of the instructions, information and data needed to understand and proceed through the programme in an organized fashion. Goal sheets and guidelines for testing are explained to the patient in an effort to set reasonable goals since much ground must be covered within a short time. This is important since many patients enter the ECU with the unrealistic idea that they will be able to test every inhalant, food and chemical to which they could be exposed.

Group meetings

Group meetings form the second stage of education. Patients are usually able to think more clearly and retain more information after fasting has been completed. Lectures deal with diet, immunotherapy and environmental control. Instructors stress the importance of eating less chemically contaminated food and provide information on obtaining organically grown foods.

The home 'oasis'

Patients are taught how to construct an oasis in the home. Within the realm of economic feasibility, patients should use hard surface flooring, high-quality air filters that remove up to 96% of air contaminants, formaldehyde-free furnishings, safe uncontaminated linens and electrical or hot water heating systems that eliminate the use of natural gas inside the home. Making at least one room in the house an 'oasis' is an absolute necessity for the environmental patient.

Before leaving

Each patient is interviewed by nutrition, testing and psychological specialists, who summarize results of challenge, intradermal testing and psychological testing. These interviews are recorded on a tape cassette and given to the patient to assist them in treating their illness at home.

STRESS MANAGEMENT

The importance of reducing total load in all aspects of life makes controlling emotional stress a necessary treatment goal for the environmental patient in the ECU. Patients have the opportunity, both individually and in group training sessions, to learn new coping skills.

Exercise

An exercise programme often proves beneficial for improved muscle tone, increased energy levels and heightened feelings of self-control and accomplishment. The simple prescription of a daily brisk walk around the unit corridors can make a significant difference to an overwhelmed patient.

Biofeedback

Biofeedback is used in those cases where patients are very tense or anxious. Tense muscle groups or cardiovascular changes (i.e. reduced circulation in extremities or heart palpitations) provide cues that stress levels are high. Simple relaxation procedures help the patient to diminish such symptoms and to cope with the stress on their bodies.

Group therapy

Group sessions involve training in such areas as communication skills and time management. Often, patients experience great difficulty in explaining their illness to others and may incite hostility in family members and friends simply by the manner in which they make requests or restrict living conditions. A general goal is to help them show consideration and concern for others by using more effective verbal and non-verbal communication.

Behavioural studies

Behavioural studies yield a definitive psychological profile of the environmental patients. The following features were prominent for inpatients [3, 12]:

1 Preoccupation (perhaps to the point of obsession) with ill-health and somatic concerns which may appear delusional at times.
2 General malaise.

3 Low self-esteem with dependency and need for assurance and attention from others, but difficulty in fulfilling the needs of others.
4 Repression, denial, rationalization and other defence mechanisms.
5 Low-energy depression often accompanied by anxiety.
6 Intellectual dullness, decreased learning ability as a result of poor concentration, attention and memory deficits, perceptual motor dysfunction, poor judgment, reduced abstract ability and general inability to cope with demanding situations.
7 Decreased ego strength with a tendency to lose emotional control.
8 Cognitive dysfunctioning, often with deficits in visual motor coordination and usually perceptual distortion.
9 Feelings of unreality and difficulty in controlling strange thought processes.
10 Self-righteous behaviour in situations requiring moral or ethical judgment.
11 Self/social/emotional distancing and isolation with feelings of loneliness, emptiness and persecution originating from significant others and professionals who fail to perceive their complaints as valid.
12 Hypervigilant scanning of the environment.
13 Deterioration from a more normal level of functioning prior to onset of illness.

Intellectual changes. Intellectual changes seen with environmental treatment include improvement in memory, attentional focus, judgment and common sense, and ability to think abstractly and conceptually. An average IQ increase of 10–20 points can be expected [3]. Increased accuracy in perceiving the environment and in hand–eye coordination appears to be related to appropriate diagnosis and successful treatment of sensitivities as well as degree of patient compliance with the programme [14].

Conclusion

While food sensitivity can often be diagnosed and treated on an outpatient basis, a group of patients exists whose total environmental load precludes definitive diagnosis and treatment outside an environmentally controlled setting.

In a controlled type of setting, reduction of total environmental load is accomplished safely and rapidly. Acute nutritional deficiencies can be treated and enough competence re-established to allow determination and treatment of specific sensitivities (food, chemical and natural inhalants).

The diagnostic regimen constitutes the initial therapy. Nutritional, educational and psychological support systems can be effectively incorporated within the 2 week period. There are problems which are always associated with such a comprehensive approach; in particular, maintaining a less contaminated environment requires constant vigilance by staff and by patients. Visitors and staff from the non-controlled areas of the hospital must be educated and constantly reminded to guard against transporting pollutants into the ECU.

APPENDIX

Food challenge outline.

A step-by-step outline of procedures to follow at each mealtime:

Step 1. Check daily Meal Pattern to confirm delivery of prescribed food.
Step 2. Eat the food.
Step 3. Evaluate symptoms/pulse on Food Symptom Sheet.
Step 4. Rate food on Oral Challenge Sheet.

Criteria for rating food reactions

When trying to rate your reactions, use the following criteria as a guide. No two patients will have the same symptoms, nor will their reactions necessarily have the same ratings, but every patient should make an effort to evaluate and grade the severity of his reactions. Mental changes as well as mood changes are important clues to possible allergic reactions.

'Safe' foods are those which produce no new symptoms. They cause neither a stimulatory nor a depressive reaction. Ideally, these foods do not alter a person's state of being in any way.

Reactions will be graded on a 0–4 point scale determined by the following criteria.

0. No reaction. Considered a 'safe' food.
1. Pulse change (up or down) of 20 beats/minute. Pulse must be taken after resting 5 minutes.
2. Symptoms provoked but clear within 30–45 minutes without taking salts.
3. Symptoms are produced that require salts or neutralization for relief.
4. Symptoms are severe enough to impair individual's function or symptoms persist until the next meal. Patient will fast until clear.

REFERENCES

1 Beisel WR, Edelman R, Nauss K, Suskind RM: Single nutrient effects on immunologic function. J Am Med Assoc 1981; 245:53–8.
2 Blair JW, Fenyves EJ, Edgar RT, Rea WJ: Measurement of organic air pollutants in environmental control units. Presented at the 3rd International Conference on Indoor Air Quality and Climate, Stockholm, Sweden, August 1984.
3 Butler JR, Rea WJ, Johnson AR, Henderson L: Ecological treatment improvement effects on neuro psychological/cognitive behavior: IQ score and perceptual motor performance change. Presented at the 15th Advanced Seminar Clinical Ecology Society, Hershey, Pennsylvania, October 1981.
4 Chandra RJ: Nutrition, immunity and infection: present knowledge and future direction. Lancet 1983; i:688–91.
5 Dickey LD, ed.: Clinical ecology. Springfield: Charles C Thomas, 1976.
6 Edgar RT, Rea WJ: Comprehensive air pollution measurement in environmental control unit. Presented at the International Symposium on Indoor Air Pollution, Health and Energy Conservation, Amherst, Massachusetts, October 1981.
7 Hamblin TJ, Hussain J, Akbar AN et al: Immunological reason for chronic ill health after infectious mononucleosis Br Med J 1983; 287:85–8.
8 Johnson R: Comparison of food allergy diagnostic techniques: oral challenge, RAST and intracutaneous provocative food testing. Presented at the 16th Annual Seminar for the Society of Clinical Ecology, Banff, Canada, 1982.
9 Laseter JL, DeLeon IR, Rea WJ, Butler JR: Chlorinated hydrocarbon pesticides in environmentally sensitive patients. Clin Ecology 1983; 2:3–12.
10 Lopez de Victoria A, Rea WJ, Dart L et al: Malnutrition: a common sequelae in the chemically-sensitive patient. Presented at the 17th Advanced Seminar, Clinical Ecology Society, Colorado Springs, October 1983.
11 Mandell M, Scanlon LW: Dr Mandell's five day allergy relief system. New York: Thomas Y Crowell, 1979.
12 Milam MJ, Butler JR: The effect of food and chemical sensitivity on learning. Paper presented at the Pediatric Seminar of the Society for Clinical Ecology, New York, October 1982.
13 Miller JB: Food allergy: provocative testing and injection therapy. Springfield: Charles C Thomas, 1972.
14 Nicolette M, Milam M, Butler J: Ecological program compliance with relationship to improvement in cognitive/cerebral functioning. Presented at the 16th Advanced Seminar, Clinical Ecology Society Banff, Canada, October 1982.

15 Philpott WH, Kalita DK: Brain allergies: the psycho-nutrient connection. New Canaan: Keats, 1980.

16 Randolph TG: Food susceptibility (food allergy). In: Conn H, ed. Current therapy. Philadelphia: Saunders, 1960.

17 Randolph TG: Human ecology and susceptibility to the chemical environment. Springfield: Charles C Thomas, 1962.

18 Rea WJ: Environmentally triggered thromophlebitis. Ann Allergy 1976; 37.

19 Rea WJ: Environmentally triggered small vessel vasculitis. Ann Allergy 1977; 38:248-51.

20 Rea WJ: Cardiovascular disease triggered by foods and chemicals. In: Gerrard JW, ed. Food allergy: new perspectives. Springfield: Charles C Thomas, 1980.

21 Rea WJ, Butler JR, Laseter JL, DeLeon IR: Pesticides and brain-function changes in a controlled environment. Clin Ecology 1984; 2:145-50.

22 Rea WJ, Podell RN, Williams ML et al: Elimination of oral food challenge reaction by injection of food extract. Arch Otolaryngol 1984; 110:248-52.

23 Rinkel HJ: The management of clinical allergy. Arch Otolaryngol 1975; 76:489-90.

24 Rinkel HJ, Randolph TG, Zeller M: Food allergy. Springfield: Charles C Thomas, 1951.

25 Rowe AH: Food allergy: its manifestations and control and the elimination diets. Springfield: Charles C Thomas, 1972; 431.

26 Selyé H: The general adaptation syndrome and the diseases of adaptation. J Allergy 1946; 17:23.

27 Speer F: Migraine. Chicago: Nelson-Hall, 1977.

28 Wagstaff DJ, Street JC: Ascorbic acid deficiency and induction and hepatic microsomal hydroxylation enzymes by organochlorine pesticides. Toxicol Appl Pharmacol 1971; 19:10-19.

Chapter 56
Sublingual Testing and Treatment

Doris J. Rapp

SUBLINGUAL TESTING

Introduction

The sublingual route for the testing and treatment of allergy has been used by a relatively small number of physicians in the United States since about 1941. In spite of the paucity of scientific evidence to explain the manner by which this method is effective, a number of physicians have adopted some variation of this form of therapy for a large range of symptoms in allergic patients.

Physiology

The olfactory system is a primary defence mechanism of the body. The olfactory nerve transmits impulses directly to the brain, giving rapid warning signals of odours which may be potentially harmful to the body. The oral alarm system is another early defence mechanism. In allergic individuals, minute amounts of certain foods cause localized itching, burning, tingling or swelling which, at times, can progress to more severe systemic reactions such as throat tightening, asthma, urticaria, abdominal discomfort or anaphylaxis.

Kare et al in 1969 [18] indicated that isotopically labelled glucose placed in the ligated oropharynx of a rat passes directly into the brain by non-specific diffusion. Some of the rapid changes in affect and sensorium which have been noted with the application of sublingual antigens could be explained readily by this mechanism [20].

There is extensive venous drainage into the internal jugular vein as well as lymphatic drainage through the sublingual mucosa. Sublingual application of medications, therefore, can bypass gastric digestion and subsequent liver deactivation. Water-soluble preparations in particular can pass rapidly into the circulation, at times obviating the need for subcutaneous or intravenous therapy. Sublingual stimulation also reflexly initiates not only salivary but gastric and pancreatic enzyme activity [9].

Medical applications: routes used for treatment

Sublingual mucosa. Brunton, in 1877, was the first to describe the value of sublingually administered nitroglycerine for the treatment of angina [5]. Since that time the sublingual mucosa has been used effectively for a wide variety of medications including adrenaline, isoproterenol, steroids, progesterone, testosterone, barbiturates, insulin, heparin and a number of enzymes [9].

Nasal mucosa. The nasal mucosa recently has been found to be one route for the effective administration of ragweed pollen allergy extract [41], attenuated influenza vaccine and insulin.

Gastrointestinal tract. Orally administered vaccines of non-pathogenic intestinal bacteria have been used for about three decades in Germany to treat recurrent and chronic infections in both animals and humans [39]. Oral immunization for polio is well accepted and immunization in the gut induces antibodies in a variety of secretions (see Chapter 15). As early as 1935 the efficacy of oral food desensitization was reported [19]. Later, Black reported equivocal success with similar oral desensitization with food, pollen and dust [1, 2].

Absorption of antigen sublingually. In a double-blind study Pepys and MacKarness demonstrated that peanut allergy extract administered sublingually caused an area of erythema in a skin site previously sensitized with serum from a patient allergic to peanut (personal communication). This confirmed that the food antigen is absorbed sublingually and that the antigen can circulate and combine to a fixed antibody in the skin.

Methodology for sublingual therapy

Oral route

Sublingual antigen administration for the diagnosis and treatment of atopic disease was first suggested in 1944 [13]. Since then there have been a number of modifications to the original technique. One significant improvement has been the use of 1 : 5 rather than 1 : 10

step dilutions of antigen for testing [8] after administering sublingual glycerine and diluent as negative controls. The aim of sublingual testing is to provoke mild but obvious symptoms similar to the patient's typical complaints, with relatively strong (1 : 100 or 1 : 500 w/v) or weak (1 : 12 500 w/v) concentrations of antigen (Table 56.1). Approximately 0.1 ml of a stock allergy extract is administered sublingually and held without swallowing for 1 minute. If the patient shows no subjective or objective response to a strong concentration within 10 minutes, a weaker concentration, usually 1 : 12 500, is then administered sublingually. If the patient develops obvious signs and symptoms from either the strong (Table 56.1, column A) or weak concentration of antigen (Table 56.1, column B) the test is considered positive. If neither concentration of allergen extract elicits a change in the patient the test is considered to be negative (Table 56.1, column C) and the patient is considered to be insensitive to the antigen tested.

Dosage. The dosage which provokes symptoms is called the sublingual provocation dose. A few clinicians use this method for all allergy testing. More commonly it is used only for items such as food colouring, chocolate, mushroom or dark grains which could colour a patient's skin if injected intradermally.

Table 56.1 Simplified sublingual testing.

Antigens: dilute stock concentrates of 10 or 20% allergy extract antigens, preferably in normal saline and glycerine to obviate a reaction to standard preservatives in the diluent. Make 1 :5 w/v dilutions from the concentrate so that the first solution, 1 = 1 : 100, the second, 2 = 1 : 500, etc. The dose for sublingual testing is 0.1 ml. Some patients develop symptoms, indicating intolerance or an allergy, from overdose tests (A), others from underdose tests (B), and some respond to neither overdoses nor to underdoses of extract (C), indicating that an allergy to that test allergen is unlikely.

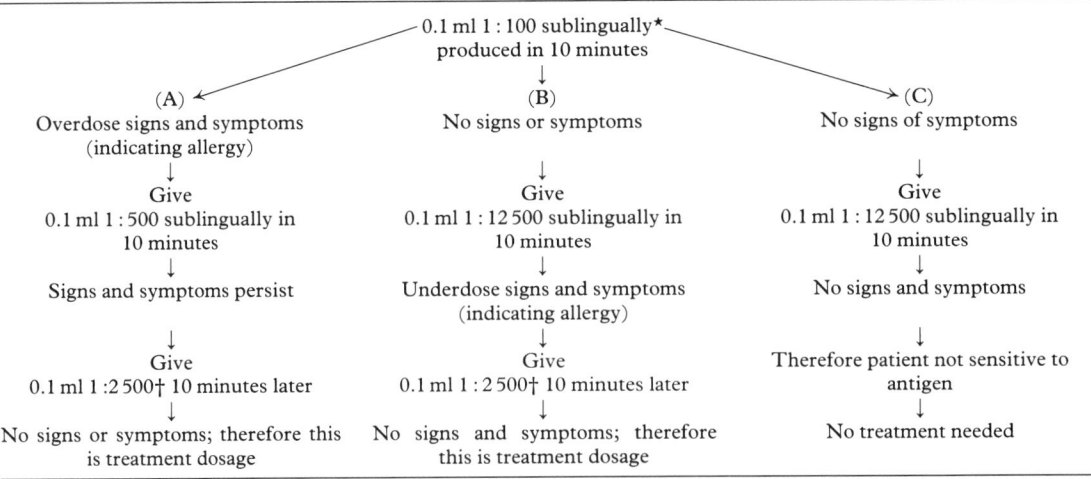

(A)	(B)	(C)
Overdose signs and symptoms (indicating allergy)	No signs or symptoms	No signs of symptoms
↓	↓	↓
Give	Give	Give
0.1 ml 1 : 500 sublingually in 10 minutes	0.1 ml 1 : 12 500 sublingually in 10 minutes	0.1 ml 1 : 12 500 sublingually in 10 minutes
↓	↓	↓
Signs and symptoms persist	Underdose signs and symptoms (indicating allergy)	No signs and symptoms
↓	↓	↓
Give	Give	Therefore patient not sensitive to antigen
0.1 ml 1 :2 500† 10 minutes later	0.1 ml 1 : 2 500† 10 minutes later	↓
↓	↓	No treatment needed
No signs or symptoms; therefore this is treatment dosage	No signs and symptoms; therefore this is treatment dosage	

*0.1 ml 1 : 100 is provocation dose.

†0.1 ml 1 : 2500 is treatment of neutralization dose. This dose can be administered either sublingually or subcutaneously for treatment.

By administering progressively weaker, or at times stronger, concentrations of stock allergy extract every 10 minutes, a dilution is often found which eliminates or neutralizes the provoked symptoms. This is called the neutralization dose. This bioassay method of testing is called the provocation–neutralization test [23].

After the bioassay, patients are requested to ingest the test-positive foods at 4-day intervals to verify sensitivity to the suspect item, as well as to afford an opportunity to document the efficacy of the treatment or neutralizing dose of allergen extract.

Foods are rarely neutralized with weak (1:325 000 w/v) concentrations [25, 38, 40]. Neutralization is more usual with dilutions of 1:500, 1:2 500 or 1:12 500 made from stock 10% allergen extract solutions.

By using the provocation–neutralization methods of allergy testing, advocates claim that it is possible in some patients to provoke and eliminate selected diverse symptoms of the type that have been attributed to food allergy since the 1930s [15, 16, 20, 22, 29, 30, 32–37] (see Table 56.2). Subjective symptoms and objective signs can be produced and eliminated by this single antigen-testing method for both RAST-positive and RAST-negative foods attributed to IgE- or non-IgE-mediated allergic reactions. A number of immunological parameters appear to change during routine provocation–neutralization testing (Table 56.3).

Table 56.2 Possible subjective symptoms produced by sublingual tests [34–37].

Skin [22, 29]
  pruritus
  urticaria
  excess perspiration
  erythema of
    ears
    nose
    cheeks

Gastrointestinal system [22, 29]
  excess salivation
  abdominal pain
  nausea
  bloating
  flatulence
  belching
  cramps
  diarrhoea
  faecal soiling

Respiratory system [22, 29]
  nasal blockage
  nasal discharge
  nasal itching
  sneezing
  postnasal discharge
  cough
  wheeze
  shortness of breath
  tight chest

Ocular symptoms [22, 29, 31, 32]
  dark eye circles
  pruritus
  erythema
  tearing
  pain
  blurred vision

Ear symptoms [22]
  pain
  popping
  tinnitus
  hearing loss
  vertigo

Cardiovascular [15, 16, 29, 34–37]
  arrhythmia
  tachycardia
  extrasystoles
  precordial pain

Nervous system [20, 27, 29, 30, 32, 33]
  headache
  hyperactivity
  fatigue
  irritability
  hostility
  agitation
  restlessness
  depression
  emotional lability
    crying
    laughter
    rapid speech
    stuttering
    obscene language
  poor coordination; inability to
    draw
    write
    read
    speak clearly

Musculoskeletal system [22, 23, 29]
  weak muscles
  painful muscles
  clumsiness
  tics
  costochondral tenderness

Genitourinary system [23, 29]
  urgency
  frequency
  involuntary micturition
  painful voiding
  genital pruritus
  vaginal discharge

Table 56.3 Possible objective signs to monitor during sublingual testing (baseline, peak of reaction, post-treatment).

Pulse	*Immunological factors*
Breathing capacity	Serotonin
peak flow meter	C3
Blood pressure	C4
Blood sugar	CH 100
Brainwave	Circulating IgG-type immune complexes
Handwriting	Sedimentation rate
Picture drawing	Prostaglandins

Intradermal provocation–neutralization

One common variation of the provocation-neutralization technique is the use of precise intradermal testing with relatively strong concentrations (1:500) of stock allergens, rather than sublingual testing to provoke symptoms [23]. Either 0.01 or 0.05 ml of the antigen, depending upon the degree of suspected sensitivity, is injected intradermally into the upper arm. The skin test site is measured and monitored carefully. If symptoms are provoked, progressively weaker 1:5 dilutions of antigen are administered every 10 minutes until the skin test site and the patient's induced signs and symptoms return to the baseline level. When indicated, the pulse, blood pressure, peak flow rate and handwriting may also be monitored every 10 minutes to help determine

in 50% glycerine and calculated so that 0.1 ml, contained in two to three drops, is equivalent to the amount of antigen which relieved the patient's symptoms. This treatment can be self-administered three times a day, either before or after meals, if the offending item cannot be avoided. It is not unusual for the patient to remain asymptomatic after ingesting small amounts of known offending food antigens within a few days following the beginning of treatment. After several months of treatment, some patients appear to require progressively less sublingual therapy while tolerating larger exposures to known previously offending food antigens. If the therapy is effective, the need for drug therapy should be significantly diminished. The advantages and disadvantages of sublingual therapy are listed in Table 56.4.

Table 56.4 Advantages and disadvantages of sublingual therapy.

Advantages	Disadvantages
Preferable for infants and children	Treatment initially required 3 times a day
Non-invasive, non-traumatic	Patient must not swallow for 60 seconds, so premature perioral swallowing is possible
Convenient	
Easy to administer	Administration of several extracts can be time consuming
Enhanced compliance	Treatment response is less rapid than by injection
Safety	Vehicle for treatment can cause sensitivity or local irritation
No intradermal irritant reaction	Excess salivation can cause dilution
Can be confirmed by other methods	False-negative reactions occur due to
Can be used to test coloured antigens (dyes, mushroom, grains, chocolate)	form of food (allergy might be due to digested food product)
Less need for drug therapy	absorptive problems in mouth
	False-positive reactions due to
	coincidence
	preservatives in extract
	environmental allergens
	antigen overload

the most efficacious dilution. The patient can then be treated either sublingually or subcutaneously with the antigen dilution which appeared to be most effective in neutralizing or relieving the symptoms, whether these are provoked by the test allergen or by actual ingestion of the problem food.

Administration of extracts. The sublingual allergy extract for treatment is usually prepared

CRITIQUE OF THE LITERATURE CONCERNING SUBLINGUAL PROVOCATION AND NEUTRALIZATION

In the last few years there have been several reviews of the efficacy of sublingual provocation and neutralization which have been critical of the usefulness of the test [10, 12, 38, 40] (Table 56.5). One major flaw in these critical

Table 56.5 Controlled studies assessing sublingual provocation or neutralization.

Author	Year published	Format	Author's interpretation	No. of patients	Blind format	Independent assessment of integrity of double-blind	Specific assessment of relevance of test antigens	Cited in 1981, 1982, 1983, review articles [12, 38, 40]
Green [11]	1974	Article	Positive	506	Single	No	Yes	Yes [38, 40]
Rapp [30]	1978	Article	Positive	1	Double	No	Yes	No
Rapp [31]	1978	Article	Positive	1	Double	No	Yes	No
Rapp [32]	1979	Article	Positive	8	Double	No	Yes	No
O'Shea and Porter [27]	1981	Article	Positive	15	Double	No	Yes	No
King [20]	1981	Article	Positive	30	Double	Yes	Yes	No
Mandell and Conte [22]	1982	Article	Positive	30	Double	No	Yes	No
Monro [24]	1983	Article	Positive	11	Double	?	Yes	No
Kailin and Collier [17]	1971	Letter to Editor	Negative	Unknown	Double	No	Yes	Yes [12, 38, 40]
Lehman [21]	1980	Article	Negative	15	Double	No	No	Yes [12, 38, 40]
Breneman et al [3]	1973	Committee report	Negative	61	Double	No	No	Yes [12, 38, 40]
Breneman et al [4]	1974	Committee report	Negative	30	Double	No	No	Yes [12, 38, 40]

Table adapted from Podell [28], with permission.

negative reviews and articles concerning provocation and neutralization [3, 4, 21] lies in the lack of verification that the patients in the trials were indeed clinically sensitive to the foods with which they were tested at the time of the study. There were admitted design faults and confounding variables in the negative experimental protocols which seriously compromised valid interpretation of the results. The major widely quoted negative references concerning sublingual therapy include two brief committee reports [3, 4] and one letter to an editor [17]. One other study [21] monitored a clinical response (colour of the nasal mucosa), which is not commonly used as a parameter to evaluate the response to sublingual testing.

One exceptionally well-controlled study by King demonstrated cognitive emotional symptoms following double-blind sublingual challenges compared with placebo ($P < 0.001$) [20]. It included repetitive pre and post base-rate trials without tests, pre and post screening trials with placebos, multiple randomized challenges with 18 allergens or placebos and agreement checks for reliability and inter-rater interpretation of symptoms. The allergens and placebos were adequately masked for odour, colour, and taste.

One single-blind [11] and six additional double-blind studies [22, 24, 27, 30–32] also strongly suggest that sublingual testing and/or treatment are both valid and effective. The sample sizes in six of these studies ranged from 8 to 506. Two of the double-blind studies were single case reports [30, 31].

A summary of both the negative and positive results is shown in Table 56.5.

Summary

Considering the serious problem in the experimental design and the limitations of the protocols, patient selection, methodology and statistical analysis in the studies quoted in the negative review articles, it would appear premature and inaccurate to state that sublingual testing is unequivocally disproven. Although the articles by the proponents of sublingual therapy appear to be somewhat better designed and executed, they provide suggestive, not definitive, evidence that these methods should be adopted. Additional studies that are both valid and reliable are clearly needed to evaluate fairly the sensitivity and the specificity of sublingual testing and/or treatment.

THE PULSE TEST

Medicine constantly searches for simple, fast and inexpensive tests which will help in the diagnosis of illness. The pulse test has been purported to aid in the detection of allergic reactions to foods, chemicals and inhalants [6]. Some physicians believe that a pulse change of greater than 16 per minute is significant. Such responses can occur within seconds to hours after a natural exposure to an antigenic food. The quality, time before onset, and duration of the response are dependent upon a large number of variables related to digestion, absorption and assimilation. By testing single foods sublingually or intradermally, it is claimed that pulse variation correlates with the onset of symptomatic, somatic and cognitive responses. Unfortunately, carefully controlled clinical studies have rarely included specific evaluation of the pulse. The value of monitoring pulse changes as an aid in the detection of the aetiology of idiopathic diseases appears to need further elucidation (see Chapter 46).

Vascular manifestations of allergy

Harkavy's text reviews the systemic manifestations of vascular allergy [15]. He clearly elucidated that many shock organs and tissues, including the cardiovascular system, respond to multiple allergenic stimuli. His work demonstrated clinical vascular pathology in both animals and humans after sensitization with specific antigens. He pointed out that reversible tachycardia, for example, could be an early harbinger of future, more serious cardiac impairment. A predisposition exists in some families for the cardiovascular systems to be a shock organ for allergic reactions. Cardiologists have noted that 34% of ventricular tachycardia, 25% of paroxysmal tachycardia and 6% of atrial fibrillation, as well as extrasystoles, occur in the absence of organic heart disease [16]. Harkavy noted that arrhythmia in persons over 40 years of age appears to be attributed frequently to underlying cardiac involvement in spite of negative clinical and electrocardiographic evidence [16]. He demonstrated that the elusive aetiology of some cardiac arrhythmias could be food sensitivities in persons with or without organic heart disease [15, 16].

Aside from a few recent studies [34–36] the extraordinary depth and quality of Harkavy's research has in my view stimulated surprisingly little impetus for further studies on the relationship between allergy and cardiovascular disease (see Chapter 42).

Pulse changes and food allergy

Food-related pulse changes were reported by Hare [14] as early as 1905. Rea et al published extensively from 1977 to 1984, documenting that the pulse increase, as well as other cardiovascular changes, can occur in response to exposure to a wide range of typical allergens and environmental chemicals.

Randolph and Rea have both noted that oral food or blinded chemical challenges in a controlled hospital environment can cause significant pulse increases in some patients to some test exposures [29, 34–37]. Rea et al recently published a study which clearly demonstrates that oral food challenges can cause pulse elevations [37]. A sample of pulse and associated handwriting changes with a single-blind mould provocation–neutralization test is shown in Fig. 56.1.

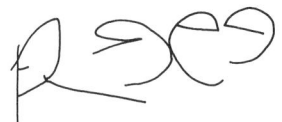

Baseline writing. Pulse 88

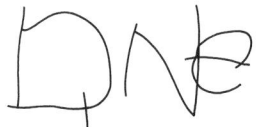

10 minutes after a 0.05 ml 1 : 25 dilution. Pulse 96

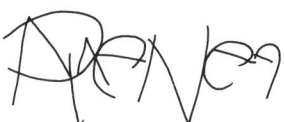

10 minutes after a 0.05 ml 1 : 125 dilution. Pulse 96. More active

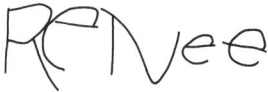

10 minutes after a 0.05 ml 1 : 625 dilution. Pulse 80. Crying, whining, hitting. Then quiet

10 minutes later. Pulse 80. Appears normal

Fig. 56.1 Pulse and associated handwriting changes with a single-blind *Alternaria* mould provocation–neutralization test in a 4-year-old white female.

In a well-controlled study by King the heart rate was measured as one objective parameter of the effect of sublingual allergens [20]. He noted that, although the mean heart rate did not change, there were more heart rate change with allergens than with the placebo challenges ($P = 0.008$).

Case report. In 1981, O'Banion reported an in-depth study of a 13-year-old male with behavioural and academic disorders [26]. He was studied by introducing single challenge foods every 4 days into his diet. His pulse was recorded periodically before and after each food was consumed. Pulse changes, as well as provoked symptoms, were used to identify specific food sensitivities. The magnitude of the pulse decreased initially and later the variability of the pulse changes subsided when the suspect foods were removed from the diet.

These findings agreed with the earlier work by Corwin et al [7] showing food-induced heart rate reactions in guinea pigs. [7]. O'Banion recommended monitoring the heart rate as an objective dependent measure for more reliable and valid results of allergic diagnosis and treatment [26].

Medical applications of the pulse test

There is little doubt that foods, inhalants, chemicals, bacteria, drugs, tobacco, foreign sera, infection and innumerable physical and emotional factors can alter the pulse. Pulse changes often reflect non-specific body responses. This vascular response can be mediated, for example, through the endocrine or nervous systems. Obvious food-related reactions, for example, can alter the gastrointestinal system by a variety of mechanisms including reflex mediation via the vagus nerve or a direct pharmacological action because a food is a cardiac stimulant or because it contains high concentrations of vasoactive amines. The challenge in medicine is to differentiate the responses that are primarily allergic or immunological in nature from those which are not.

In medical practice the value of pulse analysis is limited and not nearly as simple as indicated in the dictums outlined by Coca [6]. His observations, however, might be of value in alerting critical physicians to investigate the specific aetiology of intermittent or constant atypical pulse variations. He maintained that:

1 the pulse was not significantly changed by digestion, ordinary exercise or normal emotions;

2 the diurnal variation of the pulse should not be greater than 16 beats per minute;
3 the morning resting pulse must be the minimum daily pulse; and
4 the resting pulse should not be greater than 84 in a normal non-infected child or adult.

Limitations of the pulse test. Major limitations which preclude widespread application of his suggestions include the following:

1 Few physicians could or would spend 2 or 3 hours analysing detailed patient pulse records.
2 The interpretation of food-related pulse changes is commonly confounded by elusive delayed food reactions, as well as by prolonged reactions which can last for days.
3 A wide range of concomitant and cumulative factors can make critical pulse analysis an awesome challenge. For example, one patient described by Harkavy had atrial fibrillation during the pollen season which subsided if specific offending foods were not ingested at that time. These same foods could be ingested with impunity during non-pollen seasons.

Comparison of pulse records before and after the ingestion of individual foods or purposeful exposure to indoor or outdoor allergens, chemicals or medications might provide additional clues to help detect allergenic and non-allergenic factors related to a patient's illness. Such precise analysis may provide the insight required to design rigidly controlled, large-scale research which will answer questions related to the practical clinical value and significance of unusual diurnal pulse variations in the presence or absence of organic heart disease.

Summary

There is no doubt that a 'twitchy' vascular system can be altered in response to some antigenic challenges in some patients. If the cause of the abnormal pulse variations remains elusive, the possibility of an allergic vascular response should be considered in any thorough diagnostic evaluation. This is especially true if the patient has both a positive personal and family history of allergy.

REFERENCES

1 Black JH: The treatment of food allergy. South Med J 1942; 35:771.

2 Black JH: Treatment of respiratory allergy in children by oral administration of dust and pollen extracts. J Allergy 1950; 21:148.

3 Breneman JC, Crook WC, Deamer W et al: Report of the Food Allergy Committee on the sublingual method of provocative testing for food allergy. Ann Allergy 1973; 31:382.

4 Breneman JC et al: Final report of the Food Allergy Committee of ACA on clinical evaluation of sublingual provocative testing method for diagnosis of food allergy. Ann Allergy 1974; 33:164.

5 Brunton RL: The Goulstonian Lectures. The Royal College of Physicians. London: Macmillan, 1887.

6 Coca AF: The pulse test. New York: Lyle Stuart, 1956.

7 Corwin AH, Dukes-Dobos FN, Hamburger M: Bioassay of food allergens: food-induced reactions of the heart rate of guinea pigs. Ann Allergy 1963; 21:547–62.

8 Dickey L: Sublingual antigens. J Am Med Assoc 1971; 217:214.

9 Gibaldi M, Kanig J: Absorption of drugs through the oral mucosa. J Oral Ther Pharmacol 1965; 1:440.

10 Golbert TM: A review of controversial diagnostic and therapeutic techniques employed in allergy. J Allergy Clin Immunol 1975; 56:170–90.

11 Green M: Sublingual provocation testing for foods and F, D, and C dyes. Ann Allergy 1974; 33:274.

12 Grieco MH: Controversial practices in allergy. J Am Med Assoc 1982; 247:3106–11.

13 Hansel FK: Allergy and immunity in otolaryngology, 2nd edn. Rochester: American Academy of Ophthalmology and Otolaryngology, 1968; 134–5.

14 Hare F: The food factor in disease, Vol. I. London: Longmans, 1905; 71.

15 Harkavy J: Vascular allergy and its systemic manifestations. Washington DC: Butterworths, 1963.

16 Harkavy J: Cardiac manifestations due to hypersensitivity. Ann Allergy 1970; 28:242–51.

17 Kailin E, Collier R: 'Relieving' therapy for antigen exposure. J Am Med Assoc 1971; 217:78.

18 Kare M, Schechter P, Grossman S, Roth L: Direct pathway to the brain. Science 1969; 163:952.

19 Keston B, Waters I, Hopkins JG: Oral desensitization to common foods. J Allergy 1935; 6:431.

20 King DS: Can allergic exposure provoke psychological symptoms? A double-blind test. Biol Psychiatry 1981; 16:3–19.

21 Lehman CW: A double-blind study of sublingual provocative food testing: a study of its efficacy. Ann Allergy 1980; 45:144.

22 Mandell M, Conte A: The role of allergy in arthritis, rheumatism, and polysymptomatic cerebral, visceral, and somatic disorders: a double-blind study. J Int Acad Prevent Med 1982; July:5–6.

23 Miller JB: Food allergy. Provocative testing and injection therapy. Springfield: Charles C Thomas, 1972.

24 Monro J: Food allergy in migraine. Proc Nutr Soc 1983; 42:241.

25 Morris DL: Use of sublingual antigen in diagnosis and treatment of food allergy. Ann Allergy 1969; 27:289.

26 O'Banion DR: An ecological and nutritional approach to behavioral medicine. Springfield: Charles C Thomas, 1981:178–91.

27 O'Shea JA, Porter SF: Double-blind study of children with hyperkinetic syndrome treated with multi-allergen extract sublingually. J Learn Disabil 1981; 14:189.

28 Podell RN: Intracutaneous and sublingual provocation and neutralization. Clin Ecol 1983; II, 13–20.

29 Randolph TG: An alternative approach to allergies. New York: Lippincott & Crowell, 1980.

30 Rapp DJ: Double-blind confirmation and treatment of milk sensitivity. Med J Aust 1978; i:571.

31 Rapp DJ: Weeping eyes in wheat allergy. Trans Am Soc Ophthalmol Otolaryngol 1978; 18:149.

32 Rapp DJ: Food allergy treatment for hyperkinesis. J Learn Disabil 1979; 12:42–50.

33 Rapp DJ: Does diet affect hyperactivity? J Learn Disabil 1978; 11:56–62.

34 Rea WJ: Environmentally-triggered small vessel vasculitis. Ann Allergy 1977; 38:245–51.

35 Rea WJ: Environmentally-triggered cardiac disease. Ann Allergy 1978; 40:243–51.

36 Rea WJ et al: Recurrent environmentally-triggered thrombophlebitis: a five-year follow-up. Ann Allergy 1981; 47:338–44.

37 Rea WJ, Podell RN, Williams M et al: Elimination of oral food challenge reaction by injection of food extracts. Arch Otolaryngol 1984; 110:248–52.

38 Reisman R: American Academy of Allergy: Position statements—controversial techniques. J Allergy Clin Immunol 1981; 67:333–8.

39 Rusch V, Hyde RM, Don Luckey T: Application of S. faecalis and E. coli oral vaccines in humans and animals. Prog Food Nutr Sci.

40 Van Metre TE: Critique of controversial and unproven procedures for diagnosis and therapy of allergic disorders. Pediatr Clin North Am 1983; 30:807–17.

41 Welsh PW, Butterfield JH, Yunginger JW et al: Allergen-controlled study of intranasal immunotherapy for ragweed hayfever. J Allergy Clin Immunol 1983; 71:454.

PART V
TREATMENT OF FOOD ALLERGY

Chapter 57
Dietary Treatment of Food Allergy

C. Zanussi and E. Pastorello

Introduction

Food allergy management consists of avoiding the offending foods and of pharmacological therapy when there are adverse reactions [1, 16]. Prophylaxis is essentially based on pharmacological measures, there being until now few convincing trials of the effectiveness of specific immunotherapy [16].

Avoiding foods responsible for symptoms seems to be a very simple procedure but in practice it presents substantial problems both of a nutritional and a psychological nature. Thus it is necessary to follow some rules to have a chance of obtaining successful results.

A CORRECT DIET

The main points to consider for a correct diet can be summarized as follows:
1 Be sure of the diagnosis.
2 State how long the diet must be continued.
3 Allow amounts of offending foods according to the patient's tolerance.
4 Verify the cross-reactivity of the offending foods with other foods.
5 Maintain an adequate intake of calories, minerals and essential vitamins.

Be sure of the diagnosis

The first fundamental step is to be sure of the diagnosis, because the elimination of a food from the diet must be based on a secure diagnosis since it represents a very drastic measure for the patient. The diagnosis will be correct if the diagnostic procedure chosen is the appropriate one (see Chapters 45–48). It is important to underline the fact that the correct diagnosis of food allergy can be obtained only if the results of multiple tests agree with each other. In particular (a) history, (b) skin prick tests with commercial extracts $(1:20\,w/v)$ or with fresh foods (vegetables, fruits), (c) radioallergosorbent tests (RAST) or enzyme-linked immunosorbent assays (ELISA) to detect IgE antibody to foods in serum, (d) elimination diet and (e) open and double-blind food challenges [4, 20] should be carried out.

RAST and skin tests

It is important to remember that RAST or skin test positivity alone is not sufficient to demonstrate that a particular food is really responsible for the symptoms of the patient. We showed that only 7.9% of positive skin tests and 9.8% of positive RASTs to food allergens were concordant with symptoms in a group of urticaria/angioedema affected patients, while the other positive results were to foods that were well tolerated by the patients [18].

Skin testing extracts

We were also able to observe that in some cases the discordance between history and skin tests depends on the unreliability of the food extract: for example, in the case of apple allergy, commercial extracts are unreliable whilst fresh pulp is effective. The opposite holds true for peanuts; skin tests with fresh extracts are less reliable than those made with commercial extracts.

Finally, it is obvious and necessary to stress that a therapeutic elimination diet can only be undertaken after a clear demonstration of clinical intolerance to a certain food. It should not otherwise be attempted.

Duration of diet

The second point concerning the dietary treatment of food allergy is to state for how long the diet must be continued. In this context the natural history of food allergy is important.

Bock [2] followed 501 children from birth to 3 years of age and showed that many of them outgrow their food allergy by their third birthday. These data confirm his previous study [3] showing that the tendency to outgrow food allergy is more evident in children who have their food sensitivity diagnosed before the age of 3 years. On the other hand, Kajosaari [14] in a study of 866 Finnish children aged 1–3 and 6 years of age showed that the prevalence of food allergy increases up to 3 years of age and then decreases. Thus with the possibility of a spontaneous resolution of food allergy, a good rule is to challenge the patient at regular intervals to confirm the persistence of the adverse reactions to foods. Spontaneous resolution is not infrequent in the adult population but here it is necessary to reintroduce the eliminated foods carefully in order to avoid dangerous reactions.

The importance of breast-feeding

Breast-feeding can be useful in the prevention of atopic diseases and many authors suggest that the mother should breast-feed for as long as possible. It is important to note that breast milk is not sufficient as the sole source of food after the first 5 to 6 months of life [13, 24]. Some studies report that the prevalence of malnutrition is higher in prolonged breast-fed children and that the nutritional problems might begin after the sixth month, becoming dangerous after 12 months [6, 7].

Level of food sensitivity

Should small amounts of the offending food be included in the diet? Some food sensitivities have a very particular tolerance level. For example, some patients with lactose intolerance can drink a cup of milk containing 12 g of lac-

tose without symptoms even if they cannot tolerate the oral challenge. Many subjects with intolerance to some additives, such as tartrazine and sulphites, present a stable high threshold to provocation, as confirmed by double-blind challenge tests [17]. These patients can readily ingest foods with a low level of additive without ill-effect while the patients with a lower threshold level cannot tolerate any at all.

IgE-mediated food allergy

In many IgE-mediated food-allergic diseases it is impossible to state a practical tolerance level because the symptoms are provoked by such small quantities of the allergenic proteins, as in the case of anaphylaxis. However, in chronic IgE-mediated syndromes, double-blind challenges will reveal for some patients, a provocative dose that is high enough so that the food can be included in the diet in a small quantity.

Gastrointestinal permeability. A serious disadvantage of introducing small quantities of an offending food might be represented by the gastrointestinal diseases. Increasing gut permeability may transform the previously tolerated doses into provocative ones. Another problem is the possibility that small quantities of the offending foods might provoke subclinical effects. Some reports exist of histological abnormalities in the small intestinal mucosa from exposure to the offending food even in the absence of any clinical symptoms [21, 25].

Some authors consider that a small quantity of the offending food, even though well tolerated, could delay the outgrowing of the hypersensitivity [1]. However, the data of Bock [2] on the natural history of adverse reactions to foods do not confirm this. On the contrary, it is suggested that reintroducing tolerated quantities of offending foods should be undertaken [2, 3].

Cross-reacting foods

The fourth very important point is to decide whether it is necessary to avoid all the foods cross-reacting with the responsible foods or not. Many cross-reactions among foods have been described in allergic individuals; for example, cross-reactivity among crustaceans, such as shrimps, crab and lobster [15]; among other kinds of fish [23]; and among the different cereals [11]. Cross-reactivity between foods and pollens has also been described, particularly between grass and cereals [11], birch and apple, carrots and potatoes [8, 12] and also between mugwort and celery [19] (see Chapter 24).

Skin tests and RAST

Skin tests and RAST are not sufficient to clarify the problem. We have seen multiple positive skin tests and RAST to vegetables and fruits in 31 patients sensitive to silver birch. However, in the large majority of subjects the positive tests did not correlate with symptoms [18]. For example, in the case of apple, nine patients had positive tests without symptoms and in the case of potatoes 25 out of 31 had positive tests and no symptoms. These data clearly show that RAST and skin tests may not be indicative of a true cross-reactivity among foods.

However, it is interesting to note that Dreborg and Foucard [8] showed a good correlation between the size of the skin test wheal and the presence of symptoms for a given food so that the larger wheal could indicate a true sensitivity to that food. These studies were performed only for some foods such as apples, carrots and potatoes but could represent a new kind of approach to this difficult problem.

In order to solve the problem of cross-reactivity among foods it is necessary to make provocation challenge tests with the suspected foods.

Maintenance of adequate nutrition

The fifth and last point concerns the substitution of the offending foods with others which are not allergenic, thus maintaining the proper intake of calories, minerals and essential vitamins. The main problem is protein, especially in breast-feeding infants who develop an allergy to cow's milk.

Milk substitutes

A good substitute for milk is casein hydrolysate which contains no antigenic moieties of β-lactoglobulin, which is the main allergen of cow's milk (see Chapter 18). However, the presence of residual peptides with a molecular weight of 3850 has also been reported in this hydrolysate and these might contain some allergenicity.

Soya milk. Soya milk remains the most common substitute for cow's milk in allergic children. However, it has been shown that about one-quarter of the children allergic to cow's milk proteins and exhibiting gastrointestinal symptoms may not tolerate soya milk either.

Industrial processing of foods

Industrial processing of foods sometimes destroys the allergenic properties of food proteins as can be seen for some oils derived from vegetable seeds and margarines. Therefore, individuals allergic to peanuts should be able to ingest industrially processed peanut oils [22]. Recently the same has been demonstrated for soya bean oil [5]. It is important to test the tolerance for a particular food before adding it back fully into the diet.

Table 57.1 Daily requirements for 'reference man and woman'.

Substance	Requirements
Water	1–5 litres
Energy	2000–2700 kcal
Proteins	28–33 g
Linoleic acid	3 g
Retinol equivalents	390
Vitamin D	Sunny light
Vitamin E activity	3–6 IU
Folacin	50 μg
Niacin	9–12 mg
Riboflavin	1–1.4 mg
Thiamine	0.7–0.9 mg
Vitamin B_6	0.6–1.3 mg
Vitamin B_{12}	1 μg
Calcium (Ca)	200–400 mg
Phosphorus (P)	400 mg
Sodium (Na)	400 mg
Iron (Fe)	6.5–9 mg
Ascorbic acid	10 mg
Iodine	58–70 μg
Pantothenic acid	5 mg
Magnesium	200 mg
Zinc	8–10 mg
Copper	2 mg
Chloride	500 mg
Cobalt	0–1 μg
Chromium	200–290 μg
Manganese	2.5–2.7 mg

Source: Goodhart and Shils [10].

Daily nutritional requirements

It is important to maintain an appropriate intake of all nutrients and to prescribe a well-balanced diet related to the age and sex of the patient. A summary of the daily requirements

is shown in Table 57.1. It is particularly important to supply all the elements included in the eliminated food and not only the main ones. In order to approach this problem in a simplified and practical way we have analysed the most important elements of foods that are

Table 57.2 Characteristics of milk.

1   A high protein content, and a high amount of the eight essential amino acids
2   A high content of calcium, phosphorus, Vitamin A and riboflavin

Daily requirements of calcium and phosphorus:
  Age 3-10 : 400 mg
  Age 10-18 : 1000 mg
  Age >19 : 400 mg

Calcium content (mg) in 100 mg of:		Phosphorus content (mg) in 1000 mg of:	
Cow's milk	120	Cow's milk	120
Parmesan cheese	1200	Yeast beer	2850
Emmental cheese	700	Parmesan cheese	734
Yeast beer	240	Fontina cheese	561
Parsley	195	Egg yolk	506
Hazelnuts	183	Almonds	451
Fresh beans	64	Veal liver	333
Lettuce	50		
Carrots	41		
Green peas	30		

Riboflavin daily requirements (mg):		Riboflavin content (mg) in 100 mg of:	
Age 1-3 : 0.8		Yeast beer	7
Age 4-6 : 1.1		Veal liver	2.34
Age 7-10 : 1.2		Albumen	0.25
Age 11-14 : 1.5		Cow's milk	0.18
Age 15-22 : 1.8			
Age >22 : 1.4			

Table 57.3 Characteristics of eggs.

1   A high amount of proteins with the highest biological value
2   Important amounts of oleic acid, linoleic acid, phosphorus, iron, potassium, vitamins A, E and D and cholesterol

Daily requirements of Iron (mg):		Vitamin A (IU):	
Age 1-3 : 15		Age 1-3 : 2000	
Age 4-10 : 9		Age 7-10 : 3300	
Age 11-18 : 18		Age >11 : 4000	
Age >18 : 9			
(if women : 18)			

Iron content (mg) in 100 mg of:		Vitamin A content in 100 mg of :	
Egg yolk	6.5	Egg yolk	660
Yeast beer	28.0	Butter	1180
Veal kidney	15.0	Veal liver	6075
Veal liver	8.5	Spinach	6/12000 as carotene
Horse meat	7.0	Carrots	6075 as carotene
Dry beans	6.4		
Dry peas	5.7		
Almonds	4.1		
Spinach	3.6		
Beef	2.6		

Vitamin D daily requirements : 0.01 mg (Vitamin A shows a spontaneous increase after sunny exposure)

Vitamin content (μg) in 100 mg of:	
Egg yolk	2.5-10
Cod liver oil	2.5-15

Table 57.4 Characteristics of cereals.

Cereals are a good source of proteins such as albumin and globulins and of vitamins such as niacin, piridoxine (B_6) and thiamine (B_1)

Niacin daily requirements (mg):		Vitamin B_6 daily requirements (mg):	
Age 1–10 : 1–10		Age 1–6 : 0.6	
Age >11 : 16–20		Age 6–14 : 1.2	
		Age >15 : 1.3	

Niacin content (mg) in 100 mg of:		Vitamin B_6 content (mg) in 100 mg of:	
Wheat flour	2.6	Wheat flour	2
Rice	3.1	Dry cod	7
Veal liver	15.7	Egg yolk	7
Ham	11.8	Veal liver	5
Beef meat	8.5	Ham	2
Horse meat	8.2		
Egg yolk	4.1		

Vitamin B_1 daily requirement: 0.7–0.9 mg

Vitamin B_1 content (mg) in 100 mg of:	
Wheat flour	0.50
Maize flour	0.36
Beer yeast	10.00
Dry peas	0.69
Peanuts	0.62
Ham	0.60
Veal liver	0.38
Egg yolk	0.25

Source: Goodhart and Shils [10].

often responsible for allergic symptoms, i.e. milk, eggs and cereals.

Milk, eggs and cereals have high biological value and content of vitamins and minerals and their avoidance can lead to deficiencies. However, foods such as fruits or vegetables can be easily replaced by other similar foods without any dietary problem. The high daily requirements of calcium in young people and of iron in young women must be emphasized.

Tables 57.2–57.4 show the essential components of the above-mentioned foods and also other foods containing high quantities of

each substance. It is relatively easy to replace all the essential parts of those foods apart from calcium, which must be maintained with pharmacological preparations.

Conclusion

It is essential that after the conclusive identification of one or more foods to which the patient is allergic, a correct elimination diet is instituted before any antiallergic treatment is given.

REFERENCES

1 Bahna SL: Management of food allergy. Ann Allergy 1984; 53:678.
2 Bock SA: The natural history of food sensitivity. J Allergy Clin Immunol 1982; 69:173.
3 Bock SA: Natural history of adverse reactions to foods in children. Special Symposium on Food Allergy. 41st annual meeting of American Academy of Allergy and Immunology. New York: March 1985.
4 Bock SA., May CD: Adverse reactions to food due to hypersensitivity. In: Middleton E, Reed CE, Ellis EF, eds. Allergy principles and practise. Vol. 2. St. Louis: C V Mosby, 1983: 1415–27.
5 Bush RK, Taylor SL, Nerdlee BS, Busse WW: Soybean oil is not allergenic to soybean-sensitive individuals. J Allergy Clin Immunol 1985; 76:242–5.

6 Central Bureau of Statistics: The rural Kenyan nutrition survey. February–March 1977. Nairobi: Ministry of Finance and Planning. Soc Perspect 1977; 8:24–6.
7 Central Bureau of Statistics: Report of the child nutrition survey 1978–79. Nairobi: Ministry of Economic Planning and Development, 1977; 29–30.
8 Dreborg S, Foucard T: Allergy to apple, carrot and potato in children with birch pollen allergy. Allergy 1983; 38:167.
9 Gjesing B, Lowenstein M: Immunochemistry of food antigens. Ann Allergy 1984; 53:602–8.
10 Goodhart RS, Shils E: Modern nutrition in health and diseases. 5th edn. Philadelphia: Lea and Febiger, 1973.
11 Goodwin BFJ, Rawcliffe PM: Food allergies associated with cereal products. Food Chem 1983; 2:321.

12 Halmepuro L, Vuontela K, Kalimo K, Bjorkstein F: Cross-reactivity of IgE antibodies with allergens in birch pollen, fruits and vegetables. Int Arch Allergy Appl Immunol 1984; 74:235.

13 Jelliffe DB, Jelliffe EFP: The volume and composition of human milk in poorly nourished communities. A review. Ann J Clin Nutr 1978; 31:492–515.

14 Kajosaari M: Food allergy in Finnish children aged 1 to 6 years. Acta Paediatr Scand 1982; 71:815.

15 Lehrer SB, Waring NP, Mac Cants ML: Immunological cross-reactivity of shrimp, crab, crawfish and lobster allergens. J Allergy Clin Immunol 1984; 73:114.

16 Metcalfe DD: Food hypersensitivity. J Allergy Clin Immunol 1984; 73:749.

17 Ortolani C, Pastorello E, Fontana A, Gerosa S, Zanussi C: Chemicals and drugs as triggers of food associated disorders. Ann Allergy (in press).

18 Pastorello E: Terapia della sindrome orticaria/angioedema da allergia e intolleranza alimentare. 17 Congresso della Società Italiana di Allergologia e Immunologia Clinica. Milan: 3–5 October 1985; 273–80.

19 Pauli G, Peltre G, Bessot JC et al: Allergy to celery rot coincident with mugwort pollen sensitivity. J Allergy Clin Immunol 1984; 73:114.

20 Sampson MA: Role of immediate food hypersensitivity in the pathogenesis of atopic dermatitis. J Allergy Clin Immunol 1984; 71:473.

21 Shiner M, Ballard S, Brook CGD, Herman S: Intestinal biopsy in the diagnosis of cow's milk protein in tolerance without acute symptoms. Lancet 1975; ii:1060.

22 Taylor SL, Busse WW, Sachs MI, et al: Peanut oil is not allergenic to peanut-sensitive individuals. J Allergy Clin Immunol 1981; 63:372.

23 Tuft L, Blumesteni GI: Studies in food allergy. V. Antigenic relationship among members of fish family. J Allergy 1946; 17:329.

24 Victora CG, Vaughan JP, Martines JC, Barcelos LB: Is prolonged breast-feeding associated with malnutrition. Ann J Clin Nutr 1984; 39:307–14.

25 Vitoria JC, Aramjelo ME, Rodriguez Soriano J: Jejunal biopsy in cow's milk protein intolerance. Lancet 1978; i:722.

Chapter 58
Drug Treatment of Food Allergy and Intolerance

L. J. F. Youlten

Introduction

The use of drugs in the treatment or prevention of adverse reactions to foods or other constituents of the diet is of interest for two reasons. Firstly, the failure to identify an avoidable causal agent may require the consideration of drug therapy to prevent or relieve symptoms known or suspected to be food related. Secondly, knowledge of the mode of action of drugs effective in this condition may provide clues to the pathogenetic mechanisms of food-induced clinical reactions.

THE ROLE OF DRUG TREATMENT IN FOOD ALLERGY

Symptoms may require and respond to treatment with appropriate drugs, irrespective of the cause. Urticaria in patients where there is a clear-cut dietary trigger may respond just as well or as badly to treatment with antihistamines as that due to other causes. Such symptomatic treatment may be clinically effective but tells us little about the mechanisms of the reaction, except that histamine may be among the mediators involved. It is not proposed therefore to examine the whole range of drugs which may on occasion be indicated for the relief of food-related clinical syndromes. Such a survey would have to cover a wide area of the field of clinical therapeutics including, for example, eczema, urticaria/angioedema, asthma, rhinitis, migraine, arthritis and gastrointestinal upsets, both acute and chronic. This review will be confined to the more restricted topic of drug treatment which may have a particular experimental or specific therapeutic role in adverse reactions to foods. Most of the work in this area has, understandably, been directed to the more obviously food-related reactions, particularly those which reproducibly follow provocation testing. Since the mode of action of some of the drugs concerned is still a matter for debate, it is important not to draw too sweeping conclusions from such studies. The fact that sodium cromoglycate (SCG) inhibits mediator release from allergen-challenged mast cells does not prove, for example, that all conditions responding to this drug involve mediator release from mast cells. Other actions of SCG may be relevant to its effects, both in asthma and in food allergy.

Apart from SCG, the other drug for which claims have been made that it interferes in some more or less specific way with the genesis of food-allergic or pseudoallergic reactions is aspirin and with it the other non-steroidal anti-inflammatory drugs.

SODIUM CROMOGLYCATE

A number of studies have shown that acute adverse reactions to foods can be prevented or ameliorated by oral pretreatment with SCG. As in asthma, the efficacy of this compound seems to be most readily demonstrable in symptom-free patients subjected to provocation testing. The picture is much less clear when clinical improvement is sought in longer term studies of conditions thought to be food related. This is understandable, since such trials usually include patients in whom a dietary factor may be only one among several significant precipitating factors, or in whom an initially allergen-induced condition has produced a longstanding non-specific hyperreactivity. Such conditions may be difficult to reverse without the use of more potent drugs. Recommendations as to the dose and mode of administration of SCG have been reviewed [18].

The beneficial effect of SCG in milk intolerance was first proposed on the basis of an open study in four infants [22]. A single case of fish- or fruit-induced urticaria reproducibly blocked by cromoglycate but not by placebo in a double-blind study, was subsequently reported [27]. In a placebo-controlled cross-over study, 20 children with multiple food allergies manifest as eczema, urticaria, asthma or gastrointestinal symptoms, were treated with a dose of 100 mg four times daily. Of the 16 assessed, 10 showed improvement on SCG greater than on placebo, four showing no difference and only two preferring placebo [15]. A similar study on 16 patients including both children and adults showed a similar level of positive response [31].

Asthma

In six patients with asthma exacerbated by IgE-mediated food allergy, supported in four cases by a history of attacks precipitated by specific foods and in the other two by improvement on an elimination diet, provocation tests were performed. Pretreatment with inhaled SCG for 24 hours before the challenge was completely ineffective in preventing the response to the food concerned (soya protein, wheat or egg). In contrast, SCG administered orally at a higher dose over a similar period was effective in blocking the 25–40% fall in peak expiratory flow rate observed in all six patients after placebo. Neither route of administration was effective in preventing similar degrees of bronchoconstriction after aspirin challenge in six known aspirin-sensitive asthmatics. It was calculated that the amount of SCG absorbed was similar by both dosing routes, and it was therefore concluded that the site of action was the gastrointestinal tract [12]. This study confirmed and extended earlier work from the same authors [11,13] but similar work by others failed to show the same effect [25]. Subsequent observations seemed to support the concept that limitation of allergen absorption might account for SCG's protective effect [7, 14, 16, 34]. The failure to prevent aspirin-induced asthma may reflect the ready absorption of this drug from the normal gastrointestinal tract, or some basic difference in the nature or site of the triggering mechanism. This is of interest in view of the association of food intolerance with aspirin sensitivity in some patients with urticaria [1].

Another study involved a well-characterized group of patients in whom symptoms could be reliably induced by a specific food, in this case fish. Twenty patients who developed asthma within an hour of ingesting fish and with positive skin tests to fish extract were given 100 g of cod after three days double-blind treatment with oral placebo, SCG (400 mg four times daily) or ketotifen (1 mg twice daily). Protection was complete in eight, and partial in another eight on SCG treatment. Three of the four patients showing no protection were among the four with the highest total IgE levels [20].

Gastrointestinal allergy

Several studies on food allergy with mainly gastrointestinal manifestations have been published, but these have generally been poorly controlled and have involved few patients. However, in one placebo-controlled study, 14 children aged 2–15 years, with a history of diarrhoea within 48 hours of ingesting various foods, were treated with SCG, 50–70 mg four times daily, for two days before oral challenge with cow's milk, soya-based milk substitute or beef. In 11 of 13 trials SCG was effective in preventing or ameliorating the expected symptoms, whereas placebo was only effective in three of nine trials [28]. Such trials are difficult to find suitable patients for, since a history of a severe adverse reaction to a food often leads to a prolonged period of avoidance, during which the intolerance may well be lost spontaneously. The current degree of sensitivity always needs to be established by unprotected studies. Another problem is that an adverse reaction may be followed by a period of specific or non-specific non-responsiveness.

Eczema

The role of food allergy in eczema, particularly in childhood, has led to the investigation of SCG as a prophylactic or therapeutic agent in this condition. As in the case of urticaria, early reports were of single cases showing impressive improvement [36]. SCG has been tried topically, with mixed results [24, 40], but more frequently by the oral route. Here too results have been most clearly shown when a food factor has been identified and eliminated, and the patient then challenged against a background of low eczema activity (see Chapter 34).

Children

In an open trial of 35 children in whom foods had been established as contributing significantly to their eczema, a period of combined SCG treatment and dietary avoidance was followed by good improvement in 66%. Some, but not all, of these suffered a relapse on subsequently reintroducing the avoided foods [29].

The addition of oral SCG to the treatment programme of 22 children already on a strict exclusion diet produced no additional improvement [26]. This lent support to the view that the activity of this compound is related to the food allergy component of the eczema, which is of variable importance in different groups, probably playing a role in only a minority of adults with this condition. This is paralleled in some ways by a single-blind investigation of SCG in urticaria and angioedema, in which a higher proportion of those with an atopic background (five out of seven) showed improvement than in the non-atopic group (one of nine) [30].

Another group of 26 young children with eczema treated by food avoidance together with SCG and placebo in a cross-over design, followed in each phase by reintroduction of the avoided foods, appeared to demonstrate a strong carry-over effect in the half who received SCG before placebo [9]. If confirmed, this finding would have interesting implications, including the possibility that food administration in an allergic patient protected by SCG might induce a state of tolerance. A further, open study of 13 children under 5 years of age whose chronic eczema had improved on an elimination diet demonstrated that in about two-thirds of them SCG was effective in preventing relapse on returning to a normal diet. The stopping of SCG in these patients was subsequently followed within 2 months by relapse [10].

Adults

In adult eczema patients some studies have claimed marginal improvement but this has not generally been sufficiently encouraging to promote the widespread use of SCG in this group, reflecting perhaps the smaller role of food allergy in this age range. Even in children, however, some apparently well-designed studies have failed to show benefit [3].

Criteria of clinical improvement

Few studies in eczema have included measurements of any objective criteria which might relate to clinical improvement. These include claims that total IgE levels in the plasma can be reduced by this treatment, this effect only being observed in the patients whose skin improved on SCG. Changes in IgE do not generally accompany remissions and exacerbations of eczema, so this observation is at least a step in the direction of finding an objective index of the drug's efficacy. However, only about 15 to 20% of patients with eczema show any benefit from SCG, and the IgE changes are not sufficiently clear-cut to allow this to be a screening procedure to select suitable patients without submitting large numbers to a prolonged therapeutic trial. For example, in one large trial, only 40 of 196 patients showed a rise in IgE, and of these 19 nevertheless reported improvement. Of the 55 patients whose IgE fell, 38 showed clinical improvement, but 17 did not [19].

In another study, an open phase of 8 months oral SCG treatment (200 mg rising to 1200 mg daily) was followed by a 4-month double-blind phase in which the optimum dose for each patient was tested against placebo. Only three of 18 patients showed marked clinical improvement in the open phase, a further seven showing lesser benefit and eight none. The incidence of food allergy was similar in all three groups (three of three, four of seven and five of eight, respectively in the good, moderate and non-responders). IgE measurements in these subjects showed 20% falls in 14 of the 18, but the subsequent double-blind phase of the investigation failed to show any benefit from treatment [6].

Urticaria

In urticaria patients with evidence of food or additives (preservatives or colourings) as triggering agents, protection by SCG against provocation has also been demonstrated. In patients with chronic urticaria exacerbated by aspirin or tartrazine, the percentage increase in skin bleeding time was taken as an objective index of adverse reactions, most such patients showing a rise of 100% or more on provocation. (The 99% confidence limits for normal subjects were 52% for aspirin and 25% for tartrazine.) The provoking agent used was aspirin (50 mg, 14 patients) or tartrazine (5 mg, six patients). The dose of SCG was 800 mg 15 minutes before provocation, and the study was placebo controlled and double-blind. After SCG only six of the 14 aspirin-sensitive patients who had previously reacted gave a change over 52%, the corresponding figure for tartrazine being four of six [33].

This study, while having the merit of using an objective index of response, did not relate this to the severity of the clinical reaction, nor was it established whether bleeding time could be affected in normal subjects by oral SCG treatment. The site of action both for aspirin and SCG was proposed to be the gastric mucosa, though it seems more likely that aspirin's effect on platelets might be responsible for the effect observed on bleeding time.

Double-blind study

The same group also reported an 8-week double-blind cross-over study of 24 adults with food- and additive-induced adverse reactions, confirmed by at least two positive provocation tests after a strict exclusion diet. Increased bleeding time was again taken as an objective index of adverse reactions to foods, as well as to drugs or food additives. Symptom scores, which included skin, respiratory tract and gastrointestinal symptoms, were used to assess the patients' responses. These showed that in the fourth week of treatment there was significant advantage to the actively treated group, this being particularly noticeable in those who had received placebo in the first phase of the cross-over. This group also showed clear patient and doctor preference for SCG, but because of the small numbers involved, these reached statistical significance

only in the case of the doctors' preference, all nine patients assessed being judged better on active treatment, the corresponding figures for patient preference being 10 of 13 [2]. One significant feature of this study is the small magnitude of the effect observed. This amounted to an improvement in symptom scores of less than 30%, which while it may be statistically significant, may not be clinically significant. This is disappointing in view of the careful selection of cases for this trial. Bleeding times, which had been shown to change in an earlier study, do not appear to have been measured in the treatment phase of this investigation.

When SCG was tested in patients with positive provocation tests to food additives or drugs, it conferred no benefit in a placebo-controlled study of 15 adults [37]. Benefit was also not seen in 27 chronic urticaria patients in whom an exclusion diet had failed to elicit improvement [17]. This was in spite of the fact that the same authors were able to show clear SCG protection from multiple food-induced symptoms in two patients. The conclusion that it is specifically food-related urticaria which responds to SCG is supported by a study of 22 patients with chronic urticaria who had failed to respond to antihistamines. All had exacerbations induced by tartrazine and/or sodium benzoate. These patients showed a similar level of response (about 70%) to both dietary management and to SCG 200 mg before meals [4].

Multiple food-associated symptoms

In a number of studies, patients with a variety of symptoms ascribed to specific food allergy or intolerance have been grouped together, and here again SCG treatment seems most effective when given to patients rendered symptom-free by an avoidance diet and subsequently challenged. In 14 patients, mostly adults, with a variety of allergic symptoms, within 24 hours of food challenge, 64% of 30 food challenges produced reactions after placebo, only 8% being positive in 32 treated with SCG. Nine of the 11 patients protected against formal challenge were subsequently able to eat a full diet while on SCG without relapse [5]. In another similar study, 24 of 32 patients were protected to some extent by SCG, although there was an unusually high incidence of adverse reactions to the drug, including some of the very symptoms attributed in other cases to the food intolerance, namely urticaria, headache and gastrointestinal disturbance [23, 38]. Other similar studies have been mentioned elsewhere in this review (see e.g. [31]) and include one where no effect was observed from SCG treatment [25]. The largest group investigated was 66 patients with a variety of symptoms ascribed to single or multiple food sensitivities. Many had asthma, along with other complaints. The treatment was combined in some of the patients with partial or total dietary avoidance. Of the 21 patients reporting total suppression of symptoms, 11 were also practising dietary avoidance. The study included a placebo phase, but was not blinded. Fifteen patients reported exacerbations and 25 partial remission. Doses ranged from 300 to 2000 mg daily. The group studied was so diverse that the only conclusion to be drawn was, as in some other studies, that there might be a subgroup who benefitted from SCG, but that without dietary control the effect of the drug was only marginal [39].

Studies employing objective methods of assessment

The unsatisfactory reliance on subjective factors in many of these studies, which makes their interpretation particularly difficult when the patients have a variety of different clinical syndromes attributed to their food intolerance, gives those few studies in which objective criteria are used a particular interest. Many of these, however, have the disadvantage already mentioned that the objective criteria are not related clearly to the subjective or clinical assessment, nor is it always clear how, if at all, they are relevant to the mechanisms of adverse reactions to foods or to the mode of action of the drugs.

Polyethylene glycol

One study where SCG has shown such effects on objective criteria involved measurement of intestinal permeability. This was assessed in normal and allergic children by polyethyleneglycol (PEG) urinary excretion in the 6 hours following oral dosing with a mixture of two PEG fractions of molecular weight 400 and 1000. The dose of SCG used was 100 mg four times daily for a week and 200 mg 15 minutes before the PEG test. The allergic children with gastrointestinal manifestations showed less uptake of 'small' PEG than normal, whereas those with other allergies had greater than normal uptake. SCG reduced PEG recovery in all three groups, but variation within

groups was large. The relative excretion of the different size probe molecules was used to calculate a 'filter constant' for the intestinal barrier, and by this criterion SCG treatment clearly reduced the absorption of the smallest fractions in most (10 of 11) of the allergic, and in several of the normal group. Analysis of a calculated index related to apparent pore size of the intestinal barrier showed a change in the allergy group described as 'normalization', that is, it was consistent with reduction in pore size in those with gastrointestinal allergy, and with a rise in the 'other allergy' group [21].

Immune complexes

Immune complexes containing food proteins were detected in the serum of healthy individuals after ingesting milk, and at higher levels in two food-allergic patients (after egg). A biphasic peak was seen, and this was abolished by two prechallenge doses of SCG 500 mg, which also prevented the clinical manifestations, namely bronchospasm and itch, seen after unprotected challenge [34]. This study might have been easier to interpret if the normal subjects had received the same food challenge as the patients, and if the effects of SCG had been investigated in them too.

Neutrophil chemotactic activity

Another study in three adult subjects with milk-induced asthma showed rises in blood neutrophil chemotactic activity corresponding in time to immediate airway obstruction. A fourth subject, who developed an isolated late reaction, showed no such rise. Both neutrophil chemotactic activity rise and immediate asthmatic reaction were inhibited by the prior oral administration of SCG or of beclomethasone diproprionate [35].

ASPIRIN AND OTHER NON-STEROIDAL ANTI-INFLAMMATORY DRUGS

There has been much less investigation of the role of these cyclooxygenase inhibitors in the prophylaxis of adverse food reactions. Acute gastrointestinal and other 'allergic' reactions to foods which had previously provoked symptoms have been shown to be blocked by these drugs. The observation was made by a patient who discovered that an anti-inflammatory drug which she was taking for arthritis enabled her to eat without ill-effects shellfish, which in previous and subsequent unprotected challenge caused severe vomiting and diarrhoea. Measurement of the levels of prostaglandins E_2 and $F_{2\alpha}$ in venous blood plasma and in the stool showed high levels coinciding with the onset of the clinical reaction. The peaks were short-lasting, but measurement of a stable metabolite of $PGF_{2\alpha}$ suggested that a prostaglandin-mediated process was responsible for this type of adverse food reaction, and that inhibiting the production of cyclooxygenase products could therefore explain the protective effect observed with the aspirin-like drugs [8]. Support for this hypothesis is found in the observation that gastrointestinal disturbances, including vomiting, colic and watery diarrhoea, are among the side-effects most frequently observed during experimental or therapeutic intravenous administration of PGE_2 or $PGF_{2\alpha}$.

A study of urticaria patients who mentioned aspirin among the factors precipitating their attacks, disclosed that these patients very often had specific foods which could also cause symptoms. The induction of tolerance to aspirin by careful administration of increasing doses, and its maintenance by daily dosing, showed that this was accompanied by tolerance to the foods concerned. This incidental finding needs confirming by placebo-controlled provocation studies. In these patients, too, there was evidence of an underlying biochemical abnormality in the arachidonate pathway, since they consistently had higher than normal levels of $PGF_{2\alpha}$ [2] and histamine in blood samples taken before challenge. Paradoxically, these mediator levels fell to normal during the drug-induced reactions and the subsequent tolerant phase. Further study of this group of patients may enable their biochemical lesion to be more exactly defined, but it will not necessarily cast much light on the mechanisms of other, non-aspirin-related, types of urticaria and asthma

CONCLUSIONS

The place of drug therapy in food allergy is difficult to assess. The natural history of food-related allergic disease makes it difficult to obtain suitable patient populations for study. Food allergy or intolerance may cause a wide variety of symptoms, and these may vary greatly in one individual on different exposures, as in those with food-associated, exercise-induced anaphylaxis, to quote an extreme example. There is sometimes a lack of objective findings to support a patient's symptomatic response. When objective changes have been shown, their relevance has not always been apparent, and many studies lack critical controls to validate the tests applied. The interval between the last reported spontaneous reaction and a provocation, or between successive provocations, may profoundly affect the response. Allergen avoidance may reduce, or in other cases greatly increase, sensitivity to subsequent challenge. Food factors may be only one among several triggers in urticaria and other conditions. Few studies have involved more than a few patients, and it is often difficult to extrapolate from the formal challenge to the environmental exposure situation, or from one category of adverse reaction to another.

The efficacy of SCG is most readily demonstrated in subjects who have clear-cut symptoms precipitated acutely by the ingestion of specific foods, including those in whom there is evidence of an IgE-mediated mechanism. Attempts to treat or to elucidate the mechanisms of other, less well-defined adverse food reactions with SCG have not generally been impressive. Aspirin appears to have a specific role, related to its ability to inhibit the cyclooxygenase pathway, in those adverse food reactions which are manifest mainly as gastrointestinal upsets. The relationship between aspirin-induced urticaria or asthma, food intolerance and induced aspirin or food intolerance, suggests a central role for cyclooxygenase products as mediators or modulators in this group of conditions. It is questionable whether the findings from such clear-cut clinical syndromes as IgE-mediated food allergy or the urticaria induced by aspirin or foods, have much relevance to other forms of food intolerance. Until immunological or pharmacological clues to the mechanisms of such reactions are found treatment must remain largely empirical and symptomatic.

REFERENCES

1 Asad SI, Youlten LJF, Lessof MH: Specific desensitisation in 'aspirin sensitive' urticaria; plasma prostaglandin levels and clinical manifestations. Clin Allergy 1983; 13:459–66.

2 Asad SI, Youlten LJF, Holgate ST, Lessof MH: Plasma levels of histamine and prostaglandin in aspirin sensitive patients. (Submitted for publication.)

3 Atherton DJ, Soothill JF, Elindgo J: A controlled trial of sodium cromoglycate in atopic eczema. Br J Dermatol 1982; 106:681–5.

4 August PJ: Successful treatment of urticaria due to food additives with sodium cromoglycate and an exclusion diet. In: Pepys J, Edwards AM, eds. The mast cell: Its role in health and disease. Bath: Pitman Medical, 1979; 584–90.

5 Basomba A, Campos A, Villalmanzo IG, Pelaez A: The effect of sodium cromoglycate in patients with food allergy. Acta Allergol [Suppl] 1977; 13:95–101.

6 Benton EC, Barnetson RSC, Merrett TG, Ferguson A: Long term studies of oral sodium cromoglycate in atopic eczema. In: The Second Fisons Food Allergy Workshop. Oxford: Medicine Publishing Foundation, 1983; 123–7.

7 Brostoff J, Carini C, Wraith DG, Johns P: Production of IgE complexes by allergen challenge in atopic patients and the effect of sodium cromoglycate. Lancet 1979; i:1268–70.

8 Buisseret PD, Youlten LJF, Heinzelmann DI, Lessof MH: Prostaglandin-synthesis inhibitors in the prophylaxis of food intolerance. Lancet 1978; i:906–8.

9 Buscino L, Bernincori N, Buscino E et al: Double blind crossover study with an oral solution of sodium cromoglycate in children with atopic dermatitis due to food allergy. In: The Second Fisons Food Allergy Workshop. Oxford: Medicine Publishing Foundation, 1983; 111–5.

10 Cavagni G: Atopic dermatitis due to food allergens. Practitioner 1981; 225:1657–60.

11 Dahl R: Disodium cromoglycate and food allergy. The effect of oral and inhaled disodium cromoglycate in a food allergic patient. Allergy 1978; 33:192–4.

12 Dahl R: Oral and inhaled sodium cromoglycate in challenge tests with food allergens or acetylsalicylic acid. Allergy 1981; 36:161–5.

13 Dahl R, Zetterstrom O: The effect of orally administered sodium cromoglycate on allergic reactions caused by food allergens. Clin Allergy 1978; 8:419–22.

14 Dannaeus A, Johansson SGO: Prevention of antigen absorption in food allergic patients with oral sodium cromoglycate. In: Pepys J, Edwards AM, eds. The mast cell: Its role in health and disease. Bath; Pitman Medical 1979; 447–9.

15 Dannaeus A, Foucard T, Johansson SGO: The effect of orally administered sodium cromoglycate in asthma and urticaria due to foods. Clin Allergy 1978; 8:423–7.

16 Dannaeus A, Inganas M, Johansson SGO, Foucard T: Intestinal uptake of ovalbumin in malabsorption and food allergy in relation to serum IgG antibody and orally administered sodium cromoglycate. Clin Allergy 1979; 9:263–70.

17 Denman AM, Platts-Mills T, Brereton PJ et al: Urticaria and dietary hypersensitivity. In: Hemmings WA ed. Antigen absorption by the gut. Baltimore: University Park Press, 1978; 167–81.

18 Edwards AM: Drug management. In: The first food allergy workshop. Oxford: Medical Education Services, 1980; 95–101.

19 Edwards AM: Report on a multi centre study to examine the effects of oral sodium cromoglycate on serum IgE levels in atopic dermatitis. In: The Second Fisons Food Allergy Workshop. Oxford: Medicine Publishing Foundation, 1983; 128–31.

20 Ellul-Micallef R: Effect of oral sodium cromoglycate and ketotifen in fish-induced bronchial asthma. Thorax 1983; 38 (7):527–30.

21 Faith-Magnusson K, Kjellman NIM, Magnusson KE, Sundqvist T: Intestinal permeability in healthy and allergic children before and after sodium cromoglycate treatment assessed with different-sized polyethyleneglycols (PEG 400 and PEG 1000). Clin Allergy 1984; 14:277–86.

22 Freier S, Berger H: Disodium cromoglycate in gastrointestinal protein intolerance. Lancet 1973; i:913–5.

23 Gerrard JW: Oral cromoglycate: its value in treatment of adverse reactions to foods. Ann Allergy 1979; 42:135–9.

24 Haider SA: Treatment of atopic eczema in children: clinical trial of 10% sodium cromoglycate ointment. Br Med J 1977; i:1570–2.

25 Harries MG, O'Brien IM, Burge PS, Pepys J: Effects of orally administered sodium cromoglycate in asthma and urticaria due to foods. Clin Allergy 1978; 8:423–7.

26 Harris JM, Graham P, Hall-Smith SP, Price ML: The use of sodium cromoglycate and exclusion diets in childhood atopic eczema. In: The Second Fisons Food Allergy Workshop. Oxford: Medicine Publishing Foundation, 1983; 111–5.

27 Kingsley PJ: Oral sodium cromoglycate in gastrointestinal allergy. Lancet 1974; ii:1011.

28 Kocoshis S, Gryboski JD: Use of cromolyn in combined gastrointestinal allergy. J Am Med Assoc 1979; 242:1169–73.

29 Molkhou P, Waguet JC: Food allergy and atopic dermatitis in children: treatment with oral sodium cromoglycate. Ann Allergy 1981; 47:173–5.

30 Moneret-Vautrin DA, Claudot N: Allergie alimentaire de type I et pseudo-allergies alimentaires chez l'adulte. Effets du cromoglycate de sodium sur les manifestations cliniques. Nouv Presse Med 1980; 9:2549–52.

31 Nizami RM, Lewin PK, Baboo MT: Oral cromolyn therapy in patients with food allergy: a preliminary report. Ann Allergy 1977; 39:102–5.

32 Ortolani C, Pastorello E, Zanussi C: Prophylaxis of adverse reactions to foods. A double blind study of oral sodium cromoglycate for the prophylaxis of adverse reactions to foods and additives. Ann Allergy 1983; 50 (2): 105–9.

33 Ortolani C, Cornelli U, Bellani M et al: Sodium cromoglycate and provocation tests in chronic urticaria. Ann Allergy 1982; 48:50–2.

34 Paganelli R, Levinsky RJ, Brostoff J, Wraith DG: Immune complexes containing food proteins in normal and atopic subjects after oral challenge and effect of sodium cromoglycate on antigen absorption. Lancet 1979; i:1270–2.

35 Papageorgiou N, Lee TH, Nagakura T et al: Neutrophil chemotactic activity in milk-induced asthma. J Allergy Clin Immunol 1983; 72(1):75–82.

36 Shaw RF: Cromolyn therapy in chronic infantile eczema. Arch Dermatol 1975; 111:1537.

37 Thormann J, Laurberg G, Zachariae H: Oral sodium cromoglycate in chronic urticaria. Allergy 1980; 35:139–41.

38 Vaz GA, Tan LKT, Gerrard JW: Oral cromoglycate

in treatment of adverse reactions to foods. Lancet 1978; i:1066-8.

39 Wraith DG, Young GVW, Lee TH: The management of food allergy with diet and Nalcrom. In: Pepys J, Edwards AM eds. The mast cell: Its role in health and disease. Bath: Pitman Medical, 1979; 443-6.

40 Zachariae H, Afzelius H, Laurberg G: Topically applied sodium cromoglycate in atopic dermatitis. In: Pepys J, Edwards AM, eds. The mast cell: Its role in health and disease. Bath: Pitman Medical, 1979; 568-9.

Chapter 59
Hyposensitization

L. M. McEwen

Introduction

The wise physician practises his art as conservatively as possible. Nowhere is this so true as in the field of immunological hyposensitization in general, and in hyposensitization for food allergy in particular. The best treatment for food allergy is simple avoidance. It must be remembered that many individuals with a lifelong IgE-mediated intolerance to a single food such as egg or fish accept this from an early age. They do not consider their food intolerance an illness and the majority of these people will not proffer the information to their doctor unless specifically asked. The fact that so many individuals can accept without demur a dietary restriction enforced by food allergy should make us look very closely at our reasons for embarking on any hyposensitization to food allergens.

Indications for hyposensitization

There are really four indications which force the physician's hand to attempt hyposensitization to food.

1 The level of IgE-mediated sensitivity to a common food may be so acute that the patient cannot avoid anaphylactic accidents caused by unexpected traces of allergen.

2 The food in question may be such an essential part of the everyday enrivonment that exposure is unavoidable.
3 Hypersensitivity to multiple staple foods is usually not IgE-mediated and the penalty for accidental exposure to allergen may be less acute. Nevertheless, many sufferers must eat expensive, socially divisive and 'labour intensive' diets. Some manage well without falling victim to obsessionalism, but other patients become socially crippled and need to be set free by hyposensitization.
4 Finally, a small number of patients appear to be sensitive to such a wide range of foods that it is impossible for them to select an adequate diet and remain well, unless they can be hyposensitized.

PROBLEMS WITH IMMUNOTHERAPY

Unfortunately, immunotherapy for food allergy is generally more difficult than similar treatment for inhalant allergy. There are two reasons: anaphylactic hypersensitivity and exacerbation of coexisting allergy.

Anaphylactic hypersensitivity

Patients with anaphylactic hypersensitivity to

food often have phenomenal titres of specific antifood IgE, far in excess of the IgE levels seen in pollenosis. These are the patients most at risk from anaphylactic death following prick tests, so naturally hyposensitization is also a particularly dangerous procedure.

Exacerbation of coexisting allergy

Food allergy is often mediated by mechanisms which are not improved by conventional desensitizing injections. Allergists are familiar with the model of this difficulty: inhalant allergy in patients with atopic eczema. A minority of these people develop exacerbations of their eczema after contact with inhalants such as grass pollen or house dust and they also develop severe and sustained eczema in response to desensitizing injections. In response to this problem, allergists who wish to treat eczema or the non-atopic manifestations of food allergy by immunotherapy have been forced to develop alternative techniques.

METHODS FOR SUPPRESSION OF ALLERGIC ILLNESS

Five methods are available for the suppression of allergic illness by immunological means: graded normal exposure to allergen, graded injections, neutralizing therapy, pulse steroid therapy and enzyme-potentiated hyposensitization (Table 59.1). Only two of these

Table 59.1 Methods of immunotherapy for food allergy.

1 Graded normal exposure
2 Incremental injections
3 Neutralizing therapy
4 Pulse steroid therapy
5 Enzyme-potentiated desensitization

methods have been used chiefly for the treatment of food allergy. Much of our knowledge of the mechanisms and performance of the other three methods stems from their use for other forms of allergy. Their performance when treating food allergy cannot be considered in isolation.

GRADED NORMAL EXPOSURE

If an allergic patient is exposed to a dose of allergen by the usual route, in a dose which is too small to provoke an allergic response, and the exposure is repeated using step-wise dose increments of multiples of about 1.5, tolerance is likely to result.

Drug allergy

Aminosalicylic acid. This method has been widely used for many years to deal with allergy to drugs given by mouth, particularly during antituberculous therapy [19]. A suitable starting dose is usually between 10^{-5} and 10^{-8} of the therapeutic dose so it is necessary to start with especially prepared dilutions. The clinical situation usually dictates that the therapeutic dose is attained as quickly as possible, so the intervals at which the 30–40 steps are administered may be reduced to 2 hours. Intervals of more than a day are likely to reduce the efficacy of the method. The effect of this form of hyposensitization for drugs is not usually long-lasting so it may be used to initiate a course of therapy, but not as prophylaxis in case the drug in question is required at some unspecified time in the future.

Aspirin. Desensitization of asthmatic patients who are hypersensitive to aspirin [3] can be achieved by this method, but, as with other drugs, after desensitization has been achieved the dose of aspirin must be maintained, otherwise sensitivity will return. Although it has been suggested that maintenance of a state of unresponsiveness to aspirin results in general improvement in the patient's condition, there is no consensus on this point and the treatment is not widely advocated. From our point of view the interest lies in the fact that many aspirin-sensitive patients are also food allergic.

Inhalant allergens

Allergy to grass pollen and other inhalants can also be treated by incremental exposure. The first observations of which the author is aware were made by Herxheimer [11] who used inhalation tests to diagnose allergy in asthmatics. To avoid severe delayed reactions to these tests, patients were exposed at daily intervals to tenfold increasing doses of aerosolized allergen over a 10 000-fold range. It was noticed that some patients gave 'false-negative' responses, having been desensitized during the testing procedure. By decreasing the increments of the aerosol dose to multiples of 1.5, it was possible to achieve tolerance to specific allergens in a useful proportion of patients.

The results of this work differ from the results of oral desensitization to drugs. When drug allergy is being treated, the desentization appears to be systemic but when the airways are exposed to incremental doses of allergen, the desensitization is thought to be a local phenomenon, although there may also be a systemic effect. Another important difference is that the desensitization produced by the inhaled allergen is not so transient [21, 31]. It is quite practical to give local desensitization for grass pollen in the early spring and then wait for the pollen to come into the air. To allow the same time-lapse between oral drug desensitization and a subsequent full dose would often lead to disaster.

Food allergy

Food allergy has been treated by this method using daily increments of the offending substance by mouth. The small initial doses necessitate the use of a diluted and preserved food extract. It is essential to ensure that the subject never ingests the food from another source in a dose which, although small, may exceed the required dose of a particular day, thereby destroying perhaps a month's effort. For this reason hyposensitization by graded exposure to a common food such as wheat flour may be difficult to achieve.

Nature of desensitization. The nature of the desensitization which is achieved by this method may be twofold. First, there is likely to be a local effect on the gut wall analogous to the effect of incremental doses of pollen on the mucosa of the airways. We know that local allergic responses in the gut wall may lead to excessive absorption of food allergen. This may be an important precursor of many expressions of food allergy [4, 7], so this local effect may be important. A systemic effect similar to that produced in the drug model is also likely. At present the relative importance of these two mechanisms is unknown. In addition, there are no published data on the long-term effects of oral desensitization to foods and, as with drugs, repeated exposure may be necessary to maintain the immunological unresponsiveness.

Clinical results of oral desensitization to foods

The concept of oral desensitization to foods as the logical extension of oral desensitization to drugs and local desensitization of the airways,

both of which are well established and reliable techniques, suggests that oral desensitization for foods should be equally effective. In fact the results are really very disappointing. True, there are reports in the literature which show that the method can be successful [29]; for instance, Patriarca et al [24], reported excellent results using this method for allergy to milk, egg and fruit. These workers carried out desensitization to one allergen at a time. Their starting dose was usually equivalent to 1 μg of the food. Their final dose was at least 10 g of the food and the incremental doses of approximately $\times 1.5$ were given daily. Nevertheless, each course of desensitization to a single food required 3 to 6 months.

In contrast to these results, others have found the method too unreliable to be useful [34]. Perhaps this explains why a method with a history stretching back 80 years to Finkelstein's first paper has never become popular [8].

Dangers of oral desensitization

Oral desensitization is particularly popular among non-medical practitioners. To them it has 'low tech' appeal. It is simple, cheap and, with the method at its crudest, no laboratory support is required. To the uninitiated, such a simple system also appears to be entirely safe, but unfortunately this is not true. Any oral dose of allergen may produce an allergic response which may be mild or life-threatening. Patriarca [24] encountered one adverse reaction which required hospital treatment. There is no doubt that oral desensitization should always be supervised by a physician.

Reactions to the treatment

As with other methods of desensitization which involve graded dosage, a reaction to an oral dose of food allergen does not mean that the attempt at desensitization must be abandoned. The dosage schedule may be resumed with a weaker dose of allergen. In Patriarca's series, it was the need to do this on many occasions which made the procedure so lengthy. As with injection therapy some patients will reach a 'sticking dose' which always provokes a reaction but which is much smaller than the dose that must be tolerated if the result is to be clinically useful.

INCREMENTAL INJECTIONS

Injections of allergen are perhaps more logical as a method of desensitization than exposure to allergen by the natural route, since the latter usually means that the allergen will be absorbed through a mucous membrane. Salvaggio [28] and his colleagues showed that an atopic subject was likely to form reaginic antibody to a powerful experimental allergen absorbed through the mucous membrane of the nose but would form non-anaphylactic antibodies and immunize just like a normal person if the antigen was administered by injection. Thus there is logic for giving parenteral injections of allergen rather than attempting desensitization by the natural route.

Graded injections for IgE-mediated food allergy are useful (see Chapter 25) but their value in non-IgE-mediated food sensitivity has not been proven.

Blind controlled trials

The first double-blind controlled trial of any method of hyposensitization was published by Frankland in 1952 [9]. He treated hay fever using injections of increasing quantities of grass pollen extract. The method was essentially the same as that established by Noon in 1911 [22], including the simple aqueous extraction method by which the vaccine was produced. Since that time, as new varieties of desensitizing vaccine have appeared, innumerable trials of injection therapy for hay fever have been published. Most have shown that the method is effective and reasonably safe. Frankland's success rate, with a benefit in 72% of subjects with hay fever and 93% of those with pollen asthma (versus a 28% control response), would be difficult to improve on (Table 59.2).

Table 59.2 Result of controlled double-blind trial of pre-seasonal hyposensitization for pollen asthma.

	Pollen extract	Placebo
Good	29	8
Moderate	0	5
Poor	2	15
Total patients	31	28

Data taken from Frankland and Augustin [9].

Purified allergen vaccines. In the past few years, vaccines prepared from freeze-dried and highly purified allergens have made their debut [10]. There seems no doubt that these are effective desensitizing agents, and for the first time, we have successful clinical trials for the treatment of allergy to domestic pets and some moulds. The treatment of allergy to insect venoms is also successful [12, 32]. The purification of allergens, both inhalant and venoms, has led to an increase in potency and an increased efficacy, but injections of allergens are never totally safe [6], and with potency comes risk. The author is already aware of at least four deaths in a single year which have followed injections of freeze-dried vaccine. (Verbal confirmation has been given by the vaccine manufacturers but as yet there is no published account of any of these accidents.) Against this background, the injection of impure food extracts into highly atopic subjects may be dangerous (see Chapter 25).

Problems with food extracts

Oxidation. Some food allergens are extremely unstable. The allergens in celery, carrot and apple oxidize very quickly [1] and to demonstrate atopic skin sensitivity it is usual to first make a scratch, then to rub into it a freshly sliced surface of the fruit or vegetable. Research on these allergens is possible only by directly extracting the raw material into a solution which contains antioxidant. It would be extremely difficult to make a reliable and standardized extract which would be suitable for injection therapy (see also Chapter 50).

Precipitation. A second difficulty is that many simple food extracts, fish and egg among them, continuously form precipitates throughout their shelf-lives. The precipitation does not reduce the potency of the allergen in the supernatant but it is unacceptable in a commercially sold vaccine. As a result, commercial food extracts are put through processes to ensure that no further precipitate will form. In the author's experience although these extracts are capable of raising a skin weal in a patient with strong atopic sensitivity to the relevant food and can be used for the radioallergosorbent test (RAST) and enzyme-linked immunosorbent assay (ELISA) techniques, their lack of standardization makes them unsuitable for injection therapy.

Multiplicity of allergens. The third problem with food allergens is that there are so many of them. Ideally, we would like a stable freeze-dried preparation of each one which was characterized and standardized to the same degree as the freeze-dried inhalant allergens which are now becoming available. Against this, injection therapy with these vaccines would still be dangerous. Their use would be limited so they would be prohibitively expensive.

NEUTRALIZING THERAPY

Bell-shaped dose–response curve

The bell-shaped dose–response curve of histamine release to allergen shown by grass pollen-sensitive leukocytes in vitro was first described by Van Arsdel et al [33]. As the dose of allergen is increased, histamine release rises to a maximum. Higher doses of allergen produce less response and a high dose can often be found which releases almost no histamine. Still higher doses provoke further histamine release which was at first believed to be 'nonspecific' (Fig. 59.1).

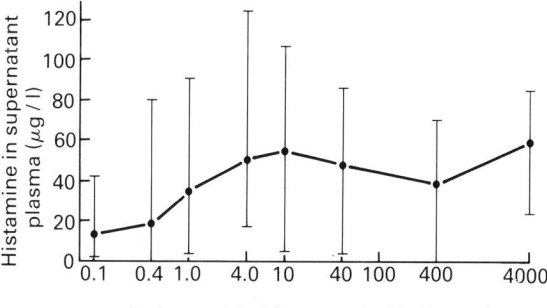

Fig. 59.1 Histamine in supernatant plasma following incubation of whole blood with varying amounts of specific antigen. These values are the means of those obtained in 29 separate experiments. From Van Arsdel et al [33].

Responses to different doses of allergen given by intradermal injection can be shown to follow a similar curve.

Underdosing. Provocation of symptoms by low concentrations of allergen injected intradermally was introduced by Rinkel as a diagnostic measure [27]. Rinkel reported that the symptoms he induced could be stopped by the injection of a higher dose of allergen. Unfortunately, this assertion seemed unreasonable to his contemporaries. Lee [13] first suggested that the high dose which abolished symptoms might be used prophylactically to protect the patient against normal exposure to allergen. The aim of this treatment is not long-term desensitization but short-term 'neutralization'. The neutralizing dose of allergen must be in-

jected at fairly frequent intervals, perhaps daily. It is possible that in some instances this treatment has a secondary late protective effect resembling conventional desensitizing injections but there is no satisfactory evidence that this is so.

Overdosing. At an early stage in the development of this technique it became clear that the clinical effects of provocation testing were usually less violent when the dose of allergen was very high indeed, and above the neutralizing dose ('overdose') rather than below it ('underdose'). The additional advantage is that the intradermal injection of an overdose usually results in a skin wheal-and-flare response in a sensitive subject (Fig. 59.2). For technical aspects of neutralization see Chapter 54.

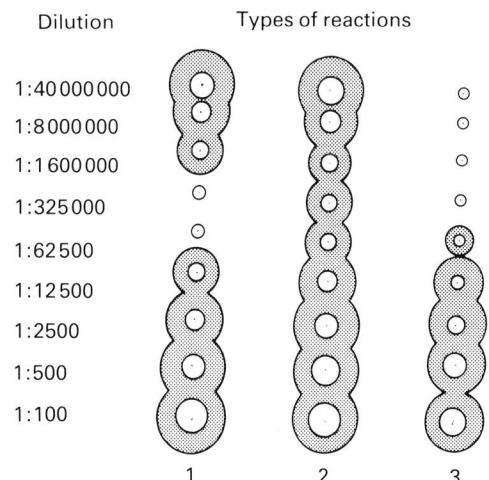

Fig. 59.2 Diagrams derived from Rinkel's original paper [26] showing different patterns of skin response to serial 1:5 dilutions of allergen injected intradermally. (1) A patient in whom underdoses and overdoses both elicit skin wheals but a range of intermediate doses do not. (2) In this patient the intermediate doses merely give reduced skin wheals. (3) The most frequent pattern of skin responses: underdoses do not elicit skin wheals. Overdoses do. Nevertheless, symptoms are more likely to be elicited by underdoses.

Safety. To the conventional allergist it is difficult to believe that this technique is not dangerous. Obviously, it would be imprudent to use it unless resuscitation equipment was available. On the other hand, the facts speak for themselves. This technique has been used by a very large group of practitioners which has been steadily increasing over the last 25 years. The number of patients who have been tested must now exceed one million. More important, a proportion of the practitioners using the technique have no training in conventional allergy and would not distinguish clearly between the risks involved in searching for the neutralizing dose of allergen in atopic and non-atopic patients. In spite of this very few deaths have been reported.

The neutralizing dose. As yet, published trials have only demonstrated that a neutralizing dose of allergen can protect the patient from natural exposure [20] or a provocation test in which allergen is administered by the natural route. Central to our understanding of the technique and possibly also to its safety is also the thesis that a neutralizing dose can abolish symptoms and skin reactions caused by the preceding overdoses. Besides this, it must be appreciated that although the description of the technique suggests that it is objective, in practice even the determination of the neutralizing point of the skin reactions is a subjective art.

Neutralization by injection. Neutralization by injection is likely to be a real phenomenon. Most of the small number of properly conducted trials which have appeared involved patients who were selected because of their known response to the therapy [2, 16, 23, 25]. More important, the neutralizing vaccines used in these trials contained just one, or a very small number of, allergens. The neutralizing doses have also been quite strong. We have already seen that it is wrong to extrapolate from trials of conventional desensitizing injections of grass pollen extract to vaccines containing mixtures of other allergens. In the same way, it is difficult to extrapolate from the trials which have been done on the neutralizing technique using one allergen to justify this therapy as it is so often practised using multiple allergens. There is no published evidence that mixtures of up to 70 different antigens could be effective. The originators of this technique were conservative in their approach. Many of their successors are not.

Conclusion

Our conclusion must be that in the restricted conditions of a trial, neutralization by injection of antigen is a demonstrable phenomenon. If used very conservatively it has clinical value. The originators of the method did use it conservatively, rarely for more than two or three allergens per patient.

PULSE STEROID THERAPY

About 1952, soon after adrenocorticotrophic hormone (ACTH) had become available as a pharmaceutical product, Houghton found that it could be used to induce tolerance to a food allergen. He administered 120 units of ACTH gel subcutaneously three times a day for 2 days. On the second day patients were instructed to eat a full meal of their allergen. On the third day all treatment was stopped. Thereafter the patient could usually tolerate the food which had previously caused reactions. By 1960 Houghton felt that the newer preparations of ACTH were less effective and he usually added oral steroid therapy in the region of 50 mg of prednisolone a day.

Houghton was a classical allergist. He only recognized quick, obvious and reproducible responses to single foods, though how many of his patients had IgE-mediated food allergy is uncertain. Houghton communicated his results on over 200 patients to the British Allergy Society at a time when proceedings were not published. So far as the author is aware he left no published account of his work.

This method possibly deserves further investigation. Very high doses of steroids given for only 2 days carry little risk. The method is best carried out in hospital but does not require the specialist expertise of an allergist and, more important, employs the offending allergen in its natural state in any 'large' dose.

ENZYME-POTENTIATED DESENSITIZATION

Animal models

The effectiveness of this method in animals and man depends solely on the way in which a small dose of β-glucuronidase can alter and enhance the sensitizing or desensitizing effect of antigen. This action of β-glucuronidase, and the cofactors which will modulate and stabilize it have been studied in laboratory animals [14, 16–18] and in dogs [5]. Throughout this experimental work in animals the treatment was given by subcutaneous injection.

Clinical administration

Clinically, the β-glucuronidase–allergen mixture is administered in a small plastic 'cup' strapped over a scarification on the forearm. The formulation also contains hyaluronidase which aids absorption of the dose. This method of delivery has been chosen in preference to injection chiefly because of its inherent safety.

Advantages. Enzyme-potentiated desensitization has a number of advantages. First, economy of dosage. A single dose each year is adequate for the control of hay fever. For food allergy three or four doses per annum are sufficient. Second, safety. The extremely small doses of allergen required and the slow absorption of the dose through the scarification greatly reduce the likelihood of an anaphylactic reaction to the treatment.

Grass pollen allergy as the paradigm for immunotherapy

As always, the treatment of grass pollen hay fever is the yardstick by which we compare

different methods of immunotherapy. Ortolani's group have recently reviewed the results of their use of enzyme-potentiated desensitization for the treatment of hay fever. They have given just over 1400 doses, spread over 4 years. This group also treats very large numbers of hay fever patients with conventional desensitization injections and they are able to compare the two methods (Ortolani, personal communication). The results of therapy using classical desensitization and enzyme-potentiated desensitization show a similar failure rate (approximately 17%) but the enzyme-potentiated method gives a greater percentage of *total* relief of symptoms (13% versus 5%) (Fig. 59.3).

Conventional injections produced local reactions at the site of injection in 15% of patients and a further 5% experienced a generalized reaction such as asthma and urticaria. In contrast, the enzyme-potentiated method elicited 5% of local reactions, and no general reactions (Fig. 59.4). This method has

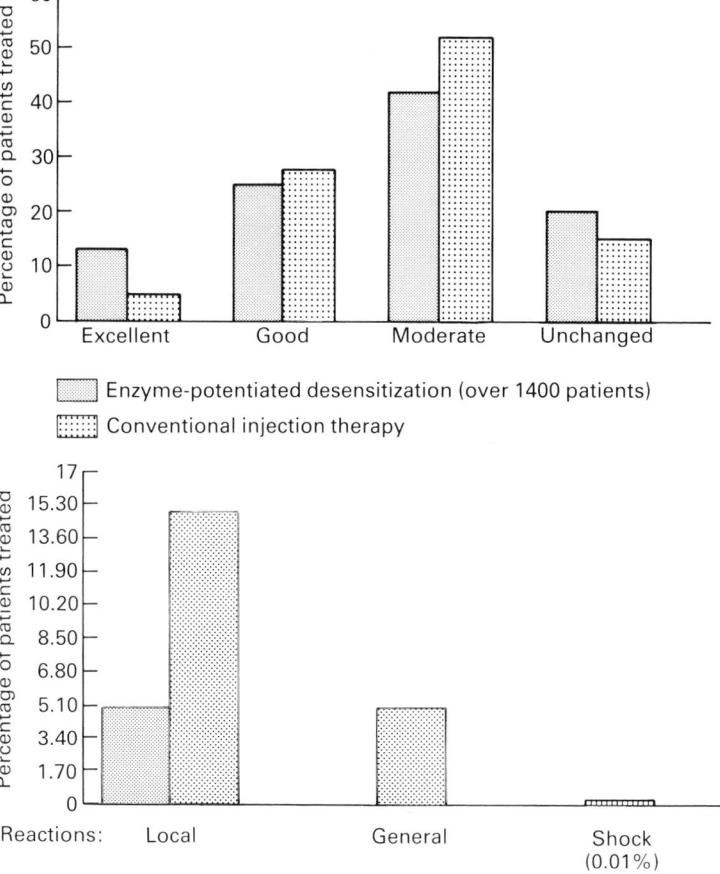

Enzyme-potentiated desensitization (over 1400 patients)
Conventional injection therapy

Fig. 59.3 Comparison of enzyme-potentiated desensitization and conventional injection therapy for grass pollen desensitization (Ortolani, personal communication).

Enzyme-potentiated desensitization
Conventional injection therapy

Fig. 59.4 Side-effects of a season's treatment by enzymepotentiated desensitization or conventional injection therapy for grass pollen desensitization.

Table 59.3 Randomized double-blind trial of enzyme-potentiated desensitization for hay fever: 3 weeks after a single treatment subjects received an intranasal dose of 1000 Noon units of grass pollen extract. Results expressed as subjects experiencing a full attack of hay fever.

	Protected	Not protected
Treated	13	6
Placebo	0	6

Fisher's exact test: $P = 0.01$.
Modified from McEwen et al [18].

Table 59.4 Double-blind trial of enzyme-potentiated desensitization to mixed food antigen in ulcerative colitis: patients with grade 3 sigmoidoscopy at some time during 14-month follow-up period.

	Group size	Sigmoidoscopy grade 3
Treated	27	1
Control	30	8

Fisher's exact test: $P < 0.025$.

been shown to be effective by a double-blind clinical trial [18] (Table 59.3) and it would seem that for hay fever this method of immunotherapy is likely to be the treatment of choice.

Use in ulcerative colitis

This method of desensitization has been subjected to the most severe test of all: a placebo-controlled double-blind trial using mixed food antigen in a group of patients who had not been subjected to allergy testing or dieting but were merely proved by biopsy to be suffering from ulcerative colitis. After 28 months, when the code was broken, it was found that in the 14-month follow-up period, eight control patients had shown grade three sigmoidostomy changes (bleeding mucosa ahead of the sigmoidoscope) while only one patient who had received active treatment was similarly affected (Table 59.4). The difference is statistically significant ($P < 0.025$). Other features, such as the numbers of patients who reported bleeding in the stools at the start of

the follow-up period (1 versus 6, $P = 0.025$) and the consumption of oral prednisolone, which was very different in the two groups (Fig. 59.5), supported the conclusion that the active treatment was beneficial. In contrast to the work on hay fever, in this trial it seems likely that the treatment did cause mild reactions in the early stages when there was an excess of patients suffering from mild inflammation (sigmoidoscopy grade 1 or less) in the treated group.

These results suggest that enzyme-potentiated desensitization may be used with mixed allergens as a 'blanket therapy' to protect patients from allergies which have not been accurately diagnosed. This is a surprising and disturbing conclusion which obviously requires confirmation. If true, it is to be hoped that the new method will not be misused.

Mechanism of action. The mechanism by which enzyme-potentiated desensitization protects the patient remains uncertain. Specific antigen will cause leukocyte migration inhibition in a serum-free system using the blood from patients who exhibit late hypersensitivity

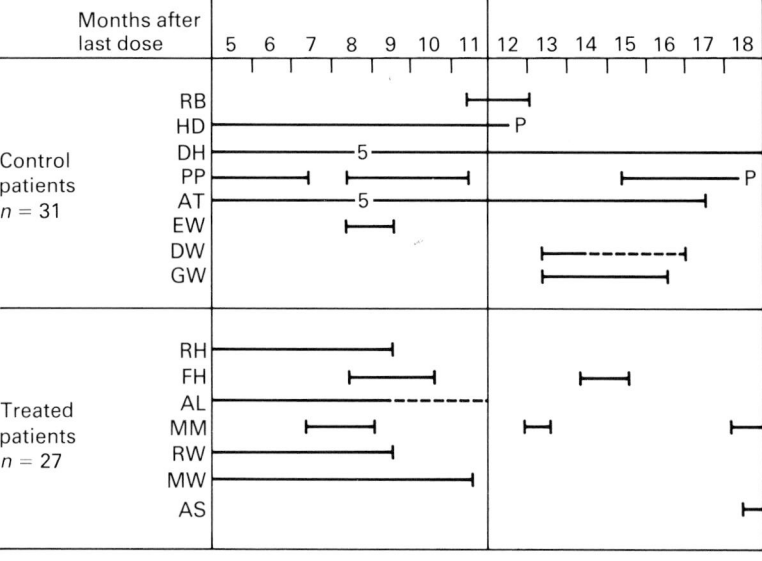

Fig. 59.5 Double-blind trial of enzyme-potentiated desensitization for ulcerative colitis. Effect on consumption of oral prednisone during 14-month follow-up. (——), prednisone therapy; (- - -), <5 mg/day; 5, emergency '5-day regime' for severe colitis; P, emergency protocolectomy. A third control patient underwent proto-colectomy for dysplasia.

responses to certain foods. In two patients who were successfully treated for milk sensitivity, milk no longer inhibited migration of the patient's leukocytes in vitro (Brostoff, personal communication). Starr and Weinstock, in parallel with their work on blocking antibody in hay fever patients treated by conventional desensitizing injections [30], showed that hay fever patients who had been relieved of their symptoms by enzyme-potentiated desensitization neither produced blocking antibody nor was there any change in their serum IgE (personal communication).

A case history. A young woman of 26 suffered from widespread atopic eczema and multiple acute IgE-mediated food allergies. Accidental ingestion of foods to which she was sensitive had resulted in anaphylactic collapse and necessitated intensive care on a number of occasions. She was anaphylactically sensitized to a very wide range of foods including most fruit, nuts, milk, cheese and egg. She also suffered less frightening reactions after exposure to many more foods including grains. Her total IgE was 3800 units, and her RAST results were positive grade two to the foods which caused less dramatic illness, grade four to foods which caused anaphylactic collapse.

Two years after the start of enzyme-potentiated desensitization this patient was almost free of eczema and was able to eat all the foods which had previously provoked anaphylactic attacks in almost normal quantities. Nevertheless, her total IgE was still 2800 units/ml, and her RAST results for many of the foods which she could now eat perfectly well were still grade four. Perhaps it should also be pointed out that this patient was treated safely by enzyme-potentiated desensitization as an outpatient. She only required five doses in the first year of treatment and four in the next. In the third year of treatment her interval between doses is 5 months. Like many other severely allergic patients it is unlikely that she will ever be able to stop maintenance doses but the intervals between them are likely to be extended to 1 year. A number of other case reports of patients suffering from different varieties of food sensitivity have already been published [15].

Conclusion

Enzyme-potentiated desensitization for food allergy has three advantages: greater safety, economy of dosage and proven efficacy when used with mixed food antigens. It seems likely that this method, or a development of it, will ultimately supersede other methods of immunotherapy. It is almost certain that the stimulus delivered to the immune system by β-glucuronidase could be reproduced by a drug if industrial research was focused in this direction and due to the pressures of commerce this may be the direction which immunotherapy will take. On the other hand, the ability to manipulate the immune system with a natural enzyme in a dose which can be extracted from a few millilitres of blood is such an attractive concept that the present method may survive.

REFERENCES

1 Bjorksten F, Halmepuro L, Hannuksela M, Lahti A: Extraction and properties of apple allergens. Allergy 1980; 35:671.
2 Boris M et al: Bronchoprovocation blocked by neutralisation therapy. J Allergy Clin Immunol 1983; 7:92.
3 Dor PJ, Vervloet D, Baldocchi G, Charpin J: Aspirin intolerance and asthma: induction of tolerance and long term monitoring. Clin Allergy 1985; 15:37–42.
4 Dumont GCL, Beach RC, Menzies IS: Gastrointestinal permeability in food-allergic eczematous children. Clin Allergy 1984; 14:55–9.
5 Eaton KK: Personal communication.
6 Ewan PW: Anaphylatic reaction to desensitisation. Br Med J 1980; 281:1069.
7 Falth-Magnusson K, Kjellman NIM, Magnusson KE, Sundquist T: Intestinal permeability in healthy and allergic children before and after sodium cromoglycate treatment assessed with different sized polyethylene-glycols (Peg 400 and Peg 1000). Clin Allergy 1984; 14:277–86.
8 Finkelstein H: Kuhmilch ab ursache Erhahrumstorungen bei Sauglingen. Monatsschr Kinderheilkd 1905; 4:65–72.
9 Frankland AW, Augustin R: Prophylaxis of summer hay fever and asthma. Controlled trial comparing crude grass-pollen extracts with isolated main pollen component. Lancet 1954; i:1055.
10 Frostad AB, Grimmer O, Sandviit L et al: Clinical effects of hyposensitisation using a purified allergen preparation from Timothy pollen as compared to crude aqueous extracts from Timothy pollen and a four-grass pollen mixture respectively. Clin Allergy 1983; 13:337–57.
11 Herxheimer HGJ: Bronchial hyposensitisation in man. Int Arch Allergy Appl Immunol 1951; 2:27–40.
12 Hunt KJ, Valentine MD, Sobotka AK et al: A con-

trolled trial of immunotherapy in insect hypersensitivity. N Engl J Med 1978; 299:257–61.

13 Lee CH, Williams RI, Binkley EL Jr: Provocative testing and treatment for foods. Arch Otolaryngeal 1969; 90:87.

14 McEwen LM: Enzyme potentiated hyposensitisation. II. Effects of glucose, glucosamine, N-acetylaminosugars and gelatin on the ability of beta glucuronidase to block the anamnestic response to antigen in mice. Ann Allergy 1973; 31:79–83.

15 McEwen LM: Enzyme potentiated hyposensitisation. V. Five case reports of patients with acute food allergy. Ann Allergy 1975; 35:98–103.

16 McEwen LM, Starr MS: Enzyme potentiated hyposensitisation. I. The effect of pre-treatment with beta glucuronidase, hyaluronidase, and antigen on anaphylactic sensitivity of guinea-pigs, rats and mice. Int Arch Allergy 1972; 42:152–8.

17 McEwen LM, Nicholson M, Kitchen I, White S: Enzyme potentiated hyposensitisation. III. Control by sugars and diols of the immunological effect of beta glucuronidase in mice and patients with hay fever. Ann Allergy 1973; 31:543–50.

18 McEwen LM, Nicholson M. Kitchen I et al: Enzyme potentiated hyposensitisation. IV. Effect of protamine on the immunological behaviour of beta glucuronidase in mice and patients with hay fever. Ann Allergy 1975; 34:290–5.

19 Madigan DG, Griffiths LL, Lynch MJG et al: Para aminosalicylic acid in tuberculosis: clinical and pharmacological aspects. Lancet 1950; i:239–45.

20 Miller JB: A double blind study of food extract injection therapy: a preliminary report. Ann Allergy 1977; 38:185.

21 Nichelson JA, Georgitis JW, Meuller UR et al: Local nasal immunotherapy for ragweed-allergic rhinitis. III. A second year of treatment. Clin Allergy 1983; 13:509–20.

22 Noon L: Prophylactic inoculation against hay fever. Lancet 1911; i:1572.

23 O'Shea JA, Porter SF: Double blind study of children with hyperkinetic syndrome treated with multiallergen extract sublingually. J Learning Disabilities 1981; 14:189–91.

24 Patriarca G, Venuti A, Schiavina D, Romano A: In: Zanussi C, Ortolani C, Torzuoli P, eds. Food allergy. Milano: Massom Italia, 1979; 131–4.

25 Rea WJ, et al: Elimination of oral food challenge reaction by injection of food extracts. Arch Otolaryngol 1984; 110:248–52.

26 Rinkel HJ: Inhalant allergy. I. Ann Allergy 1949; 625–30.

27 Rinkel HJ, Lee CH, Brown DW Jr et al: The diagnosis of food allergy. Arch Otolaryngol 1964; 79:71.

28 Salvaggio E, Cavanach SSD, Lowell FC, Leskowitz S: A comparison of the immunologic responses of normal and atopic individuals to intranasally administered antigen. J Allergy 1964; 35:62.

29 Shenassa MM, Perelmutter L, Gerrard DM: Desensitisation to peanut. J Allergy Clin Immunol 1985; 75:177.

30 Starr MS, Weinstock M: Studies in pollen allergy. III. Int Arch Allergy 1970; 38:514–21.

31 Taylor G, Shivalkar PR: Arthus-type reactivity in the nasal airways and skin in pollen sensitive subjects. Clin Allergy 1971; 1:407–14.

32 Urbanek R, Karitzky D, Forster J: Hyposensitisation therapy with pure bee venom. Dtsch Med Wochenschr 1978; 103:1656–60.

33 Van Arsdel PP Jr, Middleton E Jr, Sherman WB, Buchwald H: A quantitative study on the in vitro release of histamine from leucocytes of atopic persons. J Allergy 1958; 29:429–37.

34 Zanussi C: Food allergy treatment. Clin Immunol Allergy 1982; 2:221–40.

Chapter 60
Transfer Factor and Allergies

Alan S. Levin

Historical considerations

The passive transfer of delayed-type hypersensitivity with cellular elements from an immune individual to a naive individual was initially described in animals by Landsteiner and Chase in 1940 [26]. Later Lawrence demonstrated this phenomenon in humans [27]. At that time, the passive transfer of delayed hypersensitivity was thought to be effected by viable donor cells in the recipient. In 1955, Lawrence demonstrated that this transfer of immunity was effected by low molecular weight fragments from disrupted leukocytes [28]. The theory that specific transfer of immune reactivity could be effected by low molecular weight compounds drew a great deal of resistance from the immunological community. At that time, transfer factor was considered controversial.

Transfer factor therapy

Transfer factor remained a controversial laboratory curiosity until the first reported attempt to use transfer factor therapeutically in a patient with the Wiskott–Aldrich syndrome, a genetically determined immunodeficiency disorder [36]. Since that time, numerous reports have appeared in the medical literature describing studies involving the use of transfer factor therapy in immunodeficiency disorders [3, 4, 17, 19, 23, 31–33, 39, 47, 50, 59, 60, 62, 63, 72], cancer [6, 11–13, 18, 24, 30, 34, 35, 37, 38, 54–58, 61, 66], autoimmune disease [5, 10] and infectious diseases [20, 29, 43, 53, 64]. Controlled single-blind [5, 39] and double-blind trials [43, 53, 64] have demonstrated the safety and efficacy of this therapeutic modality in autoimmune disease and infectious diseases (Fig. 60.1).

BIOCHEMICAL CHARACTERIZATION

Active moieties

Increased interest in lymphokine therapy in the treatment of immunologically mediated disease has resulted in a large number of investigations into the active moieties of transfer factor. These efforts were initially hindered by the lack of reliable in vitro and animal models of transfer factor [22, 46]. With newer technologies, several animal models [2, 21, 22, 46, 48, 70] and in vitro assays [1, 16, 51, 52, 68, 69, 71] have been developed which aid in the characterization of transfer factor.

It is now clear that transfer factor, as derived from dialysable human leukocyte extract, represents a mix of immunopotentiators.

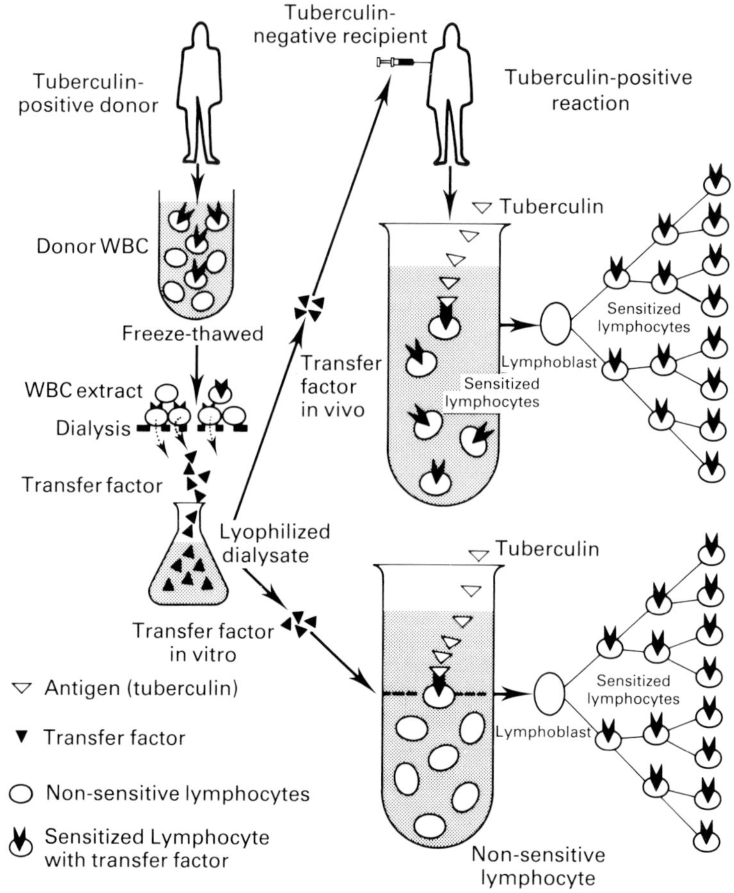

Fig. 60.1 Ability of dialysable transfer factor (TF) to confer sensitivity on a specific antigen either in vivo or in vitro is demonstrated in these experiments. Preparation of TF from leukocytes of tuberculin-sensitive individuals is shown on the left. When injected into tuberculin-negative recipient (top centre), the dialysable TF converts to tuberculin-positive state. Lymphocytes from such a TF-sensitized person, when incubated with antigen, can produce a clone of specifically sensitized lymphocytes in vitro (bottom centre) which induces lymphoblast transformation that leads to production of a clone of tuberculin-sensitive cells. From Patterson R, Norman P, Van Metre T: Immunotherapy-immunomodulation. JAMA 1982; 248:2759–72. © 1982, American Medical Association.

These include antigen-specific and non-antigen-specific helper and suppressor factors.

Antigen specific factors

Borkowsky and Lawrence [7, 8] demonstrated that antigen-specific activity can be deleted from leukocyte extract containing transfer factor by specific antigen coated on polystyrene. This antigen-specific activity can be recovered by elution from the polystyrene using either 8 M urea or low pH glycine·HCl buffer (Fig. 60.2). This transfer factor activity has a molecular weight between 2500 and 16 000 and appears to originate from helper T cells but binds to suppressor T cells and macrophages. The inducer activity also reacts with a variety of sera directed at a framework of residues in the variable region of immunoglobulins as well as sera directed at T cell immunoglobulin-like molecules.

T cell receptor fragment

This led Borkowsky and Lawrence to hypothesize that that active moiety of transfer

factor represents a fragment of T cell receptor molecule which perhaps functions to enhance immune reactivity by blocking suppressor T cell activity.

Inhibitory activity. Other in vitro experiments demonstrate a second class of molecules in transfer factor, also with molecular weights between 2500 and 16 000, which specifically inhibits the inducer moiety in the transfer factor preparations (Fig. 60.2), as well as inhibiting the capacity of sensitized lymphocytes to respond appropriately in vitro to antigen. These inhibitory molecules bind specifically to antibody directed at the related antigen epitopes in response to which transfer factor induces reactivity and to which immune lymphocytes react. These suppressor moieties originate from suppressor T cells and bind to helper T cells and macrophages.

Suppressor T cell receptor fragment

These properties led Borkowsky and Lawrence to postulate that this class of molecules represents a fragment of suppressor T

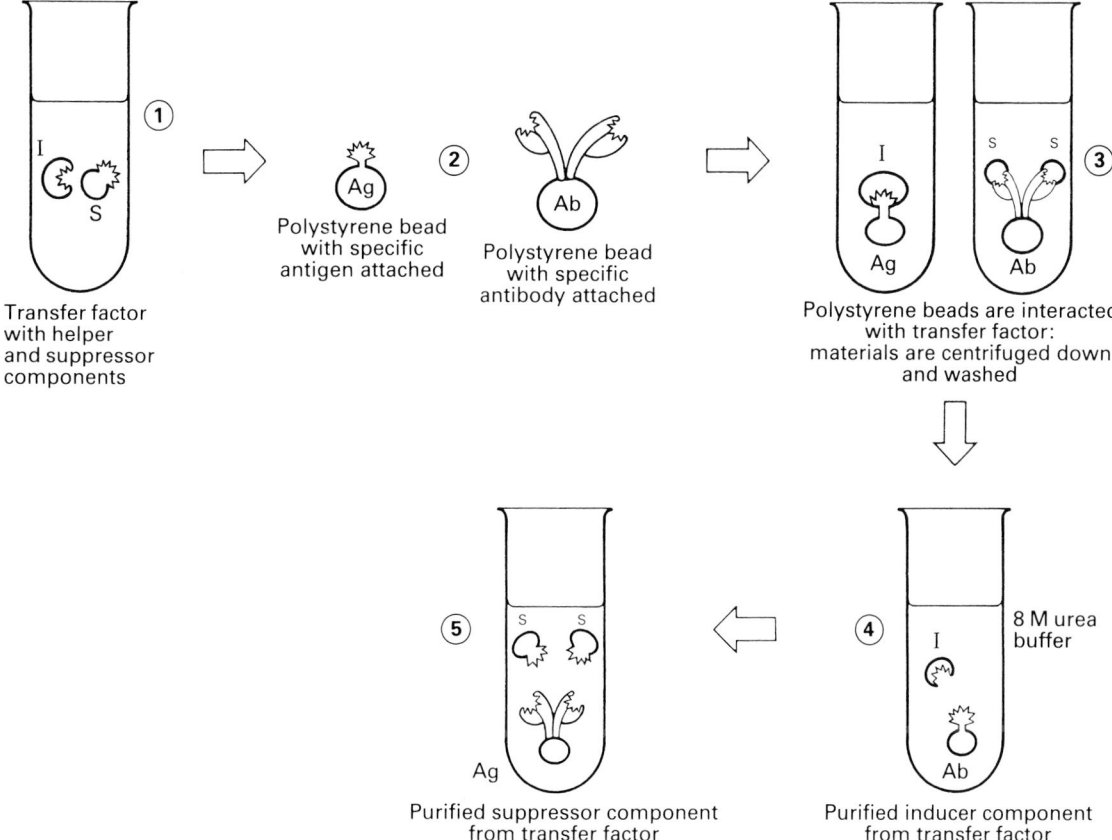

Fig. 60.2 Purification of suppressor and inducer components of transfer factor.

cell receptor [8]. Further characterization of dialysable leukocyte extract transfer factor has been performed by Fudenberg and Wilson [16]. These investigators have isolated and characterized at least 35 different active components in human dialysable transfer factor.

RATIONALE FOR TRANSFER FACTOR THERAPY IN FOOD ALLERGY

Suppressor cells in food allergy

Currently the general consensus of immunological opinion asserts that inappropriate responses to environmental agents (allergies) and self-antigens (autoimmunity) are a result of the inability of the host to suppress these reactions [9, 40, 65]. The acquired loss of suppressor cell activity is presently thought to be a major component in the development of autoimmune reactivity and allergies.

Oral tolerance

Animal studies have demonstrated that feeding of protein antigens causes the activation of suppressor cells in gut-associated lymphoid tissue (GALT). This suppressor cell activity can be abrogated with cyclophosphamide pretreatment [44]. Feeding of antigen causes suppressor T cells to mask Peyer's patch B cell priming to that orally administered antigen [41] (see Chapter 15). Miller and Hanson [42] showed that feeding mice with ovalbumin induced the development of antigen-specific suppressor cells in the gut mucosa. Specific immune unresponsiveness could be passively transferred with T suppressor cells from these ovalbumin-fed donors. This is a clear demonstration that non-responsiveness to food protein antigens is mediated, at least in part, by suppressor T cells.

Suppressor T cell deficiency and IgE

In humans, suppressor T cell deficiency and circulating IgE elevation were found to correlate positively with atopic eczema and food intolerance. Food-specific IgE levels to milk and eggs were found to be significantly elevated in this population. It was suggested that this population of humans, with atopic eczema, suffered this disorder because of the absence of suppressor T cell activity on food-reactive IgE-producing B cells [73]. Cow's milk protein hypersensitivity in young humans may be due to delayed maturation of suppressor cell populations [67].

Evidence that immunomodulators can act as 'normalizing agents'

T cell markers

Evidence in the current immunological literature indicates that some immunomodulatory agents act by normalizing T cell numbers and function. That is, these agents tend to raise depressed function into the normal range without causing supranormal activity or without themselves acting as a mitogen or antigen. This type of activity has been shown with thymosin fraction V in humans [49] and with whole thymosin in the spleen and lymph nodes of thymectomized guinea pigs [14].

Helper/suppressor ratios

In addition to the enhancement of helper activity, thymosin fractions have been shown to normalize, in vitro, the helper/suppressor ratios of systemic lupus erythematosus (SLE) patients who have decreased numbers of T suppressor cells [25]. Similar findings have been reported in vivo in SLE patients [15]. Transfer factor has also been shown to normalize lymphocyte marker profiles in immune-compromised patients suffering from disseminating herpes zoster [45].

CLINICAL EXPERIENCE WITH TRANSFER FACTOR IN FOOD ALLERGY

Since transfer factor has been shown to be a normalizing agent and has both helper and suppressor activities, it is reasonable to presume that therapy with transfer factor will normalize aberrant immunological responses in allergic patients. Since allergy patients most often react adversely to multiple environmental triggers, we elected to use transfer factor derived from pools of normal donors because this group is most likely to contain specificities

necessary to normalize the inappropriate immunological reactions of our patients.

Administration of transfer factor

Transfer factor was obtained from buffy coat preparations of 100 normal blood bank donors by the techniques described previously [37]. One dose of transfer factor is 1 ml containing that material derived from 5×10^8 lymphocytes. This material is administered as a subcutaneous injection every other week. Our protocol for treating patients with food and inhalant allergies with transfer factor is as follows.

Patient selection

Patients with food and inhalant allergies documented by history, skin test and in many cases diet challenge who are refractory to conventional treatment modalities were considered for the treatment.

History. Patients with food allergies commonly report having a history of recurrent ear infections as a young child. Chief complaints as an adult usually involve chronic nonspecific bowel complaints, migraine headaches, chronic skin rashes and on occasion asthma.

Skin tests. Food allergy skin testing involves injecting 0.1 ml of a 1:5 dilution of commercial food antigen intradermally. Reactions are read as positive if there is greater than a 2 mm growth in wheal size. Reactions are read at 10 minutes to assess immediate reactivity (IgE and/or IgG4), 24 hours to assess IgG1, IgG2 type reactivity and 48 hours to assess delayed hypersensitivity (T cell) type immunity.

Diet challenge. Patients are asked to strictly avoid the food to be tested for at least 48 hours, preferably for 2 weeks. They are asked to keep a meal and symptom diary. At the time of challenge, the patients are asked to eat a substantial portion of the food and keep track of symptoms. A positive test is one in which a clear-cut onset of symptoms can be identified within 48 hours of challenge. If patients encounter a positive challenge test, they are asked to repeat the test to verify its validity.

Conventional treatment. This includes dietary and environmental avoidance, drug therapy (β-agonists, antihistamines and corticosteroids) and immunotherapy with traditional build-up injections of antigens.

No age or sex restrictions apply to transfer factor therapy. It has been used successfully in young infants and elderly adults.

Immunological assessment

Baseline B and T lymphocyte assessments were performed initially using the E rosette assay [72] and subsequently using commercially available monoclonal antibodies (Ortho), with T cell subsets and helper/suppressor ratios (OKT4/OKT8) also being measured. Along with the immunological assessment, routine blood chemistry and haematology examinations were also performed. Immunological and haematological parameters were followed quarterly.

Symptom assessment

Patients were evaluated every 2 weeks and response to treatment was assessed both by the patient and the physician.

Results

A total of 88 patients have been treated, 35 males and 53 females. The ages ranged from 5 to 72 with a mean age of 34. The racial characteristics were relatively uniform with 85 Caucasians, two Blacks and one Oriental.

Table 60.1 summarizes the clinical responses of the patients. As can be seen from the table, the clinical responses were similar in males and females with 43% reporting marked improvement in symptoms. Among this group are three males and two females who were steroid-dependent asthmatics with treatment histories of 5–16 years of dependence on oral corticosteroid therapy who now remain free of symptoms and off steroids for between 5 months and 1.5 years.

Approximately 33% reported improvement in symptoms making an aggregate of 76% positive responses to transfer factor therapy. Approximately 20% of patients reported no change in symptoms and 4.5% reported they were definitely made worse by transfer factor. In all cases of adverse reactions, the response could be reversed by short courses of oral steroids (40 mg of prednisone orally per day for 3 days).

As can be seen from Table 60.2, patients reporting clinical improvement had a statistically significant increase in total T cells with no significant change in helper/suppressor ratio, while those reporting no clinical change had no changes in their immunological profiles. Patients reporting marked improvement tended to have lower total T cells at the

Table 60.1 Clinical response to treatment with transfer factor in 88 food-allergic patients.

Response*	Males	Females
Marked improvement	12	26
Improvement	12	17
No change	7	10
Worse	1	3

* Assessed by the patient.

Table 60.2 Immunological profiles in food-allergic patients treated with transfer factor.

	Average total T cells	t value* P value	Average helper/ suppressor ratio	t value P value
Patients reporting marked improvement ($n=10$)				
Pretreatment	744	$t=-2.939$ $P=0.0165$	1:1	$t=-1.51$ $P=0.227$
Post-treatment	1700	S	1:3	NS
Patients reporting improvement ($n=9$)				
Pretreatment	1027	$t=-3.382$ $P=0.0096$	1:1	$t=0.676$ $P=0.547$
Post-treatment	1763	S	1:2	NS
Patients reporting no change ($n=4$)				
Pretreatment	840	$t=-0.709$ $P=0.53$	1:2	$t=0.731$ $P=0.662$
Post-treatment	1021	NS	1:2	NS

* Student's *t*-test.
S = statistically significant to the 0.05 level.
NS = not statistically significant to the 0.05 level.

initiation of treatment and enjoyed a greater increase in these cells than did those reporting improvement of a lesser degree. The difference between the marked improvement group and the improvement group becomes insignificant when the five steroid-dependent asthmatics are removed from the data.

Case reports

Two representative cases are presented. In each case, treatment included diet control and environment control in addition to transfer factor therapy. Clinical improvement was coincident with an improvement in immunological parameters.

Case 1: disabling food and inhalant allergies

Clinical history. S.S., a 39-year-old heterosexual male accountant presented a chief complaint of disabling food and inhalant allergies. His illness started approximately 3 years previously when he suffered a 4-month viral syndrome. The acute phases of the illness were characterized by symptoms of low-grade fever, lymphadenopathy and malaise. Mono spot tests (for Epstein-Barr-associated infectious mononucleosis) were negative. After recovering from the acute illness, there was a resolution of the lymphadenopathy and fevers but the patient continued to suffer from malaise. He also noted an intolerance to alcoholic beverages, milk and milk products, corn and scented chemicals. He noted symptoms of headache and confusion while passing through the detergent aisle of supermarkets. Perfumes caused similar symptoms. Foods containing corn and milk products caused headaches and violent diarrhoea. The patient found that avoiding these foods allowed him to function with minimum discomfort but he suffered an unacceptable weight loss from his normal of 175 lb to 135 lb.

Past medical history. The patient was the product of a normal pregnancy and delivery and his early childhood medical history was non-contributory. He was, however, treated for 5 years between ages 11 and 16 with tetracycline for acne. He recalled a mild hay fever problem as a young boy but this never caused him to consult a physician. The rest of the past medical history was non-contributory.

Family history. Family history was significant in that his mother suffered from rheumatoid arthritis and his father had psoriasis and colitis. The patient was an only child. He is married and at the time had one infant child who was asymptomatic.

The patient was initially treated by an internist who effectively ruled out metabolic, malignant and connective tissue disease. He was referred by an allergist who found the patient to have atopic disease but traditional build-up therapy was not beneficial.

Clinical examination. Physical examination revealed a thin, alert, White male in no acute distress. Physical and neurological examinations were non-contributory. Immunological assessment revealed OKT11$^+$ cells at 1231 per ml (normal = 1000–2500), surface Ig$^+$ cells at 120 per ml (normal = 250–500) and a OKT4$^+$/OKT8$^+$ ratio of 1.1 (normal = 1.4–2.3).

Treatment. After treatment including seven 1-ml injections of transfer factor (that material derived from 500 million leukocytes) given subcutaneously every other week, the patient reported increased tolerance to aerosolized petrochemicals such as automobile exhaust fumes, perfumes and scented chemicals. He also noted a substantial decrease in the frequency and severity of headaches as well as an increased tolerance to foods. He was able to eat more foods and noted a weight gain to 160 lb. Repeat immunological assessment revealed OKT11$^+$ cells at 1767, surface Ig$^+$ cells at 484 and an OKT4$^+$/OKT8$^+$ ratio of 1.6.

Case 2: steroid-dependent asthma

Clinical history. E.H., a 57-year-old medically retired military pilot had severe life-threatening asthmatic attacks precipitated by foods and aerosolized petrochemicals for the previous 5 years. Three of these episodes required emergency resuscitation and one hospitalization with endotracheal intubation and mechanical respiration.

Past medical history. The patient had mild 'bronchial problems' as a youngster as well as measles, mumps, chicken pox and pertussis. As a young adult, however, he was healthy enough to pass many rigorous flight physicals in the United States Air Force. He served as a jet fighter pilot and was exposed to very high levels of kerosene fumes with no apparent physical problems. He noted initial problems with hay fever while serving in Alaska. These were successfully treated with injection therapy.

During the Viet Nam war, he flew 10 missions in a small spotter airplane above the large cargo ships dropping Agent Orange. He recalls no significant exposure to that herbicide. He does recall suffering from a malaria-type disorder with chills and high fevers which resolved over a 6-week period with no apparent sequela.

Upon return from South-East Asia, the patient began to notice increasing difficulty with sinusitis and postnasal drip in the spring while serving in the mid-west of the United States. At this time, several courses of allergy desensitization were unsuccessful in reducing symptoms. Symptoms worsened and a bronchospastic component developed requiring medical retirement from the military. His condition worsened until he required continual treatment with inhaled steroids and oral prednisone varying from 10 to 60 mg every other day for 5 years prior to starting transfer factor therapy.

Clinical examination. Physical examination revealed a well-developed, well-nourished White male with mildly laboured respirations of 20 per minute. The examination was significant in that there was bilateral nasal polyposis with bluish and boggy nasal mucosa. Examination of the chest revealed mild diffuse wheezes with no rales. The rest of the examination was non-contributory.

Initial immunological assessment revealed OKT11$^+$ cells at 1164 per ml, surface Ig$^+$ cells at 314 and an OKT4$^+$/OKT8$^+$ ratio of 2:1.

Treatment. The patient had been treated with prednisone for the previous 5 years when he was started on treatment of 1 ml of transfer factor every other week. After 10 injections the patient had been off all oral and inhaled steroids for 12 weeks.

Follow-up immunological assessment revealed OKT11$^+$ cells at 1817, surface Ig$^+$ cells at 288 and an OKT4$^+$/OKT8$^+$ ratio of 1.6.

CONCLUSION

Transfer factor, as derived from dialysates of leukocytes, is a mix of low molecular weight immunomodulatory agents with antigen-specific inducer and suppressor activities as well as non-antigen-specific suppressor factors. When given to humans, it appears to normalize immunoreactivity without producing supranormal responses and without acting as an antigen. The side-effects of this treatment are those of the enhancement of immunoreactivity. If the patient is 'living in peaceful co-existence' with a pathogenic agent such as the cytomegalovirus, enhanced reactivity may cause unwanted inflammation in a vital organ like the kidney or brain. Fortunately, those cells which are enhanced by transfer factor are exquisitely sensitive to oral corticosteroids and adverse reactions can be reversed quickly if detected at an early stage.

Since transfer factor is a blood product, the question of acquired immunodeficiency syndrome (AIDS) is commonly brought up. Since AIDS is a viral illness and since there has never been a report of viral illness transmitted by transfer factor, transfer of AIDS is extremely unlikely.

Clinical improvement

Data derived from our clinical experience suggest that transfer factor therapy produces a clinical improvement in symptoms in 76% of allergic patients treated. This improvement was associated with a statistically significant increase in total T cells with no significant change in helper/suppressor ratios. Nineteen per cent of the patients reported no change in symptoms following transfer factor therapy. This group showed no statistically significant change in their total T cells or helper/suppressor ratios. Approximately 5% of the patients reported being made more symptomatic from transfer factor therapy. All adverse reactions could be reversed with short courses of prednisone given orally.

The evidence derived from the literature and the above reported clinical experience indicates that transfer factor may be a helpful adjunct to the management of otherwise refractory food and inhalant allergy patients.

REFERENCES

1 Arala-Chaves MP, Porto MT, Kauppinen HL: Study of the immunopotentiator effects of dialyzable leukocyte extracts obtained out of leukocytes previously used for interferon production. Vox Sang 1982; 43:233–42.

2 Ashorn RGI, Marnela KM, Uotila A, Krohn KJE: Augmentation of delayed-type hypersensitivity in antigen-primed guinea pigs by human dialyzable leukocyte extract. Chromatographic and enzymatic characterization of the active principle. Acta Pathol Microbiol Immuno Scand 1982; 90:331–7.

3 Ballow M, Good RA: Report of a patient with T-cell deficiency and normal B-cell function: a new immunodeficiency disease with response to transfer factor. Cell Immunol 1975; 19:219–29.

4 Ballow M, Dupont B, Good RA: Autoimmune hemolytic anemia in Wiskott–Aldrich syndrome during treatment with transfer factor. J Pediatr 1973; 83:772–80.

5 Basten A, Pollard JD, Stewart GJ: Transfer factor in treatment of multiple sclerosis. Lancet 1980; ii:931–4.

6 Blume M, Rosenbaum E, Cohen R et al: Adjuvant immunotherapy of high risk stage I melanoma with transfer factor. Cancer 1981; 47:882–90.

7 Borkowsky W: Transfer factor—25 years later. A. Harvey Neidorff Memorial Lecture at the American Association for Clinical Immunology and Allergy Grossinger Forum. April 29, 1984.

8 Borkowsky W, Lawrence HS: Deletion of antigen-specific activity from leukocyte dialysates containing transfer factor by antigen-coated polystyrene. J Immunol 1981; 126:486–9.

9 Brostoff J, Hudspith BN, Boot JR: Influence of mediators of type I hypersensitivity on lymphocyte function in atopics and normals. In: Steffen C, Ludwig H, eds. Developments in immunology, clinical immunology and allergology. Amsterdam: Elsevier/North-Holland Biomedical Press, 1981:357–62.

10 Bukowski RM, Deodhar S, Hewlett J: Immunotherapy of human neoplasm with transfer factor. In: Ascher MS, Gottlieb AA, Kirkpatrick C, eds. Transfer factor: basic properties and clinical applications. New York: Academic Press, 1976:542–8.

11 Byers VS, Levin AS, Hackett AJ, Fudenberg HH: Tumor specific cell mediated immunity in household contacts of cancer patients. J Clin Invest 1975; 55:500–17.

12 Byers VS, LeCam L, Levin AS et al: Osteogenic sarcoma: immunotherapy of clinically disease free patients with transfer factor: long-term followup. Cancer Immunol Immunotherapy 1979; 6:243–51.

13 Byers VS, Levin AS, Hackett AJ et al: Tumor specific transfer factor therapy in osteogenic sarcoma. A two-year followup study. Ann NY Acad Sci 1976; 277:621–7.

14 Chebotarev VF: The effect of late thymectomy and thymosin on the quantity of antibody forming cells in the spleen and lymph nodes of guinea pigs. Mikrobiol Epidemiol Immunobiol 1976; 5:126–8.

15 Chen Z, Zhanc C, Wu Q: Disseminated lupus erythematosus and the transfer factor. Rhumatologie (France) 1981; 11:443–6.

16 Fudenberg HH, Wilson GB: Dialyzable transfer factor: clinical uses and studies on purification of the activity. In: Natelson S, Pesce AJ, Dietz AA, eds. Clinical immunochemistry. New York: American Association for Clinical Chemistry 1978:228–50.

17 Fudenberg HH, Spitler LE, Levin AS: Treatment of immune deficiency disorders. Am J Pathol 1972; 69:529–36.

18 Fudenberg HH, Levin AS, Spitler LE et al: Therapeutic uses of transfer factor. Hosp Pract 1974; 9:95–104.

19 Griscelli C, Revillard JP, Beutel H et al: Transfer factor therapy in immuno-deficiencies. Biomedicine 1973; 18:220–7.

20 Jose DJ, Ford GW, Welch JS: Therapy with parent's lymphocyte transfer factor in children with infection and malnutrition. Lancet 1976; i:263–6.

21 Kelsius PH, Fudenberg HH: Bovine transfer factor. In vivo transfer of cell-mediated immunity to cattle with alcohol precipitates. Clin Immunol Immunopathol 1977; 238–46.

22 Kirkpatrick CH: Transfer of cellular immunity with transfer factor. J Allergy Clin Immunol 1979; 63:71–3.

23 Kirkpatrick CH, Smith TK: Chronic mucocutaneous candidiasis: immunologic and antibiotic therapy. Ann Intern Med 1974; 80:310–20.

24 Kirsh MM, Orringer MB, McAuiliffe S et al: Transfer factor in the treatment of carcinoma of the lung. Ann Thorac Surg 1984; 38:140–5.

25 Koriyama KK, Daniels JC: In vitro effects of thymosin on T-cell subsets in systemic lupus erythematosus. J Immunopharmacol 1980; 2:381–96.

26 Landsteiner K, Chase MW: Experiments on transfer of cutaneous sensitivity to simple chemical compounds. Proc Soc Exp Biol Med 1942; 49:688–90.

27 Lawrence HS: The cellular transfer of cutaneous hypersensitivity to tuberculin in man. Proc Soc Exp Biol Med 1949; 71:516–22.

28 Lawrence HS: The transfer in humans of delayed skin sensitivity to streptococci M substance and to tuberculin with disrupted leukocytes. J Clin Invest 1955; 34:219–30.

29 Leser PG, Margarido L, Belda W et al: Cell mediated immunity in patients with Virchowian hanseniasis before and after treatment with transfer factor. Hansenol Int 1980; 5:3–27.

30 Levin AS: Transfer factor therapy: current status. South Med J 1975; 68:1465–6.

31 Levin AS, Spitler LE, Fudenberg HH: Immune deficiency states. Feingold B, ed. Introduction to clinical allergy. Springfield, Illinois: C C Thomas, 1973;346–59.

32 Levin AS, Spitler LE, Fudenberg HH: Transfer factor therapy in immune deficiency states. Annu Rev Med 1973; 24:175–208.

33 Levin AS, Spitler LE, Fudenberg HH: Transfer factor 1. Methods of therapy. In: Bergsma D, Good RA, eds. Birth defects: original article series. New York: Sinauer, 1975.

34 Levin AS, Byers VS, Fudenberg HH, Wybran J: Immunologic parameters for monitoring immunotherapy with tumor specific transfer factor. Trans Assoc Am Physicians 1974; 87:153–8.

35 Levin AS, Byers VS, LeCam LM, Johnston JO: An unusual metastasis in an osteogenic sarcoma patient on tumor specific transfer factor therapy. New York: Academic Press, 1976; 537–42.

36 Levin AS, Spitler LE, Stites DP, Fudenberg HH: Wiskott–Aldrich syndrome, a genetically determined cellular immunologic deficiency: clinical and laboratory responses to therapy with transfer factor. Proc Natl Acad Sci USA 1970; 67:821–8.

37 Levin AS, Byers VS, Fudenberg HH et al: Osteogenic

sarcoma: immunologic parameters before and during therapy with tumor specific transfer factor. J Clin Invest 1975; 55:487–99.

38 Levin AS, Byers VS, Hackett AJ et al: Tumor specific transfer factor therapy in osteogenic sarcoma. Chicago, Illinois: Immunotherapy in Cancer, Proceedings of ITR, 1975.

39 Littman BH, Rocklin RE, Parkman R, David JR: Combination transfer factor-amphotericin B therapy in a case of chronic mucocutaneous candidiasis-A controlled study. In: Ascher MS, Gottlieb AA, Kirkpatrick CH, eds. Transfer factor: basic properties and clinical applications. New York: Academic Press, 1976; 495–49.

40 Lydyard PM, Brostoff J, Pack S, Parry HF: Evidence of diminished suppressor T cell activity in patients with atopy and systemic lupus erythematosus. Immunobiology 1981; 158:173–81.

41 MacDonald TT: Immunosuppression caused by antigen feeding. II. Suppressor T cells mask Peyers patch B cell priming to orally administered antigen. Eur J Immunol 1983; 13:138–42.

42 Miller SD, Hanson DG: Inhibition of specific immune responses by feeding protein antigens. Evidence for tolerance and specific active suppression of cell-mediated immune responses to ovalbumin. J Immunol 1979; 123:2344–50.

43 Motszko CS, Marx Jr JJ, Halsby RC et al: A randomized trial of transfer factor therapy in the treatment of Herpes zoster infections. Immunol Allergy Pract 1985; 7:37–43.

44 Mowat FM, Ferguson A: Hypersensitivity in the small intestinal mucosa. V. Induction of cell-mediated immunity to a dietary antigen. Clin Exp Immunol 1981; 43:574–82.

45 Peetoom F, Florey MJ: Lymphocyte marker testing in relation to the clinical use of dialyzed leukocyte extract containing transfer factor (DLE-LTF). Haematologica (Pavia) 1980; 13:225–37.

46 Peterson EA, Greenberg LE, Manzara T, Kirkpatrick CH: Murine transfer factor. I. Description of the model and evidence for specificity. J Immunol 1981; 126:2480–4.

47 Rachelefsky GS, Stiehm ER, Amman AJ et al: T-cell reconstitution by thymus transplantation and transfer factor in severe combined immunodeficiency. J Pediatr 1975; 55:114–18.

48 Rifkind D, Frey JA, Petersen EA, Dinowitz M: Delayed hypersensitivity to fungal antigens in mice. III. Characterization of the active component in immunogenic RNA extracts. J Infect Dis 1976; 133:533–7.

49 Schafer LA, Goldstein AL, Gutterman JU, Hersh EM: In vitro and in vivo studies with thymosin in cancer patients. Ann NY Acad Sci 1976; 277:609–20.

50 Sheehy MJ, Miller NJ, Rappeport JM et al: A patient with post-hepatitis B immune deficiency: nonspecific helper factor partially restores the in vitro immune response. Vox Sang 1981; 40:346–51.

51 Schindler TE, Baram P: Transfer factor: specific and nonspecific effects and chemical characteristics of dialyzable leukocyte lysates (DLL). III. Biochemical characterization. Allergol Immunopathol (Madr) 1980; 8:203–12.

52 Shindler TE, Venton DL, Baram P: In vivo effects of human dialyzable leukocyte lysate. III. Modulation of spleen cell proliferative response to antigen by components of leukocyte dialysates and an initial characterization of an ampliative nucleoside. Cell Immunol 1983; 80:130–42.

53 Shulman ST, Hutto JH, Ayoub EM: A double-blind

evaluation of transfer factor therapy of HB(s)Ag-positive chronic aggressive hepatitis: preliminary report of efficacy. Cell Immunol 1979; 43:352–61.

54 Silva J, Allern J, Wheeler R et al: Transfer factor therapy of disseminated neoplasms. In: Ascher MS, Gottlieb AA, Kirkpatrick C, eds. Transfer factor: basic properties and clinical applications. New York: Academic Press, 1976; 573.

55 Spitler L: BCG, Levamisole and transfer factor in the treatment of cancer. Prog Exp Tumor Res 1980; 25:178–81.

56 Spitler LE, Levin AS, Fudenberg HH: Human lymphocyte transfer factor. In: Busch H, ed. Methods in cancer research. New York: Academic Press, 1973.

57 Spitler LE, Levin AS, Fudenberg HH: Transfer factor. In: Good RA, Bach, eds. Clinical immunology. Vol. 2. New York: Academic Press, 1974.

58 Spitler LE, Levin AS, Fudenberg HH: The Wiskott-Aldrich syndrome. In: Dietschy JM, Early LE, Fudenberg HH et al, eds. The science and practice of clinical medicine. New York: Academic Press, 1974.

59 Spitler LE, Levin AS, Fudenberg HH: Transfer factor. II. Results of therapy. In: Bergsma D, Good RA, eds. Birth defects: original article series. New York: Sinauer, 1975.

60 Spitler LE, Levin AS, Fudenberg HH: The Wiskott-Aldrich syndrome: immunological studies in patients and family members. Cell Immunol 1975; 19:201–18.

61 Spitler LE, Levin AS, Wybran J: Adjuvant immunotherapy for malignant melanoma with BCG and transfer factor. Cell Immunol 1976; 21:119.

62 Spitler LE, Levin AS, Huber H, Fudenberg HH: Prediction of results of transfer factor therapy in the Wiskott–Aldrich syndrome by monocyte IgG receptors. Proc. Sixth Leukocyte Culture Conference. New York: Academic Press, 1972; 795–803.

63 Spitler LE, Levin AS, Stites DP et al: The Wiskott-Aldrich syndrome. Results of transfer factor therapy. J Clin Invest 1972; 51:3216–24.

64 Steele RW, Myers MG, Vincent MM: Transfer factor for the prevention of varicella-zoster infection in childhood leukemia. N Engl J Med 1980; 303:355–9.

65 Turner MW, Brostoff J, Mowbray JF, Skelton A: The atopic syndrome: in-vitro immunological characteristics of clinically defined subgroups of atopic subjects. Clin Allergy 1980; 10:575–84.

66 Wagner G, Gitsch E, Havelec L: Transfer factor therapy in invasive cervical cancer patients. Report of a doubleblind study. Wien Klin Wochenschr 1983; 95:738–42.

67 Weil S, Kuperman O, Ilfeld D et al: Nonspecific suppressor cell activity and lymphocyte response to beta-lactoglobulin in cow's milk protein hypersensitivity. J Pediatr Gastroenterol Nutr 1982; 1:389–93.

68 Wilson GB, Fudenberg HH: Effects of dialyzable leukocyte extracts with transfer factor activity on leukocyte migration in vitro. II. Separation and partial characterization of the components in DLE producing the antigen-dependent and antigen-independent effects. J Lab Clin Med 1979; 94:819–37.

69 Wilson GB, Smith CL, Fudenberg HH: Effects of dialyzable leukocyte extracts (DLEs) with transfer factor activity on leukocyte migration in vitro. III. Characterization of the antigen-independent migration inhibition factor in DLEs as a neutrophil immobilizing factor. J Allergy Clin Immunol 1979; 64:56–66.

70 Wilson GB, Welch TM, Fudenberg HH: Tx: a component in human dialyzable transfer factor that induces cutaneous delayed hypersensitivity in guinea pigs. Clin Immunol Immunopathol 1977; 7:187–202.

71 Wilson GB, Welch TM, Knapp DR, Fudenberg HH: Characterization of Tx, an active subfraction of human dialyzable transfer factor. I. Identification of the major component in TFg, a precursor of Tx, as hypoxanthine. Clin Immunol Immunopathol 1977; 8:551–68.

72 Wybran J, Levin AS, Spitler LE, Fudenberg HH: Rosette forming cells, immunological diseases and transfer factor. N Engl J Med 1973; 228:710–13.

73 Zachary CB, MacDonald DM: Quantitative analysis of T-lymphocyte subsets in atopic eczema, using monoclonal antibodies and cytofluorimetry. Br J Dermatol 1983; 108:411–22.

Chapter 61
Prevention of Food Allergy

J. F. Soothill

THE SCOPE OF THE PROBLEM

Food allergy is often obvious when ingestion is followed by the rapid onset of urticaria or angioedema. This was objectively established by the studies of Präusnitz on his food-allergic friend, Küstner. Food allergy is common, and commonly underdiagnosed, especially in children. The fact that it is more common in infants and children suggests that they are especially prone to sensitization to foods, but that many recover. Indeed there is evidence that, in the newborn period, genetically vulnerable individuals are especially prone to sensitization to a wide range of antigens, both inhaled and ingested.

Food allergy and atopy

Food allergy is more common in atopic subjects, that is the 30% of the population [23] who react to one or more of a range of common allergens by an immediate response to skin prick test, but it is not confined to them. Food intolerance (an adverse reaction to a food in quantities not damaging to the majority) may be due to mechanisms other than allergy, such as primary or secondary enzyme defects, which may be termed food idiosyncrasy (see Fig. 61.1). Both forms of food intolerance may produce local (gastrointestinal) or systemic effects and they may occur together (e.g. cow's milk allergy with associated lactose intolerance).

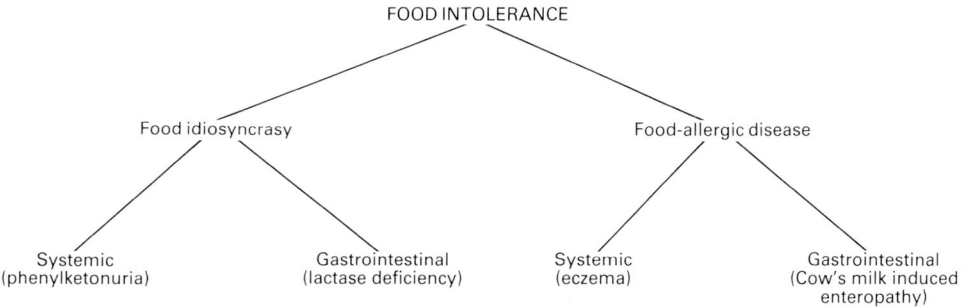

Fig. 61.1 The various mechanisms by which food or its additives can cause disease.

Mechanisms of damage

The mechanisms of food-allergic damage are far from clear (see Chapter 13) but there is some evidence that all of the hypersensitivity mechanisms defined by Coombs and Gell[14] may be involved. Coeliac disease, the most well-recognized food intolerance, is thought to be a food allergy, possibly mediated by T cells[18]. Its early recognition, and the characteristic jejunal biopsy appearance of subtotal villus atrophy, led to the assumption that wheat gluten is particularly damaging. The recognition that infection and other foods such as cow's milk can provoke similar if less severe lesions[41] strengthens the view that it is allergic in origin. However, by no means all food allergy, gastrointestinal or other, is associated with villus atrophy.

DIAGNOSIS

Food provocation test

Food-allergic disease can affect many organs and cause many symptoms. Goldman et al[24] recommended that, to establish the diagnosis for research purposes, the food should be given three times with the induction of symptoms, and the patient should recover when the food is withdrawn. Recognized idiosyncrasy should be excluded. However, giving food three times is rarely justified for clinical diagnosis; a single double-blind provocation to confirm the history is usually sufficient. Even a single challenge may be contraindicated in those who have had anaphylactic response or laryngeal oedema.

Some symptoms for which Goldman's criteria for diagnosis have been satisfied are shown in Table 61.1, classified by the affected organ; many others are suspected[20]. For some symptoms (e.g. anaphylaxis and eczema) there is plenty of evidence of immunological upset to justify the diagnosis of allergy, whether the onset is quick or slow, but, as with other allergy, the mechanisms involved have not been established by the only valid

method, passive transfer. For the diseases that are manifested quickly after low doses of antigen there is a significant increase of IgE antibody to causative foods[46], but for the more slowly induced symptoms, such as migraine[17], there is not.

Presumption of allergy

The presumption that these symptoms are allergic in origin springs from the remarkable range of foods, in virtually any combination, that can provoke symptoms: foods provoking symptoms together are associated by antigenicity rather than chemical similarity (as would be predicted by idiosyncrasy). Circumstantial evidence such as an excess of atopy and atopic diseases in patients or first degree relatives also supports an allergic aetiology. The passive transfer of eczema by parental bone marrow graft in severe combined immunodeficiency strongly points to an allergic cause for this slow onset food allergy, but for many of the other diseases this view is only inferential.

In vitro tests

Unfortunately, in vitro tests are still of limited value in diagnosis of food-allergic disease (see Chapter 50) but they may play a part in distinguishing allergy from idiosyncrasy.

PREVENTION OF FOOD ALLERGY

Food-allergic disease may be prevented at four stages[33].
1 Avoidance of damaging sensitization.
2 Avoidance of the food to which the patient is already sensitized.
3 Avoidance of entry of the food allergen into the circulation.
4 Modification of a damaging state of sensitization.

Symptomatic treatment by drugs and general management are important in some food-allergic disease (e.g. eczema). However, preven-

Table 61.1 Symptoms of food allergy for which Goldman's criteria for diagnosis have been satisfied (classified by the affected organ).

Systemic	Anaphylaxis, sudden death
Gastrointestinal	Vomiting, diarrhoea, abdominal pain
Secondary to intestinal disease	Anaemia, oedema, failure to thrive
Skin	Urticaria, angioedema, eczema
Respiratory	Rhinitis, asthma
Central nervous systems	Migraine, behaviour disorder, fits

tion by avoidance of food to which the patient is sensitized is much easier than avoidance of inhalant allergens, and is the mainstay of patient management and of diagnosis (see also Chapters 46 and 57). Hyposensitization is not established for food allergy (but see Chapter 59). Avoidance of damaging sensitization is the main topic of this chapter, and is especially important in the neonatal period when the common food allergens are first met. In addition, the quality of infant feeding may affect not only the development of allergy to the antigens in the artificial infant feeds, but perhaps also sensitivities to other antigens, including non-food antigens. Much of this effect may be antigen-non-specific.

Breast-feeding

The principal measure for avoiding damaging sensitization is exclusive breast-feeding and this is desirable for all infants for nutritional and other reasons. Sensitizing food antigens (such as certain artificial infant feeds) should be avoided not only in the newborn period, but also at other times of special vulnerability to sensitization, such as after gastro-enteritis [27,43].

FACTORS PREDISPOSING TO FOOD ALLERGY

Atopy

Food allergy most commonly occurs in atopic subjects, who can be identified by a positive immediate (20 minutes) wheal and flare reaction to prick tests with one or more of a number of inhalant or food allergen extracts (see Chapter 50). This test for identifying atopics depends on an IgE-mediated reaction, but atopics are sensitized in other systems too, so the pathogenesis of any particular disease with which atopics are associated is far from clear. Atopy is strongly familial [64]; about half the offspring of one atopic parent are atopic (even more if both parents are atopic), but the particular atopic syndromes (eczema, asthma, urticaria, etc.) differ not only between families but also among individuals in the same family. This suggests multifactorial pathogenesis, including polygenic inheritance. Observed concordance of atopic disease and of IgE levels in identical twins is considerably less than 100% [5,38] so environmental factors must contribute as well [55].

Atopy and immunodeficiency

The observation that immunodeficient children often have allergic diseases, including atopy, led to the suggestion that atopics and other patients with immunopathological diseases might also have common minor immunodeficiencies [54]. Persistent overactivity of an ordinarily protective mechanism may occur as a result of failure of effective antigen handling by another.

IgA deficiency. Kaufman and Hobbs [36] found that a significantly increased proportion of atopic subjects had abnormally low serum immunoglobulins (<mean −2SD) especially serum IgA. Transient immunodeficiency, especially of IgA, is a common cause of recurrent infections in infancy; a prospective study of newborn offspring of atopic parents showed that before symptoms had developed, those who later became atopic (most developed eczema) had lower IgA levels than those who did not develop symptoms, although the difference between the two subgroups had disappeared by 1 year [59] (Fig. 61.2 and 61.3).

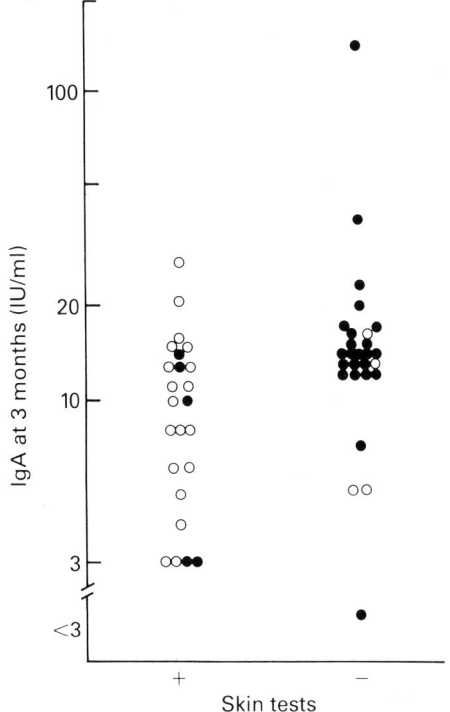

Fig. 61.2 Serum IgA concentration at 3 months of infants who at 1 year of age were either skin test positive or skin test negative. More children with eczema (○) were skin test positive and they also had lower serum IgA than those children without eczema (●). From Soothill et al [56], with permission.

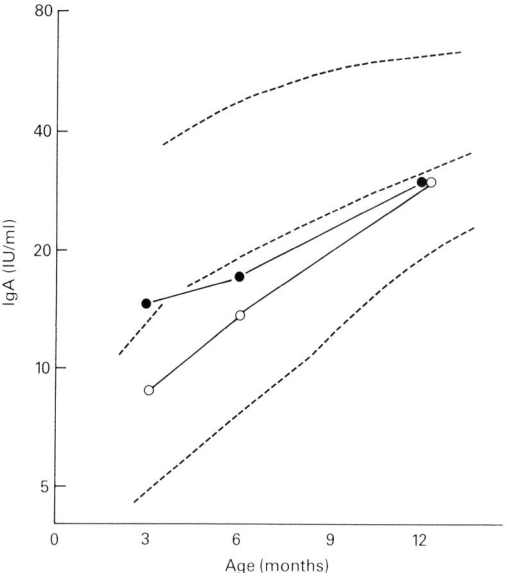

Fig. 61.3 Children who were skin test positive (○) tended to have lower serum IgA levels than those who were skin test negative (●). From Soothill et al [56], with permission.

This suggests that the IgA deficiency was associated with the development of atopic disease, since it was present first. It also strengthens the view that neonatal antigen experience in an immunodeficient host may be important for subsequent allergic sensitization. A number of subsequent studies have not detected this association but there are abnormally few IgA-containing B lymphocytes in intestinal submucosa in infants with cow's milk enteropathy [66]. This points to the importance of a local IgA reaction to foods in the gastrointestinal tract, perhaps antigen exclusion, in the protection against allergy, but the non-inflammatory hepatic clearance of complexes containing dimeric IgA [49] may also be important.

Abnormal C2 and yeast opsonization. Other immunodeficiencies associated with atopic disease include defects of yeast opsonization, and of the second component of complement. The defect in yeast opsonization is associated with an abnormality of a so-far undefined component of the complement pathways. This defect occurs in 5% of the general population, but in 27% of atopic individuals; C2 tends to be abnormally low in about 1.5% of the general population, but in 22% of atopic subjects [63].

Support for the fact that these defects are primary and not secondary to atopic disease comes from the finding that they are mutually exclusive; in an atopic child, if one is defective, the other is normal. Children with a rarer defect of neutrophil mobility associated with hyperimmunoglobulin E are also often atopic [29]. The association of atopy with this range of defects supports the view that defective antigen handling may be the general basis of atopy.

Suppressor T cells. Another immunodeficiency, possibly related causally to atopy, is that of T suppressor cells, which are known to be relevant for the experimental induction of IgE antibody [58]. Increased IgE antibody formation might result from defective T cell suppression in atopic individuals, and T cell abnormalities in the neonatal period have been demonstrated [35]. Reports of low levels of T suppressor cells in human atopic disease, determined by mitogen-driven assays [32] or by monoclonal antibodies [11] support the view that such systems may be relevant.

Food-allergic subjects take up more of an antigen to which they are sensitized and they incorporate it into IgE and IgG (complement-fixing) complexes, rather than IgA complexes [7, 50]. The relevant abnormality appears to be of antigen handling, and possibly of IgA.

Atopy and tissue type

Many immunopathological diseases including atopy are linked to particular tissue types. Marsh et al [44] reported weak linkages between certain tissue types and the IgE antibody response to minor antigenic determinants of pollen. However, although the antibody response was associated with tissue types, atopy and atopic disease (e.g. hay fever) were not. Such association might not be expected since the atopic state is antigen nonspecific. On the other hand, Thorsby et al [60] reported that atopic disease was linked to HLA-A1 and -B8, but Krain and Teresaki [39] reported linkage to HLA-A3 and -B7. This apparent disagreement was clarified by studying tissue types of patients presenting with different syndromes. Turner et al [62] found that whereas HLA-A1 and -B8 were more frequent in individuals with eczema, HLA-A3 and -B7 were more frequent in those

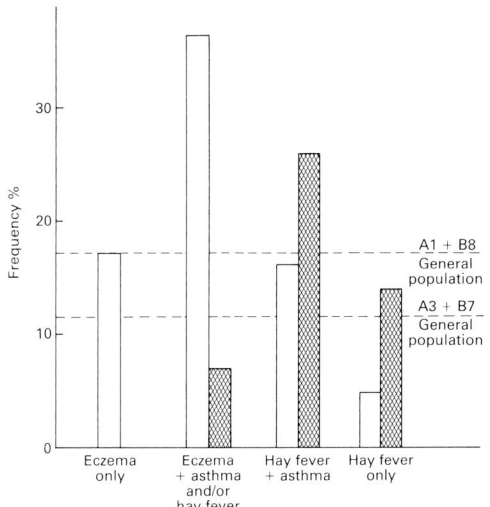

Fig. 61.4 Frequencies of the HLA antigen combination A1 + B8 (solid columns) and A3 + B7 (shaded columns) in atopic patients classified by clinical manifestations. The general population frequencies for these antigens are indicated by the horizontal lines, there being a trend for A1 + B8 to be increased in eczema patients and for A3 + B7 to be increased in those with hay fever + asthma. From Turner et al [62], with permission.

with hay fever (Fig. 61.4). This supports the view that atopy is transmitted by polygenic inheritance, and may explain the varied syndromes in atopy. Thus, any one of several mechanisms of immunodeficiency may cause atopy, but the different syndromes of atopy are independently genetically controlled, for example by tissue type.

NEONATAL ENVIRONMENTAL FACTORS

The transient IgA deficiency and the frequent non-concordance in infancy of the eczema-asthma syndrome in identical twins, suggests that neonatal environmental factors are important in the development of atopic allergy, including food allergy. With inhalant allergy there is other evidence that neonatal environmental factors are important. Atopic disease is less common in developing than developed countries [22]. Morrison-Smith's study [48] of immigrants to Britain confirmed that compared with indigenous children there was a lower incidence of asthma in children of African origin born outside Britain who come to

Britain in early childhood, but a similar incidence in offspring of parents of African origin who were born in Britain (Table 61.2). This suggests that the difference in incidence of asthma between the two groups of African children is due to neonatal environmental factors.

Table 61.2 Percentage of 19 995 Birmingham school-children with asthma, classified by race and place of birth.

	n	Percentage with asthma
White	19 033	4.3
Negro		
Born in UK	689	6.8
Born elsewhere	273	1.1

Data from Morrison-Smith [48].

Month of birth

Similarly, asthma occurs more frequently in children born in Europe in late Autumn [56] (Fig. 61.5) which suggests that seasonal differ-

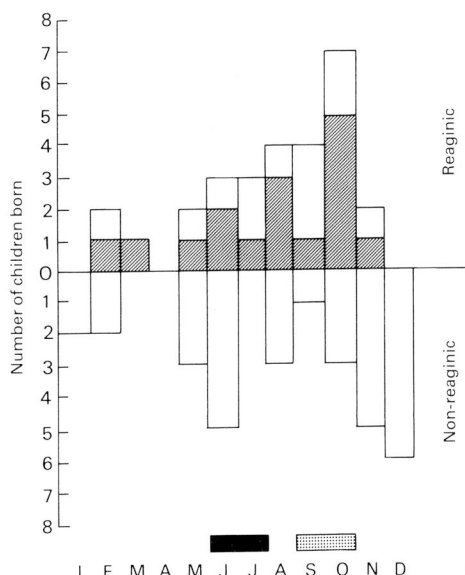

Fig. 61.5 Month of birth of infants who were subsequently classified as reaginic or non-reaginic according to skin tests. Infants giving positive skin test reactions for *Dermatophagoides* are indicated by cross-hatching. The pollen season (black bar) and the mite season (stippled bar) are also indicated. Skin reaction to any antigen was more common in those infants born in September and October (in England) than those born in the rest of the year. From Soothill et al [56], with permission.

ences in neonatal antigen contact are important for the development of atopic disease, but the fact that not only pollen but also dander allergy is maximal in boys born in both Spring and Autumn [6] suggests that the mechanism may be complex.

Other associations

Further evidence comes from the association of asthma with obstetric complications and with neonatal surgery [34, 53]. However, sensitization can also occur in later life, if the stimulus is strong enough. Parental smoking is related to the frequency of allergic diseases [37] so it is likely that non-specific factors may operate both in infancy and later.

INFANT FEEDING

The immunological aspects of infant feeding are complex [55]. Ingested antigens (food and bacterial) gain entry to the circulation and are important in stimulating the immune response in the neonate. Immune responses include local and systemic antibody formation (especially IgA), partial tolerance [13] and specific reduction of subsequent antigen entry through the intestinal mucosa, i.e. immune exclusion of antigens [65] (see Chapter 11). Though all these responses occur simultaneously to the same antigen stimulus, they show independent genetic variation, even to the same antigen [57].

Avoidance of cow's milk feeds

It is clear that imbalance of these complex responses could lead to allergy to food. This has led to a hypothesis that certain infant foods that are regarded as especially allergenic may be particularly important in the general development of allergy. Following the report of Grulee and Sandford [25] that eczema became more frequent with the increase of artificial infant feeding which occurred in the 1930s, Glaser and Johnstone [21] reported that avoidance of cow's milk and dairy products by using alternative foods (especially soya) prevented respiratory allergy in artificially fed genetically susceptible children. These differences were presumably a result of antigen avoidance and the same may apply to the presumably non-antigenic response to human milk, but there is evidence for an antigen-non-specific protection too.

Role of breast-feeding

Several prospective studies have shown that regimens which include exclusive breast-feeding reduce the prevalence of eczema in infants of atopic parents [10, 12, 26, 45] and some have reported a reduction of respiratory allergy too.

The effect is not absolute; negative retrospective studies [40] should not be considered important, since early supplements are often given without the mother's knowledge. It is possible that small amounts of supplementary feeds given early may be even more sensitizing than full bottle feeding [19, 51] (Figs. 61.6 and 61.7). This is consistent with the experimental observation of Jarrett and Hall [30] that small quantities of oral antigen are more sensitizing than larger quantities.

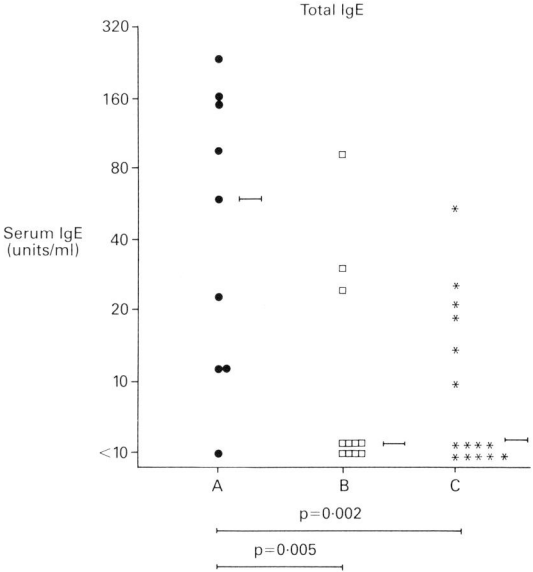

Fig. 61.6 Total serum IgE concentrations in the two patient groups and controls measured by PRIST. A = Milk-restricted patients with allergy to cows' milk. B = Non-milk-restricted patients with allergy to cows' milk. C = Age-matched controls. Total serum IgE was significantly higher in group A than in groups B or C. From Firer et al [19], with permission.

Duration of breast-feeding

Important points of uncertainty are the duration of exclusive breast-feeding, and what to do if it fails. The choice of 4 months for introduction of other feeds by Matthew et al [45] was arbitrary, but is consistent with currently recommended normal infant feeding policy for nutritional reasons [15]. It is likely that individuals differ in the length of exclusive and

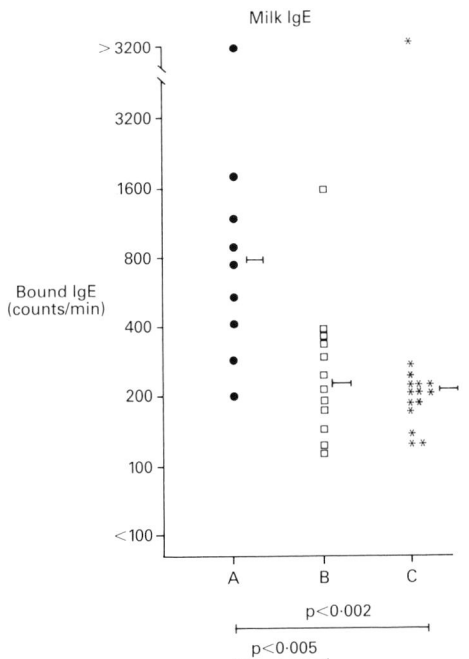

Milk IgE

Bound IgE (counts/min)

p<0·002

p<0·005

Fig. 61.7 Milk-specific IgE antibodies in the two patient groups and controls measured by radioallergosorbent tests. Values in group A were significantly higher than those in groups B or C (see Fig. 61.6). From Firer et al [19], with permission.

for an arbitrary period, say until 1 year [21], especially in those infants whose atopic parents are allergic to cow's milk or eggs. The recommendation for exclusive breast-feeding for 4 months can be made for all full-term normal babies, but especially for the offspring of atopic parents. However, abnormal infants, such as the grossly premature, hypoglycaemic or the jaundiced, for example, may have special requirements precluding this. Where alternatives are needed, expressed human milk, feeds based on casein hydrolysates or soya-based preparations, are probably the most rational. A number of alternatives to exclusive breast-feeding are listed in Table 61.3.

Breast-feeding and eczema. In the prospective study of Matthew et al [45] the beneficial effect of breast-feeding on susceptibility to eczema seemed more sustained than the effect on serum IgE level. IgE antibody and allergic disease are not synonymous, but there is experimental evidence that supplementary feeds do have an antigen-non-specific effect on the IgE antibody response. The subsequent IgE response to ovalbumin of suckled rat pups given supplements of a cow's milk-based infant feed (which contained no ovalbumin) was greater than that of unsupplemented controls [51].

Breast-feeding and intestinal flora. Many studies have reported that artificially fed babies have a mainly Gram-negative intestinal flora with a predominance of *Escherichia coli*, as compared with breast-fed babies, who have mainly Gram-positive bifidobacteria [8, 9]

partial breast-feeding required to protect them. The data of Saarinen et al [52] suggest that very much longer periods (up to 18 months) of partial breast-feeding may be of additional help, but inevitably this study was poorly controlled.

It seems reasonable to avoid highly sensitizing foods such as cow's milk products and eggs

Table 61.3 Breast-feeding substitutes in the prevention and treatment of food allergy.

Type	Examples	Application
Human milk	Expressed own mother's milk Expressed milk from other mothers	Very ill, food-allergic children
Infant feeds containing cow's milk protein	SMA Gold Cap liquid concentrate	Infants who are not cow's milk allergic—perhaps less sensitizing than other such infant feeds
Infant feeds containing hydrolysed cow's milk protein	Pregestamil Nutramigen (>3 months)★ Flexical (>2 years)★	Cow's milk-allergic infants, infants of atopic parents whose mothers cannot breast-feed them, and ?post-gastroenteritis
Infant feeds containing soya protein	Cow and Gate Formula S Prosobee New Velactin Wysoy	Cow's milk-allergic infants and infants of atopic parents whose mothers cannot breast-feed
Goat's or ewe's milk (boiled)		Cow's milk-allergic children (>1 year)★
Elemental	Vivonex	Allergy to many foods (>12 years)★

★ Preparations not nutritionally satisfactory for infants and children below the age shown.

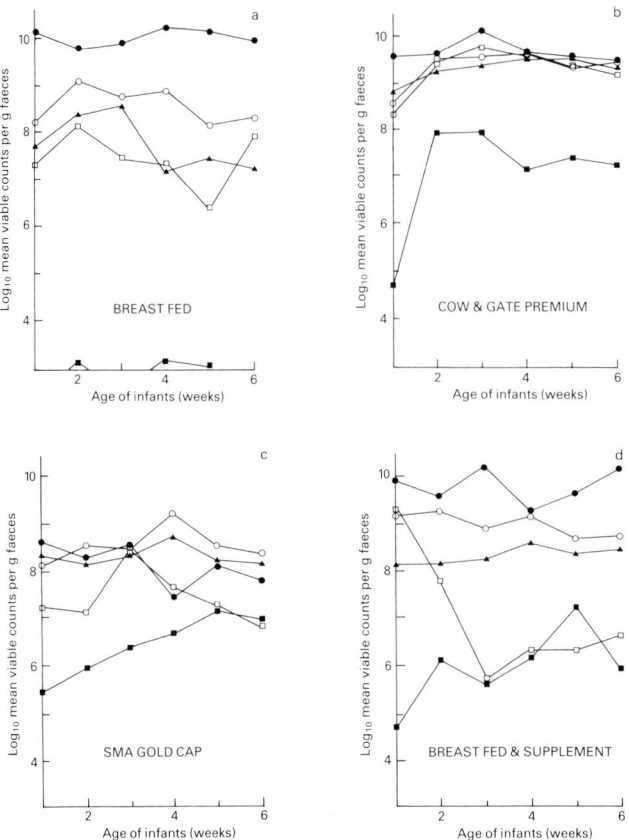

Fig. 61.8 Mean viable counts of faecal organisms isolated from (a) 13 breast-fed infants, (b) nine infants fed Cow and Gate Premium milk, (c) 10 infants fed SMA Gold Cap milk, and (d) 15 infants fed breast milk plus supplement. ●——● = Bifidobacteria; ○——○ = coliform bacilli; ▲——▲ = *Streptococcus faecium*; □——□ = bacteroides; and ■——■ = clostridia. Of note is that none of the breast-fed children had clostridia whereas all the others did. From Bullen et al [8], with permission.

(Fig. 61.8). It is not known whether immunodeficiency influences this effect. An effective way of producing IgE antibodies in an experimental animal is to administer very small doses of antigen, even by mouth, at the same time as a strong adjuvant [30]. *E. coli* endotoxin is a powerful adjuvant and perhaps an artifically fed, slightly immunodeficient child may fail to control the *E. coli* endotoxin. This may in turn act as a potent adjuvant, resulting in IgE antibody formation to environmental allergens, foods and other normally swallowed substances.

Feeding and post-gastroenteritis food allergy

Clinical confirmation of this multifactorial view comes from the observation that gastrointestinal cow's milk allergy may develop in infants after gastroenteritis (bacterial or viral) if they are given cow's milk based feeds during recovery [27]. Anderson et al [2] reported that different cow's milk based infant feeds had different sensitizing potentials for guinea pigs, and Manuel and Walker-Smith [43] have shown that similar differences in sensitization risk occur in infants after gastroenteritis. These findings support the antigen-specific mechanisms of food allergy avoidance, as well as the antigen non-specific ones outlined above. Pure human milk is the safest food, but food antigens from the mother's diet transmitted to her milk will undoubtedly elicit food-allergic symptoms, and may possibly sensitize some infants (see Chapter 18). Soya feeds [21] and hydrolysed cow's milk protein feeds [43] are less sensitizing than conventional cow's milk-based feeds. However, exclusive breast-feeding would probably have prevented the gastroenteritis, and so avoided the risk, as well as reduced the liability to sensitization.

Selection of vulnerable infants for protection

Exclusive breast-feeding for 4 months is appropriate management for all infants[15], as is avoidance of smoking in the household. The strength of the urging of these and other measures (house dust and pet avoidance) recommended by the World Health Organization (WHO) Working Party (1985) is influenced by evidence of predisposition. The highly familial nature of atopic disease[37] provides an easy mode of selection for many. The chances increase with multiple affected first degree relatives, though one is probably enough. However, many atopics have no such relative and it is perhaps in these that cord blood IgE determinations which predict the development of atopic disease [37, 47] might be useful. Screening every neonate is hardly feasible, and the additional probability indicated in infants with affected relatives is perhaps too small to be useful.

Sensitization via breast-feeding

Two other important questions are whether sensitization ever occurs in utero and whether foods transmitted in the mother's milk can ever primarily sensitize.

Antigens in breast milk

Examples of allergic disease in exclusively breast-fed infants suggest that sensitization can occur (see Chapter 18). Glaser and Johnstone[21] recommended that mothers should avoid dairy products during pregnancy as well as postnatally, but there is no evidence that this does protect against food allergy in the infant. In addition, the dangers of therapeutic or preventative diets (other than exclusive breast-feeding) cannot be overstressed, especially in infancy[61] as they can be dangerously nutritionally inadequate. Diets require specialist dietetic supervision.

Breast-feeding and coeliac disease. Breast-feeding may prevent other food-allergic diseases besides atopic ones. There has been a recent apparent reduction in the prevalence of coeliac disease in Britain[42] which followed the trend for breast-feeding and cessation of the early (before 4 months) introduction of solid feeds. This suggests that non-atopic food allergy may be prevented or delayed as well as possibly atopic disease not provoked by foods.

Ulcerative colitis. The association of ulcerative colitis with a history of artificial feeding [1, 67] first led to the suggestion that this too may be a food allergy. This is true of some cases of ulcerative colitis, particularly below the age of 1 year [31], but most adult cases are probably not due to food allergy, although both may be prevented by exclusive breast-feeding.

FOOD ALLERGEN AVOIDANCE

The other approaches to prevention of food-allergic disease are dealt with in detail elsewhere [33]. Avoidance of the food to which the patient is sensitized constitutes the main line of management of severely food-allergic patients, particularly children, though mildly affected ones may be treated symptomatically. Food allergy is much more common in children than in adults and usually gets better, so the important thing is to make life tolerable until this happens. The failure to achieve this has resulted from irrational scepticism, despite the obvious association of symptoms with food in patients who develop symptoms quickly, or after a single food (e.g. urticaria induced by egg or tomato). A slow response after exclusion diet in the relief of childhood eczema, for example, is much more difficult for the uninitiated to understand.

Atopic eczema and other symptoms

In atopic eczema, scepticism of the role of food allergy has been refuted by a double-blind controlled trial entailing comparisons of the effect of empirical food avoidance in groups of patients[4]. The theory of slow food allergy suggests that any combination of any foods could provoke any symptom, and there is no evidence that available tests help in selection of the relevant foods, but all must be avoided if the disease is to be prevented. Much eczema, clearly an allergic disease, benefits from this approach[3] but so do diseases in which the immunopathogenesis is less well established, such as migraine[17] or the hyperkinetic syndrome[16]. Repeated double-blind controlled provocation[24] has confirmed the role of food allergy in many other diseases involving all systems of the body and, since many children grow out of allergy, it is likely that such studies will underestimate the true frequency. Methods of handling such patients by diet are outlined in Chapter 57.

Oral sodium cromoglycate

Oral sodium cromoglycate reduces the uptake of antigen by food-allergic subjects and is of some benefit in patients with food allergy partly successfully treated by diet. The drug is especially useful in minimizing the effect of breaks of the diet for parties and so on[10]. One special use is for the food-allergic breast-fed infant, whose disease is triggered by foods eaten by the mother and passively transferred to the infant in her milk. This may be prevented by properly supervised maternal diet, but when such a mother wishes to eat an allergen-containing meal, oral sodium cromoglycate taken before the meal may prevent the disease in the child (Stratton, 1982, personal communication).

Beclomethasone. Beclomethasone taken orally has been shown by controlled trial to be effective in controlling eczema[28]; its effect may also be local in the gastrointestinal tract.

A PRACTICAL APPROACH TO PREVENTION OF DAMAGING SENSITIZATION TO FOODS

Who is susceptible?

Newborn offspring of atopic parents are particularly susceptible; however, the initial management should be applied, wherever possible, to all healthy full-term babies.

What should be done?

Exclusive breast-feeding (with thirst satisfied by extra water or dextrose solution) is recommended for 4 months. Weaning should then be started with rice, meats, vegetables, fruits and so on and, if desired, a soya-based milk substitute (Table 61.2). Vitamin supplements (colourless), etc., may then be started, but cow's milk-derived foods (including butter and cheese), eggs and wheat should be avoided until 1 year of age. Foods to which the parents are allergic may be avoided too. Partial breast-feeding should be maintained for several more months, possibly even into the second year. Infants with special problems (premature, jaundiced, hypoglycaemic, etc.) will require special appropriate management. Respiratory irritants (smoking) and common allergens (house dust mite, pets, etc.) should also be avoided.

What should be done if this fails?

If the mother cannot breast-feed, a nutritionally adequate infant feed based on hydrolysed casein (Pregestamil) or perhaps soya (see Table 61.2) may be given, with weaning as above.

Postgastroenteritis. Giving one of the less sensitizing feeds (see Table 61.2) after severe gastroenteritis will reduce the chance of cow's milk sensitization.

REFERENCES

1 Acheson ED, Truelove SC: Early weaning in the aetiology of ulcerative colitis. Br Med J 1961; ii: 929.

2 Anderson KJ, McLaughlin P, Devey ME, Coombe RRA: Anaphylactic sensitivity of guinea pigs drinking different preparations of cow's milk and infant formuli. Clin Exp Immunol 1979; 35: 454.

3 Atherton DJ: Allergy and atopic eczema. II. Clin Exp Dermatol 1981; 6: 317.

4 Atherton DJ, Sewell M, Soothill JF et al: A double blind cross-over trial of an antigen avoidance diet in atopic eczema. Lancet 1978; i: 402.

5 Bazaral M, Orgel HA, Hamburger RN: Genetics of IgE and allergy; serum IgE levels in twins. J Allergy Clin Immunol 1974; 54: 288.

6 Bjorksten F, Suoniemi I: Early allergen contacts, adjuvant factors and subsequent allergy. In: Kerr JW, Ganderton MA, eds. Proc of XI International Congress of Allergology and Clinical Immunology. London: MacMillan 1983; 145.

7 Brostoff J, Carini C, Wraith DG, Johns P: Production of IgE complexes by allergen challenges in atopic patients and the effect of sodium cromoglycate. Lancet 1979; i: 1268.

8 Bullen CL, Tearle PV, Steward MG: The effect of 'humanized' milks and supplemented breast feeding on the faecal flora of infants. J Med Microbiol 1977; 10: 403.

9 Bullen JJ: Iron-binding proteins and other factors in milk responsible for resistance to *Escherichia coli*. Ciba Found Symp 1976; 42:

10 Businco L, Marchetti F, Pellegrini G et al: Prevention of atopic disease in 'at risk newborns' by prolonged breast feeding. Ann Allergy 1983; 51: 296.

11 Butler M, Atherton DJ, Levinsky RJ: Quantitative and qualitative defects of T cell suppression in patients with atopic eczema. Clin Exp Immunol 1982; 50: 49.

12 Chandra RK: Prospective studies of the effect of breast

feeding on incidence of infection and allergy. Act Paediatr Scand 1979; 68: 691.

13 Chase MW: Inhibition of experimental drug allergy by prior feeding of the sensitizing agent. Proc Soc Exp Bio Med 1946; 61: 257.

14 Coombs RRA, Gell PGH: Classification of allergic reactions responsible for clinical hypersensitivity and disease. In: Gell PGH, Coombs RRA, Lachmann PJ, eds. Clinical aspects of immunology. Oxford: Blackwell Scientific, 1975.

15 Department of Health and Social Security: Present day practice in infant feeding. Report on health and social subjects, No. 20, London: HMSO, 1980.

16 Egger J, Carter CM, Gumley D et al: A controlled trial of oligoantigenic treatment in the hyperkinetic syndrome. Lancet 1985; i: 540.

17 Egger J, Carter CM, Wilson J, et al: Is migraine food allergy? Lancet 1983; ii:865–9.

18 Ferguson A, Parrott DMV: Histopathology and time course of rejection of allografts of mouse small intestine. Transplantation 1973; 15: 546.

19 Firer MA, Hosking CS, Hill DJ: Effect of antigen load on development of milk antibodies in infants allergic to milk. Br Med J 1981; 283: 693.

20 Gerrard JW: Food allergy–new perspectives. Springfield, Illinois: Charles C Thomas, 1980.

21 Glaser J, Johnstone DE: Prophylaxis of allergic disease in newborns. J. Am Med Assoc 1953; 153: 620.

22 Godfrey RC: Asthma and IgE levels in rural and urban communities of the Gambia. Clin Allergy 1975; 5: 201.

23 Godfrey RC, Griffiths M: The prevalence of immediate positive skin tests to *Dermatophagoides pteronyssimus* and grass pollen in school children. Clin Allergy 1976; 6: 79.

24 Goldman AS, Anderson DW, Sellars WA et al: Milk allergy. I. Oral challenge with milk and isolated milk proteins in allergic children. Pediatrics 1963; 32: 425.

25 Grulee C, Sandford H: The influence of breast feeding and artificial feeding in infantile eczema. J Pediatr 1936; 9: 223.

26 Hamberger RN, Heller S, Mellon MH et al: Current status of the clinical and immunologic consequences of a prototype allergic disease prevention programme. Ann Allergy 1983; 51: 281.

27 Harrison M, Kilby A, Walker-Smith JA et al: Cows' milk protein intolerance, possible association with gastroenteritis, lactose intolerance and IgA deficiency. Br Med J 1976; 1: 1501.

28 Heddle RJ, Soothill JF, Bulpitt CJ, Atherton DJ: Combined oral and nasal beclomethasone diproprionate in children with atopic eczema; a randomised controlled trial. Br Med J 1984; 289: 651.

29 Hill HR, Quie P: Raised serum IgE levels and defective neutrophil chemotaxis in three children with eczema and recurrent bacterial infection. Lancet 1974; i: 183.

30 Jarrett EE, Hall E: Selective suppression of IgE antibody responsiveness by maternal influence. Nature 1979; 280: 145.

31 Jenkins HR, Pincott JR, Soothill JR et al: Food allergy; the major cause of infantile colitis. Arch Dis Child 1984; 59: 326.

32 Jensen JR, Cramers M, Threstrup-Pedersen K: Subpopulations of T lymphocytes and non-specific suppression cell activity in patients with atopic dermatitis. Clin Exp Immunol 1981; 45: 118.

33 Johnstone DE, Soothill JF: Prevention of allergic disease. In: Bierman CW, Pearlman DS, eds. Allergic diseases of infancy, childhood and adolescence. Philadelphia: WB Saunders: 1980.

34 Johnstone DE, Roghmann KL, Pless IB: Factors associated with the development of asthma and hay fever in children. Pediatrics 1975; 56: 398.

35 Juto R, Strannegard O: T Lymphocytes and blood eosinophils in early infancy in relation to heredity for allergy and type of feeding. J Allergy Clin Immunol 1979; 64: 38.

36 Kaufman H, Hobbs JR: Immunoglobulin deficiencies in an atopic population. Lancet 1970; ii: 1061.

37 Kjellman NIM, Johansson SGD: IgE and atopic allergy in newborns and infants with a family history of atopic disease. Acta Paediatr Scand 1976; 65: 495.

38 Konig P, Godfrey S: Exercise-induced bronchial liability in monozygotic (identical) and dizygotic (non-identical) twins. J Allergy Clin Immunol 1974; 54: 280.

39 Krain LS, Teresaki PI: HLA antigens in atopic dermatitis. Lancet 1973; i: 1059.

40 Kramer MS, Moroz B: Do breast feeding and delayed introduction of solid foods protect against subsequent atopic eczema? J Pediatr 1981; 98: 546.

41 Kuitunen P, Rapola J, Savilahti E, Visikorpi JKV: Response of the jejunal mucosa to cow's milk in the malabsorption syndrome with cow's milk intolerance. Acta Paediatr Scand 1973; 62: 585.

42 Littlewood JM, Crollick AJ, Richards IDG: Childhood coeliac disease is disappearing. Lancet 1980; ii: 1359.

43 Manuel PD, Walker-Smith J: A comparison of three infant feeding formulae for the prevention of delayed recovery after infantile gastroenteritis. Acta Paediatr Belg 1981; 34: 13.

44 Marsh DG, Fiso SH, Hussain R et al: Genetics of human immune response to allergens. J Allergy Clin Immunol 1980; 65: 322.

45 Matthew DJ, Taylor B, Norman AP et al: Prevention of eczema. Lancet 1977; i: 321.

46 May CD, Remigo L, Bock SA: Usefulness of measurement of antibodies in serum in diagnosis of sensitivity to cows milk and soy proteins in early childhood. Allergy 1980; 35: 301.

47 Michel FB, Bousquet J, Greillien P et al: Comparison of cord blood immunoglobulin E concentrations and maternal allergy for the predictor of atopic diseases in infancy. J Allergy Clin Immunol 1980; 65: 422.

48 Morrison-Smith J: Skin tests and atopic allergy in children. Clin Allergy 1973; 3: 269.

49 Orlans E, Peppard J, Reynolds J, Hall JG: Rapid active transport of immunoglobulin A from blood to bile. J Exp Med 1978; 147: 588.

50 Paganelli R, Levinsky RJ, Atherton DJ: Detection of specific antigen within immune complexes. Validation of the assay and its application to food antigen–antibody complexes in healthy and food allergic subjects. Clin Exp Immunol 1981; 46: 44.

51 Roberts SA, Soothill JF: Provocation of allergic response by supplementary feeds of cow's milk. Arch Dis Child 1982; 57: 127.

52 Saarinen VM, Kajosaari H, Backman A, Siimes MA: Prolonged breast feeding as prophylaxis for atopic disease. Lancet 1979; ii: 163.

53 Salk L, Grellong BA, Straus W, Dietrich J: Perinatal complications in the history of asthmatic children. Am J Dis Child 1974; 127: 30.

54 Soothill JF: Some intrinsic and extrinsic factors predisposing to allergy. Proc R Soc Med 1976; 69: 1439.

55 Soothill JF: The atopic child. In: Soothill JF, Hay-

ward AH, Wood CBS, eds. Paediatric immunology, Chapter 15. Oxford: Blackwell Scientific, 1983.

56 Soothill JF, Stokes CR, Turner MW et al: Predisposing factors and the development of reaginic allergy in infancy. Clin Allergy 1976; 6: 305.

57 Swarbrick ET, Stokes CR, Soothill JF: The absorption of antigens after oral immunization and the simultaneous induction of specific systemic tolerance. Gut 1978; 20: 121.

58 Tada T: Regulation of reaginic antibody formation in animals. Prog Allergy 1975; 19: 122.

59 Taylor B, Norman AP, Orge HA et al: Transient IgA deficiency and pathogenesis of infantile atopy. Lancet 1973; ii: 111.

60 Thorsby E, Engeset A, Lie SO: HLA antigens and susceptibility to diseases. A study of patients with acute lymphoblastic leukaemia, Hodgkin's disease and childhood asthma. Tissue Antigens 1971; 1: 147.

61 Tripp JH, Francis DEM, Knight JA, Harries JT: Infant feeding practices; a cause for concern. Br Med J 1979; 2: 707.

62 Turner MW, Brostoff J, Wells RS et al: HLA in eczema and hay fever. Clin Exp Immunol 1977; 27: 43.

63 Turner MW, Mowbray JF, Harvey BAM et al: Defective yeast opsonization and C2 deficiency in atopic patients. Clin Exp Immunol 1978; 34: 253.

64 Van Arsdel PP, Motulsky AG: Frequency and hereditability of asthma and allergic rhinitis in college students. Acta Genet 1959; 9: 101.

65 Walker WA, Isselbacher KJ, Bloch KJ: Intestinal uptake of macromolecules; effect of oral immunization. Science 1972; 177: 608.

66 Walker-Smith JA: Cows' milk intolerance as a cause of post-enteritis diarrhoea. J Pediatr Gastroenterol Nutr 1982; 1: 163.

67 Whorwell PJ, Holdstock G, Whorwell GM, Wright R: Bottle feeding, early gastroenteritis, and inflammatory bowel disease. Br Med J 1979; i: 382.

To make the world a better place to live in is an ambition not falsified or diminished by the propensity of those who seek the reputation of having finely critical minds to say knowingly, 'Ah, but what do you mean by better?' It is philosophic naivety to suppose that a single, simple, uncontroversial and general form of words can represent all that is connoted by such particular declarations, not likely to be challenged individually, as that good drains are better than bad and that good books are better than bad, which are true even if people may not agree completely about what in a book entitles it to be classified in the one category or the other. Again, it is better to be well than sick and alive than dead. It is in a compendium of these and other possible particular meanings that we can say the purpose of science is to make the world a better place to live in and that—in Bacon's words—the 'Dignity and proficiency' of science rest upon its ability to promote that wholly admirable ambition.

Sir Peter Medawar
The Limits of Science
Oxford University Press, 1985
(Reproduced with permission)

Index